T0406084

The Diabetes Textbook

Joel Rodriguez-Saldana

Editor

The Diabetes Textbook

Clinical Principles, Patient Management
and Public Health Issues

Second Edition

Volume II

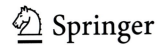 Springer

Editor
Joel Rodriguez-Saldana
Mexico City, Mexico

ISBN 978-3-031-25518-2   ISBN 978-3-031-25519-9   (eBook)
https://doi.org/10.1007/978-3-031-25519-9

© The Editor(s) (if applicable) and The Author(s), under exclusive license to Springer Nature Switzerland AG 2019, 2023

This work is subject to copyright. All rights are solely and exclusively licensed by the Publisher, whether the whole or part of the material is concerned, specifically the rights of translation, reprinting, reuse of illustrations, recitation, broadcasting, reproduction on microfilms or in any other physical way, and transmission or information storage and retrieval, electronic adaptation, computer software, or by similar or dissimilar methodology now known or hereafter developed.

The use of general descriptive names, registered names, trademarks, service marks, etc. in this publication does not imply, even in the absence of a specific statement, that such names are exempt from the relevant protective laws and regulations and therefore free for general use.

The publisher, the authors, and the editors are safe to assume that the advice and information in this book are believed to be true and accurate at the date of publication. Neither the publisher nor the authors or the editors give a warranty, expressed or implied, with respect to the material contained herein or for any errors or omissions that may have been made. The publisher remains neutral with regard to jurisdictional claims in published maps and institutional affiliations.

This Springer imprint is published by the registered company Springer Nature Switzerland AG
The registered company address is: Gewerbestrasse 11, 6330 Cham, Switzerland

Preface to the Second Edition

For Andy and Ashley, lighthouses of my life

The first edition of *The Diabetes Textbook* was the result of more than three decades of endeavors in outpatient diabetes management, starting with the creation of a diabetes clinic in a public hospital in Mexico City in 1990. Shortly afterwards, we met Dr. Donnell Etzwiler and his colleagues from the International Diabetes Center in Minneapolis. Don was an advocate of structured diabetes care using a scientifically based, cost-effective and patient-centered approach [1]. He was also aware of the need to improve the quality of diabetes care based on principles established by Shewhart, Deming, Juran, and many other brilliant minds in the history of quality in industry. Don was a highlight in our efforts to develop and implement an outpatient diabetes model that has benefited thousands of people with diabetes, mostly from undeserved communities. Starting in 1991, we have presented an international diabetes conference in which we have assembled a large faculty of experts from all over the world, including basic science, public health, and clinical management. Many of them became longtime friends, collaborators of *The Diabetes Textbook*, and strong supporters of its creation. We have come to understand that communication, collaboration, and hard work are crucial to confront "the largest epidemic in human history" in the words of Professor Paul Zimmet [2]. The COVID-19 pandemic has confirmed the crucial link of globalization and social determinants of health in outcomes and prognosis; diabetes is a clear example of the persisting consequences of health disparities [3].

The second edition of *The Diabetes Textbook* recognizes the importance of multidisciplinary management. I am extremely grateful for the contributions and enthusiasm of almost two hundred experts from five continents. Their expertise in the most diverse professional areas reflects the complexities of diabetes care and the multiple needs for its management. New chapters have increased the scope and enriched the previous edition, and comprehensive updates have been carried out in the original version. All the coauthors are kindly and forever recognized, but special thanks are directed to Sanjay Kalra and Maggie Powers, and very especially to Victoria Serhiyenko, who in the midst of a national tragedy provided her invaluable support. Above all, this book is devoted to persons with diabetes and their families [1]. The burden on suffering continues to be huge, and every day we honor our commitment to support them to achieve a successful life with diabetes.

Mexico City, Mexico   Joel Rodriguez-Saldana
2023

References

1. Etzwiler DD. Don't ignore the patients. Diabetes Care. 2001;24:1840–1.
2. Zimmet PZ. Diabetes and its drivers: the largest epidemic in human history? Clin Diabetes Endocrinol. 2017;31:1.
3. Khunti K, Aroda VR, Aschner P, Chan JCN, Del Prato S, Hambling CE, et al. The impact of the COVID-19 pandemic on diabetes services: planning for a global recovery. Lancet Diabetes Endocrinol. 2022;10:890–900.

Contents

Part VII

Cardiovascular Risk Factors

Diabetes and Hypertension

39

Hasan Syed, Sowjanya Naha, Dharshan Khangura, Michael Gardner, L. Romayne Kurukulasuriya, and James R. Sowers

Objectives
- To explore the contemporary understanding of the pathophysiology of HTN complicating diabetes
- To review large scale clinical trials assessing HTN treatment goals and outcomes in diabetes
- Identify the indications for ambulatory BP monitoring
- Interpret HTN guidelines from different organizations
- To review glycemic lowering drugs that can reduce BP

Introduction

According to the United States (US) Centers for Disease Control and Prevention 2020 National Diabetes Statistics Report, 68.4% of patients over the age of 18 diagnosed with diabetes mellitus (DM) also have hypertension (HTN). A total of 34.2 million people or 10.5% of the US population has diabetes. DM has been diagnosed in 8.2% or 26.9 million. This is an underestimate due to under diagnosis of DM. Therefore, 7.3 million people or 21.4% were undiagnosed. Thus, a significant portion of the population has both DM and HTN, which predisposes them to

H. Syed · S. Naha · D. Khangura · M. Gardner
Division of Endocrinology Diabetes and Metabolism, Department of Medicine, University of Missouri, Columbia, MO, USA
e-mail: Hmsnf7@health.missouri.edu; nahas@health.missouri.edu; gardermj@health.missouri.edu

L. R. Kurukulasuriya (✉)
Division of Endocrinology Diabetes and Metabolism, Department of Medicine, University of Missouri, Columbia, MO, USA

Harry S Truman VA Hospital, Columbia, MO, USA
e-mail: kurukulasuriyar@health.missouri.edu

J. R. Sowers
Division of Endocrinology Diabetes and Metabolism, Department of Medicine, University of Missouri, Columbia, MO, USA

Dalton Cardiovascular Center Research Center, Columbia, MO, USA
e-mail: sowersj@health.missouri.edu

© The Author(s), under exclusive license to Springer Nature Switzerland AG 2023
J. Rodriguez-Saldana (ed.), *The Diabetes Textbook*, https://doi.org/10.1007/978-3-031-25519-9_39

cardiovascular disease (CVD) and chronic kidney disease (CKD) [1]. In patients with DM and HTN, CVD is the key cause of premature morbidity and mortality and is the greatest contributor to health care costs. Therefore, the importance of screening for HTN is paramount and should be done at every routine office visit [2]. Indeed, the 2020 Canadian HTN guidelines also recommend that newly diagnosed patients with HTN be screened for diabetes using a fasting glucose and/or hemoglobin A1c. They also consider recommending an intensive systolic blood pressure (BP) target of <120 in appropriate patients with CKD. In the Centers for Disease Control and Prevention National Diabetes Statistics Report, HTN was defined as BP greater than or equal to 140/90 mmHg or taking prescription medications for treatment of HTN [3]. Independent of other CVD risk factors, HTN shows a significant increase in CVD that is incremental with each 20 mmHg rise of systolic BP and 10 mmHg rise of diastolic BP across the range from 115/75 to 185/115 mmHg. Patients with DM typically have additional risk factors apart from DM itself such as dyslipidemia, obesity, physical inactivity, vascular stiffness, and microalbuminuria, which further elevate CVD and CKD risk [4].

Pathophysiology

The pathophysiology of HTN in DM is multifactorial, involving multiple organ systems, metabolic signaling pathways, and environmental and genetic factors. Adipose tissue, when located disproportionately in the abdomen (visceral adiposity), is associated with insulin resistance, HTN, hyperglycemia, and a pro-inflammatory state [4]. Bioactive molecules and hormones referred to as adipokines have altered secretion in obesity, which contributes to obesity-related insulin resistance and HTN. Angiotensinogen, aldosterone-stimulating factor, dipeptidyl peptidase, leptin, adiponectin, resistin, tumor necrosis factor (TNF), interleukin 6, and complement-C1q TNF-related protein 1 (CTRP1) are examples of such pro-inflammatory adipokines that are increased with increased visceral adiposity [5, 6].

Insulin resistance is strongly associated with endothelial dysfunction, which results in impaired vascular relaxation and arterial stiffness, which is a biomarker for increased CVD. Impaired insulin metabolic signaling in insulin-resistant states such as obesity and type 2 DM is characterized by impaired serine phosphorylation of insulin receptor substrate-1 (IRS-1) and downstream phosphionositide

3-kinase, protein kinase B activation leading to reduced endothelial nitric oxide (NO) synthase activation and NO bioavailability in the vasculature. In insulin resistance, there is impairment of insulin growth factor signaling with activation of extracellular signal-regulated kinase (ERK1/2) and upregulation of endothelin-1, which contributes to increased vascular contraction and maladaptive growth and remodeling [5, 6].

The systemic and tissue renin-angiotensin-aldosterone system (RAAS) is often inappropriately activated in insulin-resistant states. In part, this is related to increased angiotensin II (Ang II) and aldosterone production by omental adipose tissue. Ang II and aldosterone may also inhibit insulin metabolic signaling in endothelial cells and vascular smooth muscle cells, as well as classical insulin sensitive tissues such as skeletal muscle, adipose, and liver tissue. There is increasing evidence that the inappropriate activation of RAAS is a major contributor to progression of CVD and chronic kidney disease (CKD) as it relates to endothelial dysfunction and arterial stiffness in insulin-resistant states [7].

Angiotensinogen and Ang II are produced in increased amounts in adipose tissue under oxidative stress and chronic low-grade inflammation. CTRP1 in rodent models of obesity and insulin resistance promotes the production of aldosterone [5]. Ang II and aldosterone activate nicotinamide adenine dinucleotide phosphate (NADPH) oxidase, a major source of reactive oxygen species, which promotes oxidative stress and impaired NO-mediated vasodilation. Furthermore, aldosterone has been shown to increase epithelial sodium channel (eNaC) expression on the endothelial cell surface, thereby promoting endothelial cell cytoskeleton cortical stiffness. Increased uric acid, as a result of consumption of diets rich in fructose, also appears to contribute to immune and inflammatory responses leading to RAAS activation, endothelial dysfunction, and increased vascular stiffness [5, 7].

At the level of the nephron, the sodium-glucose cotransporter-2 (SGLT2) is a low-affinity, high-capacity transporter that is primarily responsible for plasma glucose reabsorption in the proximal convoluted tubule. In DM, glucose reabsorption is increased due to increased expression of SGLT2 associated with glomerular hyperfiltration causing glucose toxicity along with sodium reabsorption and retention [6]. Hyperinsulinemia may also cause sodium retention via increased expression of sodium transporters like eNaC in the distal nephron and increased activation of the sodium hydrogen exchanger in the proximal tubule (Fig. 39.1) [5].

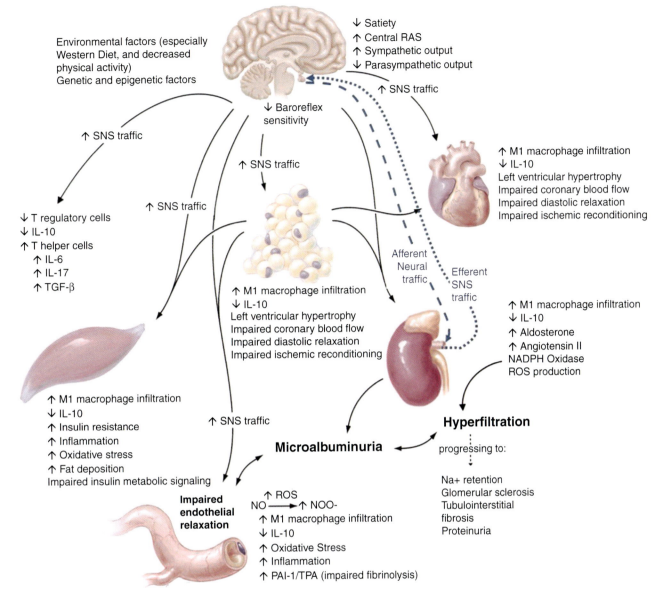

Fig. 39.1 Systemic and metabolic factors that promote coexistent diabetes mellitus, hypertension, cardiovascular, and chronic kidney disease. (Used with permission from Sowers JR. Recent advances in hypertension. J Am Heart Assoc. 2013;61:943–947)

Large-Scale Trials Assessing HTN

- United Kingdom Prospective Diabetes Study (UKPDS)
- Hypertension Optimal Treatment (HOT)
- The Action in Diabetes and Vascular disease, PreterAx and DiamicroN MR Controlled Evaluation (ADVANCE)
- Appropriate Blood Pressure Control in Diabetes (ABCD)
- Systolic Hypertension in Europe (Syst-Eur)
- The Action to Control Cardiovascular Risk in Diabetes (ACCORD)
- The International Verapamil SR—Trandolapril (INVEST)
- The Ongoing Telmisartan Alone and in Combination with Ramipril Global Endpoint Trial (ONTARGET)
- Veterans Affairs Diabetes Trial (VADT)

- Systolic Hypertension in the Elderly Program (SHEP)
- Systolic Blood Pressure Intervention Trial (SPRINT)

Review of the Evidence

Evidence of the management of HTN in diabetic patients was sparse prior to the Hypertension in Diabetes Study (HDS) in 1998. Since then, there have been many large-scale trials that have examined BP control and CVD outcomes. The United Kingdom Prospective Diabetes Study (UKPDS) aimed to study the intensity of BP control and its effect on clinical outcomes in a subset of the group. Comparisons were made of intensive control with a goal of <150/85 mmHg versus less intensive control with a goal of <180/105 mmHg. The median follow-up was 8.4 years, and mean BP in the intensive group was 144/82 mmHg compared to 154/87 mmHg in the less intensive group. A significant reduction in diabetes-related death, stroke, heart failure, and microvascular disease such as retinopathy was seen in the intensive group [8]. The ADVANCE study showed that reducing systolic BP by 5.6 mmHg and diastolic BP by 2.2 mmHg compared to placebo conferred a risk reduction of 8% for macrovascular events, 9% for microvascular events, and 18% for CVD death. The intervention in this study was adding a fixed dose perindopril/indapamide to existing standard therapy. The ABCD study treated DM patients with HTN and high normal BP with goal systolic BP of <130 mmHg. The HTN group's mean BP was 132 mmHg, and the high normal group achieved a mean BP of 128 mmHg. The HTN group had reduced total mortality, and the high normal group had reduced incidence of stroke and decreased progression of nephropathy. The Syst-Eur study showed a decrease in overall mortality and morbidity related to CVD events in diabetic and nondiabetic populations by lowering systolic BP [9].

The ACCORD study compared intensive BP control (<120 mmHg systolic) versus standard BP control (<140 mmHg systolic) and found no statistically significant difference in CVD but did see a reduction in stroke in the intensive group. However, the intensive group was associated with increased risk of hypotension, bradycardia, hyperkalemia, and renal impairment [10]. After observational analysis, the INVEST study showed that the group with goal systolic BP <130 mmHg compared to goal 130–139 mmHg had marginally increased all-cause mortality, and the group with systolic BP of <110 mmHg had significant increase in all-cause mortality (hazard ratio 2.18) [11]. The ONTARGET study examined CVD risk reduction with particular attention to baseline BP. They found significant reduction in CVD with a baseline systolic BP >140 mmHg [12], less reduction if baseline was <130 mmHg, but continued benefit for stroke reduction with lower baseline BP. The VADT study along with the ONTARGET study showed an increased risk of myocardial infarction and CVD events with low diastolic BP. In the VADT study group, diastolic BP was <70 mmHg with a systolic BP 130–139 mmHg [13]. The SPRINT trial aimed for a target systolic BP of 120 mmHg in adults 50 years of age or older with HTN and saw a significant reduction in CVD. This trial showed an associated 33% reduction of heart attack, heart failure, and stroke and a 25% reduction of death compared to a target systolic BP of 140 mmHg. Diabetic patients and patients with a history of previous stroke were excluded from this trial [14].

Guidelines and BP Targets

The most recent National Committee on Prevention, Detection, Evaluation, and Treatment of High BP (JNC 8) was released in 2014. They based their recommendations on evidence from randomized control trials (RCT), expert opinion, and the quality of evidence, which differed from the JNC 7 panel that included observational trials. JNC 8 recommends initiating pharmacological therapy to lower BP to a goal of <140/90 mmHg in patients age > 18 with DM. The ACCORD-BP study supported this lower systolic BP goal of <140 mmHg in the diabetic population compared to <150 mmHg in the nondiabetic population. Major trials such as Syst-Eur, UKPDS, and SHEP studies supported the conclusion that treatment to a systolic BP of <150 mmHg lowers mortality and improves CVD and cerebrovascular health outcomes. The HOT trial found that a diastolic BP reduced to <80 mmHg was associated with a reduction in major cardiovascular events when compared to <90 mmHg and < 85 mmHg by 51% and 24%, respectively. However, JNC 8 determined that this study was not of sufficient quality to recommend a lower diastolic goal, as it was a post hoc analysis of a small subgroup of the study population [9].

The European Society of Cardiology and European Association for the Study of Diabetes recommends systolic BP(SBP) of 130 or below for diabetics treated for hypertension if tolerated. In patients 65 or older, the SBP target range of 130–140 mmHg is recommended if tolerated. In all patients with DM, SBP should not be lowered to <120 mmHg. Diastolic blood pressure (DBP) should be lowered to <80 mmHg but not <70 mmHg. If office SBP is ≥140 mmHg and/or DBP is ≥90 mmHg, drug therapy is recommended in combination with non-pharmacological therapy [15].

The European Society of Hypertension and European Society of Cardiology as part of their 2018 guidelines recommend that antihypertensives should be started in diabetics, when office BP is ≥140/80 mmHg, aiming at an SBP of 130 mmHg. If treatment is well tolerated, treated SBP values of <130 mmHg should be considered because of the benefits on stroke prevention. SBP values of <120 mmHg should be avoided. In patients over 65 years of age, treating to a target SBP range of 130–139 mmHg is recommended. They recommend targeting DBP < 80 mmHg, but not <70 mmHg. In diabetic or nondiabetic patients with CKD, it is recommended to lower SBP to a range of 130–139 mmHg [16].

The International Society of Hypertension Global Hypertension Practice Guidelines recommend that blood pressure should be lowered if BP is ≥140/90 mmHg and treated to a target of <130/80 mmHg (< 140/80 in elderly patients) in diabetics [17].

The American Diabetes Association (ADA 2021 guidelines) recommends a BP goal of less than 130/80 for individuals with diabetes and hypertension at higher cardiovascular risk (existing atherosclerotic cardiovascular disease [ASCVD] or 10-year ASCVD risk ≥15%) if it can be safely attained. In diabetics with hypertension at lower risk for cardiovascular disease (10-year atherosclerotic cardiovascular disease risk <15%), ADA guidelines recommend a blood pressure target of <140/90 mmHg. In pregnant patients with diabetes and preexisting hypertension, a blood pressure target of 110–135/85 mmHg is suggested to reduce the risk for accelerated maternal hypertension and minimizing impaired fetal growth [2]. The American Association of Clinical Endocrinology (AACE) and American College of Endocrinology (ACE), in their 2015 clinical practice guidelines, recommend a goal of approximately 130/80 mmHg in pre-DM and DM patients with HTN. They also indicate that the goal should be individualized based on patient age, duration of disease, and comorbidities. If patients have complex comorbidities, are frail, or experience adverse effects of medications, a more relaxed goal is supported. If this can be achieved safely without adverse medication effects, a more intensive goal of 120/80 can be used [18].

The appropriate target goal for BP In the diabetic population has been the subject of much debate, as control is related to reduction in CVD and kidney disease. There have been many large-scale trials with discrepant results, which have led to confusion. The JNC 7 advocated a target of 130/80 mmHg; however, the trials that used these parameters rarely achieved the target systolic BP and were limited to only a few studies. Consideration of more recent trials such as SPRINT, post hoc analysis of ACCORD, and meta-analysis suggest that a more aggressive systolic BP target of <130 mmHg may be more appropriate than the systolic target of 140 mmHg that was recommended by JNC 8. Wu et al. analyzed a large Chinese cohort of 101,510 individuals with data from 2006 to 2014. The study involved patients with established DM and excluded those who had a BP >140/90 mmHg, were taking antihypertensives, were previously diagnosed with HTN, or had baseline CVD or cancer, in an effort to reduce confounding of mortality outcomes. This left them with 2311 diabetic, normotensive patients whom they examined whether BP of <120/80 mmHg had increased mortality. Their data suggested an increase in CVD events in patients with BP <120/80 mmHg [19]. It is important to note that in this study the participants were predominantly male and had early-stage DM without complications, whereas the ACCORD and SPRINT trials included high-risk hypertensive patients treated to a goal. Based on the collective data from all of the above trials, it appears that there may be a sweet spot to target between 120 and 135 mmHg systolic BP and that a more aggressive target of <120/80 mmHg may be considered for select diabetic patients at the highest risk for stroke [20]. An individual patient tolerance of medications and comorbidities must be considered when managing HTN.

Lifestyle Modification

Approach to weight loss and maintenance based on National Institutes of Health (NIH) clinical guidelines for treatment of obesity [21, 22]:

- Low calorie diet (800–1200 kcal/day): 8% weight loss over 6 months, reduces abdominal fat.
- Very low calorie diet (250–800 kcal/day): similar long-term weight loss, greater initial weight loss compared to low calorie diet.
- Aerobic exercises: Modest weight loss, improve cardiorespiratory fitness, may reduce abdominal fat.
- Physical activity + reduced caloric intake: greater weight loss than either alone.
- Add behavioral therapy to weight loss approach: additional short-term benefits.
- Initial weight loss goal: 10% reduction from baseline weight.
- Target weight loss: 1–2 pounds/week for 6 months.
- Start with moderate physical activity: 30–45 min at least 3–5 days/week.
- Bariatric surgery: BMI > 40 kg/m^2 or > 35 kg/m^2 with high-risk obesity-related morbidity and failed less invasive measures.

The most important therapy whether initial or in combination with pharmacotherapy is lifestyle modification. This involves reduced dietary sodium intake (<2 g/day), weight loss, physical activity, and moderation of alcohol intake. Moderation of alcohol intake is defined as less than two drinks or less in a day for men and one drink or less for women [23]. In the United States, one standard drink contains roughly 14 g of pure alcohol, which is found in 12 oz. of regular beer, 5 oz. of wine, 8–9 oz. of malt liquor, and 1.5 oz. of distilled spirits such as vodka, rum, gin, tequila, and whiskey [24]. In the NIH-funded Look AHEAD (Action for Health in Diabetes) trial, the impact of intensive lifestyle modification (ILI) including diet, physical activity, and behavioral modification on adults with DM type 2 was evaluated [25]. They compared their intervention to that of usual care of DM using diabetes support and education. At 1 year, the ILI group lost 8.6% of their initial body weight compared to 0.7%, decreased mean hemoglobin A1c −0.64 compared to −0.14, decreased systolic BP −6.8 mmHg compared to −2.8 mmHg and had a larger decrease in metabolic syndrome 93.6–78.9% compared to 94.4–87.3%, all of which were statistically significant [26].

Evidence demonstrates that excess dietary consumption of sodium impacts not only one's BP but also several other BP-independent effects. Sodium can affect multiple organ systems in the body, including neurologic, cardiac, renal, and vascular. It has been shown that high sodium intake is also associated with increased glucocorticoid production, insulin resistance, and metabolic syndrome [27]. In many countries, public health recommendations include sodium restriction to less than 5–6 g per day. However, the Cochrane systemic review and multi-study meta-analysis demonstrated that a further reduction in sodium will lower BP even further [28]. The Dash-Sodium study, a multicenter, 14-week randomized feeding trial, followed three different dietary intakes of sodium for 1 month: (3.3 g, 2.4 g, and 1.5 g). The greatest BP drop was noticeable within the group with the greatest sodium restriction [29]. The US Department of Agriculture and Department of Health and Human Services currently recommend consumption of 2.3 g or less of sodium per day in adults.

In addition to sodium restriction, diet modification can have a positive impact on not only BP but also in the treatment of obesity. Two specific diets that have shown to be particularly effective are the Dietary Approaches to Stop HTN (DASH) diet and the Mediterranean diet. The DASH diet is based on the premise of a diet high in whole grains, fish, poultry, fruits, vegetables, low-fat dairy products, and reduced saturated and total fats. In essence, the diet is rich in potassium, magnesium, calcium, protein, and fiber. In the original DASH studies, carbohydrates supplied 55% of calories, total fats 27% of calories, proteins 18%, and saturated fats 6% [30]. The diet should consist of at least six to eight daily servings of grains, less than six servings of lean meats (poultry and fish), four to five daily servings of fruits and vegetables, two to three servings of low-fat milk products and fats and oils, and five or less servings per week of sweets, nuts, seeds, and legumes [31].

The first DASH feeding trials resulted in participants having lower BP and LDL cholesterol endpoints with statistical significance. Systolic BP was reduced on average by 11.4 mmHg ($P < 0.001$), and diastolic BP was reduced on average by 5.5 mmHg ($P < 0.001$). Seventy percent of participants had normal BP (goal SBP <140 and DBP <90 mmHg) at the end of the trial compared to 23% on the control diet [32]. Compared to controls, the DASH diet also reduced the estimated 10-year CVD risk by 18%. The relative risk ratio compared to controls at 8 weeks with baseline 10-year CVD risk was 0.82 (95% CI, 0.75–0.90, $P < 0.001$). In other studies, the DASH diet also decreased pulse wave velocity (PWV) over time ($p = 0.014$) reaching significance after 2 weeks ($p = 0.026$) [33]. Additional information on PWV will be provided later in this chapter.

The Mediterranean diet embodies the Mediterranean culture and lifestyle. Although there are now many variants of this diet, the traditional premise comprises low amounts of saturated fats, meat and meat products, and consumption of high amounts of olive oil, fruits, vegetables, cereals, legumes, nuts, moderate amounts of fish and dairy products, and wine in moderation [34]. Unlike the DASH diet, the Mediterranean diet has an increased consumption of the total amount of fats, up to 40% of caloric intake, with less than 7–8% of caloric intake consisting of saturated fats [35]. In the Greek European Prospective Investigation into Cancer and Nutrition (EPIC) prospective cohort study, lower consumption of meat and meat products, higher consumption of vegetables and fruits, and minimization of saturated fats with more monounsaturated fats were considered most beneficial with a higher predictive score of lower mortality [36]. In addition to diet, regular physical activity and culture-specific psychosocial support played an integral part in the Mediterranean diet. Meals were often consumed with others with frequent rest after meals that presumably reduced overall stress. In addition, mealtime interactions can also be correlated with dietary adherence (Fig. 39.2) [37].

The Mediterranean diet is associated with reduced all-cause mortality and reduced cardiovascular mortality in addition to improved health. A systematic review of 2824 studies with eight meta-analyses and five randomized controlled trials (RCTs) was done in 2015 that compared the Mediterranean diet to a control diet in patients with DM2 and prediabetic states. These studies demonstrated remission of metabolic syndrome, favorable effects on body weight, total and LDL cholesterol, and overall reduced risk of future diabetes by 19–23% [38]. The Prevencion con Dieta Mediterranea trial (PREDIMED) was a parallel-group, multicenter, randomized trial that studied primary cardiovascular prevention when comparing Mediterranean diets to a low-fat control diet. Although there was not a noted effect on all-cause mortality, results were suggestive of a protective effect with noted unadjusted hazard ratios of 0.7 ($p = 0.015$) when compared to the control diet. There was an absolute risk reduction in approximately three major cardiovascular events per 1000 person-years [39].

Combining the Mediterranean diet with a healthy lifestyle, avoidance of tobacco products and regular exercise has shown to have a positive outcome with reduced mortality rate. The Healthy Ageing Longitudinal study in Europe (HALE) project was conducted between 1988 and 2000 that showed a 50% lower rate of all-cause and cause-specific mortality in individuals aged 70–90 years of age who adhered to the Mediterranean diet with a heathy lifestyle [40]. In the exercise and nutrition intervention for cardiovascular health (ENCORE) study, combining the DASH diet with weight management resulted in larger BP reductions with improved secondary outcomes in vascular and autonomic function and reduced left ventricular mass. Up to 12.5 mmHg systolic and 5.9 mmHg diastolic reduction in BP was observed in the DASH diet combined with a behavioral weight management program [41].

Aerobic exercise is not only effective in weight loss but also thought to lower BP independent of weight loss [42]. According to the recommendations from American College

Fig. 39.2 Mediterranean diet pyramid

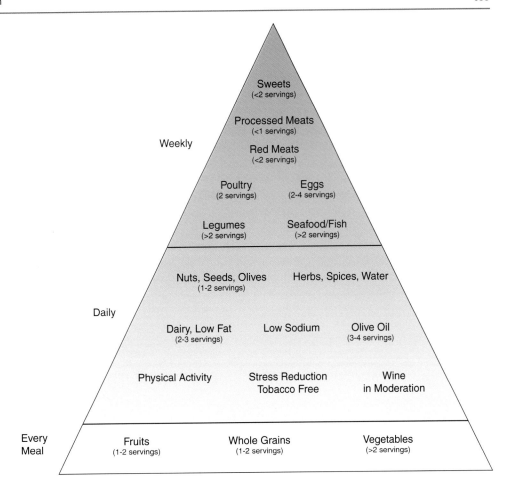

Sweets
(<2 servings)

Processed Meats
(<1 servings)

Red Meats
(<2 servings)

Weekly

Poultry
(2 servings)   Eggs
(2-4 servings)

Legumes
(>2 servings)   Seafood/Fish
(>2 servings)

Nuts, Seeds, Olives
(1-2 servings)   Herbs, Spices, Water

Daily

Dairy, Low Fat
(2-3 servings)   Low Sodium   Olive Oil
(3-4 servings)

Physical Activity   Stress Reduction
Tobacco Free   Wine
in Moderation

Every
Meal

Fruits
(1-2 servings)   Whole Grains
(1-2 servings)   Vegetables
(>2 servings)

of Sports Medicine and American Heart Association, all healthy adults should engage in moderate-intensity aerobic physical exercise for minimum of 30 min for 5 days per week, vigorous-intensity activity minimum of 20 min for 3 days per week or combination of moderate, and vigorous-intensity activity [43]. Moderate-intensity physical activity should target a heart rate of 50–70% of his or her maximum heart rate (MHR). The MHR (calculated as 220 minus your age) is the upper limit of what your cardiovascular system can handle during exercise. For example, a 40-year-old patient should sustain heart rate between 90 and 126 for 30 min (0.5 or 0.7 × [220–40]). Vigorous-intensity physical activity should target 70–85% of his or her MHR. However, a 2011 review suggests that the MHR prediction in adults that are overweight or obese can be more accurately determined using a MHR equation: 208–0.7 × age [44]. Per the American College of Sports Medicine Position Stand, a minimum of 150 min of moderate-intensity activity per week with an energy deficit of 500–1000 kcal per day is recommended for continued weight loss. With a structured and supervised exercise program, weight loss can be maximized [45].

There are multiple ways in which lifestyle modification can be implemented; however, the common ingredient is significant determination and effort on the part of the patient with the support of a multidisciplinary team. Not only is it effective, as was evidenced by the Look AHEAD trial, but it could also reduce financial burden and adverse events as a result of fewer medications needed for treatment. At 9.6 years of follow-up, the ILI group used less insulin, antihypertensives, and statins compared to the control group [26].

DM Medications

The following are diabetes medications/classes shown to reduce BP:

- Thiazolidinedione
- Glucagon-like peptide-1 (GLP-1) receptor agonist
- Dipeptidyl diphosphatase 4 (DPP-4) inhibitor
- Sodium–glucose cotransport 2 (SGLT2) inhibitor
- Bromocriptine mesylate

GLP-1 receptor agonist exenatide had a significant effect on BP reduction [46]. When studied in 120 patients, after 52 weeks, there was a decrease in BP with a greater effect observed when the baseline BP was higher. In patients with a baseline systolic BP >130 mmHg, there was a reduction of 11.4 mmHg in systolic BP and a reduction of 3.6 mmHg in diastolic BP. In patients with a mean BP of 128/78, there was a reduction of 6.2 mmHg in systolic BP and a reduction of 2.8 mmHg in diastolic BP. These reductions were independent of both weight loss and medication changes. Exenatide has the benefit of once weekly dosing and causes weight loss in a dose-dependent fashion. It has been shown to cause weight loss in 75% of patients at 30 weeks with average loss of 4 kg, and like its effect on BP, greater effect is seen with patients with a higher BMI (>30 kg/m²) at baseline [47]. Exenatide is thought to have both natriuretic and vasodilator properties [48, 49]. In a case series of 12 patients who took exenatide over a 12-week period, noticeable increases in plasma concentrations of vasodilators, cyclic guanosine monophosphate (cGMP), cyclic adenosine monophosphate (cAMP), and atrial natriuretic peptide (ANP) while suppressing the RAAS suggest vasodilator and natriuretic properties [50]. Further evidence suggests that exenatide may also have diuretic and renal vasodilator effects. Liraglutide Effect and Action in Diabetes: Evaluation of Cardiovascular Outcome Results (LEADER) trial demonstrated a sustained decrease in BP (SBP/DBP –1.2/–0.6 mmHg) with a slight increase in heart rate (3 bpm.) [51]. In a meta-analysis of 25 trials with once a week exenatide and daily liraglutide, it was shown that GLP-1 receptor agonists had beneficial effects on systolic and diastolic BP [52].

Insulin resistance intervention after strole (IRIS) III study showed that addition of 30 mg of pioglitazone for 20 weeks to the existing medication regimen of 2092 diabetics with A1c between 6.6% and 9.9% reduced systolic BP from 141 to 137 mmHg and diastolic BP from 83 to 81 mmHg. Interestingly, fewer or even no antihypertensives were needed in 25% of previously hypertension-treated patients at the end of the study [53]. Thiazolidinedione's mechanism of action is through activation of peroxisome proliferator-activated nuclear receptors (primarily PPARγ receptor) and subsequent upregulation of genes decreasing insulin resistance. Studies have shown that lowering the expression of PPARγ receptors increased BP [54]. Some evidence suggests vasodilatory effects through inhibition of arginine vasopressin and norepinephrine responses and direct vascular effect through inhibition of calcium uptake of vascular smooth muscle [55, 56].

The DPP4 inhibitors, in addition to hyperglycemic control, have been shown to have a modest effect on BP, as well as a favorable effect on atherosclerosis, stroke and CVD. Sitagliptin, a DPP4 inhibitor, was used in a small study and showed a statistically significant reduction of –2.0 mmHg to –2.2 mmHg in systolic BP and –1.6 mmHg to –1.8 mmHg in diastolic BP [57]. One proposed mechanism includes upregulation of GLP-1, increasing NO bioavailability and therefore improving overall endothelial function in HTN [58, 59].

SGLT2 inhibitors have been reported to be associated with weight loss and to act as osmotic diuretics, resulting in lower-ing of BP [60]. One meta-analysis indicated a significant reduction in systolic and diastolic BP with a weighted mean difference of –2.46 mmHg in SBP and weighted mean differences of –1.46 mmHg for DBP. The weighted mean difference for the effect of SGLT2 inhibitors on body weight was –1.88 kg across all studies. There were no heart rate changes [61]. Another metanalysis with clinical trials with a duration of at least 12 weeks comparing SGLT-2 inhibitors with placebo or active drugs showed that patients on SGLT-2 inhibitors had statistically significant –1.2 reduction in systolic BP and –1.9 reduction in diastolic BP [62]. Clar et al. reported that dapagliflozin treatment was associated with a reduction in SBP ranging from –1.3 to –7.2 mmHg in the patients treated with doses of 10 mg [63]. Rosenstock et al. reported a reduction in SBP in response to canagliflozin treatment ranging from –0.9 mmHg with 50 mg once daily to –4.9 mmHg with 300 mg once daily (compared to –1.3 mmHg with placebo and –0.8 mmHg with sitagliptin) [64]. Inhibitors of sodium-glucose co-transporter-2 reduce BP beyond the projected impact of weight reduction on BP. A large-scale multicenter RCT has demonstrated that treatment with an SGLT-2 inhibitor, empagloflozin, was associated with small reductions in systolic/diastolic BP, weight, waist circumference, and uric acid levels compared to placebo. Results also indicated reduced risk of death from CVD, nonfatal myocardial infarction, nonfatal stroke, and death from all causes [65].

Large randomized controlled trials have reported statistically significant reductions in cardiovascular events for three of the SGLT-2 inhibitors (empagliflozin, canagliflozin, and dapagliflozin) and four GLP-1 receptor agonists (liraglutide, dulaglutide, semaglutide, and albiglutide) [2]. We now have data from several trials that indicate CV benefits from the use of glucose-lowering drugs in patients with CVD or at very high/high CV risk. The results obtained from these trials strongly suggest using both GLP1-RAs (LEADER, SUSTAIN-6, Harmony Outcomes, REWIND, and PIONEER 6) and SGLT2 inhibitors (EMPA-REG OUTCOME, CANVAS, DECLARE-TIMI 58, and CREDENCE), in patients with T2DM with prevalent CVD or very high/high CV risk [15]. Meta-analyses of the trials reported to date suggest that in type 2 diabetes with established ASCVD, GLP-1 receptor agonists, and SGLT2 inhibitors reduce risk of atherosclerotic major adverse cardiovascular events to a comparable degree [66]. SGLT2 inhibitors also appear to reduce risk of heart failure hospitalization and progression of kidney disease in patients with established ASCVD, multiple risk factors for ASCVD, or diabetic kidney disease [67]. It is unknown whether the use of both classes of drugs will provide an additive cardiovascular outcomes benefit [2].

Bromocriptine Mesylate quick release (Cycloset) is a quick release dopamine receptor agonist indicated for treatment of type 2 diabetes. This is a micronized formulation. Proposed mechanism of actions is reestablishing morning brain dopamine D2 receptor activity, reducing sympathetic tone, and increasing insulin sensitivity. These actions lead to improved post prandial hyperglycemia. Study with 15 poorly controlled diabetics on metformin and GLP-1 agonist showed that bromocriptine mesylate caused a significant reduction in blood pressure compared to placebo. Systolic (134 ± 4 vs. 126 ± 6 mmHg), diastolic (78 ± 3 vs. 73 ± 4 mmHg), and mean arterial blood pressure (97 ± 5 vs. 90 ± 4 mmHg) all decreased significantly ($P < 0.05$) [68]. Some patients may end up with orthostatic hypotension. Another study with 1791 patient on metformin addition of bromocriptine Mesylate has shown to reduce cardiovascular risk compared to placebo [69].

Addition of hypoglycemic agents with antihypertensive effects should be done cautiously in hypertensive diabetics well controlled on antihypertensives. The need may arise to reduce the doses of antihypertensive drugs. Patients should be warned about the blood pressure lowering effects of these drugs.

Antihypertensive Medications

Medication classes used to treat HTN:

- ACEI (ACE inhibitor)
- ARB (angiotensin receptor blocker)
- CCB (calcium channel blocker)
- Diuretics
- Alpha/beta-adrenergic blockers
- Beta-adrenergic blockers
- Alpha blockers
- Alpha-2 agonists
- Mineralocorticoid receptor (MR) blockers
- Vasodilators
- Renin inhibitors

When initiating pharmacotherapy for the treatment of HTN, it is important to consider patient characteristics, medication tolerability, and desirable protective effects. The preferred initial medication according to the ADA and AACE/ACE is a RAAS blocker (ACEI or ARB) in patients with DM due to the beneficial effect on cardiovascular outcomes. If BP is not controlled, other classes of medications should be added until goal BP is obtained [4]. Evidence including systematic reviews and meta-analysis has shown that RAAS blockers not only are comparable to other classes of medications in efficacy for treatment of HTN but also reduce the risk of microalbuminuria and creatinine doubling. This suggests that RAAS blockers may be preferred to other antihypertensive agents, as it is well documented that both HTN and DM are associated with the development of CKD [70, 71]. The combination of an ACEI and ARB is not recommended, as they were associated with increased risk of hypotension, syncope, and renal failure in Ongoing Telmisartan Alone and in combination with Ramipril Global enspoint Trial (ONTARGET) [56]. In the

JNC 8 guidelines, there was no preference given to a particular agent, and it was recommended that a thiazide-type diuretic, CCB, ACEI, or ARB be used as the initial antihypertensive medication. These guidelines were derived solely from RTCs, which are considered the gold standard for evidence-based medicine [9].

Amlodipine, a CCB, has been compared to other medications in large-scale clinical trials in patients with DM and HTN. The Avoiding Cardiovascular Events through Combination Therapy in Patients Living with Systolic Hypertension (ACCOMPLISH) trial compared the combination of benazepril/amlodipine to benazepril/hydrochlorothiazide and found a 21% relative risk reduction in cardiovascular events with the amlodipine-containing combination. The Anglo-Scandinavian Cardiac Outcomes Trial (ASCOT) found a 14% reduction in cardiovascular events with amlodipine compared to atenolol. CCBs are well tolerated, do not have unfavorable effects on metabolism, and may be the best medication to add to a RAAS blocker if combination therapy is required to reach BP goals in the diabetic population [72].

Diuretics, in particular the thiazide-type diuretics, are a common first choice for the treatment of HTN; however, there are some disadvantages to their use in the diabetic population. They can cause metabolic derangements such as hyperuricemia, dyslipidemia, insulin resistance, and hyperglycemia. Despite these side effects, diuretics have been shown to be as effective as CCBs and ACEIs in decreasing the risk of CVD events and have a significant role in the treatment of HTN in DM [72].

Beta-blockers have been associated with metabolic derangements including dyslipidemia, increased insulin resistance, and weight gain. Beta-blockers can mask hypoglycemia symptoms. Like diuretics, beta-blockers have a significant role in the treatment of HTN in DM, particularly when patients have had a previous myocardial infarction, rhythm disorder, or heart failure. The Glycemic Effects in Diabetes Mellitus: Carvedilol-Metoprolol Comparison in Hypertensives (GEMINI) trial studied patients already on a RAAS blocking agent. Results suggested that if a beta-blocker is indicated, carvedilol might be superior to metoprolol as it was not associated with the increase in hemoglobin A1c or dyslipidemia that was seen with metoprolol [72, 73].

Combination therapy is often necessary in diabetics with HTN and lead to more patients achieving goals when compared to monotherapy, regardless of the baseline BP. In the UKPDS study, three or more medications were required to achieve goals in up to one third of patients [74]. It was the recommendation of the JNC 7 that if BP was more than 20 systolic and more than 10 mmHg diastolic above goal that combination therapy be initiated [75].

When patients are not at goal on optimal doses of three antihypertensive agents including a diuretic, it is referred to as resistant HTN. Resistant HTN is common in patients with diabetes and obesity. Secondary causes of HTN should be excluded and referral to a HTN specialist should be considered in resistant cases. There is a hypothesis that resistant hypertension occurs due to excess sodium retention. Thus, additional diuretic action by adding a mineralocorticoid receptor (MR) blocker may be beneficial. Spironolactone and eplerenone are steroidal MR blockers, and the newer Finerenone is a nonsteroidal MR antagonist. Since Eplerenone and Finerenone are more selective mineralocorticoid receptor blockers, they are not associated with gynecomastia and menstrual irregularities seen with spironolactone. A study showed that spironolactone was superior to placebo, doxazosin, and bisoprolol in patients with resistant HTN; however, this was not done in a solely diabetic population, and patients with CKD with a GFR <45 mL/min were excluded. MR blockers should be used cautiously, as they can lead to hyperkalemia, especially in the DM population, in which CKD is more common [76]. In the Finerenone trial for reducing kidney failure and disease progression in diabetic kidney disease (FIDELIO- DKD) showed that when finerenone is added to treatment of patients with CKD and type 2 diabetes already on maximum tolerable doses of renin angiotensin system blockers it resulted in lower risks of CKD progression and cardiovascular events than placebo [77]. Finerenone is indicated to reduce the risk of sustained eGFR decline, end-stage kidney disease, cardiovascular death, nonfatal myocardial infarction, and hospitalization for heart failure in adult patients with chronic kidney disease (CKD) associated with type 2 DM.

Aliskiren is the only renin inhibitor out in the market. It is an effective antihypertensive agent that is well tolerated. In the air versus oxygen in myocardial infraction trial (AVOID), Aliskerin plus losartan showed a 20% greater reduction in proteinuria compared to losartan and placebo. This study showed that the reno protective effect of Aliskerin was independent of the BP lowering effect in diabetic and hypertensive patients with nephropathy on losartan [78]. The Aliskiren Trial in Type 2 Diabetes using Cardiorenal end points (ALTITUDE) was done to determine the safety and effectiveness of direct renin inhibitors compared with placebo with respect to fatal and nonfatal renal and cardiovascular events in patient with type 2 diabetes who were on an ACE inhibitors or ARB. This study did not show a statistically significant difference in cardiovascular events with addition of Aliskerin, but the addition of Aliskerin caused a higher incidence of hyperkalemia and hypotension [79]. At his point, addition of Aliskiren to ACE inhibitor and ARB therapy is not recommended (Fig. 39.3).

Fig. 39.3 Flow chart for the treatment of HTN in diabetes

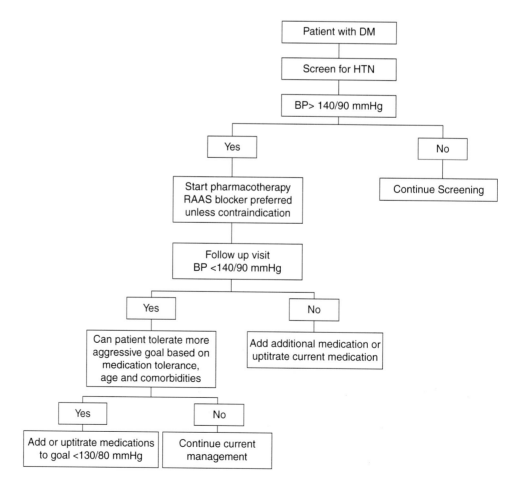

Other Monitoring Modalities

Screening and monitoring of treatment for HTN has traditionally been based on evaluation in the healthcare setting. Out-of-office BP monitoring has been used in European guidelines; as of April 2021, the US Preventive Services Task Force (USPSTF) has endorsed its use for diagnosis and management of HTN. Ambulatory BP monitoring (ABPM) involves placement of a BP cuff on the nondominant arm that measures BP over the course of a 24-h period by taking measurements every 15–30 min. Compared to in-office BP measurement, ABPM is of higher prognostic value for CKD, CVD, and mortality risks [80].

Suspected white coat HTN, evaluation of resistant HTN, episodic HTN, suspected episodes of hypotension, and evaluation of treatment efficacy are indications for ABPM. Patients with DM who have BP excursions on 24-h monitoring are at increased risk of complications even before the diagnosis of HTN. Both Type 1 DM and Type 2 DM in comparison with controls without DM have been found to have higher mean BP values. These elevated means were associated with higher rates of nephropathy, albuminuria, retinopathy, and increased left ventricular mass. BP normally has a physiologic circadian rhythm in which BP drops >10% during the night relative to daytime BP. Patients in which BP decreases by <10% are said to have a non-dipping pattern, which was observed to be more prevalent in those with DM. This non-dipping pattern has been associated with cardiovascular autonomic neuropathy; its contribution to progression of chronic DM complications however is more controversial. Studies thus far have shown some mixed results and may be more relevant and add information to other BP values when related to outcomes with retinopathy. Hyperglycemia has exhibited a role in normal nocturnal BP fall, likely related to its effect on modifying circulating plasma volume, interfering with blood flow distribution and renal hemodynamics. Decreased BP means and increased BP fall during the night have been seen after 1 week of improved glycemic control in type 1 DM. Patients with normal office BP measurements (<140/90 mmHg) with elevated ABPM measurements (>135/85 mmHg) are referred to as having masked HTN. Type 2 DM patients have been shown to have a higher prevalence of masked HTN at 30% versus 10–20% in those without DM. Masked HTN has been associated with increased cardiovascular risk and when studied in Type 2 DM patients was associated with albuminuria and increased left ventricular wall thickness. ABPM appears to add significant information that can be used in risk stratification in the DM population and should be utilized more frequently. However, additional clinical study is needed to further explore the parameters obtained with ABPM and their effects on the complications of DM and to develop treatment strategies to benefit such patients [81].

PWV is a noninvasive measure of arterial stiffness with carotid-femoral PWV considered the reference standard measurement of aortic stiffness. It is not used clinically in the United States; however, it is suggested in Europe by expert consensus that carotid-femoral PWV greater than 10 m/s is a cardiovascular risk factor for middle-aged adults with HTN. Studies have shown an association between DM and aortic stiffness measured by PWV, which did not vary by gender but was significantly stronger in Caucasians as compared to African Americans. In more advanced DM, present for more than 10 years, albuminuria and elevated glycosylated hemoglobin were all associated with higher aortic stiffness measured by PWV. This suggests that PWV measurement may contribute to the currently available methods to risk stratify patients who have more risk of developing cardiovascular events and mortality related to complications of DM. However, further clinical studies are needed to help delineate how this modality for the measurement of arterial stiffness can specifically be used in the diabetic population and if treatment targeting arterial stiffness can improve outcomes [82].

COVID-19 and Antihypertensive Therapy in Individuals with Diabetes

The ongoing novel SARS-CoV-2 coronavirus (COVID-19) pandemic has had a disproportionate impact on individuals with multiple medical comorbidities. For instance, a large observational study from China revealed that up to 23.7% of patients with severe infection had a history of hypertension and 16.2% were known diabetics compared to patients with nonsevere infection of whom just 13.4% and 5.7% had a history of hypertension and diabetes, respectively [83]. Likewise, studies in the United States have shown as much as 78% of patients admitted to ICU with COVID-19 have diabetes and that diabetics are more than twice as likely as nondiabetics to get admitted to a hospital with COVID-19 after adjusting for other comorbidities [84]. It is now believed that diabetic individuals have an exaggerated immune response to infection with COVID-19 leading to increased production of inflammatory cytokines and reactive oxygen species. This cascade ultimately results in greater end organ injury and excess mortality [85]. These individuals also have a higher prevalence of heart failure and chronic kidney disease that predispose to complications from COVID-19. Moreover, it has been observed that many patients with hypertension and diabetes share common underlying socioeconomic themes such as lack of access to quality healthcare and healthy foods that increases their risk for adverse outcomes [86].

Extensive research into COVID-19 infection in this subset of patients has led to questions on the role of ACE inhibitors and ARBs in its pathogenesis. Specifically, the observation that the novel coronavirus binds to human cells via the angiotensin-converting enzyme 2 raised concerns that medications such as ACE inhibitors and ARBs might accelerate infection with the novel coronavirus by increasing the levels of this enzyme. However, currently, there is no clinical evidence to support this hypothesis. The European Society of Cardiology Council on Hypertension, the American College of Cardiology (ACC)/American Heart Association (AHA)/Heart Failure Society of America (HFSA) and the American Society of Hypertension have all released policy statements strongly recommending that patients continue treatment with their usual antihypertensive regimen [87]. Therefore, at this time, recognizing the multiple benefits obtained with these classes of medications in patients with diabetes and hypertension, it is not advisable to discontinue therapy simply because of COVID-19 infection [88].

Future Considerations

There should be more awareness about HTN complicating diabetes. Healthcare systems should have more aggressive screening to diagnose these conditions. Every new hypertensive patient should be screened for diabetes. Lifestyle modifications are the cornerstone for management of these two interrelated medical conditions and should be emphasized at a younger age. Schools should have more programs that advocate healthy living.

Most of current HTN studies are based on office BP monitoring. ABPM and home BP monitoring should be used more frequently. This technique is a very useful tool in white coat HTN (high BP in clinic but normal in other settings) and masked HTN (normal BP in clinic and high BP at other settings). Additionally, it is also helpful in resistant HTN, episodic HTN, autonomic dysfunction, and hypotension while taking antihypertensive medications. ABPM also identifies patients who have nocturnal HTN dipper versus non-dippers. This has important implications since non-dippers are at higher cardiovascular risk. Some experts believe that home BP monitoring should be done several times a day and dosage of BP medications adjusted based on BP at a given time similar to finger stick blood glucose monitoring and adjustment of insulin dosing.

There should be more American Society of Hypertension certified HTN centers that are focused on treating patients who have more complex issues with HTN and related complications so that patients can be referred to these centers for more comprehensive care. Internal medicine and related residency and fellowship training programs should encourage more trainees to become hypertension specialists. More research should be done on genetic analysis to provide more individualized medicine, which will help

determine the appropriate medication/medications for any given patient. The low efficacy of some therapies could be related to interindividual genetic variability. Genetic studies of families have suggested that heritability accounts for 30–50% of interindividual variation in blood pressure (BP). Genome-wide studies have confirmed that genetic factors are related not only to BP elevation but also to interindividual variability in response to antihypertensive treatment. Due to the polygenic nature of hypertension, a single locus cannot be used as a relevant clinical target for all individuals. Therefore, the analysis of complex traits, such as drug response phenotypes, should involve the assessment of interactions among multiple loci. Genome-wide association studies (GWASs) have led to the discovery of variants associated with drug efficacy and adverse drug reactions. However, due to the multigenic and multifactorial nature of the drug response phenotypes, further research in this area is required to establish reliable recommendations [89].

Conclusion

Over 20 million people in the United States have both HTN and DM. Diagnosis and treatment of these conditions is very important to decrease the risk of CVD, which is a major cause of morbidity, mortality, and healthcare cost. The pathophysiology of HTN in DM is complex with the inappropriate activation of the RAAS system, the endocrine action of adipose tissue, oxidative stress, and maladaptive effects on the vascular endothelium being involved. The western diet and obesity play an important role in inducing a pro-inflammatory state contributing to metabolic derangement. There have been multiple large-scale clinical trials that have examined BP control in DM and its effect on CVD outcomes. The data from these studies suggests that targeting a systolic BP between 120 mmHg and 135 mmHg would be most appropriate, reserving a more aggressive target of <120/80 mmHg in select patients that are at highest risk of stroke and can tolerate the target without adverse effects. Lifestyle modification remains the most important intervention including a reduced sodium diet, weight loss, exercise, and moderation of alcohol intake. When treating DM in patients with HTN, it is important to note that the choice of DM medications can have an impact on BP control. ACEI or ARB should be considered preferred initial therapy for diabetics with HTN due to beneficial effect on CVD and renal outcomes. Adding medications or titrating existing medications should be done until BP goals are met. ABPM should be used for further evaluation in cases of resistant HTN, episodic HTN, and suspected white coat HTN or episodes of hypotension. PWV may be an additional tool that can be used to identify patients at risk for developing CVD and complications of DM. There continues to be further studies contributing to the knowledge of these interrelated conditions.

Concluding Remarks: Diabetes and hypertension are frequent co-existing risk factors that are promoted by obesity and increase the risk for both CVD and CKD. There is increasing evidence that treatment of both conditions should be individualized based on various factors such as age and duration of diabetes. Emerging evidence suggests that an optimal goal for blood pressure control is less than 130/85 mmHg for most patients with diabetes.

Multiple Choice Questions

1. Which one of the following studies showed that combination of angiotensin converting enzyme inhibitor and angiotensin receptor blockers were associated with and increased risk of renal failure?
   (a) UKPD
   (b) **ONTARGET**
   (c) ADVANCE
   (d) VADT
   (e) SPRINT

   The ONTARGET trial-Ongoing Telmisartan Alone and in combination with Ramipril global endpoint trial showed that the combination was associated with increased risk of hypotension, syncope, and renal failure.

2. Ambulatory BP monitoring will be helpful in all the following conditions except:
   (a) 45 year with uncontrolled HTN on maximum dose of three medications including a diuretic
   (b) **60 year old with well-controlled HTN on 2 BP medications**
   (c) 35 year with good BP at home and local store but high at the physician office
   (d) 45-year-old diabetic who complains of orthostatic symptoms
   (e) To evaluate masked HTN (normal office BP with elevated Home BP)

   Ambulatory BP monitoring should be considered in suspected white coat HTN, resistant HTN, episodic HTN (i.e., pheochromocytoma), autonomic dysfunction, or suspected episodes of hypotension.

3. All of the following antidiabetic medications will lower BP except:
   (a) Exanetide
   (b) Sitagliptin
   (c) Pioglitazone
   (d) Empagloflozin
   (e) **Insulin.**

   Antidiabetic medications GLP-1 agonists, DPP4 inhibitors, SGLT-2 inhibitors, Bromocriptine mesylate QR, and thiazolidinediones have shown to reduce BP.

4. All of the following are true about DASH diet except:
   (a) Has as a positive impact on BP
   (b) DASH diet is high in whole grains, fish, poultry, fruits, and vegetables
   (c) Has shown to reduce cardiovascular risk
   (d) **Has been shown to increase pulse wave velocity**
   (e) DASH diet will lower LDL cholesterol

   DASH diet has shown a positive impact on BP, obesity, and LDL cholesterol. DASH diet has also been shown to reduce cardiovascular risk and reduce pulse wave velocity.

5. When treating diabetics with HTN, which of the following is correct?
   (a) **American Diabetic Association and American Association of Clinical Endocrinologists recommend RAAS blockers as first line treatment.**
   (b) JNC 8 recommends a BP goal of less than 120/80 for all diabetics.
   (c) Use of thiazide diuretics are not recommended due to associated metabolic derangements.
   (d) Metoprolol is preferred over carvedilol.
   (e) There is no additional benefit of using RAAS blockers over other antihypertensives.

   AACE and ADA recommend RAAS blockers as the first line of treatment for diabetics due to beneficial effects on cardiovascular outcome. In addition, it reduces microalbuminuria and the risk of creatinine doubling. JNC 8 recommends a BP goal of <140/90. Despite metabolic derangements associated with thiazide diuretics, they are still used to treat diabetics. Diuretics have shown to reduce cardiovascular risk. Unlike metoprolol, carvedilol will not increase blood sugar or lipids.

6. The 2020 Canadian HTN guidelines recommend that newly diagnosed patients with HTN be screened for which of the following cardiovascular risk factors?
   (a) Kidney disease
   (b) Dyslipidemia
   (c) Diabetes mellitus
   (d) b and c
   (e) a, b and c.

   The 2020 Canadian HTN guidelines recommend that newly diagnosed patients with HTN be screened for diabetes with a fasting glucose and/or hemoglobin A1c, as well as hyperlipidemia with labs for serum total cholesterol, LDL, HDL, non-HDL cholesterol, and triglycerides, as well as kidney disease with urinalysis, assessment of albumin excretion in diabetics.

7. What is the initial weight loss goal from baseline weight in the National Institutes of Health clinical guidelines for treatment of obesity?
   (a) 5%
   (b) 20%
   (c) 30%
   (d) **10%**
   (e) 25%

Approach to weight loss and maintenance based on National Institutes of Health clinical guidelines for treatment of obesity recommends an initial weight loss goal of a 10% reduction from baseline weight.

8. All of the following are nondesirable side effects of beta blockers in diabetics except:
   (a) Masking of hypoglycemia symptoms
   (b) **Lowering of heart rate**
   (c) Dyslipidemia
   (d) Weight gain
   (e) Insulin resistance

   Beta-blockers have been associated with metabolic derangements including dyslipidemia, increased insulin resistance, and weight gain and can mask hypoglycemia symptoms.

9. The following have been postulated to be involved in the pathophysiology of HTN in DM except:
   (a) Sodium retention due to hyperfiltration
   (b) Reduced nitric oxide bioavailability
   (c) Deranged metabolic signaling of insulin.
   (d) **Reduced sympathetic nervous system activation**
   (e) Inappropriate activation of the RAAS system

   The pathophysiology of HTN in DM is multifactorial, involving multiple tissues, organ systems, metabolic signaling pathways, and environmental and genetic factors.

10. Lowering systolic BP to less than what number was shown in multiple major trials to lower mortality and improves CVD outcomes?
    (a) 160
    (b) **150**
    (c) 140
    (d) 130
    (e) 120

    Major trials such as Syst-Eur, UKPDS, and SHEP studies supported the conclusion that treatment to a systolic BP of <150 mmHg lowers mortality and improves CVD and cerebrovascular health outcomes.

11. All of the following statements are true of finerenone except
    (a) It is a non-steroidal mineralocorticoid receptor antagonist
    (b) Contraindicated in patients with adrenal insufficiency
    (c) **Best taken on an empty stomach**
    (d) Only Mineralocorticoid receptor antagonist indicated to reduce the risk of sustained eGFR decline, end stage kidney disease, cardiovascular death, nonfatal myocardial infarction, and hospitalization for heart failure in adult patients with chronic kidney disease (CKD) associated with type 2 diabetes
    (e) No relevant affinity to androgen, progesterone, and estrogen receptors

Finerenone is a nonsteroidal mineralocorticoid receptor blocker that can be taken with or without food. It is contraindicated in adrenal insufficiency and with concomitant use with strong CYP3A inhibitors. It is the only MR blocker indicated to reduce the risk of sustained eGFR decline, end-stage kidney disease, cardiovascular death, nonfatal myocardial infarction, and hospitalization for heart failure in adult patients with chronic kidney disease (CKD) associated with type 2 diabetes. No relevant affinity to androgen, progesterone, and estrogen receptors. It can be taken with or without food.

References

1. Centers for Disease Control and Prevention. National diabetes statistics report: estimates of diabetes and its burden in the United States, 2020. Atlanta, GA: U.S. Department of Health and Human Services; 2020.
2. American Diabetes Association. Chapter 10. Cardiovascular disease and risk management. Diabetes Care. 2021;44(Supplement 1):S125–50.
3. Rabi D, et al. Hypertension Canada's 2020 comprehensive guidelines for the prevention, diagnosis, risk assessment, and treatment of hypertension in adults and children. Can J Cardiol. 2020;36(5):596–624.
4. Karuparthi PR, Yerram P, Lastra G, Hayden MR, Sowers JR. Understanding essential hypertension from the perspective of the cardiometabolic syndrome. J Am Soc Hypertens. 2007;1(2):120–34.
5. Lastra G, Syed S, Kurukulasuriya RL, Manrique C, Sowers JR. Type 2 diabetes mellitus and hypertension: an update. Endocrinol Metab Clin North Am. 2014;43(1):103–22.
6. DeMarco VG, Aroor AR, Sowers JR. The pathophysiology of hypertension in patient with obesity. Nat Rev Endocrinol. 2014;10(6):364–76.
7. Jia J, Sowers JR. Hypertension in diabetes: an update of basic mechanisms and clinical disease. Hypertension. 2021;78:1197–205.
8. Williams B. The hypertension in diabetes study (HDS): a catalyst for change. Diabet Med. 2008;25(Suppl. 2):13–9.
9. James PA, Oparil S, Carter BL, et al. 2014 evidence-based guideline for the management of high blodd pressure in adults: report from the panel members appointed to the eighth joint national committee (JNC 8). JAMA. 2014;311(5):507–20.
10. The ACCORD study group. Effects of intensive blood pressure control in patients with type 2 diabetes. N Engl J Med. 2010;362:1575–85.
11. Pepine CJ, Handberg EM, Cooper-DeJoff RM, For the INVEST investigators, et al. A calcium antagonist vs a non-calcium antagonist hypertension treatment strategy for patients with coronary artery disease: the international verapamil-tandolapril study (INVEST): a randomized controlled trial. JAMA. 2003;290(21):2805–16.
12. The ONTARGET Investigators. Telmisartan, Ramipril, or both in patients at high risk for vascular events. N Engl J Med. 2008;358:1547–59.
13. Duckworth W, Abraira C, Moritz T, et al. VADT investigators. Glucose control and vascular complications in veterans with type 2 diabetes. N Engl J Med. 2009;360:129–39.
14. The SPRINT Research group. A randomized trial of intensive vs standard blood pressure control. N Engl J Med. 2015;373:2103–16.

15. Cosentino F, et al. 2019 ESC guidelines on diabetes, pre-diabetes, and cardiovascular diseases developed in collaboration with the EASD. Eur Heart J. 2020;41(2):255–323.

16. Williams B, et al. 2018 ESH/ESC guidelines for management of arterial hypertension. Eur Heart J. 2018;39:3021–104.

17. Unger T. 2020 International society of hypertension global hypertension practice guidelines. Hypertension. 2020;75(6):1334–57.

18. Handelsman Y, Bloomgarden ZT, Grunberger G, et al. American Association of Clinical Endocrinologists and American College of endocrinology—clinical practice guidelines for developing a diabetes mellitus comprehensive care plan—2015. Endocr Pract. 2015;21(4):413–37.

19. Zhijun W, Jin C, Vaidya A, Jin W, Huang Z, Shouling W. Xian Ga longitudinal pattern of longitudinal patterns of blood pressure, cardiovascular events, and all-cause mortality in normotensive diabetic people. Hypertension. 2016;68:71–7.

20. Whaley-Connell A, Sowers JR. Blood pressure-related outcomes in a diabetic population. Hypertension. 2016;68(1):71–7.

21. Clinical Guidelines on the Identification. Evaluation, and treatment of overweight and obesity in adults—the evidence report. National Institutes of health. Obes Res. 1998;6(suppl 2):51S–209S.

22. Jindal A, Brietzke S, Sowers JR. Obesity and the Cardiorenal metabolic syndrome: therapeutic modalities and their efficacy in improving cardiovascular and renal risk factors. Cardiorenal Med. 2012;2:314–27.

23. U.S. Department of Health and Human Services. (n.d.). Drinking levels defined. National Institute on alcohol abuse and alcoholism. https://www.niaaa.nih.gov/alcohol-health/overview-alcohol-consumption/moderate-binge-drinking.

24. U.S. Department of Health and Human Services. (n.d.). What is a standard drink? National Institute on Alcohol Abuse and Alcoholism. https://www.niaaa.nih.gov/alcohols-effects-health/overview-alcohol-consumption/what-standard-drink.

25. Look AHEAD Research Group. Reduction in weight and cardiovascular disease risk factors in individuals with type 2 diabetes: one-year results of the look AHEAD trial. Diabetes Care. 2007;30(6):1374–83.

26. The Look AHEAD Research Group. Cardiovascular effects of intensive lifestyle intervention in type 2 diabetes. N Engl J Med. 2013;369:145–54.

27. Baudrand R, Campino C, Carvajal CA, et al. High sodium intake is associated with increased glucocorticoid production, insulin resistance and metabolic syndrome. Clin Endocrinol (Oxf). 2014;80(5):677–84.

28. He FJ, Li J, Macgregor GA. Effect of longer term modest salt reduction on blood pressure: Cochrane systematic review and meta-analysis of randomised trials. BMJ. 2013;346:f1325.

29. Sacks FM, Svetkey LP, Vollmer WM, et al. Effects on blood pressure of reduced dietary sodium and the dietary approaches to stop hypertension (DASH) diet. DASH-sodium collaborative research group. N Engl J Med. 2001;344(1):3–10.

30. Miller ER, Erlinger TP, Appel LJ. The effects of macronutrients on blood pressure and lipids: an overview of the DASH and OmniHeart trials. Curr Atheroscler Rep. 2006;8:460–5.

31. Your guide to lowering your blood pressure with DASH. U.S. Department of Health and Human Services. National Institutes of Health. National Heart, Lung, and Blood Institute.

32. Conlin PR, Chow D, Miller ER, et al. The effect of dietary patterns on blood pressure control in hypertensive patients: results from the dietary approaches to stop hypertension (DASH) trial. Am J Hypertens. 2000;13(9):949–55.

33. Lin PH, Allen JD, Li YJ, Yu M, Lien LF, Svetkey LP. Blood pressure-lowering mechanisms of the DASH dietary pattern. J Nutr Metab. 2012;2012:472396, 1.

34. Dernini S, Berry EM. Mediterranean diet: from a healthy diet to a sustainable dietary pattern. Front Nutr. 2015;2:15.

35. Willett WC, Sacks F, Trichopoulou A, et al. Mediterranean diet pyramid: a cultural model for healthy eating. Am J Clin Nutr. 1995;61(6 Suppl):1402S–6S.

36. Trichopoulou A, Martínez-gonzález MA, Tong TY, et al. Definitions and potential health benefits of the Mediterranean diet: views from experts around the world. BMC Med. 2014;12:112.

37. Patton SR, Dolan LM, Powers SW. Mealtime interactions relate to dietary adherence and glycemic control in young children with type 1 diabetes. Diabetes Care. 2006;29(5):1002–6.

38. Esposito K, Maiorino MI, Bellastella G, Chiodini P, Panagiotakos D, Giugliano D. A journey into a Mediterranean diet and type 2 diabetes: a systematic review with meta-analyses. BMJ Open. 2015;5(8):e008222.

39. Estruch R, Ros E, Salas-salvadó J, et al. Primary prevention of cardiovascular disease with a Mediterranean diet. N Engl J Med. 2013;368(14):1279–90.

40. Knoops KT, De Groot LC, Kromhout D, et al. Mediterranean diet, lifestyle factors, and 10-year mortality in elderly European men and women: the HALE project. JAMA. 2004;292(12):1433–9.

41. Blumenthal JA, Babyak MA, Hinderliter A, et al. Effects of the DASH diet alone and in combination with exercise and weight loss on blood pressure and cardiovascular biomarkers in men and women with high blood pressure: the ENCORE study. Arch Intern Med. 2010;170(2):126–35.

42. Fletcher GF, Balady G, Blair SN, Blumenthal J, Caspersen C, Chaitman B, Epstein S, Sivarajan Froelicher ES, Froelicher VF, Pina IL, Pollock ML. Statement on exercise: benefits and recommendations for physical activity programs for all Americans. Circulation. 1996;94:857–62.

43. Haskell WL, Lee IM, Pate RR, et al. Physical activity and public health: updated recommendation for adults from the American College of Sports Medicine and the American Heart Association. Med Sci Sports Exerc. 2007;39(8):1423–34.

44. Franckowiak SC, Dobrosielski DA, Reilley SM, Walston JD, Andersen RE. Maximal heart rate prediction in adults that are overweight or obese. J Strength Cond Res. 2011;25(5):1407–12.

45. Donnelly JE, Hill JO, Jacobsen DJ, et al. Effects of a 16-month randomized controlled exercise trial on body weight and composition in young, overweight men and women: the Midwest exercise trial. Arch Intern Med. 2003;163(11):1343–50.

46. Bergenstal R, Kim T, Trautmann M, et al. Exanatide once weekly elicited improvements in blood pressure and lipid profile over 52 weeks in patients with type 2 diabetes (abstract no. 1239). Circulation. 2008;1:18LS1086.

47. Kurukulasuriya LR, Sowers JR. Therapies for type 2 diabetes: lowering HbA1c and associated cardiovascular risk factors. Cardiovasc Diabetol. 2010;9:45.

48. Mendis B, Simpson E, Macdonald I, Mansell P. Investigation of the haemodynamic effects of exenatide in healthy male subjects. Br J Clin Pharmacol. 2012;74(3):437–44.

49. Irace C, De Luca S, Shehaj E, et al. Exenatide improves endothelial function assessed by flow mediated dilation technique in subjects with type 2 diabetes: results from an observational research. Diab Vasc Dis Res. 2013;10(1):72–7.

50. Endocrine Society's 96th Annual Meeting and Expo, June 21–24, 2014—Chicago LBSU-1074: Exenatide Induces an Increase in Vasodilatory Mediators.

51. Marso SP, et al. LEADER steering committee; LEADER trial investigators. Liraglutide and cardiovascular outcomes in type 2 diabetes. N Engl J Med. 2016;375:311–22.

52. Vilsbøll T, et al. Effects of glucagon-like peptide-1 receptor agonists on weight loss: systematic review and meta-analyses of randomised controlled trials. BMJ. 2012;344:d7771.

53. Schöndorf T, Forst T, Hohberg C, Pahler S, Link C, Roth W, Pfützner A, Lübben G, Link C, Pfützner A. The IRIS III study: pioglitazone improves metabolic control and blood pressure in patients with type 2 diabetes without increasing body weight. Diabetes Obes Metab. 2007;9(1):132–3.

54. Auclair M, Vigouroux C, Boccara F, et al. Peroxisome proliferator-activated receptor-γ mutations responsible for lipodystrophy with severe hypertension activate the cellular renin–angiotensin system. Arterioscler Thromb Vasc Biol. 2013;33:829–38.

55. Buchanan TA, Meehan WP, Jeng YY, et al. Blood pressure lowering by pioglitazone. Evidence for a direct vascular effect. J Clin Invest. 1995;96(1):354–60.

56. Verma S, Bhanot S, Arikawa E, Yao L, Mcneill JH. Direct vasodepressor effects of pioglitazone in spontaneously hypertensive rats. Pharmacology. 1998;56(1):7–16.

57. Mistry GC, Maes AL, Lasseter KC, et al. Effect of sitagliptin, a dipeptidyl peptidase-4 inhibitor, on blood pressure in nondiabetic patients with mild to moderate hypertension. J Clin Pharmacol. 2008;48:592–8.

58. Liu J, Wong WT, et al. Dipeptidyl peptidase 4 inhibitor sitagliptin protects endothelial function in hypertension through a glucagon-like peptide 1-dependent mechanism. Hypertension. 2012;60(3):833–41.

59. Mason RP, Jacob RF, Kubant R, Ciszewski A, Corbalan JJ, Malinski T. Dipeptidyl peptidase-4 inhibition with saxagliptin enhanced nitric oxide release and reduced blood pressure and sICAM-1 levels in hypertensive rats. J Cardiovasc Pharmacol. 2012;60(5):467–73.

60. Oliva RV, et al. Blood pressure effects of sodium-glucose co-transport 2 (SGLT2) inhibitors. J Am Soc Hypertens. 2014;8:330–9.

61. Mazidi M, et al. Effect of sodium-glucose cotransport-2 inhibitors on blood pressure in people with type 2 diabetes mellitus: a systematic review and meta-analysis of 43 randomized control trials with 22 528 patients. J Am Heart Assoc. 2017;6(6):6e00407.

62. Monami M, et al. Efficacy and safety of sodium glucose co-transport-2 inhibitors in type 2 diabetes: a meta-analysis of randomized clinical trials. Diabetes Obes Metab. 2014;16:457–66.

63. Clar C, Gill JA, Court R, Waugh N. Systematic review of SGLT2 receptor inhibitors in dual or triple therapy in type 2 diabetes. BMJ Open. 2012;2:e001007.

64. Rosenstock J, Aggarwal N, Polidori D, Zhao Y, Arbit D, Usiskin K, Capuano G, Canovatchel W, Group CDS. Dose-ranging effects of canagliflozin, a sodium-glucose cotransporter 2 inhibitor, as add-on to metformin in subjects with type 2 diabetes. Diabetes Care. 2012;35:1232–8.

65. Zinman B, Wanner C, Lachin JM, et al. Empagliflozin, cardiovascular outcomes, and mortality in type 2 diabetes. N Engl J Med. 2015;373:2117–28.

66. Zelniker TA, et al. Comparison of the effects of glucagon-like peptide receptor agonists and sodium-glucose cotransporter 2 inhibitors for prevention of major adverse cardiovascular and renal outcomes in type 2 diabetes mellitus. Circulation. 2019;139:2022–31.

67. Zelniker TA, et al. SGLT2 inhibitors for primary and secondary prevention of cardiovascular and renal outcomes in type 2 diabetes: a systematic review and meta-analysis of cardiovascular outcome trials. Lancet. 2019;393:31–9.

68. Alatrach M, Agyin C, Adams J, Chilton R, Triplitt C, DeFronzo RA, Cersosimo E. Glucose lowering and vascular protective effects of cycloset added to GLP-1 receptor agonists in patients with type 2 diabetes. Endocrinol Diabetes Metab. 2018;1(4):e00034.

69. Chamarthi B, Ezrokhi M, Rutty D, Cincotta AH. Impact of bromocriptine-QR therapy on cardiovascular outcomes in type 2 diabetes mellitus subjects on metformin. Diabetes Obes Metab. 2011;13(10):880–4.

70. Vijakama P, Thakkinstain A, Lertrattananon D, et al. Renoprotective effects of renin-angiotensin system blockade in type 2 diabetic patients: a systematic review and network meta-analysis. Diabetologia. 2012;55:566–78.

71. Wu HY, Huang JW, Lin HJ, et al. Comparative effectiveness of renin-angiotensin system blockers and other antihypertensive drugs in patients with diabetes: systamitic review and Bayesian network meta-analysis. BMJ. 2013;347:f6008.

72. Grossman E, Messerli FH. Management of blood pressure in patients with diabetes. Am J Hypertens. 2011;24(8):863–75.

73. Reboldi G, Gentile G, Angeli F, et al. Optimal therapy in hypertensive subjects with diabetes mellitus. Curr Atheroscler Rep. 2011;13:176–85.

74. Sowers JR, Lastra G, Roca R, et al. Initial combination therapy compared with monotherapy in diabetic hypertensive patients. J Clin Hypertens (Greenwich). 2008;10:668–76.

75. National High Blood Pressure Education Program. The Seventh report of the Joint National Committee on Prevention detection evaluation and treatment of high blood pressure. Bethesda, MD: National Heart, Lung, and Blood Institute (US); 2004. NIH Publication No4–5230.

76. Williams B, MacDonald TM, Morant S, et al. For the British hypertension Society's PATHWAY studies group. Spironolactone versus placebo, bisoprolol, and doxazosin to determine the optimal treatmet for drug-resistant hypertension (PATHWAY-2): a randomized, double-blind, crossover trial. Lancet. 2015;386(10008):2059–68.

77. Bakris GL, Agarwal R, Anker SD, Pitt B, Ruilope LM, Rossing P, Kolkhof P, Nowack C, Schloemer P, Joseph A, Filippatos G, FIDELIO-DKD Investigators. Effect of finerenone on chronic kidney disease outcomes in type 2 diabetes. N Engl J Med. 2020;383:2219–29.

78. Parving HH, Persson F, Lewis JB, Lewis EJ, Hollenberg NK, AVOID Study Investigators. Aliskiren combined with losartan in type 2 diabetes and nephropathy. N Engl J Med. 2008;358(23):2433.

79. Parving H-H, Brenner BM, McMurray JJV, de Zeeuw D, Haffner SM, Solomon SD, Chaturvedi N, Persson F, Desai AS, Nicolaides M, Richard A, Xiang Z, Brunel P, Pfeffer MA, ALTITUDE Investigators. Cardiorenal end points in a trial of aliskiren for type 2 diabetes. N Engl J Med. 2012;367:2204–13.

80. Cohen JB, Cohen DL. Integrating out-of-office blood pressure in the diagnosis and management of hypertension. Curr Cardiol Rep. 2016;18:112.

81. Leitao CB, Canani LH, Silveiro SP, Gross JL. Ambulatory blood pressure monitoring and type 2 diabetes mellitus. Arq Bras Cardiol. 2007;88(2):315–21.

82. Loehr LR, Meyer ML, Poon AK, Selvin E, Palta P, et al. Prediabetes and diabetes are associated with arterial siffness in older adults: the ARIC study. Am J Hypertens. 2016;29(9):1038–45.

83. Guan WJ, Ni ZY, Hu Y, Liang WH, Ou CQ, He JX, Liu L, Shan H, Lei CL, Hui DSC, Du B, Li LJ, Zeng G, Yuen KY, Chen RC, Tang CL, Wang T, Chen PY, Xiang J, Li SY, Wang JL, Liang ZJ, Peng YX, Wei L, Liu Y, Hu YH, Peng P, Wang JM, Liu JY, Chen Z, Li G, Zheng ZJ, Qiu SQ, Luo J, Ye CJ, Zhu SY, Zhong NS, China Medical Treatment Expert Group for Covid-19. Clinical characteristics of coronavirus disease 2019 in China. N Engl J Med. 2020;382(18):1708–20.

84. Feldman EL, Savelieff MG, Hayek SS, Pennathur S, Kretzler M, Pop-Busui R. COVID-19 and diabetes: a collision and collusion of two diseases. Diabetes. 2020;69(12):2549–65.

85. Lim S, Bae JH, Kwon HS, Nauck MA. COVID-19 and diabetes mellitus: from pathophysiology to clinical management. Nat Rev Endocrinol. 2021;17(1):11–30.

86. Mueller M, Purnell T, Mensah G, Cooper L. Reducing racial and ethnic disparities in hypertension prevention and control: what will it take to translate research into practice and policy? Am J Hypertens. 2015;28(6):699–716.

87. Naha S, Gardner MJ, Khangura D, Kurukulasuriya LR, Sowers JR. Hypertension in Diabetes. In: Feingold KR, Anawalt B, Boyce A, Chrousos G, de Herder WW, Dhatariya K, Dungan K, Grossman A, Hershman JM, Hofland J, Kalra S, Kaltsas G, Koch C, Kopp P, Korbonits M, Kovacs CS, Kuohung W, Laferrère B, EA MG, Mclachlan R, Morley JE, New M, Purnell J, Sahay R, Singer F, Stratakis CA, Trence DL, Wilson DP, editors. Endotext; 2021.

88. Hill MA, Mantzoros C, Sowers JR. Commentary: COVID-19 in patients with diabetes. Metabolism. 2020;107:154217.

89. Rysz J, et al. Pharmacogenomics of hypertension treatment. Int J Mol Sci. 2020;21(13):4709. Published 2020 Jul 1.

Further Reading

Sowers JR. Diabetes mellitus and vascular disease. Hypertension. 2013;61:943–7.

Diabetes and Atherogenic Dyslipidemia

Arshag D. Mooradian

Introduction

Despite the recent decline in the incidence of cardiovascular mortality in people with diabetes, cardiovascular disease (CVD) continues to be the leading cause of morbidity and mortality in this patient population [1–5]. The cause of accelerated atherosclerosis and premature emergence of coronary artery disease (CAD) is multifactorial. Nevertheless, dyslipidemia is an important risk factor in diabetes that is modifiable with lifestyle changes and institution of effective pharmacologic agents [6, 7].

People with diabetes can have all the variants of dyslipidemias observed in nondiabetic people [7–9]. However, in type 2 diabetes where obesity and insulin resistance are common, a typical dyslipidemia is manifested as high plasma triglyceride and low high-density lipoprotein (HDL) cholesterol concentrations and increased small dense low-density lipoprotein (LDL) cholesterol particles [8, 9].

Prevalence of Dyslipidemia in Diabetes

In the Framingham Heart Study, the prevalence of high LDL cholesterol concentrations in men and women with diabetes mellitus (9% and 15%, respectively) did not differ significantly from the rates in men and women who did not have diabetes (11% and 16%, respectively) [10]. However, people with diabetes had more often high plasma triglyceride concentrations (19% in men and 17% in women) than people without diabetes mellitus (9% of men and 8% of women). In this survey, high levels of total cholesterol, LDL cholesterol, and triglyceride were defined as values above the corresponding 90th percentile for the US population [10]. The prevalence of low plasma HDL cholesterol concentrations (defined as a value below the 10th percentile for the US popu-

lation) was 21% in men and 25% in women with diabetes, while only 12% nondiabetic men and 10% of nondiabetic women had low HDL cholesterol levels [10]. A similar increase in the prevalence of hypertriglyceridemia and low HDL cholesterol level was observed in the UK Prospective Diabetes Study (UKPDS) [11].

Pathophysiology of Dyslipidemia in Diabetes

One of the major drivers of increased plasma triglyceride concentrations in people with type 2 diabetes is the increased free fatty-acid release from insulin-resistant fat cells [7–9]. The increased flux of free fatty acids into the liver promotes triglyceride production. Subsequently, there is increased secretion of apolipoprotein B (apoB) and very low-density lipoprotein (VLDL) cholesterol.

Insulin resistance is also associated with low HDL cholesterol levels [7–9] and increased concentration of small dense LDL-cholesterol particles as VLDL-transported triglyceride is exchanged for HDL or LDL-transported cholesteryl ester through the action of the cholesteryl ester transfer protein (CETP) (Fig. 40.1). This exchange results in increased amounts of both atherogenic cholesterol-rich VLDL remnant particles and triglyceride-rich, cholesterol-depleted HDL and LDL particles. The latter triglyceride-enriched particles are hydrolyzed by hepatic lipase or lipoprotein lipase resulting in dissociated apolipoprotein A-I (apo A-I) that is filtered by the renal glomeruli and degraded in renal tubular cells (Fig. 40.1) [7–9]. The increased concentration of small dense LDL-cholesterol particles occurs by a similar lipid exchange that results in lipid depletion of the LDL particles (Fig. 40.1).

The lipid exchange pathway cannot entirely explain why low HDL cholesterol levels can also occur in people who do not have hypertriglyceridemia. In these patients, inability of insulin to upregulate the apo A-I production owing either to insulin resistance or increased inflammatory cytokines notably tumor necrosis factor (TNF) alpha might contribute to low HDL cholesterol levels [12–14].

A. D. Mooradian (✉)
Department of Medicine, University of Florida College of Medicine, Jacksonville, FL, USA
e-mail: arshag.mooradian@jax.ufl.edu

© The Author(s), under exclusive license to Springer Nature Switzerland AG 2023
J. Rodriguez-Saldana (ed.), *The Diabetes Textbook*, https://doi.org/10.1007/978-3-031-25519-9_40

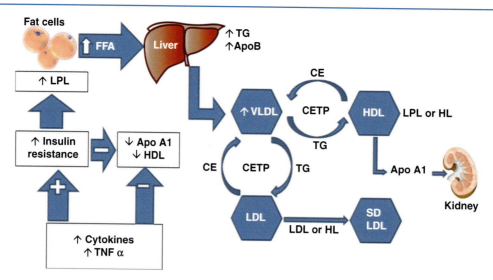

Fig. 40.1 Pathogenesis of diabetic dyslipidemia. Insulin resistance initiates the characteristic triad of high triglyceride level, low HDL cholesterol level, and high small dense LDL level. If the concentration of VLDL transported triglyceride is high, CETP promotes the transfer of LDL cholesteryl ester or HDL cholesteryl ester in exchange for triglyceride. Triglyceride-rich HDL or LDL can undergo hydrolysis by hepatic lipase or lipoprotein lipase. ↑ increased level, *TNF α* tumor necrosis factor α, *ApoA-1* apolipoprotein A-1, *ApoB* apolipoprotein B, *CE* cholesteryl ester, *CETP* cholesteryl ester transfer protein, *FFA* free fatty acid, *HL* hepatic lipase, *LPL* lipoprotein lipase, *SD LDL* small dense LDL cholesterol, *TG* triglyceride, *HDL* high-density lipoprotein, *LDL* low-density lipoprotein, *VLDL* very low-density lipoprotein. Reprinted from reference [8] with permission of the authors and the publisher

Insulin resistance is also associated with a decreased ratio of lipoprotein lipase to hepatic lipase in heparin-treated plasma, which contributes to the low HDL-cholesterol level [8, 9]. In addition, the esterification of cholesterol (mediated by lecithin-cholesterol acyl transferase) is either modestly increased or unaltered, whereas increased CETP activity depletes HDL of its cholesteryl ester and therefore contributes to the lowering of HDL cholesterol levels [8, 9].

It is noteworthy that the combination of high triglyceride and low HDL cholesterol levels is observed in familial and sporadic syndromes (e.g., familial combined hyperlipidemia and familial hypertriglyceridemia) and the onset of obesity and insulin resistance would augment the lipid abnormality phenotype in these people [9].

Atherogenicity of Dyslipidemia in Diabetes

Interventional trials with statins have proven the efficacy of these drugs in reducing cardiovascular events in people with diabetes. In these trials, the linear relationships between LDL cholesterol levels and the incidence of cardiovascular events were similar in individuals both with and without diabetes mellitus [15]. However, the role of low HDL cholesterol and increased triglyceride levels in CVD is still unproven. The association between hypertriglyceridemia and the increased risk of CVD is not as strong as the association between LDL cholesterol level and CVD risk.

Patients with elevated triglyceride levels especially in the context of familial combined hyperlipidemia or low HDL level might have increased risk for CVD. In addition, severe hypertriglyceridemia (greater than or equal to 5.65 mmol/L (500 mg/dL) increases the risk of pancreatitis.

Interventional trials that used fibrate therapy to lower triglyceride and increase HDL cholesterol levels have failed to show a reproducible reduction in cardiovascular events. In the HDL Intervention Trial (HIT), gemfibrozil treatment was associated with a 22% reduction in the risk of coronary heart disease (CHD) and a 25% reduction in the risk of stroke [16]. In the latter study, a quarter of the subjects studied had diabetes. The favorable effect of gemfibrozil in the primary prevention of CHD was also demonstrated in previous trials [17].

The Fenofibrate Intervention and Event Lowering in Diabetes (FIELD) study did not show that fenofibrate had a statistically significant effect on the primary outcome (CHD-related death or nonfatal myocardial infarction) [18, 19]. However, fenofibrate reduced the prevalence of nonfatal myocardial infarction and coronary revascularization, but it did not reduce the risk of fatal events [18, 19].

The Action to Control Cardiovascular Risk in Diabetes (ACCORD) study examined whether treatment with a statin plus a fibrate, as compared with statin alone, would decrease the risk of cardiovascular events in a population of 5518 patients with type 2 diabetes [20]. After a mean follow-up period of 4.7 years, fenofibrate with simvastatin group compared with simvastatin alone did not have reduced cardiovascular events. Further analyses suggested a possible benefit for patients with the combination of a high baseline triglyceride level and low HDL cholesterol [20]. This observation was in agreement with the previous findings in the FIELD trial [19].

The HDL has a central role in reverse cholesterol transport and possesses a number of other cardioprotective properties. However, most trials with agents known to increase HDL levels have not shown any reduction in cardiovascular events except possibly in a subgroup of patients with high serum triglycerides and low HDL cholesterol levels [21–26].

The Atherothrombosis Intervention in Metabolic Syndrome with Low HDL/High Triglycerides Impact on Global Health Outcomes (AIM-HIGH) [21] and the Heart Protection Study 2: Treatment of HDL to Reduce the Incidence of Vascular Events (HPS2-THRIVE) [22] used niacin as the HDL cholesterol-boosting agent. Four clinical trials used CETP inhibitors to increase HDL cholesterol level [23–26]. Only the Randomized Evaluation of the Effects of anacetrapib through Lipid Modification (REVEAL) trial showed favorable effects on cardiovascular outcomes, but most of the benefit was attributed to its ability to reduce non-HDL cholesterol levels [26]. It is possible that when HDL levels are increased with enhanced de novo production rather than impaired turnover secondary to CETP inhibition, the quality and functionality of HDL improve to become a more effective cardioprotective moiety [27].

Management of Dyslipidemia in Diabetes Mellitus

An integral component of the management of dyslipidemia is to exclude secondary aggravating causes notably hypothyroidism and use of hormone replacement therapy. Although most people with diabetes would require pharmacologic agents, lifestyle modifications are still important cornerstone of therapy. These include dietary restrictions, increased physical activity, and smoking cessation [7]. Glycemic control usually improves the dyslipidemia by either providing insulin or enhancing insulin action, but it may not increase the reduced HDL cholesterol levels [28]. In addition, some agents such as pioglitazone may have direct effects on lipid metabolism [8].

Medical Nutrition Therapy

Dietary interventions should be individualized based on patient's own dietary preferences [8, 9]. While the low fat diet has been the cornerstone of the dietary guidelines in the past, more recent guidelines emphasize the importance of limiting added sugars to less than 10% of total energy intake. This recommendation is based on a large body of evidence for the association between the consumption of added sugars, especially fructose from corn syrup and atherogenic lipid profile [29–32]. In addition, clinical trials using a diet enriched with monounsaturated fat such as the Mediterranean diet have shown favorable effects on cardiovascular risk [33]. When weight loss is the goal of dieting, there is not clinically meaningful difference between carbohydrate-restricted diets and fat-restricted diets. It is best to limit portion size as all calories count irrespective of their source [32, 34]. The American Diabetes Association (ADA) recommends modest weight loss for overweight individuals [35]. As little as 5% weight loss can have favorable metabolic effects, and clinical studies have shown that 7% or less of weight loss can prevent or delay the onset of diabetes in high-risk individuals [36].

Low-carbohydrate diets (LCD) can enhance weight loss in the short term although its effect is small and not sustainable [32]. In people with diabetes and insulin resistance, LCD is helpful in achieving glycemic control. However, there are untoward side effects especially when carbohydrates are severely restricted (<50 g/day) to induce ketosis. The latter curbs appetite but also may cause nausea, fatigue, and water and electrolyte losses and limits exercise capacity [32]. In addition, observational studies suggest that low-carbohydrate diets (<40% energy from carbohydrates) as well as very high carbohydrate diets (>70% energy from carbohydrate) are associated with increased mortality [32]. The available scientific evidence supports the current dietary recommendations to replace highly processed carbohydrates with unprocessed carbohydrates as well as limiting added sugars in the diet [32].

The type of fat consumed is more important than total amount of fat. A reduction in dietary saturated fat to less than 10% of total daily calories is recommended along with preferential consumption of monounsaturated fat, elimination of trans-fat intake, and limiting daily sodium consumption to less than 2300 mg [35]. Overall, Mediterranean [33] or Dietary Approaches to Stop Hypertension (DASH) [37] style diets are prudent advice to people with diabetes. Of note is that the previous recommendation of restricting dietary cholesterol intake to less than 300 mg/day has been removed from the 2015 and 2020 Dietary Guidelines for Americans [29]. People with diabetes should follow the dietary guidelines issued for the general population [35].

It is noteworthy that replacing saturated fat intake with carbohydrate lowers total cholesterol, LDL and HDL cholesterol, and may increase triglyceride level [38, 39]. On the other hand, substituting saturated fat with monounsaturated or polyunsaturated fat has favorable effect on HDL cholesterol and triglyceride levels. Dietary protein or various amino acids do not have clinically significant effects on lipoprotein profile [38, 39].

Effects of Exercise

Staying active and exercising have multiple benefits notably enhanced cardiovascular health. Increased physical activity also helps to maintain the weight loss attained with caloric restriction [40]. In addition, independent of weight loss, exercise can improve insulin sensitivity and increase HDL cholesterol levels [41, 42]. Both aerobic or resistance training improve glycemic control in type 2 diabetes, and larger improvement in glycemic control can be achieved with combined resistance and aerobic training [43].

There is a paucity of trials examining the effect of exercise on lipid changes in diabetes. In a study of postmenopausal women with type 2 diabetes, exercise without weight loss was associated with a reduction in waist circumference and improve visceral adipose tissue [44]. In another study of people with type 2 diabetes, a supervised aerobic exercise program reduced VLDL–apo B pool size [45]. Despite the limitations in these studies, it is a prudent clinical practice to encourage people with diabetes to engage in exercise to the extent possible. Overall, 30 min of walking five times a week is effective in improving insulin sensitivity and reducing the risk of diabetes in those at risk for developing diabetes [36].

Pharmacologic Interventions

Various classes of lipid-modifying agents are summarized in Table 40.1. Of these agents, statins have been consistently associated with cardiovascular event reduction [15]. Although the efficacy of statins correlates well with their ability in reducing LDL cholesterol, the potential contribution of pleiotropic effects of statin to CVD risk reduction was supported by the observation that therapeutic targeting hsCRP (highly sensitive C-reactive protein) with rosuvastatin was associated significant improvement in event-free survival, and the effect was independent of LDL cholesterol level achieved [46].

The cholesterol hypothesis in contrast to the statin hypothesis is supported by the observation that ezetimibe, a selective cholesterol absorption inhibitor, was also associated with reduction in CVD events when used in addition to statins [47]. This latter study is in contrast to earlier studies with ezetimibe, one in patients with aortic stenosis [48] and the other in those with chronic kidney disease [49]. In the latter studies, ezetimibe and statin combination did not alter mortality but had some favorable effects on secondary endpoints such as fewer coronary bypass procedures, reductions in non-hemorrhagic stroke, and arterial revascularization procedures [48, 49]. Thus, ezetimibe should be considered when maximal doses of high potency statins are not tolerated [35]. Similarly, two interventional trials with PCSK9 (pro-

protein convertase subtilisin/kexin 9) inhibitors, evolocumab and alirocumab, showed a reduction in cardiovascular events in a high-risk population with LDL cholesterol levels of 1.8 mmol/L (70 mg/dL) or higher who were receiving statin therapy [50, 51]. Another related drug soon to be available is inclisiran (Leqvio®). This investigational drug would be the first LDL cholesterol-lowering siRNA medicine. Its twice-yearly dosing by subcutaneous injection is a significant advantage in enhancing adherence to cholesterol lowering drugs [52].

An additional option is ATP citrate lyase inhibitor bempedoic acid (Nexletol®). This drug is approved for the treatment of adults with heterozygous familial hypercholesterolemia or established atherosclerotic cardiovascular disease who require additional lowering of LDL cholesterol. A single-pill combination of bempedoic acid and ezetimibe (Nexlizet®) is also available [53].

The bile acid sequestrants (BAS) have a limited role in reducing LDL cholesterol except possibly in women of reproductive age and children where safety of statins and ezetimibe is of concern. Gastrointestinal side effects, increased risk of cholelithiasis, and aggravation of hypertriglyceridemia limit the clinical utility of these agents. In general, colesevelam has a better gastrointestinal side effects profile and has favorable effects on glucose metabolism. In the glucose-lowering effect of WelChol Study (GLOWS) in patients with type 2 diabetes, colesevelam added to existing therapy with metformin- and/or sulfonylurea-lowered LDL cholesterol by 11.7% and HbA1c by 0.5% [54]. The increase in triglyceride level was not significant in the GLOWS, although in other trials, when colesevelam was added to sulfonylurea or insulin, the triglyceride levels increased by 17.7% and 21.5%, respectively ($P < 0.05$) [55–57].

Niacin lowers triglyceride, LDL cholesterol, and small dense LDL levels and raises HDL cholesterol. Thus, its pharmacologic effect is well suited to target the triad of diabetic dyslipidemia. However, the use of niacin has been limited by its side effects such as flushing, itching, gastrointestinal upset, tachycardia, hypotension, and aggravation of insulin resistance. More importantly, two large clinical trials, one the HPS-2 THRIVE and the second AIM-HIGH, failed to show any clinical benefit of adding niacin to statin therapy, and there was a possible increase in ischemic strokes with the combination therapy [21, 22]. The combination should rarely be used in patients with high risk of hypertriglyceridemia-related pancreatitis.

The role of fibrates is limited because of lack of reproducible cardiovascular benefits. However, results from the available clinical trials suggest that in the subgroup of patients with moderate dyslipidemia (high triglycerides ≥2.24 mmol/L (200 mg/dL) and low HDL cholesterol <0.9–1.0 mmol/L (35–40 mg/dL), fenofibrate treatment compared

Table 40.1 A select list of therapeutic agents available for the management of dyslipidemia

Drug or drug class	Pharmacologic effects	Side effects	Specific agents (trade name) and dosage
1. Single agent formulations			
HMG-CoA reductase inhibitors (statins)	LDL-c ↓ 18–55%	Hepatotoxicity, myopathy, risk of diabetes	Lovastatin (Mevacor®) 10–80 mg orally nightly or two divided doses
	HDL-c ↑ 5–15%		Lovastatin extended-release (Altoprev®) 10–60 mg orally nightly
	TG ↓ 7–30%		Lovastatin extended-release (Altocor®) 10–60 mg orally nightly
			Simvastatin (Zocor®) 5–80 mg orally nightly[a]
			Pravastatin (Pravachol®) 10–80 mg orally once daily
			Fluvastatin (Lescol®) 20–40 mg orally nightly
			Fluvastatin extended release (Lescol XL®) 80 mg orally up to a maximum daily dose 40 mg twice daily
			Atorvastatin (Lipitor®) 10–80 mg orally once daily
			Rosuvastatin (Crestor®) 5–40 mg orally once daily
			Pitavastatin (Livalo®) 1, 2, and 4 mg orally nightly
ATP citrate lyase inhibitor	LDL-c ↓ 17–24%	No major side effects	Bempedoic acid (Nexletol®, Nilemdo®) 180 mg orally once daily
	LDL-c ↓ 15–20%		
Ezetimibe	HDL-c ↑ 1%	No major side effects, rare myopathy	Zetia®, Ezetrol® 10 mg orally once daily
	TG ↓ 8%		
PCSK9 inhibitors	LDL-c ↓ 60%	Neurocognitive changes	Evolocumab (Repatha®) 140 mg SC Q 2 weeks or 420 mg Q month
	HDL-c ↑ 5%	Cost	Alirocumab (Praluent®) 75 mg SC Q 2 weeks or 150 mg Q month
	TG ↓ 15%		
Nicotinic acid (niacin)	LDL-c ↓ 5–25%	Flushing, hyperglycemia, hyperuricemia, hepatotoxicity	Nicotinic acid 1–2 g orally two or three times daily
	HDL-c ↑ 15–35%		Extended-release nicotinic acid (Niaspan®)
	TG ↓ 20–50%		1000–2000 mg orally nightly
	Small, dense LDL↓		Sustained-release nicotinic acid (Slo-Niacin®) 250–750 mg orally once or twice daily
			Other trade names include *B-3-50, B3-500-Gr, Niacin SR, Niacor, Niaspan ER, Neasyn-SR, Nialip, Nicocin ER*
Fibrates (fibric acid derivatives)	LDL-c ↓ 5–20%	Dyspepsia, gallstones, hepatotoxicity, myopathy	Fenofibrate, micronised (Antara™) 43 and 130 mg orally once daily
			Fenofibrate, micronised (Lofibra™) 67, 134 and 200 mg orally once daily
	HDL-c ↑ 10–35%		Fenofibrate (Tricor®) 48 and 145 mg orally once daily
			Fenofibric acid delayed release capsules (Trilipix®) 45 and 135 mg orally once daily
	TG ↓ 20–50%		Other trade names for fenofibrate include Fenoglide, Lipidil EZ, Lipidil Micro, Lipidil Supra, Lipofen, Triglide, Lipanthyl, Tricheck, Golip
			Gemfibrozil (Lopid®, Apo-Gemfibrozil®, Gen-Gemfibrozil®, PMS-Gemfibrozil®) 600mg orally twice daily Bezafibrate (Bezalip®, Bezagen®, Fibrazate®, Liparol™, Zimbacol®) 200 mg orally twice daily
	Small, dense ↓ LDL-c		Bezalip® Mono 400 mg orally once daily
			Pemafibrate (Parmodia®) 0.1–0.2 mg orally twice a day
Bile acid binding agents (or sequestrants)	LDL-c ↓ 10–20%	Gastrointestinal distress, constipation	Cholestyramine (Questran®, Prevalite®) 4–24 g orally two or three times daily
	HDL-c ↓ 1–2%		Colestipol (Colestid®) 5–30 g orally once or twice daily
	TG ↓ possible ↓ 10%		Colesevelam (Welchol®) 1.875–3.75 g orally once or twice daily

(continued)

Table 40.1 (continued)

Drug or drug class	Pharmacologic effects	Side effects	Specific agents (trade name) and dosage
Omega-3 fatty acid	TG ↓ 25–30% LDL-c ↓ 5–10% HDL-c ↑ 1–3%	Fishy aftertaste, gastrointestinal disturbances, possible association with frequent recurrences of atrial fibrillation or flutter	Lovaza® 2 g orally twice daily or 4 g once daily OTC: e.g., fish oil, Promega, Cardio-Omega 3, Marine Lipid Concentrate, MAX EPA®, SuperEPA 1200, 2–4 g/day of EPA + DHA Epanova® (omega-3-carboxylic acids) 2–4 g orally daily Vascepa® (icosapent ethyl) 4 g orally daily
2. Double agent formulations			
Simvastatin and Ezetimibe	LDL-c ↓ 45–60% HDL-c ↑ 6–10% TG ↓ 23–31%	As above for individual agents	Ezetimibe/Simvastatin (Vytorin™) 10/10 mg, 10/20 mg, 10/40 mg, and 10/80 mg orally once daily[b]
Lovastatin and nicotinic acid	LDL-c ↓ 30–42% HDL-c ↑ 20–30% TG ↓ 32–44%	As above for individual agents	Nicotinic acid/lovastatin (Advicor®) 500/20 mg, 750/20 mg, 1000/20 mg, 1000/40 mg orally nightly
Niacin extended-release/simvastatin	LDL-c ↓ 25% HDL-c ↑ 24% TG ↓ 36% Non-HDL-c ↓ 27%	As above for individual agents	Niacin extended-release/simvastatin (Simcor®) 500/20 mg to 2000/40 mg orally nightly
Simvastatin and sitagliptin	LDL-c ↓ 20–40% HDL-c ↑ 5–10% TG ↓ 10–20% Hba1c ↓ 0.5–0.07%	As above for statins	Simvastatin/sitagliptin (Juvisync®) 100/10 mg, 100/20 mg, 100/40 mg orally once daily
Atorvastatin and amlodipine	LDL-c ↓ 30–60% HDL-c ↑ or ↓ 5–10% TG ↓ 30% Anti-hypertensive	As above for statins	Atorvastatin/amlodipine (Caduet®) 2.5, 5, or 10/10, 20, 40, or 80 mg orally once daily
Bempedoic acid and ezetimibe	LDL-c ↓ 30%	As above for individual agents	Bempedoic acid/ezetimibe (Nexlizet®) 180 mg/10 mg orally once daily

Reprinted from reference [8] with some modifications and with permission of the authors and the publisher

DHA docosahexaenoic acid, EPA eicosapentaenoic acid, HDL-c high-density lipoprotein-cholesterol, LDL-c low-density lipoprotein-cholesterol, OTC over the counter, TG triglyceride

[a]The use of the 80 mg dose should be restricted to patients who have been taking simvastatin 80 mg chronically (e.g., for 12 months or more) without evidence of muscle toxicity

[b]The use of the Vytorin™ 10/80-mg dose should be restricted to patients who have been on this strength chronically (e.g., for 12 months or more) without evidence of muscle toxicity

to placebo is associated with fewer cardiovascular events [19, 20]. Fibrate use can be considered in people with elevated triglyceride level >5.6 mmol/L (500 mg/dL) along with dietary modification and improving glycemic control to prevent chylomicronemia and the associated risk of pancreatitis. When used in combination with statins, fenofibrate or bezafibrate seems to convey a minimal risk of rhabdomyolysis, while the combination with gemfibrozil should be avoided. Pemafibrate (Parmodia®) is a novel selective peroxisome proliferator-activated receptor alpha (PPARα) modulator (or fibrate) that is currently available in Japan. The ongoing clinical trial, Pemafibrate to Reduce Cardiovascular OutcoMes by Reducing Triglycerides IN patiENts With diabeTes (PROMINENT) (ClinicalTrials.gov Identifier: NCT03071692), will address the role of this fibrate in reducing cardiovascular events in people with diabetes [58].

Fish oil supplements are another option to reduce triglyceride levels. In general, daily supplements of 3–5 g of eicosapentaenoic acid (EPA) and docosahexaenoic acid (DHA) reduce serum triglyceride levels by an average of 28%. The Combination of Prescription Omega-3 Plus Simvastatin (COMBOS) trial in statin-treated patients who have persistent triglyceride levels between 200 and 499 mg/dL found that omega-3 fatty acid supplementation reduced non-HDL-c by 9% compared with 2.2% with placebo, triglycerides by 30% compared to 6% with placebo, and increased the HDL cholesterol by 3.4% [59]. Two open-label trials suggested some clinical benefits of omega-3 fatty acids. In the Gruppo Italiano per lo Studio della Infarto Miocardico (GISSI-Prevenzione) trial, mortality was reduced by 28% in people with diabetes and by 18% in nondiabetics randomized to omega-3 fatty acid supplementation [60]. Similarly, in a study of Japanese hypercholesterolemic patients, daily supplementation with 1800 mg EPA was associated with a significant reduction in nonfatal coronary events [61]. However, in subsequent large cohorts of diabetic patients, fish oil supplementation was not associated with any beneficial outcomes [62–64]. These trials used 1 g of n-3 fatty acids. The subsequent Reduction of Cardiovascular Events with Icosapent Ethyl-Intervention Trial (REDUCE-IT) found an approximately 25% relative risk reduction ($p < 0.001$) in major adverse cardiovascular events with an ethyl ester form of eicosapentaenoic acid (EPA) (Vascepa®) 4 g/day compared with placebo after a median follow-up of 4.9 years [65]. These favorable cardioprotective effects were not duplicated in the trial with omega-3 carboxylic acids (Epanova®) as the STRENGTH (a long-term outcomes study to assess STatin Residual risk reduction with EpaNova in hiGh cardiovascular risk paTients with Hypertriglyceridemia) trial was terminated early for low likelihood of demonstrating a benefit. Nevertheless, it is approved for lowering triglycerides in patients with very high levels of triglycerides. This approval was based on data from a clinical development program that included positive results from the Phase III EVOLVE (EpanoVa fOr Lowering Very high triglyceridEs) trial [66].

In rare genetic disorders with sever hypercholesterolemia such as homozygous familial hypercholesterolemia, a novel antisense oligonucleotide inhibitor of apo B100 synthesis, mipomersen (Kynamro®), was developed, but its marketing and use has been discontinued because of significant risk of liver damage [67, 68].

Lomitapide (Juxtapid®), a microsomal triglyceride transfer protein (MTP) inhibitor reduces the synthesis of chylomicrons and very low-density lipoprotein, resulting in a reduction in plasma LDL levels. The drug was approved with a boxed warning for increased the risk of hepatotoxicity. Other precautions with lomitapide include reduced absorption of fat-soluble vitamins, gastrointestinal adverse events, and numerous drug–drug interactions [69].

Another medication for the treatment of homozygous familial hypercholesterolemia is evinacumab (Evkeeza®). This monoclonal antibody against angiopoietin-like 3 (ANGPTL3) acts as an inhibitor of lipoprotein lipase and endothelial lipase. In ELIPSE HoFH trial, individuals were treated with other lipid-lowering therapies, including maximally tolerated statins, PCSK9 inhibitors, ezetimibe, LDL apheresis, and lomitapide, adding evinacumab to other lipid-lowering therapies decreased LDL cholesterol by 49% on average, compared to lipid-lowering therapies alone. The drug's prohibitive cost will limit its utility [70, 71].

Another novel medication currently in clinical trials for the treatment of familial chylomicronemia syndrome is volanesorsen (Waylivra®). This is an antisense oligonucleotide inhibitor of apo C-III mRNA. In phase 2 trials, this agent resulted in 71% decrease in triglycerides, 46% increase in HDL cholesterol, and improved blood glucose levels in type 2 diabetes [72, 73].

There is emerging evidence that diabetes is associated with increased cellular stress notably, oxidative, inflammatory, and endoplasmic reticulum stress [74, 75]. These stressors promote atherosclerosis, and in two clinical trials with anti-inflammatory drugs, canakinumab [76] and colchicine [77] reduced major adverse cardiovascular events. Targeting cellular stress with novel and safe drugs may increase the opportunities for reducing cardiovascular events in people with diabetes.

A Rational Approach to Drug Therapy

The current consensus is to recommend high-intensity statin to all patients with diabetes and atherosclerotic cardiovascular disease (i.e., secondary prevention). For those younger than 40 years of age with additional cardiovascular risk, moderate-intensity statins are recommended after the healthcare provider and the patient discuss the risks and benefits of such intervention, as there is paucity of date for individuals below age 40 or above age 75 years. For those aged over 40 years without any additional risk, moderate-intensity statin is suggested in addition to lifestyle modifications, while those with any additional risk should be on high-intensity statin (i.e., primary prevention) [35]. Various statins are categorized according to their intensity in Table 40.2. The dose and

Table 40.2 Classification of statins according to their efficacy in reducing LDL cholesterol

	High intensity	Moderate intensity
Average effect on LDL cholesterol with daily dose	Lowering of LDL cholesterol ≥50%	Lowering of LDL cholesterol 30 to <50%
Examples	(a) Atorvastatin 40–80 mg (b) Rosuvastatin 20–40 mg	(a) Atorvastatin 10–20 mg (b) Fluvastatin 40 mg twice a day or extended release 80 mg once a day (c) Lovastatin 40 mg (d) Pitavastatin 2–4 mg (e) Pravastatin 40–80 mg (f) Rosuvastatin 5–10 mg (g) Simvastatin 20–40 mg

choice of statin can be adjusted based on patient's response, side effects, and tolerability. Addition of ezetimibe to moderate-intensity statin may provide additional benefits especially in patients with acute coronary syndrome and LDL cholesterol of 1.29 mmol/L (50 mg/dL) or over or for those who cannot tolerate high-intensity statin. Combination of statin and fenofibrate may be considered in men with triglyceride levels of 2.3 mmol/L (204 mg/dL) or more and HDL cholesterol level of 0.9 mmol/L (34 mg/dL) or less. Combination of statin and niacin has no benefit beyond statin therapy, may increase the risk of stroke, and generally should be avoided. Statins are contraindicated in pregnancy [35].

Lipid profile should be measured before starting statin therapy, 4–12 week after the initiation of therapy and periodically thereafter to monitor compliance and efficacy [35]. Based on the currently available literature, an evidence-based algorithm for the drug therapy of dyslipidemia in patients with diabetes is shown in Fig. 40.2. As lowering LDL cholesterol levels are irrefutably linked to reducing cardiovascular events, the first priority for most patients with CVD should be to start statin therapy irrespective of baseline lipid levels (Fig. 40.2). High-intensity statins are recommended for those with established coronary artery disease or those who have 10-year risk of ≥20%. If the LDL cholesterol response to therapy is less than 50% in a very high-risk individual, or if the patient cannot tolerate statins, then addition of ezetimibe, bempedoic acid, and PCSK9 inhibitors such as

evolocumab and alirocumab should be considered especially if LDL cholesterol level is above 1.8 mmol/L (70 mg/dL) [35, 70, 71].

In general, cholesterol-binding resins are an option only if the patient's serum triglyceride concentration is less than 2.83 mmol/L (250 mg/dL) or less than 2.26 mmol/L (200 mg/dL) for those on sulfonylurea or insulin, as this class of agents might exacerbate hypertriglyceridemia. An attractive option is colesevelam as it has blood glucose-lowering effect in addition to its inhibition of cholesterol absorption [56]. In patients with established cardiovascular disease or for those with multiple cardiovascular risk factors, if triglyceride levels are 1.5–5.6 mmol/L (135–499 mg/dL), 4 g of icosapent ethyl can be added to reduce adverse cardiovascular events [65].

Currently, the principal rationale for targeting the triglyceride levels is to reduce the risk of pancreatitis. This serious complication rarely occurs when the serum triglyceride levels are less than 1000 mg/dL. However, individual variability in triglyceride-related risk should be taken into consideration when determining the threshold level below which the risk of pancreatitis is negligible.

When serum triglyceride level is over 5.65–11.3 mmol/L (500–1000 mg/dL) (the range is to account for differences in individual susceptibility to pancreatitis), fibrate with and without omega-3 fatty acids is recommended. An exception would be patients who have chylomicronemia associated with a profound lipolytic deficiency. It is noteworthy that the

Fig. 40.2 A suggested evidence-based algorithm for drug therapy of dyslipidemia in patients with diabetes mellitus. *LDL-c* low-density lipoprotein cholesterol, *TG* triglycerides, *CVD* cardiovascular disease. Reprinted from reference [8] with some modifications and with permission of the authors and the publisher

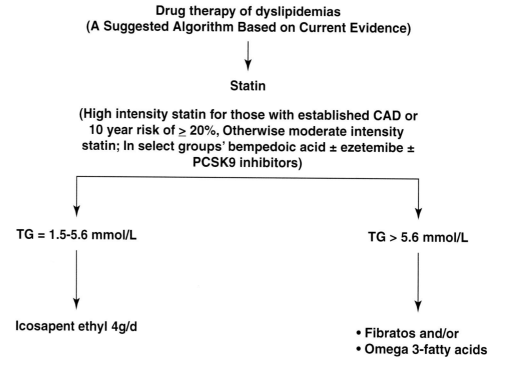

combination of a statin and a fibrate or nicotinic acid can potentiate the risk of rhabdomyolysis, and as such, these combinations should be used cautiously.

Conclusions

Type 2 diabetes is commonly associated with atherogenic dyslipidemic profile that includes high triglycerides, low HDL, and large number of small LDL particles. Lowering LDL cholesterol with statins, ezetimibe, and PCSK9 inhibitors has proven clinical benefits. In patients with established cardiovascular disease or for those with multiple cardiovascular risk factors, LDL cholesterol goal is <1.8 mmol/L (70 mg/dL). Most patients at 40–75 years of age regardless of their basal plasma cholesterol levels require statin therapy, and high-intensity statins are recommended for high-risk patients especially those with clinically established coronary artery disease. Some individuals may benefit from combination therapy with icosapent ethyl if triglyceride levels are 1.5–5.6 mmol/L (135–499 mg/dL) [65]. Use of ezetimibe and bempedoic acid in those who cannot tolerate high-intensity statins may be prudent. In select patients, PCSK9 inhibitors are an option.

In addition to proper management of the hyperlipidemia, other risk factors frequently associated with diabetes, such as hypertension, obesity, and smoking, should be addressed.

Multiple Choice Questions

1. One of the major drivers of increased plasma triglyceride concentrations in people with type 2 diabetes is
   (a) High intake of saturated fat from animal foodstuffs
   (b) **Increased free fatty-acid release from insulin-resistant fat cells**
   (c) Inhibition of lipoprotein lipase activity
   (d) Ectopic fat distribution
   (e) All of the above

2. Diabetic dyslipidemia is characterized by
   (a) Moderate/high plasma LDL cholesterol
   (b) High plasma triglyceride levels
   (c) Low plasma HDL cholesterol levels
   (d) **All of the above**
   (e) A and B are correct

3. The increased flux of free fatty acids into the liver promotes
   (a) **Increased triglyceride, apoB, and VLDL production**
   (b) Increased total cholesterol, apo A, and LDL production
   (c) Increased triglyceride, apoA, and LDL production
   (d) Decreased triglyceride, apoB, and LDL production
   (e) Increased triglyceride, apoB, and no changes in VLDL production

4. Severe hypertriglyceridemia (greater than or equal to 5.65 mmol/L (500 mg/dL) increases the risk of
   (a) Acute myocardial infarction
   (b) Stroke
   (c) **Acute pancreatitis**
   (d) Peripheral artery disease
   (e) Acute gastritis

5. Glycemic control can be improved with:
   (a) Low carbohydrate diet
   (b) Aerobic exercise
   (c) Resistance training
   (d) Thirty minutes of walking five times a week
   (e) **All of the above**

6. Most people with diabetes would require pharmacologic agents, but lifestyle modifications are still important cornerstone of therapy when they
   (a) Include high-intensity aerobic exercise
   (b) **Achieve modest body weight loss (7%), increase physical activity and smoking cessation**
   (c) Include ketogenic diets
   (d) Increase the intake of vitamins and minerals
   (e) Are focused on dietary restrictions

7. Lowering LDL cholesterol levels is irrefutably linked to reducing cardiovascular events, the priority for most patients should be
   (a) Early insulin therapy with the goal to reduce lipolysis
   (b) **Start statin therapy irrespective of baseline lipid levels**
   (c) Additional therapy with metformin at low doses
   (d) The use of anti-platelet adhesion agents
   (e) Preparations for cardiovascular management

8. Combination therapy of statin and the following drug may increase the risk of stroke
   (a) Fenofibrate
   (b) **Nicotinic acid**
   (c) Bempedoic acid
   (d) PCSK9 inhibitors
   (e) Ezetimibe

9. In patients with established cardiovascular disease or for those with multiple cardiovascular risk factors, if triglyceride levels are 1.5–5.6 mmol/L (135–499 mg/dL)
   (a) Icosapent ethyl, 1 g/day should be added
   (b) Fenofibrate should be added
   (c) **Icosapent ethyl, 4 g/day can be added to reduce adverse cardiovascular events**
   (d) Omega-3 carboxylic acids 4 g/day can be added to reduce adverse cardiovascular events.
   (e) Recommend low carbohydrate diet

10. While statins have well established cardiovascular benefits, the following agents are also shown to be associated with reduced cardiovascular adverse events
   (a) Bempedoic acid

(b) **PCSK9 inhibitors**
(c) **Niacin**
(d) Omega-3 fatty acids
(e) Antioxidant vitamins such as vitamin E and C

References

1. Gregg EW, Li Y, Wang J, Burrows NR, Ali MK, Rolka D, Williams DE, Geiss L. Changes in diabetes-related complications in the united states, 1990–2010. N Engl J Med. 2014;370:1514–23.
2. Cheng YJ, Imperatore G, Geiss LS, Saydah SH, Albright AL, Ali MK, Gregg EW. Trends and disparities in cardiovascular mortality among U.S. adults with and without self-reported diabetes, 1988–2015. Diabetes Care. 2018;41:2306–15.
3. Rawshani A, Rawshani A, Franzen S, et al. Risk factors, mortality, and cardiovascular outcomes in patients with type 2 diabetes. N Engl J Med. 2018;379:633–44.
4. GBD 2017 Causes of Death Collaborators. Global, regional, and national age-sex-specific mortality for 282 causes of death in 195 countries and territories, 1980-2017: a systematic analysis for the Global Burden of Disease Study 2017. Lancet. 2018;392:1736–88.
5. Dagenais GR, Leong DP, Rangarajan S, et al. Variations in common diseases, hospital admissions, and deaths in middle-aged adults in 21 countries from five continents (PURE): a prospective cohort study. Lancet. 2020;395:785–94.
6. Yusuf S, Joseph P, Rangarajan S, et al. Modifiable risk factors, cardiovascular disease, and mortality in 155 722 individuals from 21 high-income, middle-income, and low-income countries (PURE): a prospective cohort study. Lancet. 2020;395:795–808.
7. Mooradian AD. Evidence based cardiovascular risk management in diabetes. Am J Cardiovasc Drugs. 2019;19:439–48.
8. Chehade JM, Gladysz M, Mooradian AD. Dyslipidemia in type 2 diabetes: prevalence, pathophysiology and management. Drugs. 2013;73:327–39.
9. Hachem SB, Mooradian AD. Familial dyslipidaemias: an overview of genetics, pathophysiology and management. Drugs. 2006;66:1949–69.
10. Jacobs MJ, Kleisli T, Pio JR, Malik S, L'Italien GJ, Chen RS, Wong ND. Prevalence and control of dyslipidemia among persons with diabetes in the United States. Diabetes Res Clin Pract. 2005;70:263–9.
11. U.K. Prospective Diabetes Study 27. Plasma lipids and lipoproteins at diagnosis of NIDDM by age and sex. Diabetes Care. 1997;20:1683–7.
12. Mooradian AD, Haas MJ, Wehmeier KR, Wong NC. Obesity related changes in high density lipoprotein metabolism. Obesity. 2008;16:1152–60.
13. Mooradian AD, Albert SG, Haas MJ. Low serum high-density lipoprotein cholesterol in obese subjects with normal serum triglycerides: the role of insulin resistance and inflammatory cytokines. Diabetes Obes Metab. 2007;9:441–3.
14. Haas MJ, Mooradian AD. Regulation of high-density lipoprotein by inflammatory cytokines: establishing links between immune dysfunction and cardiovascular disease. Diabetes Metab Res Rev. 2010;26:90–9.
15. Cholesterol Treatment Trialists' (CTT) Collaborators. Efficacy of cholesterol-lowering therapy in 18,686 people with diabetes in 14 randomized trials of statins: a meta-analysis. Lancet. 2008;371:117–25.
16. Rubins HB, Robins SJ, Collins D, et al. Gemfibrozil for the secondary prevention of coronary heart disease in men with low levels of high-density lipoprotein cholesterol. Veterans Affairs High-Density Lipoprotein Cholesterol Intervention Trial Study Group. N Engl J Med. 1999;341:410–8.
17. Frick MH, Elo O, Haapa K, Heinonen OP, Heinsalmi P, Helo P, et al. Helsinki Heart Study: primary prevention trial with gemfibrozil in middle-aged men with dyslipidemia. Safety of treatment, changes in risk factors, and incidence of coronary heart disease. N Engl J Med. 1987;317:1237–45.
18. Keech A, Simes RJ, Barter P, Best J, Scott R, Taskinen MR, et al. Effects of long-term fenofibrate therapy on cardiovascular events in 9795 people with type 2 diabetes mellitus (the FIELD study): randomized controlled trial. Lancet. 2005;366:1849–61.
19. Scott R, O'Brien R, Fulcher G, Pardy C, D'Emden M, Tse D, et al. Effects of fenofibrate treatment on cardiovascular disease risk in 9,795 individuals with type 2 diabetes and various components of the metabolic syndrome: the Fenofibrate Intervention and Event Lowering in Diabetes (FIELD) study. Diabetes Care. 2009;32:493–8.
20. ACCORD Study Group, Ginsberg HN, Elam MB, Lovato LC, Crouse JR III, Leiter LA, Linz P, et al. Effects of combination lipid therapy in type 2 diabetes mellitus. N Engl J Med. 2010;362:1563–74.
21. AIM-HIGH Investigators, Boden WE, Probstfield JL, Anderson T, Chaitman BR, Desvignes-Nickens P, Koprowicz K, et al. Niacin in patients with low HDL cholesterol levels receiving intensive statin therapy. N Engl J Med. 2011;365:2255–67.
22. HPS2-THRIVE Collaborative Group, Landray MJ, Haynes R, Hopewell JC, Parish S, Aung T, Tomson J, et al. Effects of extended-release niacin with laropiprant in high-risk patients. N Engl J Med. 2014;371:203–12.
23. Barter PJ, Caulfield M, Eriksson M, Grundy SM, Kastelein JJ, Komajda M, ILLUMINATE Investigators, et al. Effects of torcetrapib in patients at high risk for coronary events. N Engl J Med. 2007;357:2109–22.
24. Schwartz GG, Olsson AG, Abt M, Ballantyne CM, Barter PJ, Brumm J, et al. Effects of dalcetrapib in patients with a recent acute coronary syndrome. N Engl J Med. 2012;367:2089–99.
25. Lincoff AM, Nicholls SJ, Riesmeyer JS, et al. Evacetrapib and cardiovascular outcomes in high-risk vascular disease. N Engl J Med. 2017;376:1933–42.
26. The HPS3/TIMI55-REVEAL Collaborative Group. Effects of anacetrapib in patients with atherosclerotic vascular disease. N Engl J Med. 2017;377:1217–27.
27. Mooradian AD, Haas MJ. Targeting high-density lipoproteins: increasing de novo production versus decreasing clearance. Drugs. 2015;75:713–22.
28. Hollenbeck CB, Chen YD, Greenfield MS, Lardinois CK, Reaven GM. Reduced plasma high density lipoprotein-cholesterol concentrations need not increase when hyperglycemia is controlled with insulin in noninsulin-dependent diabetes mellitus. J Clin Endocrinol Metab. 1986;62:605–8.
29. Dietary Guidelines Advisory Committee. Scientific report of the 2020 dietary guidelines. Advisory report to the Secretary of Agriculture and the Secretary of Health and Human Services. Washington, DC: U.S. Department of Agriculture, Agricultural Research Service; 2020. https://www.dietaryguidelines.gov/2020-advisory-committee-report. Accessed 22 March 2021.
30. Mooradian AD, Smith M, Tokuda M. The role of artificial and natural sweeteners in reducing the consumption of table sugar: a narrative review. Clin Nutr ESPEN. 2017;18:1–8.
31. Mooradian AD. In search for an alternative to sugar to reduce obesity. Int J Vitam Nutr Res. 2019;89:113–7.
32. Mooradian AD. The merits and the pitfalls of low carbohydrate diet: a concise review. J Nutr Health Aging. 2020;24:805–8.

33. Nordmann AJ, Suter-Zimmermann K, Bucher HC, Shai I, Tuttle KR, Estruch R, Briel M. Meta-analysis comparing Mediterranean to low-fat diets for modification of cardiovascular risk factors. Am J Med. 2011;124:841–51.

34. Alexandraki I, Palacio C, Mooradian AD. Relative merits of low-carbohydrate versus low-fat diets in managing obesity. South Med J. 2015;108:401–6.

35. American Diabetes Association. 10. Cardiovascular care and risk management. Standards of Medical Care in Diabetes-2021. Diabetes Care. 2021;44(Suppl 1):S125–50.

36. Knowler WC, Barrett-Connor E, Fowler SE, Hamman RF, Lachin JM, Walker EA, Nathan DM, Diabetes Prevention Program Research Group. Reduction in the incidence of type 2 diabetes with lifestyle intervention or metformin. N Engl J Med. 2002;346(6):393–403.

37. Sacks FM, Svetkey LP, Vollmer WM, et al. Effects on blood pressure of reduced dietary sodium and the Dietary Approaches to Stop Hypertension (DASH) diet. DASH-Sodium Collaborative Research Group. N Engl J Med. 2001;344:3–10.

38. Lichtenstein AH. Thematic review series: patient oriented research. Dietary fat, carbohydrate, and protein: effects on plasma lipoprotein patterns. J Lipid Res. 2006;47:1661–7.

39. Mooradian AD, Haas MJ, Wong NC. The effect of select nutrients on serum high-density lipoprotein cholesterol and apolipoprotein A-I levels. Endocr Rev. 2006;27:2–16.

40. Mooradian AD. Obesity: a rational target for managing diabetes mellitus. Growth Horm IGF Res. 2011;11(Suppl A):S79–83.

41. Wilund KR, Ferrell RE, Phares DA, Goldberg AP, Hagberg JM. Changes in high-density lipoprotein-cholesterol sub-fractions with exercise training may be dependent on cholesteryl ester transfer protein (CETP) genotype. Metabolism. 2002;51:774–8.

42. Halverstadt A, Phares DA, Ferrell RE, Wilund KR, Goldberg AP, Hagberg JM. High-density lipoprotein cholesterol, its subfractions, and responses to exercise training are dependent on endothelial lipase genotype. Metabolism. 2003;52:1505–11.

43. Sigal RJ, Kenny GP, Boulé NG, et al. Effects of aerobic training, resistance training, or both on glycemic control in type 2 diabetes: a randomized trial. Ann Intern Med. 2007;147:357–69.

44. Giannopoulou I, Ploutz-Snyder LL, Carhart R, Weinstock RS, Fernhall B, Goulopoulou S, Kanaley JA. Exercise is required for visceral fat loss in postmenopausal women with type 2 diabetes. J Clin Endocrinol Metab. 2005;90:1511–8.

45. Alam S, Stolinski M, Pentecost C, Boroujerdi MA, Jones RH, Sonksen PH, Umpleby AM. The effect of a six-month exercise program on very low-density lipoprotein apolipoprotein B secretion in type 2 diabetes. J Clin Endocrinol Metab. 2004;89:688–94.

46. Ridker PM, Danielson E, Fonseca FA, Genest J, Gotto AM Jr, Kastelein JJ, et al. Rosuvastatin to prevent vascular events in men and women with elevated C-reactive protein. N Engl J Med. 2008;359:2195–207.

47. Cannon CP, Blazing MA, Giugliano RP, McCagg A, White JA, Theroux P, et al. Ezetimibe added to statin therapy after acute coronary syndromes. N Engl J Med. 2015;372:2387–97.

48. Rossebø AB, Pedersen TR, Boman K, Brudi P, Chambers JB, Egstrup K, et al. Intensive lipid lowering with simvastatin and ezetimibe in aortic stenosis. N Engl J Med. 2008;359:1343–56.

49. Baigent C, Landray MJ, Reith C, Emberson J, Wheeler DC, Tomson C, et al. The effects of lowering LDL cholesterol with simvastatin plus ezetimibe in patients with chronic kidney disease (Study of Heart and Renal Protection): a randomised placebo-controlled trial. Lancet. 2011;377:2181–92.

50. Sabatine MS, Giugliano RP, Keech AC, et al. Evolocumab and clinical outcomes in patients with cardiovascular disease. N Engl J Med. 2017;376:1713–22.

51. Schwartz GG, Steg PG, Szarek M, et al. Alirocumab and cardiovascular outcomes after acute coronary syndrome. N Engl J Med. 2018;379:2097–107.

52. Ray KK, Wright RS, Kallend D, et al. Two phase 3 trials of inclisiran in patients with elevated LDL cholesterol. N Engl J Med. 2020;382:1507–19.

53. https://www.acc.org/latest-in-cardiology/articles/2020/02/24/10/09/fda-approves-bempedoic-acid-for-treatment-of-adults-with-hefh-or-established-ascvd. Accessed 22 March 2021.

54. Zieve FJ, Kalin MF, Schwartz SL, Jones MR, Bailey WL. Results of the Glucose-Lowering effect of Welchol Study (GLOWS): a randomized, double-blind, placebo-controlled pilot study evaluating the effect of colesevelam hydrochloride on glycemic control in subjects with type 2 diabetes. Clin Ther. 2007;29:74–83.

55. Bays HE, Goldberg RB, Truitt KE, Jones MR. Colesevelam hydrochloride therapy in patients with type 2 diabetes mellitus treated with metformin: glucose and lipid effects. Arch Intern Med. 2008;168:1975–83.

56. Fonseca VA, Rosenstock J, Wang AC, Truitt KE, Jones MR. Colesevelam HCl improves glycemic control and reduces LDL cholesterol in patients with inadequately controlled type 2 diabetes on sulfonylurea-based therapy. Diabetes Care. 2008;31:1479–84.

57. Goldberg RB, Fonseca VA, Truitt KE, Jones MR. Efficacy and safety of colesevelam in patients with type 2 diabetes mellitus and inadequate glycemic control receiving insulin-based therapy. Arch Intern Med. 2008;168:1531–40.

58. Pradhan AD, Paynter NP, Everett BM, et al. Rationale and design of the Pemafibrate to Reduce Cardiovascular Outcomes by Reducing Triglycerides in Patients with Diabetes (PROMINENT) study. Am Heart J. 2018;206:80–93.

59. Davidson MH, Stein EA, Bays HE, Maki KC, Doyle RT, Shalwitz RA, et al. COMBination of prescription Omega-3 with Simvastatin (COMBOS) Investigators. Efficacy and tolerability of adding prescription omega-3 fatty acids 4 g/d to simvastatin 40 mg/d in hypertriglyceridemic patients: an 8-week, randomized, double-blind, placebo-controlled study. Clin Ther. 2007;29:1354–67.

60. Marchioli R, Schweiger C, Tavazzi L, Valagussa F. Efficacy of n-3 polyunsaturated fatty acids after myocardial infarction: results of GISSI-Prevenzione trial. Gruppo Italiano per lo Studio della Sopravvivenza nell'Infarto Miocardico. Lipids. 2001;36(Suppl):S119–26.

61. Yokoyama M, Origasa H, Matsuzaki M, Matsuzawa Y, Saito Y, Ishikawa Y, et al. Effects of eicosapentaenoic acid on major coronary events in hypercholesterolaemic patients (JELIS): a randomised open-label, blinded endpoint analysis. Lancet. 2007;369:1090–8.

62. ORIGIN Trial Investigators, Bosch J, Gerstein HC, Dagenais GR, Díaz R, Dyal L, Jung H, et al. n-3 fatty acids and cardiovascular outcomes in patients with dysglycemia. N Engl J Med. 2012;367:309–18.

63. Bowman L, Mafham M, ASCEND Study Collaborative Group. Effects of n-3 fatty acid supplements in diabetes mellitus. N Engl J Med. 2018;379:1540–50.

64. Manson JE, Cook NR, Lee IM, et al. Marine n-3 fatty acids and prevention of cardiovascular disease and cancer. N Engl J Med. 2019;380:23–32.

65. Bhatt D, Steg PG, Michael Miller M, et al. Cardiovascular risk reduction with icosapent ethyl for hypertriglyceridemia. N Engl J Med. 2019;380:11–22.

66. Kastelein JJ, Maki KC, Susekov A, Ezhov M, Nordestgaard BG, Machielse BN, Kling D, Davidson MH. Omega-3 free fatty acids for the treatment of severe hypertriglyceridemia: the EpanoVa fOr Lowering Very high triglyceridEs (EVOLVE) trial. J Clin Lipidol. 2014;8:94–106.

67. Fogacci F, Ferri N, Toth PP, et al. Efficacy and safety of mipomersen: a systematic review and meta-analysis of randomized clinical trials. Drugs. 2019;79:751–66.

68. https://go.drugbank.com/drugs/DB05528. Accessed 22 March 2021.

69. Gryn SE, Hegele RA. Novel therapeutics in hypertriglyceridemia. Curr Opin Lipidol. 2015;26:484–91.

70. Patel RS, Scopelliti EM, Savelloni J. Therapeutic management of familial hypercholesterolemia: current and emerging drug therapies. Pharmacotherapy. 2015;35:1189–203.

71. Takata K, Nicholls SJ. Tackling residual atherosclerotic risk in statin-treated adults: focus on emerging drugs. Am J Cardiovasc Drugs. 2019;19:113–31.

72. Yang X, Lee SR, Choi YS, Alexander VJ, Digenio A, Yang Q, et al. Reduction in lipoprotein-associated apoC-III levels following volanesorsen therapy: phase 2 randomized trial results. J Lipid Res. 2016;57:706–13.

73. Esan O, Wierzbicki AS. Volanesorsen in the treatment of familial chylomicronemia syndrome or hypertriglyceridaemia: design, development and place in therapy. Drug Des Devel Ther. 2020;14:2623–36.

74. Mooradian AD. Therapeutic targeting of cellular stress to prevent cardiovascular disease. A review of the evidence. Am J Cardiovasc Drugs. 2017;17:83–95.

75. Mooradian AD. Targeting select cellular stress pathways to prevent hyperglycemia-related complications: shifting the paradigm. Drugs. 2016;76:1081–91.

76. Ridker PM, Everett BM, Thuren T, et al. Antiinflammatory therapy with canakinumab for atherosclerotic disease. N Engl J Med. 2017;377:1119–31.

77. Nidorf SM, Fiolet ATL, Mosterd A, et al. Colchicine in patients with chronic coronary disease. N Engl J Med. 2020;383:1838–47.

Obesity and Diabetes: Clinical Aspects

41

Sean Wharton, Rebecca A. G. Christensen,
Christy Costanian, Talia Gershon,
and Joel Rodriguez-Saldana

Objectives

1. To contrast the utility of assessments of obesity and their accuracy in determining health risk
2. To discuss genetic, social, and environmental causes of obesity and diabetes
3. To summarize different treatment methods for obesity and diabetes

Introduction

The worldwide prevalence of obesity has been increasing since the 1980s, and by 2014, 600 million adults had obesity [1]. There are region-specific variations in these rates; nonetheless, rates of obesity have been increasing in both developing and developed nations [1]. Furthermore, it has been estimated that the rates of obesity will continue to rise and reach over 40% of adults in the United Kingdom and over 50% of adults in the United States by 2030 [2].

Obesity has been recognized as a major public health concern owing to the considerable increases in health risks associated with excess weight. Having obesity is associated with an increased risk of having chronic [3] and communicable diseases [4]. Furthermore, having obesity is associated with 4.7 to 13 years of life lost [5, 6], with the greatest decrease in life expectancy for individuals with a body mass index ≥ 45 kg/m^2 [5]. This places a considerable burden on healthcare systems.

It has been estimated that more than $100 billion is spent annually in the United States for direct healthcare costs associated with obesity [7, 8]. These costs can affect people both individually and systemically. For example, a study observed that patients with overweight and obesity paid considerably more (22–41%) for an emergency department visit precipitated by shortness of breath and chest pains than those with normal weight, with cost increasing per BMI category [9]. Furthermore, obesity can have considerable costs in relation to loss of productivity. Results from a large observational study in the United States observed that individuals with excess weight are 32–118% more likely to report missing work in the past year with the likelihood increasing with each BMI category [10].

Type 1 diabetes was traditionally associated with individuals with lower weight. However, with improvements in glycemic control and increasing use of insulin, a weight-promoting hormone, now many patients with type 1 diabetes also have obesity [11]. Weight management has been challenging in this group, as insulin is the primary treatment [12], and the fear of hypoglycemic can promote excessive calorie intake [13]. Type 1 diabetes and obesity are not well studied at this stage; therefore, this chapter will focus on type 2 diabetes (T2D).

Assessment of Obesity

Body Mass Index (BMI)

Body mass index (BMI) is the most commonly used method for classifying individuals as having obesity and is calculated by dividing weight in kilograms by height in meters squared. The World Health Organization (WHO) has pro-

S. Wharton
The Wharton Medical Clinic, Hamilton, Canada

School of Kinesiology and Health Science, York University, Toronto, ON, Canada

R. A. G. Christensen · T. Gershon
The Wharton Medical Clinic, Hamilton, Canada

C. Costanian
School of Kinesiology and Health Science, York University, Toronto, ON, Canada

J. Rodriguez-Saldana (✉)
Multidisciplinary Diabetes Centre Mexico, Mexico City, Mexico

© The Author(s), under exclusive license to Springer Nature Switzerland AG 2023
J. Rodriguez-Saldana (ed.), *The Diabetes Textbook*, https://doi.org/10.1007/978-3-031-25519-9_41

Table 41.1 World Health Organization's weight categories according to body mass index

Category	Body Mass Index
Normal weight	18.5–24.9 kg/m^2
Overweight	25.0–29.9 kg/m^2
Obesity class I	30.0–34.9 kg/m^2
Obesity class II	35.0–39.9 kg/m^2
Obesity class III	≥40 kg/m^2

vided guidelines for using BMI to categorize individuals as having underweight, normal weight, overweight, or obesity (Table 41.1). BMI is meant to be a measure of health, and research has suggested that increasing levels of BMI are associated with poorer health outcomes [1]. As such, obesity can be further subcategorized as: Class I: 30.0–34.9 kg/m^2, Class II: 35–39.9 kg/m^2, and Class III: ≥40 kg/m^2.

Although BMI is currently used to track trends in obesity, there are criticisms for its lack of utility in determining body composition, as well as in predicting morbidity and mortality. Additionally, due to differences in the accumulation of central adiposity, BMI thresholds may not be appropriate for all ethnicities. Indeed, a WHO expert committee [14] and other international organizations [15, 16] have recognized this issue and recommend lowering thresholds by 2.5 kg/m^2 for individuals of Asian descent. However, there is considerably variability in the health risk associated with a given BMI in all ethnic groups. For example, individuals who identify as White in the United States have a lower body fat percentage for a given BMI than those in Europe [17]. Thus, to avoid confusion and due to the lack of sufficient concise evidence, WHO guidelines still use the cutoff of a BMI ≥30 kg/m^2 for obesity [14]. Moreover, BMI does not consider a subject's body composition when classifying their health risk [18] and therefore may not be an accurate predictor of cardiovascular disease and other conditions that correlated with adipose percentage, adipose type, and location. Morbidity and mortality staging systems, such as Edmonton obesity staging system (EOSS), have been proposed for use instead of or along with BMI.

Body Circumference(s)

Waist Circumference

Excess abdominal adiposity is associated with a greater risk of death [19] and having chronic conditions such as T2D [20, 21] irrespective of BMI. As such, waist circumference can be used to assess health. However, there is considerable disagreement regarding the most optimal site to measure waist circumference. WHO recommends measuring a person's waist circumference at the midpoint between the lower margin of the last palpable rib and the top of the iliac crest [22].

The National Institutes of Health (NIH) has identified waist circumferences ≥102 cm for men and ≥88 cm for women as an indication of increased risk of morbidity and mortality [22]. However, these thresholds have been criticized due to known ethnic differences in abdominal fat distribution [23]; therefore, ethnic-specific thresholds have been proposed to address this limitation. For example, the use of lower thresholds (87–90 cm for men, 54–77 cm for women) is recommended for South Asians as it was observed that these thresholds were more strongly associated with ill-health in this population [24]. There has also been criticism regarding the use of universal waist circumference thresholds for all BMI categories, since the NIH waist circumference thresholds were developed by taking the average waist circumference for a large sample of White men and women with a BMI of 30 kg/m^2 [25]. Therefore, the NIH thresholds may be more of a surrogate measure for BMI rather than an assessment of health risk. To address this limitation, Ardern et al. [26] developed BMI-specific waist circumference thresholds that are more strongly related to poor health. These new thresholds range from 87 cm (normal weight) to 124 cm (class II obese) in men and 79 cm (normal weight) to 115 cm (class II obese) in women.

Waist-to-Hip Ratio

Waist-to-hip ratio is another tool used to measure body fat distribution and evaluate health risks associated with excess weight [27]. Waist-to-hip ratio is calculated by dividing an individual's waist circumference by their hip circumference [18]. While there is no agreement regarding the most optimal site to measure waist circumference, in general protocols recommend that hip circumference be measured around the widest portion of the buttocks. Waist-to-hip ratios are meant to build on solely waist circumference measurements as hip circumferences are thought to provide information regarding key measures of body composition like muscle mass, while waist circumference is used to assess abdominal adiposity [28]. The WHO recommends that waist-to-hip ratios of ≥0.9 for men and ≥0.85 women be used to identify a substantially increased risk of ill-health [27].

Several criticisms regarding the utility of waist-to-hip ratio in assessing body composition and health have been made. To begin, changes in weight are not consistently correlated with changes in waist-to-hip circumferences. For example, when individuals gain or lose weight, their waist-to-hip ratio tends to increase and decrease, respectively. However, patients can have increases in their waist-to-hip ratio, while their weight remaining weight stable [29]. Research has also suggested that changes in waist-to-hip ratios independent of changes of weight are not associated with improvements in cardiovascular health risk [30]. Thus, it may be the change in weight that contributes to the changes in waist-to-hip ratio that is associated with a risk of ill-health rather than changes in the ratio itself [31].

Body Fat

Two types of body fat are present: subcutaneous and visceral. Subcutaneous fat is located directly under the skin and is not associated with poor health [30]. On the other hand, visceral fat, also known as organ fat, surrounds the organs, and when in excess, it is closely associated with metabolic complications [32]. The total of both subcutaneous and visceral fat is considered when measuring an individual's body fat content, which is usually given as a percentage of total body mass. Many methods exist for evaluating body fat, and these methods include, but are not limited to, skinfold thickness, bioelectrical impedance analysis (BIA), dual energy X-ray absorptiometry (DEXA), and the 4-compartmental model. While there is criticism regarding the use of universal cutoffs due to ethnic differences in body composition [33, 34], cutoffs of ≥25% and ≥35% are proposed for men and women, respectively [35]. Various methods of measuring body fat are described in further detail below.

Skinfold Thickness

Skinfold thickness is measured using a caliper. The caliper is used to measure the thickness of subcutaneous adipose tissue. Measurements should be taken when an individual is standing in a relaxed position. The caliper is then used to take skinfold measurements, typically along the right side of the body, at various points such as the bicep, tricep, subscapular, and supra-iliac areas. These values are then entered into prediction equations that convert skinfold measures to body fat percentages. However, there can be considerable variability in body fat distribution based on differences in sex [36, 37], ethnicity [23], and age [37]. Thus, rather than universal thresholds, such as those recommended for BMI categorization, various population-specific equations have been suggested [38–41], such as the sex-specific equations proposed by Jackson and Pollock.

Bioelectrical Impedance Analysis (BIA)

Lean tissue is highly conductive due to its increased electrolyte and water content compared to fat, which is more of an insulator. BIA uses these differences in the flow of electric current through body tissues to estimate body fat. An electrical current is sent through your body, and based on the rate it returns, an individual's total body water can be calculated. This total body water value is then used to estimate fat free (muscle, bone, tissue) and fat mass [42].

BIA is an easy, inexpensive, and quick way to assess body fat. However, many factors can affect the accuracy of this measurement and should be controlled for when using BIA to assess body fat. Dehydration and moderate exercise increases the body's electrical resistance leading to an overestimation of body fat, and consumption of a meal decreases electrical resistance, therefore resulting in lower estimates of body fat [43]. Additionally, having excess weight is associated with greater amounts of extracellular fluids. Thus, BIA may not be an appropriate tool to assess body fat in individuals with overweight or obesity as extracellular fluids will contribute to an underestimation of body fat [43].

Dual Energy X-Ray Absorptiometry (DEXA)
DEXA was initially developed for the measurement of total bone mineral since it uses X-rays to distinguish between and measure three major bodily components: bone mineral, fat mass, and non-bone lean tissue. The advantages of using DEXA are that it operates with a safe radiation level for a whole-body scan [44] and provides a more accurate assessment of body fat than the other methods outlined above [45, 46]. However, the cost associated with the equipment and expertise to run the test often makes the use of DEXA to assess body fat prohibitive. There are also machine specifications that limit the use of DEXA for assessing body fat in individuals with severe obesity. For example, the maximum weight that most machines can hold is 300 pounds with a width of 60 cm [47]. Additionally, DEXA determines an individual's body fat based on underlying assumptions regarding the distribution of bone mineral, fat, and non-bone lean tissue, which may be inaccurate due to person-to-person variability. Similar to other tools used to assess body fat, factors such as level of hydration and age can lead to an altered body composition distribution.

The Four-Compartmental Model
To assess an individual's body fat using the four-compartment model, four measurements must be taken: (1) body weight, (2) body density, (3) total body water, and (4) total body mineral [48, 49]. Various tools can be used to measure these four factors such as water displacement tests or DEXA. Each factor is then put into a prediction equation to estimate body fat. While this method is considered more accurate than other methods for assessing body fat discussed in this chapter and is frequently used to validate more simplistic measures [49], similar to DEXA, specialized laboratory equipment costs and technician expertise mean that this method is often not practical or feasible for the rapid assessment of body fat [49].

Causes of Obesity

In the most basic terms, obesity develops as a result of an energy imbalance, in which an individual consumes a greater amount of calories than they expend. However, obesity is a complex, multifactorial disease, and there are many avenues that contribute to this energy imbalance, without one definitive cause. A system map referred to as the "spaghetti map" was constructed to describe the interplay of factors that result in the development of obesity [50]. Sixteen thematic clusters are represented on this map, which include categories such as the influence media, social, and psychological factors. Each cluster has various sub-factors, which make up this diagram, the description of which is far beyond the scope of this textbook and chapter. As such, this section will focus on the factors that are most salient to the development of obesity and T2D.

Hereditable Factors

While obesity is often viewed as a condition resulting from disordered eating or other patient choice-related cause(s), genetics play a key role in the development of obesity. Genome studies have identified over 200 genes that are associated with body weight and adiposity in mice [51]. In humans, a single-gene mutation in 11 genes was found to be responsible for the development of over 150 cases of obesity. A deficiency of the melanocortin 4 receptor (MC4) gene [52] and Prader Willi chromosomal abnormalities [53] is the most common congenital single gene mutations leading to obesity. Furthermore, genes associated with hyperphagia, a characteristic typically defined as a behavioral cause of obesity, have been identified [54]. Taken together, this evidence suggests there is likely a variety of genes and genetic mutations that have contributed to the development of obesity [51, 55].

Population studies have provided additional evidence that supports the notion of a strong hereditable component to obesity. For example, research suggests that children who have one or both parents with a BMI greater than 30 kg/m^2 are at a 2.5 to 10.4 times greater risk of having childhood obesity [56]. Moreover, studies conducted on monozygotic twins further support the influence of genes on obesity development. Studies have observed a strong correlation in the BMI of separately reared monozygotic twins ranging from 0.61 to 0.70 [57, 58]. However, this is not to discount the effects of environmental factors on the development of obesity. Indeed, when comparing the BMIs of monozygotic and dizygotic twins reared in the same environment, their BMIs were more strongly correlated than those reared apart [57].

Environmental Factors

Diet

Obesity has been referred to as over nutrition in comparison to the energy expenditure, which alludes to the importance of dietary factors in the development of this chronic disease. As energy expenditure is challenging to modify, diet frequently becomes the key modifiable risk factor. An increase in caloric consumption has been observed in most high-income countries from the 1980s through the mid-1990s that appears concomitant with increases in the prevalence of obesity [59]. There were country-specific trends in caloric consumption that further support this notion. For example, the United States had one of the largest increases in BMI over the 10-year period (1.5 kg/m^2 on average) as well as the largest increase in caloric consumption per capita (314 kcal/day). Nonetheless, researchers state that changes in absolute caloric intake alone cannot explain the increase in the rates of obesity that has been occurring over the past four decades [60]. Thus, other factors, such as the macronutrient content of an individual's diet, may also contribute to changes in weight.

The influences of individual macronutrients, such as sugar and fats, have previously been explored with equivocal results. For example, when controlling for differences in total caloric and sugar consumption, each 100 kcal increase in dietary fat has been associated with a 0.21 kg/m^2 increase in BMI [59]. Additionally, research suggests that high dietary fat intake in women with overweight or obesity who have a familial history of obesity is associated with significant increases in their BMI [61]. Conversely, a large meta-analysis observed that increased sugar intake was associated with a 0.75 kg/m^2 increase in BMI. These results are in line with the WHO recommendations to decrease the intake of free sugars to <10% of total caloric intake to decrease an individual's likelihood of having overweight or obesity and to decrease sugar intake to <5% for greater health benefits [62]. Thus, while it still remains unclear exactly how macronutrients contribute to the development of obesity, both the quantity and type of caloric intake appear to play a role.

Physical Activity

When energy expenditure is lower than caloric intake, the balance leans toward increased weight. Theoretically, increases in energy expenditure through the participation in physical activity could result in sufficient caloric deficits to delay or prevent disease onset. Indeed, increased physical activity is often associated with decreases in weight [63] and greater weight loss maintenance over the long term [64]. However, research suggests that individuals with overweight and obesity complete significantly less steps per day than their normal weight counterparts [65]. Moreover, individuals with obesity are unlikely to meet basic public health physical activity recommendations of 30 min/day of moderate to vigorous physical activity a minimum of 5 days/week, completing only an average of 17.3 min of moderate and 3.2 min of vigorous physical activity a day.

Physical inactivity is becoming a major health concern worldwide. While individuals with overweight and obesity participate in less physical activity on average than those with normal weight, overall less than 5% of adults in the United States meet public health physical activity recommendations [65]. While purposeful physical activity, also referred to as exercise, plays a role in weight management, nonpurposeful physical activity may also be contributing to the increased rates of obesity. Indeed, adults spend more than half of their day being sedentary [65]. This is likely in part due to shifts in occupational demands during the twentieth century, which led to a decrease in physically intensive jobs, such as labor jobs, and increase in the rate of jobs with significant sedentary time, such as office managers [66]. These trends had the unintended side effect of decreasing the amount of structured nonpurposeful physical activity and therefore decreasing caloric expenditure throughout the course of a work day. Moreover, it is important to consider changes to the built environment, which has also occurred over this time period that may further contribute to physical inactivity. Research suggests that individuals who live in more walkable neighbors participate in more physical activity and are less likely to have overweight or obesity [67]. Thus, it appears that other factors, beyond personal choices, have contribute to low physical activity levels, and by extension, increase in the rates of obesity.

Type 2 Diabetes (T2D)

Obesity and a genetic predisposition are well-known risk factors for T2D [68]. The relationship between obesity and T2D is mostly described as being interdependent with obesity significantly increasing the risk of T2D, since over 90% of patients with T2D are obese [69]. Four prospective cohort studies examining the role of obesity in cardiovascular risk factors and disease concluded that children with overweight or obesity and who also had overweight or obesity as adults had increased risks of developing T2D, hypertension, dyslipidemia, and carotid-artery atherosclerosis. The risks of these outcomes among children with obesity who became non-obese by adulthood were similar to those among children who were never obese [70].

A strong association between increasing BMI and glucose intolerance exists [71]. It has been established that insulin action declines as a function of BMI. This relationship is approximately linear in both men and women, and so obesity can be considered as being in an insulin-resistant state.

Moreover, a long duration of obesity is associated with lower fasting insulin levels, indicating pancreatic β-cell exhaustion. Those who had class III obesity and insulin resistance need a very large amount of insulin to maintain glucose tolerance. It is clear that individuals with obesity and insulin-resistance impose a large stress on pancreatic β-cells, and this is maintained for prolonged periods of time [71].

It must be noted that the strong associations between excess body fat and T2D do not necessarily indicate that being overweight or obese will cause T2D, since not all individuals with obesity develop diabetes and not all individuals with T2D have obesity [69]. Therefore, obesity alone is not sufficient to cause T2D. Furthermore, obesity, insulin resistance, and eventually T2D share common risk factors, as they are included in the continuum of risk factors for cardiometabolic disease. Thus, the fundamental shared risk factors for obesity and T2D at the individual level may be poor diet and physical inactivity [72]. The relationship between obesity and T2D is affected by several modifying factors, such as duration of obesity, distribution of body fat, physical activity, diet, and genetics/ethnicity [73]. In the last half century, lifestyles, including dietary habits, have changed across the world, accompanied by the global obesity epidemic. While physical activity has decreased in many regions, especially in low-income countries, in high-income countries such as the United States, overall physical activity has remained stable or even increased over the last 30 years as the obesity epidemic has mounted [72, 74]. This suggests that the main driver of the obesity epidemic in the United States may be a worsening diet, while in most low-income countries, it is likely a combination of decreased physical activity and worsening diet [72, 75, 76].

The excess adiposity accompanying T2D, particularly in a central or visceral location, is thought to be part of the pathogenic process [73]. The pathophysiological mechanism between obesity and T2D relates primarily to the adipose tissue, which has been recognized as an endocrine organ that secretes hormones and communicates with the central nervous system to regulate appetite and metabolism [73]. The increased adipocyte mass leads to increased levels of circulating free fatty acids (FFA) and other fat cell products, called adipokines. Adipocytes secrete a number of biologic products (nonesterified free fatty acids, retinol-binding protein 4, leptin, TNF-, resistin, and adiponectin). Again, studies have generally suggested that circulating levels of these products are elevated in individuals with T2D [73]. In addition to regulating body weight, appetite, and energy expenditure, adipokines also modulate insulin sensitivity. The increased production of free fatty acids and some adipokines may cause insulin resistance in skeletal muscle and liver [73] . For example, free fatty acids impair glucose utilization in skeletal muscle, promote glucose production by the liver, and impair beta cell function. In contrast, the production by adipocytes of adiponectin, an insulin-sensitizing peptide, is reduced in obesity, and this may contribute to hepatic insulin resistance [73]. Adipocyte products and adipokines also produce an inflammatory state and may explain why markers of inflammation such as IL-6 and C-reactive protein are often elevated in T2D [73]. Adipose tissue also can cause insulin resistance by elevating leptin levels [77]. Leptin is a protein produced by adipocytes. The main role of leptin is to regulate food intake and energy expenditure by reducing food intake and increasing sympathetic nervous system outflow, therefore inducing weight loss. Recent evidence showed that leptin levels fall during weight loss and increase brain activity in areas involved in emotional, cognitive, and sensory control of food intake [78]. Restoration of leptin levels maintains weight loss and reverses the changes in brain activity. Thus, leptin is a critical factor linking reduced energy stores to eating behavior. In obesity, the actions of both leptin and insulin within the liver are resistant. Therefore, in individuals with obesity, leptin levels are elevated, and this has been found to positively correlate with insulin resistance [78]. Leptin can impair the production of insulin and reduce the effects of insulin on the liver.

Treatment for Obesity and T2D

A modest weight loss of 5–10% has been shown to result in improvements in morbidity and mortality risks among individuals with overweight and obesity [79]. Thus, weight loss is typically prescribed to individuals with overweight and obesity. Obesity and T2D are comorbid conditions with approximately 85% of patients with T2D having overweight or obesity [69]. Moreover, excess weight has been associated with elevated blood glucose levels [80, 81]. Weight loss has been shown to result in improvements in glucose levels [82–86] and even complete remission of T2D [83, 84]. Therefore, treatments for obesity are often also prescribed for T2D. Treatment options for obesity and T2D are categorized into three domains: lifestyle, pharmacological, and surgical interventions.

Lifestyle Intervention

As with T2D, lifestyle intervention is the first-line treatment option for weight management. Lifestyle interventions for weight management consist of dietary, physical activity, or combined interventions with variable success (range: 2–13% of initial body weight loss [87, 88]). While in the short-term (<6 months), dietary and combined interventions appear to be equally more effective than those that are purely physical in nature, over the long term (≥1 year), combined interventions seem to have greater weight loss success [88–90].

The benefits of combined lifestyle interventions for glycemic control in individuals with impaired glucose tolerance (IGT) [91, 92] and T2D [93, 94] have been well established in large-scale randomized control trials. Specifically, the *Diabetes Prevention Program* (DPP) in the United States and *Finnish Diabetes Prevention study* (DPS) enrolled IGT patients and randomized them to an intensive combined lifestyle intervention program, or control, with the DPP program including a third arm prescribed metformin. Patients participating in the intensive lifestyle intervention had greater improvements in key glycemic indicators such as fasting plasma glucose [91, 92] and glycated hemoglobin [92] than controls. Moreover, a smaller proportion of patients progressed to T2D in intensive lifestyle intervention group than controls [91, 92] or those prescribed metformin [91]. In patients who already have T2D, combined lifestyle intervention can also result in significant improvements in glycemic control. The Look AHEAD study randomized patients with T2D to receive an intensive combined lifestyle intervention or a diabetes support and education group and also observed greater decreases in weight and glycated hemoglobin after 1 [93, 94] and 4 year(s) [94] of treatment in the intensive combined intervention group. Unfortunately, these improvements due to the lifestyle intervention decreased overtime [93, 94].

Currently, there is considerable disagreement regarding what is the most optimal diet, or physical activity type for weight management. For example, dietary recommendations for weight management once focused on decreasing not only caloric intake but also the intake of dietary fat as this macronutrient was thought to be associated with ill-health. However, results from several meta-analyses suggest that at 1 year there is no significant difference in the weight loss achieved by patients prescribed a low fat versus low carbohydrate diet [95–97]. When taking into consideration the management of T2D, certain types of diets may be more optimal as they are associated with not only weight loss but also improvements in glycemic control. Specifically, individuals who consumed a low carbohydrate diet had greater decreases in their glycated hemoglobin [95] than participants consuming a low fat diet.

Physical activity can be categorized as aerobic or anaerobic. Aerobic, also referred to as cardio, includes activities like running and dancing. Anaerobic, also referred to as resistance, is a type of activities that can only be performed in short bursts due to the muscle oxygen demand, such as weight lifting or sprinting. Research suggests that either aerobic or anaerobic exercise interventions can result in improvements in glycated hemoglobin; however, combined exercise interventions resulted in greater improvements than solely aerobic or anaerobic interventions [98]. Owing to the health benefits associated with physical activity, the American College of Sports Medicine and the American Diabetes Association has released a joint statement that advocates for individuals with T2D participate in both aerobic and anaerobic physical activity weekly. Specifically, they recommend individuals with T2D participate in a minimum of 3 days/week of aerobic and 2–3 days/week of anaerobic activities for improvement in blood sugar [99]. For weight management, participating in both anaerobic and aerobic physical activity is also more beneficial than aerobic or resistance alone [100, 101]. Furthermore, a greater amount (>250 min/week vs. 150 min/week) of moderate to vigorous physical activity is recommended for significant weight loss [101].

Patients are able to achieve clinically significant improvements in their T2D and weight when implementing behavioral changes. Yet, these improvements are often transient in nature as patients are prone to regaining weight, or returning to previous habits [88, 102, 103]. This can be especially detrimental for patients with T2D as weight (re)gain is associated with a concomitant increases in glycated hemoglobin in populations with [104] and without T2D [105, 106]. Thus, the use of other interventions that can directly counteract physiological changes that make individuals prone to regaining weight, such as pharmacological or surgical interventions, may be advantageous.

Pharmacological Interventions

Pharmacological intervention is recommended for individuals who have attempted and previously failed at losing weight and have a BMI $\geq$30, or BMI $\geq$27 with at least one other medical condition [107]. Pharmaceuticals have a distinct advantage over lifestyle interventions as they directly target physiological changes that occur with and may inhibit weight loss and weight maintenance. Pharmaceutical intervention for weight can also provide additional benefits in the management of T2D beyond weight loss. Research suggest that taking weight management pharmaceuticals is associated with greater improvements in blood glucose levels and other metabolic parameters such as waist circumference and blood pressure than lifestyle intervention alone [108–110]. Moreover, patients who take weight management pharmaceuticals are also less likely to develop T2D [110], and patients with T2D have a greater rate of remission [85, 86]. Thus, effective interventions for weight management should commence as soon as T2D, or impaired glucose tolerance or abdominal obesity, is diagnosed.

Options for weight management for pharmaceuticals remain limited with only two agents available worldwide. Orlistat (Xenical), which has been available for over two decades, is the most widely approved weight management pharmaceutical. Its side effects include oily stools and fecal incontinence, which contribute to the high attrition rates (33–77% [111, 112]) observed among patients taking this agent. Patients prescribed orlistat lose significantly more weight than those just participating in lifestyle interventions, with T2D patients losing on average 4.6–6.2% of their initial body weight and significantly greater improvements in key diabetes indicators such as glycated hemoglobin and fasting blood glucose [113]. However, it is unclear whether these improvements in T2D indicators are due to the medication's effects, or to the amount of weight loss achieved.

A GLP1 analogue, liraglutide 3.0 mg (Saxenda), has been approved for use within the United States, Canada, Mexico, the United Arab Emirates, and most European countries. Several large randomized control trials, referred to as the *Satiety and Clinical Adiposity–Liraglutide Evidence in Non-Diabetic and Diabetic People* (SCALE), have examined the efficacy of this pharmaceutical for weight management. The only SCALE study that examined individuals with T2D observed that after 56 weeks of treatment, individuals taking the medication had a greater weight loss (6% vs. 2% weight loss) and improvements in glycemic control than those taking the placebo [114]. It is important to note that liraglutide 3.0 mg was initially prescribed and still remains on the market as a T2D medication (Victoza) at the maximum therapeutic dose of 1.8 mg, which may allude to greater beneficial effects in respective to the management of T2D compared to other weight management pharmaceuticals. Only one study has directly compared the efficacy of orlistat, liraglutide, and lifestyle modification for weight management, but it excluded individuals with T2D [109]. Nevertheless, patients in this study who were prescribed liraglutide 3.0 mg lost more weight and had greater improvements in their blood glucose than patients prescribed orlistat or just a lifestyle intervention after 20 and 56 weeks of treatment [109].

Other pharmaceuticals available for weight management include a phentermine and topiramate combination (Qsymia), a bupropion and naltrexone combination (Contrave), and lorcaserin (Belviq). However, these pharmaceuticals are only approved for weight management in the United States and are under review in Canada, Europe, and other countries. Several studies have examined the efficacy of these medications for glycemic control and weight management in individuals with T2D. All three of these medications resulted in significantly greater weight loss (lorcaserin: −9.3 vs. −7.5 kg [82], phentermine/topiramate: −9.1 vs. −2.6 kg [85], and bupropion/naltrexone: −5.3 vs. −1.9 kg [86]) than placebo. Moreover, patients with T2D had greater improvements in their glycated hemoglobin and required the addition of less T2D medication to control their blood sugars than those just participating in the lifestyle intervention [82, 85, 86].

The prescription of pharmaceuticals is much more common in the treatment of T2D than weight. This may be due to the more acute detrimental effects that high blood glucose can have on a patient when the effects of excessive weight tend to occur over the long term. Diabetes medications can have a beneficial (i.e., metformin, liraglutide) or detrimental (i.e., insulin, secretagogues) effect on a patient's ability to lose weight [107, 115, 116]. Thus, it is important to consider the effects that these medications can have on a patient's weight prior to prescribing them. This is in line with recommendations from The Endocrine Society, which recommended weight-losing and weight-neutral medications as first- and second-line agents for T2D management in patients with overweight or obesity [107]. Further, if insulin therapy is necessary, it is recommended to co-prescribed a diabetes medication with weight negative properties to mitigate the weight gain typically associated with insulin [107]. Given the association between weight gain and elevated blood glucose levels [80, 81], it may be advantageous to prescribe weight neutral and weight negative T2D medications as first- and second-line treatment of diabetes in lean populations as well as overweight and obese.

Surgical Intervention

Compared to lifestyle and pharmaceutical interventions, patients who undergo bariatric surgery lose more weight and maintain a greater proportion of this loss over the long term, making bariatric surgery the most effective treatment for obesity [117]. However, there are lifelong dietary changes and potential complications that accompany this intervention [117–119], which had meant that until recently, bariatric surgery was reserved for individuals with severe obesity. Multiple international organizations [15, 16] recommend bariatric surgery for individuals who had previously failed at weight loss and have a BMI ≥40 kg/m^2 or a BMI ≥35 kg/m^2 with at least one comorbidity. However, with bariatric surgery being recognized as a metabolic surgery due to the reduction in cardiometabolic risk factor levels observed post-surgery, as well as due to the differences for disease risk attributed to excess weight by ethnicity, these organizations now recommend consideration of patients with lower (i.e., <35 kg/m^2) BMIs for this surgery.

The International Federation for the Surgery of Obesity and Metabolic Disorders surveyed national organizations in 56 countries to determine trends in bariatric surgery. This survey contained 16 possible procedures. Sleeve gastrectomy was the most common procedure (45.9%), followed by roux-en-y gastric bypass (39.6%), and then gastric banding (7.4%), with no other procedure accounting for greater than 2% of procedures performed worldwide [120]. Below is a brief description of the three most common surgical procedures:

- Roux-En-Y gastric bypass: A small portion of the upper stomach is made into a pouch and is attached to the jejunum, bypassing a portion of the digestive system and making a y shape, which gives this procedure its name [117]. This procedure is referred to as both a restrictive and malabsportive weight loss procedure. It is considered restrictive as the resizing of the stomach restricts the amount of food that a patient can consume and malabsorptive, as bypassing part of the stomach and intestine results in decreased absorption of nutrients.
- Sleeve gastrectomy: A large portion of the stomach is removed, and the remainder is stapled closed resulting in a smaller tubular shaped stomach [119]. This is a purely restrictive as the new smaller size of the stomach decreases the amount of calories the patient can consume [121], but no bypassing of the digestive system takes place to result in malabsoprtion.
- Gastric banding: A small, thin band, typically made of a flexible material such as silicon, is placed around the upper stomach to create a pouch [117]. Similar to the sleeve gastrectomy, this is a purely restrictive procedure. For the majority of patients, frequent adjustments to the band are necessary within the first 2 years to promote and maintain weight loss [122].

Bariatric surgery is a relatively safe procedure, with 30-day mortality rates ranging from 0.05% to 0.5% [119, 123] and 30-day complication rates of 1.4–5.9% [119]. One-year post-surgery, patients who underwent sleeve gastrectomy (range: 68.2–69.7% excess weight [123, 124]) and roux-en-y (60.5–62.6% excess weight [118, 123, 124] appear to lose comparable amounts of weight, and patients who underwent gastric banding (42.6–47.5% excess weight [118, 123]) have considerably less weight loss.

Bariatric surgery may be one of the best tools for the management and treatment of T2D. Patients with T2D typically lose less weight than nondiabetic populations in lifestyle and pharmaceutical interventions. However, a meta-analysis observed that patients in the T2D sub-sample lost more weight than the full sample of patients with and without T2D. This may suggest the lower mean weight loss in the full sample was due to less optimal weight outcomes in patients without T2D [84]. Moreover 86.6% of patients with T2D experience improved or complete resolution of their diabetes post-surgery [84]. Over half of patients with T2D that undergo bariatric surgery have complete resolution of their diabetes regardless of the procedure; however, the proportion of patients who go into remission is significantly greater for those with sleeve gastrectomy (79.7%) and roux-en-y (80.3%) than those with gastric banding (56.7%) [84]. Lastly, patients who undergo bariatric surgery can have additional benefits beyond significant weight loss and improvements or resolution of their T2D or IGT, such as a decrease in mortality risk [125–127] and risk of T2D complications [126, 127].

Gastric banding is now being recognized as an inferior bariatric surgery procedure, likely due to the decreased weight loss and improvements in comorbidities. Furthermore, due to complications and insufficient weight loss, over half of patients who undergo gastric banding will need band removal and conversion to another type of bariatric procedure [128]. Owing to these suboptimal outcomes, the Canadian Diabetes Association has recommended against the use of the gastric band [12]. This may mean that other procedures will increase in popularity as gastric banding falls into disuse. For example, a less common surgery that is gaining traction is the bilio-pancreatic diversion with the duodenal switch. This procedure is more invasive than the other three procedures discussed but has better results in terms of diabetes remission and long-term weight loss than the more common alternatives (i.e., roux-en-y bypass and gastric banding) [84].

Conclusion

Obesity is a chronic disease categorized by excessive weight with ill-health effects. BMI is the most common tool to categorize obesity, with a recommended threshold of ≥30 kg/m². There are many different methods to assess obesity; however, due to considerable differences in the associations of excess weight and ill-health based on age, sex, and ethnicity, heavy criticism exists regarding the use of universal thresholds. Nonetheless, these measurements remain in use due to their ability to assess the potential health impacts of excess weight.

Obesity is a chronic, multifactorial disease. Multiple factors have been identified that are associated with developing obesity, with genetics, diet, and physical activity being the factors that are most salient to obesity and T2D. Mechanistic studies have determined the presence of several genes associated with having obesity, and epidemiological studies have further supported this evidence. Increased caloric intake, macronutrient content, and lack of physical activity also play a role in the development of obesity, but these are modifiable risk factors, which can be manipulated in the treatment of these conditions.

Treatment options for obesity, as with T2D, can be categorized as lifestyle,

Pharmacological, or surgical. Lifestyle intervention is a first line of treatment; however, treatment benefits are often not maintained over the long term. Thus, medications and surgery provide additional opportunities for weight management and have been shown to have greater efficacy for weight loss and improvements in comorbidities than lifestyle interventions alone.

Concluding Remarks

1. Obesity is a chronic medical characterized by excess weight associated with ill-health effects. For trend analysis and owing to the ease of measurement, a BMI ≥ 30 kg/m² is the most frequently used definition.

2. A multitude of factors contribute to the development of obesity; however, genetics, diet, and physical activity are the most important. T2D is closely linked to obesity and share similar biological processes and epidemiology.

3. Lifestyle, pharmaceutical, and surgical treatment options all have the potential to improve and eliminate the negative health effects of T2D or excess weight; however, surgical interventions are the most successful.

Multiple Choice Questions

1. Body mass index is a tool commonly used to classify an individual as having obesity. What threshold is used to define obesity?
   (a) Greater than or equal to 27.5 kg/m²
   (b) **Greater than or equal to 30 kg/m²**
      Although there is variability in the ill-health effects associated with a given BMI based on ethnicity, the World Health Organization still recommends a threshold of 30 kg/m² to define obesity.
   (c) Greater than or equal to 35 kg/m²
   (d) Greater than or equal to 40 kg/m²
   (e) No threshold exists

2. Which of the following are methods used to assess obesity?
   (a) Skinfold measures
   (b) Dual Energy X-ray Absorptiometry (DEXA)
   (c) Forehead circumference
   (d) **A & B**
      Many circumference measurements are used to assess obesity such as waist, hip, and neck circumferences, but forehead circumference is not one of them.
   (e) All of the above

3. What are some common demographics that make the use of absolute thresholds for the assessment of obesity and its ill-health effects difficult?
   (a) Age
   (b) Sex
   (c) Ethnicity
   (d) **All of the above**
      Age, sex, and ethnicity can all change the association that excess weight can have with ill-health.

For example, some excess weight may actually be beneficial to elderly populations as it has been shown to decrease frailty. Women are able to have higher body fat percentages than men without ill-health effects. Furthermore, certain ethnicities, for example, people of Asian descent, start to have exhibit ill-health effects at lower levels of body fat than White counterparts.

   (e) None of the above

4. Which of the following is true regarding the notion that there is hereditary component to the development of obesity?

   (a) Children who have one parent with obesity are at a greater risk for developing obesity than those with two

   (b) BMIs of monozygotic and dizygotic twins raised together are more similar than those raised apart

   (c) Genes have been found that are associated with hypophagia

   (d) All of the above

   (e) **None of the above**

   Children who have two parents with obesity are at a greater risk of having obesity, and genes have been identified associated with hyperphagia (excessive eating). Furthermore, while it is true that the BMI of twins reared together are more similar than those raised apart, there is still a strong association in the BMIs of twins reared apart.

5. Which of the following are patient modifiable risk factors associated with the development of obesity?

   (a) **Physical activity**

   Physical activity is the only factor that listed that individuals have control over. While it is possible for the built environment to be modified to encourage more physical activity, this is not something that an individual would be able to change by themselves.

   (b) The built environment

   (c) Genetics

   (d) Type 2 diabetes

   (e) A & B

6. Which of the following diet and physical activity factors contribute to the development of obesity?

   (a) Excessive caloric intake

   (b) Being sedentary

   (c) Macronutrient content of diet

   (d) Employment

   (e) **All of the above**

   Beyond the typical modifiable factors that are addressed in the treatment of obesity, such as diet and physical activity, other factors, such as your employment, can contribute to weight gain. This is due to occupational shifts that have occurred during the twentieth century that have resulted in an increase in management and decrease in labor type jobs.

7. Adipokines secreted by adipocytes, regulate body weight, appetite, and energy expenditure. They also contribute to increasing insulin resistance by?

   (a) Increasing lipid production

   (b) Decreasing leptin levels

   (c) **Modulating insulin sensitivity**

   In addition to regulating body weight, appetite, and energy expenditure, adipokines also modulate insulin sensitivity. The increased production of free fatty acids and some adipokines may cause insulin resistance in skeletal muscle and liver.

   (d) Promoting beta cell function

   (e) Reducing markers of inflammation

8. Which of the following statements is true regarding low fat and low carbohydrate diets?

   (a) Low fat diets are more beneficial for weight loss, but low fat and low carbohydrate diets are equally effective for managing diabetes management.

   (b) Low carbohydrate diets are more beneficial for weight loss, but low fat and low carbohydrate diets are equally effective for diabetes management.

   (c) Low fat and low carbohydrates are equally beneficial for weight loss, but low fat diets are more beneficial for diabetes management.

   (d) **Low fat and low carbohydrates are equally beneficial for weight loss, but low carbohydrate diets are more beneficial for diabetes management**.

   While low fat and low carbohydrates do appear to be equally effective for weight management, diets low in carbohydrates appears to be more beneficial for patients with T2D. Indeed, research has suggested that T2D consuming diets lower in carbohydrates will have greater improvements in glycemic control than consuming a low fat diet.

   (e) Low fat and low carbohydrate diets are equally effective in the management of obesity and diabetes.

9. Which of the following statements is false regarding weight management medications:

   (a) **Weight management medications decrease weight, but do not provide any benefits for the management of diabetes**

   Each of the available weight management medications have been tested in populations with T2D, and all have been shown to improvement glycemic control. Furthermore, these patients typically require the addition of less glycemic medication than those given a placebo.

   (b) Liraglutide 3.0 mg is more effective for glycemic control than orlistat.

(c) All approved weight management medications are associated with greater improvements in glycated hemoglobin than lifestyle intervention alone.

(d) Patients prescribed weight management medications lose significantly more weight than those participating in only lifestyle interventions.

(e) Liraglutide, a weight management medication, is also available as a T2D medication at a lower therapeutic dose.

10. Which of the following correctly lists the three treatment options for obesity and T2D in order from most to least effective?

(a) Medication, lifestyle, and surgical

(b) Lifestyle, medication, and surgical

(c) **Surgical, medication, lifestyle**

Patients who undergo surgical intervention lose more weight and have greater rates in T2D remission than patients taking weight management medications or just lifestyle intervention. Furthermore, patients taking weight management medications have greater improvements than lifestyle alone.

(d) Surgical, lifestyle, medication

(e) They are all equally effective treatments for weight and diabetes management.

Glossary

Bariatric Surgery It is a type of surgical procedure that decreases the amount of calories a patient can consume and/or digests to result in significant weight loss. Types of bariatric surgery include roux-en-y gastric bypass, sleeve gastrectomy, and gastric banding.

Body Fat It is the amount of subcutaneous and visceral fat in a person's body that can be presented as an absolute value or percentage.

Body Mass Index It is the most common tool to assess obesity. It is calculated by dividing weight in kilograms by height in meters squared.

Malabsorptive Bariatric Surgery It is a bariatric surgery procedure that alters a patient's digestive tract to decrease the amount of nutrients they can absorb from calories consumed. Examples of types of bariatric surgery that use this technique include the roux-en-y gastric bypass and bilio-pancreatic diversion with the duodenal switch.

Metabolic Surgery It is a newer term used to refer to bariatric surgery owing to the drastic improvements in metabolic conditions that have been observed post-surgery.

Obesity It is excess body weight associated with ill-health. Multiple objective methods exist to classify obesity, with a BMI greater than or equal to 30 kg/m^2 the most common.

Restrictive Bariatric Surgery It is a bariatric surgery procedure that decreases the amount of calories a patient can consume by decreasing the size of the stomach. Examples of types of bariatric surgery that use this technique include the sleeve gastrectomy and gastric banding.

Subcutaneous Fat It is the type of body fat located just beneath the skin and can be felt by pinching the skin.

Visceral Fat It is the type of body fat located internally around the organs. As such, visceral fat is also called organ fat.

References

1. World Health Organization. Overweight and obesity. Geneva: WHO; 2015. [cited 2017 Oct 8]. http://www.who.int/mediacentre/factsheets/fs311/en/
2. Wang YC, McPherson K, Marsh T, Gortmaker SL, Brown M. Health and economic burden of the projected obesity trends in the USA and the UK. Lancet. 2011;378(9793):815–25.
3. Wilson PWF, D'Agostino RB, Sullivan L, Parise H, Kannel WB. Overweight and obesity as determinants of cardiovascular risk: the Framingham experience. Arch Intern Med. 2002;162(16):1867–72.
4. Christensen RAG, Raiber L, Macpherson AK, Kuk JL. The association between obesity and self-reported sinus infection in non-smoking adults: a cross-sectional study. Clin Obes. 2016;6(6):389–94.
5. Fontaine KR, Redden DT, Wang C, Westfall AO, Allison DB. Years of life lost due to obesity. JAMA. 2003;289(2):187–93.
6. Chang SH, Pollack LM, Colditz GA. Life years lost associated with obesity-related diseases for U.S. non-smoking adults. PLoS One. 2013;8(6):e66550.
7. Tsai AG, Williamson DF, Glick HA. Direct medical cost of overweight and obesity in the USA: a quantitative systematic review. Obes Rev. 2011;12(1):50–61.
8. Kim DD, Basu A. Estimating the medical care costs of obesity in the United States: systematic review, meta-analysis, and empirical analysis. Value Heal. 2016;19(5):602–13.
9. Peitz GW, Troyer J, Jones AE, Shapiro NI, Nelson RD, Hernandez J, et al. Association of body mass index with increased cost of care and length of stay for emergency department patients with chest pain and dyspnea. Circ Cardiovasc Qual Outcomes. 2014;7(2):292–8.
10. Cawley J, Rizzo JA, Haas K. Occupation-specific absenteeism costs associated with obesity and morbid obesity. J Occup Environ Med. 2007;49(12):1317–24.
11. Conway B, Miller RG, Costacou T, Fried L, Kelsey S, Evans RW, et al. Temporal patterns in overweight and obesity in Type 1 diabetes. Diabet Med. 2010;27(4):398–404.
12. Clement M, Harvey B, Rabi DM, Roscoe RS, Sherifali D, Canadian Diabetes Association 2013. Clinical practice guidelines for the prevention and management of diabetes in Canada. Can J Diabetes. 2013;37(Suppl.1):S20–5. https://doi.org/10.1016/j.jcjd.2013.01.014.
13. Goebel-Fabbri AE. Disturbed eating behaviors and eating disorders in Type 1 diabetes: clinical significance and treatment recommendations. Curr Diab Rep. 2009;9(2):133–9.
14. World Health Organization Expert Consultation. Appropriate body-mass index for Asian populations and its implications for policy and intervention strategies. Lancet. 2004;363(9403):157–63.
15. Dixon JB, Zimmet P, Alberti KG, Rubino F. Bariatric surgery: an IDF statement for obese Type 2 diabetes. Diabet Med. 2011;28(6):628–42.

16. Rubino F, Nathan DM, Eckel RH, Schauer PR, Alberti KGMM, Zimmet PZ, et al. Metabolic surgery in the treatment algorithm for Type 2 diabetes: a joint statement by international diabetes organizations. Diabetes Care. 2016;39(6):861–77.

17. Deurenberg P, Yap M, van Staveren WA. Body mass index and percent body fat: a meta analysis among different ethnic groups. Int J Obes Relat Metab Disord. 1998;22(12):1164–71.

18. Dobbelsteyn CJ, Joffres MR, MacLean DR, Flowerdew G. A comparative evaluation of waist circumference, waist-to-hip ratio and body mass index as indicators of cardiovascular risk factors. The Canadian Heart Health Surveys. Int J Obes Relat Metab Disord. 2001;25(5):652–61.

19. Zhang C, Rexrode KM, Van Dam RM, Li TY, Hu FB. Abdominal obesity and the risk of all-cause, cardiovascular, and cancer mortality: sixteen years of follow-up in US women. Circulation. 2008;117(13):1658–67.

20. Wang Y, Rimm EB, Stampfer MJ, Willett WC, Hu FB. Comparison of abdominal adiposity and overall obesity in predicting risk of Type 2 diabetes among men. Am J Clin Nutr. 2005;81(3):555–63.

21. Janssen I, Katzmarzyk PT, Ross R. Body mass index, waist circumference, and health risk: evidence in support of current National Institutes of Health guidelines. Arch Intern Med. 2017;162(18):2074–9.

22. National Institutes of Health. The Practical Guide 2000 Identification, evaluation, and treatment of overweight and obesity in adults. NIH, Bethesda, MD. NIH Publ Number 00-4084. October:26–7.

23. Carroll JF, Chiapa AL, Rodriquez M, Phelps DR, Cardarelli KM, Vishwanatha JK, et al. Visceral fat, waist circumference, and BMI: impact of race/ethnicity. Obesity (Silver Spring). 2008;16(3):600–7.

24. Bodicoat DH, Gray LJ, Henson J, Webb D, Guru A, Misra A, et al. Body mass index and waist circumference cut-points in multi-ethnic populations from the UK and India: the ADDITION-Leicester, Jaipur heart watch and New Delhi cross-sectional studies. PLoS One. 2014;9(3):1–6.

25. Lean ME, Han TS, Morrison CE. Waist circumference as a measure for indicating need for weight management. BMJ. 1995;311(6998):158–61.

26. Ardern CI, Janssen I, Ross R, Katzmarzyk PT. Development of health-related waist circumference thresholds within BMI categories. Obes Res. 2004;12(7):1094–103.

27. World Health Organization. Waist circumference and waist-hip ratio: report of a WHO expert consultation. Geneva: World Health Organization; 2008; (December):8–11.

28. Molarius A, Seidell J. Selection of anthropometric indicators for classification of abdominal fatness—a critical review. Int J Obes Relat Metab Disord. 1998;22(8):719–27.

29. Caan B, Armstrong MA, Selby JV, Sadler M, Folsom AR, Jacobs D, et al. Changes in measurements of body fat distribution accompanying weight change. Int J Obes Relat Metab Disord J Int Assoc Study Obes. 1994;18(6):397–404.

30. Taksali SE, Caprio S, Dziura J, Dufour S, Calı AMG, Goodman TR, et al. High visceral and low abdominal subcutaneous fat. Diabetes. 2008;57(2):367–71.

31. Wing RR, Jeffery RW, Burton LR, Thorson C, Kuller LH, Folsom AR. Change in waist-hip ratio with weight loss and its association with change in cardiovascular risk factors. Am J Clin Nutr. 1992;55(6):1086–92.

32. Matsuzawa Y, Shimomurn I, Nakumura T, Keno Y, Kotani K. Pathophysiology and pathogenesis of visceral fat obesity. Obes Res. 1995;3(Suppl 2):187S–94S.

33. Deurenberg-Yap M, Chew SK, Deurenberg P. Elevated body fat percentage and cardiovascular risks at low body mass index levels among Singaporean Chinese, Malays and Indians. Obes Rev. 2002;3(3):209–15.

34. Deurenberg P. Universal cut-off BMI points for obesity are not appropriate. Br J Nutr. 2001;85(2):135–6.

35. World Health Organization (WHO). Obesity: preventing and managing the global epidemic. Report of a WHO consultation. World Health Organ Tech Rep Ser. 2000;894(i-xii):1–253. http://www.ncbi.nlm.nih.gov/pubmed/11234459

36. Sloan A, Burt J, Blyth C. Estimation of body fat in young women. J Appl Physiol. 1962;17:967–70.

37. Durnin JV, Womersley J. Body fat assessed from total body density and its estimation from skinfold thickness: measurements on 481 men and women aged from 16 to 72 years. Br J Nutr. 1974;32(1):77–97.

38. Slaughter MH, Lohman TG, Boileau RA, Horswill CA, Stillman RJ, Van Loan MD, et al. Skinfold equations for estimation of body fatness in children and youth. Hum Biol. 1988;60(5):709–23.

39. Jackson AS, Pollock ML, Ward A. Generalized equation for predicting body density of women. Med Sci Sport Exer. 1980;12(3):175–82.

40. Jackson AS, Pollock ML. Generalized equations for predicting body density of men. Br J Nutr. 1978;40(3):497–504.

41. Durnin JV, Rahaman MM. The assessment of the amount of fat in the human body from measurements of skinfold thickness. Br J Nutr. 1967;21(3):681–9.

42. Kushner RF. Bioelectrical impedance analysis: a review of principles and applications. J Am Coll Nutr. 1992;11(2):199–209.

43. Sun SS, Chumlea WC, Heymsfield SB, Lukaski HC, Schoeller D, Friedl K, et al. Development of bioelectrical impedance analysis prediction equations for body composition with the use of a multicomponent model for use in epidemiologic surveys 1–4. Am J Clin Nutr. 2003;77(22):331–40.

44. Roubenoff R, Kehayias JJ, Dawson Hughes B, Heymsfield SB. Use of dual-energy x-ray absorptiometry in body composition studies: not yet a gold standard. Am J Clin Nutr. 1993;58(5):589–91.

45. Bosy-Westphal A, Later W, Hitze B, Sato T, Kossel E, Glüer CC, et al. Accuracy of bioelectrical impedance consumer devices for measurement of body composition in comparison to whole body magnetic resonance imaging and dual X-ray absorptiometry. Obes Facts. 2008;1(6):319–24.

46. Wattanapenpaiboon N, Lukito W, Strauss BJ, Hsu-Hage BH, Wahlqvist ML, Stroud DB. Agreement of skinfold measurement and bioelectrical impedance analysis (BIA) methods with dual energy X-ray absorptiometry (DEXA) in estimating total body fat in Anglo-Celtic Australians. Int J Obes Relat Metab Disord. 1998;22(9):854–60.

47. Rothney MP, Brychta RJ, Schaefer EV, Chen KY, Monica C. Body composition measured by dual-energy X-ray absorptiometry half-body scans in obese adults. Obesity. 2009;17(6):1281–6.

48. Chouinard LE, Schoeller DA, Watras AC, Clark RR, Close RN, Buchholz AC. Bioelectrical impedance vs. four-compartment model to assess body fat change in overweight adults. Obesity. 2007;15(1):85–92.

49. Lee SY, Gallagher D. Assessment methods in human body composition. Curr Opin Clin Nutr Metab Care. 2008;11(5):566–72.

50. Butland B, Jebb S, Kopelman P, McPherson K, Thomas S, Mardell J, et al. Foresight tackling obesities: future choices—project report. Gov Off Sci. 2007;1–161.

51. Rankinen T, Zuberi A, Chagnon YC, Weisnagel SJ, Argyropoulos G, Walts B, et al. The human obesity gene map: the 2005 update. Obesity. 2006;14(4):529–644.

52. Mergen M, Mergen H, Ozata M, Oner R, Oner C. A novel melanocortin 4 receptor (MC4R) gene mutation associated with morbid obesity. J Clin Endocrinol Metab. 2001;86(7):3448–51.

53. Cassidy SB, Schwartz S, Miller JL, Driscoll DJ. Prader-Willi syndrome. Genet Med. 2012;14(1):10–26.

54. Farooqi IS, O'Rahilly S. New advances in the genetics of early onset obesity. Int J Obes. 2005;29(10):1149–52.

55. Farooqi IS, O'Rahilly S. Genetic factors in human obesity. Obes Rev. 2007;8(Suppl 1):37–40.

56. Reilly JJ, Armstrong J, Dorosty AR, Emmett PM, Ness A, Rogers I, et al. Early life risk factors for obesity in childhood: cohort study. BMJ. 2005;330(7504):1–7.

57. Stunkard AJ, Harris JR, Pedersen NL, McClearn GE. The body-mass index of twins who have been reared apart. N Engl J Med. 1990;322(21):1483–7.

58. Price RA, Gottesman II. Body fat in identical twins reared apart: roles for genes and environment. Behav Genet. 1991;21(1):1–7.

59. Silventoinen K, Sans S, Tolonen H, Monterde D, Kuulasmaa K, Kesteloot H, et al. Trends in obesity and energy supply in the WHO MONICA project. Int J Obes. 2004;28(5):710–8.

60. Brown RE, Sharma AM, Ardern CI, Mirdamadi P, Mirdamadi P, Kuk JL. Secular differences in the association between caloric intake, macronutrient intake, and physical activity with obesity. Obes Res Clin Pract. 2015;10(September):1–13.

61. Heitmann BL, Lissner L, Sorensen TIA, Bengtsson C. Dietary fat intake and weight gain in women genetically predisposed for obesity. Am J Clin Nutr. 1995;61(6):1213–7.

62. World Health Organization. Guideline: sugars intake for adults and children. Geneva: World Health Organization-WHO; 2014. p. 48.

63. Jeffery RW, Wing RR, Sherwood NE, Tate DF. Physical activity and weight loss: does prescribing higher physical activity goals improve outcome? Am J Clin Nutr. 2003;78(4):684–9.

64. Wing RR, Hill JO. Successful weight loss maintenance. Annu Rev Nutr. 2001;21:323–41.

65. Tudor-Locke C, Brashear MM, Johnson WD, Katzmarzyk PT. Accelerometer profiles of physical activity and inactivity in normal weight, overweight, and obese U.S. men and women. Int J Behav Nutr Phys Act. 2010;7:60.

66. Wyatt ID, Hecker DE. Occupational changes during the 20th century. Mon Labor Rev. 2006;129(3):35–57.

67. Frank LD, Sallis JF, Conway TL, Chapman JE, Saelens BE, Bachman W. Many pathways from land use to health: associations between neighborhood walkability and active transportation, body mass index, and air quality. J Am Plan Assoc. 2006;72(1):75–87.

68. Ali O. Genetics of Type 2 diabetes. World J Diabetes. 2013;4(4):114.

69. Astrup A, Finer N. Redefining Type 2 diabetes: "diabesity" or "obesity dependent diabetes mellitus"? Obes Rev. 2000;1(2):57–9.

70. Juonala M, Magnussen CG, Berenson GS, Venn A, Burns TL, Sabin MA, et al. Childhood adiposity, adult adiposity, and cardiovascular risk factors. Obstet Gynecol Surv. 2012;67(3):156–8.

71. Ferrannini E, Camastra S. Relationship between impaired glucose tolerance, non-insulin-dependent diabetes mellitus and obesity. Eur J Clin Investig. 1998;28 Suppl 2:3-6-7.

72. Mozaffarian D, Wilson PWF, Kannel WB. Beyond established and novel risk factors lifestyle risk factors for cardiovascular disease. Circulation. 2008;117(23):3031–8.

73. Al-Quwaidhi A, Critchley J, O'Flaherty M, Pearce M. Obesity and Type 2 diabetes mellitus: a complex association. Saudi J Obes. 2013;1(2):49.

74. Murray CJL, Atkinson C, Bhalla K, Birbeck G, Burstein R, Chou D, et al. The state of US health, 1990-2010: burden of diseases, injuries, and risk factors. JAMA. 2013;310(6):591–608.

75. Mozaffarian D. Foods, obesity, and diabetes—are all calories created equal? Nutr Rev. 2017;75:19–31.

76. Lim SS, Vos T, Flaxman AD, Danaei G, Shibuya K, Adair-Rohani H, et al. A comparative risk assessment of burden of disease and injury attributable to 67 risk factors and risk factor clusters in 21 regions, 1990–2010: a systematic analysis for the Global Burden of Disease Study 2010. Lancet. 2012;380(9859):2224–60.

77. Lazar MA. How obesity causes diabetes: not a tall tale. Science. 2005;307(5708):373–5.

78. Ahima RS. Revisiting leptin's role in obesity and weight loss. J Clin Invest. 2008;118(7):2380–3. http://www.ncbi.nlm.nih.gov/pubmed/18568083.

79. Wing RR, Lang W, Wadden TA, Safford M, Knowler WC, Bertoni AG, et al. Benefits of modest weight loss in improving cardiovascular risk factors in overweight and obese individuals with Type 2 diabetes. Diabetes Care. 2011;34(7):1481–6.

80. Vittal BG, Praveen G, Deepak P. A study of body mass index in healthy individuals and its relationship with fasting blood sugar. J Clin Diagn Res. 2010;4(6):3421–4. http://www.jcdr.net/article_fulltext.asp?id=990

81. Innocent O, ThankGod OO, Sandra EO, Josiah EI. Correlation between body mass index and blood glucose levels among some Nigerian undergraduates. HOAJ Biol. 2013;2(1):4.

82. Magkos F, Nikonova E, Fain R, Zhou S, Ma T, Shanahan W. Effect of lorcaserin on glycemic parameters in patients with Type 2 diabetes mellitus. Obesity. 2017 May;25(5):842–9.

83. Mottalib A, Sakr M, Shehabeldin M, Hamdy O. Diabetes remission after nonsurgical intensive lifestyle intervention in obese patients with Type 2 diabetes. J Diabetes Res. 2015;2015(2015):4.

84. Buchwald H, Estok R, Fahrbach K, Banel D, Jensen MD, Pories WJ, et al. Weight and Type 2 diabetes after bariatric surgery: systematic review and meta-analysis. Am J Med. 2009;122(3):248–256 e5.

85. Garvey WT, Ryan DH, Bohannon NJV, Kushner RF, Rueger M, Dvorak RV, et al. Weight-loss therapy in Type 2 diabetes: effects of phentermine and topiramate extended release. Diabetes Care. 2014;37(12):3309–16.

86. Hollander P, Gupta AK, Plodkowski R, Greenway F, Bays H, Burns C, et al. Effects of naltrexone sustained-release/bupropion sustained-release combination therapy on body weight and glycemic parameters in overweight and obese patients with Type 2 diabetes. Diabetes Care. 2013;36(12):4022–9.

87. Dakour Aridi HN, Wehbe M-R, Shamseddine G, Alami RS, Safadi BY. Long-term outcomes of roux-en-Y gastric bypass conversion of failed laparoscopic gastric band. Obes Surg. 2017;27(6):1401–8.

88. Curioni CC, Lourenço PM. Long-term weight loss after diet and exercise: a systematic review. Int J Obes. 2005;29(10):1168–74.

89. Johns DJ, Hartmann-Boyce J, Jebb SA, Aveyard P. Diet or exercise interventions vs combined behavioral weight management programs: a systematic review and meta-analysis of directcomparisons. J Acad Nutr Diet. 2014;114(10):1557–68.

90. Miller WC, Koceja DM, Hamilton EJ. A meta-analysis of the past 25 years of weight loss research using diet, exercise or diet plus exercise intervention. Int J Obes. 1997;21(10):941–7.

91. Knowler WC, Barrett-Connor E, Fowler SE, Hamman RF, Lachin JM, Walker EA, et al. Reduction in the incidence of Type 2 diabetes with lifestyle intervention or metformin. N Engl J Med. 2002;346(6):393–403.

92. Lindstrom J, Louheranta A, Mannelin M, Rastas M, Salminen V, Eriksson J, et al. The Finnish Diabetes Prevention Study (DPS). Diabetes Care. 2003;26(12):3230–6.

93. Look AHEAD Research Group LAR, Pi-Sunyer X, Blackburn G, Brancati FL, Bray GA, Bright R, et al. Reduction in weight and cardiovascular disease risk factors in individuals with Type 2 diabetes: one-year results of the look AHEAD trial. Diabetes Care. 2007;30(6):1374–83.

94. Look AHEAD Research Group, Wing RR. Long-term effects of a lifestyle intervention on weight and cardiovascular risk factors in individuals with Type 2 diabetes mellitus: four-year results of the Look AHEAD trial. Arch Intern Med. 2010;170(17):1566–75.

95. Nordmann AJ, Nordmann AJ, Briel M, Keller U, Yancy WS Jr, Brehm BJ, et al. Effects of low-carbohydrate vs low-fat diets on weight loss and cardiovascular risk factors: a meta-analysis of randomized controlled trials. Arch Intern Med. 2006;166(3):285–93.

96. Tobias DK, Chen M, Manson JAE, Ludwig DS, Willett W, Hu FB. Effect of low-fat diet interventions versus other diet interventions on long-term weight change in adults: a systematic review and meta-analysis. Lancet Diabetes Endocrinol. 2015;3(12):968–79.

97. Hu T, Mills KT, Yao L, Demanelis K, Eloustaz M, Yancy WS, et al. Effects of low-carbohydrate diets versus low-fat diets on metabolic risk factors: a meta-analysis of randomized controlled clinical trials. Am J Epidemiol. 2012:S44–54.

98. Davidson LE, Hudson R, Kilpatrick K, Kuk JL, McMillan K, Janiszewski PM, et al. Effects of exercise modality on insulin resistance and functional limitation in older adults. Arch Intern Med. 2009;169(2):122–31.

99. Colberg SR, Sigal RJ, Fernhall B, Regensteiner JG, Blissmer BJ, Rubin RR, et al. Exercise and type 2 diabetes: the American College of Sports Medicine and the American Diabetes Association: joint position statement. Diabetes Care. 2010;33(12):e147–67.

100. Arciero PJ, Gentile CL, Martin-Pressman R, Ormsbee MJ, Everett M, Zwicky L, et al. Increased dietary protein and combined high intensity aerobic and resistance exercise improves body fat distribution and cardiovascular risk factors. Int J Sport Nutr Exerc Metab. 2006;16(4):373–92.

101. Donnelly JE, Blair SN, Jakicic JM, Manore MM, Rankin JW, Smith BK. Appropriate physical activity intervention strategies for weight loss and prevention of weight regain for adults. Med Sci Sports Exerc. 2009;41(2):459–71.

102. Brownell KD, Jeffery RW. Improving long-term weight loss: pushing the limits of treatment. Behav Ther. 1987;18(4):353–74.

103. Jeffery RW, Drewnowski A, Epstein LH, Stunkard AJ, Wilson GT, Wing RR, et al. Long-term maintenance of weight loss: current status. Health Psychol. 2000;19(1S):5–16.

104. Jacob AN, Salinas K, Adams-Huet B, Raskin P. Weight gain in Type 2 diabetes mellitus. Diabetes Obes Metab. 2007;9(3):386–93.

105. Kroeger CM, Hoddy KK, Varady KA. Impact of weight regain on metabolic disease risk: a review of human trials. J Obes. 2014;2014(2014):8.

106. Beavers KM, Case LD, Blackwell CS, Katula JA, Goff DC, Vitolins MZ, et al. Effects of weight regain following intentional weight loss on glucoregulatory function in overweight and obese adults with pre-diabetes. Obes Res Clin Pract. 2015;9(3):266–73.

107. Apovian CM, Aronne LJ, Bessesen DH, McDonnell ME, Murad MH, Pagotto U, et al. Pharmacological management of obesity: an endocrine society clinical practice guideline. J Clin Endocrinol Metab. 2015;100(2):342–62.

108. Padwal R, Li SK, Lau DCW. Long-term pharmacotherapy for overweight and obesity: a systematic review and meta-analysis of randomized controlled trials. Int J Obes Relat Metab Disord. 2003;27:1437–46.

109. Astrup A, Carraro R, Finer N, Harper A, Kunesova M, Lean MEJ, et al. Safety, tolerability and sustained weight loss over 2 years with the once-daily human GLP-1 analog, liraglutide. Int J Obes. 2012;36(6):843–54.

110. Pi-Sunyer X, Astrup A, Fujioka K, Greenway F, Halpern A, Krempf M, et al. A randomized, controlled trial of 3.0 mg of liraglutide in weight management. N Engl J Med. 2015;373(1):11–22.

111. Rucker D, Padwal R, Li SK, Curioni C, Lau DCW. Long term pharmacotherapy for obesity and overweight: updated meta-analysis. BMJ. 2007;335(7631):1194–9.

112. Vray M, Joubert J-M, Eschwège E, Liard F, Fagnani F, Montestruc F, et al. Results from the observational study EPIGRAM: management of excess weight in general practice and follow-up of patients treated with orlistat. Therapie. 2005;60(1):17–24.

113. Hollander PA, Elbein SC, Hirsch IB, Kelley D, McGill J, Taylor T, et al. Role of orlistat in the treatment of obese patients with Type 2 diabetes: a 1-year randomized double-blind study. Diabetes Care. 1998;21(8):1288–94.

114. Davies MJ, Bergenstal R, Bode B, Kushner RF, Lewin A, Skjoth TV, et al. Efficacy of liraglutide for weight loss among patients with Type 2 diabetes: the SCALE diabetes randomized clinical trial. JAMA. 2015;314(7):687–99.

115. Hermansen K, Mortensen LS. Bodyweight changes associated with antihyperglycemic agents in Type 2 diabetes mellitus. Drug Saf. 2007;30(12):1127–42.

116. Van Gaal L, A S. Weight management in Type 2 diabetes: current and emerging approaches to treatment. Diabetes Care. 2015;38(6):1161–72.

117. American Society for Metabolic and Bariatric Surgery. Story of obesity surgery. 2004. [cited 2017 Mar 27]. https://asmbs.org/resources/story-of-obesity-surgery.

118. Garb J, Welch G, Zagarins S, Kuhn J, Romanelli J. Bariatric surgery for the treatment of morbid obesity: a meta-analysis of weight loss outcomes for laparoscopic adjustable gastric banding and laparoscopic gastric bypass. Obes Surg. 2009;19(10):1447–55.

119. Hutter MM, Schirmer BD, Jones DB, Ko CY, Cohen ME, Merkow RP, et al. First report from the American College of Surgeons Bariatric Surgery Center Network: laparoscopic sleeve gastrectomy has morbidity and effectiveness positioned between the band and the bypass. Ann Surg. 2011;254(3):410–22.

120. Angrisani L, Santonicola A, Iovino P, Vitiello A, Zundel N, Buchwald H, et al. Bariatric surgery and endoluminal procedures: IFSO worldwide survey 2014. Obes Surg. 2017;27(9):2279–89.

121. Buchwald H, Williams SE. Bariatric surgery worldwide 2003. Obes Surg. 2004;14(9):1157–64.

122. Flint RS, Coulter G, Roberts R. The pattern of adjustments after laparoscopic adjustable gastric band. Obes Surg. 2015;25(11):2061–5.

123. Buchwald H, Avidor Y, Braunwald E, Jensen MD, Proies W, Fahrbach KSK. Bariatric surgery: a systematic review and meta-analysis. JAMA. 2004;292(14):1724–7.

124. Karamanakos SN, Vagenas K, Kalfarentzos F, Alexandrides TK. Weight loss, appetite suppression, and changes in fasting and postprandial ghrelin and peptide-YY levels after roux-en-Y gastric bypass and sleeve gastrectomy. Ann Surg. 2008;247(3):401–7.

125. MacDonald KG, Long SD, Swanson MS, Brown BM, Morris P, Dohm GL, et al. The gastric bypass operation reduces the progression and mortality of non-insulin-dependent diabetes mellitus. J Gastrointest Surg. 1996;1(3):213–20.

126. Flum DR, Dellinger EP. Impact of gastric bypass operation on survival: a population-based analysis. J Am Coll Surg. 2004;199(4):543–51.

127. Christou NV, Sampalis JS, Liberman M, Look D, Auger S, McLean APH, et al. Surgery decreases long-term mortality, morbidity, and health care use in morbidly obese patients. Ann Surg. 2004;240(3):416–24.

128. DeMaria EJ, Sugerman HJ, Meador JG, Doty JM, Kellum JM, Wolfe L, et al. High failure rate after laparoscopic adjustable silicone gastric banding for treatment of morbid obesity. Ann Surg. 2001;233(6):809–18.

Further Reading

Astrup A, Finer N. Redefining Type 2 diabetes: "Diabesity" or "Obesity Dependent Diabetes Mellitus"? Obes Rev. 2000;1(2):57–9. Explores the relationship between obesity and T2D.

Butland B, Jebb S, Kopelman P, McPherson K, Thomas S, Mardell J, et al. Foresight tackling obesities: future choices—project report. Gov Off Sci.. 2007;1–161. Section 5 includes an in-depth discussion of the development and treatment of obesity according to the spaghetti map.

Sharma AM, Kushner RF. A proposed clinical staging system for obesity. Int J Obes. 2009;33(3):289–95. Seminal text on the Edmonton Obesity Staging System (EOSS) to evaluate the morbidity and mortality associated with excess weight.

Wharton S, Serodio KJ. Next generation of weight management medications: implications for diabetes and CVD risk. Curr Cardiol Rep. 2015;17(5):35. Discusses the mechanism of action for weight management medications, and their use in the context of diabetes.

Wharton S, Sharma A, Lau D, Canadian Diabetes Association 2013. Clinical practice guidelines for the prevention and management of diabetes in Canada: weight management in diabetes. Can J Diabetes. 2013;37(suppl 1):S61–8. Provides a more in-depth discussion of weight management options for patients with diabetes, including graphical representations of common bariatric procedures.

Metabolic and Bariatric Surgery in Diabetes Management

42

Luis Zurita Macías Valadez, María E. Frigolet,
Raúl Marín Dominguez, Radu Pescarus, Carlos Zerrweck,
Vanessa Boudreau, Aristithes Doumouras, Tyler Cookson,
and Mehran Anvari

Objectives

1. To describe the types and principles of the distinct bariatric surgical techniques
2. To define the clinical outcomes of most performed bariatric procedures
3. To illustrate the molecular and other mechanisms that explain metabolic outcomes of bariatric surgery
4. To explain the evolving bariatric techniques

Introduction

Bariatric surgery is the conjunct of surgical techniques to induce weight loss and metabolic health in morbidly obese patients. The recommendations for bariatric surgery are BMI ≥ 40 kg/m² or BMI 35–39.9 kg/m² with at least one comorbidity associated to obesity or clinical condition with impaired quality of life [1] (Table 42.1).

Bariatric surgery is currently the most effective treatment for severe obesity. Its effects are defined according to the amount of weight loss (surgery success has been defined as

≥50% excess weight loss [2]), mortality, quality of life, and social function, which are all positively modified as observed in several studies [3].

Bariatric surgery first evolved from a bowel resection [4], and the first Roux-en-Y gastric bypass (RYGB) [5] was intended for the treatment of obesity [4, 5]. Since then, numerous techniques have been introduced, and technology has migrated the open-surgery approach to the endoscopic, laparoscopic, and robotic approaches. Such minimally invasive methodologies and the enhanced recovery aim after bariatric surgery have significantly reduced risks and complications driven by the surgery.

Throughout time, metabolic improvements after bariatric surgery were responsible for shifting bariatric surgery to metabolic surgery, a concept first proposed by Buchwald and Varco in 1978 [6, 7]. For instance, type 2 diabetes (T2D) and other various metabolic abnormalities were resolved or remitted shortly after surgery. Metabolic surgery has been proved by randomized controlled trials to be safe and a more effective treatment for obesity and T2D compared with conventional medical multidisciplinary approach (lifestyle changes or pharmacotherapy) [8–10].

In fact, metabolic surgery could be considered in obesity class 1 (BMI 30–34.9 kg/m²) and diabetic subjects when hyperglycemia is inadequately controlled despite medical treatment [11]. Thus, since 2016, the American Diabetes Association (ADA) includes metabolic/bariatric surgery in their Standards of Care for Diabetes algorithm [12].

Different recommendations in this regard are still valid, and consensus should be gained in years to come. Finally, bariatric surgery and its metabolic effects represent, to date, the most effectual tool for obesity treatment. Importantly, the investigation of the mechanisms associated with massive weight loss and metabolic improvements will enlighten the medical community toward the understanding of processes involved in the development of obesity and related diseases.

L. Z. M. Valadez (✉) · R. M. Dominguez
Clínica de Sobrepeso y Obesidad (CISO), Mexico City, Mexico

M. E. Frigolet
Laboratorio de Enfermedades Metabólicas: Obesidad y Diabetes, Hospital Infantil de México Federico Gómez, Mexico City, Mexico

R. Pescarus
Department de Chirurgie bariatrique, CIUSSS Du-Nord-De-Lile-De-Montreal, Universite de Montreal, Montreal, QC, Canada

C. Zerrweck
Clínica Integral de Cirugía para la Obesidad y Enfermedades Metabólicas, Hospital General Tláhuac, Mexico City, Mexico

V. Boudreau · A. Doumouras · T. Cookson · M. Anvari
McMaster University, Hamilton, ON, Canada
e-mail: boudreav@mcmaster.ca; doumoua@mcmaster.ca; tcookson@stjoes.ca; anvari@mcmaster.ca

© The Author(s), under exclusive license to Springer Nature Switzerland AG 2023
J. Rodriguez-Saldana (ed.), *The Diabetes Textbook*, https://doi.org/10.1007/978-3-031-25519-9_42

Table 42.1 Obesity-related comorbidities to indicate bariatric surgery in patients with a BMI of 35–39.9 kg/m²

T2D	Obesity-hypoventilation syndrome
High risk of T2D-insulin resistance, prediabetes, and/or metabolic syndrome	Pickwickian syndrome
Nonalcoholic fatty liver disease (NALFD)	Idiopathic intracranial hypertension
Nonalcoholic steatohepatitis (NASH)	Gastroesophageal reflux disease (GERD)
Obstructive sleep apnea (OSA)	Severe venous stasis disease
Osteoarthritis (knee/hip)	Impaired motility due to obesity
Urinary stress incontinence	Considerably impaired quality of life

Types of Bariatric Surgery

Traditionally, bariatric procedures have been characterized as restrictive [laparoscopic adjustable gastric banding (LAGB), sleeve gastrectomy (SG)]; malabsorptive [biliopancreatic diversion with duodenal switch (BPD-DS), single anastomosis duodeno-ileal bypass with sleeve gastrectomy (SADI-S)]; and mixed procedures [Roux-en-Y gastric bypass (RYGB)] [1]. However, now we know that not only energy restriction and nutrient absorption explain profound weight loss, but other mechanisms are involved. Here, we describe the most common techniques and their mechanisms of action as well as their influence on improved metabolism.

Laparoscopic Adjustable Gastric Band (LAGB)

In this procedure, a silicone band is placed around the gastric cardias, creating a small gastric pouch (approximately 30 mL) and restricting food intake. The band is connected to a port that is fixed at the abdominal wall [13]. Through this port, sterile saline is injected to adjust the inner diameter of the band. The reduction of this diameter decreases the gastric pouch emptying and consequent food intake. The adjustment of the band can be changed over time depending on the evolution of the patient (Fig. 42.1a).

Sleeve Gastrectomy (SG)

SG was initially performed as the first step of the laparoscopic biliopancreatic diversion to reduce the high morbidity in super-obese and/or high-risk patients [14]. Because of adequate weight loss in this group of patients, SG was accepted in 2012 by the American Society for Metabolic and Bariatric Surgery (ASMBS) as an independent bariatric procedure [15]. SG is currently the most common procedure performed in the United States [16] and worldwide [17, 18]. The latter is because while it offers adequate success rates, it is also a less technically challenging procedure, representing lower morbidity and mortality compared with the RYGB [19].

The SG technique consists of the dissection of the greater curvature of the stomach. This is performed from 2 to 6 cm proximal to the pylorus toward the angle of His. Then, an orogastric bougie (32–36 Fr) is placed and used as a guide for vertical gastric transection. Approximately 80% of the body and gastric fundus is resected and removed, leaving a tubular pouch or sleeve-shaped stomach [19, 20] (Fig. 42.1b).

Roux-en-Y Gastric Bypass (RYGB)

Currently, RYGB is considered the "gold-standard" weight loss surgery and was, until recent years, the most frequently performed bariatric surgery [17]. The procedure has several components: gastric remnant, gastric pouch, gastrojejunal and jejunojejunal anastomosis, alimentary limb, biliopancreatic limb, and common limb. A small gastric pouch (30–50 mL) is constructed by dividing the gastric cardias from the rest of the stomach. Then, the jejunum is divided 40–150 cm distally to the ligament of Treitz, creating two limbs. The proximal limb is called biliopancreatic limb (BPL) (from the excluded stomach to the proximal division of the jejunum) and distal limb, which will be connected to the gastric pouch (gastrojejunal anastomosis). The biliopancreatic limb is anastomosed to the jejunum (from 75 to 150 cm distally to the gastrojejunal anastomosis). This anastomosis will divide the distal limb into alimentary limb (from GJA to JJA) and common limb. The distal intestine is called common limb (from JJA to terminal ileum) [21] (Fig. 42.1c).

Biliopancreatic Diversion with Duodenal Switch (BPD-DS)

BPD-DS is the most effective surgical treatment for severe obesity and T2D [8, 22]. Nevertheless, because it is a technically challenging surgery with the highest postoperative complication rate, this is the most infrequent procedure [23]. The technique consists of two stages, which may be performed in one or two surgeries depending on the presence of super-obesity and, thus, the patients' risk. During the first stage, an SG is performed. In the second stage, the duodenum is transected, and its proximal part is anastomosed at 250 cm proximal to the ileocecal valve (alimentary limb). The excluded limb (biliopancreatic limb) is connected, creating an ileal-ileal anasto-

Fig. 42.1 (**a**) Laparoscopic adjustable gastric band (LAGB). (**b**) Sleeve gastrectomy (SG). (**c**) Roux-en-Y gastric bypass (RYGB). (**d**) Biliopancreatic diversion with duodenal switch (BPD-DS). *GJA* gastrojejunal anastomosis, *JJA* jejunojejunal anastomosis, *AL* alimentary limb, *BPL* biliopancreatic limb, *CL* common limb, *DIA* duodeno-ileal anastomosis, *IIA* ileoileal anastomosis

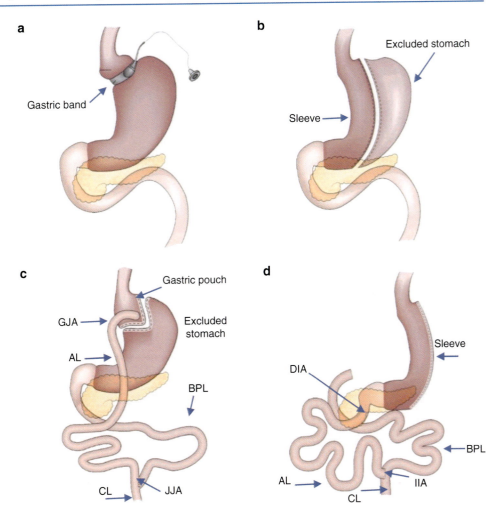

mosis, 100 cm proximal to the ileocecal valve, generating a common limb in a *Roux-en-Y* configuration. The main difference between a BPD-DS and an RYGB is the length of the small intestine bypassed, which, in the case of BPD-DS, is substantially greater than RYGB, resulting in increased malabsorption of nutrients (Fig. 42.1d).

One Anastomosis Gastric Bypass (OAGB)

OAGB, initially named mini-gastric bypass, was introduced in 2001 by Rutledge et al. as a simple and effective treatment for morbid obesity [24]. In 2005, Carbajo et al. proposed a modification of this technique and changed the name to one anastomosis gastric bypass [25]. There is currently an increasing number of OAGB performed worldwide [26–29]. OAGB is not yet accepted as a treatment for morbid obesity in the United States due to a lack of prospective and long-term follow-up studies [29].

The OAGB technique begins with the construction of a long sleeve-like gastric pouch using a 36 Fr bougie as a guide. Then, this gastric pouch is anastomosed to the jeju-

num (from 200 to 300 cm distally to the ligament of Treitz) in a Billroth II-like style [30, 31].

Single Anastomosis Duodeno-ileal Bypass with Sleeve Gastrectomy (SADI-S)

SADI-S is a relatively new surgical technique, introduced in 2007 by Sanchez Pernaute et al., described as a modification of BPD-DS in an effort to simplify the technique and reduce the complications associated to a long anesthetic procedure [32]. In 2020, the ASMBS accepted the SADI-S technique as an appropriate metabolic bariatric surgery [24].

The SADI-S technique comprises two stages. First, a tubular gastric pouch is created, wider than an SG, using a 54 Fr bougie. Second, the duodenum is sectioned, and its distal part is anastomosed with the ileum (200–300 cm proximal to the ileocecal valve). This Billroth II-like configuration in comparison to the *Roux-en-Y* decreases by half the number of anastomosis and has no mesentery opening, reducing operative time and the risk of intestinal obstruction [32].

Mechanisms of Action of Bariatric Surgery

Despite the effectiveness of bariatric surgery for the treatment of morbid obesity and associated metabolic diseases [9, 33, 34], its underlying mechanisms of action remain unclear. Several mechanisms have been related to bariatric/metabolic surgery, from food intake restriction and malabsorption, hormone release, and gut microbiota composition modifications, all of which influence metabolism.

Gastric Volume Restriction

Over the years different gastric restriction techniques have been performed, varying from 15 to 200 mL gastric capacity; nevertheless, no correlation has been found between stomach volume and weight loss [35]. Other mechanisms like gastric emptying speed, increase of intragastric pressure, as well as changes in gastrointestinal hormones may be involved in weight loss in the gastric restrictive bariatric procedures.

Malabsorption

The malabsorption of nutrients is achieved after bypassing distinct lengths of the small intestine. In 2010, Odstrcil et al. reported that malabsorption accounted for approximately 6% and 11% of the total reduction in combustible energy absorption at 5 and 14 months after RYGB, secondary to fat malabsorption with little or no malabsorption of proteins and carbohydrates [36].

Enteroendocrine Modifications

Since several hormones that control appetite and satiety processes are derived from the gastrointestinal tract, and bariatric surgery modifies the size and capacity of the stomach and/or the gut, then metabolic changes driven by the surgery have been found associated with altered pancreatic and gut peptide profiles [37]. Here, we will review the peptides that have been investigated and related to the metabolic outcomes of bariatric surgery.

Ghrelin

Ghrelin is secreted by the gastric and duodenal enteroendocrine cells and is not fully activated until acetylated. Once acetylated due to the action of ghrelin-O-acyltransferase (GOAT), it exerts an orexigenic action at the central nervous system (CNS), increasing food intake. In fasting conditions, ghrelin is acetylated, which is able to activate the growth hormone secretagogue receptor (GHSR) found in the hypothalamus and pituitary glands [38]. During obesity, the acetylated levels of ghrelin are apparently higher compared to those levels of ghrelin in lean subjects [39].

After bariatric surgery, mixed results regarding the circulating levels of ghrelin have been found, depending on the surgical technique. While gastric banding has been associated with increased ghrelin concentrations [40], RYGB and SG have been related to decreased levels of the hormone [41–43]. This could be attributed to the fact that RYGB excludes the gastric fundus, reducing the contact between ghrelin-producing cells and ingested food. However, further research is needed to elucidate the involvement of ghrelin in the short- and long-term effects of bariatric and metabolic surgery.

Incretins

Interestingly, weight loss or regain following combined restrictive-malabsorptive bariatric surgery is not predictive of diabetes remission, and glycemic control has been observed to improve soon after surgery, before clinically significant weight loss [44–47]. Due to the timing of these observations following surgery, other mechanisms related to the anatomical reconstruction of the GI tract are likely present to account for this. One explanation for such rapid responses relies on the variable concentrations of incretins after surgery.

Incretins are intestinal peptides known for stimulating insulin production after food intake. The main incretins are GIP (glucose-dependent insulinotropic polypeptide) and GLP-1 (glucagon-like peptide-1), which are specifically secreted from K cells in the small intestine and L cells in the ileum and colon, respectively [48]. Some clinical reports have described reduced fasting and postprandial concentrations of GIP after bariatric surgery [49, 50]. However, other groups have not found the same, and it is possible that these controversies rely on the type of procedure and diabetes diagnosis before surgery [51–53].

On the other hand, GLP-1 has shown, more consistently, that its concentrations are modified shortly after bariatric surgery and that this peptide represents a possible and partial explanation for some metabolic consequences of the surgery. Although using a small cohort, a prospective study found that total GLP-1 levels and the incretin effect were dramatically increased within 1 month of RYGB surgery and prior to clinically significant weight loss [52].

Indeed, analogs of GLP-1 (i.e., liraglutide, semaglutide) have been used for the treatment of both obesity and diabetes, establishing weight loss reductions of 5–10% and improved glucose tolerance in patients with T2D [54]. Acute and marked increases of circulating GLP-1 after LAGB, RYGB, and SG have been reported by several [55–57], and such increases are not achieved by patients that lose similar amounts of weight due to energy restriction [52]. Furthermore, it has also been suggested that higher serum concentrations of GLP-1 are associated with better weight loss results 1 year after the surgery [42].

Mechanisms that possibly explain rises in GLP-1 after surgery highlight the "hindgut hypothesis" versus the "foregut hypothesis" [58, 59]. The former states that improved glucose homeostasis is caused by the delivery of nutrients to the distal part of the small intestine to enhance the secretion of factors involved in glucose metabolism, and the latter adjudicates the lower glucose concentrations to the exclusion of the duodenum and jejunum from their interaction with nutrients. The main candidate molecule supporting the hindgut hypothesis is GLP-1, which exerts its effects via several pathways. First, the peptide decreases appetite and gastrointestinal motility in humans, reducing food consumption [60]. Also, the insulinotropic properties of GLP-1 are associated with increased insulin gene transcription and biosynthesis, as well as increased *glucokinase* and *Glut2* gene expression [61, 62]. Finally, GLP-1 has been associated with increased beta cell proliferation and decreased apoptosis [63].

Although the effects of GLP-1 account for some of the observed consequences of bariatric surgery, additional mechanisms are involved. For instance, humans using the specific GLP-1 receptor antagonist exendin 9-39 and animal models that lack GLP-1 receptor expression and, thus, have GLP-1 ablated response show similar weight loss after RYGB and SG [64], evidencing the influence of other factors in the process.

Other gut hormones that have been found implicated in the metabolic changes after bariatric surgery are cholecystokinin (CCK), pancreatic peptide YY (PYY), pancreatic polypeptide (PP), and secretin, among others. CCK is a hunger suppressant and a stimulator of digestion, which apparently increases after SG more than after RYGB [65, 66]. PYY delays gastric emptying, alters colon motility, and regulates appetite centrally [67–69]. Seemingly, PYY increases postprandially after bariatric surgery independent of the type of procedure [55]. Despite the extensive research and recent findings, further research is needed to better understand the role of these gut hormones in bariatric surgery.

Adipokines

Several adipokines (molecules that are released from adipose tissue) have been explored regarding their concentrations and influence over metabolic surgery. The most well-known adipokines are leptin and adiponectin. Leptin represents the communicator between adipose tissue and the CNS to suppress food intake during energy sufficiency [70]. During obesity conditions, resistance to the action of leptin concurs with hyperleptinemia. Adiponectin acts on peripheral tissues, exerts anti-inflammatory and insulin-sensitizing actions, and is decreased in serum of obese subjects [71]. In fact, the secretion of this adipokine is considered to be a hallmark of healthy adipocyte function [72]. After bariatric surgery, leptin decreases and adiponectin increases, which suggests gain of adequate function of the adipose tissue [73–77]. Interestingly, some groups found that adiponectin production was significantly increased 2 weeks after the surgery when weight loss has not occurred yet, meaning that adipokine promotion is independent of massive weight loss [78].

Along with adipokine secretion modifications, adipocyte size and adipose tissue structure have also been reported different after surgery [79]. The surgery-derived modifications in adipose tissue could be contributing to decreased chronic inflammation, which is thought to be one of the most important mediators of metabolic improvement after surgery. However, the global contribution of adipose tissue and derived hormones on metabolic improvements mediated by bariatric surgery needs to be revealed yet.

Gut Microbiota

The human intestinal tract contains an extraordinary conjunct of microorganisms, namely, the bacterial component of the human gut microbiota. The number of genes in the human gut microbiota exceeds the human genome by 150-fold [80], and it confers metabolic advantages such as vitamin and fatty acid generation, carbohydrate fermentation, and bile acid metabolism.

It has been shown that in addition to weight loss and glucose tolerance, RYGB modifies gut microbiota composition and diversity within 3 months and later, during a long-term period [81]. Compared with controls, and at the phylum level, RYGB increased the abundance of Proteobacteria and Bacteroidetes and decreased Firmicutes [82–84].

Although SG has also been related to microbiota modifications, RYGB has more robust effect on the composition of gut microbiota. One possible reason for this difference is that compared with RYGB, SG induces relatively mild physical manipulations of the intestinal tract. Additionally, with exposure of the luminal contents of the intestine to an aerobic environment during prolonged surgery or increased concentrations of swallowed air reaching the gut with RYGB compared to SG, the survival of obligate anaerobic bacteria is threatened, and it may contribute to the expansion of aerobic bacteria populations in the gut microbiota following bariatric/metabolic surgery.

Bile Acids

Bile acids play a role in glucose and lipid homeostasis. The bile acid receptor FXR not only regulates bile acid synthesis but also stimulates glycogen synthesis, decreases gluconeogenesis, and increases glycolysis [85]. Bile acid receptor TGR5 activation has been associated with gallbladder filling, modulation of energy expenditure, GLP-1 release from L cells, reduction of inflammatory mediators, and suppression of hepatic glycogenolysis [72, 86–89]. Multiple studies have reported increased fasting and postprandial bile acid concentrations following RYGB [90–92]. The mechanisms involved have not been identified. Several physiologic processes altered by metabolic surgery are associated to elevated concentrations of bile acids. Whether these processes are modified by the change in bile acid concentrations remains unclear.

Histological and Anatomical Changes

Alterations in pancreatic and hepatic tissue and blood flow can be seen after bariatric surgery. Immonen et al. reported that diabetic patients subjected to bariatric surgery experienced a normalization of hepatic fat content and a decrease in liver volume, as well as an increase in insulin-mediated hepatic glucose uptake, which was negatively correlated with liver fat content without any changes in BMI, suggesting a direct impact in hepatic glucose regulation [93]. Honka et al. reported that patients that underwent bariatric surgery had a decreased pancreatic lipid content and pancreatic blood flow. Glucose tolerance was found to be inversely correlated to pancreatic fat and decreased pancreatic blood flow associated to improvement of β-cell function [94].

In summary, the improvements in systemic metabolism and mainly in T2D after bariatric surgery are due to histological changes, modifications in several hormonal factors, gut microbiota composition, and their interaction. This is still under investigation, and so far, we can point out to some gut and adipose molecules as well as the microbiome, which have been associated with the amelioration of metabolic syndrome that accompanies bariatric surgery. Finally, the complex interaction between bariatric surgery, weight loss, and metabolic improvements reveals that the restriction or malabsorption components are no longer applicable to explain by themselves the effects of the surgery.

Outcomes After Metabolic Surgery

Bariatric surgery's main indication is for weight loss in individuals with obesity. Through manipulating the GI tract, bariatric surgery causes a plethora of effects that achieve substantial weight loss in a high proportion of patients. Importantly, this GI tract manipulation has effects beyond weight loss and has effects on several important metabolic disorders. In this way, bariatric surgery is a potential option for treatment for individuals with diabetes of all weights. Accordingly, this section will discuss the weight and diabetes outcomes following metabolic surgery and the implications of bariatric and metabolic surgery on other obesity-related comorbidities using an evidence-based approach.

Weight Loss After Metabolic Surgery

The weight loss component of metabolic surgery remains its most widespread indication and is the clear gold standard in the treatment of severe obesity. Patients that undergo metabolic surgery show both statistically and clinically significant weight loss soon after surgery that is maintained for several years [9, 33, 44, 95–99]. Specifically, total body weight loss at 1 year after metabolic surgery is about 25–30%, compared to 5–10% weight loss with medical therapy, and is accompanied by large reductions in body mass index (BMI) and waist circumference [33, 44, 96, 98]. At 1 year, reductions in BMI range from 19.6% to 27.6% for surgical patients compared to 1.81% to 10.14% for medical therapy patients; at 2–3 years, reductions range from 19.1% to 33.8% for surgical patients and 4.4% to 4.7% for medical therapy patients; and at 5 years, reductions range from 18.6% to 21.9% for surgical patients compared to 6.59% for medical therapy patients [9, 33, 44, 95–99]. Similarly, reductions in waist circumference at 1 year range from 17.5% to 22.8% for surgical patients and 3.6% to 7.2% for medical therapy patients; at 2–3 years, reductions range from 12.8% to 20.7% for surgical patients compared to 1.5% to 7.7% for medical therapy patients; and at 5 years, reductions range from 12.2% to 14.7% for surgical patients and 1.3% for medical therapy alone [9, 33, 44, 95, 96, 98, 99]. One of the most eminent trials in this area is the STAMPEDE trial, which randomized 150 obese patients with uncontrolled T2D to receive either intensive medical therapy alone or intensive medical therapy plus RYGB or SG [33]. A 5-year follow-up to the STAMPEDE trial showed a total body weight loss of 18% for SG and 22% for RYGB compared to 6% for medical therapy alone [9]. Moreover, metabolic surgery is much more successful than medical therapy at initiating and maintaining weight loss in morbidly obese patients with long-standing T2D.

Diabetes Remission and Main Diabetes-Associated Abnormalities Following Metabolic Surgery

Although bariatric surgical techniques have been established for the treatment of obesity by promoting weight loss and reshaping intestinal hormone signals responsible for postprandial satiety, nutrient absorption, and insulin sensitivity, the use of these techniques for the primary purpose of treating obesity-related comorbidities is still not as widely accepted compared to use primarily for weight loss. There is, however, evidence to support the use of bariatric surgical techniques in patients with T2D. With data showing that diabetic patients with obesity had increased remission rates following bariatric surgery, investigations focused on bariatric surgery to specifically manage T2D. Compiling this data in 2009, a large meta-analysis ultimately consisting of 3188 T2D patients showed that diabetes completely resolved in 78.1% of patients and either improved or resolved in 86.6% of patients following bariatric surgery [100].

Evidence from Randomized Controlled Trials

Currently, it is difficult to compare remission rates between studies as they often use different definitions of diabetes remission and different methodologies, such as variable follow-up periods. These studies are further limited by relatively small sample sizes. While studies struggle to agree on the definitions of diabetes remission, most studies would agree that a percent glycated hemoglobin (%HbA1c) level less than 6.5% without the use of antidiabetic medication represents a T2D patient in remission. Several randomized controlled trials (RCTs) have described statistically and clinically significant differences in diabetes markers, including HbA1c, fasting plasma glucose, and homeostatic model assessment for insulin resistance (HOMA-IR) scores, between patients that receive metabolic surgery and those that receive intensive medical therapy [8, 33, 96, 101]. These studies primarily examined RYGB, biliopancreatic diversion with duodenal switch (BPD-DS), or SG in which their 1-year diabetes remission rates range from 35% to 44% for surgical patients compared to 0% to 9% for medical therapy patients, their 2-year remission rates range from 21.6% to 89.5% for surgical patients compared to 0% to 5.9% for medical therapy patients, and their 5-year remission values were also extremely variable with rates ranging from 18.8% to 50% for surgical patients compared to 0% for medical therapy patients [8, 9, 33, 95, 96, 101]. However, in spite of the large variation in remission rates, metabolic surgery consistently outperforms intensive medical therapy alone for the management of T2D in these RCTs.

Renal Changes and Micro-/Macrovascular Complications

When looking at diabetes-related complications, the STAMPEDE trial showed that there were either minimal or no changes to the measures of renal function, such as glomerular filtration rate (GFR), albuminuria, or creatinine-to-albumin ratio [95]. Conversely, Du et al. found that in patients with class 2 or 3 obesity, hyperuricemia was either resolved or improved in about 73% of patients following metabolic surgery, compared to 4% of class 1 obese patients [102]. These results would suggest that higher BMI subjects could benefit more from metabolic surgery in terms of positive renal changes; however, there is little evidence to validate this finding.

Microvascular complications, including retinopathy, nephropathy, and neuropathy, and macrovascular complications, including coronary artery disease, cerebrovascular disease, and peripheral artery disease, can occur in T2D patients with long-standing disease. Prospectively collected data on the attenuation or reduced risk of micro- and macrovascular complications is limited. However, among the 603 patients with T2D in the Swedish Obese Subjects (SOS) study, there were a 56% and a 32% decreased incidence of micro- and macrovascular complications, respectively, following bariatric surgery compared to the medical therapy group at a 15-year follow up [103]. Similarly, the incidence of microvascular complications was 59% lower in bariatric surgery patients compared to nonsurgical controls in a retrospective matched cohort study including 4024 surgical patients with a median follow-up of 4.3 years [104]. Further, a 2021 meta-analysis found that bariatric surgery reduced macrovascular complications by 50% with a mean follow-up time of 10.96 years [105].

Outcomes of Other Comorbidities Associated with Obesity and Metabolic Syndrome Following Metabolic Surgery

In addition to diabetes, there is evidence that metabolic surgery improves other obesity-related comorbidities, such as hypertension, dyslipidemia, and cardiovascular diseases. The research into the effect of bariatric surgery on these other comorbidities is often secondary to diabetes outcomes. As such, one cannot state conclusively whether metabolic surgery improves these conditions and whether the amelioration of these conditions is strictly due to weight loss or is also dependent on weight loss-independent mechanisms. We can, however, comment on the current state of knowledge regarding the impact of metabolic surgery on various test parameters, including blood pressure and serum lipid levels, to preliminarily assess the potential of metabolic surgery in attenuating obesity-related comorbidities.

Hypertension

Hypertension is one of the components that comprise "metabolic syndrome." As a major risk factor for cardiovascular and renal diseases, blood pressure management is imperative to prevent the development of other complications. Prevention or management of high blood pressure can be achieved by also managing weight. Metabolic surgery generally decreased systolic blood pressure (SBP) with reductions ranging from 12 mmHg to 34 mmHg [44, 96, 97, 99], while diastolic blood pressure (DBP) had reductions ranging from 5 mmHg to 10 mmHg [44, 96, 99]. A retrospective study found that metabolic surgery resolved or improved hypertension in 60% of class 2 or 3 obese subjects and 20% of class 1 obese subjects at 3 years postoperatively [102]; however, due to the small sample size, these results were not significant. In the STAMPEDE trial, neither SBP nor DBP was reduced by metabolic surgery at 1, 3, or 5 years, but there was a significant decrease in the number of antihypertensive medications required to manage the disease [9, 33, 95]. Similar results were found in a small RCT with no changes in SBP or DBP at 1 year following metabolic surgery [98], and another RCT showed reductions in antihypertensive medications following RYGB [97]. Any changes in blood pressure following metabolic surgery are still controversial, yet it appears that those who receive metabolic surgery require less medical management of hypertension.

Obstructive Sleep Apnea

Obstructive sleep apnea (OSA) is an obesity-related disorder that increases the risk of hypertension development. Several studies have found that a large proportion of bariatric surgery patients show improvement in the number of sleep disturbances, sleep efficiency, and the severity of OSA [106–109] while others show no change in polysomnographic variables in the years after bariatric surgery [10]. A systematic review of OSA outcomes following bariatric surgery including 69 studies and 13,900 patients saw that BPD-DS, followed by SG, RYGB, and finally LAGB, had the most improvement in OSA postoperatively [107]. In fact, 99% of BPD-DS patients saw improvement in their OSA, compared to 85.7% for SG, 79.2% for RYGB, and 77.5% for LAGB [107]. Bariatric surgery has quite promising results in attenuating OSA symptoms. While unlikely to be the primary objective for performing bariatric surgery, improvement of OSA is a favorable secondary effect.

Dyslipidemia

Abnormal serum lipid levels are also a condition of metabolic syndrome. Typically, we see higher low-density lipoprotein (LDL) cholesterol and triglycerides (TG) and lower high-density lipoprotein (HDL) cholesterol in metabolic syndrome. In articles that categorically assessed dyslipidemia incidence before and after metabolic surgery, dyslipidemia was resolved in about 50% of patients at 1 year and 59% at 3 years [98, 102]. Within the first 1–5 years following metabolic surgery, there are consistent results of elevated HDL cholesterol to acceptable levels (≥45 mg/dL or 1.17 mmol/L) and decreased TGs to optimal levels (<150 mg/dL or 1.7 mmol/L), which is not observed in the medical therapy group [9, 33, 44, 96, 97, 110]. In regard to LDL cholesterol, the results are discrepant between studies. Several studies did not observe any changes in LDL cholesterol from baseline to their respective follow-up period in either the metabolic surgery recipients or those receiving medical therapy [9, 95, 96]. However, appropriate LDL reductions have also been observed following metabolic surgery in other studies [44, 97]. Particularly, one study showed that BPD-DS reduced LDL cholesterol and TGs to clinically optimal levels (<2.6 mmol/L or 100 mg/dL for LDL cholesterol), but this was not observed in the patients that received RYGB surgery. Reductions in LDL cholesterol following BPD-DS have also been reported in other studies [110, 111]. While some techniques, including RYGB, may normalize serum lipid levels

apart from LDL cholesterol, it is possible that BPD-DS can achieve optimal LDL cholesterol reductions. At the 1-, 3-, and 5-year follow-ups in the STAMPEDE trial, the use of lipid-lowering medications by metabolic surgery recipients decreased by 60%, 56%, and 43% from baseline, respectively, with no changes in lipid-lowering medications by the patients receiving medical therapy only [9, 33, 95].

Cardiovascular Disease

Cardiovascular disease (CVD) is the leading cause of death worldwide, and both obesity and T2D can greatly increase the risk for CVD development. A group from the United States sought to determine if metabolic surgery can protect obese T2D patients from CVD with their retrospective cohort study of over 2200 diabetic patients with obesity undergoing metabolic surgery compared to over 11,000 matched controls. Looking specifically at major adverse cardiovascular events (MACE) over an 8-year period, this group found that metabolic surgery recipients had a hazard ratio of 0.61 compared to controls [112]. This suggests that metabolic surgery patients with both obesity and diabetes were about 40% less likely to experience a MACE in the first 8 years after surgery. A 2021 propensity score matched study of 2638 patients assessing bariatric surgical patients and nonsurgical controls with severe obesity and cardiovascular disease showed similar success with a hazard ratio of 0.58 for surgical patients compared to the nonsurgical controls [113]. In subgroup analyses of patients with a history of heart failure or ischemic heart disease, bariatric surgery reduced the incidence of MACE by 56% and 40%, respectively [113]. In addition to this, in terms of individual cardiovascular events, metabolic surgery patients had a much lower incidence of heart failure, coronary artery disease, cerebrovascular disease, nephropathy, and atrial fibrillation [112]. Moreover, the use of antidiabetic, antihypertensive, and lipid-lowering medications was significantly reduced in metabolic surgery patients [112], further corroborating the observations of the STAMPEDE trial.

Special Topics

Apart from the conventional use for metabolic surgery in T2D patients with a BMI ≥ 35 kg/m², physicians have started to apply these surgical techniques to different populations, such as in T2D patients with a BMI < 35 kg/m² or in type 1 diabetic (T1D) patients. Moreover, current studies are aiming to identify which type of bariatric surgery is the most effective for diabetes remission and to determine the long-term outcomes following metabolic surgery. These special topics serve as the future of metabolic surgery research and application to target populations.

The Use of Metabolic Surgery in Type 2 Diabetes Patients with a BMI < 35 kg/m²

Bariatric/metabolic surgery is typically only performed in patients with a BMI ≥ 35 kg/m² and long-standing diabetes. While the use of metabolic surgery is still controversial in overweight and class 1 obese patients, the idea that metabolic surgeries may be used to manage uncontrolled T2D in these patients is becoming more popular. In metabolic surgery patients with a BMI < 35 kg/m², clinically significant reduction in BMI, weight, and waist circumference has been observed as early as 6 months after surgery [114]. This effect is seen following various metabolic surgery techniques, including RYGB [98, 102, 114–120], BPD [121], SG [114, 122], one anastomosis gastric bypass (OAGB), [122] and LAGB [98, 114, 123]. Additionally, a reduced BMI is often maintained for several years following metabolic surgery in class 1 obese patients [102, 117, 121, 122]. Most studies that compare metabolic surgery to other anti-obesity or antidiabetic standard-of-care treatments, such as GLP-1 analogs, intensive medical therapy, lifestyle interventions, and SGLT2 inhibitors, also show marked reductions in anthropometric variables with metabolic surgery compared to the pharmacological or lifestyle interventions [98, 114, 116, 123].

What should be noted, however, are the comparisons between class 1 obesity and class 2/3 obesity weight outcomes following metabolic surgery. The changes in weight loss are not absolute in obesity patients. Instead, all three classes of obesity tend to exhibit comparable BMIs for several years following surgery [102]. While remaining clinically significant, it appears that patients with a higher preoperative BMI achieve greater anthropometric effects postoperatively compared to overweight or class 1 obese metabolic surgery patients. Thus, to assess and compare the benefits of metabolic surgery between different classes of obesity, we must explore the outcomes of diabetes following surgery in this population.

A retrospective review found no difference in diabetes remission rates between class 1 and class 2/3 obese patients at 1- or 3-year follow-up [102]. However, while some may argue that metabolic surgery is more efficacious for the management of diabetes in patients with a higher preoperative BMI, it needs to be determined whether metabolic surgery is also reasonably more effective than standard medical and lifestyle interventions in patients with a BMI lower than 35 kg/m². From data in RCTs and prospective studies in this population, diabetes remission rates within 1 year of surgery range from 51 to 65% and somewhere around 26 and 84% between 18 months and 5 years after surgery [102, 114, 115, 118, 120–122]. In the few studies that compared remission rates after metabolic surgery to medical therapy, the diabetes remission rates in the medically treated groups were either nonexistent or significantly lower at 0–6% [114, 118, 120].

Notably, these studies are limited by small sample sizes and poor follow-up. Regardless, although there is debate on whether higher classes of obesity may or may not exhibit greater benefits from metabolic surgery than lower classes, these preliminary results show that the benefits that are observed in T2D patients with a BMI < 35 kg/m² remain superior to medical therapies. Instead of comparing between classes of obesity, a "cut-off point," which defines a certain weight category that no longer attains higher diabetes remission rates than medical therapies, should be determined.

Metabolic Surgery in Type 1 Diabetics

Obesity is common in T2D patients and increases the risk for the development of diabetes [124]. However, obesity is rarer in T1D patients, although a subset of T1D patients is overweight [125]. Moreover, intense insulin treatment may make patients more susceptible to weight gain [126, 127]. By examining the outcomes of bariatric surgery in obese patients with T1D, we can begin to assess the viability of metabolic surgery in this population. A systematic review and meta-analysis of outcomes following bariatric surgery in obese T1D patients show clinically significant weight loss [128]. In addition to this, although bariatric surgery reduced daily insulin requirements, insulin therapy was still required [128]. This can be explained since T1D patients have little to no β-islet cell activity to produce their own insulin. Bariatric surgery also decreased HbA1c levels, but only to 7.9 ± 1.1% [128]; these levels remain quite elevated and are not indicative of diabetes remission, in spite of the statistically significant improvement. Further investigation into the efficacy of metabolic surgery in T1D patients is warranted, but based on these preliminary results, the efficacy of surgery is unclear and may be considered draconian relative to the extent of diabetes remission.

The suggested mechanisms for improved glycemic control and reduced insulin requirements are similar to those in T2D metabolic surgery patients. Weight may ameliorate obesity-related insulin resistance via reduced lipotoxicity and inflammation [128]. Although studies in this area are small and limited, there is some evidence to suggest that insulin requirements following bariatric surgery are not directly correlated to weight loss, indicating that there are other mechanisms for improved glycemic control independent of weight loss [129]. Reduced insulin requirements may be simply due to decreased caloric intake and glycemic load. Further, increased incretin release due to the hindgut hypothesis may inhibit the actions of glucagon and even potentiate insulin activity in patients with residual β-islet cell function [130]. Regardless, mechanisms that reduce insulin sensitivity and potentiate the actions of insulin will allow for the mitigation of excessive exogenous insulin use. Kirwan et al.

report that bariatric surgery results in the remission or improvement of many obesity-related comorbidities, including hypertension and dyslipidemia [128]. A single, small retrospective study comparing BPD-DS and SG recipients found that T1D and T2D patients had similar remission rates of hypertension and dyslipidemia [131]. Therefore, although the use of metabolic surgery to induce remission of diabetes in T1D patients is contentious, there is currently no contraindication for the use of these techniques in obese patients with T1D or obesity-related comorbidities.

Diabetes Remission and Relapse Using Different Types of Metabolic Surgery

With such a wide array of different bariatric surgical techniques, it is difficult to parse out which may be the most effective in terms of diabetes remission based on the hundreds of studies with consistent or contradictory findings. The 2009 meta-analysis by Buchwald et al. showed that diabetes remission rates are maintained at a 2-year follow-up with BPD-DS at 95.1%, RYGB at 80.3%, then gastroplasty at 79.7%, and finally LAGB at 56.7% [100]. The relationships between different techniques are echoed in a 2020 network meta-analysis of RCTs evaluating diabetes remission following metabolic surgery in patients with follow-ups greater than 3 years with rank probabilities of remission at 91.3% for BPD-DS, 84.2% for OAGB, 58.4% for RYGB, 39.9% for SG, and 24.9% for LAGB [132]. Notably, the remission rates for RYGB and LAGB were substantially lower in the 2020 study compared to the study conducted in 2009.

Using RCTs, we can also evaluate the relapse rates of diabetes for the various techniques. BPD-DS had a 37% relapse rate between postoperative years 2 and 5 [8]. RYGB had moderate relapse rates with 25% relapse between years 1 and 2 [101], 53% relapse between years 2 and 5 [8], and 47.6% relapse between years 1 and 5 [9, 33]. On the other hand, SG had 60% diabetes relapse between postoperative years 1 and 2 [101] and about 46% relapse between years 1 and 5 [9, 33].

Even though LAGB is not performed as widely as it was a decade ago, this technique can be compared to the more modern surgeries. While diabetes remission does not typically correlate directly to weight loss following metabolic surgery as stated earlier in this chapter, RCTs using LAGB to attenuate diabetes have shown weight loss is the major force promoting diabetes remission [123, 132, 133], likely due to a lack of considerable anatomical reconstruction of the GI tract. This may also explain why surgeries like BPD-DS, RYGB, and SG typically perform better than LAGB.

Patients appear to exhibit the highest diabetes remission rates and the lowest relapse following BPD-DS compared to the other surgical techniques. In a 2005 review of 312 obese

T2D BPD-DS patients, over 99% of patients achieved diabetes remission at 1 year, and there was only a 2% relapse rate over 10 years [110]. These values are drastically higher than those reported in the RCTs and meta-analyses; regardless, BPD-DS is consistently the most effective in terms of both weight loss and diabetes remission rates; however, this technique is not used as frequently worldwide due to its inherent technical challenges and there is also a higher risk of complications including nutritional deficiencies when the proximal small intestine is bypassed [134]. While more research into this area is definitely needed, there is a strong potential for successful treatment of diabetes using bariatric surgical techniques.

Long-Term Outcomes of Metabolic Surgery

One of the strongest available long-term studies on T2D remission is the SOS study [103]. This prospective matched cohort study examined diabetes remission for non-adjustable gastric banding (NGB), vertical banded gastroplasty (VBG), and RYGB versus standard diabetes and obesity care over a 15-year period. T2D remission rates at 2 years after surgery were 16.4% for medical therapy patients and 72.3% for bariatric surgery patients. At 15 years, diabetes remission rates decreased to 6.5% for medical therapy patients and to 30.4% for bariatric surgery patients. There is a high relapse in diabetes remission from 2 to 5 years; however, remission rates were still much greater in the bariatric surgery group compared to the medical therapy group. In addition to this, the risk of both macro- and microvascular complications was significantly reduced in those that had bariatric surgery.

A recent retrospective study of insulin-treated T2D patients that received BPD-DS showed substantial diabetes remission rates 10 years after metabolic surgery with up to 68% of patients in complete remission [135]. Importantly, those with a shorter disease duration at the time of surgery were more likely to achieve complete diabetes remission compared to those with longer disease duration [135]. As metabolic surgery is seldom going to be a primary management strategy for diabetes, earlier diagnosis and treatment will be an important factor in order for patients to have the best chances of achieving remission with metabolic surgery.

Complications After Bariatric/Metabolic Surgery

Bariatric/metabolic surgery is considered extremely safe nowadays, even as safe as a laparoscopic cholecystectomy [136]. Morbidity and mortality rates have decreased dramatically since the introduction of the laparoscopic approach, as well as the evolution of technology, understanding of associated diseases, and perioperative management of patients [137]. In order to standardize the way in which complications in bariatric surgery should be reported, their classification by temporality and severity has been established [138]. Early complications are those that occur within the first 30 days, and after that, they are considered late complications. By severity, they are divided into minor and major, with the major generally being those that cause early reintervention, bleeding that requires blood transfusions, need for ICU, and hospital stay longer than 7 days. The most common complications appear during this period, being mainly bleeding (intra-abdominal or gastrointestinal), leak/fistula, and stenosis, which is observed in approximately 2–19% of cases (there is variability depending on the type of procedure [139, 140]). Deep vein thrombosis (DVT) and pulmonary embolism (PE) can also occur within this period but are less frequent. Mortality should not exceed 0.1–0.5% [136]. In terms of late complications, the RYGB has been associated with a greater cause of readmissions and a greater number of complications compared to SG [141]. The most observed pathologies during follow-up are cholelithiasis, marginal ulcers, internal hernias, reflux, and nutritional deficiencies. Some of the factors associated to higher morbidity are open procedures, extreme obesity, previous DVT/PE, sleep apnea, revisional surgery, and surgeries performed at low-volume hospitals [142].

Even though bariatric surgery, with the upcoming technologies, has proved to be a safer procedure, less invasive and novel patient-targeted approaches are being developed in order to decrease current rates of complications, morbidity, and mortality.

Evolving Technologies for Metabolic Treatment

The prevalence of obesity is continuously increasing worldwide with an accentuation during the current COVID-19 pandemic. Currently, bariatric surgery represents the best option for the treatment of obesity and its related metabolic comorbidities. Importantly, only a small fraction of the eligible population undergoes bariatric surgeries even in those countries with well-established bariatric surgery centers.

Recently, various endoscopic treatments have evolved with the goal of offering minimally invasive options for a greater number of patients suffering from obesity as well as diabetes [143]. Although not currently FDA approved, these interventions might represent viable options in the future somewhere in the continuum of care between bariatric surgery and pharmacotherapy and lifestyle interventions. These metabolic endoscopic interventions may offer a different therapeutic perspective than the well-established gastric space-occupying devices and endoscopic gastric suturing procedures.

Currently, there are three main types of endoscopic small bowel interventions that could have a significant impact in patients with metabolic syndrome: endoscopic anastomosis systems, duodenal mucosal resurfacing systems, and finally endoluminal bypass liner systems.

Endoscopic Magnetic Compression Anastomotic Devices

Endoscopic therapies trying to replicate the weight loss and metabolic results of the SADI-S procedure have been described. The Incisionless Magnetic Anastomosis System (IMAS-GI Windows, West Bridgewater, MA, United States) relies on a magnet that is introduced through the working channel of the endoscope and takes its final octagonal form when deployed into the lumen. A recent case series of eight patients with a BMI of 35–47 and T2D illustrated the feasibility of a combined laparo-endoscopic procedure [144]. The proximal magnet was inserted endoscopically and positioned 2 cm distal to the pylorus, while the distal magnet was inserted laparoscopically through a 5 mm enterotomy 300 cm proximal to the ileocecal valve. The magnets were expelled per rectum at a median of 29.5 days post procedure with no complications. All anastomoses were patent at 1 year. The baseline HbA1c was reduced below 7% in 75% of patients, and greater than 5% of total body weight loss was seen in 87.5% of patients at 12 months [144].

The Magnamosis device (Magnamosis Inc.) is a pair of rare earth magnets encased in a polycarbonate shell [145]. Following multiple successful animal studies, a first-in-human trial was published in 2017. This case series included five patients. The surgical procedures were performed through laparotomy in complex urology cases requiring the creation of an ileal conduit. One small bowel side-to-side anastomosis was created in each case with a central hole being performed surgically to obtain immediate patency. No complications such as anastomotic leaks, bleeding, or stenosis were noted during the 13-month median follow-up (range: 6–18 months). Although no metabolic interventions were attempted to date using this device, Magnamosis Inc. has recently been awarded an NIH grant to study the effect of a Magnetic Duodeno-Ileal Bypass (DIPASS) on T2D in a primate model [146].

Finally, a third device, EasyByPass (EasyNOTES) [147], uses neodymium rare earth magnets that are placed endoscopically to create a gastrojejunal anastomosis under fluoroscopy and with the help of a large external magnet [143]. A few weeks following the creation of the new anastomosis, a pyloric plug is inserted endoscopically to divert the gastric contents through the new gastrojejunostomy [147]. There is currently no published data on the use of this device in animal or human studies.

Duodenal Mucosal Resurfacing

The Revita duodenal mucosal resurfacing (DMR) procedure is a minimally invasive endoscopic procedure in which the mucosa distal to the ampulla of Vater is thermally ablated using a specially designed catheter (Fractyl Laboratories, Lexington, MA, United States) that is advanced over a guidewire under endoscopic guidance. Following a mucosal saline lift, a sequential ablation of the duodenal mucosa is performed for about 10 cm distal to the ampulla [148]. In a recent international multicenter study, the effect of DMR was studied in patients with T2D treated with at least one oral hypoglycemic medication and with a BMI ranging from 24 to 40 kg/m² [149]. The procedure was completed in 80% of patients. There was only one significant adverse event: fever with spontaneous resolution. Mean HbA1c was 10 mmol/mol (0.9%) lower at 1 year post DMR compared to baseline. There was some weight loss at 4 weeks post procedure with weight stabilization afterward. No correlation between the weight loss and glycemic control was noted.

Another DMR device, DiaGone (Digma Medical, Petah Tikva, Israel), uses a precisely controlled laser technology to target the duodenal submucosal neural plexi [150]. The results of a small multicenter feasibility study were published in an abstract in 2019 [151]. Nine patients with a BMI of 34.0 ± 4.6 kg/m² and T2D with insufficient glycemic control on metformin were enrolled. A significant decrease ($p < 0.01$) in fasting glucose (12.4 mmol/L baseline to 9.5 and 9.7) and HbA1c (7.83% mmol/mol baseline to 6.4% and 6.48%) was noted at 3 and 6 months following the procedure. No adverse events nor change in weight was noted during the 6-month follow-up [151].

Endoluminal Bypass Liners

Currently, there are two types of endoluminal "sleeve" systems that share the same mechanism of prevention of contact between the gastric contents and the proximal small bowel and possibly alterations in gut microbiota [143, 152] (Table 42.2).

Duodenal-Jejunal Bypass Liner

The first system is the duodenal-jejunal bypass liner EndoBarrier (DJBL – GI Dynamics, Lexington, MA, USA). EndoBarrier is a 60 cm fluoropolymer liner that is placed under endoscopic and fluoroscopic control. The proximal nitinol anchor is deployed in the duodenal bulb with the liner

Table 42.2 Current endoscopic metabolic interventions targeting the small intestine [143]

Endoscopic small bowel interventions	Clinical options
Endoscopic anastomotic devices	IMAS: Incisionless Magnetic Anastomosis System (GI Windows) Magnamosis (Magnamosis Inc.) EasyByPass incisionless anastomosis device (EasyNOTES)
Duodenal mucosal resurfacing systems	Revita (Fractyl Laboratories) DiaGone (Digma Medical)
Endoluminal bypass liner systems	Duodenal-jejunal bypass liner (DJBL – GI Dynamics) Gastro-duodenal bypass liner (ValenTx Endoluminal Bypass)

released distally into the small bowel [150]. It is removed endoscopically after 3–12 months. A meta-analysis published in 2018 that included 17 studies evaluating EndoBarrier has shown an overall 18.9% total body weight loss and a 1.3% reduction in HbA1c. The weight loss was shown to be still significant at the 12-month follow-up post device explantation [153].

Notwithstanding the excellent results published in the previous studies, a multicenter controlled trial in the United States had to be terminated early when 3.5% of patients developed hepatic abscesses [154]. Recently, the largest multicenter randomized controlled study of DJBL was published [155]. The study enrolled 170 patients with inadequately controlled T2D and obesity that were subsequently randomized to intensive medical care with or without DJBL. Interestingly, there was no significant difference in the percentage of patients achieving a HbA1c reduction of ≥20% at 12 months (primary outcome). There was, however, greater weight loss in the DJBL group (24% of patients achieved ≥15% weight loss in the DJBL group compared to only 4% in the intensive medical care group at 12 months). Better reduction in systolic blood pressure, cholesterol levels, and alanine transaminase was noted at 12 months. There were 19 early explantations of the DJBL, and these were caused by seven cases of migration of the device, abdominal pain in five patients, upper gastrointestinal bleeding in two patients, cholecystitis in two patients, and a single case of liver abscess, anticoagulation, or withdrawal of consent. The hepatic abscess resolved following explantation of the device and percutaneous drainage of the abscess. One explantation had to be performed laparoscopically as the endoscopic removal failed [155]. Although there was no improved glycemic control, the improvement in weight and other comorbidities together with the lower rate of hepatic abscess (1.3%) is encouraging. The large US STEP-1 FDA-approved trial is currently actively recruiting patients, and this will hopefully generate valuable information about the efficacy and safety profile of DJBL.

Gastro-duodenal Bypass Liner

The second system is the gastro-duodenal bypass liner system (ValenTx Endoluminal Bypass, Maple Grove, MN, USA). This device has twice the size of the DJBL (120 cm) with the proximal part being anchored at the gastroesophageal junction. It is designed to reproduce some of the restrictive and hypoabsorptive characteristics of a classic laparoscopic gastric bypass. The initial human experience reported in 13 patients showcased impressive results with a 54% excess weight loss and >70% improvement in associated comorbidities after 12 months [156]. Only four of these patients had T2D; 3/4 had more than 1% improvement in Hb1Ac, and 1/4 had significant improvement *with cessation of hypoglycemic treatment* [156]. Despite these encouraging results, early device removal was necessary due to odynophagia and intolerance in 17% and 23% of cases, respectively [156, 157]. In a more recent multicenter international study, 32 patients with a mean BMI of 42.3 kg/m^2 were enrolled into a single-arm feasibility trial [158]. Eighty-eight percent of devices remained implanted after 12 months, with notable adverse events including knotting of the sleeve in two patients, distal migration of the device requiring removal through laparotomy in one patient, and esophageal food impaction in one patient. Although no metabolic data was published, subjects lost on average 17.6% total body weight and 44.8% excess body weight at 12 months. Ongoing device development and further clinical investigations are currently underway.

Multiple Choice Questions

1. What is the gold standard bariatric/metabolic surgery?
   (a) LAGB
   (b) SG
   (c) **RYGB**
   (d) BPD-DS

2. What is the most commonly performed bariatric surgery worldwide?
   (a) LAGB
   (b) **SG**
   (c) RYGB
   (d) BPD-DS

3. What are the main surgeries that promote decreased ghrelin and an increase of GLP-1 and YY?
   (a) LAGB and SG
   (b) SG and RYGB
   (c) **RYGB and BPD-DS**
   (d) BPD-DS and LAGB

4. What is the main orexigenic hormone that is suppressed after sleeve gastrectomy?
   (a) Adiponectin
   (b) Leptin
   (c) **Ghrelin**
   (d) PYY-GLP-1

5. What hormone, which increases after RYGB, is associated with insulin resistance and appetite?
   (a) Adiponectin
   (b) Leptin
   (c) Ghrelin
   (d) **GLP-1**

6. Which of the following is an indication for bariatric surgery?
   (a) Obesity class 1
   (b) Obesity class 2 without comorbidities associated
   (c) **Obesity class 3 even when no comorbidities are associated**
   (d) BMI > 30 kg/m^2 and metabolic syndrome

7. According to the Standards of Care for Diabetes algorithm, when can metabolic surgery be considered?
   (a) Obesity class 1
   (b) **Diabetic subjects with inadequately controlled hyperglycemia despite medical treatment in subjects with a BMI ranging from 30 to 34.9 kg/m^2**
   (c) Overweight patients with uncontrolled diabetes
   (d) Metabolic surgery is not currently considered as an option for treatment

8. What changes in the composition of gut microbiota are associated after RYGB?
   (a) **Increased presence of Proteobacteria and Bacteroidetes**
   (b) Increase in Bacteroidetes and Firmicutes
   (c) Decrease in Firmicutes and Proteobacteria
   (d) Increase in *Lactobacillus* and Firmicutes

9. What is the adipokine that communicates between adipose tissue and the CNS to suppress food intake during energy sufficiency and decreases after bariatric surgery?
   (a) Adiponectin
   (b) GLP-1
   (c) **Leptin**
   (d) PYY

Glossary

Adipokines Hormones that are released from adipose tissue. The most well-known adipokines are leptin and adiponectin.

Bariatric Surgery Type of surgery that involves changes in the digestive system (restriction or redirection) in order to achieve weight loss and metabolic improvement

Incretins Intestinal peptides known for stimulating insulin production after food intake. The main incretins are PYY and GLP-1.

Laparoscopic surgery Minimal invasive surgery where trough small incisions (5–10 mm), ports are placed, CO_2 is insufflated, a camera (that transmit imagen from abdominal cavity to a monitor) and specialized instruments are inserted to perform a surgery. This type of surgery has the advantage to be faster and less invasive compared to open approach and facilitates a faster recovery.

Obesity Abnormal or excessive fat accumulation that presents a risk to health. It is considered when BMI is ≥30 kg/m².

Obesity Class 1 Patients with a BMI ranging from 30 to 34.9 kg/m²

Obesity Class 2 Patients with a BMI ranging from 35 to 39.9 kg/m²

Obesity Class 3 Patients with a BMI of 40 kg/m² or greater

Roux-en-Y Gastric Bypass Gold standard bariatric surgery that involves a re-routing of the passage of food. A small gastric pouch is created and connected to the jejunum, "bypassing" the stomach, the duodenum, and the first portion of the jejunum. After the surgery, a decrement in ghrelin and GIP and an increase of GLP-1 and PYY are observed.

Sleeve Gastrectomy Vertical transection of the stomach, starting at the greater curvature at 6 cm proximal to the pylorus toward the angle of His. It is performed with a laparoscopic stapler, guided over a 32Fr orogastric tube. It decreases the amount of food intake, ghrelin concentrations, and appetite and increases intragastric pressure.

References

1. Mechanick JI, Apovian C, Brethauer S, Timothy Garvey W, Joffe AM, Kim J, et al. Clinical practice guidelines for the perioperative nutrition, metabolic, and nonsurgical support of patients undergoing bariatric procedures - 2019 update: cosponsored by American Association of Clinical Endocrinologists/American College of Endocrinology, the Obesity Society, American Society for Metabolic and Bariatric Surgery, obesity medicine association, and American Society of Anesthesiologists. Obesity (Silver Spring). 2020;28(4):O1–O58.
2. Reinhold RB. Critical analysis of long term weight loss following gastric bypass. Surg Gynecol Obstet. 1982;155(3):385–94.
3. Warholm C, Marie Oien A, Raheim M. The ambivalence of losing weight after bariatric surgery. Int J Qual Stud Health Well-being. 2014;9:22876.
4. Henrikson V. Can small bowel resection be defended as therapy for obesity? Obes Surg. 1994;4:54.
5. Mason EE, Ito C. Gastric bypass in obesity. Surg Clin North Am. 1967;47(6):1345–51.
6. Buchwald H. The evolution of metabolic/bariatric surgery. Obes Surg. 2014;24(8):1126–35.
7. Buchwald H, Buchwald JN. Metabolic (bariatric and nonbariatric) surgery for Type 2 diabetes: a personal perspective review. Diabetes Care. 2019;42(2):331–40.
8. Mingrone G, Panunzi S, De Gaetano A, Guidone C, Iaconelli A, Nanni G, et al. Bariatric-metabolic surgery versus conventional medical treatment in obese patients with Type 2 diabetes: 5 year follow-up of an open-label, single-centre, randomised controlled trial. Lancet. 2015;386(9997):964–73.
9. Schauer PR, Bhatt DL, Kirwan JP, Wolski K, Aminian A, Brethauer SA, et al. Bariatric surgery versus intensive medical therapy for diabetes—5-year outcomes. N Engl J Med. 2017;376(7):641–51.
10. Dixon JB, Schachter LM, O'Brien PE, Jones K, Grima M, Lambert G, et al. Surgical vs conventional therapy for weight loss treatment of obstructive sleep apnea: a randomized controlled trial. JAMA. 2012;308(11):1142–9.
11. Rubino F, Nathan DM, Eckel RH, Schauer PR, Alberti KG, Zimmet PZ, et al. Metabolic surgery in the treatment algorithm for Type 2 diabetes: a joint statement by international diabetes organizations. Diabetes Care. 2016;39(6):861–77.
12. American Diabetes A. Standards of medical care in diabetes-2016 abridged for primary care providers. Clin Diabetes. 2016;34(1):3–21.
13. Ren CJ, Fielding GA. Laparoscopic adjustable gastric banding [lap-band]. Curr Surg. 2003;60(1):30–3.
14. Silecchia G, Rizzello M, Casella G, Fioriti M, Soricelli E, Basso N. Two-stage laparoscopic biliopancreatic diversion with duodenal switch as treatment of high-risk super-obese patients: analysis of complications. Surg Endosc. 2009;23(5):1032–7.
15. Committee ACI. Updated position statement on sleeve gastrectomy as a bariatric procedure. Surg Obes Relat Dis. 2012;8(3):e21–6.
16. English WJ, DeMaria EJ, Brethauer SA, Mattar SG, Rosenthal RJ, Morton JM. American Society for Metabolic and Bariatric Surgery estimation of metabolic and bariatric procedures performed in the United States in 2016. Surg Obes Relat Dis. 2018;14(3):259–63.
17. Ponce J, Nguyen NT, Hutter M, Sudan R, Morton JM. American Society for Metabolic and Bariatric Surgery estimation of bariatric surgery procedures in the United States, 2011-2014. Surg Obes Relat Dis. 2015;11(6):1199–200.
18. Ozsoy Z, Demir E. Which bariatric procedure is the most popular in the world? A bibliometric comparison. Obes Surg. 2018;28(8):2339–52.
19. Rosenthal RJ, International Sleeve Gastrectomy Expert P, Diaz AA, Arvidsson D, Baker RS, Basso N, et al. International sleeve gastrectomy expert panel consensus statement: best practice guidelines based on experience of >12,000 cases. Surg Obes Relat Dis. 2012;8(1):8–19.
20. Baltasar A, Serra C, Perez N, Bou R, Bengochea M, Ferri L. Laparoscopic sleeve gastrectomy: a multi-purpose bariatric operation. Obes Surg. 2005;15(8):1124–8.
21. Higa KD, Ho T, Boone KB. Laparoscopic Roux-en-Y gastric bypass: technique and 3-year follow-up. J Laparoendosc Adv Surg Tech A. 2001;11(6):377–82.
22. Buchwald H, Avidor Y, Braunwald E, Jensen MD, Pories W, Fahrbach K, et al. Bariatric surgery: a systematic review and meta-analysis. JAMA. 2004;292(14):1724–37.
23. Buchwald H, Estok R, Fahrbach K, Banel D, Sledge I. Trends in mortality in bariatric surgery: a systematic review and meta-analysis. Surgery. 2007;142(4):621–32; discussion 32-5.
24. Rutledge R. The mini-gastric bypass: experience with the first 1,274 cases. Obes Surg. 2001;11(3):276–80.
25. Carbajo M, Garcia-Caballero M, Toledano M, Osorio D, Garcia-Lanza C, Carmona JA. One-anastomosis gastric bypass by laparoscopy: results of the first 209 patients. Obes Surg. 2005;15(3):398–404.
26. Chevallier JM, Arman GA, Guenzi M, Rau C, Bruzzi M, Beaupel N, et al. One thousand single anastomosis (omega loop) gastric bypasses to treat morbid obesity in a 7-year period: outcomes show few complications and good efficacy. Obes Surg. 2015;25(6):951–8.
27. Kular KS, Manchanda N, Rutledge R. A 6-year experience with 1,054 mini-gastric bypasses-first study from Indian subcontinent. Obes Surg. 2014;24(9):1430–5.
28. Mahawar KK, Jennings N, Brown J, Gupta A, Balupuri S, Small PK. "mini" gastric bypass: systematic review of a controversial procedure. Obes Surg. 2013;23(11):1890–8.

29. Parikh M, Eisenberg D, Johnson J, El-Chaar M, American Society for M, Bariatric Surgery Clinical Issues C. American Society for Metabolic and Bariatric Surgery review of the literature on one-anastomosis gastric bypass. Surg Obes Relat Dis. 2018;14(8):1088–92.

30. Carbajo MA, Luque-de-Leon E, Jimenez JM, Ortiz-de-Solorzano J, Perez-Miranda M, Castro-Alija MJ. Laparoscopic one-anastomosis gastric bypass: technique, results, and long-term follow-up in 1200 patients. Obes Surg. 2017;27(5):1153–67.

31. Mahawar KK, Himpens J, Shikora SA, Chevallier JM, Lakdawala M, De Luca M, et al. The first consensus statement on one anastomosis/mini gastric bypass (OAGB/MGB) using a modified Delphi approach. Obes Surg. 2018;28(2):303–12.

32. Sanchez-Pernaute A, Rubio Herrera MA, Perez-Aguirre E, Garcia Perez JC, Cabrerizo L, Diez Valladares L, et al. Proximal duodenal-ileal end-to-side bypass with sleeve gastrectomy: proposed technique. Obes Surg. 2007;17(12):1614–8.

33. Schauer PR, Kashyap SR, Wolski K, Brethauer SA, Kirwan JP, Pothier CE, et al. Bariatric surgery versus intensive medical therapy in obese patients with diabetes. N Engl J Med. 2012;366(17):1567–76.

34. Angrisani L, Santonicola A, Iovino P, Vitiello A, Higa K, Himpens J, et al. IFSO worldwide survey 2016: primary, endoluminal, and revisional procedures. Obes Surg. 2018;28(12):3783–94.

35. Wang Y, Guo X, Lu X, Mattar S, Kassab G. Mechanisms of weight loss after sleeve gastrectomy and adjustable gastric banding: far more than just restriction. Obesity (Silver Spring). 2019;27(11):1776–83.

36. Mahawar KK, Sharples AJ. Contribution of malabsorption to weight loss after Roux-en-Y gastric bypass: a systematic review. Obes Surg. 2017;27(8):2194–206.

37. Meek CL, Lewis HB, Reimann F, Gribble FM, Park AJ. The effect of bariatric surgery on gastrointestinal and pancreatic peptide hormones. Peptides. 2016;77:28–37.

38. Delhanty PJ, Neggers SJ, van der Lely AJ. Des-acyl ghrelin: a metabolically active peptide. Endocr Dev. 2013;25:112–21.

39. Barazzoni R, Zanetti M, Nagliati C, Cattin MR, Ferreira C, Giuricin M, et al. Gastric bypass does not normalize obesity-related changes in ghrelin profile and leads to higher acylated ghrelin fraction. Obesity (Silver Spring). 2013;21(4):718–22.

40. Safatle-Ribeiro AV, Petersen PA, Pereira Filho DS, Corbett CE, Faintuch J, Ishida R, et al. Epithelial cell turnover is increased in the excluded stomach mucosa after Roux-en-Y gastric bypass for morbid obesity. Obes Surg. 2013;23(10):1616–23.

41. Jacobsen SH, Olesen SC, Dirksen C, Jorgensen NB, Bojsen-Moller KN, Kielgast U, et al. Changes in gastrointestinal hormone responses, insulin sensitivity, and beta-cell function within 2 weeks after gastric bypass in non-diabetic subjects. Obes Surg. 2012;22(7):1084–96.

42. Dirksen C, Jorgensen NB, Bojsen-Moller KN, Kielgast U, Jacobsen SH, Clausen TR, et al. Gut hormones, early dumping and resting energy expenditure in patients with good and poor weight loss response after Roux-en-Y gastric bypass. Int J Obes. 2013;37(11):1452–9.

43. Yousseif A, Emmanuel J, Karra E, Millet Q, Elkalaawy M, Jenkinson AD, et al. Differential effects of laparoscopic sleeve gastrectomy and laparoscopic gastric bypass on appetite, circulating acyl-ghrelin, peptide YY3-36 and active GLP-1 levels in non-diabetic humans. Obes Surg. 2014;24(2):241–52.

44. Mingrone G, Panunzi S, De Gaetano A, Guidone C, Iaconelli A, Leccesi L, et al. Bariatric surgery versus conventional medical therapy for Type 2 diabetes. N Engl J Med. 2012;366(17):1577–85.

45. Pories WJ, Caro JF, Flickinger EG, Meelheim HD, Swanson MS. The control of diabetes mellitus (NIDDM) in the morbidly obese with the Greenville gastric bypass. Ann Surg. 1987;206(3):316–23.

46. Cohen RV, Pinheiro JC, Schiavon CA, Salles JE, Wajchenberg BL, Cummings DE. Effects of gastric bypass surgery in patients with Type 2 diabetes and only mild obesity. Diabetes Care. 2012;35(7):1420–8.

47. Astiarraga B, Gastaldelli A, Muscelli E, Baldi S, Camastra S, Mari A, et al. Biliopancreatic diversion in nonobese patients with Type 2 diabetes: impact and mechanisms. J Clin Endocrinol Metab. 2013;98(7):2765–73.

48. McIntosh CH, Widenmaier S, Kim SJ. Glucose-dependent insulinotropic polypeptide (gastric inhibitory polypeptide; GIP). Vitam Horm. 2009;80:409–71.

49. Guidone C, Manco M, Valera-Mora E, Iaconelli A, Gniuli D, Mari A, et al. Mechanisms of recovery from Type 2 diabetes after malabsorptive bariatric surgery. Diabetes. 2006;55(7):2025–31.

50. Clements RH, Gonzalez QH, Long CI, Wittert G, Laws HL. Hormonal changes after Roux-en Y gastric bypass for morbid obesity and the control of Type-II diabetes mellitus. Am Surg. 2004;70(1):1–4. discussion-5.

51. Laferrere B, Heshka S, Wang K, Khan Y, McGinty J, Teixeira J, et al. Incretin levels and effect are markedly enhanced 1 month after Roux-en-Y gastric bypass surgery in obese patients with Type 2 diabetes. Diabetes Care. 2007;30(7):1709–16.

52. Laferrere B, Teixeira J, McGinty J, Tran H, Egger JR, Colarusso A, et al. Effect of weight loss by gastric bypass surgery versus hypocaloric diet on glucose and incretin levels in patients with Type 2 diabetes. J Clin Endocrinol Metab. 2008;93(7):2479–85.

53. Rubino F, Forgione A, Cummings DE, Vix M, Gnuli D, Mingrone G, et al. The mechanism of diabetes control after gastrointestinal bypass surgery reveals a role of the proximal small intestine in the pathophysiology of Type 2 diabetes. Ann Surg. 2006;244(5):741–9.

54. Nuffer WA, Trujillo JM. Liraglutide: a new option for the treatment of obesity. Pharmacotherapy. 2015;35(10):926–34.

55. Dimitriadis GK, Randeva MS, Miras AD. Potential hormone mechanisms of bariatric surgery. Curr Obes Rep. 2017;6(3):253–65.

56. Hutch CR, Sandoval D. The role of GLP-1 in the metabolic success of bariatric surgery. Endocrinology. 2017;158(12):4139–51.

57. Holst JJ, Madsbad S, Bojsen-Moller KN, Svane MS, Jorgensen NB, Dirksen C, et al. Mechanisms in bariatric surgery: gut hormones, diabetes resolution, and weight loss. Surg Obes Relat Dis. 2018;14(5):708–14.

58. Mason EE. History of obesity surgery. Surg Obes Relat Dis. 2005;1(2):123–5.

59. Rubino F, Gagner M. Potential of surgery for curing Type 2 diabetes mellitus. Ann Surg. 2002;236(5):554–9.

60. Larsson H, Holst JJ, Ahren B. Glucagon-like peptide-1 reduces hepatic glucose production indirectly through insulin and glucagon in humans. Acta Physiol Scand. 1997;160(4):413–22.

61. Fehmann HC, Goke R, Goke B. Cell and molecular biology of the incretin hormones glucagon-like peptide-I and glucose-dependent insulin releasing polypeptide. Endocr Rev. 1995;16(3):390–410.

62. Wang Y, Perfetti R, Greig NH, Holloway HW, DeOre KA, Montrose-Rafizadeh C, et al. Glucagon-like peptide-1 can reverse the age-related decline in glucose tolerance in rats. J Clin Invest. 1997;99(12):2883–9.

63. Buteau J, El-Assaad W, Rhodes CJ, Rosenberg L, Joly E, Prentki M. Glucagon-like peptide-1 prevents beta cell glucolipotoxicity. Diabetologia. 2004;47(5):806–15.

64. Vidal J, de Hollanda A, Jimenez A. GLP-1 is not the key mediator of the health benefits of metabolic surgery. Surg Obes Relat Dis. 2016;12(6):1225–9.

65. Mans E, Serra-Prat M, Palomera E, Sunol X, Clave P. Sleeve gastrectomy effects on hunger, satiation, and gastrointestinal hormone and motility responses after a liquid meal test. Am J Clin Nutr. 2015;102(3):540–7.

66. Peterli R, Steinert RE, Woelnerhanssen B, Peters T, Christoffel-Courtin C, Gass M, et al. Metabolic and hormonal changes after laparoscopic Roux-en-Y gastric bypass and sleeve gastrectomy: a randomized, prospective trial. Obes Surg. 2012;22(5):740–8.

67. Batterham RL, Cowley MA, Small CJ, Herzog H, Cohen MA, Dakin CL, et al. Gut hormone PYY(3-36) physiologically inhibits food intake. Nature. 2002;418(6898):650–4.

68. Witte AB, Gryback P, Holst JJ, Hilsted L, Hellstrom PM, Jacobsson H, et al. Differential effect of PYY1-36 and PYY3-36 on gastric emptying in man. Regul Pept. 2009;158(1-3):57–62.

69. Batterham RL, Cohen MA, Ellis SM, Le Roux CW, Withers DJ, Frost GS, et al. Inhibition of food intake in obese subjects by peptide YY3-36. N Engl J Med. 2003;349(10):941–8.

70. Sainz N, Barrenetxe J, Moreno-Aliaga MJ, Martinez JA. Leptin resistance and diet-induced obesity: central and peripheral actions of leptin. Metabolism. 2015;64(1):35–46.

71. Kadowaki T, Yamauchi T, Kubota N, Hara K, Ueki K, Tobe K. Adiponectin and adiponectin receptors in insulin resistance, diabetes, and the metabolic syndrome. J Clin Invest. 2006;116(7):1784–92.

72. Frikke-Schmidt H, O'Rourke RW, Lumeng CN, Sandoval DA, Seeley RJ. Does bariatric surgery improve adipose tissue function? Obes Rev. 2016;17(9):795–809.

73. Abdennour M, Reggio S, Le Naour G, Liu Y, Poitou C, Aron-Wisnewsky J, et al. Association of adipose tissue and liver fibrosis with tissue stiffness in morbid obesity: links with diabetes and BMI loss after gastric bypass. J Clin Endocrinol Metab. 2014;99(3):898–907.

74. Lee YJ, Heo YS, Park HS, Lee SH, Lee SK, Jang YJ. Serum SPARC and matrix metalloproteinase-2 and metalloproteinase-9 concentrations after bariatric surgery in obese adults. Obes Surg. 2014;24(4):604–10.

75. Chen J, Pamuklar Z, Spagnoli A, Torquati A. Serum leptin levels are inversely correlated with omental gene expression of adiponectin and markedly decreased after gastric bypass surgery. Surg Endosc. 2012;26(5):1476–80.

76. Kim MJ, Marchand P, Henegar C, Antignac JP, Alili R, Poitou C, et al. Fate and complex pathogenic effects of dioxins and polychlorinated biphenyls in obese subjects before and after drastic weight loss. Environ Health Perspect. 2011;119(3):377–83.

77. Bobbioni-Harsch E, Morel P, Huber O, Assimacopoulos-Jeannet F, Chassot G, Lehmann T, et al. Energy economy hampers body weight loss after gastric bypass. J Clin Endocrinol Metab. 2000;85(12):4695–700.

78. Sams VG, Blackledge C, Wijayatunga N, Barlow P, Mancini M, Mancini G, et al. Effect of bariatric surgery on systemic and adipose tissue inflammation. Surg Endosc. 2016;30(8):3499–504.

79. Cancello R, Zulian A, Gentilini D, Mencarelli M, Della Barba A, Maffei M, et al. Permanence of molecular features of obesity in subcutaneous adipose tissue of ex-obese subjects. Int J Obes. 2013;37(6):867–73.

80. Qin J, Li R, Raes J, Arumugam M, Burgdorf KS, Manichanh C, et al. A human gut microbial gene catalogue established by metagenomic sequencing. Nature. 2010;464(7285):59–65.

81. Palleja A, Kashani A, Allin KH, Nielsen T, Zhang C, Li Y, et al. Roux-en-Y gastric bypass surgery of morbidly obese patients induces swift and persistent changes of the individual gut microbiota. Genome Med. 2016;8(1):67.

82. Zhang H, DiBaise JK, Zuccolo A, Kudrna D, Braidotti M, Yu Y, et al. Human gut microbiota in obesity and after gastric bypass. Proc Natl Acad Sci U S A. 2009;106(7):2365–70.

83. Damms-Machado A, Mitra S, Schollenberger AE, Kramer KM, Meile T, Konigsrainer A, et al. Effects of surgical and dietary weight loss therapy for obesity on gut microbiota composition and nutrient absorption. Biomed Res Int. 2015;2015:806248.

84. Tremaroli V, Karlsson F, Werling M, Stahlman M, Kovatcheva-Datchary P, Olbers T, et al. Roux-en-Y gastric bypass and vertical banded gastroplasty induce long-term changes on the human gut microbiome contributing to fat mass regulation. Cell Metab. 2015;22(2):228–38.

85. Cipriani S, Mencarelli A, Palladino G, Fiorucci S. FXR activation reverses insulin resistance and lipid abnormalities and protects against liver steatosis in Zucker (fa/fa) obese rats. J Lipid Res. 2010;51(4):771–84.

86. Li T, Holmstrom SR, Kir S, Umetani M, Schmidt DR, Kliewer SA, et al. The G protein-coupled bile acid receptor, TGR5, stimulates gallbladder filling. Mol Endocrinol. 2011;25(6):1066–71.

87. Watanabe M, Houten SM, Mataki C, Christoffolete MA, Kim BW, Sato H, et al. Bile acids induce energy expenditure by promoting intracellular thyroid hormone activation. Nature. 2006;439(7075):484–9.

88. Potthoff MJ, Potts A, He T, Duarte JA, Taussig R, Mangelsdorf DJ, et al. Colesevelam suppresses hepatic glycogenolysis by TGR5-mediated induction of GLP-1 action in DIO mice. Am J Physiol Gastrointest Liver Physiol. 2013;304(4):G371–80.

89. Habib AM, Richards P, Rogers GJ, Reimann F, Gribble FM. Co-localisation and secretion of glucagon-like peptide 1 and peptide YY from primary cultured human L cells. Diabetologia. 2013;56(6):1413–6.

90. Ahmad NN, Pfalzer A, Kaplan LM. Roux-en-Y gastric bypass normalizes the blunted postprandial bile acid excursion associated with obesity. Int J Obes. 2013;37(12):1553–9.

91. Albaugh VL, Flynn CR, Cai S, Xiao Y, Tamboli RA, Abumrad NN. Early increases in bile acids post Roux-en-Y gastric bypass are driven by insulin-sensitizing, secondary bile acids. J Clin Endocrinol Metab. 2015;100(9):E1225–33.

92. De Giorgi S, Campos V, Egli L, Toepel U, Carrel G, Cariou B, et al. Long-term effects of Roux-en-Y gastric bypass on postprandial plasma lipid and bile acids kinetics in female non diabetic subjects: a cross-sectional pilot study. Clin Nutr. 2015;34(5):911–7.

93. Immonen H, Hannukainen JC, Iozzo P, Soinio M, Salminen P, Saunavaara V, et al. Effect of bariatric surgery on liver glucose metabolism in morbidly obese diabetic and non-diabetic patients. J Hepatol. 2014;60(2):377–83.

94. Honka H, Koffert J, Hannukainen JC, Tuulari JJ, Karlsson HK, Immonen H, et al. The effects of bariatric surgery on pancreatic lipid metabolism and blood flow. J Clin Endocrinol Metab. 2015;100(5):2015–23.

95. Schauer PR, Bhatt DL, Kirwan JP, Wolski K, Brethauer SA, Navaneethan SD, et al. Bariatric surgery versus intensive medical therapy for diabetes—3-year outcomes. N Engl J Med. 2014;370(21):2002–13.

96. Ikramuddin S, Korner J, Lee WJ, Connett JE, Inabnet WB, Billington CJ, et al. Roux-en-Y gastric bypass vs intensive medical management for the control of Type 2 diabetes, hypertension, and hyperlipidemia: the diabetes surgery study randomized clinical trial. JAMA. 2013;309(21):2240–9.

97. Liang Z, Wu Q, Chen B, Yu P, Zhao H, Ouyang X. Effect of laparoscopic Roux-en-Y gastric bypass surgery on Type 2 diabetes mellitus with hypertension: a randomized controlled trial. Diabetes Res Clin Pract. 2013;101(1):50–6.

98. Courcoulas AP, Goodpaster BH, Eagleton JK, Belle SH, Kalarchian MA, Lang W, et al. Surgical vs medical treatments for Type 2 diabetes mellitus: a randomized clinical trial. JAMA Surg. 2014;149(7):707–15.

99. Halperin F, Ding SA, Simonson DC, Panosian J, Goebel-Fabbri A, Wewalka M, et al. Roux-en-Y gastric bypass surgery or lifestyle with intensive medical management in patients with Type 2 diabetes: feasibility and 1-year results of a randomized clinical trial. JAMA Surg. 2014;149(7):716–26.

100. Buchwald H, Estok R, Fahrbach K, Banel D, Jensen MD, Pories WJ, et al. Weight and Type 2 diabetes after bariatric surgery: systematic review and meta-analysis. Am J Med. 2009;122(3):248–56 e5.

101. Kashyap SR, Bhatt DL, Wolski K, Watanabe RM, Abdul-Ghani M, Abood B, et al. Metabolic effects of bariatric surgery in patients with moderate obesity and Type 2 diabetes: analysis of a randomized control trial comparing surgery with intensive medical treatment. Diabetes Care. 2013;36(8):2175–82.

102. Du X, Fu XH, Shi L, Hu JK, Zhou ZG, Cheng Z. Effects of laparoscopic Roux-en-Y gastric bypass on Chinese Type 2 diabetes mellitus patients with different levels of obesity: outcomes after 3 years' follow-up. Obes Surg. 2018;28(3):702–11.

103. Sjostrom L, Peltonen M, Jacobson P, Ahlin S, Andersson-Assarsson J, Anveden A, et al. Association of bariatric surgery with long-term remission of Type 2 diabetes and with microvascular and macrovascular complications. JAMA. 2014;311(22):2297–304.

104. O'Brien R, Johnson E, Haneuse S, Coleman KJ, O'Connor PJ, Fisher DP, et al. Microvascular outcomes in patients with diabetes after bariatric surgery versus usual care: a matched cohort study. Ann Intern Med. 2018;169(5):300–10.

105. Hussain S, Khan MS, Jamali MC, Siddiqui AN, Gupta G, Hussain MS, et al. Impact of bariatric surgery in reducing macrovascular complications in severely obese T2DM patients. Obes Surg. 2021;31(5):1929–36.

106. Priyadarshini P, Singh VP, Aggarwal S, Garg H, Sinha S, Guleria R. Impact of bariatric surgery on obstructive sleep apnoea-hypopnea syndrome in morbidly obese patients. J Minim Access Surg. 2017;13(4):291–5.

107. Sarkhosh K, Switzer NJ, El-Hadi M, Birch DW, Shi X, Karmali S. The impact of bariatric surgery on obstructive sleep apnea: a systematic review. Obes Surg. 2013;23(3):414–23.

108. Nastalek P, Polok K, Celejewska-Wojcik N, Kania A, Sladek K, Malczak P, et al. Impact of bariatric surgery on obstructive sleep apnea severity and continuous positive airway pressure therapy compliance-prospective observational study. Sci Rep. 2021;11(1):5003.

109. Peromaa-Haavisto P, Tuomilehto H, Kossi J, Virtanen J, Luostarinen M, Pihlajamaki J, et al. Obstructive sleep apnea: the effect of bariatric surgery after 12 months. A prospective multicenter trial. Sleep Med. 2017;35:85–90.

110. Scopinaro N, Marinari GM, Camerini GB, Papadia FS, Adami GF. Specific effects of biliopancreatic diversion on the major components of metabolic syndrome: a long-term follow-up study. Diabetes Care. 2005;28(10):2406–11.

111. Piche ME, Martin J, Cianflone K, Bastien M, Marceau S, Biron S, et al. Changes in predicted cardiovascular disease risk after biliopancreatic diversion surgery in severely obese patients. Metabolism. 2014;63(1):79–86.

112. Aminian A, Zajichek A, Arterburn DE, Wolski KE, Brethauer SA, Schauer PR, et al. Association of metabolic surgery with major adverse cardiovascular outcomes in patients with Type 2 diabetes and obesity. JAMA. 2019;322(13):1271–82.

113. Doumouras AG, Wong JA, Paterson JM, Lee Y, Sivapathasundaram B, Tarride JE, et al. Bariatric surgery and cardiovascular outcomes in patients with obesity and cardiovascular disease: a population-based retrospective cohort study. Circulation. 2021;143(15):1468–80.

114. Parikh M, Chung M, Sheth S, McMacken M, Zahra T, Saunders JK, et al. Randomized pilot trial of bariatric surgery versus intensive medical weight management on diabetes remission in Type 2 diabetic patients who do NOT meet NIH criteria for surgery and the role of soluble RAGE as a novel biomarker of success. Ann Surg. 2014;260(4):617–22; discussion 22-4.

115. Espinosa O, Pineda O, Maydon HG, Sepulveda EM, Guilbert L, Amado M, et al. Type 2 diabetes mellitus outcomes after laparoscopic gastric bypass in patients with BMI <35 kg/m(2) using strict remission criteria: early outcomes of a prospective study among Mexicans. Surg Endosc. 2018;32(3):1353–9.

116. Bhandari M, Mathur W, Kumar R, Mishra A, Bhandari M. Surgical and advanced medical therapy for the treatment of Type 2 diabetes in class i obese patients: a short-term outcome. Obes Surg. 2017;27(12):3267–72.

117. Boza C, Valderas P, Daroch DA, Leon FI, Salinas JP, Barros DA, et al. Metabolic surgery: roux-en-Y gastric bypass and variables associated with diabetes remission in patients with BMI <35. Obes Surg. 2014;24(8):1391–7.

118. Chong K, Ikramuddin S, Lee WJ, Billington CJ, Bantle JP, Wang Q, et al. National differences in remission of Type 2 diabetes mellitus after Roux-en-Y gastric bypass surgery-subgroup analysis of 2-year results of the diabetes surgery study comparing Taiwanese with Americans with mild obesity (BMI 30-35 kg/m(2)). Obes Surg. 2017;27(5):1189–95.

119. Billeter AT, Kopf S, Zeier M, Scheurlen K, Fischer L, Schulte TM, et al. Renal function in Type 2 diabetes following gastric bypass. Dtsch Arztebl Int. 2016;113(49):827–33.

120. Cummings DE, Arterburn DE, Westbrook EO, Kuzma JN, Stewart SD, Chan CP, et al. Gastric bypass surgery vs intensive lifestyle and medical intervention for Type 2 diabetes: the CROSSROADS randomised controlled trial. Diabetologia. 2016;59(5):945–53.

121. Adami GF, Camerini G, Papadia F, Catalano MF, Carlini F, Cordera R, et al. Type 2 diabetes remission and control in overweight and in mildly obese diabetic patients at long-term follow-up after biliopancreatic diversion. Obes Surg. 2019;29(1):239–45.

122. Lee WJ, Chong K, Lin YH, Wei JH, Chen SC. Laparoscopic sleeve gastrectomy versus single anastomosis (mini-) gastric bypass for the treatment of Type 2 diabetes mellitus: 5-year results of a randomized trial and study of incretin effect. Obes Surg. 2014;24(9):1552–62.

123. Wentworth JM, Playfair J, Laurie C, Ritchie ME, Brown WA, Burton P, et al. Multidisciplinary diabetes care with and without bariatric surgery in overweight people: a randomised controlled trial. Lancet Diabetes Endocrinol. 2014;2(7):545–52.

124. Al-Goblan AS, Al-Alfi MA, Khan MZ. Mechanism linking diabetes mellitus and obesity. Diabetes Metab Syndr Obes. 2014;7:587–91.

125. Sibley SD, Palmer JP, Hirsch IB, Brunzell JD. Visceral obesity, hepatic lipase activity, and dyslipidemia in Type 1 diabetes. J Clin Endocrinol Metab. 2003;88(7):3379–84.

126. Reichard P, Berglund B, Britz A, Cars I, Nilsson BY, Rosenqvist U. Intensified conventional insulin treatment retards the microvascular complications of insulin-dependent diabetes mellitus (IDDM): the Stockholm diabetes intervention study (SDIS) after 5 years. J Intern Med. 1991;230(2):101–8.

127. Holl RW, Swift PG, Mortensen HB, Lynggaard H, Hougaard P, Aanstoot HJ, et al. Insulin injection regimens and metabolic control in an international survey of adolescents with Type 1 diabetes over 3 years: results from the Hvidore study group. Eur J Pediatr. 2003;162(1):22–9.

128. Kirwan JP, Aminian A, Kashyap SR, Burguera B, Brethauer SA, Schauer PR. Bariatric surgery in obese patients with Type 1 diabetes. Diabetes Care. 2016;39(6):941–8.

129. Middelbeek RJ, James-Todd T, Patti ME, Brown FM. Short-term insulin requirements following gastric bypass surgery in severely obese women with Type 1 diabetes. Obes Surg. 2014;24(9):1442–6.

130. Kielgast U, Krarup T, Holst JJ, Madsbad S. Four weeks of treatment with liraglutide reduces insulin dose without loss of glycemic control in Type 1 diabetic patients with and without residual beta-cell function. Diabetes Care. 2011;34(7):1463–8.

131. Robert M, Belanger P, Hould FS, Marceau S, Tchernof A, Biertho L. Should metabolic surgery be offered in morbidly

obese patients with Type I diabetes? Surg Obes Relat Dis. 2015;11(4):798–805.

132. Ding SA, Simonson DC, Wewalka M, Halperin F, Foster K, Goebel-Fabbri A, et al. Adjustable gastric band surgery or medical management in patients with Type 2 diabetes: a randomized clinical trial. J Clin Endocrinol Metab. 2015;100(7):2546–56.

133. Dixon JB, O'Brien PE, Playfair J, Chapman L, Schachter LM, Skinner S, et al. Adjustable gastric banding and conventional therapy for Type 2 diabetes: a randomized controlled trial. JAMA. 2008;299(3):316–23.

134. Gracia JA, Martinez M, Aguilella V, Elia M, Royo P. Postoperative morbidity of biliopancreatic diversion depending on common limb length. Obes Surg. 2007;17(10):1306–11.

135. Kapeluto JE, Tchernof A, Masckauchan D, Biron S, Marceau S, Hould FS, et al. Ten-year remission rates in insulin-treated Type 2 diabetes after biliopancreatic diversion with duodenal switch. Surg Obes Relat Dis. 2020;16(11):1701–12.

136. Bockelman C, Hahl T, Victorzon M. Mortality following bariatric surgery compared to other common operations in Finland during a 5-year period (2009-2013). A Nationwide registry study. Obes Surg. 2017;27(9):2444–51.

137. Nguyen NT, Hinojosa M, Fayad C, Varela E, Wilson SE. Use and outcomes of laparoscopic versus open gastric bypass at academic medical centers. J Am Coll Surg. 2007;205(2):248–55.

138. Brethauer SA, Kim J, El Chaar M, Papasavas P, Eisenberg D, Rogers A, et al. Standardized outcomes reporting in metabolic and bariatric surgery. Obes Surg. 2015;25(4):587–606.

139. Guilbert L, Joo P, Ortiz C, Sepulveda E, Alabi F, Leon A, et al. Safety and efficacy of bariatric surgery in Mexico: a detailed analysis of 500 surgeries performed at a high-volume center. Rev Gastroenterol Mex (Engl Ed). 2019;84(3):296–302.

140. Lim R, Beekley A, Johnson DC, Davis KA. Early and late complications of bariatric operation. Trauma Surg Acute Care Open. 2018;3(1):e000219.

141. Hu Z, Sun J, Li R, Wang Z, Ding H, Zhu T, et al. A comprehensive comparison of LRYGB and LSG in obese patients including the effects on QoL, comorbidities, weight loss, and complications: a systematic review and meta-analysis. Obes Surg. 2020;30(3):819–27.

142. White GE, Courcoulas AP, King WC, Flum DR, Yanovski SZ, Pomp A, et al. Mortality after bariatric surgery: findings from a 7-year multicenter cohort study. Surg Obes Relat Dis. 2019;15(10):1755–65.

143. McCarty TR, Thompson CC. Bariatric and metabolic therapies targeting the small intestine. Tech Innov Gastrointest Endosc. 2020;22(3):145–53.

144. Schlottmann F, Ryou M, Lautz D, Thompson CC, Buxhoeveden R. Sutureless duodeno-ileal anastomosis with self-assembling magnets: safety and feasibility of a novel metabolic procedure. Obes Surg. 2021;31(9):4195–202.

145. Graves CE, Co C, Hsi RS, Kwiat D, Imamura-Ching J, Harrison MR, et al. Magnetic compression anastomosis (magnamosis): first-in-human trial. J Am Coll Surg. 2017;225(5):676–81.e1.

146. Harrison MR. Magnetic duodeno-ileal bypass for metabolic syndrome in rhesus monkeys: project 1R44DK112453-01A1.

147. EasyNOTESMedical. www.easynotes-medical.com

148. Winder JS, Rodriguez JH. Emerging endoscopic interventions in bariatric surgery. Surg Clin North Am. 2021;101(2):373–9.

149. van Baar ACG, Holleman F, Crenier L, Haidry R, Magee C, Hopkins D, et al. Endoscopic duodenal mucosal resurfacing for the treatment of Type 2 diabetes mellitus: one year results from the first international, open-label, prospective, multicentre study. Gut. 2020;69(2):295–303.

150. McCarty TR, Thompson CC. The current state of bariatric endoscopy. Dig Endosc. 2021;33(3):321–34.

151. Mraz M, Marcovitch I, Lankova I. 1131-P: endoscopic duodenal submucosal laser ablation for the treatment of Type 2 diabetes mellitus: results of first-in-human pilot study. Arlington: American Diabetes Association: Diabetes; 2019.

152. Ruban A, Ashrafian H, Teare JP. The endobarrier: duodenal-jejunal bypass liner for diabetes and weight loss. Gastroenterol Res Pract. 2018;2018:7823182.

153. Jirapinyo P, Haas AV, Thompson CC. Effect of the duodenal-jejunal bypass liner on glycemic control in patients with Type 2 diabetes with obesity: a meta-analysis with secondary analysis on weight loss and hormonal changes. Diabetes Care. 2018;41(5):1106–15.

154. Kaplan L, Buse, JB, Mullin, C, editors. EndoBarrier therapy is associated with glycemic improvement, weight loss and safety issues in patients with obesity and Type 2 diabetes on oral antihyperglycemic agents. In: Proceedings of the 76th scientific sessions; 2016 Jun 10–14; New Orleans, LA; 2016.

155. Aruchuna R. Duodenal-Jejunal bypass liner for the management of Type 2 diabetes mellitus and obesity. A multicenter randomized controlled trial. Ann Surg. 2022;275(3):440–7.

156. Sandler BJ, Rumbaut R, Swain CP, Torres G, Morales L, Gonzales L, et al. One-year human experience with a novel endoluminal, endoscopic gastric bypass sleeve for morbid obesity. Surg Endosc. 2015;29(11):3298–303.

157. Sandler BJ, Rumbaut R, Swain CP, Torres G, Morales L, Gonzales L, et al. Human experience with an endoluminal, endoscopic, gastrojejunal bypass sleeve. Surg Endosc. 2011;25(9):3028–33.

158. Sandler BJ, Biertho L, Anvari M, Rumbaut R, Morales-Garza LA, Torres-Barrera G, et al. Totally endoscopic implant to effect a gastric bypass: 12-month safety and efficacy outcomes. Surg Endosc. 2018;32(11):4436–42.

Diabetes and Smoking: The Burden of Evidence

43

Sameer Aggarwal, Deepak Khandelwal, Deep Dutta, Sanjay Kalra, and Yatan Pal Singh Balhara

Introduction

Smoking has been identified as the leading preventable risk factor for premature mortality and morbidity. Large volumes of literature are now available linking smoking with cardiovascular morbidity and mortality, diabetes, vascular damage, cancers, and neurocognitive dysfunction, among others. It will not be erroneous to state that every system of the body is affected by smoking. Smokers die on average 8–10 years younger than nonsmokers. This chapter intends to highlight the complex relationship between smoking and the occurrence and the associated morbidity related to diabetes.

Smoking and Diabetes: Incidence and Mechanism

The impact of smoking on glycemia is complex. Smoking is strongly linked with both increased incidence and severity of diabetes. Smoking cessation, at least in the short term, is associated with weight gain, which is also associated with increased incidence of diabetes.

The risk of developing diabetes in smokers has been found to be dose dependent. A meta-analysis of 25 studies reported that heavy smokers (smoking ≥ 20 cigarettes/day) were more likely to develop diabetes (relative risk (RR) = 1.61; 95% CI = 1.43–1.80) as compared to light smokers (RR = 1.29; 95% CI = 1.13–1.48) and former smokers (RR = 1.23; 95% CI = 1.14–1.33). A study on industrial workers in a large cohort of individuals in Taiwan showed that compared to never-smokers, both current smokers and ex-smokers in their first 2 years of abstinence had higher odds ratios (ORs) for newly diagnosed diabetes mellitus (never-smokers 3.6%, OR = 1; current smokers 5.5%, OR = 1.499, 95% CI = 1.147–1.960, and $p = 0.003$; ex-smokers in their first year of abstinence 7.5%, OR = 1.829, 95% CI = 0.906–3.694, and $p = 0.092$; and ex-smokers in their second year of abstinence 9.0%, OR = 2.020, 95% CI = 1.031–3.955, and $p = 0.040$) [1]. This higher incidence of diabetes in ex-smokers was independent of the associated weight gain [1].

Smoking is found to cause diabetes by insulin resistance as well as decreased insulin release due to pancreatic β-cell damage by inflammatory and oxidative pathway mechanisms. Another concerning fact is that fetal exposure to smoking (maternal smoking during pregnancy) is associated with increased risk of diabetes later in life [2]. The silver lining is the observation that a healthy lifestyle intervention can go a long way in reducing this risk of diabetes among these persons [2].

Smoking is associated with increased and differential DNA methylation of type 2 diabetes genes, especially the ANPEP, KCNQ1, and ZMIZ1 genes, which may explain how smoking is associated with long-term increased diabetes risk [3].

S. Aggarwal
Division of Endocrinology, Department of Medicine, Pandit Bhagwat Dayal Sharma Post-graduate Institute of Medical Sciences (PGIMS), Rohtak, Haryana, India

D. Khandelwal
Department of Endocrinology, Maharaja Agrasen Hospital, New Delhi, India

D. Dutta
Department of Endocrinology, Venkateshwar Hospital, New Delhi, India

S. Kalra (✉)
Department of Endocrinology, Bharti Hospital, Karnal, Haryana, India

Y. P. S. Balhara
Department of Psychiatry, National Drug Dependence Treatment Centre (NDDTC), All India Institute of Medical Sciences (AIIMS), New Delhi, India

© The Author(s), under exclusive license to Springer Nature Switzerland AG 2023
J. Rodriguez-Saldana (ed.), *The Diabetes Textbook*, https://doi.org/10.1007/978-3-031-25519-9_43

Smoking and Non-microvascular or Non-macrovascular Complications

Smoking is an independent predictor of atherosclerosis. It has a stronger association with postprandial dyslipidemia and not fasting lipid values. It has been linked with postprandial hypertriglyceridemia [4].

Smoking and Microvascular Complications of Diabetes

Smoking increases the risk for microvascular complications of diabetes, probably via its metabolic effects in combination with increased inflammation and endothelial dysfunction [5]. This association is strong in type 1 diabetes patients and seen for all microvascular complications. However, the association of smoking with microvascular complications in type 2 diabetes is comparatively weaker except for nephropathy. Studies have clearly supported the negative impact of smoking on diabetic kidney disease in type 2 diabetes too, but its independent influence on retinopathy and neuropathy in type 2 diabetes remains unclear [5].

Smoking and Diabetic Nephropathy

Several studies have demonstrated that smoking promotes the development and progression of diabetic nephropathy in persons with both type 1 and type 2 diabetes, and smoking is an independent risk factor for diabetic kidney disease. Also, smoking is associated with an increased risk for end-stage renal disease and decreased survival on commencement of dialysis. In a 13-year follow-up study by Biesenbach et al., the progression of diabetic nephropathy was clearly increased in smokers. Other prospective studies have also confirmed more frequent diabetic nephropathy in smokers than non-smokers. Continued smoking has shown to be associated with further poor renal outcome as compared to persons who quit smoking. Smoking adversely affects renal hemodynamics and protein excretion even in subjects without apparent renal disease. In addition, it impairs the prognosis for renal function in patients with nondiabetic renal disease. Factors implicated in the pathogenesis of smoking-induced renal function impairment are the sympathetic activation, increased endothelin production, increased oxidative stress, and impaired endothelial cell-dependent vasodilation [6]. Cessation of smoking has been associated with slower progression of the nephropathy and, as an alone measure, may reduce the risk of progression by 30% in patients with type 2 diabetes.

Smoking and Diabetic Retinopathy (DR)

Smoking has a profound negative impact on overall eye health in diabetes [5]. Smoking has been implicated in the development and progression of numerous ocular diseases, including age-related macular degeneration, glaucoma, and cataracts. Chronic smoking has been shown to be associated with decreased retinal circulation as well as abnormalities in the retinal vessel parameters. Smoking leads to a higher incidence of and accelerated progression of diabetic retinopathy (DR) in patients with type 1 diabetes. However, in type 2 diabetes, evidence is controversial in context of smoking and DR. The Hoorn study demonstrated a nonsignificant trend for increased DR incidence in cigarette smokers as well as ex-smokers. Another, 25-year follow-up study showed a nonsignificant trend of developing more proliferative DR in current smokers. However, there was no statistically significant association between smoking status or pack-years of smoking and proliferative DR. In the same study, mild NPDR was more common among current smokers than former smokers, which may suggest that smoking is indeed related to early forms of diabetic retinopathy. However, many studies have reported no association with smoking and retinopathy in type 2 diabetes. Rather the United Kingdom Prospective Diabetes Study (UKPDS) study demonstrated a protective effect of smoking on both new development and progression of DR. Thus in type 2 patients, the effects of smoking on DR is more complex and yet to be fully elucidated [6].

Smoking and Diabetic Neuropathy

Like the association of smoking and retinopathy, there is evidence that smoking is an independent risk factor of peripheral neuropathy in patients with type 1 diabetes [7]. However, the association of smoking with neuropathy in type 2 diabetes is not clear. Surprisingly, a protective effect of smoking has been reported in few studies. In other studies with patients with type 2 diabetes, smoking was not a risk factor for the polyneuropathy or sensory neuropathy as diagnosed by symptoms and signs. A meta-analysis including 10 prospective and 28 cross-sectional studies has found that smoking had an unadjusted odds ratio of 1.26 for prospectively developing diabetic sensory polyneuropathy. In the cross-sectional studies, the pooled odds ratio for diabetic sensory polyneuropathy due to smoking was 1.42. However, for both analyses, evidence was graded as low strength. More studies are needed to evaluate the association between smoking and neuropathy [7].

Smoking and Macrovascular Complications of Diabetes

Smoking has been shown to be a significant risk factor for all-cause mortality, and for mortality due to cardiovascular disease (CVD) and coronary heart disease (CHD) in patients with diabetes.

Coronary Artery Disease

Smoking is a major risk factor for CVD in nondiabetic subjects, as well as diabetic subjects. In the London cohort of the 8-year prospective, World Health Organization Multinational Study of Vascular Disease in Diabetes, it was shown that smoking is significantly associated with an increased risk for coronary heart disease (CHD) in type 1 and type 2 diabetes patients [8]. In the Diabetes Control and Complications Trial (DCCT), designed to study the role of intensive insulin treatment and optimized glycemic control in type 1 diabetes, smoking was not a significant risk factor for macrovascular complications [9, 10]. The subjects participating in this study were young, and, thus, the DCCT was not optimally designed to study the role of tobacco use in macrovascular complications [9, 10]. Other studies in slightly older type 1 subjects with diabetes have shown that smoking does increase the risk for CHD. In type 2 subjects with diabetes, the UKPDS clearly showed that cigarette smoking is a significant and independent risk factor for CHD, stroke, as well as peripheral vascular disease [11]. In the Nurses' Health Study, in women with type 2 diabetes, it was demonstrated that smoking was associated in a dose-dependent manner with an increased mortality and CHD. The risk for mortality from all causes was 1.64 in diabetic women who smoked 15 to 34 cigarettes per day and 2.19 in women who smoked more than 34 cigarettes per day [12]. Ten years after having stopped smoking, the risk for mortality has normalized when compared with nonsmoking diabetic women. Another data has shown that compared with never-smokers, the relative risks for CHD were 1.66 for current smokers of 1 to 14 cigarettes per day and 2.68 for current smokers of 15 or more cigarettes per day [12].

A meta-analysis in the Asia-Pacific region, in men with diabetes, the hazard ratio for CHD comparing current smokers with nonsmokers was 1.42 [13]. Cigarette cessation strategies can be beneficial in terms of reducing the burden of CVD in men with diabetes [14].

A large prospective study by Chaturvedi et al. studied the effects of smoking cessation on cardiovascular risk in diabetic patients [15]. Mortality risks in previous smokers with diabetes were compared with risks for subjects who have never smoked. All-cause mortality risks were around 50% higher for patients who stopped smoking during the past 1–9 years and 25% higher in individuals who quit smoking before that, when compared with subjects who have never smoked [15]. The results from this study show that stopping smoking reduces mortality risk in diabetes, but risks still remain high several years after quitting smoking. The mortality risk with smoking in diabetes is dependent on the duration of smoking.

Smoking and Cerebrovascular Accident/ Stroke

Smoking also increases the risk of stroke in patients with diabetes, but the association may not be as strong as CHD. Smoking and HbA1c are predictors of stroke among the type 2 diabetes patients without a history of a previous stroke. In the London cohort of the 8-year prospective World Health Organization Multinational Study of Vascular Disease in Diabetes, it was shown that smoking was not significantly associated with stroke [16]. In a study using the general practice research database in the United Kingdom, smoking was an additional risk factor for stroke in type 2 diabetes patients [17]. In the Nurses' Health Study, in smokers who smoked 1 to 14 cigarettes per day, the risk was significant for CHD but not for stroke [12]. In those who smoked 15 cigarettes or more per day, the relative risks for CHD and stroke were 2.68 and 1.84, respectively [12]. Similar trends were shown in a Swedish study, in which the relative risk of smoking was higher in myocardial infarction (2.33) than for stroke (1.12) in 30- to 59-year-old patients [18].

Smoking cessation should be a main target for the prevention of CVDs in patients with type 2 diabetes and is also very cost-effective. Smoking cessation should be integrated in a multiple-risk-factor control program [19]. This was shown in the Steno-2 trial, where a decrease in smoking rate was combined with a successful decrease in other risk factors in the intensively treated group [20].

Smoking and Peripheral Artery Disease

Smoking is associated with exacerbation of peripheral artery disease in diabetes. Smoking per se is a risk factor for peripheral artery disease (Buerger's disease). The peripheral artery disease associated with smoking per se primarily affects the medium-sized arteries. In contrast, diabetes per se affects the more distal arteries and arterioles. The presence of smoking in the background of diabetes has a synergistic effect on the peripheral artery disease occurrence and progression [21]. Smoking at least one pack of cigarettes per day ([OR] 2.5; 95% CI 1.1, 6.0) was associated with a significant increase in the occurrence of symptomatic peripheral artery disease [22]. The presence of diabetes was the strongest predictor of peripheral artery disease in smokers in that study [22]. Ankle brachial index (ABI) assessment has an important role in disease severity assessment as well as prognostication (predicting cardiovascular and all-cause mortality) [21].

Smoking Cessation, Diabetes, and Technology

One of the aims of the comprehensive management plan for diabetes is to include smoking cessation plan for the patients with support from the family, friends, diabetic educator, and physician. The "5 A's"—ask, assess, advise, assist, and arrange—are five intervention steps suggested to help patients quit smoking (Box 43.1). Also, interventions to prevent relapse should be undertaken with patients who have quit smoking. Counseling and behavior therapy remain most important in helping patients quit smoking. Pharmacotherapy is often helpful with the use of nicotine replacement therapy (including nicotine patches, gum, and lozenges) and sustained-release bupropion. Patients receiving bupropion must be closely monitored for seizures and hyperglycemia. There is evidence supporting the safety and efficacy of varenicline in smokers with diabetes. However, the glycemic status must be monitored carefully in patients receiving varenicline as case reports of severe hypoglycemia in patients with type 1 diabetes exist. A meta-analysis reported that delivering structured smoking cessation interventions or medication for smoking cessation was found to have significantly better smoking abstinence rates compared to counselling or optional medication.

Box 43.1 Five Intervention Steps to Help Patients Quit Smoking

Ask: Identify active smoker/ex-smoker at each visit.
   Assess: Determine person's willingness to quit smoking.
   Advise: Strongly advise all tobacco users to quit.
   Assist: Assist patients in quitting smoking.
   Arrange: Arrange follow-up visits.

It must be highlighted that the weight gain and the associated transient mild increase in the risk of diabetes in patients who quit smoking should not be a deterrent for stopping smoking. It must be clearly highlighted to the smokers that quitting overall has a beneficial effect of quality of life and

survival. In a large community-based cohort (Framingham Offspring Study data collected from 1984 through 2011), smoking cessation was associated with a lower risk of coronary artery disease events among participants without diabetes, and weight gain that occurred following smoking cessation did not modify this association, which supports a net cardiovascular benefit of smoking cessation, despite subsequent weight gain [23].

The diagnosis and treatment of diabetes or any of its complication are potential "teachable moments" for smoking cessation as at the time of diagnosis, patients were found to have significantly higher motivation to quit.

Recent reports have suggested that the use of Internet and mobile phone-based technology (mHealth) can go a long way in promoting healthy lifestyle habits and institute positive feedback mechanism, which can help in smoking cessation as well as ensuring better glycemic control in patients with diabetes [24].

Multiple-Choice Questions

1. Which of the following is the correct statement regarding the relationship of smoking and glycemia?
   (a) Smoking is linked with increased incidence of diabetes.
   (b) Smoking is linked with increased severity of diabetes.
   (c) The risk of developing diabetes in smokers has been found to be dose dependent.
   (d) All of the above.
2. Smoking is associated most evidently with which microvascular complications in type 2 diabetes?
   (a) Retinopathy
   (b) Nephropathy
   (c) Neuropathy
   (d) Gastroparesis
3. Other than retinopathy, smoking has been implicated in the development and progression of which other ocular diseases?
   (a) Age-related macular degeneration
   (b) Glaucoma
   (c) Cataract
   (d) All of the above
4. Which of the following is a false statement regarding mortality risks in smokers with diabetes?
   (a) Remains high even several years even after quitting smoking
   (b) Dependent on duration of smoking
   (c) Increases only in type 2 diabetes persons, not in type 1 diabetes persons
   (d) Dose dependent
5. What parts are primarily affected by the peripheral artery disease associated with smoking per se?
   (a) Medium-sized arteries

(b) Distal arteries and arterioles

(c) Large arteries

(d) Capillaries

6. What parts are primarily affected by the peripheral artery disease associated with diabetes per se?

(a) Medium-sized arteries

(b) Distal arteries and arterioles

(c) Large arteries

(d) Capillaries

7. What pharmacological agents are helpful in quitting smoking?

(a) Nicotine gums/patches

(b) Sustained-release bupropion

(c) Varenicline

(d) All of the above

8. Varenicline use for smoking cessation in type 1 diabetes persons has been reported with which adverse event?

(a) Hypoglycemia

(b) Hyperglycemia

(c) Hypokalemia

(d) Hyponatremia

9. What might be associated with smoking cessation in short term?

(a) Weight gain

(b) Weight loss

(c) Increased risk of diabetes

(d) A and C

10. Which of the following statement is incorrect regarding cessation of smoking?

(a) Smoking cessation may lead to transient increase in body weight.

(b) Smoking cessation may be associated with transient mild increase in the risk of diabetes.

(c) Smoking cessation may lead to transient increased risk of coronary artery disease.

(d) B and C.

Answers

1. Option D
2. Option B
3. Option D
4. Option C
5. Option A
6. Option B
7. Option D
8. Option A
9. Option D
10. Option C

References

1. Sung YT, Hsiao CT, Chang IJ, Lin YC, Yueh CY. Smoking cessation carries a short-term rising risk for newly diagnosed diabetes mellitus independently of weight gain: a 6-year retrospective cohort study. J Diabetes Res. 2016;2016:3961756.

2. Chang CH, Chuang LM. Fetal exposure to parental smoking and the risk of type 2 diabetes: are lifestyle-related factors more important? J Diabetes Investig. 2016;7(4):472–5.

3. Ligthart S, Steenaard RV, Peters MJ, van Meurs JB, Sijbrands EJ, Uitterlinden AG, Bonder MJ, BIOS consortium, Hofman A, Franco OH, Dehghan A. Tobacco smoking is associated with DNA methylation of diabetes susceptibility genes. Diabetologia. 2016;59(5):998–1006.

4. Valdivielso P, Hidalgo A, Rioja J, Aguilar I, Ariza MJ, González-Alegre T, González-Santos P. Smoking and postprandial triglycerides are associated with vascular disease in patients with type 2 diabetes. Atherosclerosis. 2007;194(2):391–6.

5. Chang SA. Smoking and type 2 diabetes mellitus. Diabetes Metab J. 2012;36(6):399–403.

6. Haire-Joshu D, Glasgow RE, Tibbs TL. Smoking and diabetes. Diabetes Care. 1999;22(11):1887–98.

7. Ford SK, Shilliday BB. Smoking and diabetes: helping patients quit. Clin Diabetes. 2006;24:133–7.

8. Effect of intensive diabetes management on macrovascular events and risk factors in the diabetes control and complications trial. Am J Cardiol. 1995;75:894–903.

9. Sinha RN, Patrick AW, Richardson L, et al. A six-year follow-up study of smoking habits and microvascular complications in young adults with type 1 diabetes. Postgrad Med J. 1997;73:293–4.

10. Moy CS, LaPorte RE, Dorman JS, et al. Insulin-dependent diabetes mellitus mortality. The risk of cigarette smoking. Circulation. 1990;82:37–43.

11. Turner RC, Millns H, Neil HA, Stratton IM, Manley SE, Matthews DR, Holman RR. Risk factors for coronary artery disease in non-insulin dependent diabetes mellitus: United Kingdom prospective diabetes study (UKPDS: 23). BMJ. 1998;316:823–8.

12. Al-Delaimy WK, Willett WC, Manson JE, Speizer FE, Hu FB. Smoking and mortality among women with type 2 diabetes: the Nurses' health study cohort. Diabetes Care. 2001;24:2043–8.

13. Al-Delaimy WK, Manson JE, Solomon CG, Kawachi I, Stampfer MJ, Willett WC, Hu FB. Smoking and risk of coronary heart disease among women with type 2 diabetes mellitus. Arch Intern Med. 2002;162:273–9.

14. Kengne AP, Nakamura K, Barzi F, Lam TH, Huxley R, Gu D, Patel A, Kim HC, Woodward M Asia Pacific Cohort Study Collaboration. Smoking, diabetes and cardiovascular diseases in men in the Asia Pacific region. J Diabetes. 2009;1:173–81.

15. Chaturvedi N, Stevens L, Fuller JH. Which features of smoking determine mortality risk in former cigarette smokers with diabetes? The World Health Organization multinational study group. Diabetes Care. 1997;20:1266–72.

16. Giorda CB, Avogaro A, Maggini M, Lombardo F, Mannucci E, Turco S, Alegiani SS, Raschetti R, Velussi M, Ferrannini E, DAI Study Group. Incidence and risk factors for stroke in type 2 diabetic patients: the DAI study. Stroke. 2007;38:1154–60.

17. Mulnier HE, Seaman HE, Raleigh VS, Soedamah-Muthu SS, Colhoun HM, Lawrenson RA, De Vries CS. Risk of stroke in people with type 2 diabetes in the UK: a study using the general practice research database. Diabetologia. 2006;49:2859–65.

18. Nilsson PM, Cederholm J, Eeg-Olofsson K, Eliasson B, Zethelius B, Fagard R, Gudbjornsdottir S, Swedish National Diabetes Register. Smoking as an independent risk factor for myocardial infarction or stroke in type 2 diabetes: a report from the Swedish National Diabetes Register. Eur J Cardiovasc Prev Rehabil. 2009;16:506–12.

19. Hokanson JM, Anderson RL, Hennrikus DJ, Lando HA, Kendall DM. Integrated tobacco cessation counseling in a diabetes self-management training program: a randomized trial of diabetes and reduction of tobacco. Diabetes Educ. 2006;32:562–70.

20. Gaede P, Lund-Andersen H, Parving HH, Pedersen O. Effect of a multifactorial intervention on mortality in type 2 diabetes. N Engl J Med. 2008;358:580–91.

21. Vogt MT, McKenna M, Wolfson SK, Kuller LH. The relationship between ankle brachial index, other atherosclerotic disease, diabetes, smoking and mortality in older men and women. Atherosclerosis. 1993;101:191–202.

22. Eason SL, Petersen NJ, Suarez-Almazor M, Davis B, Collins TC. Diabetes mellitus, smoking, and the risk for asymptomatic peripheral arterial disease: whom should we screen? J Am Board Fam Pract. 2005;18:355–61.

23. Clair C, Rigotti NA, Porneala B, Fox CS, D'Agostino RB, Pencina MJ, Meigs JB. Association of smoking cessation and weight change with cardiovascular disease among adults with and without diabetes. JAMA. 2013;309:1014–21.

24. Rehman H, Kamal AK, Sayani S, Morris PB, Merchant AT, Virani SS. Using mobile health (mHealth) technology in the management of diabetes mellitus, physical inactivity, and smoking. Curr Atheroscler Rep. 2017;19:16.

25. Gupta N, Gupta ND, Garg S, Goyal L, Gupta A, Khan S, Moin S. The effect of type 2 diabetes mellitus and smoking on periodontal parameters and salivary matrix metalloproteinase-8 levels. J Oral Sci. 2016;58(1):1–6.

Hyperglycemic Crises: Diabetic Ketoacidosis

Bobak Moazzami, Zohyra E. Zabala, and Guillermo E. Umpierrez

Diabetic ketoacidosis (DKA) most often occurs in patients with type 1 diabetes, but many patients with type 2 diabetes may develop ketoacidosis under stressful medical and surgical conditions [1]. In contrast to popular belief, DKA is more common in adults than in children. Data from the T1D Exchange Clinic Network including 2561 patients shows that young adults (18–25 years) have the highest occurrence of DKA (~5%) defined as ≥1 event in the prior 3 months [2]. In community-based studies [1, 2], more than 40% of patients with DKA are older than 40 years, and more than 20% are older than 55 years. Worldwide, infection is the most common precipitating cause for DKA, occurring in 30–50% of cases. Other precipitating causes are intercurrent illnesses (i.e., surgery, trauma, myocardial ischemia, pancreatitis), psychological stress, and noncompliance with insulin therapy.

Treatment of patients with DKA and hyperosmolar hyperglycemic syndrome (HHS) is associated with substantial mortality and healthcare costs. DKA is the leading cause of mortality among children and young adults with T1D, accounting for ~50% of all deaths in diabetic patients younger than 24 years of age [3]. In the United States, the overall inpatient DKA mortality is <1% [3, 4], but a higher rate is reported among elderly patients with life-threatening illnesses [3–6]. Mortality increases substantially with aging, with mortality rates for those over 65–75 years reaching 20–40%. The cause of death in patients with DKA rarely results from the metabolic complications of hyperglycemia or metabolic acidosis but relates to the underlying medical illness (i.e., trauma, infection) that precipitated the ketoacidosis.

In up to 25% of patients, the initial presentation consists of combined features of DKA and HHS. Over 30% of patients have features of both DKA and HHS with most recent evidence confirming that about one out of four patients will have both conditions at the time of presentation with hyperglycemic crisis [7]. Patients presenting with this phenotype have shown to have a worse prognosis and have a higher risk of mortality (8%) compared to those with isolated hyperglycemic crises (3% for isolated DKA and 5% for isolated HHS) [8].

Pathogenesis

DKA is characterized by uncontrolled hyperglycemia, metabolic acidosis, and increased circulating total body ketone concentration. Ketoacidosis results from the lack of, or ineffectiveness of, insulin with concomitant elevation of counterregulatory hormones (glucagon, catecholamines, cortisol, and growth hormone) [9, 10]. In individuals with and without diabetes, insulin controls hepatic glucose production by suppressing hepatic gluconeogenesis and glycogenolysis. In insulin-sensitive tissues such as muscle, insulin promotes protein anabolism, glucose uptake, and glycogen synthesis and inhibits glycogenolysis and protein breakdown. In addition, insulin inhibits lipolysis, ketogenesis, and free fatty acid (FFA) [1, 10]. In contrast, counter-regulatory hormones (glucagon, catecholamines, cortisol, and growth hormone) promote metabolic pathways opposite to insulin action, both in the liver and peripheral tissues, leading to altered glucose production and disposal and increased lipolysis and the production of ketone bodies.

The pathophysiologic basis for hyperglycemia and ketoacidosis in DKA is shown in Fig. 44.1 [11]. Hyperglycemia results from increased hepatic glucose production and impaired glucose utilization in peripheral tissues. Increased gluconeogenesis results from the high availability of gluco-

B. Moazzami · Z. E. Zabala · G. E. Umpierrez (✉)
Division of Diabetes, Endocrinology and Metabolism, Emory University, Atlanta, GA, USA
e-mail: bobak.moazzami@emory.edu; zohyra.zabala@emory.edu; geumpie@emory.edu

© The Author(s), under exclusive license to Springer Nature Switzerland AG 2023
J. Rodriguez-Saldana (ed.), *The Diabetes Textbook*, https://doi.org/10.1007/978-3-031-25519-9_44

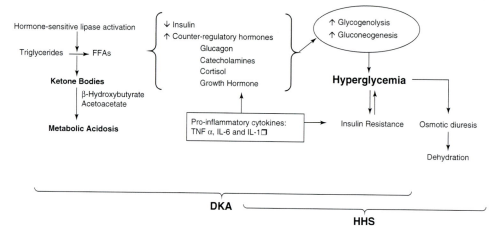

Fig. 44.1 Pathogenesis of hyperglycemic emergencies [11]. Hyperglycemia and the accumulation of ketone bodies result from a relative or absolute insulin deficiency and excess counter-regulatory hormones (glucagon, cortisol, catecholamines, and growth hormone). *Increased ketone bodies and ketoacidosis.* Decrease in insulin levels combined with increase in counter-regulatory hormones, particularly epinephrine, causes the activation of hormone-sensitive lipase in adipose tissue and breakdown of triglyceride into glycerol and free fatty acids (FFAs). In the liver, FFAs are oxidized to ketone bodies, a process predominantly stimulated by glucagon. The two major ketone bodies are β-hydroxybutyrate and acetoacetic acid. Accumulation of ketone bodies leads to a decrease in serum bicarbonate concentration and metabolic acidosis. Higher insulin levels present in HHS inhibit ketogenesis and limit metabolic acidosis. *Increased glucose production in DKA and HHS.* When insulin is deficient, hyperglycemia develops because of three processes: increased gluconeogenesis, accelerated glycogenolysis, and impaired glucose utilization by peripheral tissues. Hyperglycemia causes osmotic diuresis that leads to hypovolemia, decreased glomerular filtration rate, and worsening hyperglycemia

neogenic precursors (alanine, lactate, and glycerol) and from the increased activity of gluconeogenic enzymes (phosphoenolpyruvate carboxykinase (PEPCK), fructose-1,6-bisphosphatase, and pyruvate carboxylase) [10]. In addition, both hyperglycemia and high ketone levels cause an osmotic diuresis leading to hypovolemia and decreased glomerular filtration rate; the latter further aggravates hyperglycemia [11].

The mechanisms that underlie the increased production of ketones have been recently discussed in several reviews [1, 11]. The association of insulin deficiency and increased concentration of catecholamine, cortisol, and growth hormone causes the activation of hormone-sensitive lipase in adipose tissue. This enzyme causes endogenous triglyceride breakdown with subsequent release of large amounts of fatty acids into the circulation. Elevated FFAs are transported into the hepatic mitochondria, where they are oxidized to ketone bodies, a process predominantly stimulated by glucagon. Glucagon lowers the hepatic levels of malonyl coenzyme A (CoA), the first committed intermediate in the synthesis of long-chain fatty acids (lipogenesis) and a potent inhibitor of fatty acid oxidation. Malonyl CoA inhibits carnitine palmitoyl acyltransferase (CPTI), an enzyme that regulates the movement of FFA into the mitochondria. Therefore, reduction in malonyl CoA leads to stimulation of CPTI and effectively increases ketoacid production. In addition to increased ketone body production, there is also evidence that decreased clearance of ketoacids also contributes to the development of DKA.

Precipitating Causes

DKA is the initial manifestation of diabetes in 20–30% of patients with type 1 diabetes. In known diabetic patients, precipitating factors for DKA include infections, intercurrent illnesses, psychological stress, and noncompliance with therapy (Table 44.1). Infection is the most common precipitating factor for DKA, occurring in 30–50% of cases [1]. Urinary tract infection and pneumonia account for most infections. Other acute conditions that may precipitate DKA include cerebrovascular accident, alcohol abuse, pancreatitis, pulmonary embolism, myocardial infarction, and trauma. Drugs that affect carbohydrate metabolism such as corticosteroids, thiazides, and sympathomimetic agents may also precipitate the development of DKA.

One large retrospective review from the UK reported that hyperglycemic emergencies occurred at a rate of 1–2 per 1000 person-years following initiation of antipsychotics [13]. Of the antipsychotics, olanzapine and risperidone were associated with the highest risk [13]. Anticancer medications including immune checkpoint inhibitors such as ipilimumab, nivolumab, and pembrolizumab have been associated with newly diagnosed diabetes and DKA. Around 1% of patients taking these medications develop diabetes with half of them presenting with DKA as the first manifestation of diabetes. Patients with beta-cell autoimmunity are more susceptible to develop diabetes while taking anticancer medications [14–16].

Recently, the use of sodium glucose co-transporter 2 (SGLT2) inhibitors, a new class of oral antidiabetic agents that

Table 44.1 Causes of DKA and HHS

Precipitating cause	% of admissions	
	DKA[a]	HHS[b]
Infection	30–35	40–60
Failure to take insulin	15–40	0–35
New onset diabetes	20–25	20–25
Medical illnesses	10–20	10–15
Unknown	2–10	–

[a]Data are from refs. 2, 7, 12
[b]Data are from refs. 2, 7, 11

lowers plasma glucose by inhibiting proximal tubular reabsorption of glucose in the kidney, has been associated with DKA in patients with T1D and T2D [17–21]. An atypical presentation of DKA, which can lead to delayed recognition and treatment, has been referred to as "euglycemic DKA" due to only mild to moderate elevations in blood glucose reported in many cases. Compiled data from randomized studies with the use of SGLT2 inhibitors reported a very low incidence of DKA in patients with T2D (~0.07%) [22, 23]; however, the risk of ketosis and DKA is higher in patients with T1D. About 10% of patients with T1D treated with SGLT2 inhibitors develop ketosis, and 5% require hospital admission for DKA. Potential mechanisms have been proposed, including higher glucagon levels, reduction of daily insulin requirement leading to a decrease in the suppression of lipolysis and ketogenesis, and decreased urinary excretion of ketones [1].

The importance of noncompliance and psychological factors in the incidence of DKA has been emphasized in recent studies [24–26]. In a survey of 341 female patients with type 1 diabetes, Polonsky et al. reported that psychological problems complicated by eating disorders were a contributing factor in 20% of recurrent ketoacidosis in young women. In addition, eating disorders are reported in up to one-third of young women with type 1 diabetes. Factors that may lead to insulin omission in young subjects included fear of gaining weight with good metabolic control, fear of hypoglycemia, rebellion from authority, and diabetes-related stress. Lack of insulin treatment adherence is reported as a major precipitating cause for DKA in urban black and medically indigent patients. Many studies have reported that in urban black patients, poor compliance with insulin accounted for more than 50% of DKA cases admitted to a major urban hospital [1, 27]. Limited resources and lack of health insurance increase hospitalization rates for DKA by two- to threefold higher than comparable rates among diabetic persons with private insurance.

Although the use of continuous subcutaneous insulin infusion by an insulin pump was associated with an increased risk of DKA, recent mechanical improvements in such devices and the use of frequent home glucose monitoring have reduced this complication considerably [1]. In one of the largest prospective studies for therapy and follow-up of type 1 diabetes, the Diabetes Control and Complications Trial, the incidence of DKA was quite low in patients treated with continuous insulin infusion devices.

Ketosis-Prone Diabetes

A growing number of ketoacidosis cases have been identified in adult individuals with clinical features of type 2 diabetes that are not accompanied by precipitating factors [28]. This variant of type 2 diabetes has been referred to as ketosis-prone diabetes [29]. Patients with ketosis-prone diabetes are usually obese, have a strong family history of diabetes, and have a low prevalence of autoimmune markers [28]. The age of onset of ketosis-prone diabetes is usually in the fourth or fifth decade of life; however, the incidence has been increasing in the pediatric population. The prevalence is two- to threefold higher in men compared to women. While this entity has been reported across different ethnicities worldwide, people of African origin and Hispanics appear to have the highest risk [30]. Most patients present with a few weeks of polyuria, polydipsia, and weight loss and are found to have severe hyperglycemia accompanied with urinary ketonuria or frank DKA [31]. The clinical course of patients with ketosis-prone diabetes is different than those with chronic insulin dependence from type 1 diabetes with DKA. Many obese subjects with ketosis-prone diabetes experience near-normoglycemic remission off insulin therapy within the first few months of treatment. While at the beginning, these patients show impairments in both insulin secretion and insulin action, aggressive diabetes management results in significant improvement in β-cell function and insulin sensitivity that is usually sufficient to allow discontinuation of insulin therapy in almost 70% of individuals within a few months of treatment [32, 33].

COVID-19 and DKA

With the recent coronavirus disease 2019 (COVID-19) pandemic, there is now accumulating evidence that suggests a higher frequency and severity of DKA among those with COVID-19. A higher number of DKA admissions occurred during the COVID-19 pandemic, which was mostly seen among those with type 2 diabetes and newly diagnosed diabetes and less frequently in patients with type 1 diabetes [12]. Possible reasons for this increased DKA incidence during the pandemic include social restrictions, less access to medical care, and an increased prevalence in a sedentary lifestyle. Results from a large cohort of patients with DKA during the COVID-19 pandemic showed that patients with COVID-19 had a higher body mass index, higher insulin requirements, prolonged time to resolution of DKA, and a sixfold higher rate of mortality compared with patients without COVID-19 [34].

Diagnosis

Symptoms and Signs

Symptoms of hyperglycemia including polyuria, polydipsia, and weight loss are usually present for several days prior to the development of DKA [3, 11]. Two-thirds of patients present with weakness, nausea, vomiting, and abdominal pain [35]. Abdominal pain, sometimes mimicking an acute abdomen, is especially common in children; although the cause has not been elucidated, delayed gastric emptying and ileus induced by electrolyte disturbance and metabolic acidosis have been implicated as possible causes of abdominal pain.

Physical examination reveals signs of dehydration, including loss of skin turgor, dry mucous membranes, tachycardia, and hypotension. Mental status can vary from full alertness to profound lethargy; however, fewer than 20% of patients are hospitalized with loss of consciousness [10]. Acetone on breath and labored Kussmaul respiration may also be present on admission, particularly in patients with severe metabolic acidosis.

Laboratory Findings

The syndrome of DKA consists of the triad of hyperglycemia, ketosis, and acidemia (Table 44.2) [10]. Diagnostic criteria for DKA accepted by the American Diabetes Association are a blood glucose greater than 250 mg/dL, pH lower than 7.3, serum bicarbonate lower than 15 mEq/L, and a moderate degree of ketonemia (hydroxybutyrate and acetoacetic acid greater than 3 mmol) [3]. The key diagnostic feature is the elevation in circulating total blood ketone concentration.

Table 44.2 Diagnostic criteria for DKA

	DKA		
	Mild	Moderate	Severe
Plasma glucose (mg/dL)	>250	>250	>250
Arterial pH	7.25–7.30	7.00–<7.24	<7.00
Serum bicarbonate (mEq/L)	15–18	10–<15	<10
Urine ketone[a]	Positive	Positive	Positive
Serum ketone	Positive	Positive	Positive
Effective serum osmolality[b]	Variable	Variable	Variable mOsm/kg
Anion gap	>10	>12	>12
Alteration in sensorium	Alert	Alert/drowsy	Stupor/coma

Modified with permission from Diabetes Care from the American Diabetes Association Consensus Statement on Hyperglycemic Crises, 2009 [3]

[a] Nitroprusside reaction

[b] Effective serum osmolality: 2[measured Na$^+$ (mEq/L)] + glucose (mg/dL)/18

Table 44.3 Useful formulas for the evaluation of DKA

1. Calculation of anion gap (AG):
$$AG = [Na^+] - [Cl^- + HCO3^-]$$
2. Total and effective serum osmolality:

$$Total = 2[Na^+] + \frac{glucose(mg/dL)}{18} + \frac{BUN(mg/dL)}{2.8}$$

$$Effective = 2[Na^+] + \frac{glucose(mg/dL)}{18}$$
3. Corrected serum sodium:

$$Corrected\ [Na+] = \frac{1.6 \times glucose(mg/dL) - 100}{100} + [measured\ Na+]$$
4. Total body water (TBW) deficit:

$$TBW\ deficit = [wt\ (kg) \times 0.6] - \left[\frac{corrected\ Na^+}{140}\right] - 1$$

Assessment of ketonemia can be performed by the nitroprusside reaction, which provides a semiquantitative estimation of acetoacetate and acetone levels, or by direct measurement of beta-hydroxybutyrate, the main ketoacid in DKA.

Accumulation of ketoacids results in an increased anion gap metabolic acidosis. The anion gap is calculated by subtracting the sum of chloride and bicarbonate from the sodium concentration [Na-(Cl + HCO$_3$)]. The normal anion gap is 12 ± 2 mEq/L (Table 44.3).

Not all patients who present with ketoacidosis have DKA. Patients with chronic ethanol abuse with a recent binge culminating in vomiting and acute starvation may develop alcoholic ketoacidosis (AKA). The key difference between AKA and DKA is the concentration of blood glucose. DKA is characterized by severe hyperglycemia; the presence of ketoacidosis without hyperglycemia in an alcoholic patient suggests AKA. In addition, some patients with decreased food intake lower than 500 calories/day may present with starvation ketosis. The diagnosis of starvation ketosis is suggested by a history of poor intake and the fact that it rarely presents with a serum bicarbonate concentration less than 18 mEq/L [10].

The following laboratory findings should be kept in mind in patients admitted with suspected or confirmed DKA. Leukocytosis is present in most patients with DKA; however, a leukocyte count greater than 25,000 mm^3 or the presence of greater than 10% neutrophil bands is seldom seen in the absence of bacterial infection [10]. The admission serum sodium is usually low because of the osmotic flux of water from the intracellular to the extracellular space in the presence of hyperglycemia. An increase in serum sodium concentration in the presence of hyperglycemia indicates a rather profound degree of water loss. To assess the severity of sodium and water deficit, serum sodium may be corrected by adding 1.6 mg/dL to the measured serum sodium for each 100 mg/dL of glucose above 100 mg/dL [36]. The admission serum potassium concentration is usually elevated in patients with DKA. These high levels occur because of a shift of potassium from the intracellular to the extracellular space due to acidemia, insulin deficiency, and hypertonicity.

Treatment

The American Diabetes Association algorithm for the management of hyperglycemic emergencies is shown in Fig. 44.2 [3]. Successful treatment of DKA requires frequent monitoring of patients, correction of hypovolemia and metabolic disorder, and careful search for the precipitating cause for DKA. Most patients with uncomplicated DKA can be treated in the emergency department or in step-down units, if close nursing supervision and monitoring are available. Several studies have failed to demonstrate clear benefits in treating DKA patients in the intensive care unit (ICU) compared to step-down units [37–39]. The mortality rate, length of hospital stay, and time to resolve ketoacidosis are similar between patients treated in ICU and non-ICU settings. In addition, ICU admission has been associated with more laboratory testing and higher hospitalization cost in patients with DKA [37, 40].

Patients with mild to moderate DKA can be safely managed in the emergency department or in step-down units, and only patients with severe DKA or those with a critical illness as precipitating cause (i.e., myocardial infarction, gastrointestinal bleeding, sepsis) [3, 41] should be treated in the ICU. Patients with altered mental status and comatose state have higher mortality than alert patients and should be managed in the ICU.

Fluid Therapy

All patients with DKA are volume depleted (fluid deficit ~5–8 L) requiring aggressive fluid resuscitation to restore intravascular volume and renal perfusion. Isotonic saline (0.9% NaCl) is infused at a rate of 500–1000 mL/h during the first 2 h, but larger volume may be required in patients with hypovolemic shock to restore normal blood pressure and tissue perfusion. After intravascular volume depletion has been corrected, the rate of normal saline infusion should be reduced to 250 mL/h or changed to 0.45% saline depending upon the serum sodium concentration. The free water deficit can be estimated, based on corrected serum sodium concentration, using the following equation: water deficit = (0.6)(body weight in kilograms) × (1 − [corrected sodium/140]) [10]. The goal is to replace half the estimated water deficit over a period of 12–24 h.

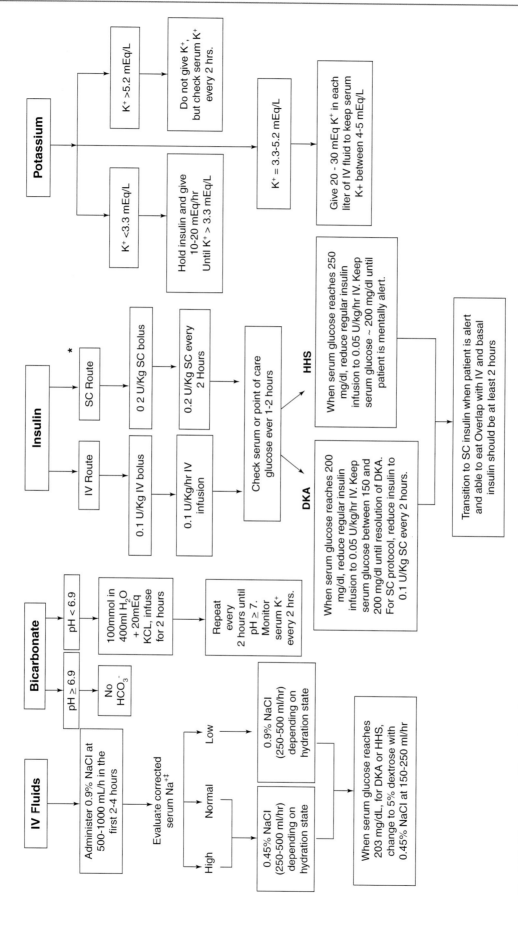

Fig. 44.2 Management of hyperglycemic emergencies [3]. *Subcutaneous Insulin Protocol has not been validated for HHS (Modified with permission from Diabetes Care from the American Diabetes Association Consensus Statement on Hyperglycemic Crises, 2009 [3])

Once the plasma glucose reaches 250 mg/dL, replacement fluids should contain 5–10% dextrose to allow continued insulin administration until ketonemia is controlled while avoiding hypoglycemia [3]. An important aspect of fluid management in patients with DKA is to replace the volume of urinary losses. Failure to adjust fluid replacement for urinary losses may delay the correction of electrolytes and water deficit.

Capillary blood glucose testing should be determined during treatment every 1–2 h at the bedside using a glucose oxidase reagent strip; and blood should be drawn every 4 h for determination of serum electrolytes, glucose, blood urea nitrogen, creatinine, magnesium, phosphorus, and venous pH until resolution of ketoacidosis.

Insulin Therapy

Insulin therapy is the cornerstone of DKA management. Insulin lowers blood glucose concentration by increasing peripheral glucose utilization and reducing hepatic glucose production. In addition, insulin therapy inhibits lipolysis and the release of free fatty acid from adipose tissue and decreases ketogenesis.

Regular insulin given intravenously by continuous infusion remains the drug of choice. Intermittent infusion or hourly boluses of low-dose intravenous insulin should be avoided because of regular insulin's [3] short half-life. The American Diabetes Association recommends an initial intravenous bolus of regular insulin of 0.1 units/kg of body weight, followed by a continuous infusion of regular insulin at a dose of 0.1 units/kg per hour until blood glucose levels reach 250 mg/dL [1]. Once glucose is lower than 250 mg/dL, dextrose should be added to intravenous fluids, and the insulin infusion rate is reduced to 0.05 units/kg per hour. Thereafter, the rate of insulin administration should be adjusted to maintain glucose levels at approximately 150–200 mg/dL and continued until ketoacidosis is resolved. Resolution of hyperglycemia takes about 4–6 h, but resolution of ketoacidosis takes longer (~10–14 h); thus, dextrose is needed to allow insulin infusion and the prevention of hypoglycemia [10].

Several studies and a meta-analysis have reported that the administration of hourly or every 2 h doses of subcutaneous rapid-insulin analogs (lispro and aspart) represents an effective alternative to the intravenous infusion of regular insulin [42–44]. The administration of an insulin subcutaneous bolus of 0.2–0.3 U/kg followed by 0.1–0.2 U/kg every 1–2 h, respectively, until glucose is <250 mg/dL. The dose is then reduced by half to 0.05 U/kg every 1 h or 0.01 U/kg every 2 h until resolution of DKA [42, 45]. Using scheduled subcutaneous insulin allows for safe and effective treatment in the emergency room and step-down units without the need for ICU care in patients with mild or moderate DKA. The use of intramuscular injections of rapid-acting insulin is also effective in the treatment of DKA, but this route tends to be more painful than subcutaneous injection and might increase the risk of bleeding among patients receiving anticoagulation therapy [1, 46]. The use of rapid-acting subcutaneous insulin analogs is not recommended for patients with severe and complicated DKA.

Potassium

An estimated total body potassium deficit of ~3–5 mEq/kg of body weight has been reported in adult patients with DKA [10]; however, most patients present with normal or high serum potassium. With initiation of insulin and fluid therapy, the extracellular potassium concentration invariable falls. Insulin therapy and correction of acidosis decrease serum potassium levels by stimulating cellular potassium uptake in peripheral tissues. Therefore, all patients require intravenous potassium to prevent hypokalemia.

The American Diabetes Association recommends the administration of intravenous potassium chloride (20–30 mEq/L) as soon as the serum potassium concentration is below 5.5 mEq/L. The treatment goal is to maintain serum potassium levels within the normal range of 4–5 mEq/L. A presentation with severe hypokalemia may be aggravated during insulin administration, which can induce life-threatening arrhythmias and respiratory muscle weakness. Thus, if the initial serum potassium is equal or lower than 3.0 mEq/L, potassium replacement should be given for 1–2 h at a rate of 10–20 mEq per hour, before insulin infusion is started.

Bicarbonate

Bicarbonate administration in patients with DKA is rarely indicated. Several controlled studies have failed to show any benefit from bicarbonate therapy in patients with DKA and arterial pH between 6.9 and 7.1 [3, 10]. Despite the lack of evidence, most experts in the field recommend that in patients with severe metabolic acidosis (pH < 6.9–7.0), 44.6 mEq of sodium bicarbonate should be added to a liter of hypotonic saline until pH rises to at least 7.0. In patients with arterial pH ≥ 7.0, no bicarbonate therapy is necessary.

Phosphate

Total body phosphate deficiency is present in most patients with DKA. Similar to studies with bicarbonate replacement, several studies have failed to show any beneficial effect of phosphate replacement on clinical outcome [3, 10]. Aggressive phosphate therapy may be potentially hazardous, as indicated in case reports of children with DKA who developed hypocalcemia and tetany secondary to intravenous phosphate administration. Careful phosphate replacement may be indicated in patients with cardiac dysfunction, anemia, respiratory depression, and in those with serum phosphate concentration lower than 1.0–1.5 mg/dL. If phosphate replacement is needed, it should be administered as a potassium salt, by giving half as potassium phosphate and half as potassium chloride. In such patients, because of the risk of hypocalcemia, serum calcium and phosphate levels must be monitored during phosphate infusion.

Transition to Subcutaneous Insulin

Patients with DKA should be treated with continuous intravenous or frequent subcutaneous insulin administration until ketoacidosis is resolved. Criteria for resolution of DKA include a blood glucose lower than 200 mg/dL, a serum bicarbonate level equal to or greater than 18 mEq/L, a venous pH greater than 7.3, and a calculated anion gap equal to or lower than 14 mEq/L [3, 10].

The half-life of insulin is <10 min [47]; thus, abrupt cessation of the insulin may result in rebound hyperglycemia, ketogenesis, and recurrent metabolic acidosis. Subcutaneous insulin should be given at least 2 h before discontinuing the intravenous insulin infusion [3]. The initial dose of NPH should be given 2 h before stopping insulin infusion. Earlier initiation 3–4 h before discontinuation of insulin drip should be considered when using basal insulin analogs (glargine, detemir, degludec), which have a longer delay in onset of action than NPH insulin. One randomized controlled trial evaluated the effect of co-administration of IV insulin with subcutaneous glargine shortly after the onset of treatment of DKA compared to IV insulin alone [48]. Patients who received glargine had slightly shorter time to resolution of DKA and shorter hospital stay; however, these differences were not statistically significant [48]. Another study found that the administration of basal insulin analogs early during treatment (more than 4 h) could reduce the frequency of rebound hyperglycemia after transition off insulin drip [49].

Patients with known diabetes may be given insulin at the dosage they were receiving before the onset of DKA. In patients with newly diagnosed diabetes, an initial insulin total insulin dose of 0.6 units/kg/day is usually sufficient to achieve and maintain metabolic control.

The use of insulin analogs in a basal-bolus regimen is the preferred insulin regimen and has been shown to reduce the risk of hypoglycemia compared to human insulin (NPH and regular) regimen [50]. If insulin analogs are used, the total daily dose is given 50% as basal (glargine, detemir, degludec) once daily at the same time of the day and 50% as prandial insulin 150–15 min before meals. If a patient is to be treated with NPH/regular insulin combination, the total daily dose should be given two-thirds in the morning and one-third in the evening as a split-mixed dose consisting of two-thirds of NPH and one-third of regular insulin.

Prevention

Patient education and the implementation of protocols aiming to acute and maintenance insulin administration after discharge may reduce lapses in treatment and are cost-effective ways to reduce the future risk of hospitalization for hyperglycemic emergencies [11]. Systems-based methods to reduce preventable causes of hyperglycemic emergencies may represent an important next step in reducing costs and improving patient care.

The frequency of hospitalizations for DKA has been reduced following diabetes education programs, improved follow-up care, and access to medical advice. The alarming frequency of insulin discontinuation due to economic reasons as the precipitating cause for DKA in low economic populations illustrates the need for health care legislation for reimbursement for medications to treat diabetes.

Home blood ketone monitoring, which measures beta-hydroxybutyrate levels on a fingerstick blood specimen, is commercially available ketones. Clinical studies have shown that elevation of beta-hydroxybutyrate levels is common in patients with poorly controlled diabetes and may allow early recognition of impending ketoacidosis, which may help to guide insulin therapy at home, and, possibly, may prevent hospitalization for DKA.

Multiple Choice Questions

1. Triad that is characteristic of diabetic ketoacidosis:
   (a) *Hyperglycemia, ketosis, and acidemia.*
   (b) Frequent urination, thirst, hunger.
   (c) Hyperglycemia, weight loss, fatigue.
   (d) High levels of hyperglycemia, dehydration, hyper-osmolality.
   (e) Hyperglycemia, depression of alert, unresponsiveness.
2. The key diagnostic feature of diabetic ketoacidosis:
   (a) Hyperglycemia.
   (b) Dehydration.
   (c) Confusion, stupor, and coma.
   (d) Polyuria.

(e) *Ketonemia.*

3. Which is the most common precipitating cause for diabetic ketoacidosis?
   (a) Insufficient insulin dose.
   (b) *Infection.*
   (c) Excessive food intake.
   (d) Psychological stress.
   (e) Noncompliance with therapy.

4. Ketoacidosis results from:
   (a) *Lack of or ineffectiveness of insulin and elevation of counter-regulatory hormones.*
   (b) Accelerated immune attack on beta-cells.
   (c) Increasing demands of insulin.
   (d) Low C-peptide levels.
   (e) Low compliance of patients.

5. Antidiabetic agents associated with diabetic ketoacidosis:
   (a) Metformin.
   (b) Sulfonylureas.
   (c) Glitazones.
   (d) DPP-4 inhibitors.
   (e) *SGLT2 inhibitors.*

6. Clinical symptoms of diabetic ketoacidosis include:
   (a) *Polyuria.*
   (b) *Polydipsia.*
   (c) *Weight loss.*
   (d) *Abdominal pain.*
   (e) *Labored Kussmaul respiration.*

7. The requirements for the successful treatment of diabetic ketoacidosis include:
   (a) Frequent monitoring.
   (b) Rehydration.
   (c) Insulin.
   (d) Investigating and correcting the cause.
   (e) *All of the above.*

8. The correct formula to estimate corrected serum sodium:
   (a) Corrected [Na+] = $\dfrac{6.1 \times \text{glucose}\left(\text{mg}/\text{dL}\right) + 100}{100}$ + [measured Na+].

   (b) Corrected [Na+] = $\dfrac{6.1 \times \text{glucose}\left(\text{mg}/\text{dL}\right) - 100}{100}$ + [measured Na+].

   (c) *Corrected [Na+] = $\dfrac{1.6 \times glucose\left(mg/dL\right) - 100}{100}$ + [measured Na+].*

   (d) Corrected [Na+] = $\dfrac{1.5 \times \text{glucose}\left(\text{mg}/\text{dL}\right) + 100}{100}$ + [measured Na+].

   (e) Corrected [Na+] = $\dfrac{6.1 \times \text{glucose}\left(\text{mg}/\text{dL}\right) + 200}{100}$ + [measured Na+].

9. Regarding insulin therapy, the American Diabetes Association recommends:
   (a) *An initial intravenous bolus of regular insulin of 0.1 units/kg of body weight, followed by a continuous infusion of regular insulin at a dose of 0.1 units/kg per hour until blood glucose levels reach 250 mg/dL.*
   (b) An initial intravenous bolus of intermediate-acting insulin of 0.1 units/kg of body weight, followed by a continuous infusion of long-acting insulin at a dose of 0.1 units/kg per hour until blood glucose levels reach 250 mg/dL.
   (c) An initial intravenous bolus of regular insulin of 1 units/kg of body weight, followed by a continuous infusion of regular insulin at a dose of 1 units/kg per hour until blood glucose levels reach 100 mg/dL.
   (d) An initial intravenous bolus of regular insulin of 10 units, followed by a continuous infusion of regular insulin at a dose of 1 units/kg per hour until blood glucose levels reach 150 mg/dL.
   (e) An initial intravenous bolus of insulin lispro of 1 units/kg of body weight, followed by a continuous infusion of regular insulin at a dose of 1 units/kg per hour until blood glucose levels reach 250 mg/dL.

10. Criteria for resolution of diabetic ketoacidosis include:
    (a) Blood glucose lower than 300 mg/dL, a serum bicarbonate level equal to or greater than 18 mEq/L, a venous pH greater than 3.7, and a calculated anion gap equal to or lower than 41 mEq/L.
    (b) *A blood glucose lower than 200 mg/dL, a serum bicarbonate level equal to or greater than 18 mEq/L, a venous pH greater than 7.3, and a calculated anion gap equal to or lower than 14 mEq/L.*
    (c) A blood glucose lower than 200 mg/dL, a serum bicarbonate level equal to or greater than 18 mEq/L, a venous pH greater than 7.4, and a calculated anion gap equal to or lower than 14 mEq/L.
    (d) A blood glucose lower than 150 mg/dL, a serum bicarbonate level equal to or greater than 18 mEq/L, a venous pH greater than 7.4, and a calculated anion gap equal to or lower than 14 mEq/L.
    (e) A blood glucose lower than 120 mg/dL, a serum bicarbonate level equal to or greater than 18 mEq/L, a venous pH greater than 7.4, and a calculated anion gap equal to or lower than 14 mEq/L.

References

1. Umpierrez G, Korytkowski M. Diabetic emergencies - ketoacidosis, hyperglycaemic hyperosmolar state and hypoglycaemia. Nat Rev Endocrinol. 2016;12(4):222–32.

2. Miller KM, Foster NC, Beck RW, et al. Current state of type 1 diabetes treatment in the U.S.: updated data from the T1D exchange clinic registry. Diabetes Care. 2015;38(6):971–8.

3. Kitabchi AE, Umpierrez GE, Miles JM, Fisher JN. Hyperglycemic crises in adult patients with diabetes. Diabetes Care. 2009;32(7):1335–43.

4. Centers for Disease Control and Prevention. Mortality due to Hyperglycemic crises. http://www.cdc.gov/diabetes/statistics/complications_national.htm. 11/19/2013. Accessed 2 Sept 2016.

5. Basu A, Close CF, Jenkins D, Krentz AJ, Nattrass M, Wright AD. Persisting mortality in diabetic ketoacidosis. Diabet Med. 1993;10(3):282–4.

6. Malone ML, Gennis V, Goodwin JS. Characteristics of diabetic ketoacidosis in older versus younger adults. J Am Geriatr Soc. 1992;40(11):1100–4.

7. Kitabchi AE, Nyenwe EA. Hyperglycemic crises in diabetes mellitus: diabetic ketoacidosis and hyperglycemic hyperosmolar state. Endocrinol Metab Clin N Am. 2006;35(4):725–51. viii

8. Pasquel FJ, Tsegka K, Wang H, et al. Clinical outcomes in patients with isolated or combined diabetic ketoacidosis and hyperosmolar hyperglycemic state: a retrospective, hospital-based cohort study. Diabetes Care. 2020;43(2):349–57.

9. Chupin M, Charbonnel B, Chupin F. C-peptide blood levels in keto-acidosis and in hyperosmolar non-ketotic diabetic coma. Acta Diabetol Lat. 1981;18(2):123–8.

10. Kitabchi AE, Umpierrez GE, Murphy MB, et al. Management of hyperglycemic crises in patients with diabetes. Diabetes Care. 2001;24(1):131–53.

11. Fayfman M, Pasquel FJ, Umpierrez GE. Management of Hyperglycemic Crises: diabetic ketoacidosis and hyperglycemic hyperosmolar state. Med Clin North Am. 2017;101(3):587–606.

12. Li J, Wang X, Chen J, Zuo X, Zhang H, Deng A. COVID-19 infection may cause ketosis and ketoacidosis. Diabetes Obes Metab. 2020;22(10):1935–41.

13. Lipscombe LL, Austin PC, Alessi-Severini S, et al. Atypical antipsychotics and hyperglycemic emergencies: multicentre, retrospective cohort study of administrative data. Schizophr Res. 2014;154(1–3):54–60.

14. Clotman K, Janssens K, Specenier P, Weets I, De Block CEM. Programmed cell Death-1 inhibitor-induced type 1 diabetes mellitus. J Clin Endocrinol Metab. 2018;103(9):3144–54.

15. Liu J, Zhou H, Zhang Y, et al. Reporting of immune checkpoint inhibitor therapy-associated diabetes, 2015-2019. Diabetes Care. 2020;43(7):e79–80.

16. Wright JJ, Salem JE, Johnson DB, et al. Increased reporting of immune checkpoint inhibitor-associated diabetes. Diabetes Care. 2018;41(12):e150–1.

17. Peters AL, Buschur EO, Buse JB, Cohan P, Diner JC, Hirsch IB. Euglycemic diabetic ketoacidosis: a potential complication of treatment with sodium-glucose Cotransporter 2 inhibition. Diabetes Care. 2015;38(9):1687–93.

18. Taylor SI, Blau JE, Rother KI. Perspective: SGLT2 inhibitors may predispose to ketoacidosis. J Clin Endocrinol Metab. 2015;jc20151884. https://doi.org/10.1210/jc.2015-1884

19. Bamgboye AO, Oni IO, Collier A. Predisposing factors for the development of diabetic ketoacidosis with lower than anticipated glucose levels in type 2 diabetes patients on SGLT2-inhibitors: a review. Eur J Clin Pharmacol. 2021;77(5):651–7.

20. Ata F, Yousaf Z, Khan AA, et al. SGLT-2 inhibitors associated euglycemic and hyperglycemic DKA in a multicentric cohort. Sci Rep. 2021;11(1):10293.

21. Fralick M, Redelmeier DA, Patorno E, et al. Identifying risk factors for diabetic ketoacidosis associated with SGLT2 inhibitors: a Nationwide cohort study in the USA. J Gen Intern Med. 2021;36(9):2601–7.

22. Erondu N, Desai M, Ways K, Meininger G. Diabetic ketoacidosis and related events in the Canagliflozin type 2 diabetes clinical program. Diabetes Care. 2015;38(9):1680–6.

23. Tang H, Li D, Wang T, Zhai S, Song Y. Effect of sodium-glucose Cotransporter 2 inhibitors on diabetic ketoacidosis among patients with type 2 diabetes: a meta-analysis of randomized controlled trials. Diabetes Care. 2016;39(8):e123–4.

24. Barnard KD, Skinner TC, Peveler R. The prevalence of co-morbid depression in adults with type 1 diabetes: systematic literature review. Diabet Med. 2006;23(4):445–8.

25. Canadian Diabetes Association Clinical Practice Guidelines Expert Committee, Goguen J, Gilbert J. Hyperglycemic emergencies in adults. Can J Diabetes. 2013;37 Suppl 1:S72–6.

26. Randall L, Begovic J, Hudson M, et al. Recurrent diabetic ketoacidosis in inner-city minority patients: behavioral, socioeconomic, and psychosocial factors. Diabetes Care. 2011;34(9):1891–6.

27. Umpierrez GE, Kelly JP, Navarrete JE, Casals MM, Kitabchi AE. Hyperglycemic crises in urban blacks. Arch Intern Med. 1997;157(6):669–75.

28. Smiley D, Chandra P, Umpierrez GE. Update on diagnosis, pathogenesis and management of ketosis-prone type 2 diabetes mellitus. Diabetes Manag (Lond). 2011;1(6):589–600.

29. Umpierrez GE, Woo W, Hagopian WA, et al. Immunogenetic analysis suggests different pathogenesis for obese and lean African-Americans with diabetic ketoacidosis. Diabetes Care. 1999;22(9):1517–23.

30. Lebovitz HE, Banerji MA. Ketosis-prone diabetes (Flatbush diabetes): an emerging worldwide clinically important entity. Curr Diab Rep. 2018;18(11):120–0.

31. Vellanki P, Umpierrez GE. Diabetic ketoacidosis: a common debut of diabetes among African Americans with type 2 diabetes. Endocr Pract. 2017;23(8):971–8.

32. Balasubramanyam A, Zern JW, Hyman DJ, Pavlik V. New profiles of diabetic ketoacidosis: type 1 vs type 2 diabetes and the effect of ethnicity. Arch Intern Med. 1999;159(19):2317–22.

33. Umpierrez GE. Ketosis-prone type 2 diabetes. Time to revise the classification of diabetes. Diabetes Care. 2006;29(12):2755–7.

34. Pasquel FJ, Messler J, Booth R, et al. Characteristics of and mortality associated with diabetic ketoacidosis among US patients hospitalized with or without COVID-19. JAMA Netw Open. 2021;4(3):e211091.

35. Umpierrez G, Freire AX. Abdominal pain in patients with hyperglycemic crises. J Crit Care. 2002;17(1):63–7.

36. Kinney GL, Akturk HK, Taylor DD, Foster NC, Shah VN. Cannabis use is associated with increased risk for diabetic ketoacidosis in adults with type 1 diabetes: findings from the T1D exchange clinic registry. Diabetes Care. 2020;43(1):247–9.

37. May ME, Young C, King J. Resource utilization in treatment of diabetic ketoacidosis in adults. Am J Med Sci. 1993;306(5):287–94.

38. Moss JM. Diabetic ketoacidosis: effective low-cost treatment in a community hospital. South Med J. 1987;80(7):875–81.

39. Umpierrez GE, Latif KA, Cuervo R, Karabell A, Freire AX, Kitabchi AE. Subcutaneous aspart insulin: a safe and cost effective treatment of diabetic ketoacidosis. Diabetes. 2003;52(Suppl 1):584A.

40. Javor KA, Kotsanos JG, McDonald RC, Baron AD, Kesterson JG, Tierney WM. Diabetic ketoacidosis charges relative to medical charges of adult patients with type I diabetes. Diabetes Care. 1997;20(3):349–54.

41. Glaser NS, Ghetti S, Casper TC, Dean JM, Kuppermann N, Pediatric Emergency Care Applied Research Network DKAFSG. Pediatric diabetic ketoacidosis, fluid therapy, and cerebral injury: the

design of a factorial randomized controlled trial. Pediatr Diabetes. 2013;14(6):435–46.

42. Umpierrez GE, Latif K, Stoever J, et al. Efficacy of subcutaneous insulin lispro versus continuous intravenous regular insulin for the treatment of patients with diabetic ketoacidosis. Am J Med. 2004;117(5):291–6.

43. Ersoz HO, Ukinc K, Kose M, et al. Subcutaneous lispro and intravenous regular insulin treatments are equally effective and safe for the treatment of mild and moderate diabetic ketoacidosis in adult patients. Int J Clin Pract. 2006;60(4):429–33.

44. Karoli R, Fatima J, Salman T, Sandhu S, Shankar R. Managing diabetic ketoacidosis in non-intensive care unit setting: role of insulin analogs. Indian J Pharmacol. 2011;43(4):398–401.

45. Umpierrez GE, Cuervo R, Karabell A, Latif K, Freire AX, Kitabchi AE. Treatment of diabetic ketoacidosis with subcutaneous insulin aspart. Diabetes Care. 2004;27(8):1873–8.

46. Kitabchi AE, Ayyagari V, Guerra SM. The efficacy of low-dose versus conventional therapy of insulin for treatment of diabetic ketoacidosis. Ann Intern Med. 1976;84(6):633–8.

47. Hipszer B, Joseph J, Kam M. Pharmacokinetics of intravenous insulin delivery in humans with type 1 diabetes. Diabetes Technol Ther. 2005;7(1):83–93.

48. Doshi P, Potter AJ, De Los SD, Banuelos R, Darger BF, Chathampally Y. Prospective randomized trial of insulin glargine in acute management of diabetic ketoacidosis in the emergency department: a pilot study. Acad Emerg Med. 2015;22(6):657–62.

49. Hsia E, Seggelke S, Gibbs J, et al. Subcutaneous administration of glargine to diabetic patients receiving insulin infusion prevents rebound hyperglycemia. J Clin Endocrinol Metab. 2012;97(9):3132–7.

50. Umpierrez GE, Jones S, Smiley D, et al. Insulin analogs versus human insulin in the treatment of patients with diabetic ketoacidosis: a randomized controlled trial. Diabetes Care. 2009;32(7):1164–9.

51. Benoit SR, Hora I, Pasquel FJ, Gregg EW, Albright AL, Imperatore G. Trends in emergency department visits and inpatient admissions for hyperglycemic crises in adults with diabetes in the U.S., 2006-2015. Diabetes Care. 2020;43(5):1057–64.

Hypoglycemia: Diagnosis, Management, and Prevention

45

Raquel N. Faradji, Ana C. Uribe-Wiechers, and Elena Sainz de la Maza

Objectives

To know:

- The definition and classification of hypoglycemia
- The normal physiologic counterregulatory response to hypoglycemia and glycemic thresholds
- The altered counterregulatory responses to hypoglycemia
  - T1D
  - Long-standing T2D
  - Hypoglycemia unawareness
  - Hypoglycemia-associated autonomic failure
- The epidemiology of hypoglycemia
- The detection, diagnosis, and causes of hypoglycemia
- The risk factors of hypoglycemia
- The treatment of hypoglycemia

- The strategies to reduce or prevent hypoglycemia
- The technology in the reduction and prevention of hypoglycemia
- Beta cell replacement for the treatment of severe hypoglycemia

Introduction

Hypoglycemia is one of the most important barriers to achieve optimal glycemic management in the treatment of diabetes. It may cause potentially incapacitating and life-threatening events in patients with type 1 diabetes (T1D) and long-standing type 2 diabetes (T2D). It precludes patients from reaching euglycemia, limiting the benefits of tight control. Patients may develop unawareness of hypoglycemic symptoms due to blunted responses resulting from recurrent episodes of hypoglycemia posing them into grave danger.

Hypoglycemia Definition and Classification

The ADA (American Diabetes Association) defined hypoglycemia in patients with diabetes as "all episodes of abnormally low plasma glucose concentration that expose the individual to potential harm." The International Hypoglycemia Study Group, endorsed by the ADA, and the European Association for the Study of Diabetes define hypoglycemia in three levels (Table 45.1) [1, 3, 4].

Level 1 Measurable glucose concentration of <70 mg/dL (3.9 mmol/L) or less but >54 mg/dL (3.0 mml/L). A blood glucose level concentration of 70 mg/dL has been recognized as a threshold for neuroendocrine response to falling glucose in people without diabetes. It is considered clinically important

R. N. Faradji (✉)
Clinica EnDi SC, Mexico City, Mexico

RENACED Diabetes Tipo 1, Mexico City, Mexico

Centro Medico ABC, Mexico City, Mexico

Sociedad Mexicana de Nutrición y Endocrinología, Mexico City, Mexico

A. C. Uribe-Wiechers
Clinica EnDi SC, Mexico City, Mexico

Centro Medico ABC, Mexico City, Mexico

Sociedad Mexicana de Nutrición y Endocrinología, Mexico City, Mexico

Cardiometabolic diseases, Escuela de Medicina TEC-ABC, Tecnologico de Monterrey, Mexico City, Mexico

E. S. de la Maza
Clinica EnDi SC, Mexico City, Mexico

RENACED Diabetes Tipo 1, Mexico City, Mexico

© The Author(s), under exclusive license to Springer Nature Switzerland AG 2023
J. Rodriguez-Saldana (ed.), *The Diabetes Textbook*, https://doi.org/10.1007/978-3-031-25519-9_45

Table 45.1 Levels of hypoglycemia

Level	Description	Glycemic criteria	Description
1	Hypoglycemia alert	≤70 mg/dL	Sufficiently low for treatment with fast acting carbohydrates and dose adjustment of glucose-lowering therapy
2	Clinically relevant	≤54 mg/dL	Sufficiently low to indicate serious, clinically important hypoglycemia
3	Severe hypoglycemia		Hypoglycemia associated with severe impairment requiring external assistance for recovery

Adapted from [1, 2]

Table 45.2 Clinical classification of hypoglycemia in diabetes

Severe	Requiring assistance of another individual to administer carbohydrates, glucagon, or rescue therapy.
Symptomatic	Typical symptoms of hypoglycemia are accompanied by a measured plasma glucose concentration <70 mg/dL (3.9 mmol/dL)
Asymptomatic	Not accompanied by typical symptoms of hypoglycemia but the measured plasma glucose is <70 mg/dL (3.9 mmol/dL)
Probable	Symptoms typical of hypoglycemia are present but a measured plasma glucose of <70 mg/dL (3.9 mmol/dL) could not be determined
Pseudo-hypoglycemia	A person reports symptoms of hypoglycemia, but the plasma glucose concentration is >70 mg/dL (3.9 mmol/dL)

Adapted from [4]

(independent of the severity of acute hypoglycemic symptoms) and requires attention to prevent hypoglycemia [2].

Level 2 Defined as a glucose concentration <54 mg/dL (3.0 mml/L), it indicates serious clinically important hypoglycemia. It is the threshold at which neuroglycopenic symptoms begin to occur and requires immediate action to resolve the hypoglycemic event. These low levels may lead to defective hormonal counterregulation and impaired awareness of hypoglycemia. This clinical scenario warrants investigation and review of the medical regimen.

Level 3 Defined as a severe event characterized by altered mental status and/or physical functioning that requires assistance from another person for recovery. A subgroup of severe hypoglycemia is *severe hypoglycemic coma*, which is described as a severe hypoglycemic event resulting in coma or convulsions requiring parenteral therapy [2, 5].

The clinical classification of hypoglycemia includes severe, symptomatic, asymptomatic, probable, and pseudo-hypoglycemia (Table 45.2).

Physiology of Hypoglycemia

Glucose is the predominant metabolic source of energy for the brain, as it requires a constant and adequate supply of glucose. Under normal post-absorptive conditions, the brain accounts for 65% of whole-body glucose. The brain cannot synthesize nor store glucose under normal physiologic conditions but can adapt and utilize other substrates. Thus, during periods of fasting, ketone bodies, lactate, and alanine can be used as alternative brain fuels [6, 7].

> **Decreased Glucose Uptake by the Brain**
> - When blood glucose drops to 65–70 mg/dL (3.6–3.0 mmol/L), brain glucose uptake falls.
> - At 54 mg/dL (3.0 mmol/L), the blood-to-brain glucose transport becomes rate limiting for brain glucose metabolism [7].

Normal Glucose Counterregulation

In defense against declining plasma glucose concentrations, several physiological mechanisms have evolved to prevent and correct hypoglycemia [6].

First Defense

Inhibition of endogenous insulin secretion. Insulin is the principal physiological factor that lowers plasma glucose. Insulin is secreted primarily in response to glucose, but amino acids, non-esterified fatty acids, adrenergic stimulation, and acetylcholine can also activate its secretion. Insulin secretion can be inhibited by hypoglycemia, insulin itself, somatostatin, and adrenergic activity [7].

Secondary Defense

Increased glucagon release. Glucagon is released from the alpha cells in the islet of Langerhans. The factors that stimulate its release include hypoglycemia, amino acids, catecholamines (epinephrine and norepinephrine), and free fatty acids. Inhibition of glucagon release includes insulin and somatostatin. Glucagon's physiologic actions are restricted almost exclusively by the liver, stimulating a rapid increase in hepatic production over a period of 10–15 min. The initial rise in glucose output is provided by an increase in hepatic glycogenolysis. If hypoglycemia continues, glucagon can stimulate hepatic gluconeogenesis; this can only be done if there are three carbon precursors present (glycerol, lactate, amino acids) [7].

Third Defense

Increased release of epinephrine. Similar to glucagon, epinephrine can act rapidly to increase hepatic glucose output by stimulating glycogenolysis. If hypoglycemia continues and three carbon precursors are present, epinephrine will stimulate gluconeogenesis. Epinephrine also decreases glucose utilization by directly inhibiting tissue glucose uptake and by inhibiting insulin release. Epinephrine is approximately ten times more potent than norepinephrine in producing these effects. Epinephrine stimulates glucose production directly by a beta-adrenergic mechanism and indirectly by inhibiting insulin secretion by an alpha-adrenergic mechanism. Glucose counterregulation from insulin-induced hypoglycemia is primarily by glycogenolysis during the first 2 h by gluconeogenesis thereafter. While the effect of both glucagon and epinephrine on glucose production is transient, the effect of epinephrine to limit glucose utilization is sustained [7].

Late Defense

Release of cortisol and growth hormone. Increased secretion of cortisol and growth hormone is involved in defense against prolonged hypoglycemia. Both can increase glucose through increases in gluconeogenesis. Both hormones can also inhibit insulin-stimulated peripheral glucose uptake and can increase proteolysis and lipolysis. However, prolonged hypoglycemia (3–5 h) is needed before the metabolic effects are measurable, and even at that time, they only represent 20–25% of the action of epinephrine. Thus, cortisol and growth hormone are not critical to recovery from even prolonged hypoglycemia or to the prevention of hypoglycemia after an overnight fast [7, 8].

Key Points
- The release of neuroendocrine counterregulatory hormones and the inhibition of endogenous insulin secretion occur before a healthy adult can feel any symptoms of hypoglycemia.
- In the acute phase of hypoglycemia, there is an increase in the concentrations of glucagon and epinephrine (within minutes); increases of cortisol and growth hormone occur later.
- Glucagon plays a primary role in the prevention and correction of hypoglycemia. Epinephrine is not normally critical but becomes critical when glucagon is deficient.
- Insulin, glucagon, and epinephrine play a major role in the prevention and correction of hypoglycemia. All of these three factors are impaired in diabetes (Fig. 45.1).

Glycemic Thresholds

Glycemic thresholds for the activation of counterregulatory hormones have been reported to be at or just below the lower limit of normal plasma glucose range and elicit a characteristic sequence of response (Fig. 45.1) with a defined hierarchy. Symptoms are generated at blood glucose concentrations around 50–58 mg/dL in young adults [7].

Glycemic Mechanisms

Falling plasma glucose concentrations are detected by glucose-responsive neurons in the hypothalamus and other regions of the brain. There is evidence that glucose sensors in the periphery, apart from pancreatic beta cells, have been found in the intestine, hepato-portal vein, and carotid body. Within the central nervous system (CNS), studies have identified a number of areas that contain neurons sensitive to local changes in glucose. One brain region in particular, the VMH (ventromedial hypothalamus), appears to play a crucial role during hypoglycemia. The specialized glucose-sensing neurons in the CNS have been broadly defined as either glucose exited, which increase their action potential frequency when glucose rises, or glucose inhibited, which increase their action potential frequency when glucose levels fall. These neurons are liable to react in a coordinated manner to alterations in the glucose level to which they are exposed. The neurons also respond to other metabolites such as lactate and beta hydroxybutyrate, as well as hormones such as insulin, leptin, and possibly glucagon-like peptide 1, reflecting the central role they play in responding to alterations in fuel supply and in maintaining glucose homeostasis [9].

Pathophysiology of Glucose Counterregulation in Diabetes

T1D

The physiology of glucose counterregulation is extensively impaired in patients with T1D. As endogenous insulin secretion becomes completely deficient, the first physiologic line of defense (modulation of endogenous insulin) becomes lost. As the plasma glucose concentration falls, insulin levels do not decrease. In addition, the rise in glucagon secretion (second line of defense) is lost as glucose levels decline. This is an acquired defect, but it develops early in the course of T1D. Glucagon responses to other stimuli are intact; therefore, it cannot be attributed to alpha cells and must represent a signal abnormality. The deficient glu-

Fig. 45.1 Glycemic
thresholds for hypoglycemia.
(Adapted from [6–8])

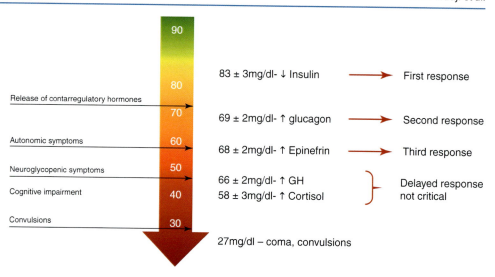

Release of contrarregulatory hormones

Autonomic symptoms

Neuroglycopenic symptoms

Cognitive impairment

Convulsions

83 ± 3mg/dl- ↓ Insulin   ⟶   First response

69 ± 2mg/dl- ↑ glucagon   ⟶   Second response

68 ± 2mg/dl- ↑ Epinefrin   ⟶   Third response

66 ± 2mg/dl- ↑ GH
58 ± 3mg/dl- ↑ Cortisol   } Delayed response not critical

27mg/dl – coma, convulsions

cagon response is tightly related to absolute insulin deficiency. Insulin levels do not fall and glucagon levels do not rise as the plasma glucose concentration falls to hypoglycemic levels (Fig. 45.2).

The epinephrine response to failing glucose concentrations is commonly attenuated. This acquired abnormality is also selective in that epinephrine response to other stimuli is intact. However, while the deficient glucagon response to hypoglycemia appears to be absolute, the deficient epinephrine response appears to be a threshold abnormality. This epinephrine abnormality has been determined to be due to previous episodes of hypoglycemia [6].

> **Additional Facts**
> - Repeated hypoglycemia produces acute reductions (30–50%) in epinephrine, pancreatic polypeptide (a marker of parasympathetic nervous system activity), and muscle sympathetic nerve activity.
> - Recent (within 24 h) antecedent hypoglycemia blunts the release of glucagon, growth hormone, adrenocorticotropic hormone (ACTH), and cortisol during subsequent hypoglycemia [7, 8].

T2D

The glucose counterregulatory mechanisms are generally intact during the initial course of T2D. Although there may be mild counterregulatory hormonal deficiencies, epinephrine secretion appears to be intact. Several studies have shown that counterregulatory hormonal release occurs at higher blood glucose levels in individuals with diabetes than in nondiabetic persons. This may confer greater protection against hypoglycemia. The glucagon response to hypoglycemia may be mildly decreased [10].

In many individuals with T2D who have insulin resistance, the lipolytic effects of epinephrine outweigh the effects of insulin on adipose tissue. Plasma free fatty acids increase in response to hypoglycemia in patients with T2D but not T1D. Epinephrine secretion in hypoglycemia may have a greater protective effect in insulin-resistant patients by promoting metabolic substrate release rather than storage. Epinephrine also stimulates the release of glucose from the kidney [10].

Nevertheless, as insulin progressively declines due to failing pancreatic endogenous secretion of insulin, glucagon response to hypoglycemia will progressively decline (Fig. 45.2).

It is important to consider the effects of aging in the response to hypoglycemia in patients with T2D as the majority of the population is elderly. With increasing age, the symptoms of hypoglycemia become less intense, and the symptom profile is modified. It has been reported that there is a modest attenuation of blood glucose recovery from hypoglycemia in the elderly nondiabetic population, in whom the rise of plasma epinephrine was slower than younger subjects. The elevation of glucagon and epinephrine occurred at lower plasma glucose levels in elderly nondiabetic patients compared to younger nondiabetic patients. The magnitude of the response is also lower in the elderly group. Also, the rate of insulin clearance from the circulation declines with increasing age, which may enhance the risk of hypoglycemia [10].

Fig. 45.2 Counterregulatory response to hypoglycemia

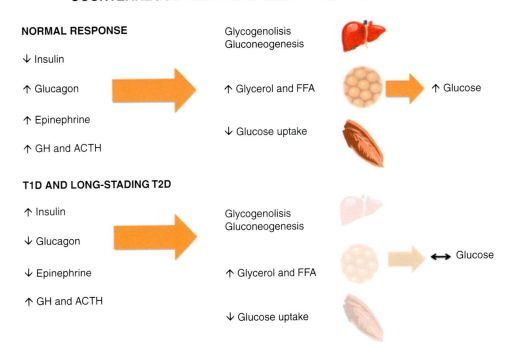

COUNTERREGULATORY RESPONSE TO HYPOGLYCEMIA

NORMAL RESPONSE

↓ Insulin

↑ Glucagon

↑ Epinephrine

↑ GH and ACTH

Glycogenolisis
Gluconeogenesis

↑ Glycerol and FFA

↓ Glucose uptake

↑ Glucose

T1D AND LONG-STADING T2D

↑ Insulin

↓ Glucagon

↓ Epinephrine

↑ GH and ACTH

Glycogenolisis
Gluconeogenesis

↑ Glycerol and FFA

↓ Glucose uptake

↔ Glucose

Hypoglycemia Unawareness

Individuals with intensive glucose control and multiple episodes of hypoglycemia find that activation of the physiologic responses to hypoglycemia is pushed to a lower plasma glucose level. This dangerous condition, called hypoglycemia unawareness, results in inability of patients to recognize falling plasma glucose until the value is <50 mg/dL (2.8 mmol/L). In some individuals, a falling plasma glucose level is not recognized at plasma glucose of 30 mg/dL (1.7 mmol/L). Thus, thresholds for the activation of physiologic defenses against hypoglycemia are labile and can change rapidly [7].

A major defect in the counterregulatory response to hypoglycemia in diabetes is a reduced autonomic response. Hypoglycemia unawareness occurs in 20% of patients with T1D and about half of the patients with long-standing T1D and is estimated to occur in about 25% of patients with long-standing T2D. As glucose declines, there is activation of the autonomic nervous system (ANS) that results in increased glucose production and decreased glucose uptake. The autonomic response is directly related to the generation of a symptomatic response to hypoglycemia. When this response becomes impaired, there is reduced awareness of the symptoms of hypoglycemia as well as reduced catecholamine release. The reduced autonomic response includes the sympathetic neural norepinephrine and acetylcholine, as well as the adrenomedullary epinephrine response (Fig. 45.3). As discussed previously, this reduced response becomes critical in patients with T1D and long-standing T2D, as there is no glucagon response, increasing the risk of hypoglycemia [9].

> **Key Points**
> - A defective autonomic response usually precedes prior episodes of hypoglycemia.
> - This sets up a vicious cycle whereby hypoglycemia increases the likelihood of subsequent hypoglycemia.
> - Hypoglycemia unawareness has been found to increase the frequency of hypoglycemia by a factor of 7 [7].

Hypoglycemia: Associated Autonomic Failure

The combination of defective glucose counterregulation (decreased glucagon release and attenuated epinephrine release) and hypoglycemia unawareness (reduced autonomic-sympathetic neural and adrenomedullary response) constitutes the clinical syndrome of hypoglycemia-associated autonomic failure (HAAF). It occurs in patients with T1D and long-standing T2D who have had recent antecedent hypoglycemia; it can also occur by sleep or prior exercise (Fig. 45.3) [11].

In patients with T1D, recent hypoglycemia has been shown to shift glycemic thresholds for autonomic and cognitive dysfunction responses to lower plasma glucose concentrations. It has been shown that avoidance of hypoglycemia

Fig. 45.3 Hypoglycemia-associated autonomic failure. (Adapted from [11])

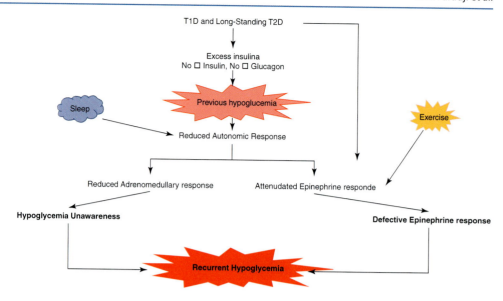

for 2–3 weeks reverses hypoglycemia unawareness and improves the reduced epinephrine defective response; nevertheless, the glucagon response is not restored [8].

> **Additional Facts**
> - Repeated episodes of relative mild <70 mg/dL (3.9 mmol/L) and only brief durations (15–20 min) of hypoglycemia can independently blunt counterregulatory responses to subsequent hypoglycemia.
> - One prolonged episode (2 h) of moderate hypoglycemia <50 mg/dL (2.8 mmol/L) is sufficient to induce HAAF within a few hours on the same day [7].

It has been proposed that repeated hypoglycemia increased cerebral glucose uptake in both healthy individuals and patients with T1D, thereby reducing the stimulus for neuroendocrine counterregulatory responses during subsequent hypoglycemia. Other mechanisms that have been proposed include activation of the hypothalamic-pituitary-adrenal axis, increases in neurotransmitters such as GABA, and changes in hypothalamic fuel sensors such as glucokinase or AMP kinase. Additionally, experimental evidence demonstrates that alcohol and opioids can downregulate subsequent ANS and neuroendocrine responses to hypoglycemia.

As mentioned above, sleep and exercise can induce HAAF. Compared to hypoglycemia during waking period, hypoglycemia during sleep (nocturnal hypoglycemia) elicits reduced counterregulatory response. Research has revealed a 60–70% reduction in epinephrine response during nocturnal hypoglycemia. Thus, exercise blunts ANS

response (by 30–50%) to subsequent hypoglycemia and vice versa. This feed-forward vicious cycle of blunted ANS responses between exercise and hypoglycemia can occur after only a few hours and persists for at least 24 h following either stress [7].

Opioid receptor blockade, via treatment with naloxone, during hypoglycemia has been shown to prevent blunting responses (epinephrine and endogenous glucagon production) to next-day hypoglycemia in individuals with T1D [7].

> **Physiologic Stimuli to Blunted Hormonal Responses to Hypoglycemia**
> - Antecedent hypoglycemia
> - Nocturnal hypoglycemia
> - Sleep
> - Alcohol
> - Opioids [7]

Epidemiology

Iatrogenic hypoglycemia is more frequent in patients with profound endogenous insulin deficiency, T1D, and advanced T2D (as its incidence increases with the duration of diabetes). The frequency of hypoglycemia is about threefold greater in T1D than in T2D. Ninety percent of all patients who receive insulin have experienced hypoglycemic episodes [12].

During the Hypoglycemia Assessment Tool (HAT) global study, which was a non-interventional, multicenter, 6-month retrospective and 4-week prospective study involving 27,585 patients with either T1D or T2D treated with insulin, in 24 countries worldwide, it was found that during the prospective period, 83% of patients with T1D and 46.5% of patients with T2D reported hypoglycemia. Overall, there were 73.3

events/patient-year of hypoglycemia in T1D and 19.3 in patients with T2D. There were 11.3 events/patient-year of nocturnal hypoglycemia in T1D and 4.9 in T2D. And finally, there were 4.9 events/patient-year of severe hypoglycemia in T1D and 2.5 events/patient-year in T2D [13].

In the United States, from 1993 to 2005, around five million emergency department visits were due to hypoglycemic events, 25% of which led to hospitalization. This is especially common in elderly patients. Additionally, the NICE-SUGAR trial demonstrated that critically ill patients who are intensively controlled had an increased risk of moderate-to-severe hypoglycemia and increased risk of death [14].

A trial involving 33,675 hospitalized patients with and without diabetes found that hypoglycemia, with either insulin or spontaneous, was associated with increased short- and long-term mortality. In this cohort of hospitalized patients to medical wards, 9% of patients had at least one episode of hypoglycemia [15].

T1D

People with T1D are bound to have hypoglycemia; as they attempt to achieve euglycemia, they will suffer numerous episodes of asymptomatic hypoglycemia. Plasma glucose concentrations may be <50 mg/dL (2.8 mmol/L) 10% of the time. They have an average of two episodes of hypoglycemia per week, thousands of such episodes over a lifetime, and an episode of severe hypoglycemia approximately once a year [7]. Population data indicate that 30–40% of people with T1D experience an average of one to three episodes of severe hypoglycemia each year. Older estimates were that 2–4% of patients with T1D die from hypoglycemia. More recent estimates are that 6–7% or 10% of those with T1D die from hypoglycemia [16].

In the DCCT (Diabetes Control and Complications Trial), severe hypoglycemia occurred in 65% of patients with T1D treated intensively and 35% of patients with T1D on the con-

ventional group over 6.5 years. There were no statistical differences in hospitalizations; however, there were two fatal motor vehicle accidents in the intensive therapy group, which may be attributed to hypoglycemia. The DCCT also confirmed that the presence of detectable endogenous insulin as measured by residual C-peptide secretion is associated with a reduced risk of hypoglycemia [17].

Ninety percent of the surviving cohort of DCCT joined the EDIC (Epidemiology of Diabetes Interventions and Complications), which was an observational follow-up study to examine the long-term effects of the original DCCT therapies. Around 50% of participants in each group reported an episode of severe hypoglycemia during the 20 years of EDIC. The main characteristics, HbA1c (glycated hemoglobin), and hypoglycemia events can be seen in Table 45.3 [18].

There was a group of participants who reported four or more episodes of hypoglycemia. During the DCCT, 54% of the intensive group and 30% of the conventional group experienced more than four episodes of severe hypoglycemia. In the EDIC, 37% of the intensive group and 33% of the conventional group experienced four or more episodes. A subset of participants (14%) experienced nearly one-half of all severe hypoglycemia in the DCCT, and 7% in the EDIC experienced almost one-third of all episodes of severe hypoglycemia. This observation exposes the possibility that there are certain individuals who are more susceptible to severe hypoglycemia [18].

In a retrospective epidemiological survey of an unselected population with T1D, the prevalence of severe hypoglycemia was reported to be 37% over a 1-year recall period, with 130 events occurring per 100 patient-years. In this report, 5% of the participants experienced 54% of all severe hypoglycemia [20].

T2D

Overall, the frequency of hypoglycemia is substantially lower in T2D than in T1D. Event rates for severe hypoglycemia are

Table 45.3 Clinical Characteristics of Patients Enrolled in the DCCT/EDIC Trial (1982-2005)

	Conventional			Intensive treatment		
	DCCT	DCCT/EDIC	EDIC	DCCT	DCCT/EDIC	EDIC
	1 year	6 years	12 years	1 year	6 years	12 years
Characteristics	(n = 730)	(n = 723)	(n = 606)	(n = 711)	(n = 698)	(n = 620)
Age (years)	27 ± 7	33 ± 7	46 ± 7	27 ± 7	34 ± 7	46 ± 7
DM duration (years)	5 ± 4	12 ± 5	24 ± 5	6 ± 4	12 ± 5	25 ± 5
BMI	24 ± 3	25 ± 3	28 ± 5	23 ± 3	27 ± 4	28 ±
HbA1c%	8.9 ± 1.6	9.1 ± 1.5	7.7 ± 1.2	8.9 ± 1.6	7.4 ± 1.1	7.8 ± 1.2
Hypoglycemia coma/seizures[a]	5.4	16.4	9.2	16.3	6.7	13.6
SH[a]	18.7	47.3	39.6	61.2	38.5	48.4

DM diabetes mellitus, *BMI* body mass index (kg/m^2), *HbA1c* hemoglobin A1c, *SH* severe hypoglycemia
Adapted from [18, 19]
[a] Events per 100 patient-years

approximately tenfold lower in T2D even during aggressive insulin therapy. They are even lower in those treated with oral hypoglycemic agents. Most episodes of hypoglycemia in T2D are considered to be mild to moderate [21].

Miller et al. performed a cross-sectional study on T2D African American population. Hypoglycemia had a prevalence of 24.5%, and severe hypoglycemia had a prevalence of 0.5%. The prevalence of hypoglycemia was highest on patients receiving triple therapy, followed by those receiving insulin alone or a single oral agent, and infrequent on those receiving hypoglycemic agents alone or diet therapy alone. In all treatment groups, the prevalence of hypoglycemia tended to increase as HbA1c decreased. The highest prevalence was seen in patients receiving insulin therapy who had HbA1c less than 7% [22].

Over 6 years in the UKPDS (United Kingdom Prospective Diabetes Study), major hypoglycemia was reported in 2.4% of T2D patients treated with metformin, 3.3% of patients treated with sulfonylurea, and 11.2% of those treated with insulin. They found a higher frequency of hypoglycemia in the intensive group compared with the conventional group. With intensive treatment, hypoglycemia occurred most frequently in the insulin-treated patients, and the prevalence of hypoglycemia was lower in the first decade of the study that in later years [8].

Oral and Injectable Agents

Hypoglycemia with oral agents medications occurs most frequently with sulfonylureas and meglitinides. Both classes of medications have increased the absolute risk of hypoglycemia by 4–9% compared to placebo or other agents. Sulfonylureas have an 11% higher risk of hypoglycemia than metformin [23].

Metformin

When used as monotherapy, metformin has minimal risk of hypoglycemia. When compared with placebo, hypoglycemia was reported in less than 5% of patients taking metformin alone. Since metformin enhances insulin sensitivity, when combined with other medications that increase circulating levels of insulin, the risk of hypoglycemia increases [24].

Alpha-Glucosidase Inhibitors

The risk of hypoglycemia is very low; however, should patients experience hypoglycemia, it cannot be treated with sucrose or fruit juice (which is hydrolyzed to glucose and fructose), since the absorption is inhibited by the mechanism of these medications. Hypoglycemic episodes must be treated with simple sugars such as oral glucose (dextrose), which can be in glucose tablets, or grapes [24].

Sulfonylureas

The risk of hypoglycemia is very common with sulfonylureas, even when administered as monotherapy. The rates of hypoglycemia differ with each sulfonylurea based on each agent's pharmacokinetic properties. Glyburide (glibenclamide) has been associated with a higher incidence of hypoglycemia when compared to glipizide. Glyburide should be avoided in patients with creatinine clearance of <50 mL/min.

In randomized clinical trials, sulfonylureas are associated with a significant greater risk of any or severe hypoglycemia when compared to insulin sensitizers or incretin-based therapies. A meta-analysis that included trials with a duration of >24 weeks, enrolling patients with T2D, comparing sulfonylurea with placebo or active drugs different from sulfonylureas, reported that hypoglycemia, including severe hypoglycemia, was frequent in patients treated with sulfonylureas. They also found that the risk of hypoglycemia with sulfonylureas is not different from that of insulin in head-to-head trials. The overall risk of severe hypoglycemia was increased more than threefold with sulfonylureas than with comparators. The cumulative incidence of hypoglycemia with sulfonylureas was 17% and for severe hypoglycemia 1.2% [25].

Amylin

Amylin analogues are associated with a high risk of hypoglycemia when they are combined with insulin therapy. Pramlintide carries a black box warning that when adding pramlintide to insulin, the prandial insulin dose must be reduced by 50% and titrated up to avoid severe hypoglycemia.

Dipeptidyl Peptidase-4 (DPP-4) Inhibitors

DPP-4 inhibitors generally do not cause hypoglycemia when used as monotherapy, are weight neutral, and are relatively well tolerated.

Sodium-Glucose Co-transporter 2 (SGLT2) Inhibitors

SGLT2 inhibitors have been shown to have a low risk of hypoglycemia with monotherapy [24].

Insulin

Glargine

Insulin glargine is a long-acting insulin analogue, which is less soluble at physiologic pH (potential of hydrogen) than human insulin. Insulin glargine reduces the risk of nocturnal hypoglycemia in T1D patients compared with insulin NPH (neutral protamine Hagedorn or isophane insulin) when taken either with prandial unmodified human insulin or rapid-acting insulin analogues [20, 26].

Detemir

This is a long-acting basal insulin that has extended duration due to molecular modifications leading to increased albumin binding. Detemir has also been associated with reduced nocturnal hypoglycemia in people with T1D compared with NPH insulin, as reported in numerous studies. In studies comparing twice-daily insulin detemir to NPH insulin, where both groups used a fast-acting insulin analogue prandially, significant reductions in hypoglycemia had been attained with detemir [20, 26].

Degludec

Insulin degludec is an ultra-long-acting insulin analogue, which forms a subcutaneous depot and is slowly released. Studies comparing insulin degludec with glargine have reported a reduced number of nocturnal hypoglycemic episodes in the degludec group.

Insulin degludec was compared with insulin glargine U100 in the SWITCH 1 and SWITCH 2 trials. Both studies used a randomized, double blind, treat-to-target, crossover design. Patients with T1D ($N = 501$; SWITCH 1) or patients with T2D ($N = 721$; SWITCH 2) who had one or more risk factors were enrolled. These patients were randomized to either insulin degludec or insulin glargine U100 for 32 weeks (16-week titration and then 16-week maintenance) and then crossed over to the alternate insulin treatment for an additional 32 weeks (16-week titration and 16 week maintenance). In SWITCH 1, the rate of overall symptomatic hypoglycemia was significantly lower with insulin degludec than insulin glargine U100 (2200.9 vs. 2462.7 episodes/100 patient-years of exposure). In SWITCH 2, the rates of severe hypoglycemia were also statistically significantly lower with insulin degludec than insulin glargine U100 (185.6 vs. 265.4 episodes/100 patient-years) [27–29].

Glargine U300

Another prolonged-acting insulin analogue is insulin glargine U300 [30, 31] (300 IU/mL). By being more concentrated, it forms a compact subcutaneous depot with a smaller surface area to produce a more gradual and prolonged release. Compared to glargine U100, it has shown lower event rates of nocturnal hypoglycemia. Glargine U300 can be injected with a 3 h flexible regimen.

There are pharmacokinetics studies [30] that compare degludec to glargine U300. The clinical studies have not shown a significant difference in the rate of hypoglycemia between the two types of insulin [32].

Fast-Acting Insulin Analogues

Fast-acting insulin analogues were developed in order to better stimulate the physiological postprandial insulin response. Data from subsequent clinical trials comparing lispro with human insulin suggest that the more physiologic

pharmacokinetics are associated with a reduced risk of nocturnal hypoglycemia. A multicenter randomized, double blind, crossover study with 90 participants demonstrated a significantly reduced severe hypoglycemia as well as improved glycemic control with insulin aspart compared with human insulin. Fast-acting insulin analogues have shown to reduce nocturnal and late postprandial hypoglycemia [20].

Clinical Manifestations

For people with diabetes, the detection of hypoglycemic symptoms is a critical tool for the recognition and treatment of hypoglycemia. Recognition of hypoglycemia is possible through self-monitoring blood glucose (SMBG), continuous glucose monitoring (CGM), and detection of hypoglycemic symptoms. Numerous biological and psychological modifiers can either facilitate or interfere with the recognition of hypoglycemia. With experience, individuals develop beliefs concerning their symptoms of hypoglycemia. Nevertheless, beliefs have a high incidence of false alarm rates; individuals with poor control may believe that they have hypoglycemia when instead they have hyperglycemia, and individuals with tight control may have hypoglycemia unawareness and not be able to recognize an episode of hypoglycemia. When blood glucose falls too low, then consciousness becomes impaired, making it difficult to accurately interpret the meaning of any symptom. Some people may deny symptoms of hypoglycemia because symptoms represent failure in their self-management [33].

Symptoms of hypoglycemia are divided into two categories (Table 45.4):

- Autonomic (neurogenic) symptoms are the result of perception of physiological changes caused by the autonomic nervous system release triggered by hypoglycemia.

Table 45.4 Symptoms of hypoglycemia

Autonomic	Neuroglycopenic
Adrenal	Slowed thinking
• Trembling	Abnormal mentation
• Shakiness	Irritability
• Palpitations	Confusion
• Nervousness	Difficulty speaking
• Anxiety	Ataxia
• Pupil dilation	Paresthesias
• Pallor	Headaches
Cholinergic	Stupor
• Clamminess	Seizures
• Sweating	Coma
• Hunger	Death (if untreated)
• Tingling	

Adapted from [34]

- Neuroglycopenic symptoms occur as a result of brain neuronal glucose deprivation. The patient usually recognizes these symptoms first.

Physical signs that result from activation of the sympathoadrenal system include pallor and diaphoresis, which are often prominent, and increased heart rate and systolic blood pressure, which are often subtler. Hypothermia is often present. Transient focal neurological deficits (diplopia, hemiparesis) occur occasionally [7].

Symptoms of hypoglycemia vary greatly among patients and depend on the individual's personal experience and sensitivity. In mild hypoglycemia, symptoms result from an ANS response and usually consist of tremors, palpitations, sweating, blurred vision, mood variations, and excessive hunger. Major cognitive deficits usually do not accompany mild reactions, so patients are generally able to self-treat. These mild symptoms usually respond to an oral ingestion of 10–15 g of carbohydrates and resolve within 10–15 min. Moderate hypoglycemia includes neuroglycopenic as well as autonomic symptoms, which usually consist of headache, mood changes, irritability, decreased attentiveness, and drowsiness. Behavioral changes such as irritability, agitation, quietness, stubbornness, and tantrums may be the prominent symptoms for the preschool child and may result from a combination of neuroglycopenic and autonomic response [5]. People often need assistance in treating themselves, and these reactions produce longer-lasting and more severe symptoms usually requiring a second dose of carbohydrates. Severe hypoglycemic symptoms are characterized by unresponsiveness, combativeness, unconsciousness, or seizures and typically require assistance from another individual. Patients who experience seizures with severe hypoglycemia are at risk for recurrence [35, 36].

Diagnosis and Detection

People may recognize hypoglycemia based on their symptoms and experience, although as discussed earlier, individuals may not be aware of an episode of hypoglycemia or may misinterpret their symptoms. It has been reported that patients who are being typically aware of their hypoglycemia, on average, recognize 50% of their hypoglycemic episodes [36]. Therefore, documentation of a low plasma glucose concentration is very helpful. A hypoglycemic episode is most convincingly documented by the Whipple's triad: symptoms compatible with hypoglycemia, a low plasma or blood glucose concentration, and restoration of those symptoms after the glucose concentration is raised to normal [8].

There are two technologies available to measure glucose in an outpatient setting: capillary measurement with point-of-care glucose meters or self-monitoring blood glucose (SMBG) and interstitial measurement with CGM, both retrospective and real time [1].

Additional Facts

- Plasma glucose samples are up to 15% higher than mixed venous whole blood glucose samples.
- Mixed venous blood glucose values can be considerably lower than arterial or capillary levels.
- Glucose meters can be imprecise, especially at low blood glucose levels [14].

Causes

The need to identify underlying causes is an important aspect of hypoglycemia evaluation and management. Looking back over the events of several hours preceding the reactions can often identify the factors precipitating an event of hypoglycemia (Table 45.5).

Table 45.5 Conventional causes of hypoglycemia

Insulin (or secretagogues or insulin sensitizers) doses are excessive, ill-timed, or of wrong type
Exogenous glucose delivery is decreased
• Missed meal
• Low carbohydrate meal
• Overnight fast
• Vomiting
Endogenous glucose production is decreased
• Alcohol ingestion
Glucose utilization is increased
• Exercise
• Sepsis, trauma, burns
Sensitivity to insulin is increased
• Late after exercise
• Weight loss
• Improved fitness
Insulin clearance is decreased
• Renal failure
• Liver failure
• Hypothyroidism

Adapted from [8]

Risk Factors and Determinants

Many factors can put T1D and T2D patients at increased risk of experiencing hypoglycemia (Table 45.6). Severe hypoglycemia is mostly associated with the use of glucose-lowering drugs, especially insulin or insulin secretagogues.

In a large retrospective cohort study involving people with T2D, severe hypoglycemia was recorded in 12 cases per 10,000 patient-years. They observed approximately six times higher incidence rate in patients using insulin during follow-up than in non-insulin users. Patients with cardiovascular disease and renal failure had approximately 1.5 times higher incidence rate of severe hypoglycemia. In this study, the current use of insulin or sulfonylureas, age ≥ 75, renal failure, and cognitive impairment/dementia were associated with a substantially increased risk of developing severe hypoglycemia in the overall population [34].

The Fremantle Diabetes Study was a longitudinal observational cohort study aimed at defining the determinants of severe hypoglycemia complicating T2D. Insulin treatment or its duration, renal impairment, peripheral neuropathy, and higher education proved to be independent predictors of first and multiple episodes of hypoglycemia. The frequency of hypoglycemia was also associated with a lower fasting serum glucose but paradoxically higher HbA1c. A prominent predictor of the first episode of hypoglycemia in this cohort was duration of insulin treatment, with each year increasing the risk by 33%. They also found that a previous history of hospitalization for severe hypoglycemia was a strong independent predictor of the first episode of hypoglycemia [37].

Physical Activity and Exercise

Physical activity may increase glucose transport and utilization by skeletal muscles, acutely and chronically. Hypoglycemia can occur during 1–2 h after exercise, or up to 17 h after exercise. Aerobic exercise results in an increase in both insulin- and non-insulin-mediated glucose uptake [38, 39].

The blood glucose response to exercise is affected by many factors including duration, intensity and type of exercise, the time of day when exercise is performed, plasma glucose, insulin levels, and the availability of supplemental and stored carbohydrates [5].

During moderate intensity exercise in nondiabetic individuals, endogenous insulin secretion is reduced by

Table 45.6 Risk factors for hypoglycemia

Insulin deficiency
Negative C peptide
Long-standing diabetes
History of severe hypoglycemia
Hypoglycemia unawareness
Extremes of age (young and elderly)
Cognitive impairment/dementia
Systemic illness
• Renal failure
• Liver failure
• Congestive heart failure
Ethanol use
Autonomic neuropathy
Glucose variability
Aggressive glycemic therapy
Peripheral neuropathy
Lower glycemic goals
Medications
• Fixed insulin regimens
• Sulfonylureas
• Salicylates
• Beta blockers
• Coumarin
• Fibrates
Nutritional factors
• Ethanol consumption
• Gastroparesis
• Fasting or missed meals
• Malnutrition
• Low-carb diets
Nocturnal hypoglycemia
Erratic schedules
Exercise (especially irregular)
Hormonal factors
• Adrenal insufficiency
• Hypothyroidism
• Hypopituitarism
• Pregnancy/breastfeeding
• Allopurinol
• Nonsteroidal anti-inflammatory drugs (NSAIDs)

40–60% [40]. The increased fuel demands on the working muscle necessitate compensatory metabolic processes in the liver and kidney. Changes in hepatic glycogenolysis and gluconeogenesis have been found to be closely coupled to the increase in glucose uptake produced by the working muscle because of the actions of the pancreatic hormones. The exercise-induced increase in glucagon secretion and the concomitant decrease in insulin secretion interact to stimulate hepatic glycogenolysis, whereas the increase in hepatic gluconeogenesis is determined primarily by glucagon's action to increase hepatic gluconeogenic precursor fractional extraction and the efficiency of intrahepatic conversion to glucose. Epinephrine and norepinephrine become important in increasing glucose production during prolonged or heavy exercise. Catecholamines can produce this effect by directly stimulating both hepatic and renal glucose production, by increasing the availability of gluconeogenic precursors (lactate, alanine, or glycerol), and by increasing lipolysis. Catecholamine-induced metabolic effects at the muscle and adipose tissue are rapid, increasing gluconeogenic precursor uptake at the liver within minutes [7].

Recent studies have demonstrated that there is a vicious cycle of counterregulatory failure between exercise and hypoglycemia. Thus, two episodes of prolonged, moderate-intensity exercise can reduce ANS and neuroendocrine responses by 50% during subsequent similar hypoglycemia. Similarly, two episodes of antecedent hypoglycemia can reduce counterregulatory responses during subsequent exercise by 40–50%. Therefore, individuals who have had a previous episode of hypoglycemia are at greater risk of hypoglycemia during exercise [40].

In a randomized crossover study involving subjects with T1D, participants were randomly assigned to morning exercise versus afternoon exercise. They found that morning exercise confers a lower risk of late-onset hypoglycemia than afternoon exercise and improves metabolic control on the subsequent day [39].

Alcohol

Ethanol induces hypoglycemia by inhibiting gluconeogenesis; as little as 50 g of alcohol might be sufficient. Alcohol excess, especially in the fasting state, is a major risk factor for severe hypoglycemia. Ethanol and its metabolism influence several pathways vital for the manufacture and production of glucose by the liver [41].

The gluconeogenesis pathway is disrupted with ethanol ingestion by

- Reduced nicotinamide adenine dinucleotide NADH/NAD ratio—as a result of the oxidation of alcohol to acetaldehyde and acetate, thus reducing the ability of the liver and kidney to oxidize lactate and glutamate to pyruvate and alpha-ketoglutarate.
- Inhibiting the release of alanine from the muscle (a vital precursor of gluconeogenesis)
- Inhibition of lactate, glycerol, and alanine uptake by the liver

Alcohol potentiates the hypoglycemic effect of insulin and sulfonylureas, and because of the inhibition of gluconeo-

genesis, glucagon and catecholamines are ineffective in raising glucose levels [7].

Moderate consumption of alcohol in the evening may predispose patients to hypoglycemia on the subsequent morning with reduced nocturnal growth hormone secretion [5].

Medications

Beta-Blockers

Propranolol and other nonselective beta-blockers decrease the ability of the liver and kidney to increase their release of glucose, enhance peripheral insulin sensitivity, and may mask the symptoms of hypoglycemia. The risk of hypoglycemia becomes even higher in the presence of renal dysfunction. The hypoglycemic effect of beta-blockers seems to be directly tied to the diminished adrenergic response to hypoglycemia and to the diminished concentration of circulating free fatty acids. Therefore, propranolol should be used with caution or, if possible, avoided in patients with renal failure. Recent studies indicate that beta-1 selective blockers do not present an increased risk for severe hypoglycemia and therefore should not be considered as being contraindicated in diabetic patients.

- Salicylates—Salicylates can act by binding hepatic glucose production and increasing insulin secretion.
- Sulfonamides—Have a chemical structure similar to sulfonylureas and have been known to have blood glucose-lowering properties.
- Angiotensin-converting enzyme inhibitors can increase insulin sensitivity and can decrease the degradation of bradykinin, which has certain insulin mimetic actions.
- Pentamidine is cytotoxic to pancreatic beta cells, and hypoglycemia occurs with the release of insulin from degenerating cells [7].

Renal Failure

Renal insufficiency is a very common predisposing condition for hypoglycemia. In fact, it is probably the second most common potentiating factor of hypoglycemia after insulin therapy. Nearly 50% of hospitalized patients who were recognized to have hypoglycemia had chronic renal failure. The mortality rate in patients with chronic renal failure may be related to the degree of hypoglycemia and to the number of risk factors for hypoglycemia. In renal failure, hypoglycemia may result from the use of insulin, antidiabetic agents, certain drugs, or a combination of the above [42].

Hypoglycemia resulting from an oral hypoglycemic agent in patients with renal failure is more likely to occur when other factors such as hepatic dysfunction, hypoalbuminemia, alcoholism, or an associated endocrine deficiency are present. It is usually manifested by neuroglycopenic symptoms rather than neurogenic symptoms, and patients may display atypical symptoms. Hypoglycemia is usually of long duration, particularly when a sulfonylurea is the causal agent.

Congestive Heart Failure

The occurrence of congestive heart failure in patients with renal failure may also precipitate hypoglycemia. The pathogenesis of hypoglycemia in heart failure is varied and involves liver dysfunction resulting from congestion, poor nutrition, cachexia, and poor blood supply to muscles and liver. Insufficient production or delivery of substrates for adequate gluconeogenesis in the liver, severe depletion of glycogen stores, possibly caused by poor dietary intake, and gastrointestinal malabsorption caused by congestive heart failure are major potentiating factors of hypoglycemia. The coexistence of renal failure and congestive heart failure may place the patient at even higher risk for hypoglycemia.

Sepsis, Trauma, and Burns

Initially, the response to the stress of infection is an increase in glucose turnover, with glucose production often exceeding glucose utilization and resulting in mild hyperglycemia. This response involves increases in both glycogenolysis and gluconeogenesis and is largely mediated by glucagon. As the infection worsens, increased release of endotoxin and its derivatives, complement activation, endoperoxide activation, and release of endogenous inflammatory mediators (tumor necrosis factor-alpha, interleukins, and other monokines) compromise cardiovascular integrity and cause central venous pooling, inadequate tissue perfusion, and microvascular protein transudation. At this stage, a decrease in splanchnic and renal blood flow occurs. Despite concomitantly reduced peripheral tissue perfusion, glucose utilization is increased. Decreased tissue oxygenation causes increased anaerobic glycolysis, which perpetuates the increased glucose utilization [7].

The inability of glucose production to keep pace with increased tissue demands results in hypoglycemia. Hepatic glycogen stores are rapidly exhausted; consequently, glucose production becomes solely dependent on gluconeogenesis. However, gluconeogenesis fails because of a reduction in ANS and neuroendocrine effects.

Glucose Variability

It has been shown that glucose variability is associated with increased risk of hypoglycemia. In an observational study involving people with T2D, they found that hypoglycemia was positively associated with glucose variability and negatively associated with mean glucose concentration. The risk of hypoglycemia was completely or virtually eliminated when the glucose variability was <30 mg/dL (<1.7 mmol/L). Therefore, lowering glycemia without reducing glucose vari-

ability should be avoided as it places the individual at greater risk of hypoglycemia [43].

Nocturnal Hypoglycemia

It has been estimated that about one-half of hypoglycemia episodes occur during sleep. Hypoglycemia, including severe hypoglycemia, occurs most commonly during the night in people with T1D.

The counterregulatory responses to hypoglycemia are attenuated during sleep, leading to HAAF syndrome; also, insulin sensitivity is enhanced during the middle of the night. Furthermore, sleep often precludes recognition of warning symptoms of developing hypoglycemia and thus appropriate response [22, 38].

Pregnancy

Normal blood glucose levels in pregnant women are 20% lower than in nonpregnant women. A great number of metabolic changes occur during pregnancy to make women more vulnerable to hypoglycemia. Pregnancy itself is associated with suppression of glucose counterregulatory responses [7].

Maternal hypoglycemia during pregnancy is a risk factor for newborns small for gestational age, which in turn is associated with increased long-term risks such as development of diabetes, coronary artery disease, and hypertension [14].

For women with T1D, severe hypoglycemia occurs three to five times more frequently in the first trimester and at a lower rate in the third trimester when compared with the incidence in the year preceding pregnancy. Risk factors for severe hypoglycemia in pregnancy include history of severe hypoglycemia, hypoglycemia unawareness, long duration of diabetes, low HbA1c in early pregnancy, glucose variability, excessive use of insulin. When pregnant and nonpregnant women are compared with CGM, mild hypoglycemia (defined by the authors as <60 mg/dL or 3.3 mmol/L) is more common in all pregnant women. For women with preexisting diabetes, insulin requirements rise throughout the pregnancy and then drop precipitously at the time of delivery of the placenta, requiring an abrupt reduction in insulin dosing to avoid post-delivery hypoglycemia.

Breastfeeding may also be a risk factor for hypoglycemia in women with insulin-treated diabetes [1].

Elderly

Hypoglycemia is a common problem in old people with diabetes. Aging modifies the cognitive, symptomatic, and counterregulatory hormonal responses to hypoglycemia. The effect of aging on increased risk of unawareness or severe episodes of hypoglycemia has also been recognized. Older individuals may have multiple risk factors for hypoglycemia such as renal impairment, chronic heart disease, malnutrition, and polypharmacy.

In older individuals, episodes of hypoglycemia are more likely to be followed by changes in the blood-brain circulation, which may further increase the risk of neurological damages in this population [12].

Severe hypoglycemia has a considerable impact on the well-being, productivity, and quality of life of old people with diabetes.

Children and Adolescents

It is now well recognized that although many physiologic responses are similar across the age groups, there can be significant developmental and age-related differences in children and adolescents. The DCCT reported a higher rate of severe hypoglycemia in adolescents as compared to adults, 86 vs. 57 events requiring assistance per 100 patient-years, despite adolescents having poorer control with HbA1c levels approximately 1% higher. There are a number of physiologic and behavioral mechanisms that contribute to this difference. First, there are behavioral factors such as variable adherence that have been clearly associated with poor glycemic control in adolescents. Second, during puberty, adolescents with or without T1D are more insulin resistant than adults. During hypoglycemia, adolescents with or without diabetes release catecholamines, cortisol, and growth hormone at higher glucose levels than adults. However, intensively treated young adults with T1D counterregulate and experience hypoglycemia symptoms at a lower glucose level, suggesting a greater susceptibility to hypoglycemia in the young [5].

Young children with T1D are noted as particularly vulnerable to hypoglycemia because of their reduced ability to recognize hypoglycemic symptoms and effectively communicate their needs [2].

Children with early-onset diabetes, particularly those diagnosed before age 6, and severe episodes of hypoglycemia have an increased range of cognitive dysfunction and brain abnormalities. Repeated hypoglycemic seizures in young children may also cause structural brain damage [12].

Hypoglycemia Impact

There are several major concerns about the risks of hypoglycemia as it may cause severe morbidity and even death. One vulnerable organ is the brain, which is markedly dependent on glucose as a fuel for normal functioning. Brain dysfunction or damage may occur, and it may cause permanent damage. Among the severe manifestations of hypoglycemia is sudden death, which may not be directly linked to the effects of hypoglycemia. Cardiovascular consequences of hypoglycemia include alteration of ventricular repolarization. Hypoglycemia creates a prothrombotic state and may predispose to ischemic injury. Additional studies have established associations between hypoglycemia and the development of cardiac arrest and cerebral ischemia and cardiac arrhythmias [38, 44].

Hypoglycemia and Cardiovascular Disease

Patients with diabetes have an increased risk of cardiovascular disease, as it is the most common cause of diabetes-related deaths. Intensive glucose control increases the risk of hypoglycemia and severe hypoglycemia. Several epidemiological studies have linked hypoglycemia to increased cardiovascular risk, as it will be discussed further [42].

Acute hypoglycemia causes pronounced physiological responses as a consequence of autonomic activation, principally of the sympathoadrenal system, and results in end-organ stimulation and a profuse release of epinephrine. This profound autonomic response provokes hemodynamic changes. The magnitude of the counterregulation is directly proportional to the depth of hypoglycemia. Blood flow is increased to the myocardium, the splanchnic circulation, and the brain. There are also an increase in heart rate and peripheral systolic blood pressure, a fall in central blood pressure (reducing peripheral resistance), and an increase in myocardial contractility, stroke volume, and cardiac output. The workload of the heart is therefore markedly increased [45].

Increased plasma viscosity occurs during hypoglycemia due to an increase in erythrocyte concentration. Also, coagulation is promoted by platelet activation and increase in factor VIII and von Willebrand factor. Endothelial function may be compromised due to an increase in C-reactive protein. Soluble vascular cell adhesion molecule 1, soluble intracellular adhesion molecule 1, and soluble E-selectin are increased from baseline under hypoglycemic conditions. Soluble P-selectin, plasminogen activator inhibitor 1, tissue plasminogen activator, von Willebrand factor, and platelet-monocyte aggregation were measured by Joy and colleagues and found to be significantly increased during hypoglycemia and returned to baseline during normoglycemia [44, 45].

Hypoglycemia in ACCORD, ADVANCE, and VADT

These three studies randomized almost 24,000 patients with long-standing T2D to standard or intensive glycemic control for up to 5 years, ensuring HbA1c levels <7%. All three trials were carried out in participants with either known cardiovascular disease or multiple risk factors. Strict glycemic control did not incur a significant cardiovascular benefit, and none of the trials demonstrated a positive effect on cardiovascular events of mortality. In fact, the ACCORD study was interrupted prematurely because of an excess mortality in the intensive group. In all three trials,

Table 45.7 Clinical Characteristics, ACCORD/ADVANCE Clinical Trials

		ACCORD		ADVANCE		VADT	
Participants		10,251		11,140		1791	
Age (years)		62		66		60	
Men/women (%)		61/39		58/42		97/33	
BMI (kg/m²)		32.2 ± 5.5		28 ± 5		6.9 ± 8.5	
Diabetes duration (years)		10		8		11.5	
History of CVD%		32		28		31	
Mean HbA1c%		8.1		7.2		9.4	
HbA1c% Intensive	HbA1c% Standard	6.4	7.5	6.5	7.3	6.9	8.5
Hypoglycemia Intensive %	Hypoglycemia Standard %	16.2	5.1	2.7	1.5	21.2	1.5
On insulin at baseline %		35		1.5		52	
Insulin Intensive %	Insulin Standard %	77	55	40	24	89	74
Mean duration of follow-up		3.5 (terminated early)		5		5.6	
CVD		35%		34%		40%	
Primary CVD end point		↓ 10% ($p = 0.16$)		↓ 6% ($p = 0.37$)		↓ 13% ($p = 0.12$)	
Mortality (overall)		↑ 22% ($p = 0.012$)		↓ 7% ($p =$ NS)		↑ 6.5% ($p = 0.12$)	
CV mortality		↑ 35% ($p = 0.02$)		↓ 12% ($p =$ NS)		↑ 25% ($p =$ NS)	

Based on [45, 46]

hypoglycemia was significantly higher in the intensive glucose-lowering arms compared with the standard arm. Symptomatic severe hypoglycemia was associated with an increased risk of death within each study arm. In the VADT study, a recent severe hypoglycemic event was an important predictor of cardiovascular death and all-cause mortality (Table 45.7) [45, 46].

It is possible that severe hypoglycemia could increase the risk of cardiovascular death in patients with underlying cardiovascular risk.

Cardiac Arrhythmias

Hypoglycemia has been known to cause electrocardiographic changes with lengthening of the corrected QT (QTc) interval and cardiac repolarization, exerting a pro-arrhythmogenic effect. Other electrocardiographic abnormalities observed during hypoglycemia include a decrease in PR interval and depressed T waves [44]. Abnormal cardiac repolarization appears to be related to the sympathoadrenal stimulation and release of catecholamines and to the hypokalemia that results from the insulin effect. In an observational study of patients with T1D, the effect of nocturnal and daytime hypoglycemia was assessed on EKG (electrocardiogram) with CGM. They found that hypoglycemia was common and had different distinct patterns in the EKG. Bradycardia was commonly seen while patients had nocturnal hypoglycemia, while with daytime hypoglycemia, they had more atrial ectopy. Prolonged QTc, T-peak to T-end interval duration, and decreased T wave symmetry were detected during nocturnal and daytime hypoglycemia [47].

Cardiovascular autonomic neuropathy or impairment is associated with increased mortality.

Cognitive Function and Dementia

Repeated severe hypoglycemia over time may impair cognitive function or damage the brain. Patients with T1D and a history of severe hypoglycemia have a slight but significant decline in intelligence scores in comparison with matched controls. Magnetic resonance imaging (MRI) in small studies of patients with T1D with no history of severe hypoglycemia when compared with patients with T1D with a history of five or more episodes of severe hypoglycemia has found cortical atrophy in nearly half of those who had a history of severe hypoglycemia. Severe hypoglycemia has been known to induce focal neurological deficits and transient ischemic attacks, which are reversible with the correction of blood glucose. Recent studies suggest that recurrent and severe hypoglycemia may predispose to long-term cognitive dysfunction and dementia [42, 44].

A number of studies have observed a relationship between dementing illness and diabetes. Both hyperglycemia and hypoglycemia potentially are implicated in the increased risk of dementing illness most commonly observed in elderly patients [12].

Dead-in-Bed Syndrome and Sudden Death

The "dead-in-bed" syndrome is an uncommon fatal event thought to be responsible for 6% of deaths of patients with

T1D who are younger than 40 years old. In 1991, Tattarsall and Gill described 22 cases of unexplained death that they labeled as dead-in-bed syndrome. Possible contributors to dead-in-bed syndrome are hypoglycemic brain damage, autonomic neuropathy, cardiac events such as arrhythmias, and electrolyte abnormalities. Nocturnal hypoglycemia is of substantial concern because patients may be "unaware" and susceptible to serious sequelae. Tanenberg reported a 23-year-old patient with T1D who died in his undisturbed bed from hypoglycemia. Postmortem download of the data in the CGM demonstrated glucose below 30 mg/dL around the time of his death and a vitreous humor glucose of 25 mg/dL [48].

Prolonged, profound hypoglycemia can cause brain death. The mechanism is thought to be sustained increased plasma glutamate release and receptor activation when plasma glucose concentrations are <18 mg/dL (1.0 mmol/L), the electroencephalogram is isoelectric, and brain glucose and glycogen levels are immeasurably low.

Quality of Life

Hypoglycemia can have a significant impact on patients' health-related quality of life, treatment satisfaction, and cost of diabetic management. The well-being of patients may be affected both directly from the effects of hypoglycemia and indirectly from fear of recurrence. Nocturnal hypoglycemia may impact one's sense of well-being on the following day because of its impact on sleep quality and quantity. Patients with recurrent hypoglycemia have been found to have chronic mood disorders including depression and anxiety. Interpersonal relationships may suffer as a result of hypoglycemia in patients with diabetes. Hypoglycemia also impairs one's ability to drive a car [1, 12].

In the UKPDS, patients reporting more frequent hypoglycemic episodes also reported increased tension, mood disturbances (anger, fatigue), and less work satisfaction. In the RECAP-DM study, participants with hypoglycemia reported significantly lower scores on scales for effectiveness, convenience, and global satisfaction than patients who did not have hypoglycemia, with concomitant barriers to treatment adherence. In this study, patients reporting symptoms of hypoglycemia were in general more markedly affected by their illness, had significantly lower self-rated general health, and had more worries about hypoglycemia than participants without hypoglycemia [49].

Fear of Hypoglycemia

When people experience hypoglycemia and its unpleasant symptoms, this has been shown to result in fear of future hypoglycemia. This concept may compromise overall glycemic control and impair quality of life. Recent, frequent, or severe hypoglycemia episodes tend to exacerbate this fear, while useful strategies to reduce the frequency of hypoglycemia, such as insulin pump adjustments or CGM, may alleviate such fear. There is clearly concern about the adverse consequences of hypoglycemia. These concerns primarily include damage to the brain and increased cardiovascular risk. Fear of hypoglycemia sometimes leads to deliberate undertreatment with insulin therapy [38].

A large study with 764 participants concluded that the frequency of severe hypoglycemia is the most important factor in the development of fear of hypoglycemia.

A retrospective study of 335 participants with either T1D or T2D found that hypoglycemia and fear of future hypoglycemia had an impact upon T1D and T2D patients. Self-treatment was the predominant means of coping with mild or moderate and severe hypoglycemia. Following mild or moderate event, neither T1D nor T2D patients utilized healthcare resources and did little more than mention the episode to their physician. Severe hypoglycemia was shown to have a considerable impact upon patient lifestyle. A major alteration to daily activities was noted with respect to fear of driving [50].

Fear of hyperglycemia is a psychological construct characterized by excessive worry about high blood glucose in combination with acceptance (and non-avoidance) of hypoglycemia—as a necessary evil to evade the development of long-term complications. It may lead to inappropriate blood glucose-lowering behaviors, including deliberate overtreatment or overzealous use of insulin, reluctance to attend to the early symptoms of hypoglycemia, and inappropriate pursuit of low blood glucose despite recurrent hypoglycemia.

Critical Illness and Hospitalization

Persons with diabetes are three times more likely to be hospitalized than those without diabetes, and approximately 25% of hospitalized patients (including people without a history of diabetes) have hyperglycemia. Inpatient hyperglycemia has been associated with prolonged hospital length of stay and with numerous adverse outcomes including mortality. Several studies have shown that aggressive lowering of glycemia in the ICU is not beneficial, markedly increases the risk of severe hypoglycemia, and may be associated with increase mortality [1].

A cohort of 33,675 hospitalized patients with and without diabetes, followed for almost 3 years, found that hypoglycemia, insulin related or non-insulin related, was associated with increased short- and long-term mortality. In this study, patients with moderate hypoglycemia during hospitalization had a more than twofold increase in mortality compared with patients without hypoglycemia. Severe hypoglycemia was associated with a threefold increase in mortality [14].

Treatment of Hypoglycemia

Treatment is aimed at restoring euglycemia, preventing recurrences, and, if possible, alleviating the underlying cause. Providers should continue to counsel patients to treat hypoglycemia with fast-acting carbohydrates at a hypoglycemia alert value of 70 mg/dL or less. This should be reviewed at each patient visit. Hypoglycemia requires ingestion of glucose or carbohydrate-containing foods. The acute glycemic response correlates better with the glucose content of food than with the carbohydrate content of food. Pure glucose is the preferred treatment, but any form of carbohydrate that contains glucose will raise blood glucose. Added fat may retard and then prolong the acute glycemic response. In T2D, ingested protein may increase insulin response without increasing plasma glucose. Therefore, carbohydrate sources high in protein should not be used to treat or prevent hypoglycemia. Ongoing insulin activity or insulin secretagogues may lead to recurrent hypoglycemia unless more food is ingested after recovery. Once glucose returns to normal, the individual should be counseled to eat a meal or snack to prevent recurrent hypoglycemia [2].

Mild Hypoglycemia

When the patient can self-treat, mild hypoglycemia is managed with the oral administration of 15–20 g of oral carbohydrate. This should be repeated every 15–20 min until glucose is >70 mg/dL (3.9 mmol/L). Treatment and follow-up testing should be repeated if hypoglycemia persists. Several sources of short-acting carbohydrate exist (Table 45.8). Employing premeasured glucose products instead of juice or food is recommended, because patients tend to consume more than

Table 45.8 Sources of carbohydrates

	Portion	Carbohydrates
Glucose products (preferred)		
Glucose tablets	1 tablet	4 g
Glucose gel	1 gel	15 g
Insta-glucose gel	1 tube	24 g
Food/beverage (if the aforementioned are not available)		
Juice	½ cup (200 mL)	15–20 g
Soft drink (regular)	½ cup (200 m)	15–20 g
Syrup or honey	1 tbsp	6 g
Sugar	2 tbsp in water	8 g

Based on [34, 38]

15 g of juice or food, and additional calories from fat or protein may cause weight gain. Commercially available glucose tablets have the added benefit of being premeasured to help prevent overtreatment [36].

The glycemic response to oral glucose is transient, typically <2 h. Therefore, ingestion of a snack or meal shortly after the plasma glucose or SMBG is raised is generally advisable [8].

> **Key Points**
> - Rule of thumb—15 g of carbohydrate will raise blood glucose at around 50 mg/dL.
> - Rule of 15 (15 × 15): 15 g of carbohydrate every 15 min until the SMBG level is >70 mg/dL (3.9 mmol/L) [40].

Moderate Hypoglycemia

Individuals with moderate reactions will often respond to oral carbohydrates but may require more than one treatment and take longer to fully recover. These patients may be alert but will frequently be uncooperative or belligerent.

Severe Hypoglycemia

Severe hypoglycemia requiring assistance of a second or third party should be assessed in the hospital setting. Patients with impaired consciousness or an inability to swallow may aspirate and should not be treated with oral carbohydrate. These patients require either parenteral glucagon or intravenous glucose. If these are not available, glucose gels, applied between the patient's cheek and gum, may be of some help until professional care arrives.

Glucagon

The use of glucagon is indicated for the treatment of hypoglycemia in people unable or unwilling to consume carbohydrates. Those in close contact with, or having custodial care of, people with hypoglycemia-prone diabetes (family members, roommates, school personnel, childcare providers, correctional institutional staff, or coworkers) should be instructed on the use of glucagon, including where the glucagon product is kept and when and how to administer it. An individual does not need to be a healthcare professional to safely administer glucagon [2].

Currently available glucagon preparations are injectable glucagon emergency kits, recently approved nasal glucagon, and liquid glucagon rescue pen. When delivered correctly, glucagon is efficacious as a rescue therapy for severe hypoglycemia [51].

Glucagon Emergency Kits

Recombinant crystalline glucagon is available as a lyophilized powder that is mixed with an aqueous diluent to a concentration of 1 mg/dL. Because aqueous glucagon is unstable, it must be used immediately; the currently available glucagon emergency kits contain powdered glucagon that must be reconstituted using a multiple-step process before the drug can be administered parenterally [5]. The dose of glucagon needed to treat moderate or severe hypoglycemia for children <5 years old is 0.25–0.50 mg; for older children (aged 5–10 years), 0.50–1 mg, and for those >10 years old, 1 mg. Glucagon should be given intramuscularly or subcutaneously in the deltoid or anterior thigh region. Glucagon can cause nausea or vomiting, and patients should be placed on their side to reduce the risk of aspiration. The effects of glucagon are delayed by approximately 10 min from the time of injection and are only inducible in those with available glycogen stores [14, 36].

Nasal Glucagon

It is a ready-to-use drug/device combination to treat severe hypoglycemia in people with diabetes aged >4 years. A 3 mg dose of nasal glucagon powder, which does not require reconstitution, is administered in the patient's nostril. Nasal glucagon is passively absorbed through the anterior nasal mucosa without the need for inhalation, making it suitable for a comatose person with profound neuroglycopenia.

The effectiveness and ease of use of nasal glucagon (3 mg) in moderate or severe hypoglycemia events were evaluated in two real-world studies involving adults, children, and adolescents with T1D. Nasal glucagon was effective in resolving 96% of hypoglycemia events in adults within 30 min. All severe events were resolved within 15 min. The time to nasal glucagon administration was <30 s for most hypoglycemic events. Most common symptoms related to nasal glucagon administration were nasal irritation and headache. Nausea and vomiting were reported in 13%.

Nasal glucagon can be delivered by a caregiver of a person experiencing a severe hypoglycemic event using a compact, portable, single-use device with no reconstitution required.

Administration of nasal glucagon is faster and has much higher success rate for the delivery of the full dose with fewer errors than injectable glucagon [5, 51].

Liquid Glucagon Rescue Pen

A novel, ready-to-use, body temperature-stable rescue pen containing liquid glucagon was recently approved for the treatment of severe hypoglycemia in people with diabetes aged 2 years and older. The glucagon rescue pen is available in two premeasured doses: 0.5 mg for pediatric use and 1.0 mg for use in adolescents and adults. Administration of glucagon with the rescue pen is a two-step process, with no need for reconstitution [51].

Emerging Rescue Therapies for Severe Hypoglycemia

BioChaperone Glucagon

A stable, ready-to-inject, aqueous formulation of human glucagon, BioChaperone glucagon (BCG) is currently being developed to treat severe hypoglycemia.

Dasiglucagon

Dasiglucagon is a novel stable peptide analogue of human glucagon in an aqueous solution at neutral pH, with improved physical and chemical stability compared with currently available glucagon formulations [51]. This formulation is being tested in the bi-hormonal closed loop system insulin pump.

> **Remember**
> - Family members or responders should avoid sublingual placement of carbohydrate in an unconscious or impaired individual because this can increase the risk of aspiration.
> - Place the patient on their side to reduce the risk of aspiration.
> - Those in close contact with people with hypoglycemia-prone diabetes should be instructed on the use of glucagon.

Intravenous Glucose

If medical staff and equipment are available, intravenous glucose should be given as a primary treatment in preference to glucagon. Comatose patients should receive intravenous glucose. The usual dose is 25 g of 50% dextrose in water (D50) over 1–3 min. D50 comes in 50 mL; therefore, administration of 25 mL is equivalent to 12.5 g of carbohydrate. Sustained intravenous infusion of dextrose 5% (D5) or dextrose 10% (D10) at 100 cm^3/h should follow, aimed at keeping the blood glucose level at approximately 80–100 mg/dL (4.4–5.6 mmol/L) to avoid hyperglycemia, causing further stimulation of insulin release and setting in motion a vicious cycle. Blood glucose levels should be monitored initially every 15–30 min for at least 2 h or longer depending on the etiology [7, 36].

Additional Facts
- D50 is an irritant, and delivery through a large gauge port and vein, followed by a saline flush, is preferable.
- Alternatively, D10 and D5 are less irritating and can be administered via a peripheral vein in a proportionally higher volume [14].

Treatment of Hypoglycemia After Exercise

Several approaches are used to minimize hypoglycemia risk with exercise. In those injecting insulins, meal insulin doses taken a few hours before exercising often are reduced by one-half for moderate activity (such as 30-min walk) to one-quarter or less for vigorous activity, such as running or swimming. Both the intensity and the duration of activity influence the need for adjustments. The meal immediately after exercising also usually will require some reduction in dose [36].

With insulin pumps, an added benefit is the ability to reduce basal rates using temporary basal infusions. During and for a period of time after vigorous exercise, reductions in 40–90% are not uncommon [36].

Snacks taken before exercise may provide protection against hypoglycemia episodes during exercise or for a short time afterward. Some people prefer not to use fast-acting carbohydrate but instead use a mixed snack with protein, fat, and carbohydrate. It is important to make the distinction between eating to prevent hypoglycemia and eating to treat hypoglycemia. Mixed snacks are less rapidly effective in raising low blood glucose and should not be preferred to pure dextrose or other rapidly effective treatment when hypoglycemia is occurring [36].

Strategies to Reduce or Prevent Hypoglycemia

Prevention

The prevention of hypoglycemia is preferable to its treatment. Improving glycemic control while minimizing hypoglycemic episodes represents a challenge but can be accomplished safely. Physicians can use this three-step strategy to minimize hypoglycemia [8]:

1. Addressing the issue of hypoglycemia in each patient encounter. This should be addressed in each patient visit.

   If patients report a history of hypoglycemia, details regarding the time of episodes need to be identified and the treatment regimen adjusted accordingly [40]. It is important to determine what the patient's symptoms were. When did they occur in relation to the patient's last meal, and what was the patient doing when the episode occurred? Was it an isolated event, or had it occurred before? How frequently do they occur? Is there any pattern to the occurrences? How long have these events been occurring? Did weight gain or weight loss occur during this period? Is the patient taking any other medication? Did the patient lose consciousness? If so, were premonitory sings present? Was the hypoglycemia documented? Did the patient recover spontaneously? What did the patient do to prevent recurrences or relieve symptoms?

2. Applying the principles of aggressive therapy. The principles of aggressive glycemic therapy include the following:
   - (a) Patient education and empowerment
   - (b) Frequent SMBG
   - (c) Flexible insulin and other drug regimens
   - (d) Individualized glycemic goals
   - (e) Professional guidance and support

   Education regarding all aspects of diabetes care is important in the prevention and treatment of hypoglycemia. Carbohydrate counting, insulin and oral medication dosing, concomitant medications, alcohol intake, exercise, and even driving should be included in the discussion. Education will help alleviate fear of hypoglycemia that may impede ideal glycemic control.

   The Blood Glucose Awareness Training (BGAT) program is a behavioral intervention designed to improve avoidance, prediction, recognition, and treatment of hypoglycemia and hyperglycemia. Classically, BGAT consists of eight weekly group sessions during which participants are trained in behavioral techniques (self-monitoring and direct feedback) and symptoms awareness and educated about food, exercise, and insulin. Studies have reported a significantly improved detection of low blood glucose and reduced frequency of hypoglycemia and hyperglycemia, particularly in people with impaired awareness of hypoglycemia from baseline to 6 months. Benefits are maintained at 12-month follow-up with significantly fewer severe hypoglycemic events. In 2008, BGAT was adapted for Internet delivery, with data demonstrating that education can be made easily accessible to large numbers [20].

Fig. 45.4 HypoCOMPaSS

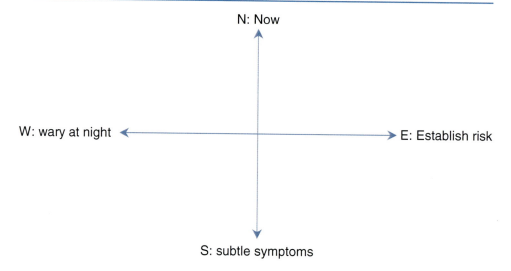

N: Now

W: wary at night

E: Establish risk

S: subtle symptoms

An education program has been developed in Germany, which focuses specifically on hypoglycemia. HyPOS consists of five weekly 90-min sessions, during which participants learn about hypoglycemia as a "vicious cycle" and are trained in symptom awareness (using diaries and SMBG). A randomized controlled trial comparing HyPOS to standard T1D education in 164 participants with impaired awareness or severe hypoglycemia found significant improvements in awareness as measured by the validated Clarke questionnaire and a modified version of the Gold score. No difference was detected in either severe hypoglycemic rate or overall glycemic control. At long-term (31 months) follow-up, incidence of severe hypoglycemia was lower in the HyPOS group with 12.5% compared with 26.5% in the controlled group [20].

The Dose Adjustment for Normal Eating (DAFNE) T1D education program that was derived from a training program developed in Düsseldorf provides a holistic approach to improving glycemic control. There is growing evidence suggesting that it reduces severe hypoglycemia and improves hypoglycemia awareness [20].

The four points of the HypoCOMPaSS (Fig. 45.4) are as follows: never delay hypoglycemia treatment, recognize personalized times of increased risk, detect subtle symptoms, and detect symptoms through regular self-monitoring, particularly for nocturnal hypoglycemia. In a multicenter randomized controlled clinical trial, the HypoCOMPaSS program was used in 110 adults with negative C-peptide T1D and impaired hypoglycemia awareness. They found that hypoglycemia awareness can be improved and recurrent severe hypoglycemia prevented in adults with long-standing T1D and impaired awareness through strategies delivered in clinical practice, targeted at rigorous avoidance of biochemical hypoglycemia without relaxation of overall control. Biochemical hypoglycemia was rapidly reduced in all

groups within the first 4 weeks, driven by the insulin dose adjustment algorithm and sustained throughout the 24-week trial [52].

3. Considering both the conventional risk factors and those indicative of compromised glucose counterregulation [8].

Hypoglycemic episodes that are not readily explained by conventional factors, for example, skipped or irregular meals, unplanned exercise, alcohol ingestion, etc., may be due to excessive doses of medications used to treat diabetes. A thorough review of blood glucose patterns may suggest vulnerable periods of the day that mandate adjustments to current medications.

A history of severe iatrogenic hypoglycemia is a clinical red flag. Unless it was the result of an obviously remediable factor, such as a missed meal after insulin administration or vigorous exercise without appropriate regimen adjustment, a substantive change in the regimen must be made. If it is not, the risk of recurrent severe hypoglycemia is unacceptably high.

In patients injecting insulin, the following strategies can help minimize hypoglycemia. With basal-bolus insulin regimen, morning fasting hypoglycemia implicates the long- or intermediate-acting insulin. Daytime hypoglycemia may be caused by the rapid, fast, or longer-acting insulins. Nocturnal hypoglycemia may also be caused by rapid and longer-acting insulins. Substitution of preprandial regular insulin with fast-acting insulin (lispro, aspart, glulisine) reduces the frequency of daytime hypoglycemia. Similarly, substitution of a long-acting insulin analogue (glargine, detemir, degludec) for intermediate-acting insulins such as NPH or premix 70/30 also reduces the frequency of nocturnal or daytime hypoglycemia [8].

With a CSII regimen using a fast-acting insulin such as lispro, nocturnal and morning fasting hypoglycemia implicate the basal insulin infusion rate, whereas daytime hypoglycemia may implicate the preprandial insulin bolus doses, the basal insulin infusion rate, or both.

Insulin secretagogues can also produce hypoglycemia related to absolute or relative insulin excess. However, sulfonylureas may pose the greatest risk of hypoglycemia in patients with altered renal or hepatic function and in older individuals. Substitution with other classes of oral agents or even GLP-1 receptor agonists (GLP-1 RA) should be considered in the event of hypoglycemia.

In patients with clinical hypoglycemia unawareness, a 2- to 3-week period of scrupulous avoidance of hypoglycemia is advisable and can be assessed by return of awareness of hypoglycemia.

Strategies to Reduce Hypoglycemia

Since the first injection of insulin in 1922, interest has increased in replacing insulin in the most physiologic manner for patients with diabetes. In the 1980s, the introduction of recombinant human insulin reduced the formation of antibodies and provided more predictable pharmacokinetic profiles. The next decade produced analogue insulins that initially were designed to provide a faster onset and shorter duration of action. These insulins (lispro, aspart, glulisine) were designed to reproduce more closely the typical physiologic prandial spikes of insulin observed following meals.

The second wave produced long-acting basal types of insulin (glargine U100, detemir) and more recently ultra-long-acting analogues (degludec, glargine U300) designed to mimic background constitutive insulin release. Studies in T1D have demonstrated that hypoglycemia (particularly nocturnal) can be reduced with fast-acting analogues rather than regular insulins. Similarly, long-acting analogues have been demonstrated to reduce hypoglycemia by 20–33% in patients with T2D when compared with NPH-based regimens. Thus, current recommendations are to use analogue-based insulin replacement whenever possible [7].

Technology in the Reduction and Prevention of Hypoglycemia

The rapid technological advances in the management of diabetes with CGM systems or integrated CGM and insulin pump use have empowered individuals with T1D to further address and reduce hypoglycemia.

Continuous Glucose Monitoring

Advances in technology have allowed the development of real-time continuous glucose monitoring (CGM) devices that can be programmed to alarm in response to failing glucose or when hypoglycemia or hyperglycemia occurs or is predicted. CGM devices provide a broad spectrum of information on real-time glucose trends. Currently available CGM devices measure interstitial glucose concentrations subcutaneously at 5- to 15-min intervals.

CGM can be divided into three categories: blinded/retrospective CGM, real-time CGM, and intermittently scanned/viewed CGM, also known as flash glucose monitoring [53].

Randomized controlled trials (RCTs) evaluating the benefit of CGM mainly focused on HbA1c as the primary outcome. Apart from the SWITCH study showing a significant effect of adding CGM to insulin pump therapy on time spent in hypoglycemia, most studies failed to demonstrate a significant or relevant reduction in mild hypoglycemia. Notably, RCTs primarily aimed at hypoglycemia prevention did demonstrate a significant reduction in mild hypoglycemia in terms of reducing the time spent in hypoglycemia by approximately 40% and reducing the number of mild hypoglycemic events per day [53].

In patients with T1D and impaired hypoglycemia awareness, data from a recent RCT and from an observational study suggested reduced severe hypoglycemia using CGM compared with SMBG.

Real-time CGM can reduce the frequency of severe hypoglycemia in people with impaired awareness of hypoglycemia and in those with long-standing T1D.

Continuous Subcutaneous Insulin Infusion (CSII)

Commonly known as insulin pump therapy, CSII has been recommended by several professional organizations as a therapeutic option for T1D complicated by problematic or severe hypoglycemia [20].

Insulin pump development began in the 1970s and over the last 20 years has become a major method of insulin replacement. Studies in children and pregnant women have demonstrated reduction in hypoglycemia when compared with MDI regimens [7].

A review and meta-analysis that only included studies of more than 6-month duration, comparing the frequency of severe hypoglycemia and the associated HbA1c during MDI and CSII, revealed a significant reduction in severe hypoglycemia in people with T1D who used CSII compared with the non-analogue-based MDI. However, most of the trials used NPH insulin as the basal insulin [54].

In multiple trials comparing CSII with multiple daily injections (MDI), there has been a modest improvement in HbA1c; however, the majority of the systematic reviews have failed to confirm a significant reduction in severe hypoglycemia. A Cochrane review found no relevant benefit of

CSII over multiple daily injections (MDI) for reducing non-severe hypoglycemic events, but data indicated a possible benefit of CSII over MDI in terms of reducing severe hypoglycemia [55]. As these meta-analyses are based on clinical trial data obtained prior to 2008, the pumps utilized are at least 10 years older than the current technology available; thus, they lack some more advanced features now available on newer pumps.

In the HypoCOMPaSS trial, the authors concluded that the restoration of hypoglycemia unawareness and the prevention of hypoglycemia could be achieved with either self-monitoring blood glucose (SMBG) and MDI or CSII and RT-CGM (real-time continuous glucose monitoring) when management is truly optimized using fast-acting and basal insulin analogues with appropriate therapeutic targets and regular SMBG including interval nighttime testing [52].

Sensor-Augmented Pumps (SAP)

SAP therapy, defined as a combination of insulin pump and CGM, represents the first step on the path toward an artificial pancreas. The first RCT to insulin pump therapy in those with T1D showed similar reductions in HbA1c after 6 months, but this was associated with significant increased hypoglycemia exposure in the insulin pump with the SMBG group.

The Sensor-Augmented Pump Therapy for A1c Reduction (STAR) 3 study randomized participants to either SAP or maintained them on MDI therapy with conventional SMBG checks for a 1-year study period and reported a greater reduction in HbA1c was associated with an increased frequency of sensor use. Those using SAP were more likely to attain the HbA1c targets and have decreased hypoglycemic exposure and decreased glycemic variability.

Sensor-Augmented Pumps with Low Glucose Suspension (Suspend on Low)

This insulin pump model is connected to a CGM that automatically suspends basal insulin delivery for a maximum of 2 h if the individual does not respond to a hypoglycemia alarm. This has been shown to reduce the duration of hypoglycemia in those with very frequent hypoglycemia at baseline, especially at night. This function also reduces moderate and severe episodes of hypoglycemia in patients with hypoglycemia unawareness. The reduction in hypoglycemia was not associated with deterioration of glucose control or ketosis [5].

The Automation to Simulate Pancreatic Insulin Response (ASPIRE) in-clinic study demonstrated that the mean duration of hypoglycemia was shorter on SAP-suspend on low and the nadir glucose was higher.

The ASPIRE in-home study reported a 37.5% reduction in the primary end point for nocturnal hypoglycemia in the SAP with low suspend vs. SAP alone. Despite this reduction in hypoglycemia, there was no deterioration in glycemic control [51].

An RCT of 247 participants showed that the use of a sensor-augmented insulin pump therapy with the threshold-suspend feature over a 3-month period reduced nocturnal hypoglycemia, without increasing HbA1c levels [56].

Sensor-Augmented Pump Therapy with Predictive Low Glucose Management (Suspend Before Low)

The Predictive Low Glucose Management system suspends basal insulin infusion with the prediction of hypoglycemia. Basal insulin infusion is suspended when sensor glucose is at or within 70 mg/dL (3.9 mmol/L) above the patient-set low limit and is predicted to be 20 mg/dL (1.1 mmol/L) above this low limit in 30 min. In the absence of patient interference, following pump suspension, the insulin infusion resumes after a maximum suspend period of 2 h or earlier if the auto-resumption parameters are met. The PLGM reduced hypoglycemia under in-clinic conditions and in short-term and long-term home studies. There was no deterioration of glycemic control with the use of the system in a 6-month randomized controlled home trial [5].

In 45 participants between the ages of 15 and 45 years, the system reduced hypoglycemia exposure by 81% and time spent <60 mg/dL (<3.3 mmol/) by 70%, while not leading into a difference in blood glucose levels in the morning [53].

Closed Loop Systems

Automated insulin delivery consists of three components: an insulin pump, a continuous glucose sensor, and an algorithm that determines insulin delivery. These systems not only suspend insulin delivery but also can increase insulin delivery based on sensor glucose values. Closed loop systems have been under development for several years with numerous algorithms and tested in clinical research centers, hotels, camps, supervised outpatient settings, and free-living conditions. Despite variable clinical and technical characteristics, artificial pancreas systems uniformly improve glucose control with a 50% relative risk reduction in hypoglycemia in outpatient settings compared to conventional pump therapy. Closed loop systems appear to hold great promise for the future as a tool to help prevent hypoglycemia in T1D [20, 53].

Fig. 45.5 Glycosylated hemoglobin compared with severe hypo rate in patient. (Adapted from [17, 36, 56])

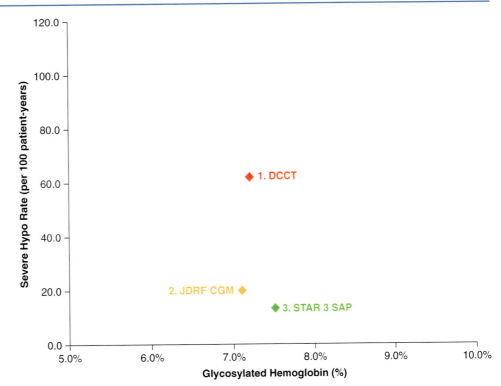

One interesting development has been the evaluation of dual-hormone delivery systems with an additional pump delivery the counterregulatory hormone dasiglucagon, potentially increasing the effect in rescuing failing blood glucose.

The development of newer technologies and devices has made it possible to achieve glycemic control while minimizing the risk of hypoglycemia, first with the CGM and then with SAP (Fig. 45.5).

Beta Cell Replacement

The transplantation of isolated islets or a whole pancreas is a potential therapy for the treatment of T1D, particularly when complicated by recurrent episodes of hypoglycemia. Patients undergoing whole pancreas transplantation require a major surgery and will be on life-long immunosuppressive therapy with a mortality rate of 3–5%. This is why it is largely performed together with kidney transplantation (simultaneous pancreas-kidney or SPK), as they will need immunosuppressive therapy [20, 57].

Both approaches can restore insulin secretion, but the transplantation of islets isolated from more than one donor pancreas is usually necessary to achieve insulin independence. The durability of insulin independence is superior following whole pancreas transplantation, especially when it is SPK.

The magnitude of the beta-cell secretory capacity responses following whole pancreas transplantation appears normal and may be sustained for more than a decade despite ongoing immunosuppression drug exposure. In the absence of immunologic graft loss, the beta-cell secretory capacity can remain stable for years during longitudinal follow-up, while first-phase insulin response to glucose may decrease coincident with lessening of glucocorticoid doses and improvement in insulin sensitivity.

In T1D recipients of intrahepatic islet transplants, there is recovery of the physiologic islet cell hormonal responses to insulin-induced hypoglycemia whereby endogenous insulin secretion is appropriately suppressed and glucagon secretion is partially restored. Rickels and colleagues have demonstrated normalization of the glycemic thresholds for counterregulatory epinephrine, autonomic symptoms, and growth hormone responses in islet transplant recipients with T1D [57].

The CIT-07 Trial (Clinical Islet Transplantation Consortium Protocol 07) was a phase 3 clinical trial of transplantation of islet products in subjects with TID, impaired awareness of hypoglycemia, and intractable severe hypoglycemia. This trial showed that 87.5% of the subjects achieved freedom of severe hypoglycemia along with glycemic control (HbA1c <7%) at 1 year post-initial islet transplantation. The subjects reported consistent, statistically significant, and clinically meaningful improvements in condition-specific health-related quality of life as well as self-assessment of overall health [58].

Pancreas transplantation has been performed in patients with T1D for >25 years. In general, hypoglycemic rates improve dramatically in the first year after transplantation. Most studies also demonstrate that counterregulatory defenses are improved after pancreatic transplantation. Most notably, glucagon response to hypoglycemia increases, accompanied at an early stage by some improvement in epinephrine and symptomatic responses [7].

> **Concluding Remarks**
> - Patients with T1D and long-standing T2D have an altered counterregulatory response to hypoglycemia, making them more susceptible.
> - Hypoglycemia is a major limiting factor in the management of diabetes; nonetheless, it is possible to improve glycemic control by acknowledging the problem, considering the risk factors, applying the principles of intensive therapy, and individualizing glycemic goals.
> - It is possible to achieve optimal glycemic control while minimizing hypoglycemia by structured patient education concerning self-monitoring and appropriate lifestyle and physiologic and flexible insulin regimen.
> - As time passes, safer and more physiologic insulin analogues are being manufactured, and novel technologies are being developed, which will facilitate achieving normoglycemia.

Multiple-Choice Questions

1. A 28-year-old T1D patient is experiencing palpitations, anxiety, shakiness, and hunger 2 h after running 10k. He checks his capillary blood glucose and it is 48 mg/dL (2.7 mmol/L). How would you classify this hypoglycemia?
   (a) **Symptomatic hypoglycemia**
   (b) Severe hypoglycemia
   (c) Moderate hypoglycemia
   (d) Hypoglycemia unawareness
   (e) Hypoglycemia-associated autonomic failure

2. An 18-year-old healthy college student is experiencing headaches, palpitations, anxiety, and hunger after a 2-h figure-skating practice; she forgot to eat breakfast before her practice. Her coach performs a capillary blood glucose with a value of 54 mg/dL (3 mmol/L). Which of the following is correct regarding the normal counterregulatory response?

   (a) Glucagon stores are depleted; therefore, cortisol and growth hormone are the principal hormonal response.
   (b) As blood glucose levels fall, there is an increased release of insulin, glucagon, and epinephrine within minutes to increase glycogenolysis and gluconeogenesis.
   (c) There is a decreased brain glucose uptake; therefore, epinephrine and cortisol will rise within minutes to increase glycogenolysis and gluconeogenesis.
   (d) **The first response is a decreased insulin level, followed by an increase in glucagon and epinephrine.**

3. A 35-year-old patient with long-standing T1D had a morning capillary blood glucose of 36 mg/dL (2 mmol/L). He denies any symptoms of hypoglycemia, although he has been having difficulty sleeping and nightmares. Which of the following statements is correct regarding his counterregulatory response to hypoglycemia?
   (a) As blood glucose levels decrease, his insulin levels will not decrease; therefore, glucagon and epinephrine become the critical response and will increase within minutes.
   (b) Cortisol and growth hormone become the principal response, since there is deficient release of glucagon and epinephrine.
   (c) **The patient is experiencing hypoglycemia unawareness, with blunted glucagon and epinephrine responses.**
   (d) Insulin levels do not decrease, and glucagon response becomes impaired; therefore, epinephrine becomes a critical response and will rise within minutes.

4. A 75-year-old patient with long-standing T2D is experiencing frequent episodes of hypoglycemia. He has background retinopathy, symmetrical neuropathy, and nephropathy with an estimated GFR of 50 mL/min. The patient states that he sometimes misses his meals. His last HbA1c was 7.5%. He is on glyburide, metformin, and bedtime insulin NPH. What changes in management will decrease his episodes of hypoglycemia?
   (a) Change insulin NPH to a more physiologic long-acting insulin analogue.
   (b) His HbA1c is at goal; ensure the patient does not skip meals and advise him to take snacks between meals.
   (c) Advise the patient to decrease the dose of his NPH by half.
   (d) **Discontinue glyburide, but continue the same dose of insulin NPH.**

5. A 35-year-old female patient with T1D had an episode of hypoglycemia on Sunday morning. Her basal insulin dose was recently increased since her fasting capillary blood glucose was not at goal. She has been experiencing abdominal cramps and fatigue as she started her menstrual period on Friday. On Saturday, she had a light dinner with two cups of wine and administered fast-acting insulin according to her carbohydrate counting. What is the most likely cause of her hypoglycemia?

(a) The increase in her basal insulin dose.

(b) Hormonal imbalance due to her menstrual period.

(c) The fast-acting insulin dose was excessive.

(d) **Alcohol intake.**

6. A 59-year-old patient with long-standing T1D with microvascular complications (diabetic proliferative retinopathy, diabetic nephropathy (estimated GFR of 45 mL/min), distal symmetric neuropathy, autoimmune hypothyroidism, dyslipidemia, and ischemic heart disease) is experiencing frequent episodes of hypoglycemia. The patient is on a flexible insulin regimen with a basal insulin analogue and a fast-acting insulin analogue, aspirin, beta-1 selective blocker, angiotensin-converting enzyme inhibitor (ACEI), and levothyroxine. His last HbA1c was 7.8%, TSH 3.2 mUI/L, and Cr 1.8 mg/dL. Which of the following confers the greatest risk for hypoglycemia?

(a) Age

(b) Background retinopathy

(c) **Diabetic nephropathy**

(d) Ischemic heart disease

(e) HbA1c level

(f) Current medications: insulin, salicylate, beta-selective blocker, ACEI

(g) Hypothyroidism

7. A 65-year-old patient with long-standing T2D with a history of background retinopathy, autonomic neuropathy, diabetic nephropathy, and ischemic heart disease is experiencing frequent episodes of hypoglycemia. He had an acute myocardial infarction with subsequent coronary artery bypass grafting (CABG) a few months ago. He is on metformin, NPH insulin, statin, beta blocker, aspirin, and angiotensin receptor blocker. His HbA1c is 7%. Which of the following is the most appropriate statement?

(a) He needs tight glycemic control to decrease the progression of microvascular complications.

(b) His HbA1c is at goal; therefore, changing insulin NPH to insulin analogue will decrease the risk of subsequent hypoglycemia while ensuring optimal glycemic control.

(c) **He has high cardiovascular risk; therefore, his HbA1c goal should be higher; consider decreasing his insulin NPH.**

(d) He has high cardiovascular risk; therefore adding an SGLT2 inhibitor will decrease his cardiovascular risk.

8. What are the clinical implications of hypoglycemia on a patient with long-standing T2D and ischemic heart disease, diabetic nephropathy, diabetic retinopathy, and peripheral neuropathy?

(a) Hypoglycemia may accelerate the progression of diabetic retinopathy to proliferative retinopathy.

(b) Hypoglycemia is associated with worsening of glomerular filtration rate and proteinuria.

(c) **Hypoglycemia can increase his cardiovascular risk by triggering arrhythmias or thromboembolic events.**

(d) Repeated hypoglycemia may worsen his peripheral neuropathy.

9. A 68-year-old patient with T2D is brought to the emergency department with altered mental status. He is awake but very confused and combative. He has a history of alcohol abuse. He is currently on basal insulin analogue, sulfonylureas, and metformin. He has a blood glucose level of 35 mg/dL. Which of the following is the most appropriate treatment for this patient?

(a) 15–20 g of carbohydrate every 15 min until his blood glucose is more than 70 mg/dL and then provide a meal.

(b) 1 mg of intramuscular glucagon, placing the patient on his side to ensure that he does not aspirate.

(c) Administer 25 g of 50% dextrose over 1–3 min, and discharge the patient when his blood glucose is more than 70 mg/dL.

(d) **Administer a bolus of dextrose 50%, and then continue with IV glucose infusion 5–10% for 2–3 days, checking blood glucose every hour.**

10. A 15-year-old patient with T1D is experiencing frequent noon and nocturnal hypoglycemia. The patient frequently misses meals, has erratic schedules, and gets confused with her insulin regimen. Which of the following strategies will most likely decrease her risk of subsequent hypoglycemia.

(a) Write down a prescription with a detailed insulin regimen and advise the patient to eat at a regular basis and avoid missing meals.

(b) Organize a meeting with her parents addressing the importance of regular meals and explain in detail and writing her insulin regimen.

(c) **Explain to the patient the importance of SMBG, explain in detail and in writing her insulin regimen, explain the importance of regular meals, and schedule an appointment with a diabetes educator.**

(d) Change the insulin regimen to a fixed dose so the patient does not get confused.

References

1. International Hypoglycaemia Study Group. Glucose concentrations of less than 3.0 mmol/L (54 mg/dL) should be reported in clinical trial: a joint position statement of the American Diabetes Association and the European Association for the Study of Diabetes. Diabetes Care. 2017;40:155–7.
2. American Diabetes Association Professional Practice Committee; American Diabetes Association Professional Practice Committee, Draznin B, Aroda VR, Bakris G, Benson G, Brown FM, Freeman R, Green J, Huang E, Isaacs D, Kahan S, Leon J, Lyons SK, Peters AL, Prahalad P, Reusch JEB, Young-Hyman D, Das S, Kosiborod M. 6. Glycemic targets: standards of medical care in diabetes-2022. Diabetes Care. 2022;45(Suppl 1):S90–2. https://doi.org/10.2337/dc22-S006. PMID: 34964868.
3. Cryer PE, Axelrod L, Grossman AB, Heller SR, Montori VM, Seaquist ER, et al. Evaluation and management of adult hypoglycemic disorders: an endocrine society clinical practice guideline. J Clin Endocrinol Metab. 2009;94:709–28.
4. Seaquist ER, Anderson J, Childs B, Dagogo-Jack S, Fish L, Heller S, et al. Hypoglycemia and diabetes: a report of a workgroup of the American Diabetes Association and the Endocrine Society. Diabetes Care. 2013;36:1384–95.
5. Abraham MB, Jones TW, Naranjo D, Karges B, Oduwole A, Tauschmann M, Maas DM. ISPAD Clinical Practice Consensus Guidelines 2018: assessment and management of hypoglycemia in children and adolescents with diabetes. Pediatr Diabetes. 2018;19(Suppl 27):178–92. https://doi.org/10.1111/pedi.12698.
6. Cryer PE. Banting lecture: hypoglycemia: the limiting factor in the management of IDDM. Diabetes. 1994;43:1378–89.
7. Davis SN, Lamos EM, Younk LM. Chapter 47 Hypoglycemia and hypoglycemic syndromes. In: Jameson JL, De Groot LJ, editors. Endocrinology: adult and pediatric. 7th ed. Philadelphia, PA: Elsevier Saunders; 2016. p. 816–838e8.
8. Cryer PE, Davis SN, Shamoon H. Hypoglycemia in diabetes. Diabetes Care. 2003;26:1902–12.
9. McCrimmon RJ, Sherwin RS. Hypoglycemia in type 1 diabetes. Diabetes. 2010;59:2333–9.
10. Zammitt NN, Frier BM. Hypoglycemia in type 2 diabetes. Diabetes Care. 2005;28(12):2948–61.
11. Cryer PE. Mechanisms of hypoglycemia-associated autonomic failure in diabetes. N Engl J Med. 2013;369(4):362–72.
12. Shaffie G, Mohajeri-Tehrani M, Pajouhi M, Larijani B. The importance of hypoglycemia in diabetic patients. J Diab Metab Disord. 2012;11(17):1–7.
13. Khunti K, Alsifri S, Aroson R, Cigrovski Berkovik M, Enters-Weijnen C, Forsen T, et al. Rates and predictors of hypoglycemia in 27 585 people from 24 countries with insulin treated type 1 and type 2 diabetes: the global HAT study. Diabetes Obes Metab. 2016;18:907–15.
14. Lamos EM, Younk LM, Davis SN. IX Glucose disorders. Chapter 25 Hypoglycemia. In: Matfin G, editor. A Clinician's guide. Endocrine and metabolic medical emergencies. 1st ed. Washington, DC: Endocrine Press Books; 2018. p. 243–58.
15. Akirov A, Grossman A, Shochat T, Simon I. Mortality among hospitalized patients with hypoglycemia: insulin related and noninsulin related. J Clin Endocrinol Metab. 2017;102(2):416–24.
16. Cryer PE. Death during intensive glycemic therapy of diabetes: mechanisms and implications. Commentary. Am J Med. 2011;124(11):993–6.
17. The DCCT Research Group. The effect of intensive treatment of diabetes on the development and progression of long-term complications in insulin-dependent diabetes mellitus. N Engl J Med. 1998;329:977–86.
18. Gubitosi-Klug RA, Braffet BH, White NH, Sherwin RS, Service FJ, Lachin JM, et al. Risk of severe hypoglycemia in type 1 diabetes over 30 years of follow-up in the DCCT/EDIC study. Diabetes Care. 2017;40:1010–6.
19. Diabetes Control and Complications Trial/Epidemiology of Diabetes Intervention and Complications (DCCT/EDIC) Research Group. Modern-day clinical course of type 1 diabetes mellitus after 30 years duration. Arch Intern Med. 2009;169(14):1307–16.
20. Little SA, Leelarathna L, Barandse SM, Walkinshaw E, Tan HK, Solomon L, et al. Severe Hypoglycaemia in type 1 diabetes mellitus: underlying drivers and potential strategies for successful prevention. Diabetes Metab Res Rev. 2014;30:175–90.
21. Cryer PE, Childs BP. Negotiating the barrier of hypoglycemia in diabetes. Diab Spectr. 2002;15(1):20–7.
22. Miller DC, Phillips LS, Zimer DC, Gallina DL, Cook CB, El-Kebbi IM. Hypoglycemia in patients with type 2 diabetes mellitus. Arch Intern Med. 2001;161:1653–9.
23. International Hypoglycaemia Study Group. Minimizing hypoglycemia in diabetes. Diabetes Care. 2015;38:1583–91.
24. Anderson M, Powell J, Campbell KM, Taylor JR. Optimal management of type 2 diabetes in patients with increased risk of hypoglycemia. Diab Metab Syndr Obes Targ Ther. 2014;7:85–94.
25. Monami M, Dicembrini I, Kundisova L, Zannoni S, Nreu B, Mannucci E. A meta-analysis of the hypoglycaemic risk in randomized controlled trials with sulphonylureas in patients with type 2 diabetes. Diabetes Obes Metab. 2014;16:833–40.
26. Little S, Shaw J, Home P. Hypoglycemia rates with basal insulin analogs. Diabetes Technol Ther. 2011;13(Suppl 1):S53–64.
27. Lane W, Bailey TS, Getery G, Grumprecht J, Philis-Tsimikas A, Thim Hansen C, et al. Effect of insulin degludec vs insulin glargine U100 on hypoglycemia in patients with type 1 diabetes. The SWITCH 1 randomized clinical trial. JAMA. 2017;318:33–44.
28. Wysham C, Bhargava A, Chaykin L, de la Rosa R, Handelsman Y, Troelsen LN, et al. Effect of insulin degludec vs insulin glargine U100 on hypoglycemia in patients with type 2 diabetes. The SWITCH 2 randomized clinical trial. JAMA. 2017;318:45–56.
29. Seaquist ER, Chow L. Hypoglycemia in diabetes. Does insulin type matter? JAMA. 2017;318:31–2.
30. Becker RHA, Dahmen R, Bergmann K, Lehmann A, Jax T, Heise T. New insulin glargine 300 units mL-1 provides a more even activity profile and prolonged glycemic control at steady state compared with insulin Glargine 100 units mL-1. Diabetes Care. 2015;38(4):637–43.
31. Bailey T, Dahmen R, Pettus J, Roussel R, Bergmann K, Maroccia M, Nassr N, Klein O, Bolli G, Heise T. Insulin glargine 300 u/ml (gla-300) provides more stable and more evenly distributed steady-state pharmacodynamic/pharmacokinetic profiles compared with insulin degludec in type 1 diabetes (T1DM). Endocr Pract. 2017;23(1):48A.
32. Rosenstock J, Cheng A, Ritzel R, Bosnyak Z, Devisme C, Cali AMG, Sieber J, Stella P, Wang X, Frías JP, Roussel R, Bolli GB. More similarities than differences testing insulin glargine 300 units/ml versus insulin degludec 100 units/ml in insulin-naive type 2 diabetes: the randomized head-to-head BRIGHT trial. Diabetes Care. 2018;41(10):2147–54. https://doi.org/10.2337/dc18-0559. PMID: 30104294.
33. Cox DJ, et al. Perceived symptoms in the recognition of hypoglycemia. Diabetes Care. 1993;16(2):519–27.
34. Bruderer SG, Bodmer M, Jick S, Bader G, Schlienger RG, Meier CR. Incidence of and risk factors for severe hypoglycaemia in treated type 2 diabetes mellitus patients in the UK – a nested case–control analysis. Diabetes Obes Metab. 2014;16:801–11.
35. Ilan G, Shamoon H. Hypoglycemia in diabetes: common, often unrecognized. Cleve Clin J Med. 2004;71(4):335–42.

36. Kaufman FR. Hypoglycemia. In: Kaufman FR, editor. Medical management of type 1 diabetes. 6th ed. Arlington, VA: United States of America. American Diabetes Association; 2012. p. 150–60.

37. Davis TM, Brown SF, Jacobs IG, Bulsara M, Bruce DG, et al. Determinants of severe hypoglycemia complicating type 2 diabetes: the Fremantle diabetes study. J Clin Endocrinol Metab. 2010;95(5):2240–7.

38. McCall AL. Chapter 40 Hypoglycemia in diabetes. In: Umpierrez GE, editor. Therapy for diabetes mellitus and related disorders. 6th ed. Arlington, VA: American Diabetes Association; 2014. p. 696–728.

39. Gomez AM, Gomez C, Aschner P, Veloza A, Muñoz O, Rubio C, Vallejo. Effects of performing morning versus afternoon exercise on glycemic control and hypoglycemia frequency in type 1 diabetes patients on sensor-augmented insulin pump therapy. J Diabetes Sci Technol. 2015;9(3):619–24.

40. Briscoe VJ, et al. Hypoglycemia in type 1 and type 2 diabetes: physiology, pathophysiology, and management. Clin Diab. 2005;24(3):115–21.

41. Arky RA. Hypoglycemia associated with liver disease and ethanol. Endocrinol Metab Clin N Am. 1989;18:175–90.

42. Desouza CV, Bolli GB, Fonseca V. Hypoglycemia, diabetes, and cardiovascular events. Diabetes Care. 2010;33(6):1389–94.

43. Monier L, Wojtusciszyn A, Collete C, Owens. The contribution of glucose variability to asymptomatic hypoglycemia in persons with type 2 diabetes. Diabetes Technol Ther. 2011;13(8):813–181.

44. Younk LM, Davis ST. Hypoglycemia and vascular disease. Clin Chem. 2011;57(2):258–60.

45. Frier BM, Schernthaner G, Heller S. Hypoglycemia and cardiovascular risks. Diabetes Care. 2011;34(2):S132–7.

46. Skyler JS, Bergenstal R, Bonow RO, Buse J, Deedwania P, Gale E, Howard B, et al. Intensive glucose control and the prevention of cardiovascular events: implications of the ACCORD, ADVANCE, and VA diabetes trials: a position statement of the American Diabetes Association and a Scientific Statement of the American College of Cardiology Foundation and the American Heart Association. Circulation. 2009;119:351–7.

47. Novodvorsky P, Chow E, Iqbal A, Sellors L, Williams S, Fawdry RA, et al. Diurnal differences in risk of cardiac arrythmias during spontaneous hypoglycemia in young people with type 1 diabetes. Diabetes Care. 2017;40:655–62.

48. Tanenberg RJ, Newton CA, Drake AJ. Confirmation of Hypoglycemia in the "Dead-in-bed" syndrome, as captured by a retrospective continuous glucose monitoring system. Endocr Pract. 2010;16(2):244–8.

49. Guisasola FA, Povedano ST, Krishnarajah G, Lyu R, Mavros P, Yin D. Hypoglycaemic symptoms, treatment satisfaction, adherence and their associations with glycaemic goal in patients with type 2 diabetes mellitus: findings from the real-life effectiveness and care patterns of diabetes management (RECAP-DM) Study. Diabetes Obes Metab. 2008;10(Suppl):25–32.

50. Leiter LA, Yale JF, Chaisson JL, Harris SB, Kleinstiver P, Sauriol L. Assessment of the impact of fear of hypoglycemic episodes on glycemic and hypoglycemia management. Can J Diabetes. 2005;29(3):186–92.

51. Thieu VT, Mitchell BD, Varnado OJ, Frier BM. Treatment and prevention of severe hypoglycaemia in people with diabetes: current and new formulations of glucagon. Diabetes Obes Metab. 2020;22(4):469–79. https://doi.org/10.1111/dom.13941. PMID: 31820562.

52. Little S, Leelarathna L, Walkinshaw E, Kai Tan H, Chapple O, Lubina-Solomon A, Chadwick TJ, et al. Recovery of hypoglycemia awareness in long-standing type 1 diabetes: a multicenter 2x2 factorial randomized controlled trial comparing insulin pump with multiple daily injections and continuous with conventional glucose self-monitoring (HypoCOMPaSS). Diabetes Care. 2014;37(8):2114–22.

53. Sherr JL, Tauschmann M, Battelino T, de Bock M, Frolenza G, Roman R, Hood KK, Maahs DM. ISPAD Clinical Practice Consensus Guidelines 2018: diabetes technologies. Pediatr Diabetes. 2018;19(Suppl 27):302–25. https://doi.org/10.1111/pedi.12731. PMID: 30039513.

54. Pickup JC, Sutton AJ. Severe hypoglycaemia and glycemic control in Type 1 diabetes: meta-analysis of multiple daily insulin injections compared with continuous subcutaneous insulin infusion. Diabet Med. 2008;25(7):765–77.

55. Little S, Chadwick T, Choudhary P, Brennand C, Stickland J, Barendse S, et al. Comparison of optimised MDI versus pumps with or without sensors in severe hypoglycaemia (the hypo COMPaSS trial). BMC Endocr Disord. 2012;12(33):1–14.

56. Bergenstal RM, et al. Threshold-based insulin-pump interruption for a reduction of hypoglycemia. N Engl J Med. 2013;369(3):224–32.

57. Rickels MR. Recovery of endocrine function after islet and pancreas transplantation. Curr Diab Rep. 2012;12:587–97.

58. Foster ED, Bridges ND, Feurer ID, Eggerman TL, Hunsicker LG, Alejandro R. Clinical islet transplantation consortium. improved health-related quality of life in a phase 3 islet transplantation trial in type 1 diabetes complicated by severe hypoglycemia. Diabetes Care. 2018;41(5):1001–8. https://doi.org/10.2337/dc17-1779.

59. Arem R. Hypoglycemia associated with renal failure. Endocrinol Metab Clin N Am. 1989;18:103–13.

Further Reading

Books

Davis SN, Lamos EM, Younk LM. Chapter 47 Hypoglycemia and hypoglycemic syndromes. In: Jameson JL, De Groot LJ, editors. Endocrinology: adult and pediatric. 7th ed. Philadelphia, PA: Elsevier Saunders; 2016. p. 816–838e8.

T1D and Hypoglycemia

Little SA, Leelarathna L, Barandse SM, Walkinshaw E, Tan HK, Solomon L, et al. Severe Hypoglycaemia in type 1 diabetes mellitus: underlying drivers and potential strategies for successful prevention. Diabetes Metab Res Rev. 2014;30:175–90.

Physiology and Pathophysiology of Hypoglycemia

Cryer PE. Banting Lecture: Hypoglycemia: the limiting factor in the management of IDDM. Diabetes. 1994;43:1378–89.

Cryer PE. Mechanisms of hypoglycemia-associated autonomic failure in diabetes. N Engl J Med. 2013;369(4):362–72.

Cryer PE, Davis SN, Shamoon H. Hypoglycemia in diabetes. Diabetes Care. 2003;26:1902–12.

McCrimmon RJ, Sherwin RS. Hypoglycemia in type 1 diabetes. Diabetes. 2010;59:2333–9.

Insulins and Hypoglycemia

Little S, Shaw J, Home P. Hypoglycemia rates with basal insulin analogs. Diabetes Technol Ther. 2011;13(Suppl 1):S53–64.

Pancreas Transplantation

Rickels MR. Recovery of endocrine function after islet and pancreas transplantation. Curr Diab Rep. 2012;12:587–96.

HRS: Hypoglycemia Risk Score

Hyporiskcore. n.d. www.hyporiskcore.com.

Hypoglycemia in ACCORD, ADVANCE, and VADT

Skyler JS, Bergenstal R, Bonow RO, Buse J, Deedwania P, Gale E, Howard B, et al. Intensive glucose control and the prevention of cardiovascular events: implications of the ACCORD, ADVANCE, and VA diabetes trials: a position statement of the American Diabetes Association and a scientific statement of the American College of Cardiology Foundation and the American Heart Association. Circulation. 2009;119:351–7.

Inpatient Management of Diabetes and Hyperglycemia

William B. Horton

Introduction

Individuals with diabetes mellitus (DM) are more likely to be hospitalized and have longer durations of hospital stay than those without DM [1]. Approximately one in four patients admitted to the hospital has a known diagnosis of DM [2, 3], and about 30% of patients with DM require two or more hospitalizations in any given year [3]. A 2007 study estimated that 22% of all hospital inpatient days were incurred by people with DM and costs associated with hospitalization for DM patients accounted for half of all healthcare expenditures for the disease [4]. Given the increasing incidence and prevalence of DM in the Unites States since that time [5], it is likely that these figures have only increased.

Recent studies show that one-third of all hospitalized patients will experience significant hyperglycemia [6], and patients without preexisting DM can even experience stress-related hyperglycemia while hospitalized [7]. Uncontrolled hyperglycemia in inpatients with or without a previous diagnosis of DM is associated with numerous adverse outcomes, including postoperative complications and mortality [2, 8–14]. This association is observed for both admission blood glucose (BG) and mean BG level throughout hospitalization [15]. Inpatient hyperglycemia has been specifically linked to increased duration of hospital stay, increased incidence of infection, increased mortality, and greater disability after hospital discharge in various studies [2, 16–20]. Observational and randomized controlled studies indicate that improved glycemic control results in lower rates of hospital complications in general medicine and surgery patients [15] and decreased length of hospital stay [7]. Moreover, inpatient glycemic control is cost-effective [1]. In the Portland Diabetic Project, initiation of continuous intravenous (IV) insulin therapy to achieve predetermined target BG values in patients with DM undergoing open-heart surgical procedures reduced the incidence of deep sternal wound infections by 66%, resulting in a total net savings of $4638 per patient [21]. In another study, intensive glycemic control in 1600 patients treated in a medical intensive care unit (ICU) was associated with a total cost savings of $1580 per patient [22]. With mounting evidence demonstrating the value of reducing both hyper- and hypoglycemia, optimizing inpatient glycemic control should be a priority for all healthcare providers.

Recognition and Diagnosis of Hyperglycemia and Diabetes on Admission

Inpatient hyperglycemia is defined as any BG value >140 mg/dL (7.8 mmol/L) [1, 15] and can occur not only in patients with known DM but also in those with previously undiagnosed DM and others who experience "stress hyperglycemia" during an acute illness or procedure [1, 15, 23, 24]. Various studies have identified hyperglycemia in 32–38% of patients in community hospitals [2, 25], 41% of critically ill patients with acute coronary syndromes [13], 44% of patients with heart failure [13], and 80% of post-cardiac surgery patients [26, 27]. In these studies, approximately one-third of non-critically ill patients and 80% of critically ill patients had no history of DM prior to admission [2, 13, 28–31].

Current guidelines recommend the initiation of BG monitoring for those with DM and those without a known history of DM who are receiving therapies associated with hyperglycemia [32]. Further sources suggest that an initial BG measurement on admission is appropriate for all hospitalized patients, regardless of the presence of preexisting DM or exposure to known inducers of hyperglycemia [15]. Guidelines also recommend that all inpatients with known DM or hyperglycemia be assessed with a laboratory measure of hemoglobin A1c (if this has not been performed in the preceding 3 months), both for diagnosis of DM and identification of patients at risk for DM [15, 32]. Hemoglobin A1c (HbA1c) values ≥6.5% suggest, in previously undiagnosed

W. B. Horton (✉)
Medicine, Division of Endocrinology and Metabolism, University of Virginia, Charlottesville, VA, USA
e-mail: WBH2N@virginia.edu

© The Author(s), under exclusive license to Springer Nature Switzerland AG 2023
J. Rodriguez-Saldana (ed.), *The Diabetes Textbook*, https://doi.org/10.1007/978-3-031-25519-9_46

patients, that DM preceded hospitalization [33]. Measurement of HbA1c during periods of hospitalization also provides the opportunity to identify patients with known DM who might benefit from intensification of their glycemic control regimen [15]. In patients with newly diagnosed hyperglycemia, HbA1c may help differentiate patients with previously undiagnosed DM from those with stress-induced hyperglycemia [34, 35].

Therapeutic Agents and Regimens for Inpatient Glycemic Control

For many reasons, inpatient hyperglycemia is best managed with insulin therapy. Patients with type 1 diabetes mellitus (T1DM) have an absolute insulin requirement and necessitate treatment with basal plus prandial insulin regimens to avoid severe hyperglycemia and ketoacidosis [15]. Patients with type 2 diabetes mellitus (T2DM) are often treated with a variety of therapies in the outpatient setting, including diet, lifestyle modifications, oral agents, non-insulin injectable medications, insulin, and/or any combination of these options [15]. However, the use of oral and other non-insulin therapies presents many challenges in the inpatient setting, as there are frequent contraindications to their use in hospitalized patients (e.g., sepsis, IV contrast dyes, pancreatic disorders, renal dysfunction, etc.) [1]. The majority of hospitalized patients will not be proper candidates for regimens other than insulin therapy, and each class of oral antidiabetic therapies possesses characteristics that may limit their desirability for inpatient use [6]. Despite these concerns, it should be noted that in certain circumstances, it may be appropriate to continue home regimens including oral glucose-lowering medications [32]. Clinical judgment should be used by the healthcare provider to evaluate patient criteria for the continued use of these agents in the hospital, including patients who are clinically stable and eating regular meals along with having no specific contraindications to the use of certain oral antidiabetic drugs [15]. Several recent randomized trials have demonstrated the potential effectiveness of glucagon-like peptide-1 (GLP-1) receptor agonists and dipeptidyl peptidase-4 (DPP-4) inhibitors in specific groups of hospitalized patients [32, 36–39]. Their inpatient use, however, remains limited by the fact that GLP-1 receptor agonists can cause nausea and should be withheld in acutely ill inpatients [6] and that a Food and Drug Administration (FDA) bulletin advised discontinuation of the DPP-4 inhibitors saxagliptin and alogliptin in patients who develop heart failure [40]. Safety and effectiveness data for sodium-glucose cotransporter-2 (SGLT2) inhibitors are currently lacking; thus, these agents are not recommended for routine inpatient use [32].

Insulin works reliably and can be quickly titrated based on changes in diet or glucose levels, making it ideal therapy in the inpatient setting [41]. For insulin-naive patients with BG levels >140 mg/dL (7.8 mmol/L) who are eating regular meals, insulin therapy can safely be initiated at a total daily dose of 0.2–0.5 units/kg body weight [42–45]. The lower starting dose is advised for leaner patients and those with renal dysfunction, while the higher starting dose is recommended for obese patients and those receiving glucocorticoids [6]. Fifty percent of the calculated total daily dose should be given as a basal component, and the remaining 50% should be split into thirds and given preprandially as the meal component [42, 43]. Patients who are NPO may receive basal insulin alone plus correctional doses with a rapid-acting analog every 4 h or regular insulin every 6 h [15, 17, 44]. Table 46.1 provides examples of basal plus prandial insulin regimens along with correctional dose protocols for inpatient glycemic control in non-critically ill inpatients.

Patients (either T1DM or T2DM) already receiving treatment with insulin prior to admission should continue treatment with a scheduled subcutaneous (SC) insulin regimen during admission [15]. These patients should have their insulin regimen modified according to clinical status both upon admission and throughout hospitalization as a way to reduce the risk for both hypo- and hyperglycemia [15]. The home total basal and prandial insulin dose should be reduced on admission for patients with poor nutritional intake, impaired kidney function, or admission BG levels <100 mg/dL (5.6 mmol/L) [15].

Finally, it should be noted that using sliding scale insulin (SSI) as the sole method for glycemic control of hospitalized patients is an ineffective therapy that should be avoided [15]. Scheduled basal plus prandial (BPP) insulin regimens mimic normal pancreas hormonal physiology and are designed to prevent hyperglycemia, whereas SSI alone only attempts to lower hyperglycemia after it has occurred [6]. SSI as sole management for inpatient hyperglycemia has routinely been shown to provide suboptimal glycemic control [46–49], and its regular use has been described as providing "action without benefit" [50]. Despite mounting evidence showing the inferiority of SSI alone, it remains ingrained in the practice of some healthcare facilities [51]. Clinician fear of hypoglycemia, clinical inertia, and resistance to institutional change have all been suggested as factors contributing to the continued use of SSI monotherapy in the inpatient setting [52]. A study comparing scheduled BPP insulin to SSI alone showed a significantly higher percentage of patients achieving goal BG levels in the BPP group than in the SSI group (66% vs. 38%) without an increase in hypoglycemia [45]. In another study [48], the risk for hyperglycemia (defined as BG >200 mg/dL or 11.1 mmol/L) was three times greater in patients managed with aggressive SSI regimens. For inpatients requiring insulin therapy to manage hyperglycemia,

Table 46.1 Basal plus prandial and correctional dose insulin regimens for glycemic control of the non-critically ill patient

A. Basal insulin orders
- Calculate TDD as follows:
  - 0.2–0.3 units/kg body weight per day in patients: aged ≥70 years and/or GFR <60 mL/min
  - 0.4 units/kg body weight per day for patients not meeting the criteria above who have BG concentrations of 140–200 mg/dL (7.8–11.1 mmol/L)
  - 0.5 units/kg body weight per day for patients not meeting the criteria above when BG concentration is 201–400 mg/dL (11.2–22.2 mmol/L)
- Distribute total calculated dose as approximately 50% basal insulin and 50% prandial insulin
- Give basal insulin once (e.g., glargine) or twice (e.g., NPH) daily, at same time each day
- Give rapid-acting (i.e., prandial) insulin in three equally divided doses before each meal. Hold prandial insulin if patient is unable to eat
- Adjust insulin doses based on bedside POCT BG measurements

B. Supplemental (correction) rapid-acting insulin analog or regular insulin

Supplemental insulin orders
- If a patient is able and expected to eat all or most of his/her meals, give rapid-acting insulin before each meal and at bedtime following the "usual" column (*Section C below*)
- If a patient is unable to eat, give regular insulin every 6 h or rapid-acting insulin every 4–6 h following the "sensitive" column (*Section C below*)

Supplemental insulin adjustment
- If fasting and premeal BG are persistently >140 mg/dL (7.8 mmol/L) in the absence of hypoglycemia, increase scale of insulin from the insulin-sensitive to the usual or from the usual to the insulin-resistant column (*Section C below*)
- If a patient develops hypoglycemia (BG <70 mg/dL or 3.8 mmol/L), decrease regular or rapid-acting insulin from the insulin-resistant to the usual column or from the usual to the insulin-sensitive column (*Section C below*)

C. Supplemental insulin scale

BG (mg/dL)	Insulin sensitive	Usual	Insulin resistant
>141–180	2	4	6
181–220	4	6	8
221–260	6	8	10
261–300	8	10	12
301–350	10	12	14
351–400	12	14	16
>400	14	16	18

TDD total daily dose, *GFR* glomerular filtration rate, *BG* blood glucose, *POCT* point-of-care testing
Adapted with permission from Reference [15]
[a] The numbers in each column of *Section C* indicate the number of units of regular or rapid-acting insulin analogs per dose. "Supplemental" dose is to be added to the scheduled insulin dose. Give half of supplemental insulin dose at bedtime. If a patient is able and expected to eat all or most of his/her meals, supplemental insulin will be administered before each meal following the "usual" column dose. Start at the insulin-sensitive column in patients who are not eating, elderly patients, and those with impaired renal function. Start at the insulin-resistant column in patients receiving corticosteroids and those treated with more than 80 units/day prior to admission. To convert mg/dL to mmol/L, divide by 18

BPP insulin regimens are superior to SSI alone and should be the preferred method utilized for glycemic control.

Glycemic Control of the Non-critically Ill Patient

Management strategies and glycemic target values vary by inpatient population and location; thus, an appropriate understanding of the protocols, procedures, and system environments needed to optimize inpatient glycemic control for various patient groups is of vital importance for all healthcare facilities and providers. Non-critically ill patients are hospitalized for management of a wide variety of issues and illnesses, though diabetes and/or hyperglycemia are often not the primary reason for admission. Nevertheless, the benefit of appropriate glycemic control should not be minimized in this scenario.

Glycemic Monitoring

Bedside capillary point-of-care testing (POCT) is the preferred method for guiding ongoing glycemic management of the non-critically ill patient [15]. Recommendations include POCT before meals and at bedtime in patients who are eating regular meals [1, 15]. Matching the timing of POCT with nutritional intake and medication administration is an important component of proper inpatient glycemic control. Premeal POCT should be obtained as close to the time of meal tray delivery as possible and no greater than 1 h before meals [53, 54]. POCT should be performed every 4–6 h in patients who are NPO or receiving continuous enteral (EN) or parenteral (PN) nutrition [1, 15]. More frequent POCT is indicated after a medication change that could affect glycemic control (e.g., glucocorticoid use or discontinuation of EN or PN) [32, 55, 56], or in patients who experience frequent episodes of hypoglycemia [17, 29].

Healthcare providers should be aware of the fact that the accuracy of most POCT meters is far from optimal [57]. Consistent BG sampling sites and methods of measurement should be used because results can vary greatly when alternating between fingerstick and alternative sites, or between samples run in the laboratory and a POCT device [15, 57]. There are also potential inaccuracies of POCT testing including intrinsic issues with technology and variability between different lots of test strips, varying tissue perfusion states and hemoglobin concentrations, and other interfering hematological factors in acutely ill patients [58–60].

Patients may be allowed to bring their personal glucometer device to the hospital, but personal meters should not be used for documentation or treatment of inpatient hyperglycemia [15]. Hospital glucometers should be used to obtain POCT results and subsequently log them into the electronic health record to allow evaluation of individual and hospital-wide trends and patterns of inpatient glycemic control [15, 61]. Real-time continuous glucose monitoring (CGM) provides frequent measurement of interstitial glucose levels as well as direction and magnitude of glucose trends [32]. Recent studies have shown that CGM provides accurate estimation of BG levels in the hospital [62, 63] and may be more effective in detecting hypoglycemic episodes [62–64]. Despite its demonstrated advantages over POCT for inpatient glycemic monitoring, CGM has not yet received full FDA approval for inpatient use. However, the FDA did grant breakthrough device designation to DexCom in March 2022 for the use of its CGM devices in the hospital setting [65]. This designation provides a more efficient and streamlined review pathway so CGM technology can hopefully get to the hospital market faster. Notably, some hospitals with established glucose management teams already allow CGM use in selected patients on an individual basis (provided both the patient and the glucose management team are well-educated in the use of this technology [32]).

Glycemic Target Values

For the majority of non-critically ill patients treated with SC insulin, a target glucose range of 140–180 mg/dL (7.8 mmol/L) is recommended [32]. Guidelines also recommend that these targets should be modified according to clinical status [1, 15]. Glucose concentrations between 180 and 250 mg/dL (10–13.9 mmol/L) may be acceptable in patients with severe comorbidities and in inpatient care settings where frequent glucose monitoring or close nursing supervision is not feasible [32]. Glycemic levels >250 mg/dL (13.9 mmol/L) may be acceptable in terminally ill patients

with short life expectancy. In such patients, less aggressive insulin regimens to minimize glucosuria, dehydration, and electrolyte disturbances are often more appropriate [32].

Consideration should be given to reassessing the insulin regimen if BG levels are consistently <100 mg/dL (5.6 mmol/L) [1, 15]. For avoidance of hypoglycemia (BG <70 mg/dL), the total basal and prandial insulin doses should be reduced if BG levels are consistently between 70 and 100 mg/dL (3.9–5.6 mmol/L) [15]. Modification of the treatment regimen is necessary when BG values fall <70 mg/dL (3.9 mmol/L) [1].

Approach to Management

As previously discussed, inpatient hyperglycemia is best managed with insulin therapy. The preferred insulin regimen for inpatient glycemic control of non-critically ill patients includes two different insulin preparations administered SC as BPP therapy [15]. The basal component requires administration of an intermediate- or long-acting insulin once or twice daily [15]. The bolus component consists of a short- or rapid-acting insulin given in conjunction with meals or nutrient delivery [15]. The safety and efficacy of BPP insulin regimens in non-critically ill patients have been demonstrated in numerous studies [44, 45, 66–68]. Correctional insulin refers to the administration of supplemental doses of short- or rapid-acting insulin together with the usual dose of bolus insulin for BG values above the target range and is usually customized to match the insulin sensitivity of each patient [15]. Table 46.1 provides examples of BPP insulin regimens along with correctional dose protocols for glycemic control in non-critically ill inpatients.

Adjustment of scheduled BPP insulin dosing can be based on total doses of correctional insulin administered in the previous 24 h [15, 45, 66]. When correctional insulin is required before most meals, it is usually the basal insulin component that should be titrated upward [15]. If BG remains consistently elevated at one time point, the dose of prandial insulin preceding that measurement should be increased [15, 43, 69]. For example, if the premeal BG at lunch is persistently elevated, it should be the breakfast dose of prandial insulin that is titrated upward. Appropriate inpatient glycemic control for many patients will often require daily insulin adjustment to reach glycemic targets while simultaneously avoiding hypoglycemia.

In patients who are NPO or unable to eat, bolus insulin should be held until nutritional intake is resumed. Basal insulin should be continued once daily (glargine or detemir) or twice daily (detemir or neutral protamine Hagedorn

[NPH]) [15]. Correctional doses of a rapid-acting insulin analog (e.g., aspart, lispro, etc.) or regular insulin can be given every 4–6 h as needed to treat BG above the desired range [15].

Medical nutrition therapy (MNT) should also be included as an essential component of any inpatient glycemic control program [15]. MNT is defined as the process of nutritional assessment and individualized meal planning in consultation with a nutrition professional [15, 70]. The goals of inpatient MNT include optimizing glycemic control, providing adequate calories to balance metabolic demands, and creating a discharge plan for follow-up care [15, 17, 32, 70–73]. Lack of attention to MNT in the hospital has been shown to contribute to unfavorable changes in BG [15, 29, 54, 74].

Many variables during hospitalization (e.g., abrupt discontinuation of meals in preparation for procedures or diagnostic studies, variability in meal intake due to acute illness, limitations in food choices, and poor coordination between insulin administration and meal delivery) can com-plicate nutritional management and create difficulties in predicting the efficacy of glycemic control strategies [15, 54]. Consistent carbohydrate (CHO) meal plans, in combination with MNT, may help facilitate inpatient glycemic control and negate some of these variables [15, 17, 32, 54]. Consistent CHO meal plans are preferred by many hospitals as they facilitate matching the prandial insulin dose to the amount of CHO consumed [32, 54] and may contribute to reductions in hypoglycemia [17, 71]. Current standards of care also recommend that if CHO counting is provided by the hospital kitchen, this option should be used in patients counting CHO at home [32, 75].

Successful inpatient glycemic control of non-critically ill patients requires a multifactorial approach that includes recognition of appropriate glycemic monitoring practices and target values along with institution of BPP insulin and MNT. Table 46.2 summarizes the procedures and strategies that should be employed to help achieve appropriate glycemic control in this patient population.

Table 46.2 Appropriate strategies for successful inpatient glycemic control in various patient populations

Patient population	Glycemic monitoring	Glycemic targets	Insulin regimen
Non-critically ill	• POCT FSG before meals and at bedtime if eating regular meals	• BG levels should generally be maintained between 140 and 180 mg/dL	• Scheduled subcutaneous basal plus prandial insulin therapy (see Table 46.1 for further details):
	• POCT FSG every 4–6 h in patients who are NPO or receiving continuous EN or PN	• Higher glycemic targets are acceptable in those who are terminally ill or have severe comorbidities	– Intermediate- or long-acting insulin (e.g., glargine, detemir, or NPH) given once or twice daily as basal component
	• More frequent POCT FSG may be considered for patients who experience or have increased risk for hypoglycemia		– Rapid-acting insulin (e.g., aspart or lispro) given in conjunction with meals as bolus component
			– Correctional doses of rapid-acting insulin given supplementally with the usual dose of bolus insulin for premeal BG values above target
Critically ill	• Patients whose severity of illness justifies invasive vascular monitoring:	• BG levels should be maintained between 140 and 180 mg/dL	• IV insulin infusion should be administered by means of validated written or computerized protocols
	– All blood samples should be drawn from an arterial line	• BG levels <110 mg/dL are not recommended and should be avoided	• Once clinically improved and/or eating regular meals, IV insulin infusion should be transitioned to SC insulin therapy (see Table 46.3 for further details)
	– If an arterial line is unavailable, sample from a venous line		
	– POCT FSG can be inaccurate and should be avoided, if possible		
	• Patients whose severity of illness does not justify invasive vascular monitoring:		
	– POCT FSG is appropriate		

(continued)

Table 46.2 (continued)

Patient population	Glycemic monitoring	Glycemic targets	Insulin regimen
Perioperative	• Determine the level of glycemic control during preoperative evaluation by checking hemoglobin A1c in patients with diabetes	• Premeal BG targets <140 mg/dL in conjunction with random BG targets <180 mg/dL in preoperative and postoperative patients who are eating regular meals	• In ambulatory patients undergoing relatively short procedures, BPP insulin therapy should be used
	• In stable patients undergoing relatively short outpatient procedures, check BG on admission, before procedure, and at discharge	• Intraoperative BG levels should be maintained between 100 and 180 mg/dL	• The day of surgery, use 75–100% of daily long-acting insulin (glargine or detemir) dose
	• For longer outpatient procedures or patients receiving intraoperative subcutaneous insulin, BG should be monitored every 1–2 h	• If a patient must be monitored in a surgical ICU post-procedure, BG should be maintained between 140 and 180 mg/dL	• Prandial insulin should be withheld while a patient is fasting
	• For extensive surgical procedures or patients receiving intravenous insulin infusion, BG should be monitored every 30 min		• Once the patient resumes eating regular meals, full BPP regimen can be resumed • IV insulin therapy is appropriate for patients undergoing long, extensive surgical procedures or those who will need to be monitored in an ICU setting post-procedure

POCT point-of-care testing, *IV* intravenous, *SC* subcutaneous, *FSG* fingerstick glucose, *ICU* intensive care unit, *EN* enteral nutrition, *BPP* basal plus prandial, *PN* parenteral nutrition, *BG* blood glucose, *NPH* neutral protamine Hagedorn

Table 46.3 Transitioning from intravenous to subcutaneous insulin in the patient who is eating regular meals

Patient data	Time (h)								
	0000	0100	0200	0300	0400	0500	0600	0700	0800
IV insulin infusion rate (units/h)	2.2	2.2	2.1	2.0	2.0	2.0	1.9	1.8	1.8
Blood glucose (mg/dL)	148	143	145	141	137	139	135	133	131

The above data demonstrates both good glycemic control and relatively stable insulin infusion rates. To calculate subcutaneous basal plus bolus insulin doses, follow these steps
1. Calculate the 24-h intravenous insulin requirement
    (a) In the example above, the patient has an average insulin infusion rate of 2 units/h
    (b) Calculated 24-h intravenous insulin requirement: 2 units/h × 24 h = 48 units
2. Calculate the subcutaneous basal insulin dose
    (a) Most sources [1, 76] recommend using 80% of the 24-h intravenous insulin requirement as the subcutaneous basal insulin dose
    (b) 80% of 48 units = 38 units
    (c) As this was calculated from an overnight period of time while the patient was not eating, the dose can be administered as 38 units of basal insulin once daily
3. Calculate the subcutaneous bolus (prandial) insulin dose using a weight-based calculation
    (a) Given the possibility of decreased appetite, starting with a conservative estimate of 0.2 units/kg for total prandial dose is appropriate
    (b) 0.2 units/kg × 80 kg = 16 units and 16 units/3 meals = approximately 5 units per meal
4. Final orders
    (a) 38 units subcutaneous daily (insulin glargine/detemir)
    (b) 5 units subcutaneous three times daily with meals (insulin lispro/aspart/glulisine)
Adapted with permission from Reference [77]
^a The patient weighs 80 kg; data extracted from an overnight period of time when the patient is not eating

Glycemic Control of the Critically Ill Patient

Hyperglycemia is common in critically ill patients, including those without a known history of DM [78]. Patients receiving treatment for critical illness develop hyperglycemia due to the effects of endogenous stress responses and the by-products of medical interventions [78]. Inflammatory cytokines and stress hormones, such as epinephrine and cortisol, inhibit insulin release and promote insulin resistance, functionally increasing BG levels by stimulating gluconeo-genesis and glycogenolysis while impeding glucose uptake in peripheral tissues [78–80]. Many medical therapies utilized in the treatment of critically ill patients also promote hyperglycemia, including administration of exogenous catecholamines and glucocorticoids, infusion of dextrose for parenteral nutrition, and even bedrest itself, which may impair glucose uptake in skeletal muscles [78, 81, 82]. In the past two decades, glycemic control among critically ill patients has been a topic of extensive study, leading to many changes in clinical practice [83].

Glycemic Monitoring

Measurement of BG concentration in critical care settings is often performed in intermittent fashion, with analysis using either POCT glucometers, laboratory blood draws, or blood gas analyzers [83]. The accuracy of glucometers has been the subject of numerous studies, with the majority concluding that they are insufficiently accurate for exclusive evaluation of BG values in the ICU [58, 83–86]. Many current glucometers are susceptible to interference from reducing substances such as ascorbic acid and acetaminophen (paracetamol), and accuracy is also affected by a patient's hematocrit levels [57, 83, 87]. The effect of hematocrit is particularly concerning in the ICU, where levels can fluctuate for many reasons. One study has demonstrated that a patient with a true BG of 80 mg/dL and a hematocrit of 0.25 may have a positive bias as great as 18 mg/dL [83, 87]. Another consideration is that BG concentration varies in different vascular beds and the site from which blood is sampled may introduce errors [83]. Sampling capillary blood in ICU patients, particularly those who are hemodynamically unstable and treated with vasopressors, can introduce large errors when compared to a reference method in which BG is measured from central venous or arterial draws [83, 84, 88]. Sampling from indwelling arterial or venous catheters in ICU patients is a reasonable option that is preferable to venipuncture, given the frequency with which BG is measured in the ICU [83].

Alternatives to the use of glucometers are measurements in the hospital's central laboratory or using a blood gas analyzer in the ICU [83]. Although central laboratory measurement is more accurate, the time delay in obtaining results makes this a less-than-ideal option in most ICU settings [83]. Using a blood gas analyzer to measure BG concentration is a practical solution but may have considerable cost implications [83]. Measurements from a properly maintained blood gas analyzer will have similar accuracy to central laboratory measurements [83, 84].

Current guidelines for BG measurement in the ICU recommend that all patients whose severity of illness justifies the presence of invasive vascular monitoring (i.e., indwelling arterial and/or central venous catheter) should have samples for measurement taken from the arterial catheter as the primary option [83]. If an arterial catheter is temporarily or permanently unavailable, blood may be sampled from a venous catheter as a secondary option (appropriate attention should be paid to maintaining sterility and avoiding contamination of the sample by flush solution in this scenario) [83]. When a patient's severity of illness does not require the presence of invasive vascular monitoring, POCT capillary BG samples obtained via glucometer are acceptable [83].

Although intermittent BG measurement is the current standard practice for critically ill patients, CGM holds great promise in this patient population. Potential advantages of CGM include the ability to observe trends in BG concentration and intervene before values enter an unacceptable range and removal of error both in timing of BG measurements and in sampling and analysis of blood [83]. Primary concerns with CGM use in the ICU relate to the effects of hemodynamic changes, pressor use, and potential interfering medications [89]. At this time, more data are needed before recommendations either for or against CGM use in critically ill patients can be made. A recent real-world preliminary analysis of the accuracy of CGM compared to POCT in 11 ICU patients with confirmed coronavirus disease 2019 (COVID-19) demonstrated early feasibility, considerable accuracy, and meaningful reduction in the frequency of point-of-care glucose testing [90]. Larger studies are needed to confirm these findings.

Glycemic Target Values

Current BG target values for critically ill patients are primarily based on results from the Normoglycemia in Intensive Care Evaluation—Survival Using Glucose Algorithm Regulation (NICE-SUGAR) study, a multicenter and multinational randomized controlled trial that tested the effect of tight glycemic control on outcomes among 6104 critically ill patients, the majority of whom (>95%) required mechanical ventilation [1, 91]. In this study, patients were randomized to intensive or conventional insulin therapy group. The glycemic target range was 81–108 mg/dL in the intensive insulin therapy group, while target BG was ≤180 mg/dL in the conventional insulin therapy group (with insulin administration reduced and then discontinued if BG levels fell below 144 mg/dL [84]). Both 90-day mortality (78 more deaths; 27.5% vs. 24.9%; $p = 0.02$) and rates of severe hypoglycemia (6.8% vs. 0.5%; $p = <0.001$) were significantly higher in the intensive versus conventional group [91]. Subsequently, several randomized controlled trials evaluating intensive insulin therapy among mechanically ventilated neurologic patients [92], patients with traumatic brain injuries [93], and critically ill pediatric patients [94] have all failed to demonstrate a clinical benefit to tight glycemic control in ICU patients [83]. Based on these findings, current guidelines for glycemic targets in critically ill patients on IV insulin therapy recommend that BG should be maintained between 140 and 180 mg/dL (7.8 and 10 mmol/L), with greater benefit potentially realized at the lower end of this range [1]. Somewhat lower glycemic targets may be appropriate in select patients, but strong evidence is currently lacking and prevents such a recommendation [1]. Targets <110 mg/dL (6.1 mmol/L) are not recommended and should be avoided [1].

Approach to Management

In the ICU setting, continuous IV insulin infusion is the most effective therapy for achieving recommended glycemic targets [17, 32]. Due to the short half-life of circulating insulin, IV delivery allows for rapid dosing adjustments to address alterations in clinical status [1]. Current guidelines recommend that IV insulin should be administered based on validated written or computerized protocols that allow for predefined adjustments in the infusion rate, accounting for glycemic fluctuations and insulin dose [32]. Several examples of published protocols are available for review [95–98]. Continued education of healthcare staff along with ongoing review of patient data and protocol results is critical for successful implementation of any insulin protocol [1, 95–98]. Table 46.2 summarizes appropriate strategies for successful inpatient glycemic control in critically ill patients.

Critically ill patients receiving IV insulin therapy will typically require transition to SC insulin once they begin eating regular meals or have clinically improved enough to be transferred to lower intensity care [1]. A safe transition requires appropriate planning and must be carried out systematically. SC basal insulin must be given at least 2–4 h prior to discontinuation of IV insulin therapy to prevent rebound hyperglycemia [76, 77]. There are currently no consensus guidelines for transitioning from IV to SC therapy, but typically 75–80% of the total daily IV infusion dose is proportionally divided into basal and prandial components [1]. The safest method is to find a several-hour period of time during which BG values are at goal and IV insulin rates are not particularly elevated or variable (i.e., the rate is reasonable and stable) [77]. The healthcare provider can then look at infusion rates during this stable period of time (ideally 6–8 h in length [99]) and extrapolate these data into a 24-h time period [77]. Utilizing this method allows for a reasonable calculation of the patient's 24-h IV insulin utilization [77]. Table 46.3 provides an example of calculating the insulin regimen necessary to transition a patient from IV to SC insulin therapy.

Glycemic Control of the Perioperative Patient

Patients with DM are more likely to undergo surgery than patients without DM [17, 44]. Surgery in DM patients is associated with longer length of hospitalization, greater perioperative morbidity and mortality, and increased rates of perioperative complications and healthcare resource utilization than in patients without DM [17, 44, 100, 101]. One retrospective observational study of 409 cardiac surgical patients demonstrated that intraoperative hyperglycemia was an independent risk factor for perioperative complications (including mortality) after adjusting for postoperative BG concentrations [102, 103]. The authors of this study also indicated that each 20 mg/dL (1.1 mmol/L) increase in BG concentration above 100 mg/dL (5.6 mmol/L) during surgery was associated with a 34% increased likelihood of postoperative complications [102]. Another retrospective cohort study of infra-inguinal vascular surgery patients showed that

the rise in BG was proportional to an increased frequency of postoperative infections [104].

Surgical patient populations pose many unique challenges to clinicians. Despite the increased risk of perioperative complications, hyperglycemia is frequently overlooked and inadequately addressed [29, 44]. Given the growing evidence linking perioperative hyperglycemia to many poor outcomes, it is imperative that healthcare providers identify and proactively address this issue.

Glycemic Monitoring

Preoperative identification of patients with DM and those at risk for perioperative dysglycemia provides a potential opportunity to reduce morbidity and mortality [105]. However, it should be noted that the incidence of preoperative hyperglycemia might not be entirely due to DM. For example, a prospective study of 493 non-DM patients undergoing elective, non-cardiac surgery found that 25% had elevated fasting plasma glucose the morning of surgery [106].

Glycemic monitoring approaches for perioperative patients are similar to those used for non-critically ill and critically ill patients, depending upon the type and length of surgery performed [103] and whether the patient is monitored in the surgical ICU, general surgical floor, or discharged home after the procedure is completed. General recommendations include determining the level of glycemic control during the preoperative evaluation by checking HbA1c values [103]. Elevated HbA1c, as a marker of poor glycemic control, correlates with increased perioperative risk in DM patients [102]. Further recommendations include checking BG levels on the patient's arrival before surgery and prior to discharge home [103]. The recommended frequency of intraoperative BG monitoring depends on many factors. In metabolically stable DM patients undergoing relatively short (i.e., less than 2 h) outpatient procedures, it is only necessary to check BG on admission, before operation, and at discharge [105]. For longer outpatient procedures or for patients receiving intraoperative SC insulin, BG should be monitored every 1–2 h at minimum [103, 105]. For higher-acuity patients undergoing extensive surgical procedures or those on intraoperative insulin infusion therapy, the American Diabetes Association recommends BG monitoring as frequently as every 30 min [32]. If the patient is observed in the hospital after the procedure, POCT is an appropriate monitoring method unless the patient is in the ICU. Once the patient is eating regular meals, recommendations for glycemic monitoring mirror those for non-critically ill patients.

Glycemic Target Values

BG goals for preoperative and postoperative patients who are eating regular meals are similar to those of non-critically ill patients and generally target values between 140 (7.8 mmol/L) and 180 mg/dL (10 mmol/L), as long as these targets can be safely achieved [1, 15]. Intraoperative BG levels should be maintained between 100 and 180 mg/dL (6–10 mmol/L), with appropriate steps taken to prevent intraoperative hypoglycemia [103, 106]. If a patient must be monitored in a surgical ICU post-procedure, glucose should be maintained between 140 and 180 mg/dL (7.8 and 10 mmol/L) [1].

Approach to Preoperative Management

Healthcare providers should have a detailed understanding of the patient's history of disease, including specific diagnosis (T1DM, T2DM, gestational DM, etc.), duration of disease, current treatment regimen, adequacy of control, and the presence and/or severity of any comorbidities [104]. Persons with DM admitted for surgical procedures should generally have their home oral antidiabetic medications discontinued [9], and it is reasonable to stop most of these medications on the morning of surgery [107, 108]. However, SGLT2 inhibitors require special attention given that the FDA now recommends that these agents should be stopped 3 days before scheduled surgeries (4 days in the case of ertugliflozin) [32] due to a higher risk of ketoacidosis. All patients with a known history of DM should be thoroughly evaluated before entering the operating room to aid in creating a successful perioperative treatment regimen. Postponing surgery in patients who present on the morning of procedure with significant dehydration, ketoacidosis, and/or hyperosmolar nonketotic states is recommended [103]. Table 46.2 summarizes recommendations for achieving appropriate inpatient glycemic control in perioperative patients.

Consensus guidelines recognize IV insulin therapy as the best method for controlling hyperglycemia in critically ill and non-critically ill surgical patients [1]; however, many logistical difficulties limit the use of this therapy in most hospital settings (particularly in non-ICU patient populations [103]). For ambulatory patients undergoing relatively short procedures, the preferable method for perioperative glycemic control is SC BPP insulin therapy. When SC insulin is continued in patients who are fasting, adjustment of their long-acting basal insulin dose is often not necessary, provided they have been receiving an adequate dose prior to admission [103, 109]. Specific recommendations include avoiding alterations of basal insulin the day before surgery unless there is report of hypoglycemia or the patient is on a diet restriction in the preoperative period [103]. On the day of surgery, use 75–100% of daily long-acting insulin dose [103]. If NPH is being used as the basal insulin, the evening dose should be reduced to 75% the day before surgery, and 50–75% of the usual morning dose should be given the day of surgery [103]. Prandial (bolus) insulin should be withheld while a patient is fasting [103]. The use of basal insulin in combination with correctional insulin can be effective at maintaining glycemic control in the desired range with low risk of hypoglycemia [44]. Once a patient is eating regular meals and monitored in a non-ICU setting, a BPP insulin regimen can be fully resumed. IV insulin therapy is appropriate for patients undergoing long, extensive surgical procedures or those who will need to be monitored in an ICU setting post-procedure [103]. IV insulin has the advantage of being quickly titratable with a rapid onset of action [105], allowing for precise glycemic control in the perioperative period. For patients treated with IV infusions, it is important to safely transition to SC insulin while maintaining glycemic control as patients transfer across different hospital units [103]. Table 46.3 details methods for converting IV therapy to an appropriate SC insulin regimen.

Special Considerations

Many special circumstances are encountered during routine inpatient care of DM patients. Not all patients are able to tolerate regular PO intake and may require EN or PN, and the approach to glycemic control of such patients is a little different than other management strategies previously described. Other special circumstances include patients who are admitted with insulin pumps and those who experience glucocorticoid-induced DM while hospitalized.

Enteral and Parenteral Nutrition

Malnutrition is reported in up to 40% of critically ill patients [75] and is associated with many poor outcomes, including increased risk of hospital complications, higher mortality rates, longer length of hospitalization, and increased healthcare costs [15, 110]. Improving the nutritional state is an important goal of inpatient care for malnourished patients; unfortunately, not all patients are able to tolerate PO intake and require EN or PN therapy. There are several retrospective and prospective studies demonstrating that the use of EN or PN therapy is an independent risk factor for the onset or aggravation of hyperglycemia independent of a prior history of DM [15, 78, 111, 112]. Early intervention to prevent and correct hyperglycemia in these patients may improve clinical outcomes [15]; however, achieving desired glycemic goals in this population poses many unique challenges [68, 78]. Current recommendations include initiating POCT in patients with or without a history of DM receiving PN or EN [15]. Several different management strategies utilizing SC insulin have been suggested, and recommendations vary by whether the patient is receiving PN or intermittent, continuous, or cycled EN [15]. For those receiving continuous EN, recommendations include administering basal insulin once (if glargine) or twice (if NPH or detemir) daily in combination with a short- or rapid-acting insulin analog in divided doses every 4 (if lispro, aspart, etc.) to 6 (if regular insulin) hours [15]. For patients on cycled EN, guidelines recommend administering basal insulin in combination with a short- or rapid-acting insulin analog upon the initiation of EN [15]. Repeating the dose of rapid-acting insulin at 4-h intervals or short-acting insulin at 6-h intervals for the duration of EN therapy is also recommended [15]. It is also preferable to give the last dose of rapid-acting insulin approximately 4 h before and short-acting insulin approximately 6 h before discontinuation of EN [15]. For those receiving bolus EN, administer short-acting or rapid-acting insulin before each bolus is delivered [15]. Finally, for patients receiving PN, regular insulin administered as part of the PN formulation can be both safe and effective [15]. Subcutaneous correctional dose insulin can be utilized in addition to the insulin that is mixed with the PN to correct any hyperglycemic excursions that may occur [15].

Glucocorticoid Therapy

Hyperglycemia is a common complication of glucocorticoid therapy, with several studies demonstrating a prevalence between 20% and 50% among patients without a previous history of DM [56, 113]. Glucocorticoid therapy increases hepatic glucose production, impairs glucose uptake in peripheral tissues, and stimulates protein catabolism with resulting increased concentrations of circulating amino acids, thus providing precursors for gluconeogenesis [114–116]. It is generally accepted that these physiological changes ultimately exacerbate postprandial hyperglycemia [117]; thus, all patients treated with glucocorticoid therapy should be evaluated for hyperglycemia whether they have a known history of DM or not. Current recommendations include initiating bedside POCT in any patient receiving treatment with glucocorticoids [15]. POCT can be discontinued in persons without DM if all BG results are <140 mg/dL (7.8 mmol/L) without insulin therapy for a period of 24–48 h [15]. Insulin therapy should be initiated in patients demonstrating persistent hyperglycemia [15]. The majority of patients with steroid-induced hyperglycemia can be treated with SC BPP regimens to achieve glycemic control, with the insulin regimen based on a starting dose of 0.3–0.5 units/kg/day [15]. Adjustment of insulin doses is often required when the glucocorticoid dose is changed [15]. During glucocorticoid tapers, insulin dosing should be proactively adjusted to avoid hypoglycemia [1].

Insulin Pumps

Patients treated with continuous subcutaneous insulin infusion (i.e., insulin pump) therapy in the outpatient setting require unique attention when hospitalized. With increasing utilization of pump therapy, many institutions allow patients on insulin pumps to continue using these devices in the hospital. Patients who utilize pump therapy in the outpatient setting can be considered for diabetes self-management while hospitalized, provided they have the mental and physical capacity to do so [1, 17, 118, 119]. In this scenario, nursing personnel should document basal rates and bolus doses (at least daily) [1]. The availability of hospital personnel with expertise in pump therapy is also vital [118, 119]. Clear policies and procedures should be established at the institutional level to guide the continued use of insulin pump technology in hospitalized patients [15].

Hypoglycemia

Hypoglycemia (both spontaneous and iatrogenic) is associated with higher risk of complications among hospitalized patients, including longer and more expensive hospital stays and increased mortality rates [120–122]. The risk for hypoglycemia is higher in hospitalized patients due to variability in insulin sensitivity related to the underlying illness, changes in counter-regulatory hormonal responses to procedures or illness, and interruptions in usual nutritional intake [123, 124]. Hospitalized patients who are elderly or severely ill are especially vulnerable to its adverse effects [120]. Given the negative outcomes associated with inpatient hypoglycemia, it is imperative that appropriate steps be taken to prevent and reduce episodes as much as possible.

Inpatient hypoglycemia is classically defined as any BG <70 mg/dL [122], as this level correlates with the initial threshold for the release of counter-regulatory hormones [15, 125, 126]. Insulin therapy is the most common preventable cause of iatrogenic hypoglycemia, followed by improper prescribing of other glucose-lowering medications, inappropriate management of the first episode of hypoglycemia, and nutrition-insulin mismatch (often related to an unexpected interruption of nutrition) [32].

For avoidance of hypoglycemia, consideration should be given to reassessing the insulin regimen if BG values <100 mg/dL are consistently noted. Modification of the regimen is necessary when BG values are <70 mg/dL, unless the event is easily explained by other factors such as a missed meal [1, 32]. Guidelines also suggest that a standardized hospital-wide, nurse-initiated hypoglycemia treatment protocol should be in place to immediately address any blood glucose <70 mg/dL (3.9 mmol/L) [32]. Additionally, the Joint Commission recommends that all hypoglycemic episodes be evaluated for a root cause and that such episodes be aggregated and reviewed to address any systemic issues [32, 127].

Emerging technologies focused on the prediction of inpatient hypoglycemia have recently been tested. While this work is in its infancy stages, early results are promising. Several groups have developed machine-learning predictive algorithms for inpatient hypoglycemia in both non-critical [128–131] and ICU [132] populations. Models like these are potentially important and, once validated for general use and prospectively tested (ideally in randomized controlled clinical trials), could provide a valuable tool to reduce rates of hypoglycemia in hospitalized patients [32]. One study has even shown that a real-time predictive informatics-generated alert, when supported by trained nurse responders, significantly reduced severe hypoglycemia among patients hospitalized on acute care medical floors [133].

Transitioning from Hospital to Home

Preparation for transition to the outpatient setting is an important goal of inpatient diabetes management and begins with hospital admission [1]. Hospital discharge itself represents a critical time for ensuring a safe transition to the outpatient setting and reducing the need for emergency department visits and rehospitalization [15], and poor coordination of patient care at the time of discharge is associated with medical errors and readmission [134]. Successful coordination of this transition requires a team approach that includes physicians, nurses, dietitians, case managers, and social workers [17]. An outpatient follow-up visit with the primary care provider, endocrinologist, or diabetes care and education specialist within 1 month of discharge is advised for all patients experiencing hyperglycemia while hospitalized [32]. If glycemic medications are changed or glycemic control is not optimal at discharge, an earlier appointment (e.g., 1–2 weeks) is preferred, and frequent contact may be needed to avoid hyperglycemia and hypoglycemia [32]. For patients discharged home on insulin therapy as a new medication, it is important that patient education and written information be provided for method and timing of insulin doses and recognition and treatment of hypoglycemia [15, 135]. Initiation of insulin administration should be instituted at least 1 day before discharge to allow assessment of safety and efficacy [15]. Measurement of HbA1c during hospitalization can assist in tailoring the glycemic management of DM patients at discharge. For patients with acceptable preadmission glycemic control (i.e., HbA1c <7%), guidelines suggest reinstitution of their preadmission insulin regimen or oral and non-insulin injectable antidiabetic medications at discharge (if there are no contraindications to continued therapy [15]). Patients with elevated HbA1c often require intensification of the outpatient regimen at discharge [15].

Conclusion

Optimal glycemic control throughout hospitalization is a goal all healthcare providers should strive to achieve. Appropriate glycemic control during the hospital stay requires effort on many levels, including provider education

to aid in ordering appropriate insulin regimens, nursing coordination on the timing of insulin administration and treatment of hypoglycemia, laboratory personnel measuring BG and reporting results promptly, and nutrition services assisting in dietary choices. Hospitals should take appropriate steps to achieve euglycemia and make patient safety in glycemic control a reality for all inpatients.

Multiple-Choice Questions

1. In the hospital, what blood glucose level is defined as representing hypoglycemia (values in mg/dL)?
   (a) <80
   (b) **<70**
   (c) <60
   (d) <50
   (e) <40

2. In the hospital, what blood glucose level is defined as representing hyperglycemia (values in mg/dL)
   (a) >100
   (b) >120
   (c) **>140**
   (d) >200
   (e) >250

3. In the hospital, what glucose range should be targeted for most patients?
   (a) 200–240
   (b) 160–200
   (c) **140–180**
   (d) 120–160
   (e) 100–140

4. Modification of the treatment regimen is necessary once any blood glucose value below what threshold is observed?
   (a) <80
   (b) **<70**
   (c) <60
   (d) <50
   (e) <40

5. Inpatient hyperglycemia is *best managed* with what form of therapy?
   (a) Metformin
   (b) Sulfonylureas
   (c) **Insulin**
   (d) GLP-1 agonists
   (e) SGLT2 inhibitors

6. In the ICU setting, what form of therapy has proven to be the *most effective* for achieving recommended glycemic targets?
   (a) Sliding scale insulin
   (b) Metformin
   (c) Sulfonylureas
   (d) **IV insulin infusion**
   (e) Basal insulin alone

7. If a patient is to initiate insulin therapy prior to hospital discharge, when should this be started to allow for assessment of safety and efficacy?
   (a) One week before discharge
   (b) After discharge
   (c) **At least 1 day before discharge**
8. What is the preferred method for blood glucose (BG) monitoring in the non-critically ill inpatient?
   (a) Continuous glucose monitoring
   (b) Venous BG sample
   (c) **Bedside capillary point-of-care testing (POCT)**
9. True or False: Patients being treated with glucocorticoid therapy should be evaluated for hyperglycemia, whether they have a known history of DM or not.
   (a) **True**
   (b) False
10. True or False: The accuracy of many glucometers can be altered by certain medications (e.g., acetaminophen [paracetamol]) and/or by a patient's hematocrit levels.
    (a) **True**
    (b) False

References

1. Moghissi ES, Korytkowski MT, Dinardo M, et al. American Association of Clinical Endocrinologists and American Diabetes Association consensus statement on inpatient glycemic control. Endocr Pract. 2009;15(4):353–69.
2. Umpierrez GE, Isaacs SD, Bazargan N, et al. Hyperglycemia: an independent marker of in-hospital mortality in patients with undiagnosed diabetes. J Clin Endocrinol Metab. 2002;87(3):978–82.
3. Jiang HJ, Stryer D, Friedman B, Andrews R. Multiple hospitalizations for patients with diabetes. Diabetes Care. 2003;26(5):1421–6.
4. American Diabetes Association. Economic costs of diabetes in the US in 2007. Diabetes Care. 2008;31(3):596–615.
5. Geiss LS, Wang J, Cheng YJ, et al. Prevalence and incidence trends for diagnosed diabetes among adult aged 20 to 79 years, United States, 1980-2012. JAMA. 2014;312(12):1218–26.
6. Levetan CS, Passaro M, Jablonski K, Kass M, Ratner RE. Unrecognized diabetes among hospitalized patients. Diabetes Care. 1998;21(2):246–9.
7. Centers for Disease Control and Prevention. Crude and age-adjusted percentage of civilian, noninstitutionalized population with diagnosed diabetes, United States, 1980–2011. Atlanta, GA: CDC; n.d.. http://www.cdc.gov/diabetes/statistics/us/index.htm. Accessed 6 Dec 2015.
8. Magaji V, Johnston JM. Inpatient management of hyperglycemia and diabetes. Clin Diab. 2011;29(1):3–9.
9. Horton WB, Weeks AQ, Rhinewalt JM, et al. Analysis of a guideline-derived resident educational program on inpatient glycemic control. South Med J. 2015;108(10):596–8.
10. Capes SE, Hunt D, Malmberg K, et al. Stress hyperglycemia and prognosis of stroke in nondiabetic and diabetic patients: a systematic overview. Stroke. 2001;32(10):2426–32.
11. Capes SE, Hunt D, Malmberg K, Gerstein HC. Stress hyperglycemia and increased risk of death after myocardial infarction in patients with and without diabetes: a systematic overview. Lancet. 2000;355(9206):773–8.
12. Falciglia M, Freyberg RW, Almenoff PL, et al. Hyperglycemia-related mortality in critically ill patients varies with admission diagnosis. Crit Care Med. 2009;37(12):3001–9.
13. Kosiborod M, Inzucchi SE, Spertus JA, et al. Elevated admission glucose and mortality in elderly patients hospitalized with heart failure. Circulation. 2009;119(14):1899–907.
14. Kosiborod M, Rathore SS, Inzucchi SE, et al. Admission glucose and mortality in elderly patients hospitalized with acute myocardial infarction: implications for patients with and without recognized diabetes. Circulation. 2005;111(23):3078–86.
15. Umpierrez GE, Hellman R, Korytkowski MT, et al. Management of hyperglycemia in hospitalized patients in non-critical care setting: an endocrine society clinical practice guideline. J Clin Endocrinol Metab. 2012;97(1):16–38.
16. Baker EH, Janaway CH, Philips BJ, et al. Hyperglycemia is associated with poor outcomes in patients admitted to hospital with acute exacerbations of chronic obstructive pulmonary disease. Thorax. 2006;61(4):284–9.
17. Clement S, Braithwaite SS, Magee MF, et al. Management of diabetes and hyperglycemia in hospitals. Diabetes Care. 2004;27(2):553–91.
18. McAlister FA, Majumdar SR, Blitz S, et al. The relation between hyperglycemia and outcomes in 2,471 patients admitted to the hospital with community-acquired pneumonia. Diabetes Care. 2005;28(4):810–5.
19. McAlister FA, Man J, Bisritz L, et al. Diabetes and coronary artery bypass surgery: an examination of perioperative glycemic control and outcomes. Diabetes Care. 2003;26(5):1518–24.
20. Pomposelli JJ, Baxter JK, Babineau TJ, et al. Early postoperative glucose control predicts nosocomial infection rate in diabetic patients. J Parenter Enter Nutr. 1998;22(2):77–81.
21. Furnary AP, Wu Y, Bookin SO. Effect of hyperglycemia and continuous intravenous insulin infusions on outcomes of cardiac surgical procedures: the Portland Diabetic Project. Endocr Pract. 2004;10(Suppl 2):21–33.
22. Krinsley JS, Jones RL. Cost analysis of intensive glycemic control in critically ill adult patients. Chest. 2006;129(3):644–50.
23. Dungan KM, Braithwaite SS, Preiser JC. Stress hyperglycemia. Lancet. 2009;373(9677):1798–807.
24. Mizock BA. Blood glucose management during critical illness. Rev Endocr Metab Disord. 2003;4(2):187–94.
25. Cook CB, Kongable GL, Potter DJ, et al. Inpatient glucose control: a glycemic survey of 126 U.S. hospitals. J Hosp Med. 2009;4(9):E7–E14.
26. Schmeltz LR, DeSantis AJ, Thiyagarajan V, et al. Reduction of surgical mortality and morbidity in diabetic patients undergoing cardiac surgery with a combined intravenous and subcutaneous insulin glucose management strategy. Diabetes Care. 2007;30(4):823–8.
27. van den Berghe G, Wouters P, Weekers F, et al. Intensive insulin therapy in critically ill patients. N Engl J Med. 2001;345(19):1359–67.
28. De La Rosa Gdel C, Donaldo JH, Restrepo AH, et al. Strict glycaemic control in patients hospitalized in a mixed medical and surgical intensive care unit: a randomized clinical trial. Crit Care. 2008;12(5):R120.
29. Inzucchi SE. Clinical practice. Management of hyperglycemia in the hospital setting. N Engl J Med. 2006;355(18):1903–11.
30. van den Berghe G, Wilmer A, Hermans G, et al. Intensive insulin therapy in the medical ICU. N Engl J Med. 2006;354(5):449–61.
31. Preiser JC, Devos P, Ruiz-Santana S, et al. A prospective randomised multi-centre controlled trial on tight glucose control by intensive insulin therapy in adult intensive care units: the Glucontrol study. Intensive Care Med. 2009;35(10):1738–48.

32. American Diabetes Association. Diabetes care in the hospital: standards of medical care in diabetes - 2021. Diabetes Care. 2021;44(Suppl 1):S211–20.

33. Saudek CD, Herman WH, Sacks DB, et al. A new look at screening and diagnosing diabetes mellitus. J Clin Endocrinol Metab. 2008;93(7):2447–53.

34. Ainla T, Baburin A, Teesalu R, Rahu M. The association between hyperglycaemia on admission and 180-day mortality in acute myocardial infarction patients with and without diabetes. Diabet Med. 2005;22(10):1321–5.

35. Norhammar A, Tenerz A, Nilsson G, et al. Glucose metabolism in patients with acute myocardial infarction and no previous diagnosis of diabetes mellitus: a prospective study. Lancet. 2002;359(9324):2140–4.

36. Fushimi N, Shibuya T, Yoshida Y, et al. Dulaglutide-combined basal plus correction insulin therapy contributes to ideal glycemic control in non-critical hospitalized patients. J Diab Invest. 2020;11(1):123–31.

37. Fayfman M, Galindo RJ, Rubin DJ, et al. A randomized controlled trial on the safety and efficacy of exenatide therapy for the inpatient management of general medicine and surgery patients with type 2 diabetes. Diabetes Care. 2019;42(3):450–6.

38. Vellanki P, Rasouli N, Baldwin D, et al. Glycaemic efficacy and safety of linagliptin compared to basal-bolus insulin regimen in patients with type 2 diabetes undergoing non-cardiac surgery: a multicentre randomized clinical trial. Diabetes Obes Metab. 2019;21(4):837–43.

39. Perez-Belmonte LM, Osuna-Sanchez J, Millan-Gomez M, et al. Glycaemic efficacy and safety of linagliptin for the management of non-cardiac surgery patients with type 2 diabetes in a real-world setting: Lina-Surg study. Ann Med. 2019;51(3–4):252–61.

40. U.S. Food and Drug Administration. FDA drug safety communication: FDA adds warnings about heart failure risk to labels of type 2 diabetes medicines containing saxagliptin and alogliptin. Silver Spring, MD: FDA; n.d.. http://www.fda.gov/Drugs/DrugSafety/ucm486096.htm. Accessed 30 Apr 2021.

41. Horton WB, Subauste JS. Top 10 facts to know about inpatient glycemic control. Am J Med. 2016;129(2):139–42.

42. Schnipper JL, Ndumele CD, Liang CL, Pendergrass ML. Effects of a subcutaneous insulin protocol, clinical education, and computerized order set on the quality of inpatient management of hyperglycemia: results of a clinical trial. J Hosp Med. 2009;4(1):16–27.

43. Maynard G, Lee J, Phillips G, et al. Improved inpatient use of basal insulin, reduced hypoglycemia, and improved glycemic control: effect of structured subcutaneous insulin orders and an insulin management algorithm. J Hosp Med. 2009;4(1):3–15.

44. Umpierrez GE, Smiley D, Jacobs S, et al. Randomized study of basal-bolus insulin therapy in the inpatient management of patients with type 2 diabetes undergoing general surgery (RABBIT 2 surgery). Diabetes Care. 2011;34(2):256–61.

45. Umpierrez GE, Smiley D, Zisman A, et al. Randomized study of basal-bolus insulin therapy in the inpatient management of patients with type 2 diabetes (RABBIT 2 trial). Diabetes Care. 2007;30(9):2181–6.

46. Baldwin D, Villanueva G, McNutt R, Bhatnagar S. Eliminating inpatient sliding scale insulin: a reeducation project with medical house staff. Diabetes Care. 2005;28(5):1008–11.

47. Umpierrez GE, Palacio A, Smiley D. Sliding scale insulin use: myth or insanity? Am J Med. 2007;120(7):563–7.

48. Queale WS, Seidler AJ, Brancati FL. Glycemic control and sliding scale insulin use in medical inpatients with diabetes mellitus. Arch Intern Med. 1997;157(5):545–52.

49. Gearhart JG, Duncan JL III, Replogle WH, et al. Efficacy of sliding scale insulin therapy: a comparison with prospective regimens. Fam Pract Res J. 1994;14(4):313–22.

50. Sawin CT. Action without benefit. The sliding scale of insulin use. Arch Intern Med. 1996;157(5):489.

51. Nau KC, Lorenzetti RC, Cucuzzella M, et al. Glycemic control in hospitalized patients not in intensive care: beyond sliding-scale insulin. Am Fam Physician. 2010;81(9):1130–5.

52. Schnipper JL, Barsky EE, Shaykevich S, et al. Inpatient management of diabetes and hyperglycemia among general medicine patients at a large teaching hospital. J Hosp Med. 2006;1(3):145–50.

53. Lubitz CC, Seley JJ, Rivera C, et al. The perils of inpatient hyperglycemia management: how we turned apathy into action. Diab Spectr. 2007;20(1):18–21.

54. Curll M, Dinardo M, Noschese M, Korytkowski MT. Menu selection, glycaemic control and satisfaction with standard and patient-controlled consistent carbohydrate meal plans in hospitalised patients with diabetes. Qual Saf Health Care. 2010;19(4):355–9.

55. Seley JJ, D'hondt N, Longo R, et al. AADE position statement: inpatient glycemic control. Diab Educ. 2009;35(Suppl 3):64S–8S.

56. Donihi AC, Raval D, Saul M, et al. Prevalence and predictors of corticosteroid-related hyperglycemia in hospitalized patients. Endocr Pract. 2006;12(4):358–62.

57. Dungan K, Chapman J, Braithwaite SS, Buse J. Glucose measurement: confounding issues in setting targets for inpatient management. Diabetes Care. 2007;30(2):403–9.

58. Scott MG, Bruns DE, Boyd JC, Sacks DB. Tight glucose control in the intensive care unit: are glucose meters up to the task? Clin Chem. 2009;55(1):18–20.

59. Vlasselaers D, Herpe TV, Milants I, et al. Blood glucose measurements in arterial blood of intensive care unit patients submitted to tight glycemic control: agreement between bedside tests. J Diabetes Sci Technol. 2008;2(6):932–8.

60. Cembrowski GS, Tran DV, Slater-Maclean L, et al. Could susceptibility to low hematocrit interference have compromised the results of the NICE-SUGAR trial? Clin Chem. 2010;56(7):1193–5.

61. Cook CB, Castro JC, Schmidt RE, et al. Diabetes care in hospitalized noncritically ill patients: more evidence for clinical inertia and negative therapeutic momentum. J Hosp Med. 2007;2(4):203–11.

62. Gomez AM, Umpierrez GE. Continuous glucose monitoring in insulin-treated patients in non-ICU settings. J Diabetes Sci Technol. 2014;8(5):940–6.

63. Gomez AM, Umpierrez GE, Munoz OM, et al. Continuous glucose monitoring versus capillary point-of-care testing for inpatient glycemic control in type 2 diabetes patients hospitalized in the general ward and treated with a basal bolus insulin regimen. J Diabetes Sci Technol. 2016;10(2):325–9.

64. Levitt DL, Spanakis EK, Ryan KA, Silver KD. Insulin pump and continuous glucose monitor initiation in hospitalized patients with type 2 diabetes mellitus. Diabetes Technol Ther. 2018;20(1):32–8.

65. Dexcom. FDA grants breakthrough device designation for Dexcom Hospital CGM system. 2022. https://investors.dexcom.com/news-releases/news-release-details/fda-grants-breakthrough-device-designation-dexcom-hospital-cgm. Press release.

66. Korytkowski MT, Salata RJ, Koerbel GL, et al. Insulin therapy and glycemic control in hospitalized patients with diabetes during enteral nutrition therapy: a randomized controlled clinical trial. Diabetes Care. 2009;32(4):594–6.

67. Umpierrez GE, Hor T, Smiley D, et al. Comparison of inpatient insulin regimens with detemir plus aspart versus neutral protamine Hagedorn plus regular in medical patients with type 2 diabetes. J Clin Endocrinol Metab. 2009;94(2):564–9.

68. Umpierrez GE, Smiley D, Hermayer K, et al. Randomized study comparing a basal-bolus with a basal plus correction insulin regimen for the hospital management of medical and surgical patients with type 2 diabetes: basal plus trial. Diabetes Care. 2013;36(8):2169–74.

69. Maynard G, Wesorick DH, O'Malley C, et al. Subcutaneous insulin order sets and protocols: effective design and implementation strategies. J Hosp Med. 2008;3(5 Suppl):29–41.

70. Schafer RG, Bohannon B, Franz MJ, et al. Diabetes nutrition recommendations for health care institutions. Diabetes Care. 2004;27(Suppl 1):S55–7.

71. Gosmanov AR, Umpierrez GE. Medical nutrition therapy in hospitalized patients with diabetes. Curr Diab Rep. 2012;12(1):93–100.

72. Schafer RG, Bohannon B, Franz MJ, et al. Translation of the diabetes nutrition recommendations for health care institutions. Diabetes Care. 2003;26(Suppl 1):S70–2.

73. Boucher JL, Swift CS, Franz MJ, et al. Inpatient management of diabetes and hyperglycemia: implications for nutrition practice and the food and nutrition professional. J Am Diet Assoc. 2007;107(1):105–11.

74. Ziegler TR. Parenteral nutrition in the critically ill patient. N Engl J Med. 2009;361(11):1088–97.

75. Draznin B, Korytkowski M, Draznin B, Drincic A. Food, fasting, insulin, and glycemic control in the hospital. In: Draznin B, editor. Managing diabetes and hyperglycemia in the hospital setting. Alexandria, VA: American Diabetes Association; 2016. p. 70–83.

76. Noschese M, Donihi AC, Koerbel G, et al. Effect of a diabetes order set on glycaemic management and control in the hospital. Qual Saf Health Care. 2008;17(6):464–8.

77. Kreider KE, Lien LF. Transitioning safely from intravenous to subcutaneous insulin. Curr Diab Rep. 2015;15(5):23.

78. Clain J, Ramar K, Surani SR. Glucose control in critical care. World J Diabetes. 2015;6(9):1082–91.

79. Kavanagh BP, McCowen KC. Clinical practice. Glycemic control in the ICU. N Engl J Med. 2010;363(26):2540–6.

80. Lena D, Kalfon P, Preiser JC, Ichai C. Glycemic control in the intensive care unit and during the postoperative period. Anesthesiology. 2011;114(2):438–44.

81. McCowen KC, Malhotra A, Bistrian BR. Stress-induced hyperglycemia. Crit Care Clin. 2001;17(1):107–24.

82. Stuart CA, Shangraw RA, Prince MJ, et al. Bed-rest-induced insulin resistance occurs primarily in muscle. Metab Clin Exp. 1988;37(8):802–6.

83. Finfer S, Wernerman J, Preiser JC, et al. Clinical review: consensus recommendations on measurement of blood glucose and reporting glycemic control in critically ill adults. Crit Care. 2013;17(3):229.

84. Kanji S, Buffie J, Hutton B, et al. Reliability of point-of-care testing for glucose measurement in critically ill adults. Crit Care Med. 2005;33(12):2778–85.

85. Hoedermaekers CW, Klein Gunnewiek JM, Prinsen MA, et al. Accuracy of bedside glucose measurement from three glucometers in critically ill patients. Crit Care Med. 2008;36(11):3062–6.

86. Finkielman JD, Oyen LJ, Afessa B. Agreement between bedside blood and plasma glucose measurement in the ICU setting. Chest. 2005;127(5):1749–51.

87. Lyon ME, Baskin LB, Braakman S, et al. Interference studies with two hospital-grade and two home-grade glucose meters. Diabetes Technol Ther. 2009;11(10):641–7.

88. Karon BS, Gandhi GY, Nuttall GA, et al. Accuracy of Roche Accu-check inform whole blood capillary, arterial, and venous glucose values in patients receiving intensive intravenous insulin therapy after cardiac surgery. Am J Clin Pathol. 2007;127(6):919–26.

89. Ehrhardt N, Hirsch IB. The impact of COVID-19 on CGM use in the hospital. Diabetes Care. 2020;43(11):2628–30.

90. Agarwal S, Mathew J, Davis GM, et al. Continuous glucose monitoring in the intensive care unit during the COVID-19 pandemic. Diabetes Care. 2021;44(3):847–9.

91. Finfer S, Chittock DR, Su SY, et al. Intensive versus conventional glucose control in critically ill patients. N Engl J Med. 2009;360(13):1283–97.

92. Green DM, O'Phelan KH, Bassin SL, et al. Intensive versus conventional insulin therapy in critically ill neurologic patients. Neurocrit Care. 2010;13(3):299–306.

93. Coester A, Neumann CR, Schmidt MI. Intensive insulin therapy in severe traumatic brain injury: a randomized trial. J Trauma. 2010;68(4):904–11.

94. Macrae D, Grieve R, Allen E, et al. A randomized trial of hyperglycemic control in pediatric intensive care. N Engl J Med. 2014;370(2):107–18.

95. Goldberg PA, Siegel MD, Sherwin RS, et al. Implementation of a safe and effective insulin infusion protocol in a medical intensive care unit. Diabetes Care. 2004;27(2):461–7.

96. Rea RS, Donihi AC, Bobeck M, et al. Implementing an intravenous insulin infusion protocol in the intensive care unit. Am J Health Syst Pharm. 2007;64(4):385–95.

97. Nazer LH, Chow SL, Moghissi ES. Insulin infusion protocols for critically ill patients: a highlight of differences and similarities. Endocr Pract. 2007;13(2):137–46.

98. DeSantis AJ, Schmeltz LR, Schmidt K, et al. Inpatient management of hyperglycemia: the Northwestern experience. Endocr Pract. 2006;12(5):491–505.

99. Furnary AP, Braithwaite SS. Effects of outcome on in-hospital transition from intravenous insulin infusion to subcutaneous therapy. Am J Cardiol. 2006;98(4):557–64.

100. Smiley DD, Umpierrez GE. Perioperative glucose control in the diabetic or nondiabetic patient. South Med J. 2006;99(6):580–9.

101. Marchant MH, Viens NA, Cook C, et al. The impact of glycemic control and diabetes mellitus on perioperative outcomes after total joint arthroplasty. J Bone Joint Surg Am. 2009;91(7):1621–9.

102. Gandhi GY, Nuttall GA, Abel MD, et al. Intraoperative hyperglycemia and perioperative outcomes in cardiac surgery patients. Mayo Clin Proc. 2005;80(7):862–6.

103. Pichardo-Lowden A, Gabbay RA. Management of hyperglycemia during the perioperative period. Curr Diab Rep. 2012;12(1):108–18.

104. Malmstedt J, Wahlberg E, Jorneskog G, Swedenborg J. Influence of perioperative blood glucose levels on outcome after infrainguinal bypass surgery in patients with diabetes. Br J Surg. 2006;93(11):1360–7.

105. Sebranek JJ, Lugli AK, Coursin DB. Glycaemic control in the perioperative period. Br J Anaesth. 2013;111(Suppl 1):i18–34.

106. Hatzakorzian R, Bui H, Carvalho G, et al. Fasting blood glucose levels in patients presenting for elective surgery. Nutrition. 2011;27(3):298–301.

107. World Health Organization. World Health Organization guidelines for safe surgery. Geneva: World Health Organization; 2009.

108. Aldam P, Levy N, Hall GM. Perioperative management of diabetic patients: new controversies. Br J Anaesth. 2014;113(6):906–9.

109. Mucha GT, Merkel S, Thomas W, Bantle JP. Fasting and insulin glargine in individuals with type 1 diabetes. Diabetes Care. 2004;27(5):1209–10.

110. Correia MI, Waitzberg DL. The impact of malnutrition on morbidity, mortality, length of hospital stay and costs evaluated through a multivariate model analysis. Clin Nutr. 2003;22(3):235–9.

111. Pancorbo-Hidalgo PL, Garcia-Fernandez FP, Ramirez-Perez C. Complications associated with enteral nutrition by nasogastric tube in an internal medicine unit. J Clin Nurs. 2001;10(4):482–90.

112. Umpierrez GE. Basal versus sliding-scale regular insulin in hospitalized patients with hyperglycemia during enteral nutrition therapy. Diabetes Care. 2009;32(4):751–3.

113. Clore JN, Thurby-Hay L. Glucocorticoid-induced hyperglycemia. Endocr Pract. 2009;15(5):469–74.

114. Felig P, Sherwin RS, Soman V, et al. Hormonal interactions in the regulation of blood glucose. Recent Prog Horm Res. 1979;35:501–32.

115. Schade DS, Eaton RP. The temporal relationship between endogenously secreted stress hormones and metabolic decompensation in diabetic man. J Clin Endocrinol Metab. 1980;50(1):131–6.

116. Umpierrez GE, Kitabchi AE. ICU care for patients with diabetes. Curr Opin Endocrinol Diab. 2004;11(2):75–81.

117. Suh S, Park MK. Glucocorticoid-induced diabetes mellitus: an important but overlooked problem. Endocrinol Metab. 2017;32(2):180–9.

118. Cook CB, Boyle ME, Cisar NS, et al. Use of continuous subcutaneous insulin infusion (insulin pump) therapy in the hospital setting: proposed guidelines and outcome measures. Diab Educ. 2005;31(6):849–57.

119. Bailon RM, Partlow BJ, Miller-Cage V, et al. Continuous subcutaneous insulin infusion (insulin pump) therapy can be safely used in the hospital in select patients. Endocr Pract. 2009;15(1):24–9.

120. Boucai L, Southern WN, Zonszein J. Hypoglycemia-associated mortality is not drug-associated but linked to comorbidities. Am J Med. 2011;124(11):1028–35.

121. Garg R, Hurwitz S, Turchin A, Trivedi A. Hypoglycemia, with or without insulin therapy, is associated with increased mortality among hospitalized patients. Diabetes Care. 2013;36(5):1107–10.

122. Turchin A, Matheny ME, Shubina M, et al. Hypoglycemia and clinical outcomes in patients with diabetes hospitalized in the general ward. Diabetes Care. 2009;32(7):1153–7.

123. Smith WD, Winterstein AG, Johns T, et al. Causes of hyperglycemia and hypoglycemia in adult inpatients. Am J Health Syst Pharm. 2005;62(7):714–9.

124. van der Crabben SN, Blumer RM, Stegenga ME, et al. Early endotoxemia increases peripheral and hepatic insulin sensitivity in healthy humans. J Clin Endocrinol Metab. 2009;94(2):463–8.

125. Cryer PE, Axelrod L, Grossman AB, et al. Evaluation and management of adult hypoglycemic disorders: an Endocrine Society Clinical Practice Guideline. J Clin Endocrinol Metab. 2009;94(3):709–28.

126. Mitrakou A, Ryan C, Veneman T, et al. Hierarchy of glycemic thresholds for counterregulatory hormone secretion, symptoms, and cerebral dysfunction. Am J Phys. 1991;260(1 Pt 1):E67–74.

127. Arnold P, Scheurer D, Dake AW, et al. Hospital guidelines for diabetes management and the Joint Commission-American Diabetes Association Inpatient Diabetes Certification. Am J Med Sci. 2016;351(4):333–41.

128. Shah BR, Walji S, Kiss A, et al. Derivation and validation of a risk-prediction tool for hypoglycemia in hospitalized adults with diabetes: the Hypoglycemia during Hospitalization (HyDHo) Score. Can J Diabetes. 2019;43(4):278–82.

129. Mathioudakis NM, Everett E, Routh S, et al. Development and validation of a prediction model for insulin-associated hypoglycemia in non-critically ill hospitalized adults. BMJ Open Diabetes Res Care. 2018;6(1):e000499.

130. Ruan Y, Bellot A, Moysova Z, et al. Predicting the risk of inpatient hypoglycemia with machine learning using electronic health records. Diabetes Care. 2020;43(7):1504–11.

131. Mathioudakis NM, Abusamaan MS, Shakarchi AF, et al. Development and validation of a machine learning model to predict near-term risk of iatrogenic hypoglycemia in hospitalized patients. JAMA Netw Open. 2021;4(1):e2030913.

132. Horton WB, Barros AJ, Andris RT, et al. Pathophysiologic signature of impending ICU hypoglycemia in bedside monitoring and electronic health record data: model development and validation. Crit Care Med. 2022;50(3):e221–30.

133. Kilpatrick CR, Elliott MB, Pratt E, et al. Prevention of inpatient hypoglycemia with a real-time informatics alert. J Hosp Med. 2014;9(10):621–6.

134. Schnipper JL, Magee M, Larsen K, et al. Society of Hospital Medicine Glycemic Control Task Force summary: practical recommendations for assessing the impact of glycemic control efforts. J Hosp Med. 2008;3(5 Suppl):66–75.

135. Lauster CD, Gibson JM, DiNella JV, et al. Implementation of standardized instructions for insulin at hospital discharge. J Hosp Med. 2009;4(8):E41–2.

Diabetes and Infection

47

Atulya Atreja, Sanjay Kalra, and Joel Rodriguez-Saldana

Whether it be the plague or influenza,
one thing that we learn at the knee of our "alma mater"
is that diabetics are more likely to get it. (Larkin and
colleagues [1])

Introduction

Before the discovery of insulin and antibiotics, it was estimated that infections were the cause of death of one in five
diabetic patients [2]. Following the discovery of insulin, a
decrease in mortality from sepsis and tuberculosis was documented since 1935 [3]; in the late 1960s, the estimated mortality from infections in people with diabetes was 5% [2].
Nevertheless, it has been shown that diabetes continues to
increase the predisposition to infections, especially bacterial,
fungal, and viral. Albeit not traditionally recognized, acute
infections are among the ten leading clinical characteristics
in patients with newly diagnosed type 2 diabetes [4]. For
example, Drivsholm and colleagues reported that the prevalence of genital itching, balanitis in men, recurrent urinary
tract and skin infections among 1137 Danish patients newly
diagnosed with type 2 diabetes was 27.2%, 12.0%, 5.7%,
and 4.3% [4]. Largely unperceived, the use and costs of antimicrobials in patients with diabetes are significantly higher
in comparison with people without diabetes [5]. Using
national registries from Finland, Reunanen et al. reported
that over 1 year, 43.6% of patients used systemic antibacterials and 4.5% had used systemic antimycotics, in comparison
with 29.1% and 1.9% respectively in people without diabetes
[5]. Until the 1980s, controversy prevailed about the

increased frequency of infections in patients with diabetes;
many clinicians believed that people with diabetes had an
increased susceptibility to infection, but this belief was not
supported by strong evidence [1, 6, 7]. Contributing factors
increasing the risk of infections in patients with diabetes
include comorbidities and chronic complications such as
foot ulcers and neurogenic bladder [6]. Beyond a disturbance
of glucose metabolism, diabetes is an inflammatory disease
in which chronic complications, including neuropathy,
chronic vascular and renal diseases alter the response to
pathogens [8].

Magnitude of Risk

The relevance of infections in the morbidity and mortality of
people with diabetes has been neglected, is not addressed or
reported in clinical trials, and is not recognized in clinical
guidelines for diabetes management [9]. Nevertheless, infections impair quality of life and impose short-time and long-
time threats on the life of people with diabetes. Despite the
general belief investigations about the epidemiology of
infections in people with diabetes are scarce [9].

The landmark specific studies—three retrospective and
three longitudinal—were carried out in Canada, Netherlands,
England, South Korea, and the United States [7, 10–14]. In
the first retrospective trial, risk ratios of infections and death
attributable to infectious disease were compared in two
groups of 513,749 non-diabetic and diabetic patients [7]. The
risk ratio for infections was equal in both groups, but the risk
ratio for infectious-related hospitalization was 2.1 and the
risk ratio for death attributable to infection was 1.92 in
patients with diabetes [7]. Risk ratios for infectious disease
hospitalization or physician claims for infectious disease
were higher in patients with diabetes; almost half of the
patients with diabetes had at least one hospitalization or physician claim [7]. In 2018, Carey, Critchley et al. published
two reports from the retrospective analysis of 102,493 pri-

A. Atreja
Department of Pulmonary Medicine, MMIMSR, Mullana, India

S. Kalra (✉)
Department of Endocrinology, Bharti Hospital, Karnal, India

J. Rodriguez-Saldana
Multidisciplinary Diabetes Center Mexico, Mexico City, Mexico

© The Author(s), under exclusive license to Springer Nature Switzerland AG 2023
J. Rodriguez-Saldana (ed.), *The Diabetes Textbook*, https://doi.org/10.1007/978-3-031-25519-9_47

mary care patients with type 1 and type 2 diabetes aged 40–89 years [10, 11]. After 5 years of follow-up, 55.0% of patients with type 1 diabetes and 56.9% of patients with type 2 diabetes had at least one infection compared with 41.3% and 46.2% of control subjects respectively [10]. They reported clear trends for increasing risk of infection at poorer levels of glycemic control and that the long-term risk of skin, cellulitis, candidiasis, bone and joint infections, endocarditis, and sepsis tended to rise at higher HbA1c levels, albeit some infections showed elevated rates among patients with diabetes with HbA1c <6.0%. In other words, even patients with good glycemic control were at higher risk of infections than people without diabetes [11]. Patients with diabetes were three times as likely to be hospitalized for infection, especially those with type 1 diabetes who were also at higher risk of death [11].

Prospective studies about the risk of infection among patients with diabetes include one of 12-month duration in which 7417 adult patients with type 1 (N = 705) or type 2 (N = 6712) diabetes were compared with 18,911 patients with hypertension [12]. Patients with diabetes had higher risks of lower respiratory tract infections, urinary tract infection, bacterial and skin and mucous membrane infection, and mycotic skin and mucous membrane infection [12]. Adjusted odds ratios were higher in every category for patients with type 1 diabetes, and the risk increased with recurrences of common infections [12]. The second study comprised a cohort of 66,426 diabetes and 132,852 age-sex-region matched non-diabetes control from the general population in South Korea [13]. Compared to non-diabetes controls, people with diabetes had a higher risk of almost all types of infections with higher adjusted incidence rate ratios for hepatic abscess, central nervous system, skin and soft tissue infections [13]. Patients with diabetes were at higher risk to intensive care unit admission and death than the general population [13]. Last but not least, Fang and colleagues conducted a 30–32-year prospective cohort analysis to investigate hospitalization for infection among 12,379 patients with diabetes, from which in 4229 infection was the cause of admission [14]. After adjusting for potential confounders, people with diabetes had a higher risk for infection (HR 1.67), especially pronounced for foot infection (HR 5.99). Overall infection mortality was low in this study (8.5%), but the adjusted risk was increased in people with diabetes (HR 1.72) [14].

Pathogenesis

The search for "an intrinsic problem" to explain the association of diabetes and infection goes back to Lassar, who postulated in 1904 that organisms thrive in a high sugar medium [1]. In 1938 Marble and colleagues stated that "patients with diabetes have less resistance to infection than normal indi-

viduals is a fact met with in the everyday experience of the clinician" and admitted that the lessened ability to cope with infection was undeniable prior to the introduction of insulin and (even) afterwards in patients with poor glycemic control [15]. In this pioneering report, Marble et al. suggested various factors as the cause of the lower resistance to infection in people with diabetes, some of which have been confirmed over the years: (1) increased sugar content of blood and tissues, (2) decreased activity of blood elements associated with resistance to infection, (3) inadequate functioning of fixed tissue cells, (4) lower capacity of tissue to react to antigenic stimuli, (5) undernutrition [15].

Diabetes and infection exemplify a vicious circle: insulin resistance and beta cell failure impair the immune response, and increased susceptibility to infections precipitates metabolic complications in patients with diabetes. Acute infections impair glycemic control, and infection is an important cause of hyperglycemic crisis, including ketoacidosis and non-hyperglycemic hyperosmolar state [16]. Large population-based observational studies have reported strong associations between higher HbA1c levels and infection risks for patients with Type 1 and Type 2 Diabetes [9]. A recent review identified 13 studies in which infections could be associated with glycemic control [8]. Except for the Diabetes Control and Complications Trial (DCCT), all the studies discussed in this review were observational either cohort or case control, identifying associations but not clearly causality [9]. Importantly, all were carried out in high income countries, but associations between diabetes and infection could be also important (and higher) in low and middle resource countries, where diabetes prevalence is rising most rapidly, and glucose control is lower [9]. Despite their limitations to measure the impact of diabetes on infection, it has been shown that hyperglycemia has negative effects on the outcomes in people with diabetes. Glycemic control is an essential goal to reduce the risk of infections and to protect maintenance of normal host defense mechanisms that determine resistance and response to infection [16]. In support of this statement, Burekovic et al. studied 450 patients with diabetes hospitalized in an intensive care unit from Bosnia and Herzegovina and they found a positive correlation between HbA1c, C-reactive protein, and HbA1c levels with acute infections [17].

The Immune Response

Specific defects in innate and adaptive immune function in people with type 1 and type 2 diabetes have been identified in multiple studies [2]. Reported abnormalities include an increase in inflammatory markers (tumor necrosis factor, interleukin-6, C-reactive protein, plasminogen activator inhibitor) and ineffective functioning of T lymphocytes, neu-

Table 47.1 Pathogenic mechanisms of infection in patients with diabetes [2, 6, 8, 9, 15–26]

Mechanism	Disorder
Leukocyte count	Increased, larger and granular; diminished levels of antioxidant genes, increased levels of proapoptotic and proinflammatory genes
Innate immunity	Macrophage dysfunction: reduced phagocytosis
	Defects in pathogen recognition; impairment in the number and activity of dendritic (antigen-presenting) cells: higher susceptibility to opportunistic infections
	Disorders in pathogen elimination, including: (1) polymorphonuclear adhesion to vascular endothelium, (2) transmigration through the vessel wall down a chemotactic gradient, (3) phagocytosis and microbial killing
	Neutrophil dysfunction including: (1) decreased phagocytosis, (2) diminished respiratory burst capacity and degranulation, (3) glucose-dependent reduction in superoxide production, (4) reduced monocyte proliferation, (4) reduced bactericidal capacity, (5) delayed bacterial clearance, (6) increased severity of infections, (7) higher susceptibility to infections, (8) apoptosis
	Downregulation of Toll-like receptors: phagocyte inhibition and killing of *Staphylococcus aureus*
	Vascular dysfunction, including (1) upregulation of intercellular cell adhesion molecule-1, vascular cell adhesion molecule-1 and selectin, resulting in limited chemotactic migration out of vessels at sites of inflammation, (2) reduced endothelial-dependent relaxation, (3) blunted nitric oxide response to bradykinin, (4) dysregulation of nitric oxide production and release of prostanoids with resulting vasoconstriction, (5) increased endothelial permeability, tissue edema
	Disorders in the complement cascade, including (1) impairment in the lectin pathway, (2) reduced attachment of C-type lectin proteins, (3) upregulation of C3 and C4 gene expression, chronic inflammatory state, (4) inhibition of complement receptor and Fc gamma receptor, (5) reduced opsonization and phagocytosis of microorganisms
	Disturbances in cell signaling pathways, activation of mitogen-activated protein kinases, including nuclear factor-kB and protein kinase C
	Non-enzymatic glycosylation of immunoglobulins
	Bacterial biofilm formation, increased survival of microorganisms
Adaptive immunity	Specific defects in T lymphocyte function
	Glycosylation and impaired functioning of antibodies in proportion to HbA1c levels
	Paradoxical hyper-reactive antigen-specific T cell inflammatory response
	Impairment in cytokine function and reduced synthesis: high levels of single and double cytokine CD4+ Th1 cells
	High levels of type 1 (tumor necrosis factor-α, IFN-γ, interleukin-2), type 2 (interleukin-5), type 17 (interleukin-17 cytokines) and other proinflammatory cytokines (interleukin-1β, interleukin-6, interleukin-18, C-reactive protein), and an anti-inflammatory cytokine (interleukin-10): oxidative stress and insulin resistance
	Low levels of IL-22
	Decreased frequency and function of natural Treg cells
	Enhanced frequencies of central memory CD4+ and CD8+ T cells resulting in disturbances on central memory, effector memory, and naïve T cells
	Diminished expression of cytotoxic markers Perforin, Granzyme B, and CD107a, decreased antigen-stimulated CD8+ T cell cytotoxic activity
	NK cell dysfunction: reduction in natural killer (NK) receptor NKG2D
	Higher levels of tissue damage in diabetic patients with tuberculosis

trophils, oxidant-antioxidant imbalance, and deficient opsonophagocytosis [18–25]. These infections are often difficult to evaluate and eradicate due to reduced humoral immune responses. Host factors like microvascular and macrovascular insufficiency, sensory and autonomic neuropathy, and mucosal colonization with *Staphylococcus aureus* and *Candida albicans* further complicate the scenario [19]. A summary of the immune responses negatively affected by diabetes and hyperglycemia is presented in Table 47.1.

Diabetes and Viral Infections

Viral infections are associated with metabolic derangements and predispose to the development of type 2 diabetes. The prevalence of type 2 diabetes in patients with hepatitis C is higher than in the general population. Hepatitis C promotes insulin resistance through multiple pathogenic mechanisms,

including (1) defects in post-receptor insulin signaling, (2) high levels of proinflammatory cytokines, (3) high levels of reactive oxygen species, (4) low levels of GLP-1, (5) diminished glucose-stimulated insulin release, and (6) beta cell apoptosis [27]. Patients infected with the human immunodeficiency virus (HIV) are also at high risk of type 2 diabetes associated with the use of combination antiretroviral therapy. The HIV virus itself has been proposed as a mechanism of hyperglycemia, but the association between obesity and diabetes is strong, as in non-infected patients [28].

The Coronavirus Pandemic and Diabetes

It appears now that a new group of viruses is emerging with members which infect the respiratory tract of birds and man.
One member of the group, strain 229E, grows and produces cytopathic effect in tissue culture. (Kennett McIntosh et al. [29])

Coronaviruses are large, enveloped, single-stranded RNA viruses found in humans and other mammals such as dogs, cats, chicken, cattle, pigs, and birds [30]. Human coronaviruses have long been considered innocuous pathogens responsible for "the common cold" in healthy people [31]. In the twenty-first century however, two highly pathogenic coronaviruses emerged from animal reservoirs to cause global epidemics with high rates of morbidity and mortality: severe acute respiratory syndrome coronavirus (SARS-CoV) in 2002 in China and Middle East respiratory syndrome coronavirus (MERS-CoV) in 2012 in Saudi Arabia [31, 32]. Clinically, flu-like symptoms are usual at the time of presentation for all three diseases, but these vary from asymptomatic to severe multisystem involvement [33]. The immune response to each of these viruses is highly complex and includes both humoral and cellular components that can have a significant impact on prognosis [33]. Global health studies confirmed higher mortality rates in persons with diabetes from infections caused by these viruses and announced the potential consequences of another emerging pandemic [24].

In December 31, 2019, a cluster of patients with pneumonia of unknown cause was linked to a seafood market selling many species of live animals in Wuhan China [31, 34]. This was reported to the World Health Organization Country Office, and the Chinese Centre for Disease Control and Prevention (China CDC) organized an intensive outbreak investigation program; by January 10, 2020, researchers from the Shanghai Public Health Clinical Center & School of Public Health released a full genomic sequence of 2019-nCoV to public databases [31, 34]. The etiology of the illness was attributed to a novel virus belonging to the coronavirus family, COVID-19, which is the acronym of "coronavirus disease 2019 [35]." COVID-19 is highly contagious and has quickly spread globally and primarily via respiratory droplets during close face-to-face contact. The average time from exposure to symptom onset is 4.6 days outside mainland China, 6.5 days in mainland China, and 5.1 days elsewhere [36, 37]. Starting with the first reports and afterwards, most of the infected patients are men and higher risk of infection is associated with comorbidities, such as diabetes, hypertension, obesity, respiratory and cardiovascular disease [32, 37, 38]. Of 120 studies with 125,446 patients, the most common comorbidities were hypertension (32%), obesity (25%), diabetes (18%), and cardiovascular disease (16%) [39]. Severity and risk of death from COVID-19 was associated with chronic kidney disease (51%), stroke (44%), and cardiovascular disease (44%) [40]. Systematic reviews and meta-analyses show that fatal outcomes associated with COVID-19 include male gender, older age, smoking, diabetes, obesity, chronic obstructive pulmonary disease, cardiovascular disease, cancer, acute kidney injury, and increased D-dimer [41]. The prevalence of comorbidities in people without diabetes is 25% [29] in comparison with 67% in people with diabetes [42], and the association with COVID-19 is more severe and conveys higher risks of mortality [42].

The World Health Organization classifies patients with COVID-19 into mild, moderate, severe, and critical disease [42]. Common symptoms include dry fever (77–90%), olfactory and/or gustatory dysfunction (64–80%), cough (64–86%), dyspnea (53–80%), myalgia (15–90%), or fatigue (38%); less common symptoms include sputum production, headache (16%), anorexia (19.4%), and diarrhea (9.42–39%) [30, 38, 43]. Clinical presentation of COVID-19 has several overlapping features with other pulmonary infections including pneumonia, chronic bronchitis, and chronic obstructive pulmonary disease [44, 45]. Mild disease is defined by patients meeting clinical and epidemiological criteria without the evidence of viral pneumonia or hypoxia, moderate disease is characterized by the evidence of pneumonia, severe disease is defined by pneumonia with a respiratory rate above 30 breaths/min or respiratory distress, and critical disease is defined by severe pneumonia complicated with respiratory distress syndrome, sepsis, or septic shock [45, 46].

Laboratory findings include a general decrease of the leukocyte count (21.5%), lymphopenia (50–83%), increased C-reactive protein level (58.3%), and high D-dimer levels (27–60%) [29, 46]. Liver function tests show increased levels of alanine aminotransferase (ALT) and aspartate aminotransferase (AST) up to 18.3% and lactate dehydrogenase (48%) [30, 43]. Additional findings in chemical chemistry include increased high-sensitivity troponin (19%), creatinine kinase (42%), ferritin (14%), and serum creatinine (22.3%) [43]. Several biomarkers have become useful tools to differentiate patients with mild to severe COVID-19 infection including procalcitonin, C-reactive protein, serum amyloid A, interleukin-6, lymphocyte count, platelet count, lactate dehydrogenase, cardiac troponin, and serum ferritin [44]. Radiologic findings include patchy shadows in the peripheral zones of both lungs with higher involvement of the lower lobe of the left lung, ground glass opacities, and consolidations [43]. Laboratory tests for diagnosing COVID-19 infection include rapid antigen tests, serological testing, nucleic acid amplification tests, and viral sequencing [47]. Rapid antigen tests have the advantages of fast detection and low cost, but their disadvantages include (1) low sensitivity and specificity and (2) inability to identify patients in the incubation period [47]. Next generation sequencing is an accurate diagnostic method, but its high cost is an obstacle for widespread use [47]. Leading diagnostic tests for COVID-19 are IgM and IgG antibodies and nucleic acid amplification tests by real-time reverse transcriptase polymerase chain reaction (PCR) [47, 48]. Antibodies measure the immune response to COVID-19 infection and are detected in all patients between the third and fourth week of clinical illness [48]. IgM antibodies are detected 3–5 days after onset and IgG antibodies are above four times higher during the recovery period [47]. IgM titers begin to decline and reach lower levels after 5 weeks whereas IgG titers persist beyond 7 weeks [48]. The PCR test is highly sensitive and specific and has become the most commonly used and reliable test for diagnosis of COVID-19 [47].

The pathology associated with symptomatic severe acute respiratory syndrome and COVID-19 involves diffuse alveolar damage [33]. Complications include acute respiratory distress syndrome (ARDS) and multisystem involvement of the heart, brain, lung, liver, kidney, and coagulopathy [38, 45]. In severe cases, a dysregulated innate host immune system can initiate a hyperinflammatory syndrome dominated by endothelial dysfunction that may lead to a hypercoagulable state with microthrombi, resulting in microvascular and macrovascular diseases in children and adults [33, 49, 50].

Since the SARS COVID outbreak in 2002, extensive structural analysis revealed key atomic interactions between human pathogenic coronaviruses and host target cells through angiotensin-converting enzyme 2 (ACE2) receptor which is highly expressed by nasal and bronchial mucosal epithelial cells and pneumocytes [30, 51]. The high transmissibility of SARS-CoV-2 is probably related to active viral replication in the upper airways in the pre-symptomatic and symptomatic phases [52]. After receptor engagement, specific proteases like the type 2 transmembrane serine protease (TMPRSS2) present in alveolar epithelial type II cells, cleave the S protein, and trigger its fusion to cells (fusogenic activity) [30, 52]. Binding of ACE2 to the viral structural spike S protein induces endocytosis of the virion, fusion of the viral envelope with the endosomal membrane to enable the release of the viral genome into the cytoplasm or alternatively at the plasma membrane after receptor engagement [52]. Severe lymphopenia occurs and the host response to the virus activates the innate and adaptive immune system, additionally impairing lymphopoiesis and increasing lymphocyte apoptosis [30]. Observational studies have demonstrated strong antibody and T cell responses in a large proportion of patients, but the humoral response appears to be proportional to COVID-19 severity [45]. In later stages of the infection, epithelial-endothelial barrier integrity is compromised; COVID-19 infects pulmonary capillary endothelial cells, increasing the inflammatory response and the influx of monocytes and neutrophils. The last stage in severe COVID-19 involves critical activation of coagulation and consumption of clotting factors, viral sepsis, organ dysfunction, and multiorgan failure [30]. Extrapulmonary manifestations of COVID-19 involve brain/nervous system, kidney, liver, gastrointestinal tract, heart/cardiovascular system, endocrine system and skin with corresponding myriad symptoms and signs [45].

According to early data reported by CDC China from more than 44,000 confirmed cases of COVID-19 infection, death rates among patients with diabetes were 7.0% compared with 0.9% in people without diabetes [34]. Impaired immune function is a clinical feature of COVID-19 infection. As already mentioned, diabetes is characterized by defects in innate and adaptive immune responses in addition to micro-angiopathic changes in the respiratory tract and other organ systems, contributing to the progression and poor prognosis of COVID-19 (Table 47.2) [24, 30, 53].

Table 47.2 Immune abnormalities against COVID-19 in diabetes

Immune response	Cell type	Abnormality
Innate	Macrophages	Lung accumulation, ↑ proinflammatory activity
	Dendritic cells	↓ Amount and function
	Neutrophils	Entrapment, ↑ ACE2 receptors
	NK cells	↓ Function
	NKT cells	↑ CD57 and CD
Adaptive immunity	B cells	Changes in number, phenotype, and function
	T cells	Targeting of CD4T cells against viral spike protein

Modified from references [24, 30, 51]

Pathophysiology of COVID-19 Infection in Hyperglycemia and Diabetes

Hyperglycemia and diabetes are long-established risk factors for viral infections and pneumonia [54]. Diabetes induces lung oxidative stress and inflammation, apoptosis of alveolar cells, persistent matrix deposition, and increases the susceptibility to viral pneumonia [55]. In addition, diabetes induces functional abnormalities in the lung, including decrease in volumes, elastic recoil and diffusion capacity, and oxidative stress injury to pancreatic beta cells [55, 56]. Compared with hospitalized patients with COVID-19 without diabetes, patients with diabetes have worse clinical profiles and outcomes including higher levels of glucose, HbA1c, leukocytes, high-sensitive C-reactive protein, procalcitonin, ferritin, D-dimer, lactic dehydrogenase, natriuretic peptide, severity of disease, higher frequency of admission to intensive care units, and mortality [55, 56]. Plasma glucose levels and diabetes are independent predictors of mortality and morbidity in patients with COVID-19 infection, and mechanisms that increase the vulnerability include increased binding affinity and efficient virus entry, reduced viral clearance, impaired T cell function, increased susceptibility to cytokine storm, cardiovascular and pulmonary preexisting disease [55]. Host-cellular protein components involved in the entry of COVID-19 [55] include angiotensin-converting enzyme-2 (ACE2), Furin, serine protease TMPRSS2, interferon-induced transmembrane proteins (IFITM), desintegrin, and metalloproteinase domain 17 proteins (ADAM17) [55]. Patients with type 2 diabetes present more severe inflammatory responses and less lymphocyte counts than patients without diabetes, are more likely to worsen from moderate to severe disease, and inflammation and lymphocyte recovery are slower [57]. Respiratory viral infections predispose to bacterial co-infections leading to increased disease severity and mortality, particularly in people with diabetes [58].

Management of Patients with COVID-19 and Diabetes

Patients with diabetes require more medical interventions and had significantly higher mortality and multiple organ injury than patients without diabetes [59]. Glucose control is associated with markedly lower mortality compared to patients with poor glycemic control (above 180 mg/dL) and is a leading goal of treatment [59]. Management of patients with diabetes and infection by COVID-19 involves general and metabolically oriented measures, summarized in Table 47.3 [46, 60–69].

Table 47.3 General management of COVID-19 infection in people with diabetes [60–72]

HbA1c: <7.0%		
Fasting plasma glucose: 72.0–144 mg/dL		
Avoid hypoglycemia: <55.0 mg/dL		
Blood pressure: <140/80 mm Hg		
Low-density lipoproteins: <100 mg/dL		
Assessment and control of comorbidities		
Stage	**Recommendation**	**Comments**
	Sensitization about the importance of optimal metabolic control	
Primary prevention	Reduce social contact	Key measure to contain the spread
	Strategies of virtual support, including telephone and telemedicine	
	Vaccination	**BNT162b2 mRNA, two dose regimen**
		Efficacy: 89.0% in preventing hospitalization from COVID-19; 90.0% in preventing admission to intensive care unit; 91.0% in preventing emergency department or urgent care visit; ranging from 81.0% to 95.0% across subgroups defined by age, sex, race, ethnicity, body mass index, and comorbidities
		Safety profile: short-term, mild to moderate pain at the injection site, fatigue, and headache
		Low incidence of serious adverse effects, similar rates in the vaccine and placebo groups
		Antibody titers decline sharply by 6 months after vaccination and decline further after 8 months
		mRNA-1273 SARS-CoV-2, two dose regimen
		Efficacy: 94.1% across key secondary analyses, including 14 days after the first dose, evidence of SARS-CoV-2 infection at baseline and in people ≥65 years old
		Safety: moderate, transient reactogenicity, serious adverse events are rare and similar in patients receiving the vaccine or placebo
		Binding and functional antibodies against variants persist in most vaccinated subjects albeit at low levels, 6 months after the first dose
		Neutralizing antibody titers significantly decreased after 8 months
		Ad26.COV2.S, one dose versus two-dose regimen
		Efficacy: 76–83% in adults 18–55 years old; 60–77% in patients ≥65 years and older; 68.0% in preventing hospitalization, 73.0% in preventing emergency department or urgent care clinic visit
		Safety: most frequent adverse events included fatigue, headache, myalgia, pain in the site of injection, and fever, especially in patients ≥65 years old
		Differential kinetics of immune responses: substantially lower median titers than mRNA vaccines at peak immunity, 4 weeks after first dose, albeit remained stable over 8 months
		Purified inactivated SARS-Cov-2, two-dose regimen
		Efficacy: 65.6% for prevention, 87.0% for preventing hospitalization, 90.3% for preventing admission to intensive care unit, 86.3% for preventing COVID-19 death
		AZD1222 (ChAdOx1 nCoV-19), two-dose regimen
		Efficacy: 74.5% overall, 83.5% in people ≥65 years old; efficacy for preventing COVID-19 infection: 64.3%
		No severe or critical symptomatic COVID-19 cases among people vaccinated
		Spike binding and neutralizing antibodies increased after the first dose and increased further when measured 28 days after the second dose
		Safety: low incidence of serious and medically attended adverse events and similar frequency with placebo; mild or moderate local and systemic reactions in both groups
		Overall waning vaccine immunity, correlates of protection not yet defined
	Wearing masks	Control the source of infection
	Hand hygiene	Protect susceptible groups
		Reduce the risk of health providers from being infected when attending to patients
		Significant inhibitory effect on the spread of respiratory viruses for healthcare providers (80%) and non-healthcare workers (47%)
	Antidiabetics	All therapeutic classes
Mild COVID-19	Isolation to contain viral transmission	On an individual basis
		Close monitoring
	Symptomatic treatment	Analgesics
		Antipyretics

Table 47.3 (continued)

	Adequate nutrition and hydration	
	Patient and family counseling	Advise about signs and symptoms of disease complications and progression including dyspnea, chest pain, and dehydration
	Antidiabetics	At usual doses:
		Metformin
		Anti-inflammatory, antithrombotic properties, reduce mortality in type 2 diabetes patients with COVID-19
		Prevention of cytokine storm
		DPP-4 inhibitors
		Prevention of coronavirus from entering host cells
		Anti-inflammatory effects
		SGLT-2 inhibitors
		Increase the expression of ACE2 in the kidney, increase susceptibility to infection
		GLP-1 receptor agonists
		Systemic anti-inflammatory properties
		Insulin
		Downregulation of ACE2 receptors
		Anti-inflammatory, antithrombotic effect
		Sulfonylureas
		A-glucosidase inhibitors
		Use with caution:
		Thiazolidinediones
		Weight gain, fluid retention, edema, increasing heart failure
Moderate COVID-19	Immediate isolation to contain viral transmission on an individual basis, depending on clinical presentation, requirements for supportive care, risk factors for severe disease and conditions at home	At health facility
		At community facility
		Self-isolation at home
	Regular monitoring	Pulse oximetry
		Temperature
		Blood pressure
	Testing and treatment for other infections causing fever	Routine use of antibiotics not advised
	Antidiabetics	At usual doses:
		DPP-4 inhibitors
		SGLT-2 inhibitors
		GLP-2 receptor agonists
		Insulin
		Use with caution
		Metformin
		A-glucosidase inhibitors
		SGLT-2 inhibitors
		Contraindicated
		Thiazolidinediones
		Sulfonylureas
Severe COVID-19	Supplemental oxygen in patients with oxygen saturation levels <90.0%	Emergency airway management, target oxygen level ≥94.0%
		Nasal cannula for flow rates up to 5 L/min
		Venturi mask for 6–10 L/min
		Face mask with reservoir bag for 10–15 L/min
	Continuous monitoring for signs of clinical deterioration	Hematological and biochemical laboratory testing
		Electrocardiogram
		Chest imaging
	Immediate supportive care	Intravenous fluids
	Antidiabetics	At usual doses:
		DPP-4 inhibitors
		Insulin
		Contraindicated:
		Metformin
		α-glucosidase inhibitors
		SGLT-2 inhibitors
		Thiazolidinediones

(continued)

Table 47.3 (continued)

Critical COVID-19	Supplemental oxygen in patients with oxygen saturation levels <90.0%	Emergency airway management, target oxygen level ≥94.0%
		Mild acute respiratory distress syndrome:
		Noninvasive ventilation through continuous positive airway pressure and bilevel positive airway pressure
		Invasive ventilation including endotracheal intubation and tracheostomy in patients with hypercapnia, hypoxemic respiratory failure, hemodynamic instability, multiorgan failure, or abnormal mental status
		Prone ventilation 12–16 h/day
	Continuous monitoring for signs of clinical deterioration	Hematological and biochemical laboratory testing
		Electrocardiogram
		Chest imaging
	Immediate supportive care	Intravenous fluids
	Antivirals	Remdesivir: 200 mg/IV on day 1, 100 mg/IV on days 2–10
	Antidiabetics	At usual doses:
		DPP-4 inhibitors
		Insulin
		Contraindicated:
		Metformin
		α-glucosidase inhibitors
		SGLT-2 inhibitors
		Thiazolidinediones
Post-COVID	Monitoring for metabolic, physical, psychosocial, and cognitive impairments	Glycemic control
		Blood pressure control
		Lipoprotein profile control
		Rehabilitation
		Vaccination prioritization

As already mentioned, diabetes is a relevant comorbidity in people with COVID-19 infection and increases the risk of severity and mortality. Glycemic and overall metabolic control are essential at every stage. Patient and family support to address the disease and its consequences in mental health is also important.

By the end of October 2021, the WHO estimated more than 243 million confirmed cases of COVID-19 globally, 4.9 million deaths, and a mortality rate of 2.03% [73]. Since the beginning of the pandemic, diabetes was identified as an important risk factor for mortality and progression to acute respiratory distress syndrome in patients with COVID-19 [74]. After 18 months, epidemiologic studies confirm that diabetes is a central contributor to severe COVID-19 morbidity and that COVID-19 has had devastating effects on people with diabetes [75]. The evidence is compelling. Patients with type 1 or type 2 diabetes (1) represent 30–40% of hospital admissions by COVID-19, (2) 21–43% of people requiring intensive care, and (3) have a mortality rate of 25% [75]. The risk of severe morbidity and mortality is 100–250% higher among people with diabetes and the impact on the general population with diabetes has been 50% higher than historical trends, more than twice that of the general population [75].

The emergence of the COVID-19 pandemic has become a landmark in the history of mankind, a mass casualty incident [76]. Its effects at the global, political, economic, and individual level have been devastating and at the end of 2021 continue to be evolving. Quantifying the overall impact and its morbidity and mortality is still not feasible until cascades of metrics including (1) population at risk, (2) population exposed, (3) people infected, (4) people diagnosed, (5) people hospitalized, (6) people with severe forms of disease, and (7) mortality can be constructed at the global, regional, and national level. Living with diabetes during the COVID-19 pandemic is challenging. The established complexities of diabetes management have been exacerbated by the scarcity of access to healthy foods, scarcity of medicines or access to medical services, and limited physical activity or exercise because of confinement [77].

Diabetes Parasitic Diseases and "The Hygiene Hypothesis"

In comparison with the high risk of bacterial, fungal, and viral infections, an inverse association between soil-transmitted helminthiasis and diabetes was initially reported by Nazligul and colleagues in 2001 [78]. The evidence is scarce and comprises six experimental studies and seven cross-sectional studies which were summarized by de Ruiter and colleagues [79]. Under the hypothesis that having diabetes would affect the susceptibility to infections, six of these studies showed that the prevalence of intestinal parasites was significantly lower among patients with diabetes; by comparison, only one small study in Brazil reported a positive association between *Strongyloides stercoralis* infection and type 2 diabetes [80]. In this study, the frequency of positive *S. stercoralis* serology in diabetics was 23% versus 7.1% in the control group ($p < 0.05$).

The odds ratio for diabetics was 3.9 (CI, 1.6–15.9, $p < 0.05$) [80]. By comparison, the remaining six studies showed a significantly lower prevalence of intestinal helminth infections in patients with type 2 diabetes, metabolic syndrome, or insulin resistance [79]. The inverse relation or "protective effect" of type 2 diabetes and helminth infections could be related to a state of cellular immune hypo-responsiveness induced by parasites mediated by a helminth-induced regulatory network involving regulatory T cells and their associated cytokines IL-10 and transforming growth factor-β [81]. These observations are related to the revised hygiene hypothesis proposed by Strachan in 1989, who proposed that improved hygiene increased the rise of allergic diseases [81]. This hypothesis states that exposure to pathogens is critical to establish immunomodulatory cells to prevent inappropriate responses [81]. Albeit strongly criticized as "a dangerous misnomer which is misleading people away from finding the true causes of the rise in allergic disease [82]" and should not diminish the importance of personal hygiene in every age group, the inverse association between helminth infections and type 2 diabetes is an interesting observation that invites further study.

Categories of Infections in Patients with Diabetes

Three categories of infections have been described: (1) common infections also occurring in persons with diabetes; (2) uncommon infections strongly associated or typical of diabetes; (3) infections related to therapeutic interventions in people with diabetes [2]. The spectrum of disease and the likely causative organisms identified in people with diabetes are presented in Table 47.4.

Table 47.4 Disease spectrum, causative microorganisms, and main clinical features

	Spectrum of infections and references	Causative microorganisms	Clinical features	Diagnostic procedure
Head and neck				
	Herpes zoster ophthalmicus [83–86]	Human herpes virus type 3	Risk ratio: 1.31 (95% CI, 1.22–1.41)	Complete medical history Ophthalmologic examination
			Represents 10–20% of herpes zoster cases, 3.2 cases per 1000 person-years	
			Peak incidence: 50–79 years, higher in patients over 80 years	
			Three clinical phases: (1) Pre-eruptive, (2) acute eruptive, (3) chronic.	
			(1) Pre-eruptive symptoms and signs: headache, fatigue, malaise, photophobia, and fever; neuralgia around the eye and forehead with pinprick anesthesia and hyperesthesia to light touch (allodynia)	
			(2) Acute eruptive phase: involves skin, eyelids, the medial canthal area, conjunctiva and cornea. Skin lesions manifest as a vesicular eruption along the ophthalmic dermatome of the trigeminal nerve, erythematous coalescing papules evolving into clear vesicles with rupture, secondary bacterial infection, and discharge, and crusting over several weeks. The Hutchinson sign refers to involvement of the tip of the nose. Eyelid involvement includes cutaneous macular rash, ptosis, and lagophthalmos. Signs of conjunctival involvement include injection and chemosis with papillary reaction, hyperemic mucopurulent conjunctivitis, and petechial hemorrhages.	
			(3) Chronic stage: cornea and anterior segment: punctuate epithelial keratitis and pseudodendrites, nummular stromal keratitis, disciform stromal keratitis, neurotrophic keratopathy corneal neovascularization, lipid extravasation, and opacification diminished corneal sensation, corneal ulceration, eye perforation, uveitis, secondary glaucoma	
			Posterior segment: acute optic neuritis, orbital phlegmon, superior orbital fissure syndrome necrotizing retinopathy, and blindness.	
			Cranial nerves: Additional compromise includes involvement of the iris, the retina, and the optic nerve, motor palsies of the third, fourth, and sixth, diplopia.	
			Late complications: postherpetic neuralgia in 20% of the patients, higher in the elderly or in patients with involvement beyond the skin	

(continued)

Table 47.4 (continued)

Spectrum of infections and references	Causative microorganisms	Clinical features	Diagnostic procedure
Malignant external otitis [2, 87–89]	*Pseudomonas aeruginosa*	Three clinical stages: (1) Infection of the external auditory canal and adjacent soft tissues	Clinical examination
	Methicillin resistant *Staphylococcus aureus*	(2) Extension of infection with osteitis of skull base and temporal bone	Ear swab culture Positive Technetium (^{99}TC) scan of failure of local treatment after more than 1 week
	Proteus mirabilis	(3) Dissemination to intracranial structures, neck spaces, and large blood vessels	Computed tomography, magnetic resonance imaging to assess progression and resolution
	Klebsiella oxytoca	Major obligatory signs: Unrelenting pain	Culture of drainage material
	Pseudomonas cepacia	Otorrhea Edema	Biopsy from the infection site
	Staphylococcus epidermidis Candida *Aspergillus fumigatus*	Granulations	Histological examination shows nonspecific inflammation and hyperplasia of squamous epithelium
	Polymicrobial infections	Microabscesses	
		Minor or occasional: Hearing loss	
		Pain at the temporomandibular joint	
		Cellulitis	
		Osteomyelitis of the skull base	
		Cranial nerve palsies: Common: facial, glossopharyngeal, vagal, spinal accessory	
		Less common: hypoglossal Rare: trigeminal, abducens, optic	
Periodontal infections [90, 91]	Most associated pathogens are indigenous to the oral cavity, but possible superinfecting microorganism may also inhabit periodontal pockets	Pain, gingival swelling	Oral examination
	Lesions usually contain a constellation of pathogens, mostly gram-negative anaerobic, but also gram-negative facultative rods		
Oral candidiasis [92]	*Candida albicans*, Pichia, Trichosporon, Geotrichum	May be asymptomatic	Dental examination
		Sore throat, dysphagia	
		White patches on the surface of the oral cavity	
		Untreated candidiasis may lead to chronic hyperplastic candidiasis: candidal leukoplakia	
Rhino-orbital or rhino-cerebral sinusitis [92–95]	Rhizopus, mucor, and absidia species	Preseptal or orbital cellulitis: Facial or ocular pain, fever, headache, nasal discharge, sinus pain	Clinical examination, culturing, magnetic resonance, histopathological evidence of fungal invasion of tissue
		Facial erythema or cyanosis	
		Sub-periosteal or orbital abscess: perinasal swelling, edema, proptosis, chemosis and even blindness	
		Facial numbness from damage to sensory branches of the fifth cranial nerve	
		Black, necrotic eschar on the palate or nasal mucosa, turbinate destruction	
		Intracranial complications: epidural and subdural abscesses, necrosis of frontal lobes, cavernous and sagittal sinus thrombosis	
		Clinical meningitis is rare	

Table 47.4 (continued)

	Spectrum of infections and references	Causative microorganisms	Clinical features	Diagnostic procedure
Respiratory system	Influenza [96, 97]	Type A influenza viruses: H1N1 and H3N2	Six times more frequent in patients with diabetes	Normal or decreased leukocyte count
			Wide range of manifestations, including: (1) asymptomatic, (2) conjunctivitis, (3) influenza-like illness, (4) viral pneumonia, (5) acute respiratory distress syndrome, (6) respiratory failure, (7) multiorgan failure	Lymphopenia and thrombocytopenia, high levels of C-reactive protein
			Sudden onset: fever, cough, malaise, wheezing, pulmonary rales, respiratory failure	Chest radiography: ground glass opacities and consolidation
				Confirmatory tests for influenza H1N1 including real-time or reverse transcriptase polymerase chain reaction
	Community-acquired pneumonia [98–110]	Outpatient: *Streptococcus pneumoniae*	Cough, fever, dyspnea, focal chest signs, respiratory failure	Clinical examination
		Mycoplasma pneumoniae	Prediction rule for diagnosis: Rhinorrhea—2, Sore throat—1, Night sweats 1, Myalgia 1, Sputum 1, Respiratory rate >25 breaths/min	Chest radiography
		Chlamydia pneumoniae	2 Temperature ≥100 °F (37.8 °C)	Pathogens are not detected in half of pneumonia episodes
		Klebsiella pneumoniae *Legionella pneumophila* *Haemophilus influenzae* Respiratory viruses Inpatient, non-intensive care unit *Streptococcus pneumoniae* *Mycoplasma pneumoniae* *Chlamydia pneumoniae* *Haemophilus influenzae* *Legionella* sp. aspiration Intensive care unit *Streptococcus pneumoniae* *Staphylococcus aureus* *Legionella pneumophila* Gram-negative bacilli *Haemophilus influenzae*	2 Positive likelihood ratio: 3 points 14.0, 1 point: 5.0, −1 point: 1.5, ≤10.2 points	Clinical indications for extensive diagnostic testing include: (1) intensive care unit admission, (2) failure of outpatient antibiotic therapy, (3) cavitary infiltrates, (4) leucopenia, (5) alcoholism, (6) chronic liver disease, (7) obstructive/structural lung disease, (8) recent travel, (9) positive Legionella urinary antigen result, (10) positive urinary antigen pneumococcal result, (11) pleural effusion
	Pulmonary tuberculosis [111–114]	*Mycobacterium tuberculosis*	Fever, night sweats, weight loss, cough, sputum, hemoptysis	Chest radiography usually shows more lung cavities and parenchymal lesions in patients with diabetes than patients without diabetes. Sputum microscopy and culture: bacilloscopy from two samples collected at the same visit
			Patients with tuberculosis and diabetes are reported to be older and heavier, and more likely to be male	Xpert MTB/RIF: *M. tuberculosis* PCR

(continued)

Table 47.4 (continued)

	Spectrum of infections and references	Causative microorganisms	Clinical features	Diagnostic procedure
	Pulmonary coccidioidomycosis [115]	*Coccidioides immitis*, *Coccidioides posadasii*	Asymptomatic or mild respiratory illness in most cases	Chest radiography showing segmental or lobar consolidations, hilar or mediastinal adenopathy, pleural effusions, residual nodules, cavities, and chronic infiltrates
			Patients with diabetes may present with diffuse pneumonia	Definitive diagnosis is serological, by means of immunodiffusion to detect immunoglobulin G and IgM-specific antibodies
			Symptoms of severe illness include fever, malaise, pneumonia, chronic structural lung disease or cardiopulmonary disease, respiratory distress syndrome	Complement fixation tests for IgG-specific antibodies are useful in immunocompetent patients
			Improvement is slow in these cases	
	Pulmonary mucormycosis [92–95]	Rhizopus, Mucor	Pneumonia refractory to antibacterials	Computed tomography
			Hemoptysis	Histopathology
			Multiple mycotic pulmonary artery aneurisms and pseudoaneurysms, bronchial obstruction, asymptomatic solitary nodules	
			Endobronchial lesions with resulting obstruction of major airways or erosion into pulmonary blood vessels	
			Less common complications include mycetomas in preexisting lung cavities or slowly necrotizing pneumonia, hypersensitivity syndromes, and allergic alveolitis	
Abdomen	Acute emphysematous cholecystitis [1, 116, 117]	*Clostridium perfringens*	Fever, right upper quadrant abdominal pain, vomiting, jaundice, peritonitis, septic shock, sepsis	Radiography
		Escherichia coli		Computed tomography
		Bacteroides fragilis		
	Pyogenic liver abscess [118–120]	Invasive *Klebsiella pneumonia* serotypes K1 and K2	Fever, chills, and abdominal pain; nausea and vomiting	Computed tomography
			Higher rates of cryptogenic etiology, gas-forming nature, thrombocytopenia, growth of *Klebsiella pneumoniae* in blood cultures, metastatic infection, and bacteremia in patients with diabetes	Isolation of *Klebsiella pneumoniae* from blood or liver abscess
			Lower rates of right upper quadrant pain, biliary origin	Multiplex PCR
	Psoas and spinal epidural abscess [121, 122]	Most frequent: *Staphylococcus aureus*, but also *Escherichia coli*, *Mycobacterium tuberculosis*, Enterobacter, and Klebsiella	May be primary, from hematogenous spread from an occult source, or secondary, by spreading from contiguous anatomical structures	Leukocytosis
			Back pain, in the flank in the buttock or in the leg, fever, malaise	Computed tomography
Genitourinary tract	Asymptomatic bacteriuria [123, 124]	*Escherichia coli*	Asymptomatic	Urine examination and culture
		Staphylococcus saprophyticus		
		Enterococcus sp.		
		Candida		
	Candiduria [125]	*Candida* sp.	Frequently asymptomatic	Clinical examination
			Rare complications include prostatitis and epididymo-orchitis	Urinary dipstick, microscopy, urinary culture
	Acute pyelonephritis [126–129]	Bacterial: *Escherichia coli* Fungal: *Candida* sp.	Presentation of symptoms is variable, ranging from fever, malaise, costovertebral angle pain and tenderness, urgency and dysuria, to intense pain, nausea, vomiting, sepsis and septic shock in severe cases	Clinical examination
				Urinary dipstick, microscopy
				A quantitative count of $\geq 10^3$ cfu/mL in the urinary culture
				Pyuria

Table 47.4 (continued)

Spectrum of infections and references	Causative microorganisms	Clinical features	Diagnostic procedure
Emphysematous pyelonephritis [129]	*Escherichia coli*	Fever, chills, abdominal and flank pain, nausea, vomiting, dysuria, pyuria	Renal ultrasound, computed tomography
	Klebsiella pneumonia	Associated with poor prognosis: thrombocytopenia, mental status changes, proteinuria	
	Proteus mirabilis		
	Pseudomonas aeruginosa		
	Citrobacter		
	Candida		
Perinephric abscess [130]	Common: *Escherichia coli*, *Enterobacter* sp., *Pseudomonas aeruginosa*, *Serratia* sp., *Citrobacter* spp.	Chronic presentation: persisting urinary infection, urine culture positive for *Proteus* spp.	Renal ultrasound, computed tomography, magnetic resonance imaging
	Less frequent: *Clostridium* spp. Bacteroides, *Actinomyces* spp., *Corynebacterium urealyticum*	Flank tenderness, localized rigidity and fullness, scoliosis, and palpable mass in some cases	
	Tuberculosis should always be considered	Signs in advanced stages: anemia, malaise empyema, psoas abscess or pyonephrosis necessitans	
	Proteus mirabilis in infected calculi	Acute: chills interspersed with high fever, loin and flank tenderness, history of bacterial skin infection	
Bacterial cystitis [123, 124, 127, 128]	*Escherichia coli*	May be asymptomatic	Medical history
		More frequent in patients treated with sodium-glucose cotransporter-2 inhibitors	Urinalysis, urine culture
		Urgency, dysuria, fever	
Fungal cystitis [125]	*Candida albicans*	Severe urgency, frequency, and nicturia	Medical history
		Sterile pyuria, microhematuria	Urine examination and culture
Emphysematous cystitis [129]	More frequent: *Escherichia coli*, *Klebsiella pneumoniae* *Enterobacter aerogenes*, *Proteus mirabilis*, *Streptococcus* sp.	From asymptomatic (7%) to severe sepsis	Clinical examination: history of neurogenic bladder, complicated urinary tract infections, bladder outlet obstruction
	Less common: *Pseudomonas aeruginosa*, *Candida albicans*, *Clostridium perfringens*, *Enterococcus faecalis*, *Staphylococcus aureus*, *Clostridium welchii*, *Candida tropicalis*, *Aspergillus fumigatus*	Common symptoms: abdominal pain (80%) and gross hematuria (60%)	Urine examination and culture
		Less common: fever (30–50%), pneumaturia, dysuria, urinary frequency and urgency (50%)	Blood culture
			Plain film of the abdomen showing curvilinear areas of increased radiolucency delineating the bladder wall and intraluminal gas
			Computed tomography
Vulvovaginal candidiasis [92, 131–136]	*Candida albicans*, *Candida glabrata*, *Candida tropicalis*	May be asymptomatic	Medical history
		Risk in patients treated with sodium-glucose cotransporter-2 inhibitors: 3–5 higher	Clinical examination of vaginal secretions including culture and wet mount, KOH microscopy, gram stain, Whiff test, pH measurement
		Acute pruritus, vaginal discharge, vaginal soreness, irritation, vulvar burning, dyspareunia, dysuria, odor, erythema, swelling of the labia and vulva	

(continued)

Table 47.4 (continued)

	Spectrum of infections and references	Causative microorganisms	Clinical features	Diagnostic procedure
	Balanoposthitis [137]	*Candida glabrata, Candida albicans, Candida tropicalis*	More frequent in uncircumcised men and in patients treated with sodium-glucose cotransporter-2 inhibitors	Medical history Physical examination
		Streptococci, Staphylococci, anaerobic bacteria, *Trichomonas vaginalis, Mycoplasma genitalis*, and herpes simplex virus have also been associated	Balanitis involves inflammation of the glans penis; posthitis is defined as inflammation of the prepuce	
	Necrotizing fasciitis [1, 2, 13]	*S. pyogenes, Clostridium* sp.	Pain, erythema, crepitation, bullous skin lesions	Medical history
			Involvement of skin, subcutaneous tissue, and superficial fascia	Clinical examination
				Plain radiography, computed tomography, or magnetic resonance imaging of the affected area
				Biopsy, gram stain, and culture
	Fournier's gangrene [138]	Mixed aerobes and anaerobes including *Escherichia coli, Klebsiella pneumoniae, Bacteroides fragilis,* Streptococcus, Enterococcus, Clostridium, Pseudomonas and Proteus	Male/female ratio: 10 to 1	Clinical examination
		Uncommon: Candida, *Lactobacillus gasseri*	Sudden pain and swelling in the scrotum	Imaging rarely necessary to ascertain extension
			Purulence or wound discharge, crepitation, fluctuance, prostration, fever	
			Necrotizing fasciitis of the external genitalia	
			Localized tenderness and wounds in genitalia and perineum	
			Fetid drainage and sloughing in affected sites	
			Sepsis, multiorgan failure	
Upper and lower extremities, skin and appendages	Hand ulceration and infection, "tropical diabetic hand syndrome" [139, 140]	*Staphylococcus* sp.	Under-reported, very few physicians are aware of its existence, resulting in late diagnosis and proper treatment	Clinical examination
			Largely reported in African countries, but also in the United States	Wound swab and culture
			More frequent in patients living in tropical and coastal areas	
			History of trauma including mild abrasions, lacerations, and insect bites; poor glycemic control, delayed presentation	
			Clinical presentation variable, ranging from localized swelling, cellulitis, and exudate, with or without ulceration, progressive hand sepsis and gangrene	
	Cutaneous zygomycosis [93, 94]	*Rhizopus* sp.	Single, painful area of erythema, induration, and cellulitis	Clinical examination
			Portals of entry include contaminated wounds, traumatic wounds, dressings, burns, and surgical sites	Skin biopsy
			Lesions secondary to trauma rapidly develop necrosis and extension to subcutaneous tissues, similar to ecthyma	
	Cellulitis [2, 6, 20, 141, 142]	*Staphylococcus aureus, Streptococcus pyogenes*, gram negatives and anaerobes less common	Painful, erythematous infection of the dermis and subcutaneous tissues presenting with warmth, edema, and advancing borders	Biopsy and histology examination
			Fever and leukocytosis	
			Most common sites include legs and digits, the face, feet, hands, torso, neck, and buttocks	

Table 47.4 (continued)

Spectrum of infections and references	Causative microorganisms	Clinical features	Diagnostic procedure
Foot ulcer infections [142–145]	Usually polymicrobial, including *Staphylococcus aureus*, *Proteus* spp., *Escherichia coli*, *Peptostreptococcus* sp., *Veilonella* sp., *Bacteroides* sp., *Escherichia coli*, *Klebsiella pneumoniae*, *Pseudomonas aeruginosa*	Contaminating ulcers in the plantar aspect of foot, tip of the toe, lateral to fifth metatarsal	Culture preferably from tissue specimens rather than swabs
		Presence of purulence or at least ≥2 classic symptoms or signs of inflammation: erythema, edema, warmth, tenderness, pain, or induration	Deep tissue sampling; curettage or tissue scraping from the base of the ulcer
		In case of neuropathy, secondary signs include discolored granulation tissue, foul odor, non-purulent discharges, delayed wound healing	Gram staining and microscopy examination
Herpes zoster [146, 147]	Varicella zoster virus	Odds ratio in patients with diabetes: 1.20 (CI 1.17–1.22)	Clinical examination
		Localized pain and paresthesia followed by erythematous macules or papules coalescing into grouped vesicular lesions or bullae usually in one dermatomal distribution, and unilateral	PCR testing for viral DNA from fluid from skin lesions
		Pustules and crusting afterwards	Direct fluorescent antibody testing on scrapings from active lesions
		Complete healing up to 4 weeks	
		Most common sites are the thoracic nerves and the ophthalmic division of the trigeminal nerve	
		Systemic symptoms include fever, headache, malaise, and fatigue	
Tinea pedis, intertrigo [92]	*Candida*	Itching and scaling of the affected skin	Clinical examination
		Plantar or intertriginal fissures	Fungal culturing of skin samples
		Paronychial inflammation of the edge surrounding skin	
Onychomycosis [92, 148, 149]	Dermatophytes: *Trichophyton rubrum*, *Trichophyton mentagrophytes*	Dystrophic, thick, brittle, and discolored nails, distal onycholysis, subungual hyperkeratosis, thickening of the nail bed and nail plate	Fungal culturing of samples from nail plates or subungual debris, direct microscopy
	Non-dermatophytes: *Candida* sp.		Histopathological examination
Hospital-acquired infections [2, 6, 20, 92, 124]			
Local	Postoperative wound infections	*Staphylococcus aureus*	7.7 higher risk	Clinical examination
			Mortality related to time with diabetes, glycemic control at hospital admission, and A1c level	Swab or biopsy examination
			Postoperative infections have been described in multiple surgical settings, including cardiothoracic, general, orthopedic, and vascular	
Systemic	Fungemia	*Candida albicans*, *Aspergillus fumigates*, *Candida glabrata*	Associated with disruption of skin barriers including injections or intravascular access	Clinical suspicion, isolation, and identification of pathogens by culturing and histopathology
	Mycosis in hemodialysis patients	*Candida* spp.	High risk in patients with onychomycosis	Clinical suspicion, isolation, and identification of pathogens by culturing and histopathology
	Urinary tract infection in post-renal transplant patients	*Escherichia coli*	Prevalence: 25–47%, higher risk in the first year post-transplant	Clinical examination, urine examination, and culture
			Additional risk factors include indwelling devices, immunosuppressive therapy and urologic abnormalities	
			May be asymptomatic or present with graft tenderness	
	Mycosis in post-transplant patients, including kidney and pancreas	*Candida* spp. *Cryptococcus neoformans*	May be asymptomatic	Clinical examination
				Blood culture

(continued)

Principles of Management

Managing infections in persons with diabetes is always a challenge for physicians. Principles of management include the following.

Awareness of Diabetes-Associated Diseases

Awareness regarding the variety and severity of diseases, in persons with diabetes, is essential for prevention and prompt treatment. Diabetes education, along with optimal glycemic control, can minimize the risk of life-threatening infections. Simple preventive measures like proper foot care can reduce disease-associated morbidity.

Adequate Choice of Antibiotics

Empirical broad-spectrum antibiotics should be used till microbiologic results can guide treatment; some infections are frequently resolved empirically. Choice of antibiotics should be based on possible causative organisms and local flora. Early suspicion of antibiotic resistance, in people with diabetes with complicated infections, can help in limiting the disease-associated morbidity and mortality. *P. aeruginosa* infections are commonly seen in hospitalized patients with cystic fibrosis, cytotoxic chemotherapy, mechanical ventilation, and broad-spectrum antibiotic therapy. Patients present with fever, shock, hypothermia, acute pneumonia, and occasionally ecthyma gangrenosum. Table 47.5 shows empirical therapies for infections in patients with diabetes, and Table 47.6 presents first

Table 47.5 Empirical selection of antimicrobial therapy and dose in adults

Infection	First choice	Alternate choice(s)
Herpes zoster ophthalmicus	Acyclovir, 800 mg PO five times daily/7–10 days	Valacyclovir 1000 mg PO three times daily/7–10 days
		Famciclovir, 500 mg PO/three times a day/7–10 days
Malignant external otitis (MEO)	Ciprofloxacin, 1.5 g IV/day plus Ceftazidime 2 g IV/8 h/10 weeks	Itraconazole, 200 mg PO or Voriconazole 200 mg PO daily/6 weeks, for MEO caused by Aspergillosis
Periodontal infections	Tetracycline, 250 mg PO/6 h or 500 mg PO/ bid Clarithromycin, 500 mg PO/day	Azithromycin, 500 mg PO/3 days
		Amoxicillin, 500 mg PO/bid/10 days
		Metronidazole, 250 mg PO/6–8 h/10 days or 500 mg PO/8 h/10 days
Oral candidiasis	Nystatin, 400,000–600,000 units PO/4 times a day after meals/7–14 days	Fluconazole, 100–200 mg PO once daily/7–14 days after clinical improvement
		Itraconazole, 200 mg PO day/7–14 days
Rhino-orbital or rhino-cerebral sinusitis	Amphotericin B, 0.25–0.3 mg/kg IV/24 h, increasing by 5–10 mg/day to a final dose of 0.5–0.7 mg/kg/day for 12 weeks	Posaconazole, oral solution, 800 mg in 4 divided doses/day for 12 weeks
		Posaconazole, oral solution, 800 mg in 4 divided doses/day
		Isavuconazole, 200 mg orally or IV, loading dose: 200 mg/8 h/2 days; 200 mg/day afterwards for 12 weeks
Influenza	Neuraminidase inhibitors	M2 Inhibitors
	Laninamivir one single inhalation of 20 mg for children <10 years, one single inhalation of 40 mg for individuals ≥10 years	Amantadine 100 mg/12 h/5 days
	Oseltamivir 75 mg/12 h/5 days	Rimantadine 100 mg/12 h/5 days
Community-acquired pneumonia	Outpatients: β-lactam (i.e., Amoxicillin 875–1000 mg/clavulanate, 62.5–125 mg PO/12 h) plus macrolide (i.e., Clarithromycin, 500 mg/day PO/5–10 days or Azithromycin, 500 mg/day PO/3 days) within 4–8 h after diagnosis	Respiratory fluoroquinolone: Moxifloxacin, 400 mg PO once daily/7–14 days
	Inpatients, non-ICU: Respiratory fluoroquinolone (i.e., moxifloxacin or levofloxacin PO or IV)	Levofloxacin, 500 mg PO once daily/10–14 days or 750 mg once daily/5–7 days or 750 mg IV/24 h/7 days
	Inpatients, ICU: A β-lactam (cefotaxime, ceftriaxone, ampicillin-sulbactam IV) plus azithromycin or respiratory fluoroquinolone (i.e., moxifloxacin, levofloxacin IV)	
	For penicillin allergic patients: a respiratory fluoroquinolone and aztreonam IM or IV	

Table 47.5 (continued)

Infection	First choice	Alternate choice(s)
Pulmonary tuberculosis	Short therapy for isoniazid sensitive TB: Isoniazid plus rifampicin PO for 6 months, plus ethambutol and pyrazinamide PO for the first 2 months	Long therapy for isoniazid mono-resistant TB: Rifampicin, ethambutol, and pyrazinamide for the first 6 months, or for 9 months with rifampicin, ethambutol, and pyrazinamide in the intensive phase and for two additional months with rifampicin and ethambutol in the continuation phase
Pulmonary coccidioidomycosis	Fluconazole, 800–1200 mg PO or IV/day	Amphotericin B, 5.0 up to 7.5–10.0 mg/kg/day IV for 12 weeks
	Inability of azoles to eradicate the fungus results in the need to continue treatment indefinitely as suppressive rather than curative therapy	Because of multiple adverse events, it should only be used in patients with refractory disease
Pulmonary mucormycosis	Amphotericin B, 5.0 up to 7.5–10.0 mg/kg/day IV for 12 weeks	Posaconazole, oral solution, 800 mg in 4 divided doses/day for 12 weeks
		Posaconazole, oral solution, 800 mg in 4 divided doses/day
		Isavuconazole, 200 mg orally or IV, loading dose: 200 mg/8 h/2 days; 200 mg/day afterwards for 12 weeks
Acute emphysematous cholecystitis	Ampicillin-sulbactam, 3 g/IV/6 h	Ampicillin 2 g/IV/6 h plus gentamicin 5 mg/kg/24 h plus clindamycin 900 mg/IV/8 h or Ceftriaxone 1–2 g IM or IV/24 h plus clindamycin or metronidazole, loading dose 15 mg/kg followed by 7.5 mg/kg IV/6 h
Pyogenic liver abscess	Multiple combination therapies have been used, including aminopenicillins, antipseudomonal penicillins, first-generation, second-generation, third-generation cephalosporins, carbapenems, fluoroquinolones, aminoglycosides, metronidazole	
Psoas and spinal epidural abscess	Nafcillin, 1000 mg IV/4 h or Oxacillin, 1000 mg/day IV every 4–6 h or Cefazolin, 100 mg/kg/day IM or IV/8 h	Ciprofloxacin 750 mg/12 h for 6 weeks
Asymptomatic bacteriuria	Screening and treatment unwarranted	
Asymptomatic candidiuria	Fluconazole, 400–800 mg PO, single dose	Caspofungin 70 mg IV loading dose → 50 mg/day
		Anidulafungin 200 mg/kg IV loading dose →100 mg/day
		Voriconazole 6 mg/kg IV/12 h; afterwards, 4 mg/kg/12 h
		Amphotericin B 0.6–0.7 mg/kg/day ± flucytosine 25 mg/kg/6 h/7–10 days
Bacterial pyelonephritis	Uncomplicated: Ciprofloxacin, 500 mg PO/bid/7 days or Tobramycin, 3–5 mg/kg IV/24 h/3 days	Uncomplicated: Levofloxacin, 250–500 mg PO/day/10 days or Ceftriaxone, 1 g/IV/24 h/3 days
	Complicated	Complicated
Emphysematous pyelonephritis	Prolonged antimicrobial therapy (i.e., Trimethoprim-sulfamethoxazole, 160/800 mg PO or IV/bid) for weeks or months plus additional surgical measures (see Table 47.5)	

(continued)

Table 47.5 (continued)

Infection	First choice	Alternate choice(s)
Bacterial cystitis	Uncomplicated: short course of antimicrobial therapy	Uncomplicated: Trimethoprim-sulfamethoxazole, 1600/800 mg/bid/3 days
	Amoxicillin, 500 mg PO/tid/7 days, or Amoxicillin/clavulanic acid, 500 mg PO/tid/7 days or Cephalexin, 250–500 mg PO/tid/7 days or Norfloxacin, 400 mg PO/bid/3 days	Nitrofurantoin, 50–100 mg/qid/7 days
	Complicated infections: prolonged antimicrobial therapy	Complicated
Fungal cystitis	Fluconazole, 400 mg IV/day/14 days	Flucytosine, 25 mg/kg/6 h/14 days or Amphotericin B 0.5–0.7 mg/kg/day/14 days
Perinephric abscess	Nafcillin, 1000 mg IV/4 h or Oxacillin, 1000 mg/day IV every 4–6 h or Cefazolin, 100 mg/kg/day IM or IV/8 h	Oxacillin, 1000 mg/day IV every 4–6 h or Cefazolin, 100 mg/kg/day IM or IV/8 h
Emphysematous cystitis	Fluoroquinolone (i.e., Levofloxacin 250 mg IV/24 h/10 days or 750 mg IV/5 days, or Moxifloxacin, 400 mg PO or IV once daily/5–14 days or Ceftriaxone, 1–2 g IM or IV/24 h/10–14 days)	Carbapenem (i.e., Cilastatin/Imipenem, 500 mg IV/6 h or 1000 mg IV/8 h) or Aminoglycoside (i.e., Gentamicin, 3 mg/kg IM or IV/8 h/day/10 days)
Vulvovaginal candidiasis	Uncomplicated: Clotrimazole, 200 mg intravaginally/3 days	Uncomplicated: Fluconazole, 150 mg, single dose
	Miconazole, 2 ovules at bedtime/3 days	Recurrent: Fluconazole, 150 mg/week/6 months
	Butoconazole, 500 mg vaginal tablet single dose	
	Recurrent: Fluconazole, 200 mg PO/8 h/1 week	
	If symptom free, fluconazole, 200 mg once a week from weeks 2 to 8, 200 mg every 2 weeks from months 3 to 6 and 200 mg every 4 weeks from months 7 to 12	
Balanoposthitis	Clotrimazole, 1–2% cream until symptoms subside	Patients with severe symptoms: Fluconazole, 200 mg single dose
Necrotizing fasciitis	Penicillin G, 24 million U IV/day plus clindamycin, 900 mg IV/8 h plus gentamicin, 5 mg/kg IV/day or Meropenem, 1 g IV/8 h plus clindamycin, 600 mg IV/8 h or lincomycin 600 mg IV/8 h	Ampicillin-sulbactam 1.5–3.0 g IV/6–8 h or Ceftriaxone, 2 g IV/24 h plus clindamycin, 900 mg IV/8 h
Fournier's gangrene	Triple antibiotic therapy including (1) a broad-spectrum penicillin or third-generation cephalosporin, (2) an aminoglycoside, (3) metronidazole or clindamycin	Alternatively, triple antibiotic therapy including (1) a broad-spectrum penicillin or third-generation cephalosporin, (2) an aminoglycoside, (3) chloramphenicol
		Vancomycin in patients infected with methicillin-resistant *S. aureus*
		Amphotericin B in patients with fungal infections
Diabetic hand syndrome	Triple antibiotic therapy to cover Staphylococcus, Gram-negative organisms and anaerobes, including (1) third-generation cephalosporin, (2) aminoglycoside, (3) metronidazole or clindamycin	Second choice therapy based on results of wound swab and culture
Cellulitis	Amoxicillin-clavulanate	Third-generation cephalosporin with or without aminoglycoside
	First-generation cephalosporin	
	Macrolides	
	Fluoroquinolone	
	Ceftriaxone	

Table 47.5 (continued)

Infection	First choice	Alternate choice(s)
Foot ulcer infections	Mild to moderate: Amoxicillin-clavulanate, 875/125 mg PO/12 h or Ampicillin/sulbactam, 3 g IV/6 h	Mild to moderate: Cephalexin, 500 mg PO/6 h plus metronidazole, 400 mg PO/8–12 h or Ciprofloxacin, 500 PO/12 h plus clindamycin, 300–450 mg PO/8 h or 600 mg IV/8 h
	Severe: Ticarcillin-clavulanate, 0.1–0.3 g IV/h or Meropenem-cilastatin 500 mg IV/8 h	Severe: Ciprofloxacin, 750 mg VO/12 h plus clindamycin, 600 mg IV/8 h or lincomycin, 600 mg IV/8 h
Herpes zoster	Acyclovir, 800 mg PO/5 times a day/7–10 days	Famciclovir, 500 mg PO/7 days Valacyclovir, 1000 mg/tid/7 days
Onychomycosis	Terbinafine, 250 mg/day PO/12 weeks	Itraconazole, 200 mg/bid/1 week on, 3 weeks of/12 weeks
	Use with caution in patients with liver or kidney disease Fluconazole, 150, 300, or 450 mg PO/week/6 months	Contraindicated in patients with congestive heart failure
Cutaneous zygomycosis	Amphotericin B, 5.0 up to 7.5–10.0 mg/kg/day IV for 12 weeks	Posaconazole, oral solution, 800 mg in 4 divided doses/day for 12 weeks Posaconazole, oral solution, 800 mg in 4 divided doses/day Isavuconazole, 200 mg orally or IV, loading dose: 200 mg/8 h/2 days; 200 mg/day afterwards for 12 weeks

Table 47.6 Choice of antimicrobial therapy by microorganisms and dose in adults

Microorganism	First line, dose, and duration		Second line, dose, and duration	
	Oral	Intramuscular or intravenous	Oral	Intramuscular or intravenous
Bacteria				
Streptococcus pneumoniae	β-lactam	Benzylpenicillin 1.2 g IV/6 h	Respiratory fluoroquinolone: Moxifloxacin, 400 mg PO once daily/7–14 days	Vancomycin, 25–30 loading dose for seriously ill patients, then 15–20 mg/kg IV/8–12 h in combination FDA approved labeling: 2 g/day IV divided either as 500 mg IV/6 h or 1 g IV/12 h
	(Amoxicillin, 500–875 mg) plus macrolide	Cefuroxime, 750–1500 mg IV/8 h; for life-threatening infections, 1.5 g IV/6 h	Gemifloxacin, Levofloxacin, 500 mg PO once daily/10–14 days or 750 mg once daily/5–7 days or 750 mg IV/24 h/7 days	Linezolid, 600 mg IV/12 h/10–14 days. Duration of treatment is 7–21 days for methicillin-resistant *Staphylococcus aureus*
	(Clarithromycin, 500 mg/day) within 4–8 h after diagnosis	Cefotaxime, for uncomplicated infections: 1 g IM or IV/12 h, for complicated infections, 2 g IV/6–8 h/7–10 days		
		Ceftriaxone, 1–2 g IM or IV/day/7–10 days, depending on clinical response		
Haemophilus influenza	Amoxicillin-clavulanate, 500–875 mg/8–12 h	Respiratory fluoroquinolone: Moxifloxacin, 400 mg PO once daily/7–14 days	Doxycycline, 100 mg/12 h day	Respiratory fluoroquinolone: Levofloxacin, 750 mg IV/24 h/7 days
		Levofloxacin, 500 mg PO once daily/10–14 days or 750 mg once daily/5–7 days	Azithromycin, 200 mg/day Clarithromycin, 500 mg/day	

(continued)

Table 47.6 (continued)

Microorganism	First line, dose, and duration		Second line, dose, and duration	
	Oral	Intramuscular or intravenous	Oral	Intramuscular or intravenous
Staphylococcus aureus	Dicloxacillin, 125–250 mg PO/6 h for moderate infections, 250–500 mg PO/6 h for severe infections	Nafcillin, 500 mg IV/4 h for moderate infections, 1000 mg IV/4 h for severe infections	Clindamycin, 150–450 mg PO/6 h	Clindamycin, 600 mg IM or IV/6–12 h up to 900 mg/8–12 h
		Oxacillin, 1 g/day IV every 4–6 h		Vancomycin, 25–30 loading dose for seriously ill patients, then 15–20 mg/kg IV/8–12 h in combination FDA approved labeling: 2 g/day IV divided either as 500 mg IV/6 h or 1 g IV/12 h
		Cefazolin, 250–500 mg/kg/IM or IV/8 h for mild to moderate infections; 100 mg/kg/day IM or IV divided every 8 h for severe infections		Linezolid, 600 mg IV/12 h/10–14 days
Mycoplasma pneumoniae	Clarithromycin, 500 mg/day	Respiratory fluoroquinolone: Moxifloxacin, 400 mg PO once daily/7–14 days		
		Levofloxacin, 500 mg PO once daily/10–14 days or 750 mg once daily/5–7 days		
Mycobacterium tuberculosis	Short therapy for isoniazid-sensitive TB: Isoniazid plus rifampicin for 6 months, plus ethambutol and pyrazinamide for the first 2 months		Long therapy for isoniazid mono-resistant TB: Rifampicin, ethambutol, and pyrazinamide for the first 6 months, or for 9 months with rifampicin, ethambutol, and pyrazinamide in the intensive phase and for two additional months with rifampicin and ethambutol in the continuation phase	
Legionella sp.	Respiratory fluoroquinolone, i.e., Moxifloxacin, 400 mg PO once daily/7–10 days or Levofloxacin, 750 mg PO once daily/5–10 days		Azithromycin, 1000 mg PO/day followed by 500 mg/day/10 days or Doxycycline, 100 mg PO/day	
Klebsiella pneumoniae		Ertapenem, 1 g IM or IV/24 h/10–14 days		Avibactam/Ceftazidime, 2.5 g (2 g Ceftazidime, 0.5 g Avibactam) IV/8 h/7–14 days
		Imipenem-Cilastatin, 1 g IV/6–8 h		
		Meropenem, 1 g IV/8 h		
Escherichia coli		Ertapenem, 1 g IM or IV/24 h/10–14 days		Aminoglycosides, i.e., Amikacin, 15 mg/kg/day IM or IV/8–12 h or Gentamicin, 3 mg/kg IM or IV/day/divided in three doses/10 days or Tobramycin, 3–6 mg/kg IM or IV/day divided in 2–3 doses
		Imipenem-Cilastatin, 1 g IV/6–8 h		
		Meropenem, 1 g IV/8 h		

Table 47.6 (continued)

Microorganism	First line, dose, and duration		Second line, dose, and duration	
	Oral	Intramuscular or intravenous	Oral	Intramuscular or intravenous
Acinetobacter		Ertapenem, 1 g IM or IV/24 h/10–14 days		Aminoglycosides, i.e., Amikacin, 15 mg/kg/day IM or IV/8–12 h or Gentamicin, 3 mg/kg IM or IV/day/divided in three doses or Tobramycin, 3–6 mg/kg IM or IV/day divided in 2–3 doses
		Imipenem-Cilastatin, 1 g IV/6–8 h		Third-generation Cephalosporins, including Cefotaxime, 1–2 g IM or IV/12 h
		Meropenem, 1 g IV/8 h		Ceftriaxone 1–2 g IM or IV/24 h
				Avibactam/Ceftazidime, 2.5 g (2 g Ceftazidime, 0.5 g Avibactam) IV/8 h
				Ampicillin-sulbactam, 1.5 g (1 g ampicillin and 0.5 g sulbactam) IM or IV/6 h
Pseudomonas aeruginosa	Levofloxacin, 250–750 mg PO/day	Cefepime, 0.5–1.0 g IM or IV or Ciprofloxacin 400 mg IV/12 h or Aztreonam, 500–1000 mg IM or IV/8–12 h		Ticarcillin-clavulanate 3.0–0.1 g IV/6 h or third-generation cephalosporin, i.e., Ceftazidime 2 g IV/8 h plus Aminoglycoside, i.e., Gentamicin, 4–6 mg/kg IV day
		Carbapenem, i.e., Imipenem/cilastatin 500–1000 mg IV/6–8 h or Meropenem, 1 g IV/8 h		Ciprofloxacin 1.5 g/day or Levofloxacin, 500 mg IV/day or Ticarcillin, 3.1 g (3 g ticarcillin and 0.1 g clavulanic acid) IV/4–6 h or Piperacillin/tazobactam, 3.375 g (3 g piperacillin and 0.375 tazobactam) IV/6 h
Fungi				
Rhizopus and *Mucor*	Amphotericin B, 5 mg/kg/day IV for 12 weeks		Posaconazole, oral solution, 800 mg in 4 divided doses/day for 12 weeks for patients who cannot tolerate or non-responders to Amphotericin B	
Candida	Oral: Nystatin 100,000 units/mL after meals	Toenail: Itraconazole, 200 mg once daily/12 weeks	Fluconazole 200 mg day/3 days	Itraconazole 200 mg day
	Toenail: Terbinafine, 250 mg once daily/12 weeks	Topical: Ciclopirox, once daily application, avoiding washing for 8 h after application		
		Efinaconazole, once daily application for 48 weeks		
		Tavaborole, once daily application for 48 weeks		

(continued)

Table 47.6 (continued)

Microorganism	First line, dose, and duration		Second line, dose, and duration	
	Oral	Intramuscular or intravenous	Oral	Intramuscular or intravenous
Aspergillus		Amphotericin B 2 g day IV/3 weeks for invasive Aspergillosis	Voriconazole 200 mg day/6 weeks, for invasive Aspergillosis	
Histoplasma capsulatum	Itraconazole	Amphotericin B 2 g day IV/3 weeks		Amphotericin B 2 g day IV/3 weeks
Coccidioides	Fluconazole, 800–1200 mg/day	Amphotericin B 2 g day IV/3 weeks for invasive Coccidioidomycosis	Voriconazole 200 mg day/6 weeks, for invasive Coccidioidomycosis	
	Warning: inability of azoles to eradicate the fungus results in the need to continue treatment indefinitely as suppressive rather than curative therapy		Posaconazole, oral solution, 800 mg in 4 divided doses/day for 12 weeks for patients who cannot tolerate or non-responders to Amphotericin B	
Viruses				
Influenza	M2 Inhibitors Amantadine 100 mg/12 h/5 days Rimantadine 100 mg/12 h/5 days Neuraminidase inhibitors Laninamivir one single inhalation of 20 mg for children <10 years, one single inhalation of 40 mg for individuals ≥10 years Oseltamivir 75 mg/12 h/5 days			
Herpes zoster	Acyclovir, 800 mg 5 times a day, 7–10 days In patients with persistent varicella DNA in the cornea, antiviral therapy may extend up to 30 days		Famciclovir, 500 mg 3 times a day, 7–10 days In patients with persistent varicella DNA in the cornea, antiviral therapy may extend up to 30 days Valacyclovir, 1 g 3 times a day, 7–10 days In patients with persistent varicella DNA in the cornea, antiviral therapy may extend up to 30 days	

and second option choices of antibacterials, antimycotics, and antivirals. Microorganisms showing increasing rates of antimicrobial resistance like Pseudomonas and Acinetobacter are effectively treated combining two antibiotics. Diabetic foot infections, skin and soft tissue infections, periodontitis along with emphysematous cholecystitis often require polymicrobial cover, especially to include anaerobes.

Glycemic Control

Poor glycemic control, especially in the presence of infection, can lead to metabolic and infection-related complica-

tions. Insulin requirements may increase during infections. Insulin is an anabolic agent, and it should be the preferred drug for glycemic control in the background of infection.

Source Control

Source control in the form of drainage or debridement of the infective focus can lead to reduction in the bacterial load, help achieve better glycemic control, and reduce the risk of complications. In addition to antimicrobials, complementary interventions for selected infections are presented in Table 47.7.

Table 47.7 Additional therapeutic measures and prognosis

Disease	Therapeutic measure	Prognosis
Herpes zoster ophthalmicus	• Oral or topical corticosteroids • Frequent artificial tears • Monitoring for signs of secondary bacterial infection • Prophylactic erythromycin ophthalmic ointment • Analgesics in the acute phase and in patients with post-herpetic neuralgia	Complications related to bad prognosis: Meningitis, brain abscess, dural sinus thrombophlebitis
Malignant external otitis	• Six weeks or longer of culture-directed antibiotic therapy, based on the 3–4-week period for bone revascularization	Reported mortality rates in recent series is 30%
	• Otolaryngology management	More aggressive strains and increasing antibiotic resistance are requiring multidrug and long-term antibiotic therapy with extended hospital stays
	• Repeated debridement of the ear, the infratemporal fossa, or skull base	Signs of disease progression and poor outcomes:
	• Radical mastoidectomy with facial nerve decompression	Lack of glycemic control
		Cranial nerve involvement
		Extension to the jugular foramen and petrous apex
		Erythrocyte sedimentation rate
		C-Reactive protein
		Causes of death:
		Meningitis, large vessel septic thrombophlebitis or rupture, septicemia, pneumonia, stroke
		Predictors of symptom resolution for fungal malignant external otitis:
		No surgical debridement
		Absence of facial paralysis
		Aspergillus as causative pathogen
		Absence of imaging findings
		Indicator of disease resolution: negative results by Ga-67 citrate scan
Periodontal infections	Systemic antibiotics are important, but only in addition to reducing the bacterial load with periodontal scaling and root planning	Because of increasing resistance, combinations of antibiotics are increasingly used
Oral candidiasis	Glycemic control Oral hygiene Avoiding tobacco use	
Rhino-orbital mucormycosis	Surgical debridement of infected tissue, including removal of the palate, nasal cartilages, and orbit as soon as possible, is crucial to prevent dissemination	Mortality rate: 25–62% Poor outcome predictors: dissemination, renal failure, inability to achieve source control, brain or cavernous sinus involvement, lack of response to antifungals
Influenza	In addition to diabetes, higher risks of complications occur in children, the elderly, and pregnant	Worldwide mortality rate for influenza from subgroups H5N1 and H7N9 of influenza A virus: 53% and 39%

(continued)

Table 47.7 (continued)

Disease	Therapeutic measure	Prognosis
Community-acquired pneumonia	Recommended actions to improve the outcomes include: (1) using a risk stratification tool like CURB-65 (confusion, urea >7 mmol/L, respiratory rate ≥30/min, low blood pressure, and older than 65), (2) procalcitonin to confirm diagnosis and assess treatment response, (3) outpatient treatment, (4) use of empirical antibiotic guidelines in accordance to local microbial etiology, (5) measure time to achieve clinical stability, step-down to oral antibiotics, early physical therapy, patient and caregiver education, appropriate venous thromboembolism prophylaxis	Odds ratio for pneumonia: 1.5
	Criteria to transition from intravenous to oral therapy: (1) absence of mental confusion, (2) ability to take oral medications, (3) hemodynamic stability (heart rate <100 beats/min, systolic blood pressure >90 mmHg), (4) respiratory rate <25 breaths/min, (5) oxygen saturation >90%	Hazard ratio for pneumonia: 2.9
	Administration of macrolides before beta-lactams is associated with a statistically significant decrease in mortality, even in hospitalized patients. Data from many countries show an increased prevalence of macrolide-resistant *Streptococcus pneumonia*. For example, in the United Sates the overall rate of macrolide-resistant *S. pneumoniae* is 50%. Nevertheless, resistance does not automatically mean treatment failure. Another important factor is the increasing awareness of respiratory viruses and atypical species as co-pathogens	Risk of invasive pneumococcal disease: 1.4–4.6, especially in individuals younger than 40 years Odds ratio for bacteremia: 1.67 Hyperglycemia is independently associated with adverse outcomes in patients with community-acquired pneumonia Preexisting diabetes and newly discovered hyperglycemia are associated with a higher risk of death, for several years. A pre-pneumonia diagnosis of diabetes is associated with a threefold increase in the risk of death up to 6 years after mild to moderate community-acquired pneumonia. Rather than disruption of the immune response, death may be related to worsening of preexisting cardiovascular and kidney disease
Tuberculosis	Although treatment schedule can be as high 95–98% under clinical trial conditions (directly observed therapy or DOT), high rates of non-adherence after 4 weeks of therapy (between 7% and 53.6%) are common. Therapeutic drug monitoring has been proposed to optimize treatment outcome and reduce drug resistance	Patients with diabetes are at a higher risk of developing active tuberculosis, drug-resistant disease, treatment failure, and mortality
	Drug-induced liver injury may be caused by isoniazid, rifampicin, or pyrazinamide, in the range of 5–33%	Compared with patients without diabetes, the risk of active tuberculosis is 1.55–3.59 higher
	Treatment of multidrug-resistant tuberculosis includes: (1) at least four drugs with proven or likely susceptibility, (2) a later generation fluoroquinolone (moxifloxacin, levofloxacin), plus an aminoglycoside (amikacin, kanamycin, capreomycin), (3) long duration of treatment (21–24 months), (4) oxazolidinones (linezolid) with monitoring for neuropathy and bone marrow toxicity, in patients with fluoroquinolone-resistant TB, (5) bedaquiline or delamanid for patients with toxicity or resistance to multidrug regimens, (6) psychological and economic support	Tuberculosis prevalence and incidence are more likely to increase in countries where diabetes prevalence has increased Death rates: for untreated smear-positive TB: 70%, for smear negative TB: 20% Patients with diabetes and tuberculosis have: (1) significantly higher rates of treatment failure and death; (2) higher risk of death during treatment and relapse following treatment; (3) remain sputum positive 2–3 months after starting TB treatment. Infection and treatment for tuberculosis impair glycemic control and peripheral neuropathy in patients receiving isoniazid

Table 47.7 (continued)

Disease	Therapeutic measure	Prognosis
Coccidioidomycosis	Exogenous adjunctive interferon-γ has been used in patients with chronic coccidioidomycosis, in addition to antifungal therapy	The disease is relatively benign in most cases but for others is debilitating and may be mortal
	Nikkomycin has shown promise as a cure in murine models of infection	Recurrence is possible in patients with benign disease
		Extrapulmonary disease occurs through hematogenous or lymphatic spread and may involve meninges, skeleton, skin, joints, glandular tissue, peritoneum, liver, pancreas, pericardium, bone marrow, kidney, bladder, and male and female reproductive organs
		In these cases treatment is prolonged, even for years with close follow-up for relapses
Emphysematous pyelonephritis	Percutaneous drainage	Delayed nephrectomy if necessary, once the patient is stable
Psoas abscess	Surgical drainage	Mortality 17%, for primary psoas abscess: 2.5%, for secondary psoas abscess: 18.9%
		Death largely related to comorbidities, delayed diagnosis, or inadequate therapy
Perinephric abscess	Percutaneous drainage	Percutaneous nephrolithotomy in case of infective stone
		In patients with chronic abscess, nephrectomy
Fungal urinary tract infections	Correct predisposing factors, including: (1) removal of indwelling devices, (2) improving urinary tract drainage, (3) discontinue systemic antibiotics, (4) treating underlying medical problems	Glycemic control is essential
		Strategies to reduce funguria include: (1) adequate hydration, (2) hygiene, (3) vaginal estrogens
Emphysematous cystitis	90% of cases are treated with medical treatment alone, 10% require medical and surgical intervention, including: bladder drainage, surgical debridement, partial cystectomy, total cystectomy, or even nephrectomy	Death rate: 7–12% from septic shock or late presentation
Necrotizing fasciitis	Surgical debridement of necrotic tissue is essential for recovery	
Fournier's gangrene	Early and aggressive surgical debridement improves survival	Wide reported mortality rate: 4.0–88.0%
	Additional interventions include negative-pressure wound therapy, hyperbaric oxygen therapy, fecal and urinary diversion, and reconstructive surgery	
Diabetic hand syndrome	Comprehensive management include: (1) hospitalization and hand elevation, (2) multiple intravenous antibiotics, (3) optimal glycemic control, (4) adequate and early surgical drainage, (5) prompt amputation if necessary, (6) rehabilitation	Life expectancy of high upper limb amputees may be lower, but the number of reported cases is low to be conclusive
Cellulitis	Most cases improve within 1 day, but thickening of the debris requires parenteral antibiotics before improvement	Recurrent cellulitis can compromise venous or lymphatic circulation and result in dermal fibrosis, lymphedema, and epidermal thickening
	Adjunctive treatment includes cool compresses, analgesics, and immobilization of the affected extremity	Prophylaxis with erythromycin, penicillin, or clindamycin is indicated in these cases

(continued)

Table 47.7 (continued)

Disease	Therapeutic measure	Prognosis
Foot ulcer infections	For mild to moderate infections, antimicrobial therapy for 1–2 weeks is adequate	Factors predicting healing include: (1) absence of exposed bone, (2) palpable pedal pulses, (3) blood pressure in the toe >45 mmHg or >80 mmHg in the ankle, (4) peripheral white cell count <12,000/mm^3, (5) lower extremity transcutaneous oxygen tension >40 mmHg
	Most severe infections and some moderate require parenteral antimicrobial therapy for 1–2 weeks with a switch to oral therapy according to clinical response	Failure to treat diabetes foot infections is associated with progressive tissue destruction, poor wound healing, amputation, sepsis, and death
	Patients with osteomyelitis not undergoing resection require 6 weeks of antimicrobial therapy	Beyond intervention, healthcare practitioners should focus on prevention in patients at high risk for diabetic foot ulcers
	Patients with osteomyelitis undergoing resection require 1 week of antimicrobial therapy	
	Urgent surgical intervention by certified specialists is necessary in case of deep abscess, compartment syndrome, and necrotizing soft tissue infections	
	Surgical intervention is advisable in cases of osteomyelitis associated with spreading soft tissue infection, destroyed soft tissue envelope, progressive bone destruction, or bone protruding through an ulcer	
Herpes zoster	Complications include post-herpetic neuralgia and secondary bacterial infections; less common complications are neurologic, and include aseptic meningitis, peripheral motor neuropathy, transverse myelitis, acute or chronic encephalitis, Guillain-Barré syndrome, and stroke symptoms resulting from vasculitis of cerebral arteries	Post-herpetic neuralgia is the most common complication; risk factors include advanced age and severity of rash and pain
Onychomycosis	Nail lacquers are an attractive option and include 8% ciclopirox, once daily/48 weeks and 5% amorolfine, once or twice weekly/6 months	Risk factors for *Candida* onychomycosis include peripheral vascular disease and female gender. Consider this diagnosis in patients with onycholysis, paronychia, or total dystrophic onychomycosis
	Unattached infected nail should be removed once a month	Onychomycosis is a significant predictor for the development of foot ulcers
	Filing of excess horny material should be done by trained professionals	Rates of mycological cure are low: 31% with azoles, 57% with terbinafine
	Patients should file away loose nail material and trim nails as directed by podologists, or every 7 days after weekly removal of medication with alcohol	
Cutaneous zygomycosis		

When to Refer

Any case which appears complex to the treating physician may be referred to a specialist. However priority referrals should be considered in case of diabetes complicating pregnancy, renal impairment, diabetic foot, life-threatening invasive mucormycosis, and coronavirus-19.

Conclusion

Hyperglycemia is associated with disorders in the immune system including lower secretion of inflammatory cytokines, impairment in neutrophile, humoral and T cell function, increased susceptibility, and delayed recovery of tissues [24]. Awareness of microvascular and macrovascular complications can help minimize the risk of infections and infection-related complications. Healthcare personnel need to be aware of unusual and severe forms of infection associated with diabetes mellitus. The use of empirical antibiotics is the same as with non-diabetics, but disease-associated complications should be anticipated and promptly treated. Immunization with influenza and pneumococcal vaccine is often recommended. Optimal glycemic control is essential for successful treatment of infections.

Multiple-Choice Questions

1. This class of drugs is associated with a higher risk of pruritis vulvae/balanoposthitis:
   (a) **SGLT2i**
   (b) Pioglitazone
   (c) Biguanides
   (d) Sulfonylureas
2. This class of drugs has an anabolic effect and is the preferred agent for glycemic control in the background of infection:
   (a) **Insulin**
   (b) GLP1RA
   (c) DPP4i
   (d) Bromocriptine
3. This parasitic infection may protect against diabetes:
   (a) **Helminthiasis**
   (b) Malaria
   (c) Mucormycosis
   (d) Lichen planus
4. Hypoglycemia may occur in all of the following setting, except
   (a) **Dengue fever**
   (b) Malaria
   (c) Insulin use
   (d) Quinine use
5. Anaerobic bacterial coverage is indicated in all of the following settings except
   (a) **Pyogenic meningitis**
   (b) Lung abscess
   (c) Infected diabetic foot
   (d) Emphysematous pyelonephritis
6. The causative organism of otitis externa is
   (a) *Klebsiella* sp.
   (b) Proteus
   (c) *Staphylococcus aureus*
   (d) **All of the above**
7. This infection is not associated with a higher risk of diabetes:
   (a) **Hepatitis A**
   (b) Tuberculosis
   (c) HIV
   (d) Hepatitis C
8. This antimicrobial drug may precipitate hypoglycemia:
   (a) **Gatifloxacin**
   (b) Azithromycin
   (c) Metronidazole
   (d) Streptomycin
9. Hyperglycemia increases the risk of COVID-19 infection because of
   (a) Oxidative stress
   (b) Inflammation
   (c) Apoptosis of alveolar cells
   (d) None of the above
   (e) **All of the above**
10. Glycemic threshold for high risk of severity and mortality from COVID-19 infection:
    (a) 120 mg/dL
    (b) 140 mg/dL
    (c) **180 mg/dL**
    (d) 200 mg/dL
    (e) 250 mg/dL

References

1. Larkin JG, Frier BM, Ireland JT. Diabetes mellitus and infection. Postgrad Med J. 1985;61:233–7.
2. Peleg AY, Weerarathna T, McCarthy JS, Davis TM. Common infections in diabetes: pathogenesis, management and relationship to glycemic control. Diabetes Metab Res Rev. 2007;23:3–13.
3. Flynn JM. The changing cause of death in diabetes mellitus. Am J Med Sci. 1935;189:157.
4. Drivsholm T, de Fine Olivarius N, Nielsen ABS. Symptoms, signs and complications in newly diagnosed type 2 diabetic patients, and their relationship to glycaemia, blood pressure and weight. Diabetologia. 2005;48:210–4.
5. Reunanen A, Kangas T, Martikainen J, Klaukka T. Nationwide survey of comorbidity, use, and costs of all medications in Finnish diabetic individuals. Diabetes Care. 2000;23:1265–71.
6. Joshi N, Caputo GM, Weitekamp MR, Karchmer AW. Infections in patients with diabetes mellitus. N Engl J Med. 1999;341:1906–12.
7. Shah BR, Hux JE. Quantifying the risk of infectious diseases for people with diabetes. Diabetes Care. 2003;26:510–3.
8. Knapp S. Diabetes and infection: is there a link? A mini-review. Gerontology. 2012;59:99–104.

9. Pearson-Stuttard J, Blundell S, Harris T, Cook DG, Critchley J. Diabetes and infection: assessing the association with glycaemic control in population-based studies. Lancet Diabetes Endocrinol. 2016;4:148–58.

10. Critchley JA, Carey IM, Harris T, DeWilde S, Hosking FJ, Cook DG. Glycemic control and risk of infections among people with type 1 or type 2 diabetes in a large primary care cohorts study. Diabetes Care. 2018;41:2127–35.

11. Carey IM, Critchley JA, DeWilde S, Harris T, Hosking FJ, Cook DG. Risk of infection in type 1 and type 2 diabetes compared with the general population: a matched cohort study. Diabetes Care. 2018;41:513–21.

12. Muller LMA, Gorter KJ, Hak E, Goudzwaard WL, Schevellis FG, Hoepelman AIM. Increased risk of common infections in patients with type 1 and type 2 diabetes mellitus. Clin Infect Dis. 2005;41:281–8.

13. Kim EJ, Ha KH, Kim DJ, Choi YH. Diabetes and the risk of infection: a national cohort study. Diabetes Metab J. 2019;43:804–14.

14. Fang M, Ishigami J, Echouffo JB, Lutsey PL, Pankow JS, Selvin E. Diabetes and the risk of hospitalization for infection: the Atherosclerosis Risk in Communities (ARIC) study. Diabetologia. 2021;64:1–8.

15. Marble A, White HA, Fernald AT. The nature of the lowered resistance to infection in diabetes mellitus. J Clin Invest. 1938;17:423–30.

16. Rayfield EJ, Ault MJ, Keusch GT, Brothers MJ, Nechemias C, Smith H. Infection and diabetes: the case for glucose control. Am J Med. 1982;72:439–50.

17. Burekovic A, Dizdarevic-Bostandzic A, Godinjak A. Poorly regulated blood glucose in diabetic patients-predictor of acute infections. Med Arh. 2014;68:163–6.

18. Mazade MA, Edwards MS. Impairment of type III group B streptococcus - stimulated superoxide production and opsonophagocytosis by neutrophils in diabetes. Mol Genet Metab. 2001;73:259–67.

19. Casqueiro J, Alves C. Infections in patients with diabetes mellitus: a review of pathogenesis. Indian J Endocr Metab. 2012;16(Suppl 1):27–36.

20. Gupta S, Koirala J, Khardori R, Khardori N. Infections in diabetes mellitus and hyperglycemia. Infect Dis Clin N Am. 2007;21:617–38.

21. Jafar N, Edriss HN. The effect of short-term hyperglycemia on the innate immune system. Am J Med Sci. 2016;351:201–11.

22. Nathella PK, Babu S. Influence of diabetes mellitus on immunity to human tuberculosis. Immunology. 2017;152:13–24.

23. Berbudi A, Rahmadika N, Tjahjadi AI, Ruslami R. Type 2 diabetes and its impact on the immune system. Curr Diabetes Rev. 2020;16:442–9.

24. Chávez-Reyes J, Escárcega-González CE, Chavira-Suárez E, León-Buitimea A, Vázquez-León P, Morones-Ramírez JR, et al. Susceptibility for some infectious diseases in patients with diabetes: the key role of glycemia. Front Public Health. 2021;9:1–18.

25. Kumar NP, Sridhar R, Banurekha VV, Jawahar MS, Fay MP, Nutman TB, et al. Type 2 diabetes mellitus coincident with pulmonary tuberculosis is associated with heightened systemic type 1, type 17, and other proinflammatory cytokines. Ann Am Thorac Soc. 2013;10:441–9.

26. Daryabor G, Atashzar MR, Kabelitz D, Meri S, Kalantar K. The effects of type 2 diabetes mellitus on organ metabolism and the immune system. Fornt Immunol. 2020;11:1–22.

27. Serfaty L. Metabolic manifestations of hepatitis C virus. Diabetes mellitus, dyslipidemia. Clin Liv Dis. 2017;21:475–86.

28. Hadigan C, Kattakuzhy S. Diabetes mellitus type 2 and abnormal glucose metabolism in the setting of human immunodeficiency virus. Endocrinol Metab Clin N Am. 2014;43:685–96.

29. McIntosh K, Dees JH, Becker WB, Zapikian AZ, Chanock RM. Recovery in tracheal organ cultures of novel viruses from patients with respiratory disease. Proc Natl Acad Sci. 1967;57:933–40.

30. Wiesinga WJ, Rhodes A, Cheng AC, Peacock SJ, Prescott HC. Pathophysiology, transmission, diagnosis, and treatment of Coronavirus Disease 2019 (COVID-19). JAMA. 2020;324:782.

31. Paules CI, Marston HD, Fauci AS. Coronavirus infections – more than just the common cold. JAMA. 2020;323:707–8.

32. Gentile S, Strollo F, Ceriello A. COVID-19 infection in Italian people with diabetes: lessons learned for our future (an experience to be used). Diabetes Res Clin Pract. 2020;162:108137.

33. Barth RF, Buja LM, Barth AL, Carpenter DE, Parwani AV. A comparison of the clinical, viral, pathologic, and immunologic features of Severe Acute Respiratory Syndrome (SARS), Middle East Respiratory Syndrome (MERS), and Coronavirus 2019 (COVID-19) diseases. Arch Pathol Lab Med. 2021;145:1194–211.

34. Zhu N, Zhang D, Wang W, Li X, Yang B, Song J, et al. A novel coronavirus from patients with pneumonia in China, 2019. N Engl J Med. 2020;382:727–33.

35. Seewoodhary J, Oozageer R. Coronavirus and diabetes: an update. Pract Diab. 2020;37:41–2.

36. Cheng C, Zhang D, Dang D, Geng J, Zhu P, Yuan M, et al. The incubation period of COVID-19: a global meta-analysis of 53 studies and a Chinese observation study of 11 545 patients. Infect Dis Poverty. 2020;10:119.

37. Lauer SA, Grantz KH, Bi Q, Jones FK, Zheng Q, Meredith HR, et al. The incubation period of coronavirus disease 2019 (COVID-19) from publicly reported confirmed cases: estimation and application. Ann Intern Med. 2020;172:577–82.

38. Huang C, Wang Y, Li X, Ren L, Zhao J, Hu Y, et al. Clinical features of patients infected with 2019 novel coronavirus in Wuhan, China. Lancet. 2020;395:497–506.

39. Yang J, Gou X, Chen Z, Guo Q, Ji R, Wang H, et al. Prevalence of comorbidities and its effects in patients infected with SARS-CoV-2: a systematic review and meta-analysis. Int J Infect Dis. 2020;94:91–5.

40. Thakur B, Dubey P, Benitez J, Torres JP, Reddy S, Shokar N, et al. A systematic review and meta-analysis of geographic differences in comorbidities and associated severity and mortality among individuals with COVID-19. Sci Rep. 2021;11:8562.

41. Dessie ZG, Zewotir T. Mortality-related risk factors of COVID-19: a systematic review and meta-analysis of 42 studies and 423,117 patients. BMC Infect Dis. 2021;21:855.

42. Emami A, Akbari A, Basirat A, Zare H, Javanmardi F, Falahati F, et al. The role of comorbidities on mortality of COVID-19 in patients with diabetes. Obes Med. 2021;25:1–5.

43. Anderson G, Casasanta D, Cocchieri A, D'Agostino F, Zega M, Damiani G, et al. Diagnostic features of SARS-covid-2-positive patients: a rapid review and meta-analysis. J Clin Nurs. 2021;30:1826–37.

44. Tabassum T, Rahman A, Araf Y, Ullah MA, Hosen MJ. Prospective selected biomarkers in COVID-19 diagnosis and treatment. Biomark Med. 2021;15:1435–49.

45. Osuchowski MF, Winkler MS, Skirecki T, Cajander S, Shankar-Hari M, Lachmann G, et al. The COVID-19 puzzle: deciphering pathophysiology and phenotypes of a new disease entity. Lancet Respir Med. 2021;9:622–42.

46. Kaye AD, Cornett EM, Brondeel KC, Lerner ZI, Knight HE, Erwin A, et al. Biology of COVID-19 and related viruses: epidemiology, signs, symptoms, diagnosis, and treatment. Best Pract Res Clin Anaestehiol. 2021;35:269–92.

47. Xiao Y, Peng Z, Tan C, Meng X, Huang X, Wu A, et al. Diagnostic options for coronavirus disease 2019 (COVID-19). Infect Control Hosp Epidemiol. 2020;41:1–2.

48. Sethuraman N, Jeremiah SS, Ryo A. Interpreting diagnostic tests for SARS-CoV-2. JAMA. 2020;323:2249–51.

49. Son MBF, Murray N, Friedman K, Young CC, Newhams MM, Feldstein LR, et al. Multisystem inflammatory syndrome in children – initial therapy and outcomes. N Engl J Med. 2021;385:23.

50. Patel P, DeCuir J, Abrams J, Campbell AP, Godfred-Cato S, Belay ED. Clinical characteristics of multisystem inflammatory syndrome in adults. A systematic review. JAMA Netw Open. 2021;4:e2126456.

51. Wan Y, Shang J, Graham R, Baric RS, Li F. Receptor recognition by novel coronavirus from Wuhan: an analysis based on decade-long structural studies of SARS. J Virol. 2020;17:e00127–0.

52. Peng R, Wu L-A, Wang Q, Qi J, Gao GF. Cell entry by SARS-CoV-2. Trends Biochem Sci. 2021;46:848–60.

53. Lu Z-H, Yu W-L, Sun Y. Multiple immune function impairments in diabetic patients and their effects on COVID-19. World J Clin Case. 2021;26:6969–78.

54. Abbasi E, Mirzaei F, Tavilani H, Khodadadi I. Diabetes and COVID-19: mechanism of pneumonia, treatment strategy and vaccine. Metabol Open. 2021;11:100122.

55. Abu-Farha M, Al-Mulla F, Thanaraj TA, Kavalakatt S, Ali H, Ghani A, et al. Impact of diabetes in patients with COVID-19. Front Immunol. 2002;11:576818.

56. Liao Y-H, Zheng J-Q, Zheng C-M, Lu K-C, Chao Y-C. Novel molecular evidence related to COVID-19 in patients with diabetes mellitus. J Clin Med. 2020;9:3962.

57. Cheng Y, Yue L, Wang Z, Zhang J, Xiang G. Hyperglycemia associated with lymphopenia and disease severity of COVID-19 in type 2 diabetes mellitus. J Diabetes Complicat. 2021;35:107809.

58. Mirzaei R, Goodarzi P, Asadi M, Soltani A, Aljabani H, Jeda AS, et al. Bacterial co-infections with SARS CoV-2. IUMB Life. 2020;72:2097–211.

59. Zhu L, She Z-G, Cheng X, Qin J-J, Zhang X-J, Cai J, et al. Association of blood glucose control and outcomes in patients with COVID-19 and pre-existing type 2 diabetes. Cell Metab. 2020;31:1–10.

60. Hao R, Zhang Y, Cao Z, Li J, Xu Q, Ye L, et al. Control strategies and their effects on the COVID-19 pandemic in 2020 in representative countries. J Biosaf Biosecur. 2021;3:76–81.

61. Polack FP, Thomas SJ, Kitchin N, Absalon J, Gurtman A, Lockhart S, et al. Safety and efficacy of the BNT162b2 mRNA Covid-19 vaccine. N Engl J Med. 2020;383:2603–15.

62. Baden LR, El Sahly HM, Essink B, Kotloff K, Frey S, Novak R, et al. Efficacy and safety of the mRNA-1273 SARS-CoV-2 vaccine. N Engl J Med. 2021;384:403–16.

63. Sadoff J, Le Gars M, Shukarev G, Heerwegh D, Truyers C, de Groot AM, et al. Interim results of a phase 1-2a trial of Ad.COV2.S Covid-19 vaccine. N Engl J Med. 2021;384:1824–35.

64. Jara A, Undurruaga EA, González C, Paredes F, Fontecilla T, Jara G, et al. Effectiveness of an activated SARS-CoV-2 vaccine in Chile. N Engl J Med. 2021;385:875–84.

65. Pegu A, O'Connell SE, Schmidt SD, O'Dell Tatana CA, Lai L, et al. Durability of mRNA-1273 vaccine-induced antibodies against SARS-CoV-2 variants. Science. 2021;373:1372–7.

66. Falsey AR, Sobieszczyk ME, Hirsch I, Sproule S, Robb ML, Corey L, et al. Phase 3 safety and efficacy of AZD1222 (ChAdOx1 nCoV-19) Covid-19 vaccine. N Engl J Med. 2021;385:2348.

67. Thompson MG, Stenehjern E, Grannis S, Ball SW, Naleway AL, Ong TC, et al. Effectiveness of Covid-19 vaccines in ambulatory and inpatient care settings. N Engl J Med. 2021;385:1355–71.

68. Collier AY, Yu J, McMahan K, Liu J, Chandrashekar A, Maron JS, Atyeo C, et al. Differential kinetics of immune responses elicited by Covid-19 vaccines. N Engl J Med. 2021;385:2010.

69. Malek RJ, Bill K, Vines CM. Clinical drug therapies and biologicals currently used or in clinical trial to treat COVID-19. Biomed Pharmacother. 2021;144:112276.

70. Bornstein SR, Rubino F, Khunti K, Mingnone G, Hopkins D, Birkenfeld AI, et al. Practical recommendations for the management of diabetes in patients with COVID-19. Lancet Diabetes Endocrinol. 2020;8:546–50.

71. Bielka W, Przezak A, Pawllik A. Therapy of type 2 diabetes in patients with SARS-CoV-2 infection. Int J Mol Sci. 2021;22:7605.

72. Steenblock C, Schwarz PE, Ludwig B, Linkermann A, Zimmet P, Kolebyakin K, et al. COVID-19 and metabolic disease: mechanisms and clinical management. Lancet Diabetes Endocrinol. 2021;9:786–98.

73. World Health Organization. COVID-19 weekly epidemiological update. 59th ed. Geneva: WHO; 2021.

74. Selvin E, Jurascheck SP. Diabetes epidemiology in the COVID-19 pandemic. Diabetes Care. 2020;43:1690–4.

75. Gregg EW, Sophiea MK, Weidegiorgis M. Diabetes and COVID-19: population impact 18 months into the pandemic. Diabetes Care. 2021;44:1916–23.

76. Gujral UP, Johnson L, Nielsen J, Vellanki P, Haw JS, Davis GM. Preparedness cycle to address transitions in diabetes care during the COVID-19 pandemic and future outbreaks. BMJ Open Diabetes Res Care. 2020;8:e001520.

77. Rose KJ, Scibilia R. The COVID19 pandemic – perspectives from people living with diabetes. Diabetes Res Clin Pract. 2021;173:108343.

78. Nazligul Y, Sabuncu T, Ozbilge H. Is there a predisposition to intestinal parasitosis in diabetic patients? Diabetes Care. 2001;24:1503–4.

79. De Ruiter K, Tahapary DL, Sartono E, Soewondo P, Supali T, Smit JWA, et al. Helminths, hygiene hypothesis and type 2 diabetes. Parasite Immunol. 2017;39:e12404.

80. Mendonca SC, Goncalves-Pires M, Rodrigues RM, Ferreira A Jr, Costa-Cruz JM. Is there an association between positive Strongyloides stercoralis serology and diabetes mellitus? Acta Trop. 2006;99:102–5.

81. Strachan DP. Hay fever, hygiene, and household size. BMJ. 1989;299:1259–60.

82. Scudellari M. Cleaning up the hygiene hypothesis. PNAS. 2017;114:1433–6.

83. Kawai K, Yawn BP. Risk factors for Herpes Zoster: a systematic review and meta-analysis. Mayo Clin Proc. 2017;92:1806–21.

84. Anderson E, Fantus RJ, Haddadin RI. Diagnosis and management of herpes zoster ophthalmicus. Dis Mon. 2017;63:38–44.

85. Vrcek I, Choudhury E, Durairaj V. Herpes Zoster ophthalmicus: a review for the internists. Am J Med. 2017;130:21–6.

86. Wollina U. Variations in herpes zoster manifestation. Indian J Med Res. 2017;145:294–8.

87. Carlton DA, Perez EE, Smouha EE. Malignant external otitis: the shifting treatment paradigm. Am J Otolaryngol. 2018;39:41–5.

88. Mion M, Bovo R, Marchese-Ragona R, Martini A. Outcome predictors of treatment effectiveness for fungal external otitis: a systematic review. Acta Otorhinolaryngol Ital. 2015;35:307–13.

89. Lee SK, Lee SA, Seon S, Jung JH, Lee JD, Choi JY, Kim BG. Analysis of prognostic factors in malignant external otitis. Clin Exp Otorhinolaryngol. 2017;3:228–35.

90. Teeuw WJ, Kosho MXF, Poland DCW, Gerdes VEA, Loos BG. Periodontitis as a possible early sign of diabetes mellitus. BMJ Open Diabetes Res Care. 2017;9:e000326.

91. Barca E, Cifcibasi E, Cintan S. Adjunctive use of antibiotics in periodontal therapy. J Istambul Univ Fac Dent. 2015;49:55–62.

92. Poradzka A, Jasik M, Karnafael W, Fiedor P. Clinical aspects of fungal infections in diabetes. Acta Pol Pharm. 2013;70:587–96.

93. Farmakoitis D, Kontoyiannis DP. Mucormycoses. Infect Dis Clin N Am. 2016;30:143–63.

94. Long B, Koyfman A. Mucormycosis: what emergency physicians need to know? Am J Emerg Med. 2015;33:1823–5.

95. Riley TT, Muzny CA, Swiatlo E, Legendre DP. Breaking the mold: a review of mucormycosis and current pharmacological treatment options. Ann Pharmacother. 2016;50:747–57.

96. Li H, Cao B. Pandemic and avian influenza A viruses in humans. Epidemiology, virology, clinical characteristics and treatment strategy. Clin Chest Med. 2017;38:59–70.

97. Ison MG. Antiviral treatments. Clin Chest Med. 2017;38:139–53.

98. Klekotka RB, Mizgata E, Król W. The etiology of lower respiratory tract infections in people with diabetes. Pneumonol Alergol Pol. 2015;83:401–8.

99. Mandell LA, Wunderink RG, Anzueto A, Bartlett JG, Campbell GD, Dean NC, et al. Infectious Diseases Society of America/American Thoracic Society Consensus Guidelines on the management of community-acquired pneumonia in adults. Clin Infect Dis. 2007;44:S27–72.

100. Prina E, Ranzani OT, Torres A. Community-acquired pneumonia. Lancet. 2015;386:1097–108.

101. Kaysin A, Viera AJ. Community-acquired pneumonia in adults: diagnosis and management. Am Fam Physician. 2016;94:698–706.

102. Lee JS, Giesler DL, Gellad WD, Fine MJ. Antibiotic therapy for adults hospitalized with community-acquired pneumonia. A systematic review. JAMA. 2016;315:595–602.

103. Waterer G. Empiric antibiotics for community-acquired pneumonia: a macrolide and a beta-lactam please! Respirology. 2017;23:450. https://doi.org/10.1111/resp.13248.

104. Torres A, Blasi F, Dartois N, Akova M. Which individuals are at increased risk of pneumococcal disease and why? Impact of COPD, asthma, smoking, diabetes, and/or chronic heart disease on community-acquired pneumonia and invasive disease. Thorax. 2015;70:984–9.

105. McAlister FA, Majumdar SR, Blitz S, Rowe BH, Romney J, Marrie TJ. The relationship between hyperglycemia and outcomes in 2,471 patients admitted to the hospital with community-acquired pneumonia. Diabetes Care. 2005;28:810–5.

106. Yende S, van der Poll T, Lee MJ, Huang DT, Newman AB, Kong L, et al. The influence of pre-existing diabetes mellitus on the host immune response and outcome of pneumonia: analysis of two multicentre cohort studies. Thorax. 2018;65:870–7.

107. Koskela HO, Salonen PH, Romppanen J, Niskanen L. Long-term mortality after community acquired pneumonia-impacts of diabetes and newly discovered hyperglycaemia: a prospective, observational cohort study. BMJ Open. 2018;4:e005715.

108. Hadfield J, Bennett L. Determining best outcomes from community-acquired pneumonia and how to achieve them. Respirology. 2017;23:138. https://doi.org/10.1111/resp.13218.

109. Mandell LA. Something new for community-acquired pneumonia? Clin Infect Dis. 2017;63:1681–2.

110. Peyrani P, Wiemken TL, Metersky ML, Arnold FW, Mattingly WA, Feldman C, et al. The order of administration of macrolides and beta-lactams may impact the outcomes of hospitalized patients with community acquired pneumonia: results from the community-acquired pneumonia organization. Infect Dis. 2018;50:13–20.

111. Dheda K, Barry CE, Maartens G. Tuberculosis. Lancet. 2015;387:1211–26.

112. Al-Rifai RH, Pearson F, Critchley JA, Abu-Raddad LJ. Association between diabetes mellitus and active tuberculosis: a systematic review and meta-analysis. PLoS One. 2017;12:e0187967.

113. Verbeeck RK, Günther G, Kibuule D, Hunter C, Rennie TW. Optimizing treatment outcome of first-line anti-tuberculous drugs: the role of therapeutic drug monitoring. Eur J Clin Pharmacol. 2016;72:905–16.

114. Riza AL, Pearson F, Ugarte-Gil C, Alisjahbana B, van de Vivjer S, Panduru NM, et al. Clinical management of concurrent diabetes and tuberculosis and the implications for patient services. Lancet Diabetes Endocrinol. 2014;2:740–53.

115. Stockamp NW, Thompson GR III. Coccidioidomycosis. Infect Dis Clin N Am. 2016;30:229–46.

116. Abengowe CU, McManamon PJM. Acute emphysematous cholecystitis. Can Med Assoc J. 1974;111:1112–4.

117. Garcia-Sancho Tellez L, Rodriguez-Montes JA, Fernandez de Lis S, Garcia-Sancho ML. Acute emphysematous cholecystitis. Report of twenty cases. Hepato-Gastroenterology. 1999;46:2144–8.

118. Thomsen RW, Jepsen P, Sorensen HT. Diabetes mellitus and pyogenic liver abscess: risk and prognosis. CID. 2007;44:1194–201.

119. Foo NP, Chen KT, Lin HJ, Guo HR. Characteristics of pyogenic liver abscess patients with and without diabetes mellitus. Am J Gastroenterol. 2010;105:328–35.

120. Siu LK, Yeh K-M, Lin J-C, Fung C-P, Chang F-Y. Klebsiella pneumoniae liver abscess: a new invasive syndrome. Lancet Infect Dis. 2012;12:881–7.

121. van den Berge M, de Marie S, Kuipers T, Jansz AR, Bravenboer B. Psoas abscess: report of a series and review of the literature. Neth J Med. 2005;63:413–61.

122. Maines E, Franceschi R, Cauvin V, d'Annunzio G, Pini Prato A, Castagnola E, et al. Iliopsoas abscess in adolescents with type 1 diabetes mellitus. Clin Case Rep. 2015;3:638–42.

123. Geerlings SE. Urinary tract infections in patients with diabetes mellitus: epidemiology, pathogenesis and treatment. Int J Antimicrob Agents. 2008;31S:S54–7.

124. Nicolle LE. Urinary tract infections in special populations. Diabetes, renal transplant, HIV infection, and spinal cord injury. Infect Dis Clin N Am. 2014;28:91–104.

125. Thomas L, Tracy CR. Treatment of fungal urinary tract infection. Urol Clin N Am. 2015;42:473–83.

126. Nicolle LE. Uncomplicated urinary tract infection in adults including uncomplicated pyelonephritis. Urol Clin North Am. 2008;35:1–12.

127. Wagenlehner FME, Weidner W, Naber KG. Antibiotics in urology – new essentials. Urol Clin N Am. 2008;35:69–79.

128. Durwood EN. Complicated urinary tract infections. Urol Clin North Am. 2008;35:13–22.

129. Amano M, Shimizu T. Emphysematous cystitis: a review of the literature. Intern Med. 2014;53:79–82.

130. Gardiner RA, Gwynne RA, Roberts SA. Perinephric Abscess. BJU Int. 2011;107(Suppl 3):20–3.

131. Hirji I, Andersson SW, Guo Z, Hammar N, Gomez-Caminero A. Incidence of genital infection among patients with type 2 diabetes in the UK General Practice Research Database. J Diabetes Complicat. 2012;26:501–5.

132. Nyirjesy P, Sobel JD. Genital infections in patients with diabetes. Postgrad Med. 2013;125:33–46.

133. Goswami R, Dadhwal V, Tejaswi S, Datta K, Paul A, Haricharan RN, et al. Species-specific prevalence of vaginal candidiasis among patients with diabetes mellitus and its relationship to their glycaemic status. J Infect. 2000;41:162–16.

134. Dovnik A, Golle A, Novak D, Arko D, Takac I. Treatment of vulvovaginal candidiasis: a review of the literature. Acta Dermatoveneorol. 2015;24:5–7.

135. Matheson A, Mazza D. Recurrent vulvovaginal candidiasis: a review of guideline recommendations. Aust N Z J Obstet Gynaecol. 2017;57:139–45.

136. Rizzi M, Trevisan R. Genitourinary infections in diabetic patients in the new era of diabetes therapy with sodium-glucose cotransporter-2 inhibitors. Nutr Metab Cardiovasc Dis. 2016;26:963–70.

137. Kalra S, Chawla A. Diabetes and balanoposthitis. J Pak Med Assoc. 2016;66:1039–41.

138. Chennamsetty A, Khourdaji I, Burks F, Killinger KA. Contemporary diagnosis and management of Fournier's gangrene. Ther Adv Urol. 2015;7:203–15.

139. Gill GV, Famuyiwa OO, Rolfe M, Archibald LK. Serious hand sepsis and diabetes mellitus: specific tropical syndrome with western counterparts. Diabet Med. 1998;15:858–62.

140. Yeika EV, Tchoumi Tantchou JC, Foryoung JB, Tolefac PN, Efie DT, Choukem SP. Tropical diabetic hand syndrome: a case report. BMC Res Notes. 2017;10:94. https://doi.org/10.1186/s13104-017-2405-3.

141. Stulberg DL, Penrod MA, Blatny RA. Common bacterial skin infections. Am Fam Physician. 2002;66:119–24.

142. Singer AJ, Tassiopoulos A, Kirsner RS. Evaluation and management of lower-extremity ulcers. N Engl J Med. 2017;377:1559–67.

143. Wijesuriya TM, Weerasekera MM, Kottahachchi J, Ranasinghe K, Dissanayake M, Prathapan S, et al. Proportion of lower limb fungal foot infections in patients with type 2 diabetes at a tertiary care hospital in Sri Lanka. Indian J Endocr Metab. 2014;18:63–9.

144. Noor S, Khan RU, Ahmad J. Understanding foot infection and its management. Diabetes Metab Syndr Clin Res Rev. 2017;11:149–56.

145. Lipski BA, Aragón-Sánchez J, Diggle M, Embil J, Kono S, Lavery L, et al. IWGDF guidance on the diagnosis and management of foot infections in persons with diabetes. Diabetes Metab Res Rev. 2016;32(Suppl 1):45–74.

146. Muñoz-Quiles C, López-Lacort M, Ampudia-Blasco J, Díez-Domingo J. Risk and impact of herpes zoster on patients with diabetes: a population-based study, 2009-2014. Hum Vacc Immunotherapeut. 2017;13:2606–11.

147. O'Connor KM, Paauw DS. Herpes Zoster. Med Clin N Am. 2013;97:503–22.

148. Cathart S, Cantrell W, Elewski BE. Onychomycosis and diabetes. J Eur Acad Dermatol Venereol. 2009;23:1119–22.

149. Zane LT, Chanda S, Coronado D, Del Rosso J. Antifungal agents for onychomycosis: new treatment strategies to improve safety. Dermatology. 2016;22:1–11.

COVID-19, Diabetes, and Cardiovascular Disease

48

Marco A. Peña Duque, Arturo Abundes Velasco,
José Carlos Núñez Gómez, Enid Andrea Islas Navarro,
and Eduardo Armando Aguilar Torres

Pathogenesis

People with chronic-degenerative diseases usually present severe COVID symptoms, as well as a higher risk of postinfection complications. These comorbidities modify metabolism by increasing the expression of the enzyme ACE-2 in infected people. ACE-2 encodes the protein through which the virus enters the cell, so the increased production of ACE-2 in patients with these diseases facilitates the entry of SARS-CoV-2 [1] and induces a great deal of impact on underlying conditions, complications of infections, and other diseases [2, 3]. It has also been observed that COVID-19 infection leads to the worsening of conditions in the presence of CVD [4, 5]. Epidemiological studies have indicated that patients with DM and COVID-19 infection require more medical interventions, have higher mortality rates [7.8% versus 2.7%, adjusted hazard ratio (HR) 1.49], and have a greater frequency of multiple-organ damage than those without DM [6].

Epidemiology

Across the United States, there were 95,235 reported deaths officially attributed to COVID-19 from March 1 to May 30, 2020. By comparison, there were an estimated 122,300 (95% prediction interval, 116,800–127,000) excess deaths during the same period. Even in situations of ample testing, deaths due to viral pathogens, including SARS-CoV-2, can occur indirectly via secondary bacterial infections or exacerbation of comorbidities, mainly CVD [7, 8]. A study published in Italy compared excess deaths from CVD and excess deaths due to the new coronavirus. The trajectory of the number of excess deaths from CVD was highly parallel to the trajectory of the number of excess deaths related to COVID-19. The number of excess deaths from DM, influenza, respiratory diseases, and malignant neoplasms remained relatively stable over time. The parallel trajectory of excess mortality from CVD and COVID-19 over time reflects the fact that essential health services for noncommunicable diseases were reduced or disrupted during the COVID-19 pandemic, and the more severe the pandemic, the heavier the impact. Many European countries have experienced sharp increases in all-cause deaths associated with the pandemic [9].

DM is associated with an increased risk of infections, especially infections of the skin and urinary and respiratory tracts. This is due to immunological dysfunction secondary to the hyperglycemic milieu of people with DM [10]. Bacterial and fungal infections have a higher incidence in patients with DM, albeit previous studies do not associate DM with an increased incidence in viral infections such as COVID-19 [11]. Nevertheless, a meta-analysis of six Chinese studies including 1527 patients hospitalized with COVID-19 demonstrated significant differences in the prevalence of hyperglycemia in severe versus non-severe cases, in addition to a prevalence of DM of 11.7% in ICU cases, in comparison with 4.0% in non-ICU cases [12]. In line with these findings, a report from the Chinese Center for Disease Control and Prevention on 44,672 COVID-19 cases, which also included nonhospitalized patients, showed a lower prevalence of DM (5.3%). But it is associated with poor prognosis [12]. A meta-analysis with 6452 patients from 30 studies showed that DM was associated with a compound poor outcome (RR 2.38 [1.88, 3.03], $p < 0.001$; I^2, 62%) [13]. A group of researchers from Mexico published an article proposing a mechanistic approach to evaluate the risk for complications and lethality attributable to COVID-19 in which they included early-onset diabetes, obesity, chronic obstructive pulmonary disease, advanced age, hypertension, immunosuppression, and chronic kidney disease [14]. Among these variables, the results of this study showed that early-onset diabetes conferred an increased risk of hospitalization and obesity conferred an increased risk for intensive care admission and intubation [14].

M. A. Peña Duque · A. A. Velasco (✉) · J. C. N. Gómez ·
E. A. I. Navarro · E. A. A. Torres
National Institute of Cardiology, Mexico City, Mexico

© The Author(s), under exclusive license to Springer Nature Switzerland AG 2023
J. Rodriguez-Saldana (ed.), *The Diabetes Textbook*, https://doi.org/10.1007/978-3-031-25519-9_48

Management of Diabetes, COVID-19, and Cardiovascular Disease

The management of DM in patients with COVID-19 infection has a remarkable impact on the mortality from this disease, according to the fact that patients with better control have fewer complications in comparison with the ones who are not in control [15]. General recommendations for DM management include increasing physical activity as part of the treatment. A study suggested that physical inactivity is correlated with a higher relative risk of COVID-19 hospitalization, even after controlling for age, sex, obesity, smoking, and alcohol intake [RR, 1.32 (95% confidence interval [CI], 1.10–1.58)] [16]. It is expected that inactivity or a sedentary lifestyle will increase to produce 11 million new patients debuting with DM2 and up to almost 2 million deaths related to metabolic syndrome leading to decreased physical activity and increased prevalence of obesity [17]. Strategies to avoid physical inactivity and reduce stress levels can promote cardiovascular protection. The promotion of physical activity is prioritized by public health agencies and has been incorporated into routine medical care [18]. A home-based training protocol could be an important and effective strategy for individuals who need to remain safe and physically active.

International guidelines have already standardized the use of a glucocorticoid, anti-inflammatory drug therapy, and prophylactic anticoagulant in patients with COVID-19 [19]. For this reason, frequent glucose monitoring in DM patients and COVID-19 is imperative. A relevant study by Lu et al. supports that less variability in glucose excursions measured as time in range was associated with a lower risk of all-cause mortality and cardiovascular mortality among patients with type 2 DM [20] . Many patients previously on oral hypoglycemic agents will require conversion to insulin during hospitalization; in severe cases of COVID-19, insulin requirements are extremely high; these patients had a worse prognosis, compared with their counterparts who had not received insulin. This finding is probably secondary to the hyperinflammatory state on insulin resistance, reflecting that insulin treatment is a marker for advanced DM [21]. The results of this review indicate that there is no reason to cease the use of antidiabetic medications, that long-term glycemic control is essential in patients with COVID-19, and that it can improve the prognosis in these patients. Although potential direct therapeutic benefits have been proposed, the safety of some glucose-lowering therapies is still questioned [22]. An observational cohort study in England to investigate the association between prescription of different classes of glucose-lowering drugs and risk of COVID-19 mortality in a population of almost three million people with type 2 diabetes showed the following hazard ratios (HR): 0.77 for metformin, 1.42 for insulin, 0.75 for meglitinides, 0.82 for SGLT2 inhibitors, 0.94 for glitazones, sulfonylureas and

GLP-1 receptor agonists, 1.07 for DPP inhibitors, and 1.26 for α-glucosidase inhibitors [23]. The study provides compelling evidence about the associations of some prescription drugs, although the differences are small and likely due to confounding [23].

Sodium-glucose cotransporter 2 (SGLT2) inhibitors have raised high expectancies because of their cardioprotective effects. The EMPA-REG OUTCOME, a randomized, double-blind, placebo-controlled trial that evaluated the effect of empagliflozin, found a significant reduction in major adverse cardiovascular outcomes including cardiovascular death, myocardial infarction, or stroke, as well as death from cardiovascular causes, death from any cause, progression of renal disease, and hospitalization for heart failure (HF) [24]. These findings were confirmed in the DAPA-HF trial in which 4744 patients with HF and a reduced ejection fraction were randomly assigned to receive either dapagliflozin or placebo in addition to standard HF therapy [25]. Of the enrolled patients, 41.8% had DM and the primary outcome of cardiovascular death or worsening HF was significantly lower in the dapagliflozin group than in the placebo group (16.3% vs. 21.2%; hazard ratio, 0.74; 95% confidence interval [CI], 0.65 to 0.85; P 0.001) [25]. This effect was not attributable to its low antihyperglycemic or natriuretic effects. Ferrannini et al. and Mudaliar et al. postulated that the action of SGLT2 inhibitors to promote ketogenesis might account for their favorable effects on the heart and kidney since enhanced ketone bodies' formation might provide an efficient fuel that could increase the energy status of organs under stress [26]. This effect would explain why this benefit is observed in patients with HF without DM. The DARE-19 trial, a randomized, double-blind, placebo-controlled trial, suggested that the SGLT2 inhibitor dapagliflozin was safe and well tolerated in patients hospitalized with COVID-19 with at least one cardiometabolic risk factor [27]. This study excluded critically ill patients, however, and did not result in a significant risk reduction in organ dysfunction or death nor an improvement in clinical status [27]. Currently there is a strong rationale to avoid treatment with metformin or SGLT2 inhibitors in patients with severe COVID-19 to reduce the risk of lactic acidosis, ketoacidosis, and volume depletion associated with the use of these drugs in the presence of severe infection [21].

Cardiovascular Complications of COVID-19 Infection

The symptoms and clinical course of COVID-19 are broad, ranging from asymptomatic to severe respiratory failure requiring mechanical ventilation. Metabolic and cardiovascular comorbidities have an important role in outcomes of patients with COVID-19 infection [15]. A meta-analysis of six published studies from China including 1527 patients with COVID-19 reported a 9.7%, 16.4%, and 17.1% prevalence of DM, cardio-cerebrovascular disease, and hypertension, respectively [11], and the increasing knowledge of COVID-19 has provided a clearer picture of its clinical evolution: The first phase is asymptomatic or primarily characterized by symptoms in the upper respiratory tract; approximately 80% of the cases are resolved. The second phase, or moderate pneumonia, occurs approximately in 15%, requiring supplementary oxygen. About 5% evolve to the third phase, or severe pneumonia, with worsening of the respiratory condition, hypoxemia, fever, and acute respiratory distress syndrome [28]. In addition to respiratory symptoms, many patients have cardiovascular symptoms, such as heart palpitations and chest tightness/pain, as the initial clinical manifestation of COVID-19 [29]. When the cardiovascular system is affected, a wide range of complications can occur, from myocardial injury and acute myocardial infarction to heart failure, myocarditis, dysrhythmias, and venous thromboembolic events [28].

Regardless of the phases in which the patient has been through, moreover, several studies also showed that COVID-19 can exacerbate preexisting cardiovascular disease and/or cause new cardiovascular injuries [30]. Increased risk for myocardial infarction, fulminant myocarditis rapidly evolving with depressed systolic left ventricle function, arrhythmias, venous thromboembolism, and cardiomyopathies mimicking STEMI presentations are the most prevalent cardiovascular complications described in patients with COVID-19 [31].

The hypothesis of the cumulative effect of previous CV disease and troponin increase was postulated due to the greater presence of ACE2 receptors in postmortem cardiac pericytes extracted from patients with heart disease compared with those without the previous disease. That explains the affinity to this system [32]. Shi et al. reported that myocardial injury may be caused by myocarditis and myocardial ischemia, which is mainly manifested by elevated troponin levels, and higher mortality rates than those in people without myocardial injury (51.2% vs. 4.5%; $p < 0.001$), being an independent risk factor for mortality [33]. Myocardial injury has also been described in 5 of the first 41 patients diagnosed with COVID-19 in Wuhan, China, with elevated serum high-sensitivity cardiac troponin I (hs-ctni) levels (>28 ng/l) [34]. However, in a cohort study of 1597 US-competitive athletes with CMR screening after COVID-19 infection, 37 (2.3%) were diagnosed with clinical and subclinical myocarditis. If cardiac testing was based on cardiac symptoms alone, only 5 athletes would have been detected for a prevalence of 0.31% [35]. Regardless of the actual incidence, acute cardiac injury has been consistently shown to be a strong negative prognostic marker in patients with COVID-19 [35].

Heart failure is an important cause of death in patients with COVID-19 and occurs as a result of different myocardial aggression mechanisms such as direct myocardial injury by viral action, indirect and direct inflammatory damage, an imbalance in oxygen supply-demand, and an increase of atherothrombotic events due to inflammatory destabilization of atheromatous plaques, which result in acute myocardial dysfunction [36]. A clinical study of 99 cases with confirmed COVID-19 from Wuhan showed that 11 (11%) patients had died, of which 2 patients had no previous history of chronic heart disease but developed heart failure and eventually died of sudden cardiac arrest [37]. Even in the absence of direct myocardial injury, patients develop disturbances in the conduction system that produce arrhythmias regardless of the previous cardiovascular state. Cardiac arrhythmias are common cardiac manifestations described in COVID-19 patients [38]. A study describing clinical profile and outcomes in 138 Chinese patients with COVID-19 reported a 16.7% incidence of arrhythmia [38].

Conclusion

Until today, the origin of SARS-CoV-2 disease and its acute repercussions have been established, but the long-term sequelae in diabetic patients with cardiovascular disease are not yet well known (long COVID). Patients with COVID-19 are at increased risk of a broad range of cardiovascular disorders including cerebrovascular disease, dysrhythmias, ischemic and non-ischemic heart disease, pericarditis, myocarditis, heart failure, and thromboembolic disease [39]. The risk and 1-year burden of cardiovascular disease in survivors of acute COVID-19 are substantial [40]. Most of these are lifelong conditions that will affect people for a lifetime and may impact their quality of life and other health outcomes [40].

Multiple Choice Questions

1. As a result of sedentary lifestyle, what is the expected amount of new patients who will develop type 2 diabetes?
   (a) 10 million
   (b) 9 million
   (c) 20 million
   (d) **11 million**
   (e) 15 million
2. What is the mortality rate from COVID-19 infection in patients with diabetes?
   (a) **7.8%**
   (b) 3%
   (c) 5.2%
   (d) 10%
   (e) 5.4%

3. What is the estimated percentage of patients with COVID-19 infection with severe pneumonia?
   (a) 80%
   (b) 15%
   (c) 45%
   (d) 100%
   (e) **5%**

4. What is the cardioprotective action attributed to SGLT2 inhibitors in patients with diabetes and heart failure?
   (a) Natriuretic effect
   (b) Low glycemic action
   (c) **Promote ketogenesis**
   (d) Lactic acidosis
   (e) Insulin sensibility

5. In severe COVID-19 infection, which classes of glucose-lowering drugs are recommended to avoid?
   (a) SGLT2 inhibitors and metformin
   (b) Insulin and SGLT2
   (c) DPP-4 inhibitors
   (d) Sulfonylureas
   (e) All are secure

6. What is the SGLT2 inhibitor that demonstrated a significant reduction in major adverse cardiovascular events and death from cardiovascular causes?
   (a) **Dapagliflozin**
   (b) Empagliflozin
   (c) Canagliflozin
   (d) Ertugliflozin
   (e) Phlorizin

7. What comorbidity is not associated with a higher prevalence of diabetes?
   (a) Parasitic
   (b) Bacterial
   (c) Fungicidal
   (d) **Viral**
   (e) Oncologic

8. In patients with CVD, the increase of which receptor is associated with a higher risk of cardiovascular complications?
   (a) CXCR4
   (b) GM2
   (c) **ACE2**
   (d) VLDLR
   (e) HLA-1

9. What is the percentage of athletes diagnosed with clinical and subclinical myocarditis after COVID-19 infection?
   (a) 0.31%
   (b) **2.3%**
   (c) 10%
   (d) 80%
   (e) 9.7%

10. What is the most prevalent comorbidity in patients with COVID-19 infection?
    (a) Diabetes mellitus
    (b) **Hypertension**
    (c) Chronic kidney disease
    (d) Parkinson's disease
    (e) Obesity

References

1. Hoffmann M, Kleine-Weber H, Schroeder S, Müller MA, Drosten C, Pöhlmann S. SARS-CoV-2 cell entry depends on ACE2 and TMPRSS2 and is blocked by a clinically proven protease inhibitor. Cell. 2020;181:271–80.

2. Steinmetz A. Treatment of diabetic dyslipoproteinemia. Exp Clin Endocrinol Diabetes. 2003;111:239–45.

3. Suri JS, Puvvula A, Biswas M, Majhail M, Saba L, Faa G, et al. COVID-19 pathways for brain and heart injury in comorbidity patients: a role of medical imaging and artificial intelligence-based COVID severity classification: a review. Comput Biol Med. 2020;124:1–15.

4. Zheng YY, Ma YT, Zhang JY, Xie X. COVID-19 and the cardiovascular system. Nat Rev Cardiol. 2020;17:259–60.

5. Suri JS, Puvvula A, Majhail M, Biswas M, Jamthikar AD, Saba L, et al. Integration of cardiovascular risk assessment with COVID-19 using artificial intelligence. Rev Cardiovasc Med. 2020;21:541–60.

6. Zhu L, She Z-G, Cheng X, Guo J, Zhang B-H, Li H. Association of blood glucose control and outcomes in patients with COVID-19 and pre-existing type 2 diabetes. Cell Metab. 2020;31:1068–77.

7. Zhu D, Ozaki A, Virani SS. Disease-specific excess mortality during the COVID-19 pandemic: an analysis of weekly US death data for 2020. Am J Public Health. 2020;111:1518–22.

8. Rizzo M, Foresti L, Montano N. Comparison of reported deaths from COVID-19 and increase in total mortality in Italy. JAMA Intern Med. 2020;180:1250–2.

9. Luk AOY, Lau ESH, Cheung KKT, Kong APS, Ma RCW, Ozaki R, et al. Glycaemia control and the risk of hospitalisation for infection in patients with type 2 diabetes: Hong Kong Diabetes Registry. Diabetes Metab Res Rev. 2017;33:1–7.

10. Hine JL, de Lusignan S, Burleigh D, Pathirannehelage S, McGovern A, Gatenby P, et al. Association between glycaemic control and common infections in people with type 2 diabetes: a cohort study. Diabet Med. 2017;34:551–7.

11. Li B, Zhao Y. Prevalence and impact of cardiovascular metabolic diseases on COVID-19 in China. Clin Res Cardiol. 2020;109:531–8.

12. Hua W, Xiaofeng L, Zhenqiang B, Jun R, Ban W, Liming L. Consideration on the strategies during epidemic stage changing from emergency response to continuous prevention and control. Zhonghua Liu Xing Bing Xue Za Zhi. 2020;41:297–300.

13. Hauang I, Lim MA, Pranata R. Diabetes mellitus is associated with increased mortality and severity of disease in COVID-19 pneumonia - a systematic review, meta-analysis, and meta-regression. Diabetes Metab Syndr. 2020;14:395–403.

14. Bello-Chavolla OY, Bahena-López JP, Antonio-Villa NE, Vargas-Vázquez A, González-Díaz A, Márquez-Salinas A, et al. Prediction mortality due to SARS-CoV-2: a mechanistic score relating obesity and diabetes to COVID-19 outcomes in Mexico. J Clin Endocrinol Metab. 2020;105:2752–61.

15. Steenblock C, Schwarz PEH, Ludwig B, Linkermann A, Zimmet P, Kulebyakin K, et al. COVID-19 and metabolic disease:

mechanisms and clinical management. Lancet Diabetes Endocrinol. 2021;11:786–98.

16. Hamer M, Kivimäki M, Gale CR, Batty GD. Lifestyle risk factors, inflammatory mechanisms, and COVID-19 hospitalization: a community-based study of 387,109 adults in UK. Brain Behav Immun. 2020;87:187–7.

17. Amini H, Habibi S, Islamoglu H, Isanejad E, Uz C, Daniyari H. COVID-19 pandemic-induced physical inactivity: the necessity of updating the global action plan on physical activity 2018-2030. Environ Health Prev Med. 2021;26:1–3.

18. Seidu S, Khunti K, Yates T, Almaqhawi A, Davies MJ, Sargeant J. The importance of physical activity in management of type 2 diabetes and COVID-19. Ther Adv Endocrinol Metab. 2021;12:1–14.

19. World Health Organization. Living guidance for clinical management of COVID-19, 2021.

20. Lu J, Wang C, Shen Y, Chen L, Zhang L, Cai J, et al. Time in range in relation to all-cause and cardiovascular mortality in patients with type 2 diabetes: a prospective cohort study. Diabetes Care. 2021;44:549–55.

21. Santos A, Magro DO, Evangelista-Poderoso R, Saad MJA. Diabetes, obesity, and insulin resistance in COVID-19: molecular interrelationship and therapeutic implications. Diabetol Metab Syndr. 2021;13:1–14.

22. Ceriello A, Prattichizzo F. Pharmacological management of COVID-19 in type 2 diabetes. J Diabetes Complicat. 2021;35:107927.

23. Khunti K, Knighton P, Zaccardi F, Bakhai E, Holman N, Kar P, et al. Prescription of glucose-lowering therapies and risk of COVID-19 mortality in people with type 2 diabetes: a nationwide observational study in England. Lancet Diabetes Endocrinol. 2021;9:293–303.

24. Steiner S. Empagliflozin, cardiovascular outcomes, and mortality in type 2 diabetes. Zeitschrift fur Gefassmedizin. 2016;13:17–8.

25. McMurray JJV, Solomon SD, Inzucchi SE, Kober L, Kosiborod MN, Martinez FA, et al. Dapagliflozin in patients with heart failure and reduced ejection fraction. N Engl J Med. 2019;381:1995–2008.

26. Packer M. SGLT2 inhibitors produce cardiorenal benefits by promoting adaptive cellular reprogramming to induce a state of fasting mimicry: a paradigm shift in understanding their mechanism of action. Diabetes Care. 2020;43:508–11.

27. Kosiborod MN, Esterline R, Furtado RHM, Oscarsson J, Gasparyan SB, Koch GG, et al. Dapagliflozin in patients with cardiometabolic risk factors hospitalised with COVID-19 (DARE-19): a randomised, double-blind, placebo-controlled, phase 3 trial. Lancet Diabetes Endocrinol. 2021;9:586–94.

28. Del Prete A, Conway F, Della Rocca DG, Biondi-Zoccai G, De Felice F, Musto C, et al. COVID-19, acute myocardial injury, and infarction. Card Electrophysiol Clin. 2022;14:29–39.

29. Wu Z, McGoogan JM. Characteristics of and important lessons from the coronavirus disease 2019 (COVID-19) outbreak in China: summary of a report of 72314 cases from the Chinese Center for Disease Control and Prevention. JAMA. 2020;323:1239–42.

30. Bansal M. Cardiovascular disease and COVID-19. Diabetes Metab Syndr Clin Res Rev. 2020;14:247–50.

31. Chung MK, Zidar DA, Bristow MR, Cameron SJ, Chan T, Harding CV, et al. COVID-19 and cardiovascular disease. From bench to bedside. Circ Res. 2021;128:1214–36.

32. Chen L, Li X, Chen M, Feng Y, Xiong C. The ACE2 expression in human heart indicates new potential mechanism of heart injury among patients infected with SARS-CoV-2. Cardiovasc Res. 2020;2020(116):1097–100.

33. Shi S, Qin M, Shen B, Cai Y, Liu T, Yang F, et al. Association of Cardiac Injury with mortality in hospitalized patients with COVID-19 in Wuhan, China. JAMA Cardiol. 2020;5:802–10.

34. Huang C, Wang Y, Li X, Ren L, Zhao J, Hu Y, et al. Clinical features of patients infected with 2019 novel coronavirus in Wuhan. China Lancet. 2020;395:497–506.

35. Daniels CJ, Rajpal S, Greenshields JT, Rosenthal GL, Chung EH, Terrin M, et al. Prevalence of clinical and subclinical myocarditis in competitive athletes with recent SARS-CoV-2 infection: results from the big ten COVID-19 Cardiac Registry. JAMA Cardiol. 2021;2021(6):1078–87.

36. Inciardi RM, Lupi L, Zaccone G, Italia L, Raffo M, Tomasoni D, et al. Cardiac involvement in a patient with coronavirus disease 2019 (COVID-19). JAMA Cardiol. 2020;5:819–24.

37. Chen N, Zhou M, Dong X, Qu J, Gong F, Han Y, et al. Epidemiological and clinical characteristics of 99 cases of 2019 novel coronavirus pneumonia in Wuhan, China: a descriptive study. Lancet. 2020;395:507–13.

38. Wang D, Hu C, Zhu F, Liu XL, Zhang J, Wang B, et al. Clinical characteristics of 138 hospitalized patients with 2019 novel coronavirus-infected pneumonia in Wuhan, China. JAMA. 2020;2020(323):1061–9.

39. Abbasi J. The COVID heart - one year after SARS-CoV-2 infection, patients have an array of increased cardiovascular risks. JAMA. 2022;327(12):1113–4.

40. Xie Y, Xu E, Bowe B, Al-Aly Z. Long-term cardiovascular outcomes of COVID-19. Nat Med. 2022;28(3):583–90.

Part IX

Chronic Complications

Biochemical Mechanisms of Vascular Complications in Diabetes

Margarita Díaz Flores, María del Carmen Cortés Ginez, and Luis Arturo Baiza Gutman

Objectives

- To analyze the biochemical and molecular mechanism of vascular diabetic complications
- To analyze the role of metabolic alterations induced by hyperglycemia in diabetic complications (altered glycolysis, diacylglycerol production, protein kinase C activation, activation of polyol and hexosamine pathways, and glycation)
- To analyze the role of oxidative stress in diabetic complications, considering reactive oxygen species production and the biochemical, metabolic, and morphological alteration induced by them
- To analyze the role of inflammation during diabetes and its participation in vascular diabetic complications
- To analyze the integrative hypothesis that explains the rise and progression of vascular diabetic complications

Diabetes and Vascular Complications

Diabetes mellitus (DM) is a heterogeneous pandemic metabolic disorder characterized by a chronically elevated blood glucose concentration (hyperglycemia) due to resistance to insulin action, defective insulin secretion, or both (insulin dysfunction). This disease affects approximately 9% of the worldwide adult population. Type 2 diabetes is diagnosed often late when already 40% of diabetics show complications. Vascular complications of diabetes are frequently responsible for morbidity and mortality in diabetic patients [1, 2].

Hyperglycemia or chronic elevation of blood glucose has been considered as the major inductor of vascular diabetic complications [1]. Persistent exposure of tissues to high concentrations of glucose can lead to damage (glucotoxicity) of endothelium and small blood vessels (microvasculature) followed by alterations of tissues and organs, including kidney (nephropathy), eyes (retinopathy), and nerves and central nervous system (peripheral and autonomic neuropathy), which are known as microvascular complications of diabetes [3, 4]. Additionally, hyperglycemia leads to damage of big blood vessels and heart or macrovascular complications, which are associated with cardiovascular diseases such as accelerated atherosclerosis, cardiomyopathy, myocardial infarction, stroke, and peripheral arterial disease [5]. There is a growing recognition that cognitive dysfunction, encephalopathy, osteopathy, liver disease, and cancer are emerging complications of diabetes.

Besides hyperglycemia, other factors are involved in the development and progression of vascular complications such as dyslipidemia and accumulation of lipid metabolites (lipotoxicity) [6], chronic inflammation, oxidative stress, hormone and cytokine levels, hypertension, and nitric oxide (NO) deficiency.

Several mechanisms involved in the pathogenesis of diabetic complications induced by hyperglycemia have been proposed; all of them consider how the high concentration of glucose is metabolized by different pathways and conduced to the accumulation of metabolites or activation of signaling molecules that induce damage of endothelium, vascular vessels, and other tissues, causing morphological and physiological impairment of several organs. The proposed mechanism includes (Fig. 49.1):

M. D. Flores (✉) · M. del Carmen Cortés Ginez
Medical Research Unit in Biochemistry, UMAE Specialty Hospital, Centro Médico Nacional Siglo XXI, Instituto Mexicano del Seguro Social (IMSS), Mexico City, Mexico

L. A. B. Gutman
Morphology and Function Unit, Faculty of Higher Studies-Iztacala, National Autonomous University of Mexico, Mexico City, Mexico
e-mail: labaiza@unam.mx

© The Author(s), under exclusive license to Springer Nature Switzerland AG 2023
J. Rodriguez-Saldana (ed.), *The Diabetes Textbook*, https://doi.org/10.1007/978-3-031-25519-9_49

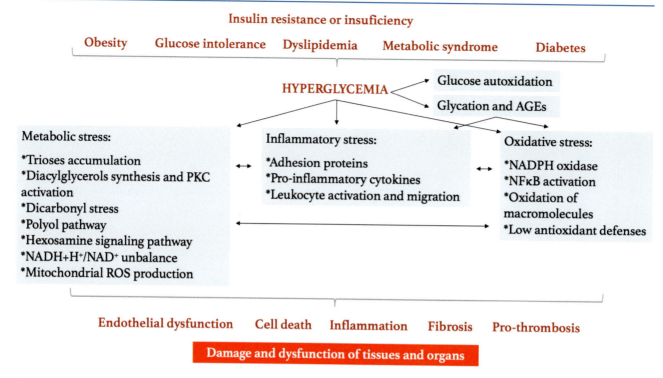

Fig. 49.1 Pathophysiological mechanisms of diabetic complications. Several chronic metabolic conditions lead to chronic or postprandial hyperglycemia, which induces metabolic, inflammatory, and oxidative stress, causing tissue and organ alterations characteristics of vascular diabetic complications. NFκB, transcription factor nuclear factor κB

1. Metabolic stress, caused by the increased flux of glucose in several metabolic pathways (Fig. 49.2), including [7]:
   (a) Glycolysis, accumulation of trioses, and generation of methylglyoxal. Trioses lead to increased formation of diacylglycerol and methylglyoxal, which are associated with the activation of protein kinase C (PKC) and intracellular glycation, respectively.
   (b) The polyol pathway and accumulation of sorbitol [7, 8].
   (c) The hexosamine signaling pathway [9].
   (d) Nonenzymatic glycation with increased formation of advanced glycation end products (AGEs) and the activation of its receptor (RAGE) [10].
2. Oxidative/reductive stress. The accumulation of reactive oxygen species (ROS) is dependent on different processes during hyperglycemia. ROS are extracellularly produced by glucose autoxidation and as a side product of glycation. Intracellularly, oxidative stress is promoted by the generation of ROS by a variety of sources such as mitochondrial electron transport chain, NADPH oxidase, xanthine oxidase, and uncoupled eNOS. An interesting point of view is that diabetic complications are majorly generated by oxidative stress driven by the NADH/NAD+ redox imbalance (reductive stress) and mitochondrial dysfunction [4].

3. Inflammatory stress. Inflammation is a common pathophysiological mechanism in many diseases, including diabetes mellitus, where several pro-inflammatory mediators are upregulated and contribute to vascular complications.

Although multiple processes contribute to vascular complications, several researchers have treated to find one mechanism that drives the other mechanisms that conduce to the vascular complications. Three major unifying hypotheses have been proposed. The more accepted hypothesis proposes that the oxidative stress induced by hyperglycemia could be a unifying and common mechanism involved in the activation of the other mechanisms; initially, the production of ROS by the mitochondria was considered as the driver of vascular complications [9]; for example, the production of O^{2-} by the mitochondria mediates the high glucose-induced increased flux in the hexosamine pathway in bovine aorta endothelial cells [9, 11]. A second hypothesis considers the dicarbonyl stress as the key to diabetic complications [12, 13]. A third hypothesis suggests that the unifying mechanism is the polyol pathway [13, 14]. The real situation of the development of vascular complications in diabetic patients is complex. Antioxidants and pharmacological agents that inhibit these pathways have shown limited clinical success

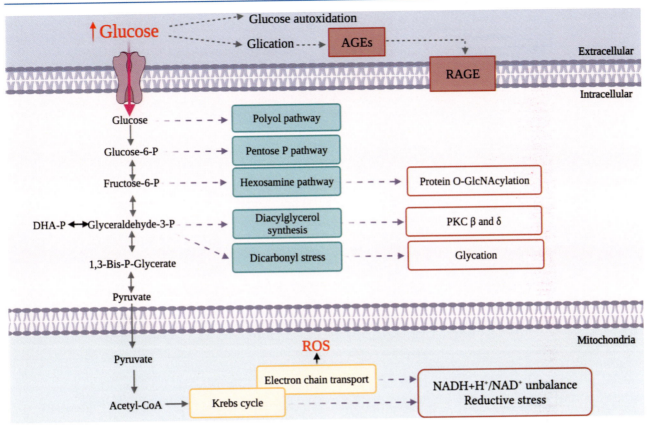

Fig. 49.2 Hyperglycemia and glucose metabolism by multiple pathways. In hyperglycemic conditions, there is an overflow of glucose uptake and metabolism in non-insulin-dependent cells, The overflow of glucose induces an NADH + H+/NAD+ imbalance and ROS production in the mitochondria, which lead to inhibition of glyceraldehyde-3-phosphate dehydrogenase and triose accumulation [dihydroxyacetone-phosphate (DHA-P) and glyceraldehyde-3-phosphate], leading to the activation of several pathways of glucose or glucose metabolites' disposal and associated with the induction of vascular complications. P, phosphate; RAGE, receptor for AGEs; O-GlcNAcylation, O-linked glycosylation with β, N-acetylglucosamine; PKC, protein kinase C

against nephropathy or retinopathy in diabetics. On the other hand, a proteomic analysis in long-duration type 1 diabetes mellitus patients (already of 50 years) found high levels of enzymes or the polyol pathway and electronic transfer chain in glomeruli of patients without nephropathy compared with glomeruli of patients with nephropathy [15, 16]; in this case also the enzymes of methylglyoxal depuration and the antioxidant enzyme superoxide dismutase were upregulated, and in some conditions, polyol pathway protects against inflammatory stress [15].

The central role of mitochondrial dysfunction as the initial driver of diabetic complications has been questioned [17, 18]. Some data indicate that reduced mitochondrial activity could be the basis of the progression of diabetic complications mediated by increased inflammation and pro-fibrotic factors [17]. However, the induction of inflammation by high glucose-induced oxidative stress in human vascular cells requires being primed with an inflammatory stimulus such as TNFα or IL-1β (inflammatory preconditioning), and it has been proposed that background of the inflammatory condition is necessary for the deleterious action of excessive glucose environment [19]. The inflammatory preconditioning stimulus promotes the ROS production inducing the overexpression of an important emergent source of O^{2-}, the NADPH oxidase, an enzyme that requires the coenzyme NADPH (reduced nicotinamide adenine dinucleotide phosphate), which also induces the expression of the major supply of this reduced coenzyme, glucose 6-phosphate dehydrogenase, increasing the flux of glucose in the pentose phosphate pathway [19]. Although mitochondria and NADPH oxidase have been considered the major sources of ROS during diabetes, several other ROS production pathways may be activated by hyperglycemia and glucose metabolites. These include glucose autoxidation, glycation, uncoupled endothelial nitric oxide synthase (NOS), xanthine oxidase, endoplasmic reticulum stress, cyclooxygenases, etc., and more studies are required to establish their role in diabetes pathogenesis [18].

Metabolic Stress

The mechanisms of glucose metabolism involved in diabetic complications include glucose autoxidation, the shunt of glucose to the polyol pathway, formation of AGEs, and elevated hexosamine pathway activity [7].

Polyol Pathway

The polyol pathway is linked with the progression of diabetic complications, especially retinopathy because of the formation of a vulnerable intermediate product during its course.

Polyol pathway is activated during hyperglycemia due to saturation of hexokinase (the enzyme that catalyzes the first step of glycolysis). This pathway is activated as blood glucose level rises and involves two enzymatic steps catalyzed by aldose reductase and sorbitol dehydrogenase, present in excess amounts in various body tissues. In the first step, glucose is converted into sorbitol, by the activity of aldose reductase 2 (ALR2), coupled to the oxidation of its cofactor NADPH. In the second step, sorbitol is further converted into fructose, by the action of sorbitol dehydrogenase, using NAD^+ as a cofactor and producing NADH.

This intracellular metabolic process results in the accumulation of sorbitol as an intermediate product because the cellular membranes are impermeable to sorbitol and prevent its efflux. Intracellular accumulation of sorbitol induces osmotic imbalance, water intake, and cellular death. Sorbitol is usually accumulated in the lens, retina, and kidney. The exact mechanism of sorbitol-induced cell death is unkwon but accounts for extensive cellular damage, leading to the progression of diabetic retinopathy, and contributes to nephropathy [7, 8]. The activation of ALR2 also leads to the overconsumption of NADPH, reducing its availability for glutathione reductase, the enzyme that restores reduced glutathione (GSH), the principal intracellular antioxidant, promoting oxidative stress [8].

Although the quantity of sorbitol remains high, sorbitol is converted into fructose in the second step of the reaction, and fructose also is overproduced due to 30% of blood glucose is consumed by the polyol pathway in diabetes. Fructose and some of its derivatives (3-deoxyglucose and fructose-3-phosphate) can glycate proteins altering their function, and in the liver, kidney, and intestine, fructose is phosphorylated to fructose-1-phosphate (F1P) by fructokinase. F1P is metabolized to dihydroxyacetone phosphate (DHAP) and glyceraldehyde 3-phosphate (G3P), which enter the glycolytic/gluconeogenic metabolite pools; these reactions depend on the fructose concentration because it lacks regulatory control, and acetyl-CoA is overproduced, leading to its overflow through the tricarboxylic acid cycle and increased reductive

stress. The overproduction of acetyl-CoA contributes to the development of liver steatosis and non-alcoholic fatty liver disease (NAFLD) and protein functional impairment because of their increased acetylation. In addition, the NADH produced during the second reaction contributes to the reductive stress and conduces to the production of more O^{2-} in the mitochondria [7].

An increase in the activity of the polyol pathway in tissues like the retina, kidney, peripheral nerves, and blood vessels occurs in diabetes because in these tissues, insulin is not required for glucose uptake. The role of the polyol pathway in diabetic retinopathy is supported because increased polyol pathway activity is observed in the retina from animal models of diabetic retinopathy and diabetic human donors with retinopathy [20]. Also, the C allele of the polymorphism at position −106 in the promoter of the *ALR2* gene *has been* associated with diabetic retinopathy [21]. However, the clinical use of an inhibitor of aldose reductase (epalrestat, sorbinil, tolrestat, fidarestat, etc.) is limited because some inhibitors fail to produce significant protection against vascular complications or present cytotoxicity [8]. The cytotoxicity is because these inhibitors frequently also inhibit ALD1, another isoenzyme of aldose reductase, which is involved in the detoxification of aldehydes 3-deoxyglucosone, hydroxynonenal, and methylglyoxal. The accumulation of these aldehydes causes cytotoxicity. Of aldose reductase inhibitors, only epalrestat is used against diabetic neuropathy in Japan, China, and India. However for safety concerns, epalrestat has not been approved yet in some countries and was withdrawn from the market of a few countries [8]. Considering that in some conditions aldose reductase has a protective role against inflammatory and oxidative stress, the use of their inhibitors for the treatment of vascular complications must be carefully evaluated [16].

Hexosamine Biosynthesis Pathway and *O*-GlcNAcylation of Proteins (Fig. 49.3)

Increased flux of glucose into the hexosamine signaling pathway has been implicated in diabetic vascular complications and is induced by hyperglycemia. In this case, glucose 6-phosphate is isomerized to fructose 6-phosphate in glycolysis, and the overproduction of fructose 6-phosphate under hyperglycemic conditions is canalized to this pathway as an alternative to glycolysis [22]. Glucosamine 6-phosphate is produced by the transference of an amino group of glutamine to fructose 6-phosphate catalyzed by the rate-limiting enzyme glutamine-fructose-6-phosphate amidotransferase (GFAT). Finally, in the hexosamine pathway, uridine nucleoside diphosphate-N-acetylglucosamine (UDP-GlcNAc) is formed by sequential enzymatic steps. UDP-GlcNAc is a donor molecule that leads

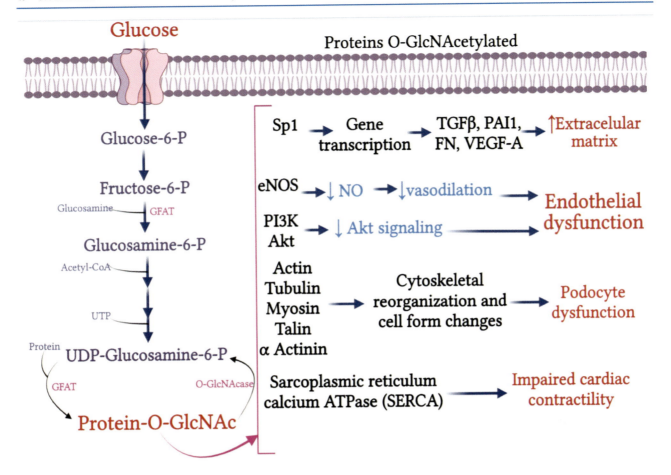

Fig. 49.3 O-GlcNAcetylated proteins and their contribution to vascular complications. The O-GlcNAcetylation of several proteins contributes to different alterations that conduce to vascular complications of diabetes. GFAT, glutamine-fructose-6-phosphate amidotransferase; Sp1, specificity protein 1; FN, fibronectin; NO, nitric oxide; P, phosphate

to O-linked glycosylation with the hexosamine-derived β, N-acetylglucosamine (O-GlcNAcylation) by the enzyme O-GlcNAc transferase (OGT) to serine and threonine residues on target proteins. Conversely, GlcNAc is removed from proteins by GlcNAcase (OGA) (Fig. 49.3).

O-linked N-acetyl glucosamine (O-GlcNAc) is highly increased in cells and tissues of diabetic animals and patients and serves as a nutrient/stress sensor since the synthesis of its donor UDP-GlcNAc depends on changes in the glucose, amino acid, fatty acid, and nucleotide concentrations. Activation of hexosamine signaling pathway mediates several deleterious effects of hyperglycemia through the O-GlcNAcylation of proteins modifying their activity. Acutely O-GlcNAc probably plays a protective function against stress-induced inflammation. However, persistent O-GlcNAcylation of proteins induced by hyperglycemia is involved in changes of gene transcription, cell signaling, vasodilatation, cytoskeletal organization, and apoptosis of endothelial cells and neurons associated with vascular complications [23]. For example, O-GlcNAcylation of endothelial nitric oxide synthase (eNOS), the protein kinase Akt, and the transcription factor specificity

protein 1 (Sp1) lead to decreased NO production, attenuated endothelial migration, and altered gene expression, respectively.

The modification of gene expression by hyperglycemia is associated with increased O-GlcNAcylation and decreased serine/threonine phosphorylation of the transcription factor Sp1 (Fig. 49.3). Sp1 induces the expression of transforming growth factor-β (TGFβ), plasminogen activator inhibitor 1 (PAI-1), and vascular endothelial growth factor A (VEGF-A) [9, 24]. The proliferation of vascular cells is triggered by VEGF-A during diabetic retinopathy. These changes in gene expression could be prevented by the inhibition of the rate-limiting enzyme GFAT or inhibitors of OGT. On the other hand, inhibition or overexpression of the enzyme that degrades N-acetyl glucosamine, O-GlcNAcase (OGA), increases the expression of VEGF-A in cultured retinal cells [24] or reverses the coronary endothelial cell dysfunction in streptozotocin-induced diabetic mice [25].

Few studies link O-GlcNAc to vasculature dysfunction in human T2DM. Arterial or venous endothelial cells obtained from patients with T2DM are characterized by endothelial insulin resistance and lower NO production. Endothelial O-GlcNAc levels are higher in T2DM patients than in non-diabetic controls and are directly correlated with serum fasting blood glucose and glycated hemoglobin A1c (HbA1c) levels. When endothelial cells from patients with T2DM are cultured in normal glucose conditions (24 h at 5 mmol/L), O-GlcNAc levels are lowered and insulin-mediated activation of endothelial nitric oxide synthase is restored. Moreover, the inhibition of the removal of O-GlcNAc from proteins using thiamet G, an O-GlcNAcase inhibitor, in endothelial cells increases O-GlcNAc levels and blunted the improvement of insulin-mediated endothelial nitric oxide synthase phosphorylation by glucose normalization. These data indicate that O-GlcNAc modification is implicated in the glucose-induced impairment of endothelial nitric oxide synthase activation in endothelial cells from patients with T2DM. O-GlcNAc protein modification may be used in the diagnosis and as a treatment target for vascular dysfunction in T2DM [26].

Synthesis of Diacylglycerols and Protein Kinase C Activation

In hyperglycemic conditions, triose phosphates and glycerolphosphate are accumulated, resulting from the inhibition of the enzyme glyceraldehyde 3-phosphate dehydrogenase (GAPDH) by the NADH overproduction and oxidative stress. Both triose phosphate and fructose (end products of the polyol pathway) lead to the formation of methylglyoxal and diacylglycerol (DAG). DAG is located in the cell membrane and activates classical isoforms of PKC (PKCα, PKCβ, and PKCδ), which induce several cell responses and lead to the production of reactive oxygen species via upregulating the expression of NADPH oxidases. PKC is also activated by ROS.

Activated PKC functions through the phosphorylation of Ser and Thr residues in its target proteins and regulates various processes related to diabetic vascular complications such as NO production, vascular permeability, angiogenesis, apoptosis, endothelial dysfunction, and basement membrane thickening. PKCδ can accelerate apoptosis of pericytes, capillary cells, resulting in the degeneration of capillaries during retinopathy. This kinase also induces the apoptosis of podocytes in culture and endothelial dysfunction in renal glomeruli of diabetic rats and mice, in a mechanism mediated by the p38 MAPK and Src homology-2 domain-containing phosphatase-1 (SHP-1) [27, 28]. The relevance of PKCδ in diabetic complications is supported by the fact that the diabetic PKCδ-knockout (Prkcd(−/−)) mice present decreased expressions of TGFβ, VEGF, and extracellular matrix and less albuminuria than diabetic PKCδ wild-type mice [28]. Poor wound healing in diabetic patients has been attributed to activation of PKCδ in fibroblasts, and pharmacologic inhibition and knockdown of PKCδ in diabetic fibroblasts improve wound healing when fibroblasts are implanted in nude mice [29].

Activation of the other isoform PKCβ in endothelial cells induces endothelin 1 expression and enhances VEGF action, increasing vascular endothelial permeability and endothelial dysfunction [27]. Clinical trials using a selective inhibitor of PKCβ ruboxistaurin that ameliorated retinal hemodynamic abnormalities in diabetic patients have not yielded very promising results; further additional clinical trials are needed using inhibitors of the PKCδ isoform.

Glycation and Advanced Glycation End Products

Glycation is defined as the no enzymatic reaction between glucose and reducing sugars with amino groups of proteins, lipids, or nucleic acids. This reaction is promoted under hyperglycemia, oxidative stress, or aging and alters the structure and function of macromolecules.

Glycation begins with the nonenzymatic reaction between aldehyde groups of glucose with amino groups in macromolecules forming first the reversible Schiff base adducts, which are rearranged to more stable, covalently bound Amadori products. Over days to weeks, early glycation products undergo further reactions such as rearrangements and dehydration to become irreversibly cross-linked, fluorescent derivatives called advanced glycation end products (AGEs), such as carboxymethyl lysine (CML), carboxyethyl lysine, pentosidine, or pyrraline derived from proteins, and N(2)-carboxyethyl-2′-deoxyguanosine (CEdG) derived from DNA [10]. AGEs are also generated in highly heated and processed foods and can be obtained from the diet.

AGEs are accumulated in several tissues of diabetic patients or experimental animals including microvasculature, aorta, retina, kidney, pancreas, colon, or skin [30, 31]. The plasma concentration of HbA1c, the Amadori adduct of the N-terminal valine of the hemoglobin β-chain, is used as a long-term biomarker of glycemic control in clinical practice; there is a linear relationship between HbA1c and mean blood glucose; however, HbA1c reflects the average glucose over ~120 days, the mean lifetime of the erythrocyte. Plasma, serum, and urinary levels of AGEs are correlated with the severity of complications in diabetic patients [32–34].

AGEs directly affect the function of macromolecules; for example, nucleotide AGEs are associated with DNA single-strand breaks and increased mutation frequencies. Also AGEs bind with AGE-binding receptors (RAGE). RAGE is a multi-ligand cell surface protein, expressed by endothelial cells, monocytes/macrophages, smooth muscle cells, neurons, podocytes, cardiomyocytes, adipocytes, podocytes, lung epithelial cells, and some cancer cells. The binding of AGEs with RAGE leads to the generation of oxidative stress, inducing proliferative, migratory, inflammatory, thrombotic, and fibrotic reactions in a variety of cells, which leads to alterations associated with diabetic vascular complications [5, 35]. Enhanced production of O^{2-} induced by hyperglycemia in vascular endothelial cells is linked with the production of AGEs and the expression of its receptor. Also, elevated levels of AGEs induce the expression of its receptor amplifying the AGE signaling [36]. The generation of ROS induced by AGEs-RAGE interaction is primarily mediated by the activation of NADPH oxidase, and further, the ROS production can be amplified in the mitochondria.

The fibrotic action of AGEs in renal and vascular cells is mediated by TGFβ-dependent and TGFβ-independent mechanisms, both are dependent on AGEs-RAGE interaction; in the first case, the expression of TGFβ is induced and TGFβ leads to the activation of the transcription factors Smads, which induce expression of pro-fibrotic proteins (ECM proteins, TGFβ receptor 1 or TGFβR1, connective tissue growth factor or CTGF, and PAI-1). In the second case, Smads are activated secondary to the activation of the ERK/p38 mitogen-activated protein kinases (MAPK) signaling pathway [37, 38].

The activation of RAGE also has been associated with sustained activation of the transcription factor NFκB (nuclear factor kappa B), resulting initially from the degradation of its inhibitor IkB and the translocation of NFκB to the nucleus and chronically by NFκB increased de novo synthesis [39].

The signaling mechanism induced by RAGE activation begins with the interaction of its highly charged cytoplasmic domain with the formin homology domain of diaphanous 1 (DAPH1). DAPH1 is required for RAGE signaling, which is blocked by the knockdown of the D*iaph1* gene. DAPH1 is a cytoplasmic actin-binding protein and after the activation of RAGE signaling leads to the activation of several effectors such as Rho GTPases (Rac 1 Cdc 42, and RHOA) and others. Rho GTPases are associated with actin cytoskeleton dynamics and the induction of cell migration in cancer and smooth muscle cells [5, 40]. Rac 1 also conducts the activation of NADPH oxidase and oxidative stress.

Recently, RAGE-DIAPH1 interaction has been considered therapeutic targets, and small molecule inhibitors of this interaction suppress the induction of migration and production of inflammatory cytokines by RAGE ligands in cultured smooth muscle cells and TH1 macrophage-like cells [41].

In addition, there are two forms of soluble RAGE: one derived from proteolytic processing of the membrane receptor or soluble RAGE (sRAGE) and another derived by alternative splicing or endogenous soluble RAGE (esRAGE).

Nuclear Factor Kappa B (NFκB)

The NFκB family of transcription factors regulates the expression of proteins involved in cell proliferation and survival, inflammation, and immune and oxidative stress responses. In physiological conditions, NFκB is induced in an adaptive response to maintain homeostasis; however, the sustained activation of NFκB is thought to have a central role in the pathogenesis of several chronic diseases including diabetes and their complications. NFκB induces the expression of several genes as a response to stressful stimuli like oxidative stress, hyperglycemia, and inflammation. The activation of NFκB is induced by a variety of stimuli including free reactive oxygen species, AGEs, pro-inflammatory cytokines, oxidized low-density lipoproteins, free fatty acids, and bacterial and viral antigens. When NFκB is not activated, it is located in the cytoplasm, forming a complex with its inhibitor IkB (inhibitor of NFκB); after the activation of the upstream signal, the inhibitor is phosphorylated by the IkB kinase (IKK) and degraded through the ubiquitin system. As a consequence, NFκB is released and translocated into the nucleus, where it activates the expression of target genes. The principal regulatory step in the activation of NFκB is the phosphorylation and activation of IKK. NFκB regulates the expression of pro-inflammatory proteins, including adhesion molecules in endothelial cells such as intracellular cell adhesion molecule (ICAM) and vascular cell adhesion molecule (VCAM), cytokines (TNFα, IL-1β), and chemokines. NFκB signaling is a potential target for therapeutic intervention, and several inhibitors of NFκB activation and signaling have been developed.

Dicarbonyl Stress, Methylglyoxal, and Endogenous Glycation

Levels of reactive aldehydes like methylglyoxal, glyoxal, and 3-deoxyglucosone are elevated in diabetes mellitus. Methylglyoxal has been related to diabetic complications for its ability to induce insulin and vascular dysfunction and to cause neuropathic pain because its generation is induced by chronic hyperglycemia. Also, its plasma concentration is elevated in diabetic patients [42]. Methylglyoxal is an α-dicarbonyl and might be the most important reactive aldehyde in diabetes and its complications. Methylglyoxal is formed as a by-product of glycolysis by fragmentation of triose phosphates accumulated in glycolysis and also is derived from the catabolism of threonine and ketone bodies, lipid peroxidation, and degradation of glycated macromolecules.

The accumulation of methylglyoxal and similar compounds also depends on their lower detoxification by the glyoxalase system. This system catalyzes the detoxification of reactive dicarbonyls in the cytoplasm, providing the principal defense against dicarbonyl glycation. The efficiency of this system is reduced by chronic hyperglycemia, because the rate-limiting enzyme, glyoxalase 1 (Glo1), is down-regulated in a high-glucose environment [12]. Glyoxalase 1 down-regulation is induced by RAGE signaling and the pro-inflammatory activation of NFκB [12]; in this case, the action of NFκB is mediated by the non-transcriptional inhibition of the antioxidant response [43].

Methylglyoxal through the glycation reaction modifies proteins and nucleic acid, being the precursor of endogenous AGEs, including arginine-derived hydroimidazolones and deoxyguanosine-derived imidazopurinones, and also induces apoptosis in vascular cells fomenting endothelial dysfunction and the progression of vascular complications including atherosclerosis [44].

Recently, it was described that the plasma concentrations of methylglyoxal and other oxo-aldehydes (glyoxal and 3-deoxyglucosone) are enhanced after carbohydrate load in type 2 diabetes, which was associated with increased risk of diabetic complications induced by elevations of postprandial glycemia [45].

NADH Overproduction or Reductive Stress

During hyperglycemia, the uptake of glucose increases in non-insulin-dependent tissues, leading to a high level of glucose metabolism as glucose entry into the cells is not limited by insulin deficiency. The increased flux of metabolites in glycolysis and the citric acid cycle in the mitochondria leads to high production of NADH, a coenzyme that receives electrons derived from oxidative degradation of glucose and provides electrons to the electron transport chain, leading to the formation of ATP and oxygen reduction. The NADH/NAD$^+$ imbalance is accentuated also by the production of NADH in the activated polyol pathway and by the consumption of NAD$^+$ by the nuclear enzyme poly ADP-ribose polymerase 1 (PARP-1) that uses NAD$^+$ as substrate.

The redox imbalance of NADH/NAD$^+$ causes initially reductive stress or pseudohypoxic stress that leads to oxidative stress. The excess of NADH promotes oxidative stress because the overflow of electrons in the electron transfer chain leads to leaking of electrons and partial reduction of oxygen with increased production of O^{2-} and other reactive oxygen species [3, 4]. Accordingly, oxidative damage triggered by redox imbalance might be a major factor contributing to the development of diabetic complications, and the prevention of NADH/NAD$^+$ redox imbalance could provide further insights for the design of novel antidiabetic strategies.

Oxidative Stress

As we discussed before, the electron overflow in the electron transport chain in non-insulin-dependent tissue under a hyperglycemic microenvironment leads to electron leaking and O^{2-} production in the mitochondria [3, 4]. The excessive production of ROS during diabetes overwhelms endogenous antioxidant defense mechanisms causing an imbalance in the production of ROS and nonenzymatic and enzymatic antioxidant mechanisms in the body, which ultimately leads to oxidative stress.

Additionally, in the production of ROS in the mitochondria, other sources of ROS have been described in diabetic condition, including NADPH oxidase, xanthine oxidase, and uncoupled eNOS, with NADPH oxidases being of special importance. There are several isoforms of O^{2-}-producing NADPH oxidase in the endothelium, smooth muscle cells, and adventitia of the vascular wall [46]. The activation and upregulation of NADPH oxidases are induced by PKCβ and PKCδ, AGEs-RAGE interaction, and inflammatory cytokines (TNFα), all of them considered as promoters of diabetic complications. NADPH oxidase is a multiprotein complex associated with the membrane.

Enhanced ROS levels induce oxidative modification of macromolecules, including lipids in the membranes (lipid peroxidation), enzymes, and nucleic acids altering their functions and cell integrity. As products of lipid peroxidation, malondialdehyde and 4-hydroxy 2-nonenals (4-HNE) are formed; when ROS react with DNA, 8-dihydro-8-oxo-2′-deoxyguanosine (8-OxodG) is produced and is removed during oxidized DNA repair and excreted in the urine. These compounds have been used as markers of oxidative stress. The highly reactive 4-HNE form covalent adducts with nucleophilic functional groups in proteins, nucleic acids, and membrane altering their functions and causing cytotoxicity or modulating a variety of signaling processes. At physiological or low concentration, 4-HNE induces cell survival or antioxidant response, becoming cytostatic and cytotoxic at higher levels. The signaling action of 4-HNE is mediated by transcription factors sensible to stress, including NFκB, nuclear factor erythroid 2-related factor 2 (Nrf2), and activating protein-1 (AP-1) [47].

Oxidative modifications of proteins (carbonylation, intermolecular dityrosine cross-linking, thiol oxidation, etc.) lead to the formation of advanced oxidized protein products (AOPPs), which induce pro-inflammatory and pro-fibrotic processes and cell death associated with progression of nephropathy and atherosclerosis. AOPPs induce inflammation by the activation of neutrophils and monocytes through NFκB activation mediated by NADPH oxidase [48]. Some actions of AOPPs are induced by their binding to RAGE in endothelial cells and podocytes [49].

DNA damage caused by oxidative stress leads to the over-activation of PARP-1. PARP-1 transfers ADP-ribose from NAD^+, leading to the formation of poly ADP-ribose (PAR) and nicotinamide; the decrease in NAD^+ and ATP levels causes energy failure and cell necrosis [3, 4]. The mechanism of cell death induced by PARP has been recently elucidated; PARP induces the release of apoptosis-inducing factor (AIF) from the mitochondria, and AIF binds to macrophage inhibitory factor (MIF), a protein with a recently discovered activity of nuclease; this complex is translocated to the nucleus, resulting in DNA fragmentation and cell death, through a caspase-independent type of cell death, designated parthanatos [50].

The activation of PARP also conduces to an inflammatory condition, since PARP-1 promotes the expression of pro-inflammatory factors, including TNFα and IL-1β, and the inhibition of PARP is a promising strategy for the prevention and treatment of diabetic complications. The inhibition of PARP ameliorates cardiovascular complications and nephropathy in an animal model of type 2 diabetes, preventing oxidative stress, inflammation, and renal fibrosis [51, 52]. It also attenuates the development of retinopathy in streptozotocin-induced diabetic rats [53] and prevents the apoptosis of cultured cardiomyocytes under high glucose concentration [54].

Although supplementation with antioxidants has been considered in the treatment of diabetic complications, interventional trials with supplemented antioxidants have failed to show significant beneficial effects. Conversely, the use of natural foods shows promising results, and the employment of a balanced "Mediterranean diet" helps in the control of free radical production and increases intracellular antioxidant defenses [55]. Early intensive glucose control is still the best strategy to avoid oxidative stress and its associated diabetic complications.

Altered Lipid Metabolism, Dyslipidemia, and Accumulation of Cytotoxic Lipids

Diabetic dyslipidemia leads to changes in systemic and local lipid metabolism that drive the pro-inflammatory and pro-apoptotic cellular changes typical of diabetic complications. Abnormalities in metabolism, accumulation, and plasma profile of lipids have been associated with insulin resistance and vascular complications [6], and several studies support the potential benefits of lipid-lowering diets and drugs, such as Mediterranean diet, omega-3 fatty acids, fibrates, and statins, for the prevention and treatment of vascular complications. A positive association between high levels of total cholesterol, low-density lipoproteins (LDL), and LDL/high-density lipoproteins (HDL) ratio and vascular complications are well established. Recently the profile of plasma ceramides has been proposed as risk factors and prognosis indica-

tors of predisposition and progression diabetes mellitus and its complications. Thus, the circulating levels of ceramide containing C16, C18, or C24 acyl chains display a superior predictive value for future adverse cardiovascular events (myocardial infarction and stroke) and plaque instability than LDL cholesterol.

Lipids and their transporting lipoproteins like LDL and HDL are glycated and/or oxidized during chronic hyperglycemia and oxidative stress. These modified lipoproteins promoted endothelial dysfunction and vascular injury due to the activation of RAGE receptors [56] and have cytotoxic, pro-inflammatory, and pro-atherogenic effects; for example, they activate the release of pro-inflammatory cytokines by retinal glial Muller cells and are cytotoxic to retinal capillary pericytes and retinal pigment epithelial cells promoting diabetic retinopathy.

Dyslipidemia and increased levels of plasmatic free fatty acids (FFA) lead to lipid peroxidation and the increased uptake of FFA in the cells. Intracellularly fatty acids are oxidized in the mitochondria producing acetyl-CoA or are used in the synthesis of di- and triacylglycerols, glycerophospholipids, and ceramide, the precursor of sphingolipids. Diacylglycerol can activate PKC, triacylglycerols can be accumulated in hepatocytes or cardiomyocytes causing steatosis and functional alterations, and ceramides have been associated with diabetic complications. The spectrum of sphingolipid actions in diabetes shifts from protective very-long chain (VLC) ceramides ($C \geq 26$) to pro-inflammatory and pro-apoptotic short-chain (SC) ceramides ($C \leq 24$). SC ceramides are mainly produced from sphingomyelins by acid sphingomyelinase (ASM), whose level increases in tissues and blood during diabetes.

SC ceramides promote intrinsic apoptosis by the increase of mitochondrial outer membrane permeability through the formation of protein-permeable ceramide channels that allow the release of cytochrome c in the cytoplasm. During diabetes, ceramides are accumulated and induce apoptosis in renal mesangial and tubular epithelial cells, contributing to diabetic nephropathy; also they induce apoptosis of retinal pericytes and contribute to the breakdown of the blood-retinal barriers and the development of retinopathy [6, 57].

Inflammatory Stress

Inflammation is induced by oxidative stress and diverse factors and is a common pathophysiological characteristic in many diseases, and diabetes is associated with a chronic pro-inflammatory condition, which is evidenced by increased serum levels of pro-inflammatory cytokines (TNFα) in diabetic patients and experimental animals [52]. Additionally, the transcription factor NFκB is activated in circulating lymphocytes of type 2 diabetic patients [58] and in a variety of tissues of diabetic animals (kidney, heart) [51, 52]. NFκB is activated by oxidative stress, TNFα, or angiotensin II (Ang II) and regulates the expression of a variety of inflammatory-related genes, including pro-inflammatory cytokines like TNFα, interleukin (IL) 1β (IL-1β), IL-6, and monocyte chemoattractant protein 1 (MCP-1); additionally, it induces the expression of cyclooxygenase-2 (COX-2), the enzyme that controls the synthesis of pro-inflammatory eicosanoids.

Ang II is a key mediator of the renin-angiotensin system (RAS), whose activation is thought to be a major mechanism underlying inflammation in diabetic complications. Ang II induces the activation of NFκB and the synthesis and release of pro-inflammatory mediators, primarily cytokines TNFα, IL-1β, and IL-6. TNFα induces macrophage recruitment and synthesis and secretion of IL-6. IL-6 stimulates the production and secretion of C-reactive protein (CRP), a key risk factor for cardiovascular diseases.

TNFα induces the expression of MCP-1 and cellular adhesion molecules in the endothelium, such as intracellular adhesion molecule-1 (ICAM-1) and vascular cell adhesion molecule-1 (VCAM-1), which leads to recruitment of leukocytes to the surface of endothelium, contributing to the endothelial dysfunction. Further leukocytes migrate across the endothelium, causing endothelial damage and inflammation in the kidney and destruction of the blood-retinal barrier, characteristics of nephropathy and retinopathy. IL-1β induces the expression of inducible nitric oxide synthase (iNOS), causing overproduction of NO, which forms peroxynitrite when it reacts with O^{2-}, amplifying the inflammatory response and producing nitrosoactive stress.

TNFα and IL-1β can induce apoptosis directly or indirectly in cardiomyocytes and neurons, contributing to cardiac dysfunction, retinopathy, and neuropathy. Additionally, TNFα is associated with cardiomyocyte hypertrophy and cardiac fibrosis, leading to heart failure.

TGFβ and Epithelial Mesenchymal Transition in Diabetic Nephropathy (Fig. 49.4)

One of the tissue changes of diabetic nephropathy is the excessive deposition of extracellular matrix (ECM) in the

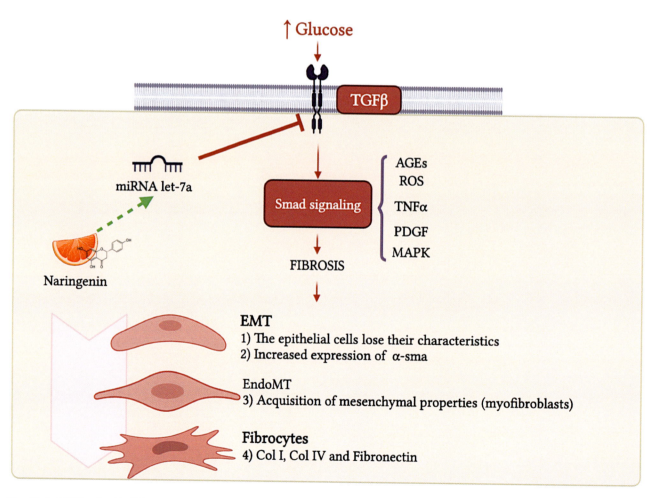

Fig. 49.4 TGFβ and epithelial mesenchymal transition in diabetic nephropathy

glomerulus and the tubular interstitium associated with the development of glomerulosclerosis and tubule interstitial fibrosis. The major source of renal ECM is myofibroblasts, whose number is increased in diabetic nephropathy. These cells are originated from different resources including activated renal fibroblasts, pericytes, epithelial-to-mesenchymal transition (EMT), endothelial-to-mesenchymal transition (EndoMT), bone marrow-derived cells, and fibrocytes [59].

EMT is one of the sources of matrix-generating fibroblast. During EMT, epithelial cells (proximal tubular cells and podocytes) lose their epithelial characteristics (downregulation of epithelial adhesion protein, E-cadherin) and acquired mesenchymal properties originating from myofibroblasts [59, 60]. During the formation of myofibroblasts, the expression of α-smooth muscle actin (α-SMA) is induced. TGFβ is a major driver for renal fibrosis, and the inhibition of TGFβ signaling significantly reduces renal fibrosis, ameliorating kidney damage and dysfunction. TGFβ induces EMT, EndoMT, and synthesis of EMC proteins (collagen I, collagen IV, and fibronectin). The promotion of fibrosis by TGFβ is mediated by the activation of the transcription factors Smads; therefore, TGFβ/Smads signaling is considered a potential therapeutic target in the prevention and treatment of renal fibrosis [59, 61]. However, Smads signaling also can be activated for other factors, including AGEs, ROS, TNFα, platelet-derived growth factor (PDGF), MAPK, and chemokines [38, 59].

Recently, it was found that the microRNA, let-7a, negatively regulates the expression of TGFβR1, preventing the induction of fibrosis by hyperglycemia on kidney mesangial cell, and naringenin (4,5,7-trihydroxy flavanone), a flavanone compound extracted from citrus fruits, upregulates let-7a and prevents the ECM deposition in the kidney of diabetic rats [62].

Endothelial Dysfunction and Nitric Oxide Deficiency

The endothelium lines the inner surface of blood vessels and modulates vascular function and structure. It controls vascular morphology, tone, permeability, inflammation, and thrombosis by the production of a variety of mediators including vasodilators (NO and prostacyclin) and vasoconstrictors (endothelin and thromboxane). This tissue is a key in the development of diabetic complications. Endothelial dysfunction is induced in diabetes by the abnormal glucose concentration and the increase of AGEs linked with plasma lipoproteins. High glucose, the activation of RAGE by AGEs-lipoproteins, and inflammatory cytokines lead to an inflammatory reaction in the vascular wall, endothelial oxidative stress, and NO deficiency, which play a major role in inducing endothelial apoptosis. Endothelial dysfunction alters the control of vascular properties by endothelium toward reduced vasodilatation and a pro-inflammatory and pro-thrombotic state [56, 63].

Reduced vasodilatation is associated with NO deficiency or reduced availability of NO, which is induced by different factors, including reduced synthesis and the reaction of NO with O^{2-}-forming peroxynitrite ($ONOO^-$) in hyperglycemia and oxidative stress conditions. Although the enzyme that synthesizes NO in the endothelium, the eNOS, is upregulated by oxidative stress (hydrogen peroxide, product of the dismutation of superoxide) or PKC [64], its essential cofactor (6R-)5,6,7,8-tetrahydrobiopterin (BH4) is oxidized by peroxynitrite. When this cofactor is oxidized, the reaction of eNOS is uncoupled, and ROS are produced instead of NO, accentuating the vascular oxidative stress [63]. Inhibitors of PKC reduce eNOS expression levels in vascular endothelium. Additionally, there is a deficiency in the substrate of NOS L-arginine due to the increase of the enzyme arginase in plasma and tissues; arginase degrades L-arginine to urea and L-ornithine [65].

Since reduced bioactivity of nitric oxide (NO) is present in diabetes, some strategies are being considered to restore NO availability; one is the promotion of NO synthesis by the supplementation of L-arginine or L-citrulline; the former is the precursor of NO production by eNOS, and its plasma concentration is decreased by diabetes, whereas L-citrulline is a neutral alpha-amino acid, found in high concentrations in watermelon. L-citrulline is an inhibitor of arginase and prevents the degradation of L-arginine; also it can be recycled to L-arginine in the mitochondria by the urea cycle; therefore L-citrulline leads to increased L-arginine bioavailability. Another strategy is to supply inorganic nitrate abundant in green leaf vegetables and beetroots, which provide NO by an unconventional via.

Oral L-arginine supplementation has been inefficient to restore NO because it is removed from the intestinal tract and liver, which does not occur with L-citrulline, and its supplementation is effective at increasing blood L-arginine and endothelial NO synthesis. L-citrulline at a dose of 2000 mg/day for 1 month increased NO levels and decreased arginase levels in the plasma of T2DM patients [65]. L-citrulline can be beneficial for diabetic patients considering these data and that L-citrulline has shown an antihypertensive action in adult patients and, in preclinical assays, L-citrulline protects the endothelial function [65]. The supplements of nitrates ameliorate or prevent the risk of diabetes and its complications in animal models; nitrate is used as a precursor for NO synthesis through serial reductions of nitrate by the nitrate-nitrite-NO pathway. This pathway acts as a backup system when NOS system is compromised during diabetes and other pathological conditions [66]. However, in human beings, nitrate-nitrite-NO pathway supplements have had poor results and probably required ascorbic acid complementation [67]. The protective action of NO has been attributed to the inhibition of NADPH oxidase activity mediated by the heme oxygenase-1 (HO-1)-dependent antioxidant mechanism, preventing the vascular oxidative stress and endothelial dysfunction [68].

When the endothelium is damaged, soluble forms of the adhesion proteins ICAM (sICAM-1), VCAM (sVCAM), and E-selectin are released from the endothelial surface, and its plasma concentration is evaluated as markers of endothelial cell dysfunction [56]. Plasma sICAM-1 concentration is increased in diabetic albuminuric patients before signals of nephropathy. Plasma ICAM-1 concentrations are negatively correlated with the vasodilatory function of the endothelium. Because oxidative stress contributes to endothelial dysfunction, a positive correlation was found between plasmatic concentrations of advanced oxidized protein products (AOPPs) and sICAM [69].

Anaerobic Metabolism and Neuropathic Pain

Nowadays, a link between anaerobic metabolism and neuropathic pain has been established. The pyruvate dehydrogenase kinase (PDK)-lactic acid axis is a critical link that connects metabolic reprogramming and neuropathic pain. Pyruvate dehydrogenase (PDH) catalyzes the irreversible oxidative decarboxylation of pyruvate to acetyl-CoA, and its activity is lost when is phosphorylated by PDK in anaerobic conditions. PDKs are upregulated in the tissues of patients and rodents with diabetes. A nociceptive role for lactate is recently recognized; lactate is the predominant end product of anaerobic glycolysis. Some tissues and organs like dorsal root ganglion are exposed to a low-oxygen condition (ischemia) during diabetes; in this condition, PDKs 2 and 4 are upregulated; these enzymes inactive PDH by phosphorylation; therefore pyruvate is transformed to lactate by lactate dehydrogenase, and the accumulation of lactate induces the expression of pain-related ion channels and neuroinflammation, leading to pain hypersensitivity and diabetic neuropathy. Suppression of *Pdk2 and Pdk4* expression attenuated the hyperglycemia-induced pain hypersensitivity and induced partial resistance to the diabetes-induced loss of peripheral nerve structure and function in streptozotocin-induced diabetic mice [70].

Concluding Remarks

- The pathophysiological mechanism leading to vascular diabetic complications includes the metabolic, oxidative, and inflammatory alterations induced by hyperglycemia.
- Increased metabolic flux of glucose leads to activation of polyol and hexosamine pathways and accumulation of trioses, dicarbonyl aldehydes, and diacylglycerols, together with $NADH/NAD^+$ redox imbalance, oxidative stress, and PKC activation.
- ROS, peroxynitrites, lipid peroxidation, and glycation cause chemical modification of macromolecules, leading to the loss of their function, nucleic acid alterations, and apoptosis.
- The interaction of AGEs with its receptor RAGE, oxidative stress, and Ang II activates different signaling pathways and transcription factors, including NFκB, which induce the expression of pro-inflammatory, pro-fibrotic, and pro-thrombotic proteins, such as TNFα, VEGF, TGFβ, and PAI-1.
- All these processes lead to endothelial dysfunction and tissue alterations (inflammation, hypertrophy, fibrosis, apoptosis, among others), as well as organ dysfunction characteristics of neuropathy, retinopathy, neuropathy, and diabetic cardiovascular disease.

Questions and Answers

1. Endothelial dysfunction is considered as the initial step in the development of vascular complications and is induced by
   (a) Low bioavailability of nitric oxide
   (b) Uncoupled of the endothelial nitric oxide synthase
   (c) **Oxidative stress and TNFα**
   (d) Glycolysis
   (e) ATP

   TNFα induces the expression of MCP-1 and cellular adhesion molecules in the endothelium, which leads to the recruitment of leukocytes to the surface of endothelium, initiating endothelial dysfunction. Oxidative stress induces the production of TNFα and ROS reacts with NO, reducing the availability of NO as a consequence of endothelial dysfunction and the reduced availability of reduced BH4, a coenzyme required for NO synthesis.

2. The activation of PKCδ caused by hyperglycemia is dependent on
   (a) Epithelial mesenchymal transition
   (b) **Increased synthesis of diacylglycerols induced by the accumulation of trioses**
   (c) Release of the apoptosis inducing factor (AIF) from the mitochondria
   (d) Increased expression of NADPH oxidase
   (e) Direct action of TGFβ

   Diacylglycerols accumulated in the membrane activate PKCβ and PKCδ; diacylglycerols are produced from trioses accumulated during glycolysis, due to the enzyme glyceraldehyde 3-phosphate dehydrogenase inactivated by oxidative stress and the low availability of its coenzyme NAD+ as a consequence of the NADH/NAD+ imbalance.

3. The fibrosis of renal glomerulus associated with diabetic nephropathy is due to
   (a) **Increased synthesis, release, and action of TGFβ**
   (b) Increased vascular permeability
   (c) Depuration of methylglyoxal
   (d) Increased activity of antioxidant enzymes
   (e) Reduced production of Ang II

   TGFβ is a major driver for renal fibrosis, and the inhibition of TGFβ signaling significantly reduces renal fibrosis. TGFβ induces the synthesis of extracellular matrix proteins. Renal fibrosis also can be induced by AGEs, TNFα, PDGF, and chemokines in a TGFβ-dependent and TGFβ-independent manner.

4. The role of the activation of the polyol pathway in the development of diabetic complications is directly due to
   (a) Formation of diacylglycerol and activation of PKC
   (b) Formation of AGEs and chemical alteration of macromolecules
   (c) Induction of the expression of TGFβ and fibrosis
   (d) **Osmotic stress by the accumulation of sorbitol and NADH/NAD+ imbalance**
   (e) Induction of the production of ROS by NADPH oxidase

   In the polyol pathway, sorbitol is accumulated as an intermediate product, because the cell membrane is impermeable to sorbitol and prevents its efflux. Sorbitol accumulation induces osmotic imbalance, water intake, and cellular death. In the second step of this pathway catalyzed by sorbitol dehydrogenase, NAD+ is reduced to NADH, contributing to NADH/NAD+ imbalance.

5. The role of the activation of the hexosamine pathway in the development of diabetic complications is mediated by
   (a) Induction of signaling by activation of RAGE
   (b) Formation of diacylglycerol and activation of PKC
   (c) Induction of the expression of TGFβ and fibrosis

(d) Osmotic stress by the accumulation of sorbitol and NADH/NAD+ imbalance
(e) **Formation of UDP-N-acetylglucosamine and O-GlcNAcylation of proteins**

Overproduced fructose 6-phosphate during glycolysis is used by the hexosamine pathway to the production of UDP-GlcNAc; the N-acetylglucosamine of this compound is transferred during O-linked glycosylation of proteins (O-GlcNAcylation), altering their functions and inducing the expression of TGFβ, PAI-1, and VEGF-A.

6. The role of glycation in the development of diabetic complications is due to
   (a) **Production of AGEs and activation of RAGE**
   (b) Formation of diacylglycerol and activation of PKC
   (c) Induction of the expression of TGFβ and fibrosis
   (d) Osmotic stress by the accumulation of sorbitol and NADH/NAD+ imbalance
   (e) Formation of UDP-N-acetylglucosamine and O-GlcNAcylation of proteins.

   The effects of AGEs are mediated by the chemical modification of macromolecules or by its interaction with their receptor RAGE. The binding of AGEs with RAGE leads to the generation of oxidative stress, inducing proliferative, migratory, inflammatory, thrombotic, and fibrotic reactions, which leads to alterations associated with diabetic vascular complications.

7. Dicarbonyl stress is associated with
   (a) Accumulation of sorbitol
   (b) Accumulation of diacylglycerols and activation of PKC
   (c) **Accumulation of glyoxal and methylglyoxal**
   (d) Production of pro-inflammatory cytokines
   (e) Production of AGEs

   Glyoxal and methylglyoxal are α-dicarbonyls and reactive aldehydes, produced as by-products of glycolysis by fragmentation of triose phosphates. These aldehydes react with proteins and nucleic acid (glycation), producing endogenous AGEs, and also induce apoptosis in vascular cells fomenting endothelial dysfunction and progression of vascular complications.

8. In a microenvironment with an excessive concentration of glucose, ROS are produced by
   (a) Aldose reductase and sorbitol dehydrogenase
   (b) **Electron transport chain and NADPH oxidase**
   (c) Glutamine-fructose-6-phosphate amidotransferase
   (d) Glyceraldehyde 3-phosphate dehydrogenase
   (e) Glucose 6-phosphate dehydrogenase

   In an excessive glucose environment, the principal sources of ROS are the electron transfer chain in the mitochondria and NADPH oxidase. ROS can be produced also by other sources such as uncoupled nitric oxide synthase and xanthine oxidase.

9. Oxidative stress contributes to vascular complications by
   (a) Activation of the transcription factor NFκB and production of TNFα
   (b) Inhibition of the glycolytic enzyme glyceraldehyde 3-phosphate dehydrogenase (GAPDH)
   (c) Oxidative modification of macromolecules
   (d) Induction of apoptosis by DNA damage
   (e) **a, b, c, and d**

   Enhanced ROS levels induce oxidative modification of macromolecules altering their functions and cell integrity. DNA damage leads to NADH/NAD imbalance and apoptosis or necrosis. Oxidation and NADH/NAD imbalance inhibit the activity of GAPDH. Also, ROS induce several signaling pathways, including the activation of NFκB and the production of TNFα.

10. TNFα contributes to diabetic complications by
    (a) NFκB activation
    (b) Induction of NADPH oxidase expression
    (c) Promoting leukocyte recruitment at the endothelial surface
    (d) Induces apoptosis in some cells
    (e) **a, b, c, and d**

    TNFα contributes to vascular complication through multiple actions, including the induction of NADPH oxidase and increased ROS production and activation of NFκB, a transcription factor that induces the expression of pro-inflammatory cytokines and MCP-1. Also, it induces the expression of adhesion molecules promoting leukocyte adhesion at the endothelial surface.

Suggested/Further Reading

1. Toma L, Stancu CS, Sima AV. Endothelial dysfunction in diabetes Is aggravated by glycated lipoproteins; novel molecular therapies. Biomedicines. 2021;9(1):18. https://doi.org/10.3390/biomedicines9010018.

   This review analyzes the role of hyperglycemia and glycated lipoproteins in the development of endothelial cell dysfunction (ECD) and the progression of diabetic vascular complications. The participation of dyslipidemia, oxidative and inflammatory stress, and epigenetic risk factors are highlighted, along with the specific mechanisms connecting them, as well as the new promising therapies to alleviate ECD in diabetes.

2. Egaña-Gorroño L, López-Díez R, Yepuri G, Ramirez LS et al. Receptor for advanced glycation end products (RAGE) and mechanisms and therapeutic opportunities in diabetes and cardiovascular disease: insights from human subjects and animal models. Front Cardiovasc Med. 2020;7:37. doi: 10.3389/fcvm.2020.00037.

   The central role of RAGE in diabetes, obesity, and cardiovascular diseases is discussed, considering its multiple ligands, its signaling mechanism, its role in macrovascular complications of diabetes, and finally the use of RAGE antagonists in preclinical and clinical studies.

3. Masaki N, Feng B, Bretón-Romero R, Inagaki E, Weisbrod RM, Fetterman JL, Hamburg NM. O-GlcNAcylation mediates glucose-induced alterations in endothelial cell phenotype in human diabetes mellitus. J Am Heart Assoc. 2020;9(12):e014046. doi: 10.1161/JAHA.119.014046.

   The linking of O-GlcNAcylation to the vasculature dysfunction in humans is analyzed in endothelial cells obtained by biopsy from a forearm vein of patients with T2DM. This study establishes that O-GlcNAc modification of proteins is implicated in the glucose-induced impairment of endothelial nitric oxide synthase activation in endothelial cells from patients with T2DM. It is suggested that O-GlcNAc protein modification may be used in the diagnosis and as a treatment target for vascular dysfunction in T2DM.

4. Qi W, Keenan HA, Li Q, Ishikado A, Kannt A, Sadowski T, et al. Pyruvate kinase M2 activation may protect against the progression of diabetic glomerular pathology and mitochondrial dysfunction. Nat Med. 2017;23(6):753-762. doi: 10.1038/nm.4328.

   This is the first proteomic analysis of glomeruli from patients with long-duration type 1 diabetes mellitus but protected from diabetic nephropathy, which allows for the identification of protective factors against the toxic effects of hyperglycemia.

5. Nigro C, Leone A, Raciti GA, Longo M, Mirra P, Formisano P et al. Methylglyoxal-glyoxalase 1 balance: the root of vascular damage. Int J Mol Sci. 2017 Jan 18;18(1). doi: 10.3390/ijms18010188.

   This review describes the metabolism of methylglyoxal and the molecular mechanism of dicarbonyl stress in the induction of endothelial dysfunction and progression of vascular damage and microvascular diabetic complications.

6. Bernardi S, Michelli A, Zuolo G, Candido R, Fabris B. Update on RAAS modulation for the treatment of diabetic cardiovascular disease. J Diabetes Res. 2016;2016:8917578.

   The role of the renin-angiotensin-aldosterone system in diabetic cardiovascular disease is analyzed, with an emphasis on the modulation of this system as the first-line therapy for the prevention of the development of cardiovascular disease in diabetic patients.

7. Román-Pintos LM, Villegas-Rivera G, Rodríguez-Carrizalez AD, Miranda-Díaz AG, Cardona-Muñoz EG. Diabetic polyneuropathy in type 2 diabetes mellitus: inflammation, oxidative stress, and mitochondrial function. J Diabetes Res. 2016;2016:3425617.

This review describes the mechanism of diabetic polyneuropathy, considering inflammation and oxidative stress as the major causes of this complication. Also, it analyzes the risk factors and methods of diagnosis and treatment of diabetic polyneuropathy.

8. Waris S, Winklhofer-Roob BM, Roob JM, Fuchs S, Sourij H, Rabbani N, Thornalley PJ. Increased DNA dicarbonyl glycation and oxidation markers in patients with type 2 diabetes and link to diabetic nephropathy. J Diabetes Res. 2015;2015:915486.

In this study, increased markers of DNA damage by glycation in plasma and urine in patients with type 2 diabetes were detected, which were further increased in patients with diabetic nephropathy.

Glossary

Advanced oxidized protein products (AOPPs) Products of oxidative modifications of proteins by ROS and hypochlorite, derived from the action of myeloperoxidase from activated leukocytes

Dicarbonyl stress Abnormal accumulation of reactive aldehydes like methylglyoxal and 3-deoxyglucosone that leads to endogenous glycation of proteins and DNA, associated with cell and tissue damage in chronic diseases and aging

Endothelial dysfunction Alteration of the regulatory function of the endothelium on the vascular tone and properties that conduce to reduced vasodilatation and a pro-inflammatory or pro-thrombotic state

Glycation The nonenzymatic reaction between glucose and reducing sugars with amino groups of proteins, lipids, or nucleic acids leads to the production of advanced glycation products or AGEs.

Hexosamine signaling pathway Pathway activated in hyperglycemic condition, where fructose-1-phosphate, an intermediate of glycolysis, is used in the formation of UDP-GlcNAc (hexosamine pathway), followed by the O-GlcNAcylation of proteins

Lipid peroxidation Oxidation of polyunsaturated fatty acids by ROS in cellular membranes through free radical chain reactions, with the formation of lipid hydroperoxides as primary products; which may decompose and lead to the formation of reactive lipid electrophiles like 4-hydroxy 2-nonenal

Reductive stress Redox imbalance between NADH and NAD^+ driven by the high metabolic flux in the citric acid cycle and the activation of the polyol pathway and poly ADP-ribose polymerase

Parthanatos Mechanism of caspase-independent type of apoptosis, where the translocation to the nucleus and activity of nucleases like the macrophage inhibitory lead to DNA fragmentation and cell death

References

1. Bailey CJ, Aschner P, Del Prato S, LaSalle J, Ji L, Matthaei S. Global partnership for effective diabetes management. Individualized glycaemic targets and pharmacotherapy in type 2 diabetes. Diab Vasc Dis Res. 2013;10(5):397–409.

2. Saeedi P, Salpea P, Karuranga S, Petersohn I, Malanda B, Gregg EW, Unwin N, Wild SH, Williams R. Mortality attributable to diabetes in 20–79 years old adults, 2019 estimates: results from the international diabetes federation diabetes atlas, 9th edition. Diabetes Res Clin Pract. 2020;162:108086. https://doi.org/10.1016/j.diabres.2020.108086.

3. Song J, Yang X, Yan LJ. Role of pseudohypoxia in the pathogenesis of type 2 diabetes. Hypoxia (Auckl). 2019;7:33–40. https://doi.org/10.2147/HP.S202775.

4. Yan L-J. NADH/NAD^+ redox imbalance and diabetic kidney disease. Biomol Ther. 2021;11(5):730. https://doi.org/10.3390/biom11050730.

5. Egaña-Gorroño L, López-Díez R, Yepuri G, Ramirez LS, Reverdatto S, Gugger PF, Shekhtman A, Ramasamy R, Schmidt AM. Receptor for advanced glycation end products (RAGE) and mechanisms and therapeutic opportunities in diabetes and cardiovascular disease: insights from human subjects and animal models. Front Cardiovasc Med. 2020;7:37. https://doi.org/10.3389/fcvm.2020.00037.

6. Chaurasia B, Summers SA. Ceramides - lipotoxic inducers of metabolic disorders. Trends Endocrinol Metab. 2015;26(10):538–50. https://doi.org/10.1016/j.tem.2015.07.006.

7. Yan LJ. Redox imbalance stress in diabetes mellitus: role of the polyol pathway. Animal Model Exp Med. 2018;1:7–13. https://doi.org/10.1002/ame2.12001.

8. Kumar M, Choudhary S, Singh PK, Silakari O. Addressing selectivity issues of aldose reductase 2 inhibitors for the management of diabetic complications. Future Med Chem. 2020;14:1327–58. https://doi.org/10.4155/fmc-2020-0032.

9. Du XL, Edelstein D, Rossetti L, Fantus IG, Goldberg H, Ziyadeh F, Wu J, Brownlee M. Hyperglycemia-induced mitochondrial superoxide overproduction activates the hexosamine pathway and induces plasminogen activator inhibitor-1 expression by increasing Sp1 glycosylation. Proc Natl Acad Sci U S A. 2000;97(22):12222–6.

10. Yamagishi S, Nakamura N, Suematsu M, Kaseda K, Matsui T. Advanced glycation end products: a molecular target for vascular complications in diabetes. Mol Med. 2015;21(Suppl 1):S32–40.

11. Giacco F, Brownlee M. Oxidative stress and diabetic complications. Circ Res. 2010;107:1058–70.

12. Nigro C, Leone A, Raciti GA, Longo M, Mirra P, Formisano P, et al. Methylglyoxal-glyoxalase 1 balance: the root of vascular damage. Int J Mol Sci. 2017;18(1):188. https://doi.org/10.3390/ijms18010188.

13. Obrosova IG, Minchenko AG, Vasupuram R, White L, et al. Aldose reductase inhibitor fidarestat prevents retinal oxidative stress and vascular endothelial growth factor overexpression in streptozotocin-diabetic rats. Diabetes. 2003;52:864–71.

14. Tang WH, Martin KA, Hwa J. Aldose reductase, oxidative stress, and diabetes mellitus. Front Pharmacol. 2012;3:87.

15. Qi W, Keenan HA, Li Q, Ishikado A, Kannt A, Sadowski T, et al. Pyruvate kinase M2 activation may protect against the progression of diabetic glomerular pathology and mitochondrial dysfunction. Nat Med. 2017;23(6):753–62. https://doi.org/10.1038/nm.4328.

16. Sarikaya M, Yazihan N, Daş Evcimen N. Relationship between aldose reductase enzyme and the signaling pathway of protein kinase C in an in vitro diabetic retinopathy model. Can J Physiol Pharmacol. 2020;98(4):243–51. https://doi.org/10.1139/cjpp-2019-0211.

17. Hallan S, Sharma K. The role of mitochondria in diabetic kidney disease. Curr Diab Rep. 2016;16(7):61. https://doi.org/10.1007/s11892-016-0748-0.

18. Iacobini C, Vitale M, Pesce C, Pugliese G, Menini S. Diabetic complications and oxidative stress: a 20-year voyage back in time and back to the future. Antioxidants (Basel). 2021;10:727. https://doi.org/10.3390/antiox10050727.

19. Peiró C, Romacho T, Azcutia V, Villalobos L, Fernández E, Bolaños JP, et al. Inflammation, glucose, and vascular cell damage: the role of the pentose phosphate pathway. Cardiovasc Diabetol. 2016;15:82.

20. Dagher Z, Park YS, Asnaghi V, Hoehn T, Gerhardinger C, Lorenzi M. Studies of rat and human retinas predict a role for the polyol pathway in human diabetic retinopathy. Diabetes. 2004;53:2404–11.

21. Katakami N, Kaneto H, Takahara M, Matsuoka TA, Imamura K, Ishibashi F, et al. Aldose reductase C-106T gene polymorphism is associated with diabetic retinopathy in Japanese patients with type 2 diabetes. Diabetes Res Clin Pract. 2011;92:e57–60.

22. Brownlee M. The pathobiology of diabetic complications: a unifying mechanism. Diabetes. 2005;54:1615–25.

23. Du X, Matsumura T, Edelstein D, Rossetti L, Zsengeller Z, Szabo C, Brownlee M. Inhibition of GAPDH activity by poly (ADP-ribose) polymerase activates three major pathways of hyperglycemic damage in endothelial cells. J Clin Invest. 2003;112:1049–57.

24. Donovan K, Alekseev O, Qi X, Cho W, Azizkhan-Clifford J. O-GlcNAc modification of transcription factor Sp1 mediates hyperglycemia-induced VEGF-A upregulation in retinal cells. Invest Ophthalmol Vis Sci. 2014;55(12):7862–73.

25. Makino A, Dai A, Han Y, Youssef KD, Wang W, Donthamsetty R, et al. O-GlcNAcase overexpression reverses coronary endothelial cell dysfunction in type 1 diabetic mice. Am J Physiol Cell Physiol. 2015;309(9):C593–9.

26. Masaki N, Feng B, Bretón-Romero R, Inagaki E, Weisbrod RM, Fetterman JL, Hamburg NM. O-GlcNAcylation mediates glucose-induced alterations in endothelial cell phenotype in human diabetes mellitus. J Am Heart Assoc. 2020;9(12):e014046. https://doi.org/10.1161/JAHA.119.014046.

27. Geraldes P, Hiraoka-Yamamoto J, Matsumoto M, Clermont A, Leitges M, Marette A, Aiello LP, Kern TS, King GL. Activation of PKC-delta and SHP-1 by hyperglycemia causes vascular cell apoptosis and diabetic retinopathy. Nat Med. 2009;15:1298–306.

28. Mima A, Kitada M, Geraldes P, Li Q, Matsumoto M, Mizutani K, et al. Glomerular VEGF resistance induced by PKCδ/SHP-1 activation and contribution to diabetic nephropathy. FASEB J. 2012;26(7):2963–74.

29. Khamaisi M, Katagiri S, Keenan H, Park K, Maeda Y, Li Q, et al. PKCδ inhibition normalizes the wound-healing capacity of diabetic human fibroblasts. J Clin Invest. 2016;126(3):837–53.

30. Jaramillo R, Shuck SC, Chan YS, Liu X, Bates SE, Lim PP, Tamae D, Lacoste S, O'Connor TR, Termini J. DNA advanced glycation end products (DNA-AGEs) are elevated in urine and tissue in an animal model of type 2 diabetes. Chem Res Toxicol. 2017;30(2):689–98.

31. Li H, Nakamura S, Miyazaki S, Morita T, Suzuki M, Pischetsrieder M, Niwa T. N 2-carboxyethyl-2′-deoxyguanosine, a DNA glycation marker, in kidneys and aortas of diabetic and uremic patients. Kidney Int. 2006;69(2):388–92.

32. Aso Y, Inukai T, Tayama K, Takemura Y. Serum concentrations of advanced glycation end products are associated with the development of atherosclerosis as well as diabetic microangiopathy in patients with type 2 diabetes. Acta Diabetol. 2000;37:87–92.

33. Aubert CE, Michel PL, Gillery P, Jaisson S, Fonfrede M, Morel F, Hartemann A, Bourron O. Association of peripheral neuropathy with circulating advanced glycation end products, soluble receptor for advanced glycation end products and other risk factors in patients with type 2 diabetes. Diabetes Metab Res Rev. 2014;30(8):679–85.

34. Waris S, Winklhofer-Roob BM, Roob JM, Fuchs S, Sourij H, Rabbani N, Thornalley PJ. Increased DNA dicarbonyl glycation and oxidation markers in patients with type 2 diabetes and link to

diabetic nephropathy. J Diabetes Res. 2015;2015:915486. https://doi.org/10.1155/2015/915486.

35. Ramasamy R, Yan SF, Schmidt AM. Receptor for AGE (RAGE): signaling mechanisms in the pathogenesis of diabetes and its complications. Ann N Y Acad Sci. 2011;1243:88–102.

36. Stefano GB, Challenger S, Kream RM. Hyperglycemia-associated alterations in cellular signaling and dysregulated mitochondrial bioenergetics in human metabolic disorders. Eur J Nutr. 2016;55(8):2339–45.

37. Lan HY. Transforming growth factor-β/Smad signalling in diabetic nephropathy. Clin Exp Pharmacol Physiol. 2012;39(8):731–8.

38. Li JH, Huang XR, Zhu HJ, Oldfield M, Cooper M, Truong LD, et al. Advanced glycation end products activate Smad signaling via TGF-beta-dependent and independent mechanisms: implications for diabetic renal and vascular disease. FASEB J. 2004;18:176–8.

39. Bierhaus A, Schiekofer S, Schwaninger M, Andrassy M, Humpert PM, Chen J, et al. Diabetes-associated sustained activation of the transcription factor nuclear factor-kappaB. Diabetes. 2001;50(12):2792–808.

40. Hudson BI, Kalea AZ, Del Mar Arriero M, Harja E, Boulanger E, D'Agati V, Schmidt AM. Interaction of the RAGE cytoplasmic domain with diaphanous-1 is required for ligand-stimulated cellular migration through activation of Rac1 and Cdc42. J Biol Chem. 2008;283(49):34457–68.

41. Schmidt AM. 2016 ATVB plenary lecture. Receptor for advanced glycation end products and implications for the pathogenesis and treatment of cardiometabolic disorders: spotlight on the macrophage. Arterioscler Thromb Vasc Biol. 2017;37:613–21.

42. Lapolla A, Flamini R, Dalla Vedova A, Senesi A, Reitano R, Fedele D, Basso E, Seraglia R, Traldi P. Glyoxal and methylglyoxal levels in diabetic patients: quantitative determination by a new GC/MS method. Clin Chem Lab Med. 2003;41:1166–73.

43. Liu GH, Qu J, Shen X. NF-kB/p65 antagonizes Nrf2-ARE pathway by depriving CBP from Nrf2 and facilitating recruitment of HDAC3 to MafK. Biochim Biophys Acta. 2008;1783:713–27.

44. Figarola JL, Singhal J, Rahbar S, Awasthi S, Singhal SS. LR-90 prevents methylglyoxal-induced oxidative stress and apoptosis in human endothelial cells. Apoptosis. 2014;19(5):776–88.

45. Maessen DE, Hanssen NM, Scheijen JL, van der Kallen CJ, van Greevenbroek MM, Stehouwer CD, Schalkwijk CG. Post-glucose load plasma α-dicarbonyl concentrations are increased in individuals with impaired glucose metabolism and type 2 diabetes: the CODAM study. Diabetes Care. 2015;8(5):913–20.

46. Mueller CF, Laude K, McNally JS, Harrison DG. Redox mechanisms in blood vessels. Arterioscler Thromb Vasc Biol. 2005;25:274–8.

47. Ayala A, Muñoz MF, Argüelles S. Lipid peroxidation: production, metabolism, and signaling mechanisms of malondialdehyde and 4-hydroxy-2-nonenal. Oxidative Med Cell Longev. 2014;2014:360438.

48. Zheng S, Zhong ZM, Qin S, Chen GX, Wu Q, Zeng JH, et al. Advanced oxidation protein products induce inflammatory response in fibroblast-like synoviocytes through NADPH oxidase-dependent activation of NF-κB. Cell Physiol Biochem. 2013;32(4):972–85.

49. Guo ZJ, Niu HX, Hou FF, Zhang L, Fu N, Nagai R, et al. Advanced oxidation protein products activate vascular endothelial cells via a RAGE-mediated signaling pathway. Antioxid Redox Signal. 2008;10(10):1699–712.

50. Wang Y, An R, Umanah GK, Park H, Nambiar K, Eacker SM, et al. A nuclease that mediates cell death induced by DNA damage and poly(ADP-ribose) polymerase-1. Science. 2016;354(6308):aad6872. https://doi.org/10.1126/science.aad6872.

51. Zakaria EM, El-Bassossy HM, El-Maraghy NN, Ahmed AF, Ali AA. PARP-1 inhibition alleviates diabetic cardiac complications in experimental animals. Eur J Pharmacol. 2016;791:444–54.

52. Zakaria EM, El-Maraghy NN, Ahmed AF, Ali AA, El-Bassossy HM. PARP inhibition ameliorates nephropathy in an animal model of type 2 diabetes: focus on oxidative stress, inflammation, and fibrosis. Naunyn Schmiedeberg's Arch Pharmacol. 2017;390(6):621–31. https://doi.org/10.1007/s00210-017-1360-9.

53. Guzyk MM, Tykhomyrov AA, Nedzvetsky VS, Prischepa IV, Grinenko TV, Yanitska LV, Kuchmerovska TM. Poly(ADP-ribose) polymerase-1 (PARP-1) inhibitors reduce reactive gliosis and improve angiostatin levels in retina of diabetic rats. Neurochem Res. 2016;41(10):2526–37.

54. Qin WD, Liu GL, Wang J, Wang H, Zhang JN, Zhang F, et al. Poly(ADP-ribose) polymerase 1 inhibition protects cardiomyocytes from inflammation and apoptosis in diabetic cardiomyopathy. Oncotarget. 2016;7(24):35618–31.

55. Ceriello A, Testa R, Genovese S. Clinical implications of oxidative stress and potential role of antioxidants in diabetic vascular complications. Nutr Metab Cardiovasc Dis. 2016;26(4):285–92. https://doi.org/10.1016/j.numecd.2016.01.006.

56. Toma L, Stancu CS, Sima AV. Endothelial dysfunction in diabetes is aggravated by glycated lipoproteins; novel molecular therapies. Biomedicine. 2021;9(1):18. https://doi.org/10.3390/biomedicines9010018.

57. Levitsky Y, Hammer SS, Fisher KP, Huang C, Gentles TL, Pegouske DJ, Xi C, Lydic TA, Busik JV, Proshlyakov DA. Mitochondrial ceramide effects on the retinal pigment epithelium in diabetes. Int J Mol Sci. 2020;21(11):3830. https://doi.org/10.3390/ijms21113830.

58. Adaikalakoteswari A, Rema M, Mohan V, Balasubramanyam M. Oxidative DNA damage and augmentation of poly (ADP-ribose) polymerase/nuclear factor kappa B signaling in patients with type 2 diabetes and microangiopathy. Int J Biochem Cell Biol. 2007;39(9):1673–84.

59. Sun YB, Qu X, Caruana G, Li J. The origin of renal fibroblasts/myofibroblasts and the signals that trigger fibrosis. Differentiation. 2016;92(3):102–7.

60. Loeffler I, Wolf G. Epithelial-to-mesenchymal transition in diabetic nephropathy: fact or fiction? Cell. 2015;4(4):631–52.

61. Meng XM, Tang PM, Li J, Lan HY. TGF-β/Smad signaling in renal fibrosis. Front Physiol. 2015;6:82.

62. Yan N, Wen L, Peng R, Li H, Liu H, Peng H, et al. Naringenin ameliorated kidney injury through Let-7a/TGFBR1 signaling in diabetic nephropathy. J Diabetes Res. 2016;2016:8738760. https://doi.org/10.1155/2016/8738760.

63. Durante W, Behnammanesh G, Peyton KJ. Effects of sodium-glucose co-transporter 2 inhibitors on vascular cell function and arterial remodeling. Int J Mol Sci. 2021;22:8786. https://doi.org/10.3390/ijms22168786.

64. Li H, Oehrlein SA, Wallerath T, Ihrig-Biedert I, Wohlfart P, Ulshöfer T, et al. Activation of protein kinase C alpha and/or epsilon enhances transcription of the human endothelial nitric oxide synthase gene. Mol Pharmacol. 1998;53:630–7.

65. Shatanawi A, Momani MS, Al-Aqtash R, Hamdan MH, Gharaibeh MN. L-Citrulline supplementation increases plasma nitric oxide levels and reduces arginase activity in patients with type 2 diabetes. Front Pharmacol. 2020;11:584669. https://doi.org/10.3389/fphar.2020.584669.

66. Schiffer TA, Lundberg JO, Weitzberg E, Carlström M. Modulation of mitochondria and NADPH oxidase function by the nitrate-nitrite-NO pathway in metabolic disease with focus on type 2 diabetes. Biochim Biophys Acta Mol basis Dis. 2020;1866(8):165811. https://doi.org/10.1016/j.bbadis.2020.165811.

67. Bahadoran Z, Mirmiran P, Kashfi K, Ghasemi A. Lost-in-translation of metabolic effects of inorganic nitrate in type 2 diabetes: is ascorbic acid the answer? Int J Mol Sci. 2021;22(9):4735. https://doi.org/10.3390/ijms22094735.

68. Tian R, Peng R, Yang Z, Peng YY, Lu N. Supplementation of dietary nitrate attenuated oxidative stress and endothelial dysfunction in diabetic vasculature through inhibition of NADPH oxidase. Nitric Oxide. 2020;96:54–63. https://doi.org/10.1016/j.niox.2020.01.007.

69. Liang M, Wang J, Xie C, Yang Y, Tian JW, Xue YM, Hou FF. Increased plasma advanced oxidation protein products is an early marker of endothelial dysfunction in type 2 diabetes patients without albuminuria 2. J Diabetes. 2014;6(5):417–26.

70. Rahman MH, Jha MK, Kim JH, Nam Y, Lee MG, Go Y, et al. Pyruvate dehydrogenase kinase-mediated glycolytic metabolic shift in the dorsal root ganglion drives painful diabetic neuropathy. J Biol Chem. 2016;291(11):6011–25.

Diabetes and Cardiovascular Disease

50

Daniel Coutiño-Castelán, Arturo Abundes-Velasco,
Félix Damas de los Santos, Eduardo A. Arias Sánchez,
Celso Mendoza González, Arturo Méndez Ortiz,
José L. Morales, José Luis Briseño de la Cruz,
César Eduardo Hernández Fonseca,
Piero Custodio Sánchez, and Joel Rodriguez-Saldana

Introduction

There are those who consider diabetes mellitus (DM) a cardiovascular disease since the most common and definitive final outcome with major sequelae is presented and depends on this system. In Mexico, the incidence of diabetic patients in the total number of patients treated by coronary intervention is higher than the world average, accounting for more than 40% of patients treated. Despite progress in contemporary pharmacological therapy in improving the management of diabetes and the more generalized use of statins and aspirin, the progression of atherosclerotic plaque and the regression percentage of the atherosclerotic plaque remains a prevalent issue among diabetic patients, as described by Raisuke [1]; see Fig. 50.1.

Since the 1980s, Colwell described the complexity of this problem in a classic paper [2] where he mentions that vascular disease in the diabetic patients is multifactorial with a wide myriad of derangements including endothelial, platelet, smooth muscle, lipoprotein, and coagulation abnormalities, all contributing to accelerated atherosclerosis, and has since proposed that a full understanding of the pathogenesis of this process could help design more effective preventive therapeutic approaches. The preventive approach with antiplatelet agents in the diabetic patient seems to be insufficient, since it is only focused on platelet function, forgetting the important contribution of the altered coagulation cascade in the diabetic, thrombo-fibrin, and resistance to fibrinolysis. That is why, currently there are multiple studies attempting to incorporate into the treatment of some component that improves fibrinolysis of the thrombus and thus increase the therapeutic spectrum that decreases the cardiovascular risk by this mechanism [3]. This is especially important in diabetic patients who undergo coronary intervention. Significant advances have been made in the knowledge of pathophysiology in relation to endothelial function, the role of inflammation, lipoproteins, and glucose metabolism, which begin to pro-

D. Coutiño-Castelán · A. Abundes-Velasco · F. D. de los Santos · E. A. Arias Sánchez
Department of Interventional Cardiology, Pan-American University, Mexico City, Mexico

C. M. González · A. M. Ortiz
Department of Adult Cardiology, Pan-American University, Mexico City, Mexico

J. L. Morales
Department of Electrocardiology, Hernandez Cardiology Clinical Specialties, Mexico City, Mexico

J. L. B. de la Cruz
Coronary Care Unit, Hernandez Cardiology Clinical Specialties, Mexico City, Mexico

C. E. H. Fonseca
Hernandez Cardiology Clinical Specialties, Mexico City, Mexico

P. C. Sánchez
National Institute of Cardiology, Mexico City, Mexico

J. Rodriguez-Saldana (✉)
Mexico City, Mexico

© The Author(s), under exclusive license to Springer Nature Switzerland AG 2023
J. Rodriguez-Saldana (ed.), *The Diabetes Textbook*, https://doi.org/10.1007/978-3-031-25519-9_50

Fig. 50.1 Progression/regression of atherosclerotic plaques with contemporary treatment in patients with and without diabetes

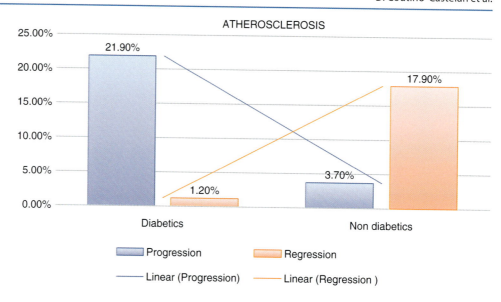

duce concrete results in the reduction of cardiovascular risk, for example, the use of inhibitors of sodium-glucose transport proteins has shown to decrease the occurrence of cardiovascular disease and mortality, compared to other types of hypoglycemic therapies [4]. It has been possible to modulate excessive vascular response and neointimal hyperplasia after the implantation of drug-eluting stents (DES) as demonstrated in multiple studies validated with ultrasound [5]; however, the main problem in the diabetic remains the progression of new plaques in sites not treated with stents. Advances in vascular intervention have been spectacular in the last few years; noninvasive and invasive imaging technology (IVUS, OCT) has greatly aided the understanding of vascular pathology in the diabetic patients and its evolution and behavior under diverse therapeutic approaches (pharmacological stents). There is no doubt that bioabsorbable stents are already a reality as current therapeutic tools [6]; however, there are certain technological improvements that will make the clinical results, especially in diabetic patients, be equated with nondiabetics. The bet on this adventure could be the search for a platform that could treat younger or incipient plaques and seek their "cure" preventing coronary lesions from reaching irreversible states in terms of anatomy and function.

We are glimpsing the future on the shoulders of giants.

Ischemic Heart Disease in Diabetic Patients

Epidemiology

Coronary artery disease is the leading cause of death in patients with diabetes mellitus [7]. Diabetes mellitus is associated with a two- to fourfold increased risk of coronary

artery disease and stroke [8–10] and with 2–3 times the risk of an acute myocardial infarction [11]. The prevalence of coronary disease increases from 2% to 4% in the general population to as high as 55% in diabetic patients [12]. The excess risk of cardiovascular disease is present in patients with type 1 diabetes mellitus and type 2 prediabetic, obese, and patients with metabolic syndrome [13]. Survival is worse in the presence of coronary artery disease, and their mortality rate is higher after myocardial infarction [14, 15]. Diabetes is present in 18–44% of patients with coronary artery disease [16–18], while in the rest, it is usual to find certain degree of dysglycemia; and previously undiagnosed diabetes can be found in up to 14–22% of patients [16]. Diabetic subjects typically have more severe coronary disease, more extensive coronary calcification, a high prevalence of left main disease, and a reduction in the recruitment of collateral circulation [19–21]. In the United States, approximately one-third of all percutaneous coronary interventions are performed in patients with diabetes, and one-quarter of patients undergoing coronary bypass surgery have diabetes [22].

Pathophysiology of Atherosclerosis (Fig. 50.2) and Endothelial Dysfunction: Metabolic Syndrome

There are several potential mechanisms through which diabetes causes accelerated formation of atherosclerotic plaques [23]; factors such as hyperglycemia, dyslipidemia, and insulin resistance lead to endothelial dysfunction [24, 25] and alterations in platelet function and coagulation [26]. All these mechanisms converge to promote plaque formation and increase its burden and complexity.

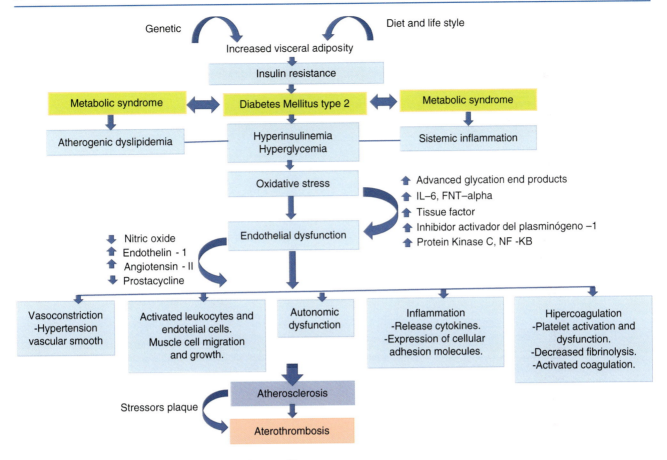

Fig. 50.2 Pathophysiology of atherosclerosis in diabetes mellitus

Treatment of Risk Factors and Its Impact on Primary Prevention

1. Hypertension Treatment: Scientific Evidence of Antihypertensive Treatment in Diabetic Patients and Lifestyle Changes and Arterial Pressure Goals in Diabetic Patients

Hypertension is twice as common in diabetic patients as in nondiabetic patients [27]; it is postulated that hyperinsulinemia, arterial stiffness, and the expansion of extracellular volume play an important role in its presentation. This association significantly increases the risk of cardiovascular (CV) death [9, 28, 29], coronary disease [30], ventricular hypertrophy [31], heart failure [32], stroke [33], retinopathy, and nephropathy [34, 35]. Clinical trials have demonstrated the benefits of improving blood pressure (BP) [36]; thus, with each sustained reduction of 10 mm Hg in systolic blood pressure, there is a 15% reduction in the risk of cardiovascular disease, a lower risk of macrovascular and microvascular disease, and a reduction in mortality [37–39]. Diabetic patients have a higher prevalence of isolated systolic hypertension and are more resistant to treatment [40–43]. In the

EUROASPIRE IV study, only 54% of patients achieved an adequate blood pressure [44]. Due to dysautonomic disorders, these patients suffer a lower reduction of nocturnal blood pressure, a higher heart rate, and a greater predisposition to orthostatic hypotension. Changes in lifestyle such as weight loss, low-sodium diet, and exercise produce beneficial effects [45]. The DASH (Dietary Approaches to Stop Hypertension) diet offers useful recommendations, such as reducing the sodium intake (<1500 mg/day), reducing the excess body weight, and increasing consumption of fruits and vegetables and low-fat foods while avoiding excessive alcohol consumption and increasing the physical activity [46]. Key management guidelines, including the Eighth Joint National Committee (JNC 8) [47] and the European Society of Hypertension and Cardiology [48], suggest that the goal of blood pressure in these patients should be less than 140/90 mmHg. Previous recommendations suggested a pressure goal of less than 130/80 mmHg. In the ACCORD-BP (Action to Control Cardiovascular Risk in Diabetes – Blood Pressure) study, they compared intensive blood pressure control (systolic blood pressure <120 mmHg) versus standard pressure control (systolic blood pressure <140 mmHg). They found a statistically significant reduction in the annual incidence of stroke in the intensive control group, but there were no differences in all-cause mortality and in the primary point of nonfatal myocardial infarction/nonfatal stroke/cardiovascular death. Serious adverse events were reported in the intensive treatment arm, such as a significant increase in serum creatinine above 1.5 mg/dL, hyperkalemia, hypotension, and syncope [49].

Contrastingly, the results of the recent SPRINT (Systolic Blood Pressure Intervention Trial) study, performed in patients with systolic blood pressure greater than 130 mm Hg and high cardiovascular risk, but without diabetes, showed a clear benefit in intensive treatment mortality. These results have again fanned the debate about the optimal blood pressure goal [50]. A meta-analysis, including 31 randomized studies and more than 71,000 hypertensive diabetics, reported that intensive blood pressure control significantly reduces the risk of stroke but fails to reduce the incidence of myocardial infarction or total mortality [51]. Although it is widely acceptable to achieve a systolic blood pressure <130/80 mm Hg in most diabetic patients and <140–150/90 mm Hg in elderly diabetic patients (>70–80 years), there is a lack of solid evidence to support this [52]. JNC 8 suggests that in adult White patients, the initial antihypertensive regimen should include any of the following drugs: a thiazide diuretic, a calcium channel blocker, an angiotensin-converting enzyme inhibitor (ACEI), and an angiotensin receptor blocker (BRA); in Black adult patients, a thiazide diuretic or a calcium channel blocker should be included [47]. It is usually suggested to start with ACE inhibitors or BRA as a first-line treatment because of its cardioprotective and nephroprotective effects. ACE inhibitors or BRAs should be included in the treatment of patients with chronic kidney disease, and they are contraindicated in pregnancy [53]. Generally patients require treatment with two or more drugs to meet the goal [54]. If treatment goals cannot be achieved despite the use of three different antihypertensive drugs (including a diuretic), then secondary hypertension should be ruled out. Finally, it is recommended that blood pressure should be closely monitored and treatment should be adjusted to avoid excessive falls in blood pressure [52].

2. Antiplatelet Treatment

Platelets have an important role in hemostasis and atherothrombotic disease. They are the first to initiate hemostasis. Three stages are recognized in the formation of the thrombus: (1) platelet adhesion; (2) extension, activation, recruitment, and aggregation; and (3) perpetuation and stabilization of the clot. The damaged endothelium exposes the subendothelial extracellular matrix and initiates the platelet activation mediated by the GP (glycoprotein) receptor complex Ib-IX-V which binds to vWF (von Willebrand factor). The exposed collagen also activates the platelets via GP VI and GP Ia/GP IIa. During the extension phase, platelet factors including ADP (adenosine diphosphate), TxA2 (thromboxane A2), epinephrine, serotonin, collagen, and thrombin are activated [55].

Aspirin. Its mechanism of action is by irreversible inhibition of COX 1 and 2, which decreases the production of TxA2 and PGI2. Mature platelets express only COX 1, releasing it when the TP (thromboxane receptor) is stimulated. Current guidelines recommend a loading dose of 150–300 mg of aspirin followed by 100 mg per day for life [56].

Clopidogrel. Eighty-five percent of the absorbed drug is hydrolyzed by the carboxylesterase in the liver and subsequently inactivated; the remainder 15% is converted by the CYP (cytochrome 450) in two active metabolites: 2-oxo-clopidogrel and R-130964. Recommended dose is 300–600 mg (loading dose) followed by 75 mg daily [57]. The use of a 150 mg daily dose was considered beneficial; however, the GRAVITAS study did not show benefit in the short or medium term with this dosage [58]. A 12-month clopidogrel treatment in diabetic patients with low bleeding risk who have a first-generation DES has shown to reduce the incidence of myocardial infarction and death [59].

Prasugrel. More efficient biotransformation depends on CYP3A4/5 and CYP2B6. The loading dose is 60 mg followed by 10 mg daily. It does not have as much variability as clopidogrel. TRITON – TIMI 38 (Trial to Assess Improvement in Therapeutic Outcomes by Optimizing Platelet Inhibition with Prasugrel – Thrombolysis in Myocardial Infarction) concluded higher efficacy when compared to clopidogrel, but with a higher bleeding rate including fatal bleeding. It is contraindicated in patients over 75 years of age who weigh less than 60 kg and have history of CVA (cerebral vascular accident) [60]. In those weighing less than 60 kg, half the dose can be given safely [61].

Ticagrelor. It is an oral reversible inhibitor of P2Y12 that inhibits red cell recapture of adenosine (which produces bradyarrhythmias). Its elimination is hepatic and is metabolized by the CYP3A. The loading dose is 180 mg followed by 90 mg every 12 h. It has other adverse effects such as dyspnea, hyperuricemia, and ventricular pauses ≥3 s in the first week, limiting its use [62]. Dyspnea can be the sole manifestation of angina in diabetic patients, so we need to be careful not to interpret it as a side effect of the drug.

Cilostazol. It inhibits PDE (phosphodiesterases) III increasing cAMP (cyclic adenosine monophosphate) levels in platelets, endothelium, and smooth muscle, acting as a vasodilator and anti-aggregant. The loading dose is

50 mg twice daily; if tolerated, it is increased to 100 mg twice daily. The benefits are more marked in diabetics and patients with diffuse lesions with many stents. It produces headache, tachycardia, palpitations, soft stools, and diarrhea leading to drug withdrawal in up to 15% of patients. It should be avoided in patients with heart failure [63].

European guidelines for myocardial revascularization recommend the use of Prasugrel and Ticagrelor over Clopidogrel, especially in diabetic patients, due to their lower variability and resistance, with a more stable and sustained therapeutic effect [57].

3. Lipid Treatment: Scientific Evidence of Lipid-Lowering Agents in Diabetic Patients

Multiple studies correlate high glucose and LDL (low-density lipoprotein) with atherosclerotic coronary disease. Statins are grouped according to their intensity: low intensity (simvastatin 10 mg, pravastatin 10–20 mg, pitavastatin 1 mg), moderate intensity (atorvastatin 10–20 mg, rosuvastatin 5–10 mg, simvastatin 20–40 mg, pravastatin 20–40 mg, pitavastatin 2–4 mg), and high intensity (atorvastatin 40–80 mg, rosuvastatin 20–40 mg).

ATP (adult treatment panel) IV guidelines recommend initiating treatment as primary prevention in diabetic patients with LDL >70 mg/dL between 40 and 75 years of age with a moderate-high dose. The goal of lipid-lowering therapy for secondary prevention is a LDL <70 mg/dL [64]. Statins have shown to reduce LDL levels by 25–35% with a 4% reduction in absolute mortality and relative risk by 30% with a 42% reduction for coronary heart disease and 37% for revascularization. There is a linear relationship between LDL reduction and cardiovascular risk [65]. The Heart Protection Study demonstrated the magnitude of benefit of statins at any LDL level, reducing the rate of cardiovascular events by 24%, including diabetic patients [66].

Statins. Intensive therapy has been shown to further decrease the risk of cardiovascular death by 1.3% for all-cause mortality. The use of statins is recommended for all patients with atherosclerotic disease. Intensive therapy reduces mortality by 16%. The risk of clinical adverse events is greater in the first six months after an ACS (acute coronary syndrome). Intensive treatment reduces risk by 24% during the early stage (15–30 days), by reducing CRP (C-reactive protein) and LDL. Patients who tolerate the intensive dose should continue this dose indefinitely [67].

Niacin. HDL (high-density lipoprotein) goal as a secondary target should be >40 mg/dL. Niacin is useful for raising HDL cholesterol. There is a 1.7% risk reduction for every 1% that the HDL is increased with niacin, but its use is limited by its adverse effects. It can decrease and even reverse atherosclerosis according to the ARBITER study [68].

Fibrates. They have little benefit. The ACCORD (Action to Control Cardiovascular Risk in Diabetes) study demonstrated that they can be combined with statins without significantly increasing adverse effects in diabetic patients, showing only benefit in nonfatal infarction and reduction of revascularization [69].

Ezetimibe. Ezetimibe binds to the Niemann-Pick receptor reducing the absorption of sterols in the intestine. It reduces LDL cholesterol by 20% when combined with statins, but there is still no evidence of benefit. So far its indication is when LDL target levels are not achieved despite intensive treatment with statins [70].

Glitazones. They stimulate the PPARG (peroxisome proliferator-activated receptor gamma) receptor improving serum glucose levels and are part of the treatment of type 2 diabetes mellitus. Pioglitazone in the PROactive (PROspective pioglitAzone Clinical Trial In macroVascular Events) study decreased LDL/HDL by 9.5% with a nonsignificant end point reduction, but relative mortality was reduced by 16%. It increases the risk of heart failure by 41% and is contraindicated when it already exists [71].

4. Hyperglycemia Treatment: Scientific Evidence of the Impact of the Glucose-Lowering Drugs on the Cardiovascular Risk of Diabetic Patients

For the purpose of this section, we will focus on drugs that have been shown to decrease cardiovascular risk in diabetic patients. Metformin, the only drug available in the biguanide class, was studied in the UKPDS (UK Prospective Diabetes Study) trial [72], which randomized 4209 patients with newly diagnosed type 2 diabetes mellitus to receive dietary restriction or sulphonylurea or insulin treatment or metformin in overweight patients. After a ten-year follow-up, there was a significant decrease in the relative risk of death from all causes of 13% with sulfonylurea or insulin versus dietary treatment and 27% with metformin versus dietary restriction. Significant reductions in the incidence of myocardial infarction were also observed in long-term follow-up. Because metformin has been shown to be safe, is well tolerated, has low risk of hypoglycemia, is low cost, and decreases cardiovascular events, it has been proposed by international associations to be the first-line drug for type 2 diabetes in the absence of contraindications and that it can be continued after starting insulin treatment [73, 74].

Sulfonylureas are the oldest glucose-lowering drugs. They have the highest rate of hypoglycemia of all oral drugs available and favor weight gain. Tolbutamide is a first-generation sulfonylurea, which has fallen into disuse because of increased cardiovascular and all-cause mortality in a randomized study [75]; the second- and third-generation sulfonylureas have not shown to have cardiovascular adverse effects [76, 77], although some have been associated with deleterious effects in the ischemic preconditioning of the myocardium [78]. One of the more recent sulfonylureas, gliclazide, has been proposed as the best in this group and the only one associated with a lower risk of major adverse cardiovascular events (MACEs) and mortality, similar to metformin [79]. Cardiovascular safety of sulfonylureas was also confirmed in the UKPDS1 primary prevention study discussed above. It is important to emphasize that when these drugs are prescribed in patients with known coronary disease, dosages should be carefully adjusted to avoid hypoglycemia, which may exacerbate myocardial ischemia [80].

Regarding the thiazolidinedione group, pioglitazone showed a 16% reduction in all-cause death, myocardial infarction, and stroke at follow-up at three years in the PROactive study [81] that included 5238 diabetic patients with evidence of macrovascular disease. The efficacy of this drug in decreasing the MACE compound was corroborated in a meta-analysis of 19 clinical trials [82], with a significantly higher incidence of severe heart failure (2.3% vs. 1.8%). Similarly, two meta-analyses showed that rosiglitazone is associated with a higher incidence of myocardial infarction and heart failure, without increasing cardiovascular mortality, which led to severe restrictions in its use in the United States and its withdrawal from the market in other countries [83, 84].

Dipeptidyl peptidase 4 (DPP-4) inhibitors have discrete hypoglycemic potency and pose a low risk of hypoglycemia. In a meta-analysis of 70 phase II clinical trials of this pharmacological group, a significant reduction in the risk of MACE (OR 0.71, 95% 0.59–0.86), myocardial infarction (OR 0.64, 95% CI 0.44–0.94), and all-cause death (OR 0.60, 95% CI 0.41–0.88), but not stroke, during a mean follow-up of 44 weeks was shown [85]. In the SAVOR-TIMI (Saxagliptin Assessment of Vascular Outcomes Recorded in Patients with Diabetes Mellitus-Thrombolysis in Myocardial Infarction) study [86] that included 16,492 diabetic patients randomly assigned to saxagliptin or placebo, the drug had no effect on MACE at follow-up at 2.1 years but significantly increased the risk of heart failure from 2.8% to 3.5%. Alogliptin also failed to reduce MACE in the EXAMINE study [87] in patients with diabetes with acute myocardial infarction or unstable angina.

Recently, an inhibitor of sodium-glucose cotransporter 2 (SGLT2) called empagliflozin is demonstrated in the EMPA-REG OUTCOME trial [88], to be superior than placebo plus standard therapy in more than 7000 patients with type 2 diabetes and established cardiovascular disease. It also proved to significantly decrease the compound of cardiovascular death, myocardial infarction, and stroke by 14% and in 38% the risk of cardiovascular death, in a median follow-up of 3.1 years.

Liraglutide, a glucagon-like peptide 1 (GLP-1) agonist receptor, was compared in the LEADER (Liraglutide Effect and Action in Diabetes: Evaluation of Cardiovascular Outcome Results) trial [89] versus placebo plus standard therapy in more than 9,000 patients with type 2 diabetes at high risk for cardiovascular disease or with cardiovascular disease and showed a 13% reduction in the primary MACE compound and 22% in cardiovascular death with a median follow-up of 3.8 years. Lixisenatide did not show a benefit when compared versus placebo in the ELIXA (Evaluation of Lixisenatide in Acute Coronary Syndrome) study [90], as it failed to decrease MACE at 25 months in patients with diabetes and acute myocardial infarction in the previous 6 months.

Inhibitors of α-glucosidase may reduce the incidence of myocardial infarction; however, the evidence is still insufficient [91]. There are other hypoglycemic drugs of new pharmacological groups, available recently or in the last phases of phase III trials [92], whose impact on cardiovascular risk is still unknown.

As for insulin, in the ORIGIN study [93], 12,537 patients with impaired fasting glucose or type 2 diabetes with known cardiovascular risk factors were randomized to receive insulin glargine or the "usual" treatment (which could be insulin, oral hypoglycemic agents, or no drugs according to local practices). The primary point of nonfatal myocardial infarction, nonfatal stroke, or death from cardiovascular causes, after a median follow-up of 6.2 years, was similar in both groups (2.94 vs. 2.85 episodes per 100 patients/year, $p = 0.63$), with higher rates of hypoglycemia and weight gain with insulin glargine and no effect on the incidence of cancer. The UKPDS [72] study also confirmed cardiovascular safety with insulin therapy. It is currently recommended to start insulin as soon as possible when blood glucose goals are not achieved with standard regimens.

The Steno-2 [94] study evaluated intensive versus conventional care strategy in the treatment of diabetic patients with microalbuminuria, with a mean follow-up of 5.5 years. The more aggressive treatment with a stepwise pharmacotherapeutic approach considering the achievement of the goals of blood glucose, blood pressure, microalbuminuria, total cholesterol and serum triglycerides, and platelet dysfunction decreased the all-cause mortality by 46% and the composite of cardiovascular events by 59%, both significantly.

In general, in diabetic patients with coronary artery disease, an HbA1c target of less than 7% is recommended according to the current ADA (American Diabetes Association) guidelines [73].

Cardiovascular Risk Evaluation in Diabetic Patients

In all patients with diabetes, the risk of atherosclerotic cardiovascular disease (ASCVD) defined as coronary death or nonfatal myocardial infarction or stroke (fatal or nonfatal) should be systematically evaluated at least every year. Among the risk factors that predispose to ASCVD are age, gender, race, diabetes, hypertension, dyslipidemia, smoking, family history of premature coronary disease (before 40 years), and the presence of albuminuria [73]. There are numerous cardiovascular risk scores, the most widely used are the American College of Cardiology/American Heart Association (ACC/AHA) ASCVD risk calculator, Framingham Risk Score, and UKPDS risk engine (which is specific for diabetic patients) named SCORE by its acronym in English Systematic Coronary Risk Evaluation. The ACC/AHA ASCVD risk tool [95] estimates the probability of having a cardiovascular event in the next ten years. It also offers treatment recommendations and is available online at http://static.heart.org/riskcalc/app/index.html.

The SCORE system [96, 97] is a simple tool that with five clinical variables estimates the risk of cardiovascular death at ten years but does not take into account diabetes since it is only considered as an independent cardiovascular risk factor after ten years of being diagnosed; this tool is available in an updated electronic version that offers treatment recommendations called HeartScore, which includes HDL cholesterol in its variables (http://www.heartscore.org).

In asymptomatic diabetic patients, routine screening studies are not recommended for coronary artery disease, as this does not improve outcomes whenever the risk factors for ASCVD are addressed [98].

Stable Ischemic Heart Disease

1. Clinical Manifestations and Risk Stratification

   Stable ischemic heart disease (SIHD) is defined as a disease that causes symptoms of angina related to stress or exercise secondary to coronary artery stenosis ($\geq 50\%$ in the case of the left main stem and $\geq 70\%$ in one or more of the major coronary arteries) [99]. At present, "angina with normal coronary arteries" also known as microvascular angina and coronary vasospasm are also included in this definition. Usually diabetic patients with SIHD present with atypical symptoms such as non-anginal chest pain or unexplained dyspnea. Some diabetic patients may have "silent ischemic heart disease" with positive ischemia tests in the absence of symptoms. All diabetic patients with suspected SIHD should be evaluated with a probability pretest, which is based on simple clinical findings such as the pain characteristics, gender, and age [100]. In general, patients with low probability (<15%) require no additional diagnostic tests; with intermediate probability (15–85%), noninvasive ischemia-inducing studies are suggested (see next section); and in patients with high probability (>85%), invasive coronary angiography (ICA) is recommended as soon as possible, especially in the presence of severe angina at a low exercise level, with decreased LVEF (left ventricular ejection fraction) (<50%) or clinical signs of high-risk events.

2. Diagnosis

   Additional studies should be performed in search of SIHD in all diabetic patients with (1) typical or atypical cardiac symptoms; (2) in the presence of signs or symptoms of concomitant vascular disease such as carotid murmur, transient ischemic attack, stroke, claudication, or peripheral arterial disease; and (3) an abnormal resting electrocardiogram (ECG) with pathological Q waves, ST-segment, or T wave alterations suggestive of myocardial ischemia. The study most widely used is exercise ECG; however, its sensitivity is only 50%, so other noninvasive ischemia-inducing studies are currently preferred, such as exercise or vasodilator stress single photon emission computed tomography (SPECT), exercise or dobutamine or vasodilator stress echocardiography, dobutamine or vasodilator stress magnetic resonance imaging (MRI), and vasodilator stress positron emission tomography (PET), whose sensitivity, specificity, and positive and negative predictive values can be consulted in the stable coronary European clinical practice guide artery disease [99]. When patients are unable to exercise or have an ECG with complete left bundle branch block or pacemaker, then pharmacological stress with vasodilators such as dipyridamole or adenosine should be considered. Coronary artery calcium can be measured with computed tomography angiography (CTA) which is a noninvasive alternative to ischemia screening that offers a sensitivity of 95–99% and a very high negative predictive value. It also offers a very close correlation with invasive coronary angiography in terms of coronary anatomy [101]. Each of these diagnostic tests can stratify the patients in low, intermediate, or high risk which guides the decision as to whether start optimal best medical therapy (BMT) or request ICA with possible revascularization, either percutaneously or surgically.

3. Therapeutic Options

   (a) Optimal medical treatment patients with type 2 diabetes mellitus have a greater risk of developing coronary artery disease (CAD) than nondiabetic patients [102]. In addition, 75% of patients with T2DM die as a result of cardiovascular diseases, including CAD [12]. In patients with T2DM, CAD tends to be more complex characterized by multivessel disease, small vessels, and calcified and diffuse lesions and are occasionally requiring additional coronary revascularization to control angina [103–105]. Current medical management emphasizes the importance of controlling risk factors, including successful blood glucose control and treatment with statins, angiotensin receptor blockers/angiotensin-converting enzyme inhibitors, and antiplatelet therapy [106]. Guidelines for the management of diabetes mellitus of the American Diabetes Association, the American College of Cardiology, and the American Heart Association recommend the following prevention strategy for coronary artery disease: blood pressure of 130/80 mm Hg or less, low-density lipoprotein cholesterol (LDL-C) below 70 mg/dL for patients with CAD, and immediate smoking cessation [107, 108]. In large-scale studies to assess clinical outcomes comparing revascularization and intensive medical management (COURAGE, BARI-2D, and FREEDOM), the one-year goal compliance rate to achieve LDL-C levels <100 mg/dL, systolic blood pressure <130 mmHg, glycosylated hemoglobin <7.0%, and smoking cessation was 18%, 23%, and 8%, respectively.

(b) Revascularization treatment. Recent advances in techniques and devices used in coronary interventional procedures have extended the indication of PCI toward more complex lesions. Drug-eluting stents (DES) have reduced restenosis and reintervention rates [108–110], although the mortality of CAD in patients with T2DM remains high.

Most clinical trials comparing the outcomes of patients with type 2 diabetes mellitus and multivessel coronary artery disease have shown that coronary artery bypass grafting (CABG) is superior to balloon angioplasty and angioplasty with bare metal stents (BMS) in terms of target vessel revascularization, myocardial infarction, and mortality.

More recently, the use of new scales to analyze angiographic and clinical variables (SYNTAX II, Euro SCORE II) has been proposed for a better decision-making process in revascularization strategies [111], particularly in patients with T2DM who will require a multidisciplinary discussion taking into account the patients' coronary anatomy, the characteristics of the lesions, age, and comorbidities.

Several clinical trials are currently being conducted in 85 centers in the USA and Europe that compare CABG with percutaneous coronary intervention (PCI) with drug-eluting stents. The "SYNergy between coronary intervention and cardiac surgery" (SYNTAX) study was a prospective randomized study comparing the efficacy of CABG and PCI with paclitaxel-releasing stents in patients with complex coronary artery disease [112]. In this study, 25.1% of the patients were diabetic. In the cohort of diabetic patients, the incidence of major coronary events and cerebrovascular disease at three years was 37.0% in the PCI group and 22.9% in the CABG group ($p = 0.002$). The incidence of target vessel revascularization was also higher in the PCI group when compared to CABG (28.0% vs. 12.9%, $p < 0.001$) [113].

In 2012, the FREEDOM study randomized a total of 1900 diabetic patients with multivessel coronary disease to CABG and PCI using mainly sirolimus-eluting stents (SES) and paclitaxel-eluting stents (PES) [114]. All-cause mortality and myocardial infarction were significantly lower in the CABG group when compared to the PCI group (18.7% vs. 26.6%). However, most patients in the PCI group were treated with first-generation DES. The use of new-generation DES, particularly everolimus-eluting stent, is changing the outcomes mainly because of a reduction in the incidence of stent thrombosis and myocardial infarction [115].

Recently, Banglore et al. published a meta-analysis of 68 randomized trials that compared the clinical outcomes of patients with CAD and diabetes revascularized with CABG versus PCI with DES, including sirolimus, paclitaxel, and everolimus-eluting stents [116]. All-cause mortality was higher in patients who were treated with sirolimus-eluting stents and paclitaxel-eluting stents compared to CABG. Meanwhile mortality rates between everolimus-eluting stents and CABG were similar. Bioabsorbable scaffolds are a new alternative that could have potential advantages over drug-eluting stents in terms of adverse coronary events. Muramatsu and colleagues compared bioabsorbable stents versus everolimus-eluting stents in diabetic patients in different clinical trials and reported that the incidence of cardiac mortality, myocardial infarction related to the treated vessel, and target vessel revascularization was similar with both types of stent (3.9% vs. 6.4%, $p = 0.38$) [117, 118].

Acute Coronary Syndromes

1. Clinical manifestations and diagnosis. Coronary disease is very common in the diabetic population; up to 32% of patients with acute coronary syndrome have diabetes mellitus [119]. Myocardial ischemia diagnosis can be challenging in diabetic patients [120, 121]. Physical

examination findings are variable and may be related to hemodynamic instability, electrical instability, or mechanical complications. Physical examination may rule out a different source of chest pain. A fundamental diagnostic aid is the 12-lead electrocardiogram, which must be acquired immediately in these patients [122]. This study may have discrete changes in more than 30% of patients and is less sensitive if there are alterations in intraventricular conduction [123, 124]. Cardiac biomarkers help in confirming the diagnosis and guiding the treatment, in addition to stratifying the risk. Troponins are more sensitive and specific, and their determination is fundamental for decision-making [125–127]. Measurement of CK-MB and copeptin is also useful [128–130]. Angiography is indicated if the suspicion of ACS is high; in other cases, coronary angiotomography may be performed. Other methods, such as echocardiography, magnetic resonance imaging, and cardiac nuclear test, complete the evaluation and diagnosis [131].

2. Risk stratification. The initial presentation characteristics are helpful markers for early prognosis; resting chest pain, heart failure, and mitral regurgitation are associated with a poorer prognosis [132]. There are many variables and scales that assess the risk of death; these scales are not always easy to apply. The TIMI risk score is a useful risk assessment tool in cases of myocardial infarction and ST-segment elevation amenable to reperfusion therapy [133]. High levels of high-sensitivity troponin are associated with an increased risk of death. A high serum creatinine and low glomerular filtration rate pose a grim prognosis to these patients; these variables are included in the Global Registry of Acute Coronary Events (GRACE) [134] and assess the risk of death or the combination of death and myocardial infarction at six months. This score showed that coronary revascularization is independently associated with better survival at one year in cases of acute coronary syndrome without high-risk ST-segment elevation; the same benefit was not observed in low- or intermediate-risk groups [135, 136]. The SYNTAX score uses angiographic criteria to make clinical decisions and thus estimate the likelihood of long-term cardiovascular and cerebral events in patients undergoing surgical or percutaneous revascularization; it predicts outcomes such as death, infarction and CVA and needs for revascularization, or the combination of all, in patients with surgical or percutaneous revascularization, based on the complexity and extent of coronary lesions. A low SYNTAX score is <22 points, intermediate from 23 to 32, and high when it is >33. Higher scores show better long-term outcomes with surgery [137, 138]. It is essential to evaluate the risk of bleeding in the treatment of myocardial infarction without ST-segment elevation. A controlled trial of patients with coronary artery disease of two or three vessels, randomized to revascularization surgery versus percutaneous treatment with drug-eluting stents, showed a significant decrease in all-cause mortality in the surgical revascularization group [139]. This finding was consistent with the SYNTAX trial. The CRUSADE scale quantifies the risk of major intrahospital bleeding [140].

3. Medical Treatment:

(a) Glucose control in the context of an ACS and glucose goals and insulin therapy. Medical treatment in the acute phase of an acute coronary syndrome is similar in patients with and without diabetes mellitus. Patients with acute coronary syndrome and diabetes mellitus are the group with the highest death rate, myocardial infarction, recurrent ischemia, and CHF (congestive heart failure) during follow-up [141]. There is a close relationship between glucose levels and mortality in this group of patients. Both hyperglycemia and hypoglycemia have adverse effects on inhospital outcomes and mortality. The NICESUGAR study showed that intensive glucose control increased mortality in adults in intensive care: serum glucose of 180 mg/dL or less resulted in lower mortality than if it was 81–108 mg/dL [142]. There is no established role for the administration of glucose-insulin-potassium infusions in NSTE (non-ST-elevated myocardial infarction)-ACS.

(b) Antiplatelet agents. Aspirin should be given to any patient with suspected or diagnosed acute coronary syndrome. When no contraindication exists, it should be started early. If there is any contraindication for its use, then clopidogrel should be started. Patients treated with early invasive reperfusion should receive the combination of aspirin with some P2Y12 inhibitor. Inhibitors of GP IIb/GP IIIa receptors in patients with acute coronary syndrome without ST-segment elevation are associated with a reduction in mortality at 30 days, particularly in patients with diabetes mellitus undergoing percutaneous revascularization. Several trials have shown the benefit of oral antiplatelet therapy in these patients with a reduction in ischemic events without an increase in bleeding complications with the use of prasugrel compared to clopidogrel [143]. In PLATO study, ticagrelor showed less ischemic events regardless of diabetic state and glycemic control, without increased bleeding than clopidogrel [144].

(c) Renin-angiotensin-aldosterone antagonists. Optimal treatment in these patients includes the use of a renin-angiotensin-aldosterone antagonist, particularly in patients with heart failure and ejection fraction less than 40%. Patients intolerant to angiotensin-converting enzyme inhibitors should receive angiotensin receptor blockers as a class I indication.

(d) Beta-blockers. They should be used in the first hours after the diagnosis of an acute coronary syndrome, provided there are no contraindications to it. If there is contraindication in the acute phase of the infarction, it can be reevaluated in the following hours.

(e) Anticoagulation. The combination of anticoagulation with antiplatelet therapy is recommended regardless of the initial treatment. Enoxaparin, bivalirudin, fondaparinux, and unfractionated heparin are among the recommended anticoagulants. Enoxaparin significantly reduces the recurrence of ischemic events and the need for invasive procedures; this benefit was sustained for up to 1 year [145], although other studies did not demonstrate a significant difference in death or myocardial infarction at 30 days when comparing this drug with unfractionated heparin [146]. Anticoagulation with bivalirudin alone suppresses ischemic events similar to the use of heparin plus glycoprotein IIb/glycoprotein IIIa inhibitors while at the same time significantly reducing the risk of bleeding complications [147–149].

(f) Statins should be initiated or continued in all patients, with and without diabetes mellitus in the context of an acute coronary syndrome, provided there is no contraindication; they reduce the recurrence of infarction, coronary disease mortality, cerebral vascular event, and the need for revascularization.

(g) Nitrates. If chest pain persists, then sublingual nitroglycerin can be administered; if there is no improvement, it can be administered intravenously, as in the case of heart failure.

(h) Calcium channel blockers. They are an alternative to avoid the recurrence of ischemia or when there is contraindication to the use of beta-blockers, provided there is no left ventricular dysfunction or altered atrioventricular conduction. They are also indicated in patients with coronary spasm [150].

4. Revascularization therapy in acute coronary syndromes:

(a) Percutaneous coronary intervention (PCI) in ST-elevated myocardial infarction (STEMI).

The frequency of coronary events requiring primary intervention is well known. The impact of diabetes mellitus on the outcomes of patients with ST-segment elevation infarction since the onset of primary angioplasty has been well established. It was first described by the Mayo Clinic and Columbia University group [151], who concluded that despite similar TIMI 3 flow rates in patients with and without diabetes, patients with diabetes are more likely to have perfusion abnormalities assessed with the reduction of the ST-segment and myocardial blush; it is also contemplated that the reduction of myocardial perfusion after primary angioplasty may contribute

to an increase in mortality in this population. Persistent ST elevation and abnormal myocardial blush in the presence of normal epicardial flow are indicative of decreased microvascular flow also known as a "non-reflux" phenomenon [152]. These alterations of the microvasculature are much more frequent in the diabetic population. Several mechanisms have been postulated for which diabetes contributes to microvascular damage. First, diabetes is associated with a prothrombotic and inflammatory state, accumulation of leukocytes, and thrombus formation in the capillaries of diabetics which leads to coronary microvascular obstruction [153].

Many studies have compared the impact of type 2 diabetes mellitus (T2DM) on prognosis in postcoronary intervention patients. In a recent meta-analysis published in 2016 [154] which included patients from the HORIZONS-AMI [155] trial and 12 other studies of which 7 were randomized controlled trials, 4163 patients were analyzed for major adverse cardiovascular events (MACE) and myocardial infarction (MI) and 17,015 patients analyzed for mortality. There was a significant increase in the rate of MACE and MI in the group of non-insulin-treated diabetes mellitus compared to the non-insulin group (OR: 1.63, 95% CI (1.17–2.27) $p = 0.04$) (OR: 1.82, 95 % CI (1.08–3.06) $p = 0.02$). These differences are also reflected in mortality. Recently published in 2017 is the largest cohort that includes patients with STEMI [156], from the UK and Wales health systems. This cohort of patients with STEMI included 281, 569 patients of which 120, 568 were patients with diabetes mellitus. STEMI with diabetes compared to patients with STEMI without diabetes were more prone to have a previous infarction (34.9 vs. 22.5%), heart failure (10.5 vs. 5.8%), and chronic renal failure (11.3 vs. 4.6%). After this cohort was adjusted for age, sex, and years of diagnosis, DM was associated with a 72% increase in the risk of mortality (1.72, 95% CI 1.66–1.79) for STEMI. The reperfusion rates managed for this cohort were 73.1% versus 79% in patients without DM.

In the final analysis, there were over 1,944,194 person years at risk, the median time to death was 2.3 (IQR 0.9–4.2) years, and 200, 360 (28.4%) died. At all-time points from hospitalization with AMI, unadjusted cumulative relative survival was significantly worse among patients with diabetes (log rank tests $p < 0.001$).

(b) Percutaneous coronary intervention (PCI) in non-ST-elevated myocardial infarction (NSTEMI).

Diabetics have a higher incidence of multivessel CAD. In the American registry CRUSADE (Can

Rapid risk stratification of Unstable angina patients Suppress ADverse outcomes with Early implementation of the ACC/AHA guidelines), the prevalence of diabetes was 33% among 46,410 patients with non-ST-elevation ACS. The PRESTO [157] trial showed that compared to NDM, patients with T2DM had an advanced age were mostly female patients and the majority had a history of heart failure and lower ejection fraction. These patients with T2DM were mainly overweight and obese and had a high rate of comorbidities. The FREEDOM [158] trial showed that in patients with diabetes and multivessel coronary artery disease, MACEs were higher in patients treated with insulin compared to patients without insulin therapy. Revascularization trends in patients with diabetes and patients with diabetes and multivessel CAD presenting with NSTEMI, ACTION Registry: 29,769 patients enrolled from July 2008 to December 2014. Overall, 36.4% were treated with CABG, 46.2% received PCI (77.2% with at least one DES), and 17.3% were treated with no revascularization. The proportion of patients receiving any kind of revascularization increased from 81.1% to 83.6% (PP < 0.0001 for trend), driven entirely by hospital-level use of CABG. Despite guidelines recommending CABG over PCI for diabetics with multivessel CAD, only about one-third of them actually receive CABG in the setting of NSTEMI. Accelerated atherosclerosis, atherosclerotic plaque rupture, and increased platelet activity, all of which increase the incidence of acute MI compared to nondiabetics. In the current propensity-matched analysis of contemporary real-life data, an early invasive strategy was associated with an increased inhospital survival in NSTE-ACS patients with concomitant DM. These results support the 2014 ACCF/AHA guideline recommendations for an early invasive strategy in diabetics, especially those with high-risk features (e.g., NSTEMI and cardiogenic shock). Meanwhile, the use of this strategy in lower-risk patients, such as those with UA (unstable angina), may not be associated with improved survival [159]. The incidence of inhospital mortality also was lower with an early invasive strategy in the secondary post-hoc analysis using a tighter match tolerance (2.5% vs. 3.7%; OR, 0.65; 95% CI, 0.56–0.75; $P < 0.0001$) and in the sensitivity analysis after excluding the patients with length of hospital stay less than 48 h in the propensity-matched cohort (2.1 vs. 3.3; OR, 0.63; 95% CI, 0.56–0.72; $P < 0.0001$). On subgroup analysis, the benefit of an early invasive strategy was demonstrated among a wide range of prespecified subgroups except in patients with UA, where there was no apparent evidence of survival benefit with an early invasive strategy (0.5% vs. 0.1%; OR, 7.86; 95% CI, 0.82–75.72; $P = 0.07$), with evidence of heterogeneity when compared to NSTEMI patients (P interaction=0.02). Diabetes was also associated with a significantly higher mortality at one year for both presentations (HR 1.7 and 1.2, respectively). At one year, patients with diabetes presenting with non-ST-elevation ACS had a risk of death that approached that of nondiabetic individuals presenting with STEMI (7.2% vs. 8.1%). In the TACTICS (Treat Angina with Aggrastat and Determine Cost of Therapy with an Invasive or Conservative Strategy)-TIMI 18 trial, an early invasive strategy was associated with a significant 22% reduction in the relative risk of death, MI, or rehospitalization for ACS at six months compared with an early conservative strategy [160].

(c) Fibrinolytic therapy in STEMI.

Regarding to fibrinolytic therapy, a meta-analysis of the Fibrinolytic Therapy Trialists' Collaborative Group, which included all the large randomized trials of fibrinolytic therapy versus placebo in STEMI, demonstrated a greater survival benefit at 35 days among diabetic patients compared with nondiabetic individuals, corresponding to 3.7 lives and 1.5 lives saved per 100 patients treated, respectively. While CABG in the setting of STEMI is typically reserved for failed PCI and for MI-related mechanical complications, primary PCI may be preferred over thrombolytic therapy in diabetic patients. However, the data to support this notion are limited [161]. A pooled analysis of individual patient data from 19 randomized trials comparing primary PCI with fibrinolysis for the treatment of STEMI included 6315 patients, 877 (14%) of whom had diabetes. The 30-day mortality rate (9.4% vs. 5.9%; $P < 0.001$) was higher in patients with diabetes. Mortality was significantly lower after primary PCI compared with fibrinolysis in both patients with diabetes (unadjusted OR 0.49; $P = 0.004$) and those without diabetes (unadjusted OR 0.69; $P = 0.001$) [162].

Complete ST resolution at 90 minutes after fibrinolytic therapy has been shown to be less prevalent between diabetic patients when compared with nondiabetic patients [163].

(d) Coronary artery bypass grafting (CABG).

The impact of diabetes on morbidity and mortality in patients undergoing surgical coronary revascularization was remarked in a retrospective analysis of the Society of Thoracic Surgery database, including 41,663 diabetic patients among a total population of 146,786. At 30 days, the mortality was significantly higher in the diabetes group (3.7% vs. 2.7%). The unadjusted and adjusted mortality OR (odds ratio) for diabetes were 1.4 and 1.2, respectively. With respect to diabetes treatments at presentation, the adjusted mortality OR for patients on oral hypoglycemic drugs and on insulin were 1.1 and 1.4, respectively. In addition, the overall morbidity and the infection rates were significantly higher among diabetic patients. Looking into long-term mortality following CABG, a prospective cohort study including 11,186 consecutive diabetic patients and 25,455 nondiabetic patients undergoing CABG from 1992 to 2001 detected a significantly higher annual mortality rate among diabetic patients (5.5%) compared with nondiabetic individuals (3.1%).The annual mortality increased to 8.4%, 16.3%, and 26.3% among diabetic patients with vascular disease, renal failure, or both, respectively. In addition to increased periprocedural morbidity and mortality as well as long-term mortality, diabetic patients must undergo repeat revascularization following CABG more frequently than their nondiabetic counterparts [164].

Heart Failure in Diabetic Patients

Introduction and Epidemiology

Cardiovascular death is the leading cause of death among patients with diabetes mellitus. The diabetic population is at higher risk of developing heart failure (HF) compared to the nondiabetic population, so diabetes mellitus (DM) is considered an independent risk factor for the development of HF, where a 1% increase in glycosylated hemoglobin increases the incidence of heart failure from 8% to 16% [165].

Bell et al. found that of 5757 patients with chronic HF treated with carvedilol, 25% had diabetes mellitus [166]. In an analysis of the European Heart Failure Pilot Survey which included 3226 patients with chronic HF, the prevalence of diabetes was 29%, and it was associated with older age, higher NYHA functional class, and predominance of ischemic HF etiology. The study concluded that DM is an independent predictor of death and hospitalization due to heart failure [167].

Pathophysiology

The development of heart failure in the diabetic patient is considered multifactorial, associated mainly with coronary disease, accelerated atherosclerosis, metabolic disorders, small vessel disease, and diabetic cardiomyopathy [168].

Diabetic cardiomyopathy was first described in 1972 when Rubler et al. [169, 170] found left ventricular dilation in the absence of ischemic heart disease in autopsies of diabetic patients. In this context, diabetic cardiomyopathy was clinically defined by the presence of structural alterations or abnormal myocardial function in the absence of hypertension, coronary disease, and valvular disease. The presence of diabetic cardiomyopathy is not essential for the development of HF in the diabetic patient.

The key for the development of HF is hyperglycemia, which leads to lipotoxicity, free fatty acid oxidation, oxidative stress, and apoptosis (apoptosis and myocardial cell necrosis is greater in the diabetic patient than in the nondiabetic patient). Other contributing factors are the constant activation of the renin angiotensin-aldosterone system, sympathetic nervous system (SNS), activation of proinflammatory cytokines, and formation of advanced glycosylation products. All of these in a greater or lesser degree lead to fibroblast proliferation and collagen deposits ultimately causing interstitial and perivascular fibrosis, the main features of diabetic cardiomyopathy [171–173]. Endomyocardial biopsy studies have found an increase in type III collagen deposits but not of type I and IV collagen in patients with type 2 DM. Others show collagen distribution patterns characterized by collagen types I and III at the perivascular level and IV at the endocardium. In both humans and animals, an increase in cardiac fibrosis has been found even before the onset of hyperglycemia [174, 175].

The end products of advanced glycosylation (EPAG) are derived from a nonenzymatic irreversible reaction between sugars and proteins, called the Maillard reaction. It is considered to play an important role in the pathophysiology of heart failure. It has been associated with endothelial dysfunction, development of atherosclerosis, diastolic dysfunction, and in advanced stages systolic dysfunction. EPAG can be covalently bonded to each other, resulting in the formation of additional bonds between matrix proteins such as collagen, laminin, and elastin. This type of binding increases the stiffness of the protein matrix and leads to diastolic dysfunction; the presence of EPAG has been associated with increased isovolumetric relaxation time and left ventricular diameter [176].

The alterations in sympathetic innervation, characteristic of diabetic neuropathy, have been associated with HF, due to alterations in the expression and activation of catecholamines and increased activation of beta 1 receptors, resulting in apoptosis, fibrosis, and ventricular dysfunction. Markers of diabetic neuropathy such as HRR (altered heart rate recovery) are associated with the development of heart failure in the diabetic patients [177].

1. Left ventricular hypertrophy (LVH) and diabetes mellitus.

    The association between left ventricular hypertrophy and DM has been controversial and has been explained by other mechanisms, such as hypertension [178]. In the Northern Manhattan Study (NOMAS) [179], ventricular mass was determined with transthoracic echocardiography. DM was shown to be an independent risk predictor for the development of left ventricular hypertrophy (adjusted odds ratio 1.46, 95% CI, 1.13–1.88, $P = 0.004$), after adjusting for age, sex, race, mass index (BMI), systolic BP, education, history of coronary artery disease (CAD), physical activity, and alcohol consumption. There was also a direct interaction between abdominal circumference and LVH ($P = 0.01$) which translates the close relationship between insulin resistance, activation of RAAS (renin-angiotensin-aldosterone system), SNS activation, and left ventricular hypertrophy in the diabetic patient with and without arterial hypertension [180, 181]. Cardiac magnetic resonance has broadened our understanding of diabetic cardiomyopathy, demonstrating fat infiltration, fibrosis, altered ventricular geometry, and ventricular mass increase. Patients with HF have higher NT-BNP (N-terminal pro-B-type natriuretic peptide) levels than nondiabetic patients, with no difference in other biomarkers.

2. From diastolic dysfunction to symptomatic HF.

The spectrum of diabetic heart disease is broad and varies from normal heart, subclinical diastolic dysfunction, and systolic dysfunction (detectable only by imaging techniques) to symptomatic heart failure.

Diastolic dysfunction is present in up to 50% of the diabetic population and has a close relationship with the levels of glycosylated hemoglobin and diabetic microangiopathy [181]. Systolic dysfunction is a late appearing condition. Fang et al. found that up to 24% of asymptomatic diabetic patients had systolic dysfunction determined with echocardiographic Doppler and Strain imaging [182].

This subclinical dysfunction in the absence of silent coronary disease and left ventricular hypertrophy has been related to glycosylated hemoglobin levels. In a study that included 219 patients, Flag et al. found that 16% had systolic dysfunction and 21% had diastolic dysfunction. The independent predictors of systolic dysfunction were glycosylated hemoglobin levels ($p < 0.001$) and lack of pretreatment with angiotensin-converting enzyme inhibitors (ACEI) ($p = 0.003$) and for diastolic dysfunction the absence of treatment with insulin ($p = 0.008$), treatment with metformin ($p = 0.01$), age ($p = 0.013$), and arterial hypertension ($p = 0.001$) [183]. Thus, the mechanisms involved with the development of heart failure depend on the control of diabetes, type of treatment implemented for both diabetes control and blockade of the renin-angiotensin-aldosterone system, and other associated factors such as age and hypertension. From et al. showed that 23% of a 1760 patient cohort had diastolic dysfunction. The cumulative five-year HF development in these patients was 36.9%, compared to 16.8% in patients without diastolic dysfunction ($p = 0.001$). Diabetic patients with diastolic dysfunction had a significantly higher mortality rate than those without diastolic dysfunction. This association was independent of the presence of arterial hypertension, coronary disease, or other echocardiographic parameters [184].

The RELAX (Phosphodiesterase-5 Inhibition to Improve Clinical Status and Exercise Capacity in Heart Failure with Preserved Ejection Fraction) trial which included diabetic and nondiabetic patients with HF and preserved systolic function showed that diabetic patients ($n = 93$) were significantly younger, obese, and more frequently males and had a higher prevalence of hypertension, renal failure, lung disease, and vascular disease. Levels of uric acid, C-reactive protein, galectin-3, collagen I, and endothelin-1 were significantly higher in diabetic patients ($p < 0.05$). Diabetic patients had lower functional capacity and a significant increase in the risk of hospitalization for renal and cardiac causes (23.7% vs. 4.9%, $p < 0.001$) [185].

BNP is a good prognostic and diagnostic marker in diabetics with HF. Van Der Horst et al. demonstrated that the diabetic population with HF has higher levels of natriuretic peptides than the nondiabetic population ($p = 0.03$), being a predictor of mortality, along with norepinephrine, in diabetic patients with advanced HF [186].

Prevention and Treatment of HF and DM

HbA1c levels > 7% are associated with an increased risk of hospitalization for HF in patients with type 2 DM [187]. The STENO II trial [94] showed that intensive glucose treatment (glycosylated Hb <6.5%) and risk factor treatment (arterial pressure <130/80 mmHg, triglycerides <150 mg/dL, total cholesterol <175 mg/dL) were associated with a reduction in CV death and infarction and need for revascularization. However, other studies such as UKPDS [188], ACCORD, ADVANCE, and VADT (Veterans Affairs Diabetes Trial) showed no benefit between intensive glucose treatment and HF [189].

The blockade of the renin-angiotensin-aldosterone system is a cornerstone in the high cardiovascular risk patient; in the HOPE study, 38% of the population was diabetic; the use of ramipril was associated with a reduction in the relative risk of HF (9.2 vs. 11.7 OR 0.77, $P < 0.001$), as well as a lesser development of de novo diabetes with a 32% risk reduction ($p = 0.002$) [190]. In the EUROPA (European Trial on Reduction of Cardiac Events with Perindopril in Patients with Stable Coronary Artery Disease) study in diabetic patients treated with perindopril, there was a reduction in hospitalization for HF [191].

Empagliflozin is a potent and selective inhibitor of sodium-glucose cotransporter (SGLT2) used in the treatment of type 2 DM. By inhibiting SGLT2, empagliflozin reduces renal glucose reabsorption and increases urinary glucose excretion. In addition to reducing hyperglycemia, empagliflozin is associated with osmotic diuresis, natriuresis, weight loss and visceral fat and blood pressure reduction, albuminuria with neutral effect on the sympathetic nervous system, and other favorable effects on the markers of arterial stiffness and vascular resistance [192]. The EMPA-REG OUTCOME study showed that empagliflozin reduced hospitalization and death from heart failure [2.8 vs. 4.5%; HR: 0.61 (0.47–0.79); $P < 0.001$] and was associated with a reduction in all-cause hospitalization [36.8% vs. 39.6%; HR: 0.89 (0.82–0.96); $P = 0.003$], arousing the discussion of HbA1c as the main therapeutic objective to reduce cardiovascular events, leaving the door open to other mechanisms involved in reducing cardiovascular death and hospitalizations for HF beyond of the strict HbA1c targets [193].

Patients with diabetes and HF in the PARADIGM-HF (Prospective Comparison of ARNI [Angiotensin Receptor Neprilysin Inhibitor] With ACEI [Angiotensin-Converting Enzyme Inhibitor] to Determine Impact on Global Mortality and Morbidity in Heart Failure) trial treated with a combination of sacubitril/valsartan had a greater long-term reduction of HbA1c than those receiving enalapril. The de novo use of insulin was 29% lower in patients receiving sacubitril/valsartan ($p = 0.0052$). These data suggest that sacubitril/valsartan may improve glycemic control in patients with diabetes and HF [194].

Pharmacological treatment of the patient with HF with and without diabetes mellitus should include ACE inhibitors, beta-blockers, and aldosterone blockers. Similar benefit has been seen in patients treated with carvedilol in both diabetic and nondiabetic patients (RRR 28% $p = 0.03$ and 37% $p < 0.001$, respectively). There was no significant difference between reducing the risk of death or NNT (number needed to treat) in patients treated with diabetes versus nondiabetics [166].

In the DIG (Digitalis Intervention Group) study, 28.4% of the patients had diabetes. In this study, the addition of digoxin to the treatment of HF reduced hospitalizations secondary to HF without a substantial increase in the risk of toxicity. However, in patients with HF treated with digoxin, it is necessary to identify predictors of toxicity, and strict control of serum levels is important to maintain their benefit [195].

Diseases of the Aorta in Diabetic Patients

Diabetes and Aortic Dissection/Aneurysm

Aortic dissection along with intramural hematoma and penetrating ulcer of the aorta comprise the acute aortic syndromes [196]. Acute aortic dissection is the result of spontaneous tear of the intima, followed by passage of blood between the intima and the aorta. This passage of blood generates a false lumen that progressively compresses the true lumen of the vessel. Clinically, it manifests as an acute and penetrating thoracic pain of sudden onset and of immediate maximum intensity with irradiation toward the back. Pathophysiologically, diabetes mellitus contributes to thickening and fibrosis of the intimal layer and degradation and apoptosis of smooth muscle cells in the media. These processes lead to necrosis and fibrosis of the elastic components of the arterial wall, which in turn produces wall stiffness and weakness, from which dissection and rupture may arise [197]. Although diabetes mellitus does not have a direct causal role in aortic dissection, its role in the development of atherosclerosis contributes to the risk of aortic dissection. Interestingly, a recent study published by Xe et al. demonstrated a paradoxical inverse relationship between DM and risk of aortic dissection in Chinese patients, suggesting that diabetes may play a protective role in the development of aortic dissection. Despite these findings, further information is necessary to elucidate the role of diabetes in aortic dissection [198, 199].

Aortic aneurysm refers to the pathologic enlargement of an aortic segment which tends to progress over time and generally cause no symptoms until they rupture. Atherosclerosis was believed to be the main factor for the development of aortic aneurysms, but recent evidence has shown that aneurysms represent a systemic disease of the vasculature associated with inflammation, smooth muscle cell apoptosis, and matrix degradation. Male gender, hypertension, smoking, and hypercholesterolemia are the main risk factors associated with aortic aneurysms [200]. Diabetic patients with aortic aneurysms are significantly less likely to present with rupture or to die from aneurysm rupture when compared to nondiabetic patients with aortic aneurysms. It is plausible that DM may have a protective effect on aortic aneurysm rupture. Again, further evidence is needed to prove this [201].

Treatment of both aortic dissection and aneurysms is complex and depends on many factors such as hemodynamic status, localization, and anatomical features, all of which are beyond the scope of this chapter.

Diabetes and Aortic Stenosis

Aortic stenosis is the most common primary valve disease in the developed world. It is characterized by a progressive narrowing of the aortic valve orifice due to degeneration, fibrosis, and calcification of the aortic leaflets [202]. This degenerative process has been associated with advanced age and atherosclerosis. Clinically, it manifests with angina, dyspnea, and syncope. A one-year survival among patients with severe aortic stenosis is approximately 50% [203].

Echocardiography is the key diagnostic tool. Aortic peak velocities >4 m/s with mean aortic gradients >40 mm Hg are consistent with severe aortic stenosis regardless of the aortic valve area (severe is >1 cm^2).

Diabetes mellitus has been associated with multiple aspects of aortic stenosis such as the following:

1. Increased inflammation: Patients with diabetes mellitus have accelerated inflammation which leads to calcification. This calcification appears earlier and is more severe than in nondiabetic patients.
2. Stenosis progression. Aortic valve area narrowing is faster in diabetic patients as a result of increased calcium and fibrotic deposits on the valve.
3. Heart failure: As mentioned previously in this chapter, diabetes contributes to left ventricular hypertrophy and with time to systolic dysfunction. The aortic valve stenosis potentiates this effect accelerating the decline in the contractile function of the heart [204].

Aortic valve replacement is the treatment of choice for patients with severe aortic stenosis. Diabetic patients with micro- and macrovascular complications (renal failure, coronary heart disease, neuropathy) have a higher surgical risk based on STS (Society of Thoracic Surgeons) score and EuroSCORE (European System for Cardiac Operative Risk Evaluation) II than nondiabetic patients. Percutaneous implant of an aortic valve (TAVI) has recently shown to be a safe and effective alternative to surgery in high-risk and intermediate-risk patients [205].

Arrhythmias in Diabetic Patients

Special Features of Arrhythmias and Atrioventricular Blocks in Diabetic Patients

In 1972, Rubler [169] introduced the term diabetic cardiomyopathy (DCM) to refer to structural and functional abnormalities of the myocardium in diabetic patients without coronary artery disease, systemic arterial hypertension, or any other morbid entity that affected the functioning of the heart. Interstitial and perivascular fibrosis is the histological landmark of the disease; hypertrophy of cardiomyocytes has also been described, although it does not appear to be a requirement [206]. The loss of normal microvasculature and remodeling of the extracellular matrix are involved and the systolic and diastolic contractile dysfunction of diabetic hearts. It is possible that in DM the increase in fibrosis is involved in the degeneration of the conduction system which may result in an increase in symptomatic bradycardias. Podlaha [207] found the presence of DM in 49.2% of patients with pacemakers

and only 38.4% in nondiabetic patients of the same age, gender, and comorbidity. Perhaps more than the degeneration of the conduction system, DCM-related interstitial fibrosis has a greater impact on the progression of ventricular remodeling, which may result in delayed left ventricular depolarization with increased QRS associated with intra- and interventricular dyssynchrony. The response to cardiac resynchronization therapy does not appear to be different between diabetic and nondiabetic patients, but mortality is higher among the first [208]. At the atria, interstitial fibrosis in patients with DCM may also be secondary to oxidative stress, growth factors, and changes in cellular binding proteins [209]. Overall, fibrosis and atrial remodeling have been identified as primary elements in the generation and maintenance of atrial fibrillation (AF) in patients with DCM [210].

Atrial fibrillation is the most frequent sustained cardiac arrhythmia in clinical practice and is one of the most important determinants of increased cardiovascular morbidity and mortality in patients with heart disease and DM. Numerous studies have shown that poorly controlled DM is associated with new-onset AF [211, 212]. Huxley et al. showed that in patients without diabetes, there is a linear trend between the presence of AF and 1% increments in the level of HbA1c [213]. In diabetic patients, HbA1c levels above 6.5% are associated with a 40% increase in the risk of AF presentation especially in women [214].

Although DCM contributes to cardiovascular disease, the one factor that directly increases the risk of mortality is the development of autonomic diabetic neuropathy (ADN). In diabetic patients with severe ADN, the sympathetic-parasympathetic innervation imbalance may contribute to death by ventricular arrhythmias both in the absence and in the presence of ischemic heart disease [215]. Also, in diabetic patients, sympathetic denervation has been shown to be predictive of sudden death, due to a decrease in the ventricular arrhythmogenic threshold, which has greater expression during events of hypoglycemia or metabolic alterations related to hyperglycemia [216]. The prevalence of ADN is estimated to be as high as 50% in diabetic patients [217]. It is possible that at the initial stages of ADN, there is an increase in sympathetic tone which manifests as tachycardia, shortening of QRS and QT interval, increase in QT dispersion, and flattening of T wave. In advanced states, neurological denervation can lead to an increase in the parasympathetic tone that subsequently increases the risk of developing bradycardia, prolongation of QTc, and other alterations in repolarization [218]. During iatrogenic hypoglycemia, prolongation of the QT interval associated with calcium overload and potassium depletion may also lead to ventricular fibrillation risk. The poor sympathetic response to hypoglycemia is not enough to counteract the electrocardiac effects; on the contrary, it may represent a synergic proarrhythmic effect by increasing repolarization alterations [219].

Multiple Choice Questions

1. Pathological mechanisms associated with increased risk of coronary atherosclerosis in patients with diabetes include:
   (a) Vasoconstriction and hypertension of vascular smooth muscle
   (b) Activation of leukocytes/endothelial cells, release of cytokines, and expression of cellular adhesion molecules
   (c) Autonomic dysfunction
   (d) Hypercoagulation
   (e) *All of the above*

2. All of the following statements about diabetic patients are true, except:
   (a) Compared to nondiabetic, patients with diabetes have two- to threefold higher rate of coronary disease and are at increased risk of myocardial infarction, congestive heart failure, and death.
   (b) Compared to nondiabetic, patients with diabetes have twofold higher rate of systemic arterial hypertension.
   (c) The current guidelines suggest that therapeutic target of blood pressure control is less than 140/90 mmHg.
   (d) Antihypertensive treatment in patients with chronic renal disease should include an angiotensin-converting enzyme inhibitor or an angiotensin receptor blocker.
   (e) *The majority of patients require only one antihypertensive drug to achieve the goal blood pressure.*

3. If a patient tolerates the intensive dose of a statin, what is the best option to do next?
   (a) Increase the dose until the patient starts with secondary effects.
   (b) *Decrease the dose until LDL is over 70 mg/dL.*
   (c) Keep the dose.
   (d) Decrease the dose until HDL starts falling.
   (e) Add ezetimibe in all cases.

4. Dyspnea may be caused by which antiplatelet agent:
   (a) Aspirin
   (b) Clopidogrel
   (c) Prasugrel
   (d) *Ticagrelor*
   (e) Ticlopidine

5. In diabetic patients, what drug has been approved as first-line hypoglycemic drug to reduce cardiovascular events?
   (a) Gliclazide
   (b) Metformin
   (c) Alogliptin
   (d) *Empagliflozin*
   (e) Pioglitazone

6. In diabetic patients with known coronary artery disease, an HbA1c target of less than ___ is recommended:
   (a) 6%
   (b) 6.5%
   (c) 6.8%
   (d) *7%*
   (e) 7.5%

7. What is the most frequent sustained cardiac arrhythmia and one of the most important factors in the increase of cardiovascular morbidity and mortality in patients with diabetes?
   (a) Ventricular fibrillation
   (b) *Atrial fibrillation*
   (c) First-degree AV block
   (d) Third-degree AV block
   (e) Atrial flutter

8. What drug was associated with a reduction in the incidence of heart failure?
   (a) Ramipril
   (b) Sacubitril/valsartan
   (c) Carvedilol
   (d) *Spironolactone (aldosterone antagonist)*
   (e) All of the above

9. Which of the following risk factors is not associated with aortic aneurysms and may have a protective effect on aortic aneurysm rupture?
   (a) Male gender
   (b) Hypertension
   (c) Smoking
   (d) Hypercholesterolemia
   (e) *Diabetes*

10. In general, what is the preferred method of coronary perfusion in patients with an acute coronary ischemic syndrome, with or without diabetes?
    (a) Fibrinolytic therapy
    (b) Coronary artery bypass grafting
    (c) *Percutaneous coronary intervention*
    (d) Aspirin
    (e) Statins

References

1. Iijima R, Ndrepepa G, Kujath V, Harada Y, Kufner S, Schunkert H, Nakamura M, Kastrati A. A pan-coronary artery angiographic study of the association between diabetes mellitus and progression or regression of coronary atherosclerosis. Heart Vessels. 2017;32:376–84.
2. Colwell JA, Lopes-Virella M, Halushka PV. Pathogenesis of atherosclerosis in diabetes mellitus. Diabetes Care. 1981;4(1):121–33.
3. Kearney K, Tomlinson D, Smith K, Ajjan R. Hypofibrinolysis in diabetes: a therapeutic target for the reduction of cardiovascular risk. Cardiovasc Diabetol. 2017;16:34.

4. Birkeland KI, Jørgensen ME, Carstensen B, Persson F, Gulseth HL, Thuresson M, Fenici P, Nathanson D, Nyström T, Eriksson JW, Bodegård J, Norhammar A. Cardiovascular mortality and morbidity in patients with type 2 diabetes following initiation of sodium-glucose co-transporter-2 inhibitors versus other glucose-lowering drugs (CVD-REAL Nordic): a multinational observational analysis. Lancet Diabetes Endocrinol. 2017;5(9):709–17. https://doi.org/10.1016/S2213-8587(17)30258-9.

5. Sakata K, Waseda K, Kume T, Otake H, Nakatani D, Yock PG, Fitzgerald PJ, Honda Y. Impact of diabetes mellitus on vessel response in the drug-eluting stent era pooled volumetric intravascular ultrasound analyses. Circ Cardiovasc Interv. 2012;5:763–71.

6. Serruys PW, Ormiston JA, Onuma Y, Regar E, Gonzalo N, Garcia-Garcia HM, Nieman K, Bruining N, Dorange C, Miquel-Hébert K, Veldhof S, Webster M, Thuesen L, Dudek D. A bioabsorbable everolimus-eluting coronary stent system (ABSORB): 2-year outcomes and results from multiple imaging methods. Lancet. 2009;373:897–910.

7. Gu K, Cowie CC, Harris MI. Mortality in adults with and without diabetes in a national cohort of the U.S. population, 1971-1993. Diabetes Care. 1998;21(7):1138–45.

8. Garcia M, McNamara P, Gordon T, Kannel W. Morbidity and mortality in diabetics in the Framingham population. Sixteen year follow – up. Diabetes. 1974;23:105–11.

9. Stamler J, Vaccaro O, Neaton J, Wentworth D. Diabetes, other risk factors, and 12 yr cardiovascular mortality for men screened in the multiple risk factor intervention trial. Diabetes Care. 1993;16:434–44.

10. Sawicki P, Berger M. Prognosis and treatment of cardiovascular disease in diabetes mellitus. J Clin Basic Cardiol. 1999;2:22–33.

11. Schnohr P, Lange P, Scharling H, Skov Jensen J. Long-term physical activity in leisure time and mortality from coronary heart disease, stroke, respiratory diseases, and cancer. The Copenhagen City Heart Study. Eur J Cardiovasc Prev Rehabil. 2006;13(2):173–9.

12. Hammoud T, Tanguay JF, Bourassa MG. Management of coronary artery disease: therapeutic options in patients with diabetes. J Am Coll Cardiol. 2000;36:355–65.

13. Lteif AA, Mather KJ, Clark CM. Diabetes and heart disease an evidence-driven guide to risk factors management in diabetes. Cardiol Rev. 2003;11:262–74.

14. Aronson D, Rayfield EJ, Chesebro JH. Mechanisms European Association for the Study of Diabetes determining course and outcome of diabetic patients who have had acute myocardial infarction. Ann Intern Med. 1997;126:296–306.

15. Donahoe SM, Stewart GC, McCabe CH, et al. Diabetes and mortality following acute coronary syndromes. JAMA. 2007;298:765–75.

16. Bartnik M, Ryden L, Ferrari R, et al. The prevalence of abnormal glucose regulation in patients with coronary artery disease across Europe. The Euro Heart Survey on diabetes and the heart. Eur Heart J. 2004;25:1880–90.

17. Gholap N, Davies MJ, Mostafa SA, Squire I, Khunti K. A simple strategy for screening for glucose intolerance, using glycated haemoglobin, in individuals admitted with acute coronary syndrome. Diabet Med. 2012;29:838–43.

18. Gyberg V, De Bacquer D, Kotseva K, et al. Screening for dysglycaemia in patients with coronary artery disease as reflected by fasting glucose, oral glucose tolerance test, and HbA1c: a report from EUROASPIRE IV--a survey from the European Society of Cardiology. Eur Heart J. 2015;36:1171–7.

19. Natali A, Vichi S, Landi P, Severi S, L'Abbate A, Ferrannini E. Coronary atherosclerosis in Type II diabetes: angiographic findings and clinical outcome. Diabetologia. 2000;43:632–41.

20. Cariou B, Bonnevie L, Mayaudon H, Dupuy O, Ceccaldi B, Bauduceau B. Angiographic characteristics of coronary artery disease in diabetic patients compared with matched non-diabetic subjects. Diabetes Nutr Metab. 2000;13:134–41.

21. Werner GS, Richartz BM, Heinke S, Ferrari M, Figulla HR. Impaired acute collateral recruitment as a possible mechanism for increased cardiac adverse events in patients with diabetes mellitus. Eur Heart J. 2003;24:1134–42.

22. Berry C, Tardif JC, Bourassa MG. Coronary heart disease in patients with diabetes: part II: recent advances in coronary revascularization. J Am Coll Cardiol. 2007;49:643–56.

23. Pasterkamp G. Methods of accelerated atherosclerosis in diabetic patients. Heart. 2013;99(10):743–9.

24. Suzuki LA, Poot M, Gerrity RG, Bornfeldt KE. Diabetes accelerates smooth muscle accumulation in lesions of atherosclerosis: lack of direct growth-promoting effects of high glucose levels. Diabetes. 2001;50(4):851–60.

25. Williams SB, Cusco JA, Roddy MA, Johnstone MT, Creager MA. Impaired nitric oxide-mediated vasodilation patients with non-insulin-dependent diabetes mellitus. J Am Coll Cardiol. 1996;27(3):567–74.

26. Vinik AI, Erbas T, Park TS, Nolan R, Pittenger GL. Platelet dysfunction in type 2 diabetes. Diabetes Care. 2001;24(8):1476–85.

27. Sowers JR. Recommendations for special populations: diabetes mellitus and the metabolic syndrome. Am J Hypertens. 2003;16:S41–5.

28. Turner RC, Millns H, Neil HA, Stratton IM, Manley SE, Matthews DR, et al. Risk factors for coronary artery disease in non-insulin dependent diabetes mellitus: United Kingdom Prospective Diabetes Study (UKPDS: 23). BMJ. 1998;316(7134):823–8.

29. Usitupa MI, Niskanen LK, Siitonen O, Voutilainen E, Pyorala K. Ten-year cardiovascular mortality in relation to risk factors and abnormalities in lipoprotein composition in type 2 (non-insulin-dependent) diabetic and non-diabetic subjects. Diabetologia. 1993;36(11):1175–84.

30. Assmann G, Schulte H. The Prospective Cardiovascular Munster (PROCAM) study: prevalence of hyperlipidemia in persons with hypertension and/or diabetes mellitus and the relationship to coronary heart disease. Am Heart J. 1988;116(6 Pt 2):1713–24.

31. Somaratne JB, Whalley GA, Poppe KK, ter Bals MM, Wadams G, Pearl A, Bagg W, Doughty RN. Screening for left ventricular hypertrophy in patients with type 2 diabetes mellitus in the community. Cardiovasc Diabetol. 2011;10:29.

32. Govind S, Saha S, Brodin LA, Ramesh SS, Arvind SR, Quintana M. Impaired myocardial functional reserve in hypertension and diabetes mellitus without coronary artery disease: searching for the possible link with congestive heart failure in the myocardial Doppler in diabetes (MYDID) study II. Am J Hypertens. 2006;19(8):851–7; discussion 858.

33. Grossman E, Messerli FH, Goldbourt U. High blood pressure and diabetes mellitus: are all antihypertensive drugs created equal? Arch Intern Med. 2000;160(16):2447–52.

34. Lea JP, Nicholas SB. Diabetes mellitus and hypertension: key risk factors for kidney disease. J Natl Med Assoc. 2002;94(8 Suppl):7S–15S.

35. Knowler WC, Bennett PH, Ballintine EJ. Increased incidence of retinopathy in diabetics with elevated blood pressure. A 6-year follow-up study in Pima Indians. N Engl J Med. 1980;302(12):645–50.

36. Zanchetti A, Ruilope LM. Antihypertensive treatment in patients with type-2 diabetes mellitus: what guidance from recent controlled randomized trials? J Hypertens. 2002;20:2099–110.

37. Stratton IM, Adler AI, Neil HA, Matthews DR, Manley SE, Cull CA, et al. Association of glycaemia with macrovascular and microvascular complications of type 2 diabetes (UKPDS 35): prospective observational study. BMJ. 2000;321(7258):405–12.

38. Barth JH, Marshall SM, Watson ID. Consensus meeting on reporting glycated haemoglobin and estimated average glucose in the

UK: report to the National Director for Diabetes, Department of Health. Ann Clin Biochem. 2008;45(Pt 4):343–4.

39. Adler AI, Stratton IM, Neil HA, Yudkin JS, Matthews DR, Cull CA, et al. Association of systolic bloo pressure with macrovascular and microvascular complications of type 2 diabetes (UKPDS 36): prospective observational study. BMJ. 2000;321(7258):412–9.

40. Fogari R, Zoppi A, Malamani GD, Lazzari P, Destro M, Corradi L. Ambulatory blood pressure monitoring in normotensive and hypertensive type 2 diabetes. Prevalence of impaired diurnal blood pressure patterns. Am J Hypertens. 1993;6:1–7.

41. Grossman E, Shemesh J, Motro M. Hypertensive patients with diabetes mellitus have higher heart rate and pulse pressure. J Hypertens. 2002;20:S60.

42. Pop-Busui R. Cardiac autonomic neuropathy in diabetes: a clinical perspective. Diabetes Care. 2010;33:434–41.

43. Ozawa M, Tamura K, Iwatsubo K, Matsushita K, Sakai M, Tsurumi-Ikeya Y, et al. Ambulatory blood pressure variability is increased in diabetic hypertensives. Clin Exp Hypertens. 2008;30:213–24.

44. Gyberg V, De Bacquer D, De Backer G, Jennings C, Kotseva K, Mellbin L, Schnell O, Tuomilehto J, Wood D, Ryden L, et al. Patients with coronary artery disease and diabetes need improved management: a report from the EUROASPIRE IV survey: a registry from the EuroObservational Research Programme of the European Society of Cardiology. Cardiovasc Diabetol. 2015;14:133.

45. American Diabetes Association. Standards of medical care in diabetes-2012. Diabetes Care. 2012;35(Supl 1):S11–63.

46. Appel LJ, Moore TJ, Obarzanek E, Vollmer WM, Svetkey LP, Sacks FM, et al. A clinical trial of the effects of dietary patterns on blood pressure. DASH Collaborative Research Group. N Engl J Med. 1997;336:1117–24.

47. James PA, Oparil S, Carter BL, Cushman WC, Dennison-Himmelfarb C, Handler J, et al. 2014 evidence-based guideline for the management of high blood pressure in adults: report from the panel members appointed to the Eighth Joint National Committee (JNC 8). JAMA. 2014;311(5):507–20.

48. Mancia G, Fagard R, Narkiewicz K, Redon J, Zanchetti A, Bohm M, et al. 2013 ESH/ESC Guidelines for the management of arterial hypertension: the task force for the management of arterial hypertension of the European Society of Hypertension (ESH) and of the European Society of Cardiology (ESC). J Hypertens. 2013;31(7):1281–357.

49. Cushman WC, Evans GW, Byington RP, Goff DC Jr, Grimm RH Jr, Cutler JA, et al. Effects of intensive blood- pressure control in type 2 diabetes mellitus. N Engl J Med. 2010;362(17):1575–85.

50. Wright JT Jr, Williamson JD, Whelton PK, Snyder JK, Sink KM, Rocco MV, Reboussin DM, Rahman M, Oparil S, Lewis CE, et al. A randomized trial of intensive versus standard blood-pressure control. N Engl J Med. 2015;373(22):2103–16.

51. Reboldi G, Gentile G, Angeli F, Ambrosio G, Mancia G, Verdecchia P. Effects of intensive blood pressure reduction on myocardial infarction and stroke in diabetes: a meta-analysis in 73,913 patients. J Hypertens. 2011;29(7):1253–69.

52. Solini A, Grossman E. What should be the target blood pressure in elderly patients with diabetes? Diabetes Care. 2016;39(Suppl 2):S234–43.

53. Scheen AJ. Renin-angiotensin system inhibition prevents type 2 diabetes mellitus. Part 2. Overview of physiological and biochemical mechanisms. Diabetes Metab. 2004;30(6):498–505.

54. Weber MA, Jamerson K, Bakris GL, Weir MR, Zappe D, Zhang Y, Dahlof B, Velazquez EJ, Pitt B. Effects of body size and hypertension treatments on cardiovascular event rates: subanalysis of the ACCOMPLISH randomised controlled trial. Lancet. 2013;381(9866):537–45.

55. Varga-Szabo D, Pleines I, Nieswandt B. Cell adhesion mechanisms in platelets. Arterioscler Thromb Vasc Biol. 2008;28:403–12.

56. Gurbel PA, Bliden KP, DiChiara J, et al. Evaluation of dose related effects of aspirin on platelet function: results from the Aspirin-Induced Platelet Effect (ASPECT) study. Circulation. 2007;115:3156–64.

57. Windecker S, Kolh P, Alfonso F, Collet JP, Cremer J, Falk V, et al. 2014 ESC/EACTS Guidelines on myocardial revascularization. Eur Heart J. 2014;35:2541–619. https://doi.org/10.1093/eurheartj/ehu278.

58. Price MJ, Berger PB, Teirstein PS, et al. Standard- vs. high-dose clopidogrel based on platelet function testing after percutaneous coronary intervention: the GRAVITAS randomized trial. JAMA. 2011;205(11):1097–105.

59. Thukkani AK, Agrawal K, Prince L, Smoot KJ, Dufour AB, Cho K, et al. Long-Term outcomes in patients with Diabetes Mellitus related to prolonging Clopidogrel more than 12 months after coronary stenting. J Am Coll Cardiol. 2015;66(10):1091–101. https://doi.org/10.1016/j.jacc.2015.06.1339.

60. Wiviott SD, Braunwald E, McCabe CH, et al. Prasugrel versus clopidogrel in patients with acute coronary syndromes. N Engl J Med. 2007;357(20):2001–15.

61. Roe MT, Goodman SG, Ohman EM, et al. Elderly patients with acute coronary syndromes managed without revascularization: Insights into the safety of long-term dual antiplatelet therapy with reduced-dose prasugrel vs. standard-dose clopidogrel. Circulation. 2013;128(8):823–33.

62. Wallentin L, Becker RC, Budaj A, Cannon CP, Emanuelsson H, Held C, et al. Ticagrelor versus clopidogrel in patients with acute coronary syndromes. N Engl J Med. 2009;361:1045–57. https://doi.org/10.1056/NEJMoa0904327.

63. Angiolillo DJ, Capranzano P, Goto S, et al. A randomized study assessing the impact of cilostazol on platelet function profiles in patients with diabetes mellitus and coronary artery disease on dual antiplatelet therapy: results of the OPTIMUS-2 study. Eur Heart J. 2008;29:2202–11.

64. Stone NJ, Robinson J, Lichtenstein AH, Merz NB, Lloyd-Jones DM, Blum CB, et al. 2013 ACC/AHA guideline on the treatment of blood cholesterol to reduce atherosclerotic cardiovascular risk in adults. J Am Coll Cardiol. 2013;63(25 Pt B):2889–934. https://doi.org/10.1016/j.jacc.2013.11.002.

65. Hulten E, Jackson JL, Douglas K, et al. The effect of early, intensive statin therapy on acute coronary syndrome: a meta-analysis of randomized controlled trials. Arch Intern Med. 2006;166(17):1814–21.

66. Heart Protection Study Collaborative Group. MRC/BHF Heart Protection Study of cholesterol-lowering with simvastatin in 5963 people with diabetes: a randomised placebo-controlled trial. Lancet. 2003;361(9374):2005–16.

67. Murphy SA, Cannon CP, Wiviott SD, et al. Reduction in recurrent cardiovascular events with intensive lipid-lowering statin therapy compared with moderate lipid-lowering statin therapy after acute coronary syndromes. J Am Coll Cardiol. 2009;54(25):2358–62.

68. Taylor AJ, Sullenberger LE, Lee HJ, et al. Arterial Biology for the Investigation of the Treatment Effects of Reducing Cholesterol (ARBITER) 2: A double-blind, placebo-controlled study of extended-release niacin on atherosclerosis progression in secondary prevention patients treated with statins. Circulation. 2004;110(23):3512–7.

69. ACCORD Study Group. Effects of combination lipid therapy in type 2 diabetes mellitus. N Engl J Med. 2010;362(17):1563–74.

70. Baigent C, Landray MJ, Reith C, et al. The effects of lowering LDL cholesterol with simvastatin plus ezetimibe in patients with chronic kidney disease (Study of Heart and Renal Protection): a randomized placebo-controlled trial. Lancet. 2011;377(9784):2181–92.

71. Saremi A, Schwenke DC, Buchanan TA, et al. Pioglitazone slows progression of atherosclerosis in prediabetes independent of changes in cardiovascular risk factors. Arterioscler Thromb Vasc Biol. 2013;33(2):393–9.

72. Holman RR, Paul SK, Bethel MA, et al. 10-year follow-up of intensive glucose control in type 2 diabetes. N Engl J Med. 2008;359(15):1577–89.

73. American Diabetes Association Standards of Medical Care in Diabetes – 2017. Diabetes Care. 2017;40(sup 1):S1–S138.

74. Inzucchi SE, Bergenstal RM, Buse JB, et al. Management of hyperglycemia in type 2 diabetes: A patient-centered approach: position statement of the American Diabetes Association (ADA) and the European Association for the Study of Diabetes (EASD). Diabetes Care. 2012;35:1364.

75. University Group Diabetes Program. Effects of hypoglycemic agents on vascular complications in patients with adult-onset diabetes. Diabetes. 1982;31(suppl 5):1–81.

76. Flynn DM, Smith AH, Treadway JL, Levy CB, Soeller WC, Boettner WA, et al. The sulfonylurea glipizide does not inhibit ischemic preconditioning in anesthetized rabbits. Cardiovasc Drugs Ther. 2005;19:337–46.

77. Mocanu MM, Maddock HL, Baxter GF, Lawrence CL, Standen NB, Yellon DM. Glimepiride, a novel sulfonylurea, does not abolish myocardial protection afforded by either ischemic preconditioning or diazoxide. Circulation. 2001;103:3111–6.

78. Cleveland JC, Meldrum DR, Brian S, Cain BS, Banerjee A, Alden H, Harken AH. Oral sulfonylurea hypoglycemic agents prevent ischemic preconditioning in human myocardium: two paradoxes revisited. Circulation. 1997;96:29–32.

79. Schramm TK, Gislason GH, Vaag A, et al. Mortality and cardiovascular risk associated with different insulin secretagogues compared with metformin in type 2 diabetes, with or without a previous myocardial infarction: a nationwide study. Eur Heart J. 2011;32(15):1900–8; Erratum in: Eur Heart J. 2012 May;33(10):1183.

80. Inzucchi SE, McGuire DK. New Drugs for the treatment of diabetes. Circulation. 2008;117:574–84.

81. Dormandy JA, Charbonnel B, Eckland DJ, Erdmann E, Massi-Benedetti M, Moules IK, et al. Secondary prevention of macrovascular events in patients with type 2 diabetes in the PROactive Study. Lancet. 2005;366:1279–89.

82. Lincoff AM, Wolski K, Nicholls SJ, Nissen SE. Pioglitazone and risk of cardiovascular events in patients with type 2 diabetes mellitus: a meta-analysis of randomized trials. JAMA. 2007;12(298):1180–8.

83. Nissen SE, Wolski K. Effect of rosiglitazone on the risk of myocardial infarction and death from cardiovascular causes. N Engl J Med. 2007;356:2457–71.

84. Singh S, Loke YK, Furberg CD. Long-term risk of cardiovascular events with rosiglitazone: a meta-analysis. JAMA. 2007;298:1189–95.

85. Monami M, Ahren B, Dicembrini I, Mannucd E. Dipeptidyl peptidase-4 inhibitors and cardiovascular risk: a meta-analysis of randomized clinical trials. Diabetes Obes Metab. 2013;15(2):112–20.

86. Scirica BM, Bhatt DL, Braunwald E, et al. Saxagliptin and cardiovascular outcomes in patients with type 2 diabetes mellitus. N Engl J Med. 2013;369:1317.

87. White WB, Cannon CP, Heller SR, et al. EXAMINE Investigators. Alogliptin after acute coronary syndrome in patients with type 2 diabetes. N Engl J Med. 2013;369(14):1327–35.

88. Zinman B, Wanner C, Lachin JM, et al. EMPA-REG OUTCOME Investigators. Empagliflozin, cardiovascular outcomes, and mortality in type 2 diabetes. N Engl J Med. 2015;373:2117–28.

89. Marso SP, Daniels GH, Brown-Frandsen K, et al. LEADER Steering Committee; LEADER Trial Investigators. Liraglutide and cardiovascular outcomes in type 2 diabetes. N Engl J Med. 2016;375:311–22.

90. Pfeffer MA, et al. Lixisenatide in patients with type 2 diabetes and acute coronary syndrome. N Engl J Med. 2015;373(23):2247–57.

91. Chiasson JL, Josse RG, Gomis R, Hanefeld M, Karasik A, Laakso M, STOP-NIDDM Trial Research Group. Acarbose treatment and the risk of cardiovascular disease and hypertension in patients with impaired glucose tolerance: the STOP-NIDDM trial. JAMA. 2003;290:486–94.

92. Mann DL, Zipes DP, Libby P, Bonow RO, Braunwald E, editors. Braunwald's heart disease: a textbook of cardiovascular medicine. 10th ed. Philadelphia, PA: Elsevier Saunders; 2015. p. 1375;Chap 61.

93. Gerstein HC, Bosch J, et al. Basal insulin and cardiovascular and other outcomes in dysglycemia. N Engl J Med. 2012;367:319–28.

94. Gaede P, Lund-Andersen H, Parving HH, Pedersen O. Effect of a multifactorial intervention on mortality in type 2 diabetes. N Engl J Med. 2008;358(6):580–91.

95. Goff DC, Lloyd-Jones DM, Bennett G, Coady S, D'Agostino RB, Gibbons R, et al. 2013 ACC/AHA cardiovascular risk assessment guideline. Circulation. 2014;129(suppl 2):S49–73. https://doi.org/10.1161/01.cir.0000437741.48606.98.

96. Conroy RM, Pyorala K, Fitzgerald AP, Sans S, Menotti A, De Backer G, et al. Estimation of ten-year risk of fatal cardiovascular disease in Europe: the SCORE project. Eur H J. 2003;24:987–1003.

97. Piepoli MF, Hoes A, Agewall S, Albus C, Brotons C, Catapano AL, et al. 2016 European Guidelines on cardiovascular disease prevention in clinical practice. Eur Heart J. 2016;37:2315–81. https://doi.org/10.1093/eurheartj/ehw106.

98. Young LH, Wackers FJT, Chyun DA, et al. DIAD Investigators. Cardiac outcomes after screening for asymptomatic coronary artery disease in patients with type 2 diabetes: the DIAD study: a randomized controlled trial. JAMA. 2009;301:1547–55.

99. Montalescot G, Sechtem U, Achenbach S, Andreotti F, Arden C, Budaj A, et al. 2013 ESC guidelines on the management of stable coronary artery disease. Eur Heart J. 2013;34:2949–3003. https://doi.org/10.1093/eurheartj/eht296.

100. Fihn SD, Gardin JM, Abrams J, Berra K, Blankenship JC, Dallas AP, et al. 2012 ACCF/AHA/ACP/AATS/PCNA/SCAI/STS guideline for the diagnosis and management of patients with stable ischemic heart disease. J Am Coll Cardiol. 2012;60(24):2564–603. https://doi.org/10.1016/j.jacc.2012.07.013.

101. Paech DC, Weston AR. A systematic review of the clinical effectiveness of 64-slice or higher computed tomography angiography as an alternative to invasive coronary angiography in the investigation of suspected coronary artery disease. BMC Cardiovasc Disord. 2011;11:32.

102. Center for Disease Control and Prevention. National diabetes fact sheet: national estimates and general information on diabetes and prediabetes in the US 2011. Washington, DC: US Department of Health and Human Services; 2011.

103. Norhammar A, Malmberg K, Diderholm E, Lagerqvist B, Lindahl B, Rydén L, Wallentin L. Diabetes mellitus: the major risk factor in unstable coronary artery disease even after consideration of the extent of coronary artery disease and benefits of revascularization. J Am Coll Cardiol. 2004;43:585–91. https://doi.org/10.1016/j.jacc.2003.08.050.

104. Creager MA, Lüscher TF, Cosentino F, Beckman JA. Diabetes and vascular disease: pathophysiology, clinical consequences, and medical therapy: part I. Circulation. 2003;108:1527–32. https://doi.org/10.1161/01.CIR.0000091257.27563.32.

105. Dagenais GR, Lu J, Faxon DP, Kent K, Lago RM, Lezama C, Hueb W, Weiss M, Slater J, Frye RL. Effects of optimal medical treatment with or without coronary revascularization on angina and subsequent revascularizations in patients with type 2 diabetes mellitus

and stable ischemic heart disease. Circulation. 2011;123:1492–500. https://doi.org/10.1161/CIRCULATIONAHA.110.978247.

106. Hlatky MA, Boothroyd DB, Bravata DM, Boersma E, Booth J, Brooks MM, Carrié D, Clayton TC, Danchin N, Flather M, Hamm CW, Hueb WA, Kähler J, Kelsey SF, King SB, Kosinski AS, Lopes N, McDonald KM, Rodriguez A, Serruys P, Sigwart U, Stables RH, Owens DK, Pocock SJ. Coronary artery bypass surgery compared with percutaneous coronary interventions for multivessel disease: a collaborative analysis of individual patient data from ten randomized trials. Lancet. 2009;373:1190–7. https://doi.org/10.1016/S0140-6736(09)60552-3.

107. American Diabetes Association. Executive summary: standards of medical care in diabetes-2012. Diabetes Care. 2012;35(Suppl 1):S4–S10.

108. Smith SC, Benjamin EJ, Bonow RO, Braun LT, Creager MA, Franklin BA, Gibbons RJ, Grundy SM, Hiratzka LF, Jones DW, Lloyd-Jones DM, Minissian M, Mosca L, Peterson ED, Sacco RL, Spertus J, Stein JH, Taubert KA. AHA/ACCF Secondary Prevention and Risk Reduction Therapy for Patients with Coronary and other Atherosclerotic Vascular Disease: 2011 update: a guideline from the American Heart Association and American College of Cardiology Foundation. Circulation. 2011;124:2458–73. https://doi.org/10.1161/CIR.0b013e318235eb4d.

109. Stone GW, Ellis SG, Cox DA, Hermiller J, O'Shaughnessy C, Mann JT, Turco M, Caputo R, Bergin P, Greenberg J, Popma JJ, Russell ME. A polymer-based, paclitaxel-eluting stent in patients with coronary artery disease. N Engl J Med. 2004;350:221–31.

110. Stone GW, Rizvi A, Newman W, Mastali K, Wang JC, Caputo R, Doostzadeh J, Cao S, Simonton CA, Sudhir K, Lansky AJ, Cutlip DE, Kereiakes DJ. Everolimus-eluting versus paclitaxel-eluting stents in coronary artery disease. N Engl J Med. 2010;362:1663–74.

111. Nashef SA, Roques F, Sharples LD, Nilsson J, Smith C, Goldstone AR, Lockowandt U. EuroSCORE II. Eur J Cardiothorac Surg. 2012;41:734–44; discussion 744-745.

112. Serruys PW, Morice MC, Kappetein AP, Colombo A, Holmes DR, Mack MJ, Ståhle E, Feldman TE, van den Brand M, Bass EJ, Van Dyck N, Leadley K, Dawkins KD, Mohr FW. Percutaneous coronary intervention versus coronary-artery bypass grafting for severe coronary artery disease. N Engl J Med. 2009;360:961–72.

113. Mack MJ, Banning AP, Serruys PW, Morice MC, Taeymans Y, VanNooten G, Possati G, Crea F, Hood KL, Leadley K, Dawkins KD, Kappetein AP. Bypass versus drug-eluting stents at three years in SYNTAX patients with diabetes mellitus or metabolic syndrome. Ann Thorac Surg. 2011;92:2140–6.

114. Farkouh ME, Domanski M, Sleeper LA, Siami FS, Dangas G, Mack M, Yang M, Cohen DJ, Rosenberg Y, Solomon SD, Desai AS, Gersh BJ, Magnuson EA, Lansky A, Boineau R, Weinberger J, Ramanathan K, Sousa JE, Rankin J, Bhargava B, Buse J, Hueb W, Smith CR, Muratov V, Bansilal S, King S, Bertrand M, Fuster V. Strategies for multivessel revascularization in patients with diabetes. N Engl J Med. 2012;367:2375–84.

115. Baber U, Mehran R, Sharma SK, Brar S, Yu J, Suh JW, Kim HS, Park SJ, Kastrati A, de Waha A, Krishnan P, Moreno P, Sweeny J, Kim MC, Suleman J, Pyo R, Wiley J, Kovacic J, Kini AS, Dangas GD. Impact of the everolimus-eluting stent on stent thrombosis: a meta-analysis of 13 randomized trials. J Am Coll Cardiol. 2011;58:1569–77.

116. Bangalore S, Toklu B, Feit F. Response to letter regarding article, "Outcomes with coronary artery bypass graft surgery versus percutaneous coronary intervention for patients with diabetes mellitus: can newer generation drug-eluting stents bridge the gap?". Circ Cardiovasc Interv. 2014;7:729.

117. Muramatsu T, Onuma Y, van Geuns RJ, Chevalier B, Patel TM, Seth A, Diletti R, García-García HM, Dorange CC, Veldhof S, Cheong WF, Ozaki Y, Whitbourn R, Bartorelli A, Stone GW, Abizaid A, Serruys PW. 1-year clinical outcomes of diabetic patients treated with everolimus-eluting bioresorbable vascular scaffolds: a pooled analysis of the ABSORB and the SPIRIT trials. JACC Cardiovasc Interv. 2014;7:482–93.

118. Onuma Y, Serruys PW. Bioresorbable scaffold: the advent of a new era in percutaneous coronary and peripheral revascularization? Circulation. 2011;123:779–97.

119. Deedwania P, Acharya T, Kotak K, Fonarow GC, Cannon CP, Laskey WK, Peacock WF, et al. On behalf of GWTG Steering Committee and Investigators. Compliance with guideline directed therapy in diabetic patients admitted with acute coronary syndrome: findings from AHA get with the guidelines – Coronary Artery Disease Program. Am Heart J. 2017;187:78–87. https://doi.org/10.1016/j.ahj.2017.02.025.

120. Mackay MH, Ratner PA, Johnson JL, Humphries KH, Buller CE. Gender differences in symptoms of myocardial ischaemia. Eur Heart J. 2011;32:3107–14.

121. Gimenez MR, Reiter M, Twerenbold R, Reichlin T, Wildi K, Haaf P, et al. Sex specific chest pain characteristics in the early diagnosis of acute myocardial infarction. JAMA Intern Med. 2014;174(2):241–9.

122. Diercks DB, Peacock WF, Hiestand BC, Chen AY, Pollack CV Jr, Kirk JD, et al. Frequency and consequences of recording an electrocardiogram >10 minutes after arrival in an emergency room in non-ST-segment elevation acute coronary syndromes (from the CRUSADE initiative). Am J Cardiol. 2006;97:437–42.

123. Savonitto S, Ardissino D, Granger CB, Morando G, Prando MD, Mafrici A, et al. Prognostic value of the admission electrocardiogram in acute coronary syndromes. JAMA. 1999;281:707–13.

124. Steg PG, James SK, Atar D, Badano LP, Blomstrom-Lundqvist C, Borger MA, et al. ESC guidelines for the management of acute myocardial infarction in patients presenting with ST-segment elevation. Eur Heart J. 2012;33:2569–619.

125. Mueller C. Biomarkers and acute coronary syndromes: an update. Eur Heart J. 2014;35:552–6.

126. Thygesen K, Mair J, Giannitsis E, Mueller C, Lindahl B, Blankenberg S, et al. How to use high-sensitivity cardiac troponins in acute cardiac care. Eur Heart J. 2012;33:2252–7.

127. Irfan A, Twerenbold R, Reiter M, Reichlin T, Stelzig C, Freese M, et al. Determinants of high-sensitivity troponin T among patients with a noncardiac cause of chest pain. Am J Med. 2012;125:491–8.

128. Raskovalova T, Twerenbold R, Collinson PO, Keller T, Bouvaist H, Folli C, et al. Diagnostic accuracy of combined cardiac troponin and copeptin assessment for early rule-out of myocardial infarction: a systematic review and meta-analysis. Eur Heart J Acute Cardiovasc Care. 2014;3:18–27.

129. Maisel A, Mueller C, Neath SX, Christenson RH, Morgenthaler NG, McCord J, et al. Copeptin helps in the early detection of patients with acute myocardial infarction: primary results of the CHOPIN trial (Copeptin Helps in the early detection Of Patients with acute myocardial infarction). J Am Coll Cardiol. 2013;62:150–60.

130. Reichlin T, Twerenbold R, Wildi K, Gimenez MR, Bergsma N, Haaf P, et al. Prospective validation of a 1-hour algorithm to rule-out and rule-in acute myocardial infarction using a high sensitivity cardiac troponin T assay. CMAJ. 2015;187:E243–52.

131. Grenne B, Eek C, Sjoli B, Dahlslett T, Uchto M, Hol PK, et al. Acute coronary occlusion in non-ST-elevation acute coronary syndrome: outcome and early identification by strain echocardiography. Heart. 2010;96:1550–6.

132. Antman EM, Cohen M, Bernink PJ, McCabe CH, Horacek T, Papuchis G, et al. The TIMI risk score for unstable angina/non-ST elevation MI: a method for prognostication and therapeutic decision making. JAMA. 2000;284:835–42.

133. Morrow DA, Antman EM, Charlesworth A, Cairns R, Murphy SA, de Lemos JA, et al. TIMI risk score for ST-elevation myocardial infarction: a convenient, bedside, clinical score for risk

assessment at presentation an intravenous nPA for treatment of infarcting myocardium early II trial substudy. Circulation. 2000;102:2031–7.

134. Fox KA, Dabbous OH, Goldberg RJ, Pieper KS, Eagle KA, de Werf V, et al. Prediction of risk of death and myocardial infarction in the six months after presentation with acute coronary syndrome: prospective multinational observational study (GRACE). BMJ. 2006;333:1091–4.

135. Cakar MA, Sahinkus S, Aydin E, Vatan MB, Keser N, Akdemir R, et al. Relation between the GRACE score and severity of atherosclerosis in acute coronary syndrome. J Cardiol. 2014;63:24–8.

136. Yan AT, Yan RT, Tan M, Eagle KA, Granger CB, Dabbous OH, et al. In-hospital revascularization and one-year outcome of acute coronary syndrome patients stratified by the GRACE risk score. Am J Cardiol. 2005;96(7):913–6.

137. Garg S, Sarno G, Serruys PW, Rodriguez AE, Bolognese L, Anselmi M, et al. Prediction of 1-year clinical outcomes using the SYNTAX score in patients with acute ST-segment elevation myocardial infarction undergoing primary percutaneous coronary intervention: a substudy of the STRATEGY (Single High-Dose Bolus Tirofiban and Sirolimus-Eluting Stent Versus Abciximab and Bare-Metal Stent in Acute Myocardial Infarction) and MULTISTRATEGY (Multicenter Evaluation of Single High-Dose Bolus Tirofiban Versus Abciximab With Sirolimus-Eluting Stent or Bare-Metal Stent in Acute Myocardial Infarction Study) trials. JACC Cardiovasc Interv. 2011;4:66–75.

138. Morice MC, Serruys PW, Kappetein P, Feldman T, Stahle E, Colombo A, et al. Five-year outcomes in patients with left main disease treated with either percutaneous coronary intervention or coronary artery bypass grafting in the SYNTAX trial. Circulation. 2014;129:2388–94.

139. Farkouh ME, Domanski M, Sleeper LA, Siami FS, Dangas G, Mack M, et al. Strategies for multivessel revascularization in patients with diabetes. N Engl J Med. 2012;367:2375–84.

140. Subherwal S, Bach RG, Chen AY, Gage BF, Rao SV, Newby LK, et al. Baseline risk of major bleeding in non–ST-segment– elevation myocardial infarction the CRUSADE (Can Rapid risk stratification of Unstable angina patients Suppress ADverse outcomes with Early implementation of the ACC/AHA guidelines) bleeding score. Circulation. 2009;119:1873–82.

141. Franklin K, Goldberg RJ, Spencer F, Klein W, Budaj A, Brieger D, et al. Implications of diabetes in patients with acute coronary syndromes. The Global Registry of Acute Coronary Events. Arch Intern Med. 2004;164:1457–63.

142. Finfer S, Chittock DR, Su SY, Blair D, Foster D, Dhingra V, et al. The NICE-SUGAR Study Investigators. Intensive versus conventional glucose control in critically ill patients. N Engl J Med. 2009;360:1283–97.

143. Wiviott SD, Braunwald E, Angiolillo DJ, Meisel S, Dalby AJ, Verheugt FW, et al. TRITON-TIMI 38 Investigators. Greater clinical benefit of more intensive oral antiplatelet therapy with prasugrel in patients with diabetes mellitus in the trial to assess improvement in therapeutic outcomes by optimizing platelet inhibition with prasugrel-thrombolysis in myocardial infarction 38. Circulation. 2008;118:1626–36.

144. James S, Angiolillo DJ, Cornel JH, Erlinge D, Husted S, Kontny F, et al. PLATO Study Group. Ticagrelor vs. clopidogrel in patients with acute coronary syndromes and diabetes: a substudy from the PLATelet inhibition and patient Outcomes (PLATO) trial. Eur Heart J. 2010;31:3006–16.

145. Goodman SG, Cohen M, Bigonzi F, Gurfinkel EP, Radley DR, Le Iouer V, et al. Randomized trial of low molecular weight heparin (enoxaparin) versus unfractionated heparin for unstable coronary artery disease: one-year results of the ESSENCE Study. Efficacy and safety of subcutaneous enoxaparin in non-Q wave coronary events. J Am Coll Cardiol. 2000;36:693–8.

146. White HD, Kleiman NS, Mahaffey KW, Lokhnygina Y, Pieper KS, Chiswell K, et al. Efficacy and safety of enoxaparin compared with unfractionated heparin in high-risk patients with non-ST-segment elevation acute coronary syndrome undergoing percutaneous coronary intervention in the Superior Yield of the New Strategy of Enoxaparin, Revascularization and Glycoprotein IIb/IIIa Inhibitors (SYNERGY) trial. Am Heart J. 2006;152:1042–50.

147. Stone GW, White HD, Ohman EM, Bertrand ME, Lincoff AM, McLaurin BT, et al. for the Acute Catheterization and Urgent Intervention Triage strategy (ACUITY) trial investigators. Bivalirudin in patients with acute coronary syndromes undergoing percutaneous coronary intervention: a subgroup analysis from the Acute Catheterization and Urgent Intervention Triage strategy (ACUITY) trial. Lancet. 2007;369:907–19.

148. Feit F, Manoukian SV, Ebrahimi R, Pollack CV, Ohman EM, Attubato MJ, et al. Safety and efficacy of bivalirudin monotherapy in patients with diabetes mellitus and acute coronary syndromes: a report from the ACUITY (Acute Catheterization and Urgent Intervention Triage Strategy) trial. J Am Coll Cardiol. 2008;51:1645–52.

149. Roffi M, Patrono C, Collet JP, Mueller C, Valgimigli M, Andreotti F, et al. 2015 ESC Guidelines for the management of acute coronary syndromes in patients presenting without persistent ST-segment elevation. Task force for the management of acute coronary syndromes in patients presenting without persistent ST-segment elevation of the European Society of Cardiology (ESC). Eur Heart J. 2016;37:267–315.

150. Amsterdam EA, Wenger NK, Brindis RG, Casey DE, Ganiats TG, Holmes DR, et al. 2014 AHA/ACC guideline for the management of patients with non-ST-elevation acute coronary syndromes. A report of the American College of Cardiology/American Heart Association Task Force on Practice Guidelines. Circulation. 2014;130:e344–426.

151. Prasad A, Sotne G, Suckey T, et al. Impact of diabetes mellitus on myocardial perfusion after primary angioplasty in patients with acute myocardial infarction. J Am Coll Cardiol. 2005;45:508–14.

152. Feldman LJ, Coste P, Furber A, et al. Optimal STenting-2 Investigators. Incomplete resolution of ST-segment elevation is a marker of transient microcirculatory dysfunction after stenting for acute myocardial infarction. Circulation. 2003;107:2684–9.

153. Biondi-Zoccai GG, Abbate A, Liuzzo G, Biasucci LM. Atherothrombosis, inflammation, and diabetes. J Am Coll Cardiol. 2003;41:1071–7.

154. Li N, Gui Y, Chen M. Comparing the adverse clinical outcomes in patients with non-insulin treated type 2 diabetes mellitus and patients without type 2 diabetes mellitus following percutaneous coronary intervention: a systematic review and meta-analysis. BMC Cardiovasc Disord. 2016;16:238.

155. Witzenbichler B, Mehran R, Guagliumi G, et al. Impact of diabetes mellitus on the safety and effectiveness of bivalirudin in patients with acute myocardial infarction undergoing primary angioplasty: analysis from the HORIZONS-AMI (Harmonizing Outcomes with RevasculariZatiON and Stents in Acute Myocardial Infarction) trial. JACC Cardiovasc Interv. 2011;4(7):760–8.

156. Alabas OA, Hall M, Rutherford MJ, el atl. Long-term excess mortality associates with diabetes following acute myocardial infarction: a population-base cohort study. J Epidemiol Community Health. 2017;71:25–32.

157. Mathew V, Gersh BJ, Williams BA, et al. Outcomes in patients with diabetes mellitus undergoing percutaneous coronary intervention in the current era: a report from the Prevention of REStenosis with Tranilast and its Outcomes (PRESTO) trial. Circulation. 2004;109(4):476–80.

158. Dangas GD, Farkouh ME, Sleeper LA, et al. Long-term outcome of PCI versus CABG in insulin and non-insulin-treated diabetic

patients: results from the FREEDOM trial. J Am Coll Cardiol. 2014;64(12):1189–97.

159. Mahmoud A, Elgendy I, Mansoor H, et al. Early invasive strategy and in-hospital survival among diabetic with non-ST-elevation acute coronary syndromes: a contemporary national Insight. J Am Heart Assoc. 2017;6:e005369.

160. Cannon CP, Weintraub WS, Demopoulos LA, et al. Comparison of early invasive and conservative strategies in patients with unstable coronary syndromes treated with the glycoprotein IIb/IIIa inhibitor tirofiban. N Engl J Med. 2001;344:1879–87.

161. Carson JL, Scholz PM, Chen AY, et al. Diabetes mellitus increases short-term mortality and morbidity in patients undergoing coronary artery bypass graft surgery. J Am Coll Cardiol. 2002;40:418–23.

162. Timmer JR, Ottervanger JP, de Boer MJ, et al. Primary percutaneous coronary intervention compared with fibrinolysis for myocardial infarction in diabetes mellitus: results from the Primary Coronary Angioplasty vs Thrombolysis-2 trial. Arch Intern Med. 2007;167(13):1353–9.

163. Angeja BG, de Lemos J, Murphy SA, et al. Impact of diabetes mellitus on epicardial and microvascular flow after fibrinolytic therapy. Am Heart J. 2002;144:649–56.

164. Leavitt BJ, Sheppard L, Maloney C, et al. Effect of diabetes and associated conditions on long-term survival after coronary artery bypass graft surgery. Circulation. 2004;110(11 Suppl 1):II41–4.

165. Kannel WB, McGee DL. Diabetes and cardiovascular disease. The Framingham study. JAMA. 1979;241:2035–8.

166. Bell DS, Lukas MA, Holdbrook FK, Fowler MB. The effect of carvedilol on mortality risk in heart failure patients with diabetes: results of a meta-analysis. Curr Med Res Opin. 2006 Feb;22(2):287–96.

167. Van Deursen VM, Urso R, Laroche C, Damman K, Dahlström U, Tavazzi L. Co-morbidities in patients with heart failure: an analysis of the European Heart Failure Pilot Survey. Eur J Heart Fail. 2014;16(1):103–1.

168. Kasznicki J, Drzewoski J. Heart failure in the diabetic population-pathophysiology, diagnosis and management. Arch Med Sci. 2014;10(3):546–56.

169. Rubler S, Dlugash J, Yuceoglu YZ, Kumral T, Branwood AW, Grishman A. New type of cardiomyopathy associated with diabetic glomerulosclerosis. Am J Cardiol. 1972;30:595–602.

170. Sharma V, McNeill JH. Diabetic cardiomyopathy: Where are we 40 years later? Can J Cardiol. 2006;22(4):305–8.

171. Aneja A, Tang WH, Bansilal S, Garcia MJ, Farkouh M. Diabetic cardiomyopathy: insights into pathogenesis, diagnostic challenges, and therapeutic options. Am J Med. 2008;121:748–57.

172. Devereux RB, Roman MJ, Paranicas M, et al. Impact of diabetes on cardiac structure and function: the Strong Heart Study. Circulation. 2000;101:2271–6.

173. Young ME, Mcnulty P, Taegtmeyer H. Adaptation and maladaptation of the heart in diabetes: part II potential mechanisms. Circulation. 2002;105:1861–70.

174. Fischer VW, Barner HB, Larose LS. Pathomorphologic aspects of muscular tissue in diabetes mellitus. Hum Pathol. 1984;15:1127–36.

175. Shimizu M, Umeda K, Sugihara N, et al. Collagen remodelling in myocardia of diabetic patients. J Clin Pathol. 1993;46:32–6.

176. Fukushima A. Lopaschuk GA Cardiac fatty acid oxidation in heart failure associated with obesity and diabetes. Biochim Biophys Acta. 1861;2016:1525–34.

177. Negishi K, Seicean S, Negishi T, Yingchoncharoen T, Aljaroudi W, Marwick TH. Relation of heart-rate recovery to new onset heart failure and atrial fibrillation in patients with diabetes mellitus and preserved ejection fraction. Am J Cardiol. 2013;111:748–53.

178. Kuch B, von Scheidt W, Peter W, Doring A, Piehlmeier W, Landgraf R, Meisinger C. Sex-specific determinants of left ventricular mass in pre-diabetic and type 2 diabetic subjects: the Augsburg Diabetes Family Study. Diabetes Care. 2007;30:946–52.

179. Eguchi K, Boden BA, Jin Z, Rundek T, Sacco R, Homma S, et al. Association between diabetes mellitus and left ventricular hypertrophy in a multi-ethnic population. Am J Cardiol. 2008;101(12):1787–91.

180. Sacco RL, Anand K, Lee H-S, Boden-Albala B, Stabler S, Allen R, Paik MC. Homocysteine and the risk of ischemic stroke in a triethnic cohort: the Northern Manhattan Study. Stroke. 2004;35:2263–9.

181. Brooks BA, Franjic B, Ban CR, Swaraj K, Yue DK, Celermajer DS, et al. Diastolic dysfunction and abnormalities of the microcirculation in type 2 diabetes. Diabetes Obes Metab. 2008;10(9):739–46.

182. Fang ZY, Schull-Meade R, Leano R, Mottram PM, Prins JB, Marwick TH. Screening for heart disease in diabetic subjects. Am Heart J. 2005;149(2):349–54.

183. Fang ZY, Schull-Meade R, Prins JB, Marwick TH. Determinants of subclinical diabetic heart disease. Diabetologia. 2005;48:394–402.

184. From AM, Scott CG, Chen HH. The development of heart failure in patients with diabetes mellitus and pre-clinical diastolic dysfunction a population-based study. J Am Coll Cardiol. 2010;55:300–5.

185. Lindman B, Dávila-Román V, Mann D, Mc Nulty S, Semigran M, Lewis G, et al. Cardiovascular phenotype in HFpEF patients with or without diabetes a RELAX Trial Ancillary Study. J Am Coll Cardiol. 2014;64:541–9.

186. Van Der Horst IC, De Boer RA, Hillege HL, Boomsma F, Voors AA, Van Veldhuisen DJ. Neurohormonal profile of patients with heart failure and diabetes. Neth Heart J. 2010;18(4):190–6.

187. American Diabetes Association. Standards of medical care in diabetes: 2008. Diabetes Care. 2008;31(suppl1):S12–54.

188. UK Prospective Diabetes Study Group. Intensive blood-glucose control with sulphonylureas or insulin compared with conventional treatment and risk of complications in patients with type 2 diabetes (UKPDS 33). Lancet. 1998;352:837–53.

189. Skyler J, Bergenstal R, Bonow R, Buse J, Deedwania P, Gale E, et al. Intensive glycemic control and the prevention of cardiovascular events: implications of the ACCORD, ADVANCE, and VA diabetes trials A position statement of the American Diabetes Association and a Scientific Statement of the American College of Cardiology Foundation and the American Heart Association. Circulation. 2009;119(2):351–7.

190. Yusuf S, Sleight P, Pogue J, et al. Effects of an angiotensin-converting-enzyme inhibitor, ramipril, on cardiovascular events in high-risk patients. The Heart Outcomes Prevention Evaluation Study Investigators. N Engl J Med. 2000;342:145–53.

191. EURopean trial On reduction of cardiac events with Perindopril in stable coronary Artery disease Investigators. Efficacy of perindopril in reduction of cardiovascular events among patients with stable coronary artery disease: randomised, double blind, placebo-controlled, multicentre trial (the EUROPA study). Lancet. 2003;362:782–8.

192. Pham D, De Albuquerque N, Darren K, Neeland I. Impact of empagliflozin in patients with diabetes and heart failure. Trends Cardiovasc Med. 2017;27:144–15.

193. Fitchett D, Zinman B, Wanner C, Lachin JM, Hantel S, Salsali A, et al. Heart failure outcomes with empagliflozin in patients with type 2 diabetes at high cardiovascular risk: results of the EMPA-REGOUTCOME trial. Eur Heart J. 2016;37:1526–34.

194. Seferovic JP, Claggett B, Seidelmann SB, Seely EW, Packer M, Zile MR. Effect of sacubitril/valsartan versus enalapril on glycaemic control in patients with heart failure and diabetes: a post-

hoc analysis from the PARADIGM-HF trial. Lancet Diabetes Endocrinol. 2017;5(5):333–40.

195. The Digitalis Investigation Group Investigators. The effect of digoxin on mortality and morbidity in patients with heart failure. N Engl J Med. 1997;336:525–33.

196. Coady MA, Rizzo JA, Elefteriades JA. Pathologic variants of thoracic aortic dissections: penetrating atherosclerotic ulcers and intramural hematomas. Cardiol Clin. 1999;17(4):637–57.

197. Nienaber CA. Pathophysiology of acute aortic syndromes. In: Baliga RR, Nienaber CA, Isselbacher EM, Eagle KA, editors. Aortic dissection and related syndromes. New York, NY: Springer; 2007. p. 17–43.

198. He X, Liu X, Liu W, Wang B, et al. Association between diabetes and risk of aortic dissection: a case-control study in a Chinese population. PLoS One. 2015;10(11):e0142697.

199. Theivacumar NS, Stephenson MA, Mistry H, Valenti D. Diabetes mellitus and aortic aneurysm rupture: a favorable association? Vasc Endovascular Surg. 2014;48(1):45–50.

200. Da Silva ES, Gornati VC, Casella IB, et al. The similarities and differences among patients with abdominal aortic aneurysms referred to a tertiary hospital and found at necropsy. Vascular. 2015;23(4):411–8.

201. Lederle FA. The strange relationship between diabetes and abdominal aortic aneurysm. Eur J Vasc Endovasc Surg. 2012;43(3):254–6.

202. Mosch J, Gleissner CA, Body S. Aikawa E Histopathological assessment of calcification and inflammation of calcific aortic valves from patients with and without diabetes mellitus. Histol Histopathol. 2017;32(3):293–306.

203. Rosenhek R, Binder T, Porenta G, Lang I, Christ G, Schemper M, Maurer G, Baumgartner H. Predictors of outcome in severe, asymptomatic aortic stenosis. N Engl J Med. 2000;343:611–7.

204. Testuz A, Nguyen V, Mathieu T, et al. Influence of metabolic syndrome and diabetes on progression of calcific aortic valve stenosis. Int J Cardiol. 2017;244:248–53.

205. Leon MB, Smith CR, Mack M, Miller DC, Moses JW, Svensson LG, Tuzcu EM, Webb JG, Fontana GP, Makkar RR, Brown DL, Block PC, Guyton RA, Pichard AD, Bavaria JE, Herrmann HC, Douglas PS, Petersen JL, Akin JJ, Anderson WN, Wang D, Pocock S. PARTNER Trial Investigators. Transcatheter aortic-valve implantation for aortic stenosis in patients who cannot undergo surgery. N Engl J Med. 2010;363:1597–607.

206. Miki T, Yuda S, Kouzu H, Miura T. Diabetic cardiomyopathy: pathophysiology and clinical features. Heart Fail Rev. 2013;18:149–66.

207. Podlaha R, Falk A. The prevalence of diabetes mellitus and other risk factors of atherosclerosis in bradycardia requiring pacemaker treatment. Horm Metab Res Suppl. 1992;26:84–7.

208. Sun H, Guan Y, Wang L, Zhao Y, Lv H, Bi X, et al. Influence of diabetes on cardiac resynchronization therapy in heart failure patients: a meta-analysis. BMC Cardiovasc Disord. 2015;15:25.

209. Zhang Q, Liu T, Ng CY, Li G. Diabetes mellitus and atrial remodeling: mechanisms and potential upstream therapies. Cardiovasc Ther. 2014;32:233–41.

210. Goudis CA, Korantzopoulos P, Ntalas I, Kallergis EM, Liu T, KetikoglouDG. Diabetes mellitus and atrial fibrillation: Pathophysiological mechanisms and potential upstream therapies. Int J Cardiol. 2015;184:617–22.

211. Benjamin EJ, Levy D, Vaziri SM, D´Agostino RB, Belanger AJ, Wolf PA. Independent risk factors for atrial fibrillation in a population-based cohort. The Framingham Heart study. JAMA. 1994;271:840–4.

212. Movahed MR, Hashemzadeh M, Jamal MM. Diabetes mellitus is a strong independent risk for atrial fibrillation and flutter in addition to other cardiovascular disease. Int J Cardiol. 2005;105:315–8.

213. Huxley RR, Alonso A, Lopez FL, et al. Type 2 diabetes, glucose homeostasis and incident atrial fibrillation: the atherosclerosis risk in communities study. Heart. 2012;98:133–8.

214. Huxley RR, Filion KB, Konety S, Alonso A. Meta-analysis of cohort and case-control studies of Type 2 diabetes mellitus anda risk of atrial fibrillation. Am J Cardiol. 2011;108:56–62.

215. Codinach Huix P, Freixa PR. Miocardiopatía diabética: concepto, función cardiaca y patogenia. An Med Interna. 2002;19:313–20.

216. Cryer PE. Death during intensive glycemic therapy of diabetes: mechanisms and implications. Am J Med. 2011;124:993–6.

217. Tesfaye S, Boulton AJM, Dyck PJ, Freeman R, Horowitz M, Kempler P, et al. Diabetic neuropathies: update on definitions, diagnostic criteria, estimation of severity, and treatments. Diabetes Care. 2010;33:2285–93.

218. Clemente D, Pereira T, Ribeiro S. Ventricular repolarization in diabetic patients: characterization and clinical implications. Arq Bras Cardioil. 2012;99:1015–22.

219. Nordin C. The case for hypoglycaemia as a proarrhythmic event: basic and clinical evidence. Diabetologia. 2010;53:1552–61.

Forrest Lowe, Wuwei Feng, and Carlos Cantú-Brito

Stroke as a Long-Term Complication of Uncontrolled Diabetes Mellitus

Introduction

The relationship between stroke and diabetes mellitus (DM) though complex is undeniable. Numerous studies have delineated a clear correlation between prediabetes, diabetes mellitus type 1, and diabetes mellitus type 2 as they relate to cerebrovascular disease with decades of research detailing the causality between hyperglycemia and stroke risk. The global prevalence of stroke continues to rise despite the advances in treatment options for cardiovascular risk factor modification such as diabetes. Diabetics represent a subset of the patients who are at 2–3 times higher risk of mortality from stroke than the general population [1]. The purpose of this chapter is to look over essential epidemiological concerns about DM and stroke and mainly to detail the microvascular and macrovascular mechanisms that promote cerebrovascular disease in diabetics which leads to stroke. Subsequently, the remarkable role of hyperglycemia in acute ischemic stroke will be revised. Additionally, the importance of glucose control for both primary and secondary stroke prevention will be discussed in terms of the role of therapeutical options for attaining normoglycemia. Finally, there will be in-depth discussion of the optimization of diabetic control as it relates to other stroke risk factors such as atherosclerosis, hypertension, and atrial fibrillation.

F. Lowe
Department of Neurology, University of Cincinnati Medical Center, Cincinnati, OH, USA

W. Feng
Department of Neurology, Medical University of South Carolina, Charleston, SC, USA

C. Cantú-Brito (✉)
Department of Neurology, National Institute of Medical Sciences and Nutrition Salvador Zubirán, Mexico City, Mexico

Epidemiological Overview of Diabetes and Stroke

In 2019, according to the global burden of disease collaborators, stroke remains as the second leading cause of death and the third leading cause of death and disability combined (as measured by disability-adjusted life-years [DALYs]) in the world [2]. DM is included within the five leading specific risk factors contributing to stroke DALYs, with a population attributable fraction (PAF) of 20.2% (95% uncertainty intervals [UIs] 13.8–29.1) of all stroke DALYs. It should be noted that among cerebrovascular diseases, DM is usually associated with the ischemic stroke type (PAF 19.5% [(10.6–34.6)]), ranking as the third most important risk factor for this type of stroke. However, in the last years, it is becoming evident that DM is also associated with hemorrhagic strokes: the PAF for intracerebral hemorrhage is 17.3% (11.2–24.8) and for subarachnoid hemorrhage of 16.8 (11.0–23.4), ranking as the fourth and five most important risk factors, respectively, for these stroke types.

The large increase in the global burden of stroke is probably not only due to population growth and aging but also because of the substantial increase in exposure to several important risk factors such as high BMI, high fasting plasma glucose, high systolic blood pressure, and low physical activity. DM is among the risk factors with an outstanding increase in the age-standardized stroke PAF from 1990 to 2019 (from 14.4% to 20.2%), corresponding to a 40.3% increase. In other words, if high fasting plasma glucose exposure were reduced to its theoretical minimum risk exposure level, there would be a 20.2% reduction in stroke in 2019 [2].

Microvascular Complications of Diabetes

Diabetes mellitus is a modifiable risk factor for ischemic stroke and is defined by one of the following: a fasting blood glucose (fbg) of ≥ 126, a hemoglobin A1C (HbA1C) of $\geq 6.5\%$, 2 h postprandial glucose of ≥ 200 mg/dL after

© The Author(s), under exclusive license to Springer Nature Switzerland AG 2023
J. Rodriguez-Saldana (ed.), *The Diabetes Textbook*, https://doi.org/10.1007/978-3-031-25519-9_51

administration of a 75 g glucose tolerance test, or a random serum glucose ≥ 200 mg/dL in a patient with classic signs of hyperglycemia/hypoglycemia [3]. The pathophysiology of DM is complex and its interrelation with the development of cerebrovascular disease is well studied. However, the microvascular and macrovascular changes that occur due to persistent hyperglycemia have not been fully elucidated. Microvascular changes within cerebrovasculature and systemic vasculature occur through multiple cellular pathways that are directly modulated by fluctuations of serum glucose.

Microvascular changes due to hyperglycemia, which are noted on both the cellular and genetic levels, occur due to a chronic, systemic, inflammatory state induced by the production of reactive oxygen species (ROS) with early changes noted on both the cellular and genetic levels. The sources of the ROS are diverse and include excess superoxide production via mitochondria, direct oxidation of serum glucose, endothelial cell nitrogen oxygen synthase (eNOS), NADPH (nicotinamide adenine dinucleotide phosphate) oxidase activation from abundance of advanced glycosylation end products (AGEs) [4], and the upregulation of mitochondrial matrix metalloproteinase (MMP-9) [5]. The dysfunction of microvascular endothelium begins to occur via these pathways in addition to many others that are far less well understood and mimic the changes found in the vasculature that is exposed to chronic inflammatory processes.

Chronic hyperglycemia causes abnormal production of ROS from normal glycolytic processes that metabolize glucose and results in excess side products including ROS which overwhelm the cellular antioxidants such as superoxide dismutase and glutathione peroxidase. To prevent continued production of ROS, many systemic cells will downregulate glucose transporters (GLUTs). However, endothelial cells normally express non-insulin-dependent GLUTs which allows for continued intracellular glycolytic generation of ROS. In addition to continued generation of ROS via glycolysis, mitochondrial dysfunction begins to occur with persistent hyperglycemia inducing a chain reaction during which multiple intracellular pathways are activated leading to further endothelial dysfunction [4].

Electron transport chain uncoupling within mitochondria propagates unmitigated binding of ROS to available intracellular oxygen further promoting oxidative stress. Indeed in numerous studies, it has been shown that inhibition of ROS production within endothelial mitochondria prevents the cumulative oxidative endothelial cell dysfunction in the setting of hyperglycemia. Apoptotic events, genetic expression of pro-inflammatory markers, and nitrogen oxide inhibition are all mitigated by inhibition of mitochondrial free radical production due to hyperglycemia [3]. In one study, Mishiro et al. demonstrated that the mitochondrial involvement in endothelial cell dysfunction is more complex than previously discerned in that hyperglycemia not only disrupts normal metabolic processes but also alters mitochondrial membrane permeability to the point of self-induced organelle apoptosis, MMP-9 production, and death of endothelial cells comprising the cerebral microvasculature [5].

Advanced glycation end products (AGEs) are byproducts of glycosylated proteins or lipids that normally occur in the presence of hyperglycemia. The exact mechanism by which AGEs are derived is via the Maillard reaction which in short produces ketoamine that form AGEs via a dual pathway. In the setting of sustained hyperglycemia such as that which exists in diabetes mellitus or even in prediabetic states, these AGEs accumulate rapidly and are deposited within various tissues. Receptors for advance glycosylation end products, RAGE, exist in normal endothelial cells and not only can prevent endothelial cell repair but also promote infiltration of the vascular endothelium by inflammatory cells. Activation of RAGE and its promoted binding to AGE in DM causes endothelial cell dysfunction which manifests in some DM patients as diabetic microangiopathy [6]. However, not all AGE-related endothelial cell dysfunction are RAGE dependent [4].

RAGE-independent endothelial dysfunction can occur due to glycation of LDL (low-density lipoprotein), extracellular cell matrix proteins, or activation of signaling proteins other than RAGE [4]. Kim et al. noted that AGE overproduction causes excessive LDL modification as well as increased expression of CD36 ligands [7]. This CD36 expression occurs predominantly in monocytes and blunts the inflammatory reaction that occurs in DM patients who experience endothelial cell injury thereby inhibiting proper endothelial repair [7]. Similarly, in the setting of hyperinsulinemia commonly present in DMII patients, macrophages derived from monocytes demonstrate insulin receptor dysfunction which is pro-atherogenic in the setting of an already compromised endothelial integrity [8].

It is also important to note that other inflammatory proteins such as monocyte chemoattractant protein-1 (MCP-1) and IL-6 are also upregulated in diabetics with the elevation of MCP-1 causing both increased macrophage recruitment and increased adipocyte insulin resistance. In fact, many inflammatory markers such as C-reactive protein (CRP), intracellular adhesion molecule 1 (ICAM-1), and vascular cell adhesion molecule 1 (VCAM-1) are overexpressed in hyperglycemia not only in the diabetic but also in normal subjects who experience impaired glucose tolerance (IGT) or postprandial hyperglycemia [9]. Persistent hyperglycemia in DMII leads to concomitant improper physiologic response yielding a state of chronic hyperinsulinemia due to insulin resistance which in and of itself is disruptive to the integrity of cerebrovascular endothelium [8].

In animal studies involving cardiac endothelium, per Bornfeldt et al., hyperinsulinemia led to downregulation of insulin-mediated endothelial pathways that promote alteration of endothelial gene expression and production of transmembranous proteins [8]. Sustained elevation of serum insulin causes saturation of insulin receptors and increased activation of 3-phosphoinositide-dependent protein kinase 1 (PDK1) which through a series of reactions promotes increased transcription of metabolic genes [8]. The epigenetic and genetic changes induced by chronic hyperglycemia can persist even years after serum glucose is controlled [10]. Consequently, these metabolic genes allow for increased rates of glycolysis, lipid synthesis, and GLUT (glucose transporter) production. Additionally, when vascular smooth muscle cells are exposed to hyperinsulinemia, they demonstrate activation of pathways influenced by insulin-like growth factor-1 receptors (IGF1R) that are known to be pro-atherogenic [8]. All of these pathways, as noted in Fig. 51.1, lead to ROS overproduction, glycolysis upregulation, and genetic modifications.

Disruption of vasculature endothelium at the microvascular level in diabetics is most commonly seen in diabetics in the form of complications such as microangiopathy, arterial retinopathy, nephropathy, and peripheral neuropathy.

Moreover, emerging evidence has demonstrated that cerebral microvascular dysfunction and damage in DM are common as depicted mainly by MRI (magnetic resonance imaging) showing typical features of cerebral small vessel disease [11]. Indeed, microvascular involvement of other known areas such as retinal microvascular abnormalities in patients with type 2 diabetes correlates with the presence of cerebral small vessel lesions [12]. Optimal brain function depends on a healthy microvasculature including the delivery of nutrients and removal of waste products in response to changes in neuronal activity maintaining the interstitial milieu for proper function of the so-called neurovascular unit (a complex interaction of several cell types including endothelial cells, astrocytes, pericytes, and neurons). In addition, cerebral microvasculature is a crucial site of the blood-brain barrier that protects the neurons from external factors and maintains the internal milieu within the CNS (central nervous system) highly regulated and also decreases and stabilizes the pulsatile hydrostatic pressure at the level of capillaries and participates in the cerebrovascular reactivity and cerebral autoregulation that regulates and maintains global brain perfusion. Cerebral microvascular dysfunction

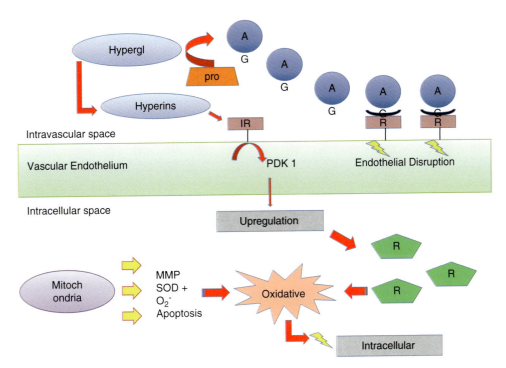

Fig. 51.1 Process of hyperglycemia-induced vascular endothelial dysfunction. Chronic hyperglycemia causes glycosylation of both fats and lipids resulting in the production of advanced glycosylated end products (AGEs). AGEs bind to receptors for advanced glycosylation end products resulting in endothelial disruption. Hyperglycemia results in concomitant hyperinsulinemia that can cause oversaturation of insulin receptors as well as overproduction of 3-phosphoinositide-dependent protein kinase (PDK1). PDK1 overproduction causes upregulation of glycolysis and subsequent overproduction of reactive oxygen species (ROS). Mitochondrial dysfunction under the influence of chronic hyperglycemia can result in overproduction of mitochondrial matrix metalloproteinase (MMP-9), superoxide dismutase, and organelle-induced apoptosis. All of these mitochondrial products as well as glycolytic-induced ROS lead to oxidative stress resulting in intracellular dysfunction, abnormal metabolic gene transcription/upregulation allowing for increased rates of glycolysis, lipid synthesis, and GLUT transporter production. *AGE* advanced glycosylated end products, *RAGE* receptor for AGEs, *PDK1* 3-phosphoinositide-dependent protein kinase, *IR* insulin receptor, *MMP* mitochondrial matrix metalloproteinase, *SOD* superoxide dismutase, and *ROS* reactive oxygen species

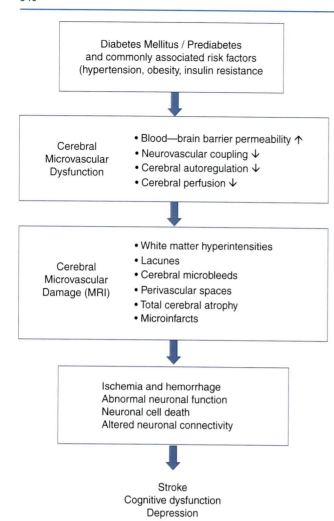

Fig. 51.2 Assumed pathway by which type DM-related cerebral microvascular dysfunction contributes to stroke and other mental disorders such as cognitive dysfunction and depression. Prediabetes and DM and commonly associated risk factors (hypertension, obesity, and insulin resistance) induce cerebral microvascular damage and dysfunction including an increase of permeability of the blood-brain barrier and decrease of neurovascular unit coupling and cerebral autoregulation as well as reduction of cerebral perfusion. These abnormalities give rise to the typical features of cerebral small vessel disease as depicted by MRI (see Fig. 51.3) and manifested clinically as stroke, cognitive disorders, and depression. (Modified from Fig. 2, [11])

may be defined as an impairment in any of these previous functions. Figure 51.2 summarized the assumed pathway by which type 2 diabetes-related cerebral microvascular dysfunction contributes to stroke and other mental disorders such as cognitive dysfunction and depression [11]. Figure 51.3 shows illustrative lesions of small vessel disease commonly observed by MRI in patients with diabetes.

Furthermore, microvascular complications were initially delineated in the landmark UK Prospective Diabetes Study (UKPDS). This was the first comprehensive study to demonstrate that strict regulation of serum glucose levels can prevent microvascular complications of hyperglycemia [13].

The data derived from this prospective study of DMII patients noted that over a period of ten years if aggressive glucose control was achieved via sulphonylurea or insulin administration, there was a significant reduction in microvascular complications regardless of intervention. Up to a 25% reduction in nephropathy and ophthalmic complications was noted in the patient arm randomized to receive intensive serum glucose control. Additionally, the final average HbA1C of patients under intensive glucose control was 11% lower with a median value of 7% which directly corresponded to an improved rate of microvascular complications in that study arm. No macrovascular benefit was observed in either study arm nor were significant deleterious macrovascular outcomes [13].

Further studies such as the Action to Control Cardiovascular Risk in Diabetes Mellitus (ACCORD) evaluated whether even more aggressive serum glucose control than that achieved by patients in UKPDS would further prevent microvascular disease. However, the ACCORD study with its target HbA1C of 6% was stopped prematurely due to a significantly increased mortality rate in the intensive therapy treatment arm [14]. Unsurprisingly, it was noted in the Heart Outcomes Prevention Evaluation (HOPE) trial that concomitant treatment of hypertension and hyperlipidemia (HLD) in diabetics leads to improved outcomes with significantly decreased frequency of microvascular complications [15]. These significant interactions between hyperglycemia and hyperlipidemia as they relate to increased risk of ischemic stroke on the microvascular level are complex and exist in both the prediabetic and diabetes mellitus patients.

As mentioned in the preceding paragraphs, persistent hyperglycemia activates the AGE/RAGE complex. Interestingly, the blockade of the excess activation of the ligand/receptor complex decreases atherosclerotic formation as well as diabetic nephropathy in hyperglycemia [9]. Increased production of vascular smooth muscle cells (VSMCs) is also encouraged during periods of hyperglycemia and has been demonstrated in DMI and DMII. Though the pathways responsible for atherosclerotic formation in diabetics are not fully understood, it is likely that vascular endothelial injury is caused by hyperglycemia which is directly responsible for creating a pro-inflammatory state promoting VSMC proliferation, microangiopathy, and microvascular changes [16]. It is this pro-inflammatory state created by hyperglycemia that forces endothelial cells such as those present in the retinal vasculature to overexpress factors such as vascular endothelial growth factor (VEGF) in order to survive in an ischemic environment [9]. According to Prasad et al., VEGF also was found in animal studies to increase vascular permeability resulting in microvascular changes as well as compromise of the blood barrier itself even in the setting of only transient hyperglycemic events [17].

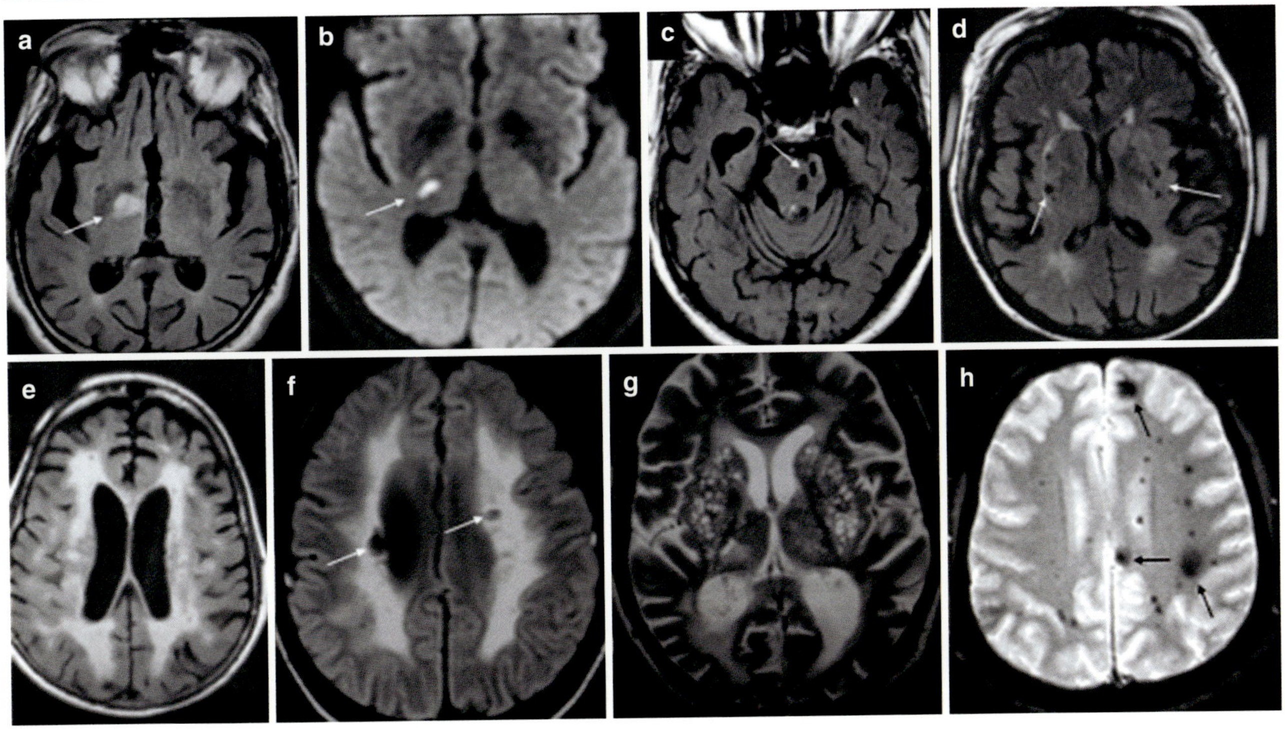

Fig. 51.3 MRI imaging characteristics of features of cerebral small vessel disease commonly seen in patients with diabetes. (**a**) FLAIR sequence depicts a thalamic lacunar infarct (arrow). (**b**) Diffusion-weighted shows a hyperintense lesion corresponding to an acute small deep (lacunar) infarct (arrow): less than 2 cm diameter. (**c**) T1-weighted imaging with a hypointense lesions in the pons corresponding to old lacunar infarcts (arrow). (**d**) FLAIR sequence showing multiple small deep lacunar infarcts (arrows). (**e**) FLAIR imaging of typical large confluent areas of white matter hyperintensities (WMH) extending from the periventricular to the center of the bilateral semioval tissues. (**f**) FLAIR imaging of WMH similar to (**e**) but including hypointense lesions (old lacunar infarcts) within the WMH (arrows). (**g**) Extensive areas of perivascular spaces on T2-weighted imaging are hyperintense because they contain CSF-like fluid, less than 3 mm diameter, seen bilaterally in the basal ganglia. (**h**) Multiple foci of microbleeds within cortex and subcortical structures on gradient-echo T2 imaging (larger lesions with arrows)

Macrovascular Complications of Diabetes

Macrovascular changes due to hyperglycemia have been shown to result in neointimal expansion after the initial endothelial injuries have begun to accumulate within the diabetic patients. Normal vascular neointimal healing and formation are adversely affected by hyperglycemia creating systemic vasculature that is abnormally thickened by abnormally proliferating VSMCs [18] leading to noncompliant vasculature, hypertension, and increased stroke risk. Involvement of multiple cerebrovascular territories including vasculature to the blood brain barrier is also compromised in the setting of hyperglycemia with dysfunction of arterial smooth muscle elasticity leading to stenosis, ischemia, and stroke [19]. Other animal studies demonstrate that cerebral arterioles likely undergo deleterious changes to endothelium more rapidly than larger cerebrovasculature such as the basilar or carotid arteries [20]. According to Zhou et al., animal studies in which arterial injury was created via balloon dilatation resulted in hyperplasia of the neointima likely due to a pro-inflammatory vascular environment from both hyperglycemia and hyperinsulinemia [21]. In summary, these animal studies demonstrating the microvascular and macrovascular effects of hyperglycemia and atherosclerosis were later partially confirmed in several human trials. The Action in Diabetes and Vascular Disease (ADVANCE) trial showed that microvascular events were significantly decreased in diabetics though the mitigation of macrovascular complication did not reach significance. The targeted HbA1C of the ADVANCE (Action in Diabetes and Vascular Disease-PreterAx and DiamicroN Controlled Evaluation) trial was 6.5% in the intensive treatment arm with the most significant benefit evident in the rate of nephropathy complications which were decreased by 21%. Later trials including the Veterans Affairs Diabetes Trial (VADT) as well as the Diabetes Control and Complications Trial (DCCT) also demonstrated similar results in short-term monitoring of the intensive treatment arms in both studies again showing significant improvement in microvascular outcomes with nonsignificant macrovascular event decrements. However, after longitudinal follow-up in the DCCT patients, it was determined that patients in the intensive glucose control arm did, in fact, demonstrate a significant reduction in ischemic cardiac diseases, strokes, or CV deaths ($n = 711$ patients in intensive treatment arm vs. $n = 730$ in conventional treatment arm, $p = 0.02$) [20]. This was in agreement with prior data that noted diabetics were up to ten times more likely to suffer CAD (coronary artery disease), peripheral vascular disease (PVD), or stroke compared to nondiabetics [22].

DM and Hyperglycemia in Acute Ischemic Stroke

One of the conditions adversely affecting outcome in patients with acute ischemic stroke is hyperglycemia. Hyperglycemic diabetic patients admitted to the hospital for acute ischemic stroke are up to two times more likely to die within the first month compared to normoglycemic patients. Lau et al. [23], in a meta-analysis of 39 studies, report a significant relationship between DM and mortality, and poor neurological and functional outcomes. They also found an association with length of hospital stay, readmission rate, and stroke recurrence. Also, the Get With The Guidelines Stroke registry found a similarly significant association between acute ischemic stroke patients with DM and mortality as well as readmission three years post-discharge in an analysis of 409,060 American patients with cerebral ischemia including transient ischemic attack [24]. Several factors may potentiate the increased risk of stroke in DM patients, including endothelial dysfunction, arterial stiffness, and systemic and local inflammation. Also, diabetes and postischemic acute hyperglycemia are likely to be associated with poor reperfusion and recanalization outcomes due to several factors including vascular injury, clot composition, and impaired collaterals; and then, hyperglycemia appears to interfere with the effi-

cacy of reperfusion therapies (Fig. 51.4) [25]. Several studies investigating the impact of thrombolysis and thrombectomy show significantly worse outcomes measure by the Modified Rankin Score between DM and non-DM groups. However, this association has not been found in several other reperfusion studies, and therefore, patients with DM and acute ischemic stroke should receive reperfusion therapy, in particular thrombolysis within a 3 h time window. Although current standards of care, indicated by the 2019 AHA (American Heart Association) guidelines, do not recommend intravenous thrombolysis treatment for patients within a 3–4.5 h time window with a history of concurrent DM and prior stroke, further large-scale studies on the relationship between DM and prior stroke properly determine its use in this population [26].

In spite that hyperglycemia is present in approximately 40% of patients with acute ischemic stroke and is associated with worse clinical outcomes, the efficacy of intensive treatment of hyperglycemia in this setting has been disappointed. Current acute stroke guidelines from the American Stroke Association suggest treating hyperglycemia to achieve a blood glucose level in the range of 140–180 mg/dL (7.8–10.0 mmol/L) and close monitoring to prevent hypoglycemia [26]. The Stroke Hyperglycemia Insulin Network Effort (SHINE) randomized clinical trial was conducted to assess the efficacy of intensive versus standard blood glucose control in 1151 patients with hyperglycemic acute ischemic stroke who received either intensive treatment of hyperglycemia (target blood glucose concentration of 80–130 mg/dL) or standard treatment of hyperglycemia (target glucose concentration of 80–179 mg/dL). Intensive compared with standard glucose control did not improve 90-day functional outcomes

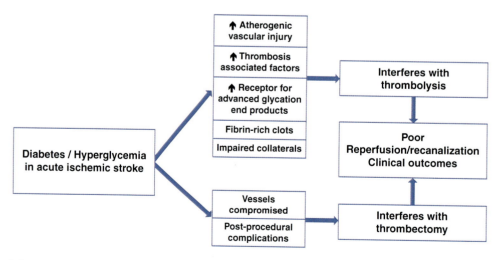

Fig. 51.4 Reperfusion outcomes in patients with diabetes and acute ischemic stroke presenting with acute hyperglycemia. Diabetes and acute hyperglycemia are likely to be associated with poor reperfusion and recanalization outcomes in patients with acute ischemic stroke, due to several factors including vascular injury, clot composition, and impaired collaterals; and then, hyperglycemia appears to interfere with the efficacy of reperfusion therapies (thrombolysis or thrombectomy). (Modified from Fig. 4, [25])

in patients with acute ischemic stroke and hyperglycemia. These findings do not support using intensive glucose control in this setting [27].

On the other hand, though the primary purpose of both parenteral insulin and oral diabetic medications is to prevent hyperglycemia, there is data that suggests that certain classes of these drugs may improve outcomes during the acute phase of an ischemic stroke, through the so-called neuroprotection process. Neuroprotection for stroke defines any strategy directly targeting brain parenchyma with the goal of antagonizing the harmful molecular and cellular events responsible for the ischemic damage thereby allowing brain cells to survive to reduced cerebral blood flow [28, 29]. White et al. noted that in a systematic review of animal studies, the administration of TZDs (thiazolidinediones) during the time of cerebral ischemic injury was associated with improved neurologic outcomes and a decrement in the overall stroke burden [30]. Though these studies have not yet been extrapolated for validity in human subjects, it is noteworthy that rosiglitazone reduced infarct volume regardless of administration before or after induction of ischemia in rat brains [28]. Interestingly, GLP-1 Ras and DPP-IVIs are endowed with a variety of pleiotropic (neuroprotective) properties demonstrated in experimental stroke models, suggesting a possible role in the treatment of acute cerebral ischemia [31]. Considering that they share several neuroprotective effects, an adequate basis exists for explorative clinical investigations on additive GLP-1 agonist plus DPP (dipeptidyl peptidase)-IVI treatment of hyperglycemia in patients with acute ischemic stroke. This strategy would assume that, while GLP-1R agonists directly interact with cerebral receptors, the action of DPP-IVIs is mediated by increasing the effects of GLP-1 including pleiotropic effects. This therapeutic option represents a basically novel strategy to confront hyperglycemia in acute ischemic stroke [31].

Diabetes and Primary Stroke Prevention

Ischemic stroke is a direct complication of diabetes with a complex interplay of multiple risk factors for cerebrovascular disease including hypertension, atherosclerosis, smoking, atrial fibrillation, and a myriad of less well-studied pathophysiological processes of contributors such as obstructive sleep apnea (Table 51.1). Macrovascular complications of hyperglycemia have been less well studied and are more difficult to directly correlate with a specific glucose control target for treatment as has been noted in UKPDS, ACCORD, and ADVANCE trials. Fortunately, microvascular complications as they relate to target HbA1C have been easier to correlate with longitudinal study data, and the cellular pathways by which hyperglycemia affects vascular endothelial cell dysfunction are beginning to be better understood. Primary prevention of ischemic stroke clearly requires hyperglycemic control, but the degree of glycemic control and its effect on other primary stroke risk factors is of equal importance for stroke prevention [32].

A review of the most current literatures reveals that primary stroke prevention is dependent on chronic control of hyperglycemia with a target HbA1C of < 7% as well as the monitoring of both fasting serum glucose and postprandial dysglycemia. What the ACCORD, ADVANCE, and VADT trials helped demonstrate was that all diabetics benefited from a target HbA1C of around 7% regardless of their baseline HbA1C, duration of disease, or baseline comorbidities. More intensive glucose control can lead to increased mortality in some subgroups while in young patients with DM disease duration of less than 15 years may in fact benefit from intensive glucose control with a lower target HbA1C [33].

The Nateglinide and Valsartan in Impaired Glucose Tolerance Outcomes Research (NAVIGATOR) trial demonstrated that patients with impaired fasting blood glucose, although not meeting diagnostic criteria for diabetes, were at increased risk of developing DM and subsequently at higher

Table 51.1 AHA/ADA guidelines for primary stroke prevention

Diabetes	Hyperlipidemia	Hypertension	Atrial fibrillation	Other risk factors
BP goal <140/90 mmHg	Statin use for patients with high CV risk	Lifestyle changes and BP screening[a]	Coumadin for CHA$_2$DS$_2$-VASc score ≥ 2[b]	Weight reduction if BMI ≥ 25
Statin use for CV risk reduction	Fibric acid derivatives only for elevated triglycerides[c]	Goal BP of <140/90, reduction more important than BP agent used	Nonvalvular AF and CHA$_2$DS$_2$-VASc of 0, no anticoagulants	Smoking cessation in all patients
No role for aspirin or fibrates	No role for statin lipid-lowering medications	Self-measurement of BP	Screening for AF in patients 65 or older with exam and EKG	40 min, three days/week moderate exercise

ADA guidelines per the following: Cefulu W et al. "American Diabetes Association: Standards of Medical Care in Diabetes—2015," *The Journal of Clinical and Applied Research and Education: Diabetes Care* 2015; 38 (1): S1–S93

[a]*BP* blood pressure, *CHA2DS2-VASc* congestive heart failure, hypertension, age, diabetes, stroke, and vascular disease, *CV* cardiovascular, *AF* atrial fibrillation, and *BMI* body mass index

[b]In patients with low hemorrhage risk and valvular AF (atrial fibrillation)

[c]No role for fibric acid derivatives in decreasing future stroke risk

risk for ischemic stroke [22]. According to Mi et al., elevated fasting blood glucose was an independent predictor for first-ever ischemic stroke or recurrent stroke [34]. Additionally, it has been surmised for years that prediabetic or diabetic patients who experience repeated episodes of dysglycemia are at higher risk of cerebrovascular disease and dysfunction of the neurovascular endothelium [35]. However, data from trials to date such as NAVIGATOR are conflicting, and it is not currently understood how to best reduce cardiovascular risks in patients with impaired fasting blood glucose or postprandial glucose [36]. What has been better studied is the impact that various antidiabetic drug classes have on benefiting patients in primary stroke prevention.

Influence of Antidiabetic Drug Classes for Primary Stroke Prevention

Though DMI patients typically use forms of synthetic insulin for glycemic control, it is well known that DMII diabetics have a wide range of oral medications available for the treatment of hyperglycemia. These diabetic drugs (Table 51.2) include multiple medications with varying mechanisms of action and benefit for treating hyperglycemia as it pertains to primary stroke prevention. In addition to reviewing these medications by drug class, it is also important to address the use of these medications around the time of an ischemic stroke as some antihyperglycemics such as thiazolidinediones can potentially improve patient outcomes [30].

The use of parenteral insulin is the most obvious and well-studied mechanism to control hyperglycemia in DMI patients. In DMI and DMII patients self-administering glargine or NPH compared to basal insulin peglispro, there has been no reported clinically significant difference in preventing future ischemic strokes or CV events. There has been associated cardiovascular benefit with insulin use and improvement of comorbid stroke risk factors outside of the documented physiologic benefits of achieving normoglycemia. Interestingly, prior studies in type 2 diabetes mellitus patients have noted that long-acting insulin formulations may be implicated in exacerbating CAD leading to increased risk of myocardial infarcts [37]. A cross-sectional, international cohort study performed by Al-Rubeaan et al. as well as studies derived by data from the Hong Kong Diabetes Registry noted clinically significant elevation in stroke risk for patients using insulin for control of hyperglycemia [38]. However, this associated stroke risk was possibly due to the fact that type 2 DM patients who are parenteral insulin users

Table 51.2 Diabetic drug classes and primary stroke prevention

Hyperglycemic medication	Mechanism of action	Stroke risk factors	Side effects	Supporting studies	Important findings
IV insulin (glargine, NPH)	Serum glucose absorption	Hyperglycemia, CAD	Hypoglycemia	UKPDS	Macrovascular outcomes similar to oral antihyperglycemics
Biguanides (metformin)	Decreased hepatic gluconeogenesis	HLD, CAD, HTN	Hypoglycemia Weight gain	UKPDS Gejl et al.	Improved outcomes in the obese
Sulfonylureas (glipizide, glyburide)	Pancreatic secretagogue	Hyperglycemia[a]	Cardiac deaths	UKPDS Azimova et al.	↓ mortality in DM patients
Meglitinides (nateglinide)	Pancreatic Secretagogue	Hyperglycemia	Hyperglycemia	NAVIGATOR Azimova et al.	No improvement in CV outcomes in IGT/DM patients
DDP-4 inhibitors (sitagliptin)	Inhibit incretin, GLP-1, GIP degradation[b]	Postprandial hyperglycemia	CKD (rare)	Azimova et al. Fisman et al. Enders et al.	↓ risk of CV outcomes Rate of MI or stroke in DM patients unchanged
Glucosidase inhibitors (acarbose)	Intestinal α-glucosidase inhibitor	Postprandial hyperglycemia HTN	GI side effects, hepatotoxicity (rare)	STOP-NIDDM	Acarbose can prevent conversion of IGT patients to DM status
Thiazolidinediones (pioglitazone)	PPAR activators	HTN	HLD CAD exacerbation	Azimova et al. White et al.	Pioglitazone ↓ risk for macrovascular events in high-risk patients
GLP-1 (exenatide, liraglutide)	Inhibits glucagon Insulin secretagogue	Weight loss, HTN, and HLD	GI side effects	Azimova et al. Mearns et al.	20% ↓ risk of CVD in DM II patients
SGL2 inhibitors (gliflozins)	Sodium glucose cotransporter inhibitor	HTN, HLD, and weight loss	AKI and CKD	Mearns et al.	Reduces SBP ↑ weight loss
Bile acid sequestrant (colesevelam)	Binds intestinal bile acids	HLD and CAD	None	Ganda et al. Porez et al.	↓ future CV events

[a]Did not reach significance for macrovascular outcomes

[b]*GLP-1* glucagon-like peptide 1 receptor, *GIP* glucose-dependent insulinotropic peptide, *DDP-4* dipeptidyl peptidase-4 inhibitors, *GLP-1* glucagon-like peptide 1, *SGL2* sodium glucose cotransporter, *GIP* gastric inhibitory polypeptide, *PPAR* peroxisome proliferator-activated receptors, *CAD* cardiac arterial disease, *HLD* hyperlipidemia, *HTN* hypertension, *CKD* chronic kidney disease, *AKI* acute kidney disease, *GI* gastrointestinal, *DM* diabetes mellitus, *CV* cerebrovascular, *IGT* impaired glucose tolerance, *MI* myocardial infarct, and *SBP* systolic blood pressure

have poorly controlled hyperglycemia [38]. Treating hyperglycemia with oral agents in DMII patients is more complex than just parenteral insulin formulations; however, many options exist for treating this patient population.

Biguanides such as metformin are a class of oral antihyperglycemics currently available for treating DMII. Metformin was used in the UKPDS trial and demonstrated a 32% relative risk reduction of cardiac ischemia and ischemic stroke in diabetics as well as 42% reduction in all macrovascular deaths related to diabetes. Interestingly, the combination of metformin and injected insulin in the same study demonstrated a significantly decreased risk for the development of macrovascular disease including ischemic stroke when patients were followed for over four years after completion of the study [39]. These data are significant in so far as that it has been documented that newly diagnosed DMII patients have a 10% increased absolute risk of stroke within five years of initial diagnosis [40]. Treatment of DMII with metformin not only decreases the increased absolute risk of ischemic stroke but also may help treat comorbid risk factors such as hypertension and hyperlipidemia, thereby further decreasing the risk of future ischemic stroke (Table 51.1) [39].

According to Gejl et al., the biguanide drug class may affect multiple stroke risk factors such as hyperglycemia and hyperlipidemia yielding a decrease in the occurrence of major cardiac or cerebral ischemic events [41]. Similarly, in large retrospective cohort studies comparing diabetics treated with metformin and diabetics treated with antihyperglycemics not including metformin, there was a significantly lower risk of stroke with an adjusted hazard ratio of 47 in the metformin group [39]. Metformin's mechanism of action in reducing cholesterol levels is not completely understood but may involve decreasing hepatic secretion of lipoproteins resulting in lower VLDL, plasma triglycerides, and LDL/HDL ratio. The cardioprotective effects of metformin in animal studies have also been well documented, and it is likely that diabetics who have an MI while on metformin have a reduction in both MI size and burden of reperfusion injury [42]. The mechanism by which metformin decreases hypertension in the diabetic is less well understood.

Sulfonylureas such as glipizide and glyburide have been long used to treat DMII, but a large body of evidence has provided conflicting data on this drug class's cardiac profile especially in patients with pre-existing CAD [39]. Per data in the UKPDS trials, intensive treatment of DMII patients with sulfonylurea monotherapy led to a significant decrease in microvascular complications though the decrease in macrovascular complications such as ischemic stroke did not reach significance [10]. Sulfonylureas likely carry an increased risk of cardiovascular complications and are still not considered a first-line monotherapy drug for any DMII patient that has concomitant underlying CAD [39].

Though meglitinides, such as repaglinide and nateglinide, are short-acting glucose-lowering drugs that do not affect lipid levels, they do lower HbA1C levels and manage hyperglycemia [39]. In prediabetics or patients with IGT, nateglinide was associated with a significant increase in episodes of hyperglycemia and unfortunately was unable to reduce the incidence of patients suffering cardiovascular or cerebrovascular ischemic events. Interestingly, it was noted that prediabetics who used nateglinide compared to placebo were not at lower risk of developing diabetes over the median five-year period of longitudinal analysis [43]. Conflicting data also exist on repaglinide's ability to decrease stroke risk in diabetics. While repaglinide did demonstrate similar efficacy in controlling hyperglycemia, metformin is more effective in decreasing the risk of CVD in DMII patients [39]. Whether meglitinides are associated with increased cardiovascular risk is not known; however, since their mode of action is similar to sulfonylureas, the same concern exists.

Dipeptidyl peptidase 4 (DDP-4) inhibitors are diabetic medications such as sitagliptin, linagliptin, alogliptin, and saxagliptin, which prolong the bioavailability of incretins, thereby better controlling postprandial hyperglycemia. Along with the regulation of postprandial glucose, these medications have been associated with decreasing vascular endothelial inflammation and improvement of endothelial dysfunction existing in diabetic vasculature as discussed earlier [39]. Gliptin-induced changes including a decrease in serum lipid levels and hypertension were also noted in animal studies [44]. However, according to Enders et al., diabetics taking DDP-4 inhibitors in combination with metformin when compared to patients taking metformin and sulfonylureas did not experience significantly reduced risk of future ischemic stroke [45]. Linagliptin was associated with a noninferior risk of a composite CV outcome in the CARMELINA (Cardiovascular and Renal Microvascular Outcome Study With Linagliptin in Patients With Type 2 Diabetes Mellitus) study [46]. Regarding CV safety of DPP-4 inhibitors (especially for heart failure), a recent meta-analysis by Mannucci et al. demonstrated a safe cardiovascular profile as its use was not associated with any major cardiovascular events [47].

Acarbose, an alpha-glucosidase inhibitor (AGI), serves a similar role in glycemic control as DDP-4 inhibitors in that they reduce postprandial hyperglycemia. Though its complete cardiovascular safety profile is not known, data from the Study to Prevent Non-Insulin-Dependent Diabetes Mellitus (STOP-NIDDM) trial reflects a positive effect of AGIs in the management of comorbid stroke risk factors with patients experiencing a hypertension relative risk reduction of 34%. STOP-NIDDM also demonstrated a nearly 50% relative risk reduction in cardiovascular events for patients taking acarbose though a head-to-head comparison study with metformin has yet to be performed [39].

Pioglitazone and rosiglitazone improve the utilization of available serum glucose and decrease the pro-inflammatory state of vascular endothelium in diabetics [39]. These two medications belong to a drug class known as thiazolidinediones. Their ability to help mitigate the oxidative injury from ROS in vascular endothelium may contribute to an overall decrease in future stroke risk in diabetics [24]. However, stroke risk in patients who take rosiglitazone remains uncertain as previous studies have implicated this medication with worsening hyperlipidemia, thereby potentially putting diabetics at increased risk of ischemic stroke. Data is conflicting concerning TZDs, especially rosiglitazone, and their role in risk development or worsening of baseline cardiac disease in diabetics. The thiazolidinediones are not recommended for use in patients with diabetes and concomitant severe congestive heart failure or prior CAD [39].

Glucagon-like peptide 1 agonists are oral antihyperglycemics with a mechanism of action similar to DDP-4 inhibitors in that they work on incretin deficiencies inherited to the pathophysiology of DMII. The GLP-1 agonists including exenatide, liraglutide, dulaglutide, albiglutide, lixisenatide, and semaglutide have been shown to significantly decrease overall HbA1C in diabetics. Additionally, the use of GLP-1 agonists in overweight diabetic patient populations has resulted in significant weight loss greater than five pounds resulting in subsequently improved control of stroke risk factors including hyperlipidemia and hypertension [48]. This class of antihyperglycemics has also been associated with cardiovascular protective effect, regulation of postprandial hyperlipidemia, and improvement of fasting LDL [39]. Recent trials (REWIND (Researching Cardiovascular Events With a Weekly Incretin in Diabetes) with dulaglutide, HARMONY with albiglutide, LEADER (Liraglutide Effect and Action in Diabetes: Evaluation of Cardiovascular Outcome Result) with liraglutide, SUSTAIN-6 (Trial to Evaluate Cardiovascular Other Long-term Outcomes with Semaglutide) with semaglutide, and EXSCEL (Exenatide Study of Cardiovascular Event Lowering Trial) with exenatide) have shown potential for GLP-1 receptor agonists in reducing cardiovascular events, including stroke [49–53]. In particular, a main reduction of stroke rate was observed for semaglutide, the oral and parenteral preparations associated with 26% and 39% reductions, and dulaglutide, associated with 24% reduction in stroke [54]; moreover, a recent systematic review with meta-analysis by Bellastella et al. regarding GLP-1RA trials involving 56,004 participants demonstrated a significant 16% reduction in stroke rates [55].

Other oral antihyperglycemics like sodium glucose co-transporter-2 (SGLT2) have similar efficacy to other oral diabetic medications in controlling HbA1C. SGLT2s are superior to sulfonylureas in improving hypertension and as a class are associated with significant weight loss in diabetics

similar to GLP-1 agonists. Compared to placebo, SGLT2s have not been implicated in hypoglycemic events among diabetics though it should be noted that a majority of the data known about their efficacy and management of hyperglycemia comes from data in which patients used them concomitantly with metformin. Data suggest that SGLT2s, when compared to placebo, have clinically significant beneficial effects on controlling major stroke risk factors including hyperlipidemia and hypertension [48]. A recent 2021 meta-analysis by Tsai et al., of five trials, including CREDENCE and CANVAS trials with canagliflozin, VERTIS CV with ertugliflozin, DECLARE-TIMI 58 with dapagliflozin, and EMPA-REG OUTCOME with empagliflozin, involving 46,969 participants showed no significant or neutral effect of SGLT2 inhibitors on the risk of stroke in DM patients [56]. In subgroup analyses, no significant effects of SGLT2 inhibitors were observed against fatal stroke, nonfatal stroke, ischemic stroke, or TIA (transient ischemic attack). However, it was found a significant 50% reduction in hemorrhagic stroke, indicating a potential protective role of SGLT2 inhibitors against hemorrhagic stroke [56]. This could be of great importance because hemorrhagic stroke is the worst stroke type.

In terms of combination therapy for control of hyperglycemia in DMII patients, bile acid sequestrants such as colesevelam have also shown to be beneficial in improving glycemic control. Clinically significant reductions in LDL have been observed with colesevelam use especially when combined with statin [57]. Bile acid sequestrants regulate multiple pathways of lipid synthesis and also appear to have an anti-inflammatory effect on endothelial cells. Some retrospective studies have noted a stroke risk reduction of 43% in patients adherent to taking colesevelam with baseline hyperlipidemia and diabetes though this relatively large risk reduction may have been skewed by confounding variables [39]. Mitigating the deleterious effects of hyperlipidemia, bile acid sequestrants have the potential to reduce the incidence of future ischemic stroke as well as cardiovascular disease [58].

Optimization of Diabetic Control and Additional Stroke Risk Factors

American Heart Association (AHA) guidelines for the primary prevention in stroke in diabetics recommend that all patients with an elevated ten-year stroke risk, which includes all diabetics, benefit from treatment with a statin [32]. Even in diabetics without comorbid cardiovascular disease, the risk of stroke is significantly elevated in patients with uncontrolled LDL compared to diabetics with LDL ≥100 mg/dL [59] with a 24% reduction in ischemic stroke occurrence associated with statin use quoted in prior studies. It is important to note that though increased LDL levels have a direct association with increased risk of ischemic stroke, there is no associated stroke risk for diabetics with elevated total cholesterol and increased HDL [32]. Trials such as the Justification for the Use of Statin in Prevention: An Intervention Trial Evaluating Rosuvastatin (JUPITER) demonstrated that stroke risk is significantly decreased with statin administration even in healthy individuals devoid of increased risk for ischemic stroke [60]. The regulation of atherosclerosis and hyperglycemia is intricately related to an interrelated, complex pathophysiology as discussed earlier in this chapter.

According to current AHA guidelines and based on data derived from the UKPDS trial, it is recommended that aggressive blood pressure management should occur in all patients with DM. The UKPDS trial demonstrated that a goal blood pressure of 140/90 is associated with a 44% relative risk reduction of future ischemic stroke in patients with either DMI or DMII [32]. Which medication regimen to use for achievement of goal blood pressure in patients with DM and baseline increased CAD risk is a point of contention as conflicting data exist as to what constitutes best medical management. Nevertheless, DM patients without additional CAD risk factors at baseline have been consistently found to have an elevated risk of future stroke due to poorly controlled hypertension alone despite AHA recommendations [59]. Per Meschia et al., prior studies such as HOPE found that ramipril administration in diabetics with CAD risk factors resulted in a significant decrease in the relative risk of future ischemic stroke (25% RR, 95% CI: 12–36, $p = 0.0004$) as well as a significant reduction in cardiovascular-related death [32]. Other studies including the Anglo-Scandinavian Cardiac Outcomes Trial (ASCOT) found that a blood pressure regimen consisting of both amlodipine and perindopril resulted in a 25% risk reduction in future strokes though more recent studies considered that successful reduction of BP is more important in reducing stroke risk than the choice of a specific agent, and treatment should be individualized on the basis of other patient characteristics and medication tolerance [32].

In the ADVANCE trial, ACE inhibitor use with concomitant indapamide administration did not result in a significant decrease in future stroke risk for DMII patients [32]. Similarly, in the diabetic subset of patients studied in the Avoiding Cardiovascular Events Through COMbination Therapy in Patients Living with Systolic Hypertension (ACCOMPLISH) trial, it was found that an ACE inhibitor plus diuretic or calcium channel blocker did not result in decreased stroke risk over the three-year follow-up period [32]. Administration of ARBs (angiotensin receptor blockers) such as valsartan has also been investigated for their ability to decrease future stroke risk in diabetics. The NAVIGATOR (Nateglinide And Valsartan in Impaired Glucose Tolerance Outcomes Research) trial, which com-

pared valsartan to placebo, demonstrated that patients with IGT and increased baseline risk for CAD did not have a significant decrease in future stroke risk [43]. Trials such as GEMINI (Genomic Medicine for III Neonates and Infants) suggest that β-blockers like carvedilol are effective and safe to use in diabetic patients to reduce blood pressures to goal. However, there have not been substantial investigations into the role of β-blockers and future stroke risk reduction in diabetics leaving this as a gap of knowledge within the literature [61].

Inflammatory changes induced by hyperglycemic states of DM patients have been shown to induce pathophysiologic changes conductive to the development of atrial fibrillation (afib). In fact, it is a commonly accepted knowledge that DM is a risk factor for the development of afib [62]. It is also known that patients with atrial fibrillation (afib) have a substantially elevated risk of ischemic stroke with diabetics at even higher risk based on the $CHADS_2$ score [32]. According to Dublin et al., treated diabetics have a 3% annual risk of developing afib that is additive based on the duration of diagnosed diabetic state [44]. A 14.9% incidence of afib exists within the diabetic population, and the incidence is nearly six times higher than that of the general population [63].

The recommendations for risk reduction of afib in diabetics are multifaceted. Depending on the $CHADS_2$ or CHADS-VASC score, patients with both DM and afib will carry at least a moderate risk of future cardioembolic, ischemic stroke [32]. As noted earlier during the discussion on diabetes and microvascular complications, the risk of peripheral arterial disease, hypertension, and aortic plaque development is elevated in all diabetics as well as those with IGT. Studies have shown that pathophysiologic changes similar to those that cause endothelial dysfunction in diabetics can also cause autonomic dysregulation which increases the risk for afib. Once these changes occur, it is important to decrease the risk of future ischemic stroke by either starting anticoagulation therapy in moderate- to high-risk patients, rate/rhythm control, or catheter ablation [64]. Unfortunately, DM patients often have neuropathy and may be unaware that they have afib, thereby making catheter ablation a less viable option due to higher rates of cardioversion failure [63]. Therefore, proper management of hyperglycemia is required to prevent changes on the cellular level that place DM patients at higher risk for the development of another ischemic stroke risk factor.

Some studies exist which have assessed whether specific oral antihyperglycemics such as metformin decrease future risk for DM to develop afib. A prospective cohort with 5.4-year median follow-up was performed by Chang et al. who noted that DM patients taking metformin had a significantly lower risk for developing afib than did DM patients not taking metformin [62]. The mechanism of benefit suggested is that metformin may reduce hyperglycemia-induced inflammatory injury to atrial myocyte, thereby preventing tachyarrhythmias known to lead to afib [62]. Moreover, it has been established that there are both increased plasma viscosity and increased activation of thrombocytes in DM patients leading to further risk of clot formation in individuals already prone to developing afib [65]. In summary, DM in patients with AF is associated with increased cardiovascular and cerebrovascular mortality. DM is a known risk factor for thromboembolic events in patients with AF and is associated with a 70% relative increase in risk of stroke [66]. The pathophysiology of diabetes-related AF is not fully understood but is related to structural, electromechanical, and autonomic remodeling. For patients with diabetes and CHA2DS2-VASc scores ≥2, direct oral anticoagulants may be recommended over warfarin, in spite that the relative safety and efficacy of direct oral anticoagulants versus warfarin were similar regardless of diabetes status [67]. Moreover, patients with longer duration of diabetes or insulin-requiring diabetes may benefit more from oral anticoagulation, even in the absence of other major risk factors included in the CHA2DS2-VASc score [66].

Directly smoking tobacco products and second-hand smoke exposure put patients at increased risk for ischemic stroke and increase progression of diseases such as hypertension and atherosclerosis [32]. Nondiabetic smokers have twice the risk of suffering a future ischemic stroke [61] while DM patients who are active smokers carry a 50% higher risk for all-cause mortality and stroke based on data derived from a large meta-analysis [68]. It is likely that smoking acutely causes hypercoagulable states within the atherosclerotic vasculature and over time causes increased rates of atherosclerotic changes within intracranial and extracranial arteries [32]. AHA recommendations for smoking cessation treatment are similar to those made by O'Keefe et al. and include counseling in combination with medications such as varenicline, clonidine, bupropion, and nicotine supplementations [61]. The differences in future stroke risk for smokers who are diabetics versus nondiabetics have not been well delineated.

A risk factor for stroke that is now becoming more recognized is abdominal adiposity more so than patient BMI. However, it should be noted that no current studies have definitively associated increased future stroke risk with increased abdominal adiposity independent of associated comorbidities such as hypertension, DM, and smoking. Olofindayo et al. conducted a prospective cohort study which found that in patients who were both obese and diabetic, the risk for future ischemic stroke was 73% higher than in age-matched individuals with only DM or central obesity alone [69]. It has also been found that regardless of diabetic status, a patient's future stroke risk nearly triples in the setting of obesity with current 2014 AHA guidelines recommending weight loss in patients with BMI ≥25 to prevent future ischemic stroke [32].

According to O'Keefe et al., waist size has proven to be an independent risk factor for the development of DM [61]. Obesity, regardless of adipocyte corporal distribution, has also been linked to the development of tachyarrhythmias with some studies noting a 4.7% increased risk of afib per increase of each unit of 1 kg/m² in BMI [65]. It is also well known that a large percentage of patients with DMII or IGT are overweight or obese placing a large percentage of DM patients overall at increased risk of future ischemic events based on BMI and waist circumference alone. Class 1 level B evidence suggests that modification of lifestyle is necessary for DM patients in order to decrease the risk of ischemic stroke with higher-level evidence denoting a clear correlation with weight loss and achieving normotension [32].

DM patients who demonstrate central adiposity and insulin resistance often have metabolic syndrome [21] though other characteristics of the syndrome including IGT (fasting serum glucose ≥ 110 mg/dL), hyperlipidemia, and hypertension can also be present [32]. Metabolic syndrome is associated with increased risk of ischemic stroke due to the presence of the risk factors which define it rather than by the existence of the syndrome itself [34]. 2014 AHA guidelines currently recognize that up to 38.5% of the general US population meets criteria for metabolic syndrome. Data from large retrospective studies have demonstrated an increased prevalence of metabolic syndrome (43.5%) in patients with a history of ischemic stroke though no direct correlation between metabolic syndrome and increased risk of stroke has been found. Additionally, prospective trials such as Stroke Prevention by Aggressive Reduction of Cholesterol Levels (SPARCL) did not find an increased risk for future stroke in the subset of 642 patients with both metabolic syndrome and prior stroke. Currently, the guidelines for primary prevention of stroke as they pertain to metabolic syndrome are that patients should focus on the management of the individual risk factors that define the disease via weight loss and proper medication regimens [32].

Other less studied risk factors such as DM and ischemic stroke include obstructive sleep apnea (OSA). OSA is not only a risk factor for future ischemic stroke but also has been suggested to have a significant association with the development of DMII. Not surprisingly, obese diabetic patients are at higher risk for developing OSA though obesity itself is an independent risk factor for OSA with some studies quoting prevalence as high as 27% in patients with BMI ≥ 30 [70]. Per Kent et al., a recent prospective cohort comprised of nearly a thousand patients found that patients with moderate to severe OSA were about three times more likely to develop DMII within an average of 2.7 years compared to non-OSA participants [71]. Other larger cohort studies with an average follow-up of nearly five years demonstrated similar results establishing a clear clinical correlation between OSA and DMII [71].

The Wisconsin Sleep Cohort Study and the Sleep Heart Health Study both demonstrated increased stroke risk in patients with OSA. The Wisconsin study was comprised of a prospective cohort which demonstrated that severe OSA conferred a triple risk for future ischemic stroke (OR, 3.09, 95% of CI: 0.74–12.81) [72]. The Sleep Heart Health Study found that when adjusting for all confounding risk factors, there was still a linear positive correlation between rising apnea-hypopnea index (AHI) and risk of stroke [73]. There have been few randomized trials to test the efficacy of OSA treatment as it relates to primary prevention of ischemic stroke though a recent study by McEvoy et al. did note that CPAP treatment versus sham treatment in patients with moderate to severe OSA and concomitant CAD/cerebrovascular disease did not result in a significant difference in cardiovascular-related deaths including stroke ($p = 0.34$; HR, 1.1; CI, 0.91–1.32) [74]. Currently, screening based on symptoms such as daytime sleepiness, snoring, and clinical suspicion is recommended [32]. However, the link between OSA and primary stroke prevention is becoming more and more clinically relevant with up to 4% of the US population now having a form of sleep apnea [32]. The final risk factor for primary stroke prevention that will be discussed is physical inactivity.

Moderate- to high-intensity physical activity has been shown to decrease risk for future cardiovascular events in patients with diabetes independent of any concomitant stroke risk factors including HLD (hyperlipidemia), HTN (hypertension), obesity, and smoking [33]. However, in the general population, some studies report that baseline low physical activity level is not associated with increased rates of future stroke when adjusting for confounding stroke risk factors [75]. Conversely, based on more recent meta-analysis derived data, the current AHA guidelines indicate that active men and women have a 30% lower annual risk of stroke than their inactive counterparts. The degree of intensity, duration, and frequency needed to achieve maximal protective effect from the development of future stroke is a point of debate. Overall, the current recommendation is for 40 min of moderate to intense, aerobic exercise at least three days per week. The data for current recommendations are derived from observational studies as clinical trials delineating clear risk reduction have not been performed [32].

Diabetes and Secondary Stroke Prevention

DM and prediabetes are present in around 30% of patients with acute ischemic stroke and are associated with increased risk for stroke recurrence [76]. Up to 95% of patient with diabetes mellitus are type II with hyperglycemia preceding DM diagnostic criteria in the form of impaired fasting glucose, impaired glucose tolerance (IGT), and episodic hyperglycemia. Wu et al.

conducted a prospective cohort study which found that after initial stroke, prediabetic patients with HbA1c $\geq$ 6.1% had a 61.3% recurrent stroke risk at three months that was still elevated at 51.1% after a year [77]. This was a significant finding due to the traditional threshold for HbA1c of 6.5% being diagnostic for DM, but in lieu of the previously discussed initial stroke risk conferred to patients that only have IGT, this is less surprising. Duration of DM diagnosis at the time of initial stroke may play a role in determining the level of glucose control needed to help prevent future strokes. According to Wu et al., patients with a long-standing history of DM did not benefit from intensive glycemic control as it relates to secondary stroke prevention [77]. However, this contrasted with the benefit found in newly diagnosed DM patients with a history of stroke who were noted to have decreased recurrent stroke risk with a goal of near normoglycemia [77].

It remains a fact that DM is highly prevalent in the global population and places patients within all age demographics at risk for poor outcomes after an initial stroke. In fact, DM is an independent predictor for both primary lacunar strokes as well as for poor prognosis for recurrent ischemic cerebrovascular events [78]. Even young adults <50 years of age with a history of DMI had a high incidence of recurrent ischemic stroke independent of concomitant risk factors [79]. Recently, in a large, cross-sectional multicenter study of DMII patients, it was noted that in the setting of poststroke recovery, only about 60% of patients achieved an HbA1c of $\leq$7.5%. Persistently, elevated HbA1c values are concerning in terms of hyperglycemia's influence on microvascular outcomes though the relativity to recurrent stroke in DM patients was again indeterminate [80].

Rigorous measures of secondary prevention are of paramount importance to avoid stroke recurrence in patients with diabetes. The main messages of the recently published AHA guidelines for secondary stroke prevention in patients with an ischemic stroke or TIA who also have diabetes include the following [76]:

- The goal for glycemic control should be individually based, and for most patients, achieving a goal of HbA1c $\leq$7% is recommended.
- Treatment of diabetes should include glucose-lowering agents with proven cardiovascular benefit to reduce the risk for future major adverse cardiovascular events (i.e., stroke, MI, cardiovascular death). As has been previously discussed, recent clinical trials [54–56] demonstrated that at least one drug in each of the three classes of glucose-lowering medications can reduce the risk for major adverse cardiovascular events in patients with DM and established atherosclerotic vascular disease, including ischemic stroke or high risk: thiazolidinediones, glucagon-like protein 1 (GLP-1) receptor agonist, and sodium glucose cotransporter 2 inhibitor.

- Considering the limited number of therapies available for prevention and treatment of stroke and the substantial attendant disability and impact on patients and their families, recent data meaningfully supports the consideration of GLP-1 receptor agonists for stroke prevention in people with type 2 diabetes at increased cardiovascular risk [54]. In patients with established atherosclerotic cardiovascular disease, including ischemic stroke, when prevention of further vascular events is the priority, GLP-1 receptor agonist therapy should be added to metformin independently of baseline HbA1c [76, 81].
- Multidimensional care (i.e., lifestyle counseling, medical nutritional therapy, diabetes self-management education and support) is indicated to achieve glycemic goals and to improve other stroke risk factors.

Around 50% of patients without diabetes with ischemic stroke have insulin resistance. Both conditions have been associated with increased risk for first ischemic stroke. The Insulin Resistance Intervention after Stroke (IRIS) trial found that insulin-resistant patients with prior stroke receiving had a 2.8% risk reduction for future stroke compared to insulin-resistant patients randomized to placebo.

Pioglitazone reduced the risk of recurrent stroke or MI by 24% (RR, 0.76 [95% CI, 0.62–0.93]), from 11.8% among placebo versus 9.0% among pioglitazone [82]. However, active treatment was associated with adverse events like weight gain and increased bone fracture risk that have restrained clinical use of pioglitazone. To date, the IRIS trial is one of the few studies to evaluate insulin-resistant patients by treatment with hypoglycemic medications with a primary endpoint of recurrent stroke or MI.

The metformin and sitagliptin in patients with impaired glucose tolerance and a recent TIA and minor ischemic stroke (MAAS) trial was aimed to assess the feasibility, safety, and effects on glucose metabolism of metformin or sitagliptin in these patients. Results revealed that metformin and sitagliptin were both effective in reducing fasting glucose and HbA1c levels in patients with recent TIA or minor ischemic stroke and IGT. However, the reduction of glucose levels and sample size was relatively small precluding any clinical relevance. A phase III trial is needed to investigate whether medical treatment, compared with lifestyle intervention, not only improves glucose metabolism in IGT but also leads to reduction of recurrent TIA or ischemic stroke in these patients [83].

Management of Additional Risk Factors and Secondary Stroke Prevention in DM

The final part of this chapter will focus on the additional secondary stroke risk factors as they relate to recurrent stroke prevention. Clearly delineated recommendations have been made for the management of recurrent stroke risk factors including hypertension, hyperlipidemia, and atrial fibrillation, among others (Table 51.3).

Hypertension is one of the most important modifiable risk factors to regulate in order to prevent the recurrence of ischemic stroke. Studies including the Post-stroke Antihypertensive Treatment Study (PATS) and Perindopril Protection Against Recurrent Stroke (PROGRESS) both noted lower rates of recurrent strokes when patients randomized to antihypertensive treatment achieved systolic blood pressures of 140 mmHg. The PROGRESS trial found that further recurrent stroke risk reduction was achieved with systolic blood pressure < 140 mmHg. Confirmation of the importance of antihypertensive administration with goal titration to blood pressures of 140/90 mmHg was found via meta-analysis of poststroke individuals though at this time there is no recommendation of specific medication regimen to achieve [76]. Of note β-blockers and diuretics have both been associated with worsening of glucose control in DM patients. A meta-analysis revealed that β-blockers not only increase fasting blood glucose (0.64 mmol) but also raise HbA1C by 0.75% in patients with DM [84]. The same study

Table 51.3 AHA/ADA guidelines for secondary stroke prevention

Diabetes	Hyperlipidemia	Hypertension	Atrial fibrillation	Other risk factors
DM testing after initial stroke	Statin for patients with stroke and LDL ≥ 100[a]	Treat HTN if patient BP ≥ 140/90 mmHg	Antithrombotic for nonvalvular afib	ASA for all ischemic stroke patients
Goal HbA1c ≤6.5% per AHA Goal HbA1c ≤7% per ADA[b]	Goal LDL < 100 mg/dL	Goal BP of ≤140/90 mmHg	Aspirin for stroke patients unable to take anticoagulants	Smoking cessation recommended for all patients
Moderate-intensity treatment for stroke prevention	Dietary and lifestyle recommended	Diet, exercise, and decreased salt intake recommended	Can delay anticoagulants for two weeks if high bleeding risk present	40 min, three days/week moderate exercise

Stroke reduction with statin use in patients with TIA or ischemic stroke of atherosclerotic etiology, high-intensity statin unless patient's age ≥ 75
[a]Treat hypertension (HTN) if BP over 140/90 mmHg for the first few days after stroke
[b]ADA guidelines differ from AHA secondary stroke prevention HbA1c goals with less stringent glycemic control recommended based on data from the ACCORD study

by Hirst et al. also demonstrated that diuretics also raised fasting blood glucose by 0.77 mmol but did not have a significant effect on HbA1C [84]. These drugs and their role as antihypertensives in patients with IGT should be taken on a case-by-case basis.

Up to 87% of both primary and recurrent strokes are ischemic. When there is regulation of both hypertension and atherosclerosis, a significant mitigation in recurrent stroke risk has been observed [67]. In accordance with findings from the SPARCL (Stroke Prevention by Aggressive Reduction in Cholesterol Levels) study, it is advised that all individuals be placed on high-dose statin. Results of the SPARCL study showed that there was an absolute risk reduction of 3.5% ($p = 0.002$) for major cardiovascular events in patients receiving high-dose statin over a five-year follow-up period. In terms of preventing recurrent stroke, patients receiving atorvastatin 80 mg daily were noted having an absolute risk reduction of 2.2% ($p = 0.03$) without significant side effects. Guidelines for secondary stroke prevention set the benchmark for lipid control with a goal LDL of $\leq$100 [76, 85]. Of note in a post hoc exploratory analysis of SPARCL, there was found to be a 28% relative risk reduction of recurrent stroke with an LDL of <70 mg/dL without increased risk for intracerebral hemorrhage. There was also a 35% risk reduction for ischemic stroke if at least a 50% reduction in LDL is achieved [86]. Considering the results of the Treat Stroke to Target study, in patients with ischemic stroke or TIA and atherosclerotic disease (intracranial, carotid, aortic, or coronary), lipid-lowering therapy with a statin and also ezetimibe, if needed, to a goal LDL-C of <70 mg/dL is recommended to reduce the risk of major cardiovascular events [76, 87].

In patients with DM, the management of hyperlipidemia is similar as regards to goal LDL, but data from randomized control trials have shown statin benefit for all DM patients at increased risk for cerebrovascular disease [76, 86]. However, the use of statins in DM patients is not without elevated risk for hyperglycemia. Macedo et al. conducted a meta-analysis of the available literature to ascertain the statins may pose a risk of DM development [88]. It was shown that there is a slightly increased risk of developing DM in patients who use statins for at least three years though the odds ratio was low (OR, 1.31; 95% CI, 0.99–1.73) and the number need to harm was 44 patients for a new diagnosis of DM. Other studies produced contrasting results with no association found between statin and DM risk though many of them were of low quality [88].

The annual risk for recurrent stroke in all patients with untreated afib who have had a recent TIA or ischemic stroke is between 7 and 10%. Anticoagulation is the optimal choice for recurrent stroke prevention regardless of diabetic status. In patients with stroke or TIA in the setting of nonvalvular AF who have anticoagulation contraindications, it may be reasonable to consider percutaneous closure of the left atrial appendage with the Watchman device to reduce recurrent stroke and bleeding [76]. The AHA/ADA recommendations for choice of anticoagulant is case dependent, and the timing to prevent recurrent stroke in the patient with afib is no different in DM patients compared to the nondiabetic patient population; however, direct oral anticoagulants may be recommended over warfarin in patients who are unable to maintain a therapeutic INR level with vitamin K antagonist anticoagulants [76]. Other risk factors for recurrent stroke prevention in diabetics include metabolic syndrome and smoking.

Patients with metabolic syndrome may not be at increased risk of recurrent stroke from the syndrome itself, but elevated fasting blood glucose does put DM patients at risk for recurrent stroke [34]. Known risk factors for both recurrent stroke and metabolic syndrome such as HLD, HTN, and DM should be modified to prevent future strokes, but screening for metabolic syndrome is not recommended. Limited data exists concerning recurrent stroke risk and smoking though the increased risk of stroke associated with smoking is generally acknowledged. However, it is less well recognized that considerable scientific evidence implicates a strong dose-response relationship between smoking and stroke risk. Shah RS and Cole JW summarize the information regarding smoking-related stroke risk, their dose-response relationship, and the costs for the individual and society [89]. The data concerning hyperglycemic control in DM patients, smoking, and recurrent stroke risk association is currently lacking.

This chapter has summarized the microvascular and macrovascular complications of DM as well as the complex pathophysiologic changes that occur at the cellular level which make diabetic patients at high risk for ischemic stroke. An overview of the epidemiological concerns about DM and stroke was discussed. Also, the remarkable role of hyperglycemia in acute ischemic stroke was revised. Primary prevention of stroke in diabetic centers around the key concept of normoglycemia maintenance which in turn leads to the indirect regulation of concomitant risk factors for ischemic stroke such as hyperlipidemia and hypertension. Optimization of glucose control via oral antihyperglycemic medications is an important facet for hyperglycemia control. Considering the limited number of therapies available for prevention and treatment of stroke and the substantial attendant disability and impact on patients and their families, recent data meaningfully supports the consideration of GLP-1 receptor agonists for stroke prevention in people with type 2 diabetes at increased cardiovascular risk [54]. In patients with established atherosclerotic cardiovascular disease, including ischemic stroke, when prevention of further vascular events is the priority, GLP-1 receptor agonist therapy should be added to metformin independently of baseline HbA1c. Secondary stroke prevention in diabetes again centers around achieving euglycemia to reduce recurrent stroke risk though there is even less evidence about optimization of risk factors than in primary stroke prevention.

Multiple Choice Questions

1. By comparison to the general population, the risk of mortality from stroke in patients with diabetes is:
   (a) Equal
   (b) Lower
   (c) **Two times higher**
   (d) **Three times higher**
   (e) Four times higher
2. Microvascular changes due to hyperglycemia occur:
   (a) Due to atherosclerosis
   (b) Due to intracapillary thrombosis
   (c) Due to production of reactive oxygen species at the cellular and genetic level
   (d) Due to persistent hyperglycemia
   (e) Due to intracapillary hypertension
3. By comparison of many systemic cells, endothelial cells:
   (a) **Express non-insulin GLUTs which allow for continued generation of ROS**
   (b) Downregulate glucose transporters to prevent continued prevention of ROS
   (c) Are highly resistant to the entrance of glucose
   (d) Express insulin-dependent GLUTs
   (e) Express unique GLUTs
4. Endothelial cell dysfunction results from:
   (a) Deposition of AGEs
   (b) Glycation of LDL
   (c) Increased expression of CD36 in monocytes
   (d) Upregulation of inflammatory proteins
   (e) **All of the above**
5. One of the first studies demonstrating that strict regulation of blood glucose prevented vascular complications was:
   (a) The DCCT trial
   (b) **UKPDS**
   (c) ACCORD
   (d) ADVANCE
   (e) VADT
6. Deleterious endothelial changes develop earlier:
   (a) In carotid arteries
   (b) In basilar arteries
   (c) **In cerebral arterioles**
   (d) In anterior cerebral arteries
   (e) In posterior cerebral arteries
7. Risk factors for ischemic stroke include the following except for:
   (a) **Microalbuminuria**
   (b) Sleep apnea

   (c) Atrial fibrillation
   (d) Hypertension
   (e) Smoking
8. Primary stroke prevention is dependent on:
   (a) An HbA1C target <7.0%
   (b) Monitoring fasting serum glucose
   (c) Monitoring postprandial glucose
   (d) **All of the above**
   (e) None of the above
9. In the UKPDS trial, patients treated with metformin showed:
   (a) A 24% relative risk reduction in ischemic stroke
   (b) **A 32% relative risk reduction in ischemic stroke**
   (c) A 40% reduction in ischemic stroke
   (d) **A 42% reduction in macrovascular deaths related to diabetes**
   (e) A 50% reduction in macrovascular deaths related to diabetes
10. Primary stroke prevention involves:
    (a) *Aggressive blood pressure management should occur in all patients with DM*
    (b) *The use of statins*
    (c) *Smoking cessation*
    (d) Screening and management of atrial fibrillation
    (e) **All of the above**

Acknowledgments We would like to thank Dr. Tarun Girotra for his generous inputs and comments to this book chapter. Dr. Feng would like to acknowledge grant supports from the National Institute of Health (P20GM109040 and HD086844), from the American Heart Association (14SDG1829003) and South Carolina Clinical and Translational Research Institute (UL1 TR001450).

References

1. Lieber B, Taylor B, Appelboom G, et al. Meta-analysis of telemonitoring to improve HbA1c levels: promise for stroke survivors. J Clin Neurosci. 2015;22:807–11.
2. GBD 2019 Stroke Collaborators. Global, regional, and national burden of stroke and its risk factors, 1990-2019: a systematic analysis for the global burden of disease study 2019. Lancet Neurol. 2021;20(10):795–820.
3. American Diabetes Association. Classification and diagnosis of diabetes. Diabetes Care. 2015;38(Suppl 1):S8–S16. https://doi.org/10.2337/dc15-S005.
4. Funk S, Yurdagul A Jr, Orr A. Hyperglycemia and endothelial dysfunction in atherosclerosis: lessons from type 1 diabetes. Int J Vasc Med. 2012;2012:569654, 19 pages.
5. Mishiro K, Imai T, Sugitani S, et al. Diabetes mellitus aggravates hemorrhagic transformation after ischemic stroke via mitochondrial defects leading to endothelial apoptosis. PLoS One. 2014;9(8):e103818. https://doi.org/10.1371/journal.pone.0103818, pages 13.
6. Kikuchi K, Tancharoen S, Ito T, et al. Potential of the angiotensin receptor blockers (ARBs) telmisartan, irbesartan, and candesartan for inhibiting the HMGB1/RAGE axis in prevention and acute treatment of stroke. Int J Mol Sci. 2013;14:18899–924.

7. Kim E, Tolhurst A, Cho S. Deregulation of inflammatory response in the diabetic condition is associated with increased ischemic brain injury. J Neuroinflammation. 2014;11:83, 9 pages.

8. Bornfeldt K, Tabas I. Insulin resistance, hyperglycemia, and atherosclerosis. Cell Metab. 2011;14(5):575–85.

9. Kitada M, Zhang Z, Mima A, et al. Molecular mechanisms of diabetic vascular complications. J Diabetes Investig. 2010;1(3):77–89.

10. Node K, Inoue T, et al. Postprandial hyperglycemia as an etiological factor in vascular failure. Cardiovasc Diabetol. 2009;8:23. https://doi.org/10.1186/1475-2840-8-23, pages 10.

11. van Sloten TT, Sedaghat S, Carnethon MR, et al. Cerebral microvascular complications of type 2 diabetes: stroke, cognitive dysfunction, and depression. Lancet Diabetes Endocrinol. 2020;8(4):325–36.

12. Zhang Y, Zhang Z, Zhang M, et al. Correlation between retinal microvascular abnormalities and total magnetic resonance imaging burden of cerebral small vessel disease in patients with type 2 diabetes. Front Neurosci. 2021;15:727998.

13. UK Prospective Diabetes Study (UKPDS) Group. Intensive blood-glucose control with sulphonylureas or insulin compared with conventional treatment and risk of complications in patients with type 2 diabetes (UKPDS 33). Lancet. 1998;352:837–53.

14. Romero J, Morris J, Pikula A. Stroke prevention: modifying risk factors. Ther Adv Cardiovasc Dis. 2008;2(4):287–303.

15. The Heart Outcomes Prevention Evaluation Study Investigators. Effects of an angiotensin-converting-enzyme inhibitor, ramipril, on cardiovascular events in high-risk patients. N Engl J Med. 2000;342(3):145–53.

16. Chen G-P, Zhang X-Q, Wu T, et al. Alteration of mevalonate pathway in proliferated vascular smooth muscle from diabetic mice: possible role in high-glucose-induced atherogenic process. J Diabetes Res. 2015;2015:379287, 11 pages.

17. Prasad S, Sajja R, Naik P, et al. Diabetes mellitus and blood-brain barrier dysfunction: an overview. J Pharm. 2014;2(2):125–38.

18. Sakaguchi T, Yan SF, Yan SD, et al. Central role of RAGE-dependent neointimal expansion in arterial restenosis. J Clin Invest. 2003;111(7):959–72.

19. Tchistiakova E, Anderson ND, Greenwood C, et al. Combined effects of type 2 diabetes and hypertension associated with cortical thinning and impaired cerebrovascular reactivity to hypertension alone in older adults. Neuroimage Clin. 2014;5:36–41.

20. Ergul A, Kelly-Cobbs A, Abdalla M, et al. Cerebrovascular complications of diabetes: focus on stroke. Endocr Metab Immune Disord Drug Targets. 2012;12(2):148–58.

21. Zhou Z, Wang K, Penn MS, et al. Receptor for AGE (RAGE) mediates neointimal formation in response to arterial injury. Circulation. 2003;107:2238–43.

22. Califf RM, Boolell M, Haffner S, et al. Prevention of diabetes and cardiovascular disease in patients with impaired glucose tolerance: rationale and design of the nateglinide and valsartan in impaired glucose tolerance outcomes research (NAVIGATOR) trial. Am Heart J. 2008;156(4):623–32.

23. Lau LH, Lew J, Borschmann K, Thijs V, Ekinci EI. Prevalence of diabetes and its effects on stroke outcomes: a meta-analysis and literature review. J Diabetes Investig. 2019;10(3):780–92.

24. Echouffo-Tcheugui JB, Xu H, Matsouaka RA, et al. Diabetes and long-term outcomes of ischaemic stroke: findings from get with the guidelines-stroke. Eur Heart J. 2018;39(25):2376–86.

25. Bradley SA, Spring KJ, Beran RG, et al. Role of diabetes in stroke: recent advances in pathophysiology and clinical management. Diabetes Metab Res Rev. 2021;38(2):e3495.

26. Warner JJ, Harrington RA, Sacco RL, Elkind MSV. Guidelines for the early management of patients with acute ischemic stroke: 2019 update to the 2018 guidelines for the early management of acute ischemic stroke. Stroke. 2019;50(12):3331–2.

27. Johnston KC, Bruno A, Pauls Q, Neurological Emergencies Treatment Trials Network and the SHINE Trial Investigators, et al. Intensive vs standard treatment of hyperglycemia and functional outcome in patients with acute ischemic stroke: the SHINE randomized clinical trial. JAMA. 2019;322(4):326–35.

28. Moretti A, Ferrari F, Villa RF. Neuroprotection for ischaemic stroke: current status and challenges. Pharmacol Ther. 2015;146:23–34.

29. Patel RAG, McMullen PW. Neuroprotection in the treatment of acute ischemic stroke. Prog Cardiovasc Dis. 2017;59:542–8.

30. White AT, Murphy AN. Administration of thiazolidinediones for neuroprotection in ischemic stroke; a preclinical systematic review. J Neurochem. 2010;115(4):845–53.

31. Ferrari F, Moretti A, Villa RF. The treatment of hyperglycemia in acute ischemic stroke with incretin-based drugs. Pharmacol Res. 2020;160:105018.

32. Meschia JF, Bushnell C, Boden-Albala B, et al. Guidelines for the primary prevention of stroke: a statement for healthcare professionals from the American Heart Association/American Stroke Association. Stroke. 2014;45(12):3754–832.

33. Low Wang CC, Reusch JEB. Diabetes and cardiovascular disease: changing the focus from glycemic control to improving the long-term survival. Am J Cardiol. 2012;110(9 Suppl):58B–68B.

34. Mi D, Jia Q, Zheng H, et al. Metabolic syndrome and stroke recurrence in Chinese ischemic stroke patients—the ACROSS-China study. PLoS One. 2012;7(12):e51406. https://doi.org/10.1371/journal.pone.0051406, pages 5.

35. Capes S, Hunt D, Malmberg K, et al. Stress hyperglycemia and prognosis of stroke in nondiabetic and diabetic patients. Stroke. 2001;32:2426–32.

36. Scheen AJ. Pharmacokinetics of dipeptidylpeptidase-4 inhibitors. Diabetes Obes Metab. 2010;12(8):648–58.

37. Hoogwerf B, Lincoff A, Rodriquez A, et al. Major adverse cardiovascular events with basal insulin peglispro versus comparator insulins in patients with type 1 or type 2 diabetes: a meta-analysis. Cardiovasc Diabetol. 2016;15:78. https://doi.org/10.1186/s12933-016-0393-6.

38. Al-Rubeaan K, Fawaz A-H, Amira MY, et al. Ischemic stroke and its risk factors in a registry-based large cross-sectional diabetic cohort in a country facing a diabetes epidemic. J Diabetes Res. 2016;2016:4132589, 9 pages.

39. Azimova K, San Juan Z, Debabrata M. Cardiovascular safety profile of currently available diabetic drugs. Ochsner J. 2014;14:616–32.

40. Jeerakathil T, Johnson J, Simpson S, et al. Short-term risk for stroke is doubled in persons with newly treated type 2 diabetes compared with persons without diabetes. Stroke. 2007;38:1739–43.

41. Gejl M, Starup-Linde J, Scheel-Thomsen J, et al. Risk of cardiovascular disease: the effects of diabetes and anti-diabetic drugs—a nested case—control study. Int J Cardiol. 2015;178:292–6.

42. Cheng Y-Y, Leu H-B, Chen T-J, et al. Metformin-inclusive therapy reduces the risk of stroke in patients with diabetes: a 4-year follow-up study. J Stroke Cardiovasc Dis. 2014;23(2):99–105.

43. Navigator Study Group. Effect of Nateglinide on the incidence of diabetes and cardiovascular events. N Engl J Med. 2010;362:1463–90.

44. Fisman EZ, Tenenbaum A. Antidiabetic treatment with gliptins: focus on cardiovascular effects and outcomes. Cardiovasc Diabetol. 2015;14:129.

45. Enders D, Kollhorst B, Engel S, et al. Comparative risk for cardiovascular diseases of dipeptidyl peptidase-4 inhibitors vs. sulfonylureas in combination with metformin: results of a two-phase study. J Diabetes Complications. 2016;30(7):1339–46.

46. Rosenstock J, Perkovic V, Johansen OE, et al. Effect of linagliptin vs placebo on major cardiovascular events in adults with type 2 diabetes and high cardiovascular and renal risk: the CARMELINA randomized clinical trial. JAMA. 2019;321(1):69–79.

47. Mannucci E, Nreu B, Montereggi C, et al. Cardiovascular events and all-cause mortality in patients with type 2 diabetes treated with dipeptidyl peptidase-4 inhibitors: an extensive meta-analysis of randomized controlled trials. Nutr Metab Cardiovasc Dis. 2021;31(10):2745–55.

48. Mearns ES, Sobieraj DM, White CM, et al. Comparative efficacy and safety of antidiabetic drug regimens added to metformin monotherapy in patients with type 2 diabetes: a network meta-analysis. PLoS One. 2015;10(4):e0125879.

49. Gerstein HC, Colhoun HM, Dagenais GR, et al. Dulaglutide and cardiovascular outcomes in type 2 diabetes (REWIND): a double-blind, randomised placebo-controlled trial. Lancet. 2019;394(10193):121–30.

50. Hernandez AF, Green JB, Janmohamed S, et al. Albiglutide and cardiovascular outcomes in patients with type 2 diabetes and cardiovascular disease (harmony outcomes): a double-blind, randomised placebo-controlled trial. Lancet. 2018;392(10157):1519–29.

51. Marso SP, Daniels GH, Brown-Frandsen K, et al. Liraglutide and cardiovascular outcomes in type 2 diabetes. N Engl J Med. 2016;375(4):311–22.

52. Marso SP, Bain SC, Consoli A, et al. Semaglutide and cardiovascular outcomes in patients with type 2 diabetes. N Engl J Med. 2016;375(19):1834–44.

53. Holman RR, Bethel MA, Mentz RJ, et al. Effects of once-weekly exenatide on cardiovascular outcomes in type 2 diabetes. N Engl J Med. 2017;377(13):1228–39.

54. Aroda V. REWIND to fast forward: time to revisit stroke prevention in type 2 diabetes? Lancet Diabetes Endocrinol. 2020;8:90–2.

55. Bellastella G, Maiorino MI, Longo M, et al. Glucagon-like peptide-1 receptor agonists and prevention of stroke systematic review of cardiovascular outcome trials with meta-analysis. Stroke. 2020;51(2):666–9.

56. Tsai WH, Chuang SM, Liu SC, et al. Effects of SGLT2 inhibitors on stroke and its subtypes in patients with type 2 diabetes: a systematic review and meta-analysis. Sci Rep. 2021;11(1):15364.

57. Ganda O. The role of bile acid sequestrants in the management of type 2 diabetes mellitus. Metab Syndr Relat Disord. 2010;8(1):S15–21.

58. Porez G, Prawitt J, Gross B, et al. Bile acid receptors as targets for the treatment of dyslipidemia and cardiovascular disease. J Lipid Res. 2012;53:1723–37.

59. Vazquez-Benitez G, Desai J, Xu S, et al. Preventable major cardiovascular events associated with uncontrolled glucose, blood pressure, and lipids and active smoking in adults with diabetes with and without cardiovascular disease: a contemporary analysis. Diabetes Care. 2015;38:905–12.

60. Ridker PM. The Jupiter trial: results, controversies, and implications for prevention. Circ Cardiovasc Qual Outcomes. 2009;2:279–85.

61. O'Keefe JH, Carter MD, Lavie CJ. Primary and secondary prevention of cardiovascular diseases: a practical evidence-based approach. Mayo Clin Proc. 2009;84(8):741–57.

62. Chang S, Wu L-S, Chiou M-J, et al. Association of metformin with lower atrial fibrillation risk among patients with type 2 diabetes mellitus: a population-based dynamic cohort and in vitro studies. Cardiovasc Diabetol. 2014;13:123.

63. De Sensi F, De Potter T, Cresti A, et al. Atrial fibrillation in patients with diabetes: molecular mechanisms and therapeutic perspectives. Cardiovasc Diagn Ther. 2015;5(5):364–73.

64. Lin Y, Li H, Lan X, et al. Mechanism of and therapeutic strategy for atrial fibrillation associated with diabetes mellitus. ScientificWorldJournal. 2013;2013:209428, 6 pages.

65. Asghar O, Alam U, Hayat SA, et al. Obesity, diabetes and atrial fibrillation; epidemiology, mechanisms and interventions. Curr Cardiol Rev. 2012;8:253–64.

66. Wang A, Green JB, Halperin JL, Piccini JP Sr. Atrial fibrillation and diabetes mellitus: JACC review topic of the week. J Am Coll Cardiol. 2019;74(8):1107–15.

67. Itzhaki Ben Zadok O, Eisen A. Use of non- vitamin K oral anticoagulants in people with atrial fibrillation and diabetes mellitus. Diabet Med. 2018;35:548–56.

68. Pan A, Wang Y, Talaei M, et al. Relation of smoking with total mortality and cardiovascular events among patients with diabetes mellitus. Circulation. 2015;132:1795–804.

69. Olofindayo J, Peng H, Liu Y, et al. The interactive effect of diabetes and central obesity on stroke: a prospective cohort study of inner Mongolians. BMC Neurol. 2015;15:65. https://doi.org/10.1186/s12883-015-0328-y, pages 7.

70. Shim U, Lee H, Oh J, et al. Sleep disorder and cardiovascular risk factors among patients with type 2 diabetes mellitus. Korean J Intern Med. 2011;26:277–84.

71. Kent B, McNicholas W, Ryan S. Insulin resistance, glucose intolerance and diabetes mellitus in obstructive sleep apnoea. J Thorac Dis. 2015;7(8):1343–57.

72. Arzt M, Young T, Finn L, Skatrud JB, Bradley TD. Association of sleep-disordered breathing and the occurrence of stroke. Am J Respir Crit Care Med. 2005;172:1447–51.

73. Redline S, Yenokyan G, Gottlieb DJ, et al. Obstructive sleep apnea-hypopnea and incident stroke: the sleep heart health study. Am J Respir Crit Care Med. 2010;182(2):269–77.

74. McEvoy R, Antic N, Heeley E, et al. CPAP for prevention of cardiovascular events in obstructive sleep apnea. N Engl J Med. 2016;375:919–31.

75. McDonnell MN, Hillier SL, Hooker SP, et al. Physical activity frequency and risk of incident stroke in a national US study of blacks and whites. Stroke. 2013;44(9):2519–24.

76. Kleindorfer DO, Towfighi A, Chaturvedi S, et al. 2021 guideline for the prevention of stroke in patients with stroke and transient ischemic attack: a guideline from the American Heart Association/American Stroke Association. Stroke. 2021;52(7):e364–467.

77. Wu S, Shi Y, Wang C, et al. Glycated hemoglobin independently predicts stroke recurrence within one year after acute first-ever non-cardioembolic strokes onset in a Chinese cohort study. PLoS One. 2013;8(11):e80690. Pages 12.

78. Palacio S, McClure L, Benavente O, et al. Lacunar strokes in patients with diabetes: risk factors, infarct locations, and prognosis: the SPS3 study. Stroke. 2014;45(9):2689–94.

79. Putaala J, Haapaniemi E, Metso A, et al. Recurrent ischemic events in young adults after first-ever ischemic stroke. Ann Neurol. 2010;68:661–71.

80. Bohn B, Schofl C, Zimmer V, et al. Achievement of treatment goals for secondary prevention of myocardial infarction or stroke in 29,325 patients with type 2 diabetes: a German/Austrian DPV-multicenter analysis. Cardiovasc Diabetol. 2016;15(1):72. https://doi.org/10.1186/s12933-016-0391-8.

81. Buse JB, Wexler DJ, Tsapas A, et al. 2019 update to: management of hyperglycemia in type 2 diabetes, 2018: a consensus report by the American Diabetes Association (ADA) and the European Association for the Study of Diabetes (EASD). Diabetes Care. 2020;43:487–93.

82. Kernan W, Viscoli CM, Furie KL, et al. Pioglitazone after ischemic stroke of transient ischemic attack. N Engl J Med. 2016;372(14):1321–31.

83. Osei E, Zandbergen A, Brouwers PJAM, et al. Safety, feasibility and efficacy of metformin and sitagliptin in patients with a TIA or minor ischaemic stroke and impaired glucose tolerance. BMJ Open. 2021;11(9):e046113.

84. Hirst A, Farmer J, Feakins B, et al. Quantifying the effects of diabetics and β-adrenoceptor blockers on glycaemic control in diabetes mellitus- a systemic review and meta-analysis. Br J Clin Pharmacol. 2014;79(5):733–43.

85. Amarenco P, Bogousslavsky J, Callahan A 3rd, et al. Stroke prevention by aggressive reduction in cholesterol levels (SPARCL) investigators. High-dose atorvastatin after stroke or transient ischemic at- tack. N Engl J Med. 2006;355:549–59.

86. Callahan A, Amarenco P, Goldstein LB, SPARCL Investigators, et al. Risk of stroke and cardiovascular events after ischemic stroke or transient ischemic attack in patients with type 2 diabetes or metabolic syndrome: secondary analysis of the stroke prevention by aggressive reduction in cholesterol levels (SPARCL) trial. Arch Neurol. 2011;68:1245–51.

87. Amarenco P, Kim JS, Labreuche J, Charles H, Abtan J, Béjot Y, Cabrejo L, Cha JK, Ducrocq G, Giroud M, et al. Treat stroke to target investigators. A comparison of two LDL cholesterol targets after ischemic stroke. N Engl J Med. 2020;382:9.

88. Macedo AF, Taylor FC, Casas JP, et al. Unintended effects of statins from observational studies in the general population: systemic review and meta-analysis. BMC Med. 2014;12:51, pages 13.

89. Shah RS, Cole JW. Smoking and stroke: the more you smoke the more you stroke. Expert Rev Cardiovasc Ther. 2010;8(7):917–32. https://doi.org/10.1586/erc.10.56.

Peripheral Arterial Disease and Diabetes Mellitus

Peripheral Arterial Disease and Diabetes Mellitus

52

Georges M. Haidar and Boulos Toursarkissian

Epidemiology

While the prevalence of PAD is not as high as that of diabetes, estimated at 5.9% among Americans age 40 and above, its prevalence is elevated to 20–30% among the diabetic population, according to National Health and Nutrition Examination Survey data. In a prospective cohort study of 48,607 men comparing diabetics and nondiabetics and the incidence of developing PAD, the relative risk was found to be 3.39. Even when adjusted for all other risk factors, the RR remained 2.61. Furthermore, the duration of diabetes was directly linked with the risk of developing PAD [1]. Diabetes has also been linked with the development of critical limb-threatening ischemia. The severity of diabetes has also been shown to correlate with PAD risk, with one study in the United Kingdom demonstrating a 28% increased risk of developing PAD with every 1% increase in glycosylated hemoglobin (HgA1c) [2]. Perhaps more importantly, diabetics with diagnosed vascular disease were found to have better management of their cardiovascular risk factors compared to diabetics with occult PAD, highlighting the importance of early recognition [3]. Other risk factors for the development of PAD include smoking, older age, male sex, hypertension, and hyperhomocysteinemia [4].

Diagnostic Challenge

Clinical detection of symptomatic PAD can be made through any number of history and physical exam findings, including claudication, diminished or absent pulses, femoral bruit, cool extremities, distal hair loss, nail thickening, or dependent rubor. Pulse exam in diabetics can be difficult to interpret, and a diminished pulse exam may simply be due to calcification of a vessel without a flow-limiting stenosis. Conversely, a palpable distal pulse does not preclude a more proximal flow-limiting stenosis. Vascular claudication is muscular pain, cramping, fatigue, or heaviness that is induced by walking, is relieved by rest, and is reproducible [5]. Clinical detection of symptomatic PAD in diabetics may be made more difficult by the presence of diabetic sensory neuropathy which may mask claudication symptoms and delay discovery of ischemic tissue loss, and motor neuropathy which may limit mobility enough that claudication is never provoked. Therefore, a careful exam and conscientious use of diagnostic studies are particularly important in the diabetic subset of PAD patients.

PAD is diagnosed and characterized through a variety of modalities inclusive of ankle-brachial index (ABI), duplex ultrasonography, continuous wave Doppler, com-

This chapter received no specific grant support from any funding agency in the public, commercial, or not-for-profit sectors.

G. M. Haidar · B. Toursarkissian (✉)
Division of Vascular and Endovascular Surgery, Department of Surgery, Long School of Medicine, University of Texas Health San Antonio, San Antonio, TX, USA

Peripheral Vascular Associates, San Antonio, TX, USA
e-mail: toursarkiss@uthscsa.edu

© The Author(s), under exclusive license to Springer Nature Switzerland AG 2023
J. Rodriguez-Saldana (ed.), *The Diabetes Textbook*, https://doi.org/10.1007/978-3-031-25519-9_52

Table 52.1 Ankle-brachial index interpretation

ABI	Interpretation
≥1.4	Non-compressible
1.0–1.39	Normal range
0.9–0.99	Borderline
0.7–0.89	Mild disease
0.5–0.69	Moderate disease
<0.5	Severe disease

puted tomography and magnetic resonance angiography, and conventional arteriography. The ABI in particular is well used for its simplicity, noninvasiveness, and reproducibility. ABI is calculated by dividing the larger of bilateral ankle systolic pressures by the larger of bilateral upper arm systolic pressures. Although ranges do not always strictly correlate with the typical interpretations, values help characterize the degree of disease present (Table 52.1).

A report of the National Health and Nutrition Examination Survey found that a value greater than 1.4 is associated with PAD as well [6]. The ABI carries a U-shaped cardiovascular and mortality risk curve, associating higher mortality with values on either side of the normal range.

The diagnostic utility of ABI in diabetics can be more difficult to interpret given that diabetic arteries are not reliably compressible compared to their nondiabetic counterparts due to medial arterial calcification (MAC) particularly in the ankles, resulting in ABI elevation and often normal ABIs in the presence of PAD [7]. In a 2010 study evaluating the validity of ABI in PAD against a multitude of patient characteristics, when compared to lower-extremity angiography, diabetic patients had a 4.36 odds ratio for a normal ABI in the presence of proven PAD [8]. Given the distal and microvascular nature of diabetic angiopathy, there is also a component of microvascular ischemia that is missed when using ABI as the sole diagnostic modality. In a study performed in the United Kingdom, microvascular cutaneous responses were measured in diabetics and nondiabetics with and without PAD, and there was a significant subset of diabetic PAD patients in whom ABIs did not capture the presence of distal microvascular functional abnormalities [9]. This highlights the importance of adjunctive diagnostic modalities in diabetics with suspected PAD despite potentially normal ABI values.

The normal triphasic waveform obtained during noninvasive Doppler testing is characterized by a swift upward wave representing antegrade flow during early systole, a downward wave representing brief retrograde flow during late systole and early diastole, and a small slow upward wave in late diastole. The three phases of the triphasic waveform represent normal antegrade flow and pressure against a compliant vessel wall. The full noninvasive vascular study provides segmental pressures, ABI, and Doppler-derived waveforms (Fig. 52.1).

Alternative modalities have been proposed as adjuncts to the ABI for more accurate and prompt diagnosis of PAD in diabetics. The toe-brachial index (TBI) and toe systolic blood pressure (TSBP) have been investigated on the premise that toe arteries are typically spared of MAC relative to ankle arteries [10]. Brooks et al. found that ABI and TBI were essentially comparable in diagnostic accuracy in diabetics except in the case of overtly calcified crural vessels, proposing that ABI be supplemented with TBI or other adjunct diagnostic modalities when ABI is greater than 1.4 [11]. A major limitation of TBI lies in its less well-defined diagnostic criteria. A review of TBIs in the diagnosis of PAD found that 0.7 is commonly recommended as the lower limit of normal and that the sensitivity of detecting PAD ranged from 90 to 100% and specificity from 65 to 100%. These values however require further large-scale studies to firmly validate these limits [12]. The TBI and TSBP have also been studied as indicators of wound healing potential and amputation risk. A TSBP below 30 mmHg is generally considered insufficient for wound healing, conferring a 3.25-fold risk of nonhealing or amputation [13].

Other noninvasive adjuncts to diagnosis and lesion localization include pulse volume recordings, continuous wave Doppler, duplex ultrasonography, and MR and CT angiography. Continuous wave Doppler, when studied against ABI and TBI, is significantly more sensitive and specific in PAD diagnosis in both diabetics and nondiabetics [14]. This is true especially in infrapopliteal disease [15].

The gold standard of PAD diagnosis had been invasive angiography, although CT angiography is growing more popular due to its less invasive nature as well as its ability to visualize beyond intraluminal defects and provide cross-sectional imaging. Interpretation of CT angiography below the knee can be very challenging in diabetic patients due to the heavy-associated calcification. Conventional angiography provides the benefit of being able to demonstrate lesions and flow dynamics in real time as well as offering the potential for intervention on the spot. However, PAD patients frequently have comorbid cardiovascular disease which puts them at higher risk of adverse outcomes with procedural sedation, not to mention associated diabetic nephropathy which limits the use of intravenous contrast. The risk of the latter can be mitigated through the use of renal protective methods or carbon dioxide angiography; however not all centers have the capability for the latter. Furthermore, CO_2 angiography's ability to demonstrate infrapopliteal lesions, more common to the diabetic population, is inferior to that of iodinated contrast in conventional angiography [16].

Fig. 52.1 Normal noninvasive study demonstrating Doppler waveforms, segmental pressures, and ABI. Normal triphasic waveforms demonstrate antegrade (1), retrograde (2), and antegrade (3) deflections observed with pulsatile flow through compliant vessels

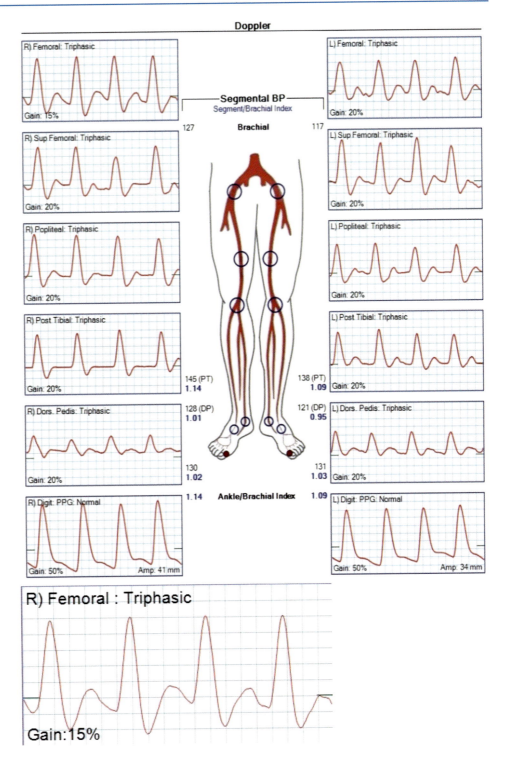

Pathophysiology, Natural History, and Outcomes

Diabetes is characterized by hyperglycemia secondary to either an autoimmune impairment of insulin production (type I) or a gradually acquired insulin resistance (type II) and results in a number of acute and chronic metabolic derangements that ultimately manifest as microvascular and macrovascular disease that closely intertwines with PAD. As noted, PAD is most commonly due to atherosclerosis, which in turn results from a combination of endothelial dysfunction, vascular inflammation, and medial smooth muscle overgrowth which contributes to the development of flow-limiting lesions [17]. Vascular homeostasis relies on a functional endothelium which is largely maintained by a steady production of nitric oxide (NO) which functions widely in vasodilatory, anti-inflammatory, antiplatelet, antioxidant, and antiatherogenic capacities. When dysfunctional, the vessel becomes vulnerable to atherosclerosis and thrombosis. Hyperglycemia promotes increased production of reactive oxygen species, which in turn blunts NO bioavailability as well as encourages smooth muscle cell hyperplasia and strongly predicts adverse cardiovascular events [17].

Not only on a cellular level do diabetes and PAD overlap, but they also demonstrate closely related clinical sequelae. Both diabetes and PAD are coronary artery disease risk equivalents and have well-established relationships with cardiovascular disease. Each disease independently as well as in conjunction increases the risk for major cardiovascular and cerebrovascular events as well as major adverse limb events. The Fremantle Diabetes Study of 1294 diabetics found that an ABI less than 0.9 was an independent predictor (HR 2.91) of first-time diabetes-related lower-extremity amputation over the mean 9.1 years of follow-up [18].

The progression of PAD follows a predictable yet not inevitable course. Two of the most commonly used tools for classifying symptomatic PAD are the Rutherford and the Fontaine classifications which aid in determining the selection of best medical therapy alone versus invasive interventions (Table 52.2).

PAD patients with diabetes are much more likely to present with more severe lower-extremity ulcers

(Fig. 52.2), and given the common presence of diabetic sensory neuropathy, these ulcers are more difficult to detect and treat at an early stage. In diabetic patients presenting with critical limb-threatening ischemia (CLTI), 50% will develop CLTI in the contralateral limb within the next 5 years [19]. In a prospective cohort study of 1244 male claudicants followed for a period of up to 15 years, diabetes and ABI were the two strongest clinical factors found to be associated with the development of CLI [20]. Both lower-extremity amputation rates and survival have been demonstrated to be significantly higher in diabetic PAD patients compared to nondiabetic PAD patients [21]. Worsened disease severity relates not only to concomitant risk factors and diabetic vasculopathy but also to the more distal nature of PAD in diabetics. Diabetics more frequently demonstrate densely calcified infrapopliteal disease, making both open and endovascular interventions more challenging. In a study published in 2016 comparing a 10-year all-cause mortality in diabetics versus nondiabetics with and without PAD, the relative risk was 2.51 after age and sex matching [22].

A population-based cohort study of 444 German subjects who underwent a first-time lower-extremity major amputation stratified by diabetes diagnosis demonstrated a time-dependent influence of diabetes on mortality. Early in follow-up, nondiabetics actually demonstrated slightly worse survival compared to diabetics; however, after 2–3 years, the survival curves crossed and diabetic mortality surpassed nondiabetic mortality. The investigators proposed that diag-

Table 52.2 Rutherford classifications of peripheral arterial disease

Grade	Classification	Description
Grade 0	Asymptomatic	Asymptomatic disease may be detected incidentally or as part of a routine screening ABI. This stage is slow and insidious in the majority of patients, and many may not progress out of this. As major limb vessels gradually narrow, a variable amount of collateral disease may develop. It is believed that for every patient with symptomatic PAD, there are six with asymptomatic disease [19]. This unearths two management gaps in that asymptomatic PAD patients with diabetes are grossly underdiagnosed and that asymptomatic PAD patients are significantly undertreated for their cardiovascular risk factors [3]
Grade 1	Mild claudication	As the degree of major limb artery narrowing increases, demand may exceed perfusion to the affected extremity and result in various degrees of intermittent claudication. Patients may begin to complain of exercise-induced cramping, fatigue, or heaviness in the buttock, thigh, or calf. Claudication is highly reproducible and is typically relieved with a couple minutes of rest. With the commonly concomitant presence of diabetes, motor neuropathy, obesity, arthritis, and other comorbidities such as heart failure and coronary artery disease, a patient with diabetes and PAD may not achieve activity levels that are adequate to provoke claudication. Claudication may also be masked by sensory neuropathy. For these reasons, patient history must be actively and thoughtfully evoked, physical exam must be critically obtained, and the comorbidities of the patient carefully must be weighed into the diagnostic algorithm
Grade 2	Moderate claudication	
Grade 3	Severe claudication	
Grade 4	Rest pain	With continued narrowing, ischemic symptoms may occur at rest which marks the beginning of critical limb ischemia. Rest pain is classically described at night when the lower extremities are elevated and perfusion is no longer assisted by gravity. Patient will describe pain with leg elevation that is relieved by dangling the extremity over the edge of the bed or by sleeping in a chair. Again, rest pain may be masked by diabetic sensory neuropathy. The end stage of PAD, beginning with mild ischemic tissue loss to ulceration and gangrene, may result with further progression of PAD or after a minor trauma or infection. Again with diabetic peripheral neuropathy, a mild injury may go unnoticed and enter a vicious cycle of poor wound healing due to poor tissue perfusion
Grade 5	Minor tissue loss	
Grade 6	Gangrene	

Fig. 52.2 Classic end-stage peripheral arterial disease. Note thickened nails, dependent rubor, and gangrene

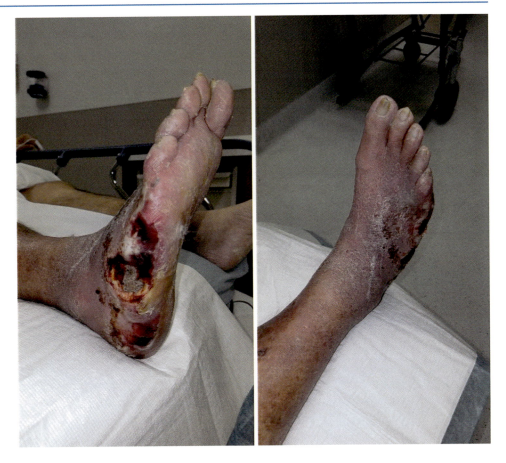

nosed diabetics had better general follow-up and were being closely monitored for their diabetes and incidentally any other comorbidities; therefore any issues with wound healing that arose may have been detected and addressed at earlier stages, suggesting that the more malignant natural history of diabetes could be held at bay with aggressive care. They also noted that the diabetic subset had more transtibial amputations, given their infrapopliteal disease, which are associated with better survival outcomes compared to transfemoral amputations [23].

Management

Better characterization of the association between diabetes and PAD strives toward earlier and more accurate diagnosis and subsequent management to achieve two major goals: improvement of lower-extremity symptoms and quality of life (inclusive of avoidance of lower-extremity amputations) as well as minimization of risk for adverse cardiovascular and cerebrovascular events. Management of PAD begins with lifestyle and risk factor modification followed by revascularization treatment algorithms when disease persists despite the former.

Risk Factor Modification

Diabetes

Interestingly, despite diabetes being one of the strongest predictors of PAD development and severity, there is no data to suggest that stringent glycemic control leads to improved outcomes or survival. In a recent meta-analysis, every 1% increase in HbA1c was associated with a 25% increase in CV disease mortality and 15% increase in all-cause mortality. Of the RCTs (randomized controlled trials) reviewed, however, intensive glycemic control never demonstrated improved CV or all-cause mortality [24]. For example, the Action to Control Cardiovascular Risk in Diabetes (ACCORD) trial was a randomized controlled trial that randomized 10,251 subjects to tight (<6.0% HbA1C) and standard (7.0–7.9% HbA1C) glycemic control arms to assess differences in cardiovascular events (nonfatal MI and CVA) and cardiovascular mortality. The tight arm was terminated after only 3.5 years due to an increased mortality rate noted in this arm [25].

Therefore to date, there is no recommendation for tight glucose control in diabetic patients, both with and without cardiovascular disease, and by extension in those with and without PAD. Current American Diabetes Association guidelines, supported by the American Heart Association, offer a tiered approach to glycemic control, noting 7.0% or lower to be appropriate for most diabetic patients. A goal of 6.5% or lower may be appropriate in younger, healthier patients with less risk factors for hypoglycemia, and conversely a less stringent goal of less than 8.0% is considered appropriate for elder, altered, more frail patients with higher risk for hypoglycemia [26]. No specific recommendations for HbA1c targets in PAD patients exist to this date.

Smoking

The association between smoking and PAD and subsequent progression to CLI, amputation, CV events, and death has been well established, and it has time and again been implicated as the strongest and most preventable risk factor for the development of PAD. The Society for Vascular Surgery practice guidelines for the management of asymptomatic PAD and claudication identify smoking cessation as a GRADE 1A recommendation [27]. Not only is there a 2.2-fold increased risk of symptomatic PAD in active smokers versus nonsmokers, but there is also a significantly increased prevalence of PAD in former smokes compared to never-smokers, thus further emphasizing the importance of prevention in addition to cessation [28].

There is also a clear survival benefit with cessation. An observational cohort study of 739 patients with symptomatic PAD followed quitters versus nonquitters after lower-extremity angiography. Thirty percent were able to quit and maintain cessation 1 year out from angiography, and at a 5-year follow-up, quitters demonstrated significantly lower all-cause mortality (14% versus 31%) and higher amputation-free survival (81% versus 60%) compared to nonquitters [29]. Furthermore, patients who smoke and do require lower-extremity revascularization of any kind are at higher risk of failed intervention and postprocedural complications. A retrospective study of 15,534 patients who underwent infrainguinal bypass found significantly increased 30-day graft failure rates in smokers versus non-smokers [8].

Despite the mountains of evidence in support of smoking cessation, tobacco use remains widely prevalent in the PAD population. From 2010 to 2015, 101,055 open and endovascular revascularization procedures were cataloged for smoking prevalence and cessation rates after intervention. At the time of intervention, 44% of patients were active smokers. Smoking was more prevalent among males, younger patients, and private insurance carriers. Smokers were also more likely to have lower overall medication compliance. At a 1-year follow-up, 36% of the smokers had quit—of these

quitters, they were more likely to be older than 70, have an ABI > 0.9, and have undergone a bypass procedure rather than a percutaneous intervention [30]. Given the demographic findings of PAD patients who are most likely to be active smokers, this gives insight into targeted opportunities for prevention of disease progression through smoking cessation efforts.

Unfortunately, cessation is difficult to achieve and maintain, as demonstrated by multiple studies observing cessation efforts. A key issue identified is the clinician's preconceived belief that long-time smokers are unlikely to quit and that therefore efforts to promote cessation are futile [31]. A cluster-randomized trial of 156 tobacco-using patients at eight vascular surgery practices compared standard counseling to protocolized cessation counseling that included surgeon-driven cessation advice, prescriptions for cessation aids, and referral to a cessation hotline. At a 3-month follow-up, the intervention group demonstrated higher interest in quitting and better knowledge of the negative health effects of smoking [32]. This demonstrated that even with minimal intervention from the surgeon, there was a significant improvement in patient mindset with regard to smoking cessation.

Positive results have been found with intensive cessation regimens targeted at PAD patients. A study in 2 Minnesota vascular centers randomized 124 active smokers with PAD who expressed a desire to quit to intensive and minimal intervention groups. The intensive intervention group included counseling from the vascular provider to quit smoking, multiple sessions with a smoking cessation counselor providing education about smoking and PAD development and progression, offers of cessation pharmacotherapy, and identification of an outside social support person to facilitate cessation efforts. The minimal intervention group received a single admonishment to quit smoking and a list of referrals for outside cessation resources. At a 6-month follow-up, the intensive intervention group had biochemically verified quit rates of 21.3% compared to 6.8% in the minimal intervention group [33].

Hypertension

Numerous large-scale studies have demonstrated an overall decrease in adverse CV events including stroke and MI, chronic kidney disease, and mortality with improved blood pressure control [34]. Hypertension is also an independent risk factor for PAD; however, the association is not as strong as that of smoking and diabetes. The treatment of hypertension is mainly aimed at reducing the risk of adverse cardiovascular and cerebrovascular events and death. That said, the Treatment of Mild Hypertension Study demonstrated that pharmacologic antihypertensive therapy in addition to dietary changes was associated with a decreased prevalence of intermittent claudication compared to dietary changes alone [35]. This is in contradiction to the theoretical concern that decreased systemic pressure may exacerbate symptomatic PAD due to decreased peripheral perfusion. The benefit of antihypertensive medications is clear; the choice of drug class is slightly murkier in the context of PAD. There existed debate about beta-blockers and their potential for worsening claudication—to date there is no clear evidence to support this, and in fact, a meta-analysis of 11 randomized trials found no association between beta-blockers and adverse effects on walking distance or claudication symptoms [36]. In the appropriate cardiac context, beta-blockers may be the preferred agent for antihypertensive control in PAD patients. That said, angiotensin-converting enzyme inhibitors (ACEIs) also demonstrate clear cardiac and renal protective effects and are potential for the improvement of claudication symptoms. The Heart Outcomes Prevention Evaluation study showed a 25% reduction of cardiac events with ramipril. A double-blind placebo-controlled trial in Australia demonstrated improvements in pain-free walk distance as well as maximum walk distance with ramipril versus placebo; however, this finding has not been reproduced in larger, long-term studies [37].

Dyslipidemia

Dyslipidemia is associated with a higher risk of adverse cardiovascular events, and reduction of cholesterol similarly reduces this risk. The Scandinavian Simvastatin Survival Study (4S) demonstrated that in patients with coronary artery disease, treatment with simvastatin was associated with a relative risk reduction of 42% for CAD-related death and 30% for all-cause mortality [38]. Many studies in the statin era have corroborated this finding and have even found cardiovascular benefits even in those patients with normal cholesterol levels. The pleiotropic effects of statins have been demonstrated in many large-scale, long-term studies.

Treatment of elevated low-density lipoprotein (LDL) has also been strongly implicated in slowing the progression of peripheral atherosclerotic disease burden as well as symptoms of PAD. In the Heart Protection Study, 6748 adults with PAD were randomized double-blindly to 40 mg of simvastatin daily versus placebo and followed for a mean of 5 years. The simvastatin arm demonstrated a 22% relative reduction in the rate of first major vascular event, defined as coronary artery events, strokes, or peripheral vascular events; and it showed a 16% relative reduction specifically for peripheral vascular events. The subgroup with normal LDL levels was

conferred protection from adverse vascular events, suggesting as before that statin therapy's benefits extend beyond lowering serum lipid levels [39]. Some of these cholesterol-independent effects involve restoring endothelial function, stabilizing atherosclerotic plaques, and decreasing oxidative stress and vessel inflammation; however, the pleiotropic effects of statin therapy are incompletely understood [40].

The use of statins has also been implicated strongly in the improvement of claudication. A prospective study of 392 patients with PAD compared lower-extremity functional performance between statin users and nonusers. When controlled for age, sex, comorbidities, health insurance, and education, statin users had significantly better lower-extremity functioning compared to statin nonusers. Leg function was measured using 6-min walking distance, 4-m walking speed, time to rise from a chair 5 times in a row, and standing balance [41]. A randomized trial of simvastatin versus placebo in symptomatic PAD patients demonstrated significant increases at 6 months and 12 months (24% and 42%, respectively) in treadmill exercise time until onset of claudication symptoms in the simvastatin arm. No significant differences in treadmill times were noted in the placebo arm at 6 or 12 months [42].

A study of 49 patients comparing 6-min walk test and treadmill exercise time until onset of claudication to real-life self-reported outdoor equivalents and noted no significant difference between the treadmill and outdoor values. Interestingly, based on subjects' responses on the Vascular Quality of Life Questionnaire, the 6-min walk test was the only test modality that correlated with quality of life assessments [43]. Unless patients notice intolerable side effects, statin use is indicated for the reduction in disease progression and mortality as well as for the improvement in quality of life and amputation-free survival in all PAD patients, regardless of serum cholesterol levels. Current recommendations provide goal LDL of less than 100 mg/dL for patients with PAD and less than 70 mg/dL for very high-risk individuals [44].

Obesity

Obesity is most frequently quantified with the body mass index (BMI), which is calculated as weight in kilograms divided by the square of the height in meters (kg/m^2). Being overweight or obese has been associated with increased all-cause mortality [45]. A compilation of 19 prospective study participants totaling 1.46 million subjects found an inverse relationship between BMI and all-cause mortality, with the lowest all-cause mortality rate in the BMI range of 20–24.9 [46]. While obesity has not been directly linked as a risk factor for PAD or adverse lower-extremity outcomes, weight loss in obese PAD patients can improve claudication symptoms by reducing weight and stress on the lower extremities.

A prospective study of 297 patients with symptomatic PAD characterized factors associated with various degrees of sedentary lifestyles and noted that the most sedentary subjects had higher BMI and diabetes prevalence as well as lower walking economy and maximum walking distance [47]. Another study of 46 symptomatic PAD patients compared subjects with normal weight and those with risk of obesity (BMI 28 or greater). Investigators compared claudication times and total walking times as well as time to recovery of baseline ABI. The risk of obesity subset had shorter times to onset of claudication as well as longer delays in recovery of baseline ABI after exercise [48]. PAD patients should be counseled to maintain healthy body weight to reduce mortality, decrease risk of diabetes, and possibly improve claudication symptoms.

Exercise

In an effort to avoid symptoms of claudication, patients may self-limit their activity level. Numerous studies have shown that sedentary lifestyle is not only linked with overall poorer outcomes, but it is also associated with decreased walking distance and quality of life [49]. A study following activity levels of subjects with PAD demonstrated that higher physical activity level was associated with lower all-cause and cardiovascular disease mortality in the studied population [50]. Simple verbal prescription of a home exercise regimen is insufficient. Patients have various obstacles including poor adherence and fear that the pain of mild claudication is deleterious which require supervision and positive feedback from a clinician vital to the success of any walking program.

Similar to smoking cessation, a simple admonishment to continue walking is not as effective as supervised exercise therapy (SET) [51]. The Claudication: Exercise Versus Endoluminal Revascularization (CLEVER) study is a multi-center randomized prospective trial comparing supervised exercise to endovascular revascularization and best medical therapy. It was found that both SET and stent revascularization improved peak walking times similarly, and both were significantly superior to best medical therapy alone in terms of improved exercise tolerance [52].

The safety of SET has been studied given PAD patients' higher baseline risk of adverse cardiovascular events and mortality. A large-scale review of clinical trials studying SET compiling a collective 82,725 h of training found that a total of 8 adverse events were reported, only 6 of which were cardiovascular in origin [53]. The safety of SET and its exceedingly low complication rate is likely related to its supervised nature.

Antiplatelets

Antiplatelet therapy is recommended to reduce risk of both fatal and nonfatal CV events in patients with symptomatic PAD. The Antiplatelet Trialists' Collaboration, an analysis of combined data from over 135,000 subjects, determined that prolonged antiplatelet therapy with aspirin was associated with a significant 25% reduction in adverse vascular events in high-risk subjects. More to the point, when looking at symptomatic PAD patients specifically, there was an association with significantly reduced overall vascular occlusion rates in the antiplatelet group versus controls (15.7% versus 24.9%), as well as when broken down to native (19.5% versus 39%) and graft (15.8% versus 23.6%) patency rates [54].

While antiplatelet use has been well supported in the literature for secondary prevention in appropriate patients, its use as a primary preventative measure in PAD and diabetes patients has not yet been as well established.

The Prevention of Progression of Arterial Disease and Diabetes (POPADAD) trial was a blinded, randomized placebo-controlled trial of aspirin and antioxidants (alone and in combination) compared to placebo in diabetics with asymptomatic PAD as defined by abnormal ABI but no symptomatic cardiovascular disease. It demonstrated no difference in primary endpoints (nonfatal MI or CVA, major amputation, death from MI or CVA) in the aspirin and non-aspirin arms, providing no evidence in support of aspirin use for primary prevention of these events in diabetics with subclinical PAD [55]. The ASCEND (A Study of Cardiovascular Events in Diabetes) trial looked at the role of aspirin for cardiovascular prevention in diabetic patients over the age of 40 and without established cardiovascular disease [56]. Aspirin use resulted in an absolute reduction of 0.17% per year in MI, stroke, TIA, and death, at the cost of an excess annual risk of bleeding of 0.13%. A 2016 meta-analysis of six studies evaluating aspirin's safety and efficacy in primary prevention of adverse vascular events was unable to find a difference between aspirin and placebo in these vascular endpoints [57]. As a result, there have been some suggestions that aspirin use be limited to those with added risk factors such as positive family history, high coronary calcium score, elevated lipoprotein A1, or other inflammatory markers [56].

A subset of PAD patients exists that continues to experience adverse vascular events despite long-term aspirin therapy. Symptomatic PAD patients on long-term aspirin were studied prospectively for aspirin responsiveness and adverse vascular outcomes for a period of up to 2 years. Aspirin responsiveness was determined by performing a platelet function test, and 25.8% of study participants were found to be aspirin-resistant. Primary adverse endpoints were more likely in the aspirin-resistant group compared to the aspirin-responsive group (32.3% versus 14.6%). The secondary endpoint of peripheral revascularization or tissue loss was not significantly different between the two groups. This study suggested that aspirin resistance is not only highly prevalent among the symptomatic PAD population but that resistance is an independent predictor of adverse vascular events and mortality, raising the question that these patients may be better served with alternative antiplatelet agents [58].

A number of alternative antiplatelet agents exist today. Clopidogrel is the oldest and most studied of these medications. The Clopidogrel Versus Aspirin in Patients at Risk of Ischaemic Events (CAPRIE) trial was a blinded, randomized trial that compared efficacy of aspirin and clopidogrel in preventing major adverse vascular events and mortality in a population of subjects with symptomatic PAD or recent MI or CVA. A relative risk reduction in these primary endpoints was noted in the clopidogrel arm compared to the aspirin arm at a mean follow-up of 1.9 years. In the subset of patients with symptomatic PAD, the relative risk reduction was 23.8% for clopidogrel compared to aspirin [59]. This suggests that clopidogrel may have better efficacy in symptomatic PAD patients.

The CHARISMA (Clopidogrel for High Atherothrombotic Risk and Ischemic Stabilization, Management, and Avoidance) [60] and CASPAR (Clopidogrel and Acetylsalicylic Acid in Bypass Surgery for Peripheral Arterial Disease) [61] trials both demonstrated the superiority of an aspirin/clopidogrel combination over aspirin alone in preventing cardiac and limb events, with no increase in major bleeding complications in patients with established cardiovascular disease. These were not primary prevention trials and were not limited to diabetic patients.

Another newer agent still is vorapaxar which prevents thrombin from binding to the PAR-1 receptor on platelets. It has been shown to be of benefit in secondary prevention in diabetic patients and decreases acute limb ischemia events as compared to other standard antiplatelets agents, at a cost of an increase in some bleeding complications [62].

Pharmacologic Treatment of Claudication

The principle that peripheral vasodilators should relieve ischemic muscular beds has been addressed with various classes of agents (e.g., calcium channel blockers, alpha-blockers, prostaglandin analogues). Effects of these agents on walking distance and claudication have been largely disappointing. The reason for failure of symptomatic relief may be related to the fact that peripheral vascular beds are already maximally dilated in patients with PAD especially during exertion. Cilostazol, on the other hand, has shown a positive impact on claudication and walking distance. A phosphodiesterase III inhibitor decreases smooth muscle tone and platelet aggregation. It is important to note that while it did

significantly reduce symptoms of claudication and increase exercise tolerance, it did not have an effect on mortality [63]. According to the 2016 AHA/ACC guidelines on PAD management, 100 mg twice daily of cilostazol is recommended for relief of claudication and improvement in exercise tolerance. The rheologic agent pentoxifylline is no longer recommended as it has failed to demonstrate any benefit in the treatment of claudication [5].

Revascularization

Indications

While most patients with symptomatic PAD generally are able to stabilize or slow disease progression with risk factor modification, 20–30% will have lifestyle-limiting or limb-threatening progression of their disease requiring invasive management [27]. Revascularization in PAD is indicated in lifestyle-limiting claudication or critical limb-threatening ischemia despite best medical therapy. The decision to perform an intervention should also be weighed against the individual patient's comorbidities, especially age and cardiac and renal functions. In claudicants, for instance, the presence of comorbidities such as arthritis, degenerative disc disease, and cardiac disease may negate any potential benefits of a vascular intervention. It is also important to note that objective measures of vascular disease correlate poorly with severity of disability. The ABI, for example, has not been found to correlate with patients' subjective assessment of quality of life [64]. Therefore, the decision to intervene should not be based solely on objective findings of disease severity but rather on the patient's reported level of disability which can then be supported by these objective findings. Invasive interventions on minimally symptomatic or asymptomatic patients are unlikely to provide significant benefit and may cause harm. According to Trans-Atlantic Inter-Society Consensus statements, a revascularization procedure should "avoid a general anesthesia, pose a lesser systemic stress, and have fewer serious complications" [65].

Furthermore, the presence of an ulcer does not always mandate intervention. Prior to revascularization, a distal wound's healing potential must be assessed based on objective parameters. This information is usually available in the patient's diagnostic workup. For instance, an ankle pressure of 70 mmHg is typically sufficient to heal a foot wound; however, in diabetics 90 mmHg might be preferred. A toe pressure of 40 mmHg in nondiabetics and 60 mmHg in diabetics is ideal [66]. Transcutaneous oxygen pressure measurements (TCOM) are also commonly utilized to determine tissue perfusion and wound healing potential. A TCOM greater than 40 mmHg is generally adequate for wound healing [67]. It is important to note that TCOM values may also be decreased due to systemic perfusion issues such as heart failure and cardiac valvular disease. Edema and infection may also lead to erroneously low values as well.

In multisegment disease, the most proximal significant lesion should be addressed first, which may relieve symptoms without distal interventions. Treatment of isolated infrapopliteal disease is not recommended for relief of intermittent claudication alone, given the higher risks of complications and recurrence. That said, treatment of infrapopliteal lesions is indicated frequently to heal ulcers. Even though these therapies often do not have long-term patency, they can allow enough perfusion to heal tissue loss or to bridge a complicated patient for optimization before more definitive surgical bypass.

Interventional Challenges

As noted previously, interventions on PAD in diabetes present a particular challenge due to disease severity, presence of other comorbidities including CAD and nephropathy, immune suppression predisposing to wound infections, and more distal heavily calcified disease that is both difficult to traverse percutaneously as well as challenging to find a suitable distal bypass target in open surgery. The presence of diabetes also is a risk factor for restenosis after percutaneous revascularization procedures [68].

Despite these challenges, revascularization in diabetics with CLTI is not only feasible but also associated with lower early amputation rates and higher survival compared to late or no intervention. An analysis of 537 diabetics with CLTI found early amputation rates to be significantly lower in those who underwent revascularization compared to those who did not (1.7% versus 51.9%), and those who did not undergo revascularization had severe CV comorbidities that precluded any type of intervention [69]. Therefore, barring any prohibitive systemic comorbidities, prompt intervention as soon as a patient fails best medical therapy is generally recommended in patients with CLTI regardless of diabetes status, given that limb salvage is significantly worse without intervention [70]. A study of 376 patients with CLI comparing diabetics to nondiabetics found that early revascularization was associated with higher amputation-free survival in both groups compared to those with delayed interventions. The accelerated form of atherosclerosis and intimal hyperplasia at intervention sites in diabetics makes early intervention critical [71].

Endovascular Versus Open

The choice of revascularization procedure is dependent on multiple factors including available resources, operator experience, and patient-specific characteristics such as location and severity of the lesions, presence of skin lesions, activity level, comorbidities, compliance, availability of adequate autogenous conduit, and personal preference. Treatment guidelines from the American Heart Association and the revised Trans-Atlantic Inter-Society Consensus document recommend endovascular therapy as the first-line treatment of focal and moderate-length lesions (Fig. 52.3), while bypass is reserved for diffuse or long-segment disease (Fig. 52.4) [72].

Fig. 52.3 Digital subtraction angiography (DSA) of crural occlusive disease (left) with restoration of inline flow to the foot after angioplasty of the posterior tibial artery (right)

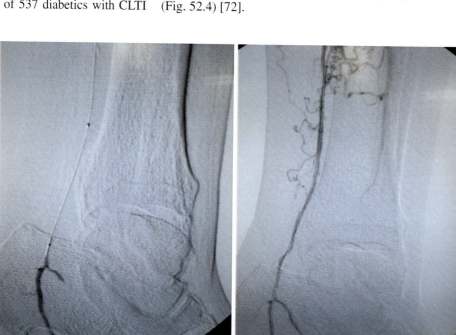

Fig. 52.4 Trans-atlantic Inter-society consensus classifications of femoropopliteal disease

Type A Lesions

- **Single Stenosis ≤10 cm in Length**
- **Single Oclusion ≤5 cm in Length**

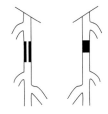

Type B Lesions

- **Multiple Lesions (Stenoses or Occlusions), Each ≤5 cm**
- **Single Stenosis or Occlusions ≤15 cm Not Involving the Infrageniculate Popliteal Artery**
- **Single or Multiple Lesions in the Absence of continuous Tibial Vessels to Improve Inflow for a Distal Bypass**
- **Heavily Calcified Occlusion ≤5 cm in Length**
- **Single Popliteal Stenosis**

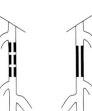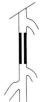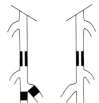

Type C Lesions

- **Multiple Stenoses or Occlusions Totaling >15 cm With or Without Heavy Calcification**
- **Recurrent Stenoses or Occlusions That Need Treatment After 2 Endovascular Interventions**

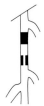

Type D Lesions

- **Chronic Total Occlusions of CFA or SFA (>20 cm, Involving the Popliteal Artery)**
- **Chronic Total Occlusion of Popliteal Artery and Proximal Trifurcation Vessels**

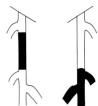

Endovascular and open surgical options should be viewed as complimentary and not necessarily competitive. For example, a patient with severe coronary artery disease with a depressed ejection fraction and poorly controlled diabetes presenting with an ischemic foot ulcer secondary to multi-segment crural disease may not have the physiologic reserve to tolerate open bypass surgery, but tibial angioplasty may provide improved flow and a chance for the ulcer to heal and avoid limb loss or sepsis while the patient undergoes coronary artery bypass and gains better glycemic control.

More recently, with the development of more advanced endovascular techniques in appropriately selected patients, the choice of revascularization modality has had no significant effect on amputation-free survival or all-cause mortality [73]. A systematic review of 57 articles encompassing 9029 patients with diabetic foot ulcers and PAD who had undergone revascularization examined outcomes and characteristics of these patients. Ulcer healing rate was 60% at a 12-month follow-up with any kind of revascularization. In three studies that utilized a PTA-first strategy, mortality and limb salvage rates were comparable to other studies that did not follow a PTA-first strategy, and there was a reported 11% failure rate of endovascular therapy requiring subsequent open bypass [70]. In one study of 1188 diabetics admitted for CLTI, PTA was performed as a first-line intervention in 993 consecutive patients. During a mean follow-up period of 26.2 months, primary patency at 5 years was 88%. The 30-day major amputation rate was 1.7%, and a 5-year survival was 74%, demonstrating in this series a comparable result to open interventions [73]. There are however many other studies that suggest that restenosis rates in diabetics undergoing endovascular interventions are high and that while adequate limb salvage can be achieved, it comes often at the cost of repeated endovascular interventions.

Similar results were demonstrated in a British study. The Bypass Versus Angioplasty in Severe Ischaemia of the Leg (BASIL) trial found that amputation-free survival and all-cause mortality were similar between PAD patients randomized to endovascular and open surgical arms; however, the surgical arm had greater morbidity in the first year. Interestingly, after 2 years, the surgical arm did surpass the endovascular arm in terms of amputation-free survival. This study reinforced that while endovascular and surgical interventions had equivalent short-term results in terms of revascularization and limb salvage, open bypass provided a more durable yet more morbid treatment option [74]. The BASIL trail was not limited to diabetic patients however.

A single-center series also from the United Kingdom found that with an aggressive multidisciplinary approach to the diabetic patient with CLTI, they were able to yield similar limb salvage and overall survival rates as in the nondiabetic patients [75]. In a retrospective study of 1977 infrainguinal open bypass patients for CLTI, inhospital mortality rates were found to be equivalent between diabetics and nondiabetics. However, rates of major adverse events (major amputations, renal insufficiency, MI, dysrhythmia, CHF, and wound infection) were significantly higher in diabetics [76]. The increased perioperative morbidity of bypass surgery must therefore be weighed against its superior long-term durability during the mindful patient selection process.

There are as of this writing two ongoing trials that specifically compare open and endovascular interventions below the knee (an area where diabetic PAD is common). These are the BASIL-2 trial and the BEST-CLI trial. Hopefully, they will help better select therapies for individual patients.

Percutaneous Therapy

Endovascular interventions continue to push the envelope. Initially only indicated for select, focal, short-segment disease, they are now often used for long-segment total occlusions (Fig. 52.5) and multifocal disease. For example, a patient with severe coronary artery disease with a depressed ejection fraction and poorly controlled diabetes presenting with an ischemic foot ulcer secondary to multi-segment crural disease may not have the physiologic reserve to tolerate open bypass surgery, but tibial angioplasty may provide improved flow and a chance for the ulcer to heal and avoid limb loss or sepsis while the patient undergoes coronary artery bypass and gains better glycemic control.

For example, a patient with severe coronary artery disease with a depressed ejection fraction and poorly controlled diabetes presenting with an ischemic foot ulcer secondary to multi-segment crural disease may not have the physiologic reserve to tolerate open bypass surgery, but tibial angioplasty may provide improved flow and a chance for the ulcer to heal and avoid limb loss or sepsis while the patient undergoes coronary artery bypass and gains better glycemic control.

Endovascular therapy options include percutaneous balloon angioplasty with or without stent placement, atherectomy, and any combination thereof. There has been some suggestion in registry data that atherectomy may be of benefit in diabetic patients in terms of a reduced restenosis rate. In general, endovascular procedures are well tolerated and result in shorter hospital stays, more rapid recovery, and less wound complications with equivalent limb salvage rates compared to open surgical revascularization in most cases. That said, as noted, endovascular interventions are generally less durable than surgical bypass and more frequently require reintervention to maintain patency [77]. A study observing 101 diabetics with CLTI who underwent endovascular infrapopliteal intervention noted successful PTA in 87.8%. The seven patients in whom PTA failed had heavily calcified, chronically totally occluded lesions that were not amenable to PTA nor to surgical bypass. The 1-year target vessel restenosis rate was 42%. However, over a mean follow-up of 2.9 years, major amputations occurred in only 7%, and all-cause mortality was 5% [78]. The major amputation rate in this series is comparable to that in another series of 508 diabetics with CLTI who underwent revascularization, with no distinction between endovascular and open, in which 10.3% underwent major lower-extremity amputation [19]. These series demonstrate the utility of endovascular interventions in terms of limb salvage despite high rates of target vessel reocclusion. Diabetes has been shown to be a risk factor for lower long-term patency rates following endovascular revascularization [79].

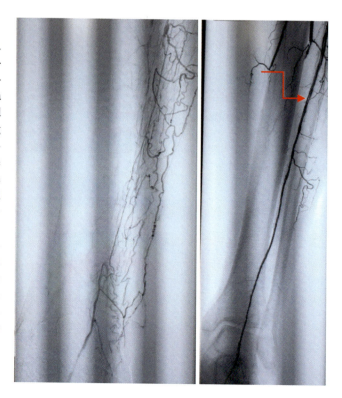

Fig. 52.5 Spidery collateralizations due to infrapopliteal occlusive disease (left). Note their disappearance after angioplasty (right) of the anterior tibial artery (arrow)

The technique of subintimal angioplasty wherein the intima is intentionally dissected and the lesion angioplastied subintimally has been used with some success in chronic total occlusions which either precluded or failed PTA or open bypass attempts. Technical success rates typically range between 80 and 90%, with notably worse outcomes in CLTI compared to claudication, and primary patency rates at 1 year range from 56 to 70% [80]. Ulcer healing rates have been excellent as well, cited at 75% over a mean 23-month follow-up for a series of 60 consecutive diabetic patients with CLTI who were deemed unfit for surgical bypass. This is comparable to ulcer healing rates with open bypass surgery [81]. A recent study in China examined the outcomes for subintimal angioplasty in diabetics with chronic distal (dorsalis pedis or plantar artery) occlusive CLI who were deemed poor candidates for open bypass or PTA. Thirty-seven such patients underwent subintimal angioplasty with an 83% success rate and 95% 1-year limb salvage rate. Complications occurred in 13% of these patients, the most common being vessel perforation followed by failed reentry [82].

Stents are sometimes needed when an angioplasty fails because of recoil or flow-limiting dissection. Critical to stent patency is the maintenance of lifestyle modifications and antiplatelet therapy. The MIRROR (Minimally Invasive IntRaceRebral HemORrhage) study, a randomized, double-blinded study of 80 patients who underwent percutaneous intervention (with and without stent placement), studied dual antiplatelet therapy (DAT) with aspirin and clopidogrel versus aspirin alone. Primary endpoints were direct measurements of two platelet activation factors from whole blood samples taken from subjects after loading doses and just before intervention as well as clinical outcome at 6 months. Markers of platelet activity were lower in the DAT group and recurrence of disease in the target lesion was lower [83]. The findings of this study favor DAT over aspirin monotherapy in PAD after endovascular stent therapy.

More recent developments in angioplasty have included the use of drug-coated angioplasty balloons to prevent restenosis. The main drug used is paclitaxel which prevents smooth muscle proliferation that causes intimal hyperplasia and recurrent stenosis. Drug-coated angioplasty has shown benefits in improving primary patency when used in the superficial femoral artery, but the results have not been as encouraging to date in the vessels below the knee (where diabetics have a high rate of atherosclerotic burden) [84].

A review of 14 randomized trials of antiplatelet therapies around the time of peripheral vascular interventions concluded that aspirin should be administered 6–24 h before PTA and continued afterward to reduce periprocedural thromboembolic events. Regarding DAT versus aspirin alone, a commonly adopted practice was noted to be indefinite use of aspirin as well as 4 weeks of post-procedural clopidogrel given the benefit noted in multiple studies with loading doses of aspirin and clopidogrel [85]. However, more long-term studies comparing dual versus monotherapy as well as long-term outcomes with newer antiplatelet agents are needed prior to making recommendation changes regarding antiplatelet therapy in PAD.

Open Surgery

Bypass surgery is the gold standard intervention for symptomatic PAD, and while it is being supplanted by the rapidly growing use of endovascular therapies, its efficacy in restoring inflow and relieving claudication symptoms and salvaging limbs is undisputed. In fact, despite the growing popularity of utilizing endovascular-first treatment algorithms, a recent retrospective analysis found that in comparing propensity-matched lower-extremity bypass versus endovascular intervention for CLTI, the former was associated with a significantly lower rate of 30-day major adverse limb events and no higher rate of 30-day major adverse cardiovascular events [85]. Therefore, it cannot be dismissed as an unjustifiably risky invasive intervention in appropriately selected patients. Lower-extremity bypass also remains the solution for lesions that are not traversable percutaneously or have failed previous percutaneous interventions. Its use is limited by severe systemic illness (e.g., severe heart failure) that may pose unacceptable operative risk, lack of adequate bypass conduit, and presence of active infection or sepsis (a commonality in diabetic CLTI patients). It is estimated that about 30% of CLTI patients will need a surgical bypass.

The best outcomes for open bypass surgery are obtained using a one-piece greater saphenous vein as the conduit. Conduit choices are as follows in order of preference: ipsilateral greater saphenous vein, contralateral greater saphenous vein, composite (spliced) vein grafts, lesser saphenous vein or arm vein, and nonautologous vein or synthetic graft. Up to 40% of bypass candidates lack adequate ipsilateral greater saphenous vein conduit and require an alternative conduit choice.

Again there exists a correlation between diabetes and treatment complications. In a cohort study of 6112 individuals who underwent open lower-extremity bypass, stratified by indication for intervention, insulin-dependent diabetes was associated with a significant 1.27 odds ratio of readmission, the majority (62.9%) of these admissions being for wound complications. This is unsurprising given diabetics' propensity for wound infection [86]. This further emphasizes the importance of perioperative glycemic control in diabetic PAD patients.

Interestingly, diabetes has not been shown to be an independent predictor of decreased bypass graft patency [87]. This finding has been demonstrated in multiple studies, including the Veterans Affairs National Surgical Quality Improvement Program (VA NSQIP) which identified 14,788 patients who underwent infrainguinal arterial bypass procedures and found that diabetes was in fact significantly protective from early graft failure [88]. The PREVENT III trial, a double-blinded randomized controlled trial of 1404 patients comparing ex vivo application of edifoligide to vein grafts versus placebo just prior to lower-extremity bypass for the prevention of graft failure, found that diabetics, while significantly more likely to present with tissue loss, did not have a higher risk of graft failure at any stage through the 12-month follow-up period [89]. Although diabetes in PAD is independently associated with a higher risk of amputation and mortality, it is not a risk factor for graft failure.

A successful graft depends on adequate inflow, outflow, and conduit quality. Bypass graft failure is classically described in three phases: early (0–30 days), intermediate (30 days to 2 years), and late (beyond 2 years). Early failure is typically attributed to technical factors or judgment error, such as poor conduit, retained venous valves, technical error, and inadequate inflow/outflow. Intermediate failure is secondary to intimal hyperplasia. Some degree of intimal hyperplasia occurs in all grafts; however, where and why this becomes pathologic and flow limiting is not well understood. There is a propensity for this to occur in areas of endothelial trauma (e.g., where a valvulotome was utilized), which strongly suggests that this process is related to a dysfunctional endothelium. Late failure is seen as a progression of the primary atherosclerotic process causing graft narrowing as well as deficiency of inflow and/or outflow.

The incidence of early graft failure is around 5%. This incidence of intermediate failure is 1–2% per month for the first year, and then it further declines to 2–4% per year thereafter. Early surveillance with duplex ultrasonography can detect stenosis before progression to occlusion. A prospective study of 68 lower-extremity vein bypasses in diabetics undergoing intensive postoperative surveillance with duplex ultrasonography found that, after a mean follow-up of 12 months, duplex US (ultrasound) could predict graft thrombosis and amputation [90].

Current literature suggests that some variation of a duplex scan should be done every 3–6 months for the first 1–2 years after bypass, with a follow-up arteriography for abnormal findings. Duplex scan is also indicated specifically if a patient has return of claudication symptoms, ABI decreases by 0.15 from highest postoperative value, or a previously palpable pulse diminishes or disappears. A peak systolic velocity (PSV) greater than 180 cm/s or velocity ratio (V_r) greater than 2 suggests a focal stenosis greater than 50%, while a mean graft velocity less than 45 cm/s indicates a low flow state that is conducive to graft thrombosis. According to Tinder et al., a PSV greater than 300 cm/s or a V_r greater than 3.5 indicates a need for graft revision, and with appropriately

tailored surveillance according to an individual graft's risk profile and postoperative duplex scan, this early detection leads to reintervention that prolongs graft patency [91]. While the most recent TASC II guidelines do not recommend routine duplex ultrasonography for lower-extremity bypass (instead they support clinical surveillance through palpation and ABI measurements every 6 months for at least the first 2 years after bypass), multiple studies have demonstrated that surveillance with duplex ultrasonography detects early lesions before progression to thrombosis [92, 93]. Tinder et al. found that more aggressive duplex surveillance for those bypasses with high-risk characteristics or an abnormal first postoperative scan was associated with higher primary-assisted patency and lower graft failure rates [94].

Patency, while important as a metric of durability, is not the only measure of a revascularization's success. Likewise limb salvage and mortality, while the typical primary outcomes, are not the only measures of patient satisfaction and quality of life. The PREVENT III trial established quality of life as a secondary endpoint and noted that after lower-extremity bypass, quality of life as assessed by the Vascular Quality of Life Questionnaire improved progressively at 0, 3, and 12 months postoperatively [89]. Another study comparing objective measures of lower-extremity function and patient perceptions of quality of life found that while objective measures such as knee flexion and extension, a 6-min walk distance, walking speed, and balance showed absolute improvements, none reached statistical significance. Despite this, there was a significant improvement of subjective quality of life and pain perception postoperatively [95].

Areas of Current Interest

Figure 52.6 summarizes a current algorithm for approaching diabetic patients with suspected peripheral arterial disease. One of the major limitations in interpreting all the studies in PAD and DM has been the inherent difficulty in having truly equivalent groups in whom to compare open and endovascular interventions. In addition to PAD, the major factors that increase the risk of limb loss are the presence of foot infection and the existence of a foot wound and its extent. In an effort to account for this, a WIFi score has been proposed, which included an assessment of the Wound, any Ischemia, and Foot infection [96]. Each category is scored from 0 to 3, and a final score is obtained allowing classification of each limb into one of four categories. Limbs staged as I are considered as low risk for limb loss while those classified as IV are considered high risk for limb loss, with known predicted limb loss rates. Each limb can be restaged following revascularization or control of infection, thereby producing a new estimated risk of limb loss. The system allows for meaningful benchmarking of results and counselling of patients.

Diabetes and PAD are not only frequently comorbid but also result in an accelerated natural history and more com-

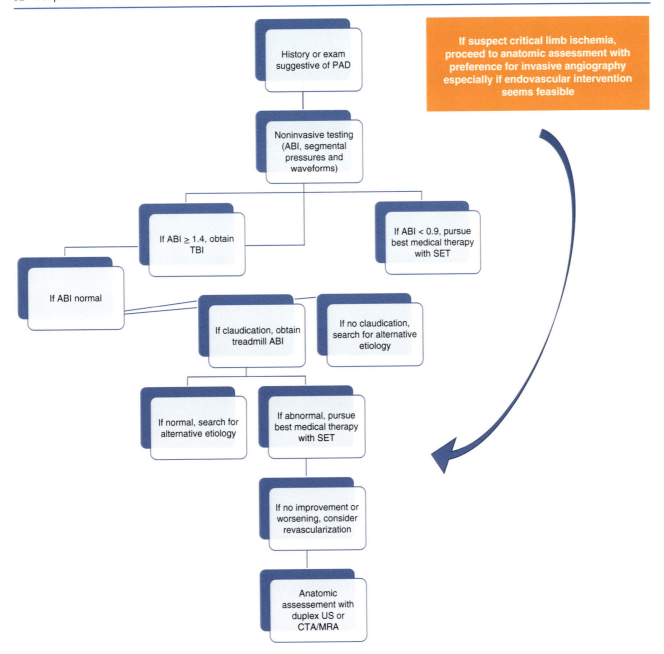

Fig. 52.6 Algorithm for suspected PAD

plicated outcomes and mortality after intervention. Therefore treatment of these patients begins with an appreciation of the significance and risk involved with their comorbidity and the importance of early intervention with lifestyle and risk factor modification. That said, once lower-extremity disease has progressed to the point of requiring an invasive intervention, the presence of diabetes should not deter attempts at revascularization. Treatment options have and continue to become more sophisticated, and with an aggressive multidisciplinary approach, they have the potential to yield noninferior outcomes in the diabetic population.

Multiple Choice Questions

1. Which of the following is *not* a known risk factor for atherosclerotic peripheral arterial disease?
   (a) Smoking
   (b) Age
   (c) Diabetes
   (d) **Trauma**
   (e) Hyperhomocysteinemia
2. According to NHANES (National Health and Nutrition Examination Survey) data, what is the prevalence of peripheral arterial disease in the general population?

(a) 1%

(b) **6%**

(c) 29%

(d) 50%

(e) 85%

3. Which of the following constitutes an abnormal ankle-brachial index?

(a) 1.0

(b) 0.6

(c) 1.5

(d) A and B

(e) **B and C**

4. History and physical exam findings of peripheral arterial disease include all of the following *except*:

(a) Lower-extremity claudication

(b) Diminished pulse exam

(c) Hair loss

(d) Dependent rubor

(e) **Pain with lower-extremity elevation**

5. Diabetics with peripheral arterial disease

(a) Should aim for a hemoglobin A1c level of 5%

(b) **Are at higher risk for limb loss than nondiabetics with peripheral arterial disease**

(c) Should have regular CT angiograms to monitor their disease burden

(d) Have reliable pulse exams for detecting the presence of flow-limiting lesions

(e) Do not benefit from supervised exercise therapy programs because of the risk of falling

6. Critical limb ischemia

(a) Is defined by the presence of rest pain and/or tissue loss secondary to a flow-limiting lesion

(b) Represents the end stage of peripheral arterial disease

(c) Risk increases with comorbid diabetes

(d) Can be masked by diabetic neuropathy

(e) **All of the above**

7. Constitutive production of nitric oxide by a functional endothelium confers upon the vessel antiplatelet, anti-atherogenic, vasodilatory, and anti-inflammatory properties.

(a) **True**

(b) False

8. Pharmacotherapy for intermittent claudication has been shown to be effective in reversing atherosclerotic disease progression.

(a) True

(b) **False**

9. Percutaneous intervention for lower-extremity peripheral arterial disease is:

(a) Reserved only for frail patients unfit for the morbidity of open surgical bypass

(b) Absolutely contraindicated in cases of completely occlusive lesions

(c) **Less durable than open bypass in the long term**

(d) Not recommended in diabetic patients due to inferior outcomes

(e) Associated with higher amputation rates compared to open surgical bypass

10. Open surgical bypass

(a) Is reserved only for severe critical limb ischemia

(b) **Requires adequate inflow and outflow as well as an appropriate conduit**

(c) Can achieve equivalent results using autogenous vein and synthetic grafts

(d) Is a definitive treatment and does not require regular surveillance

References

1. Al-Delaimy WK, et al. Effect of type 2 diabetes and its duration on the risk of peripheral arterial disease among men. Am J Med. 2004;116(4):236–40.

2. Adler AI, et al. UKPDS 59: hyperglycemia and other potentially modifiable risk factors for peripheral vascular disease in type 2 diabetes. Diabetes Care. 2002;25(5):894–9.

3. González-Clemente JM, et al. Cardiovascular risk factor management is poorer in diabetic patients with undiagnosed peripheral arterial disease than in those with known coronary heart disease or cerebrovascular disease. Results of a nationwide study in tertiary diabetes centres. Diabet Med. 2008;25(4):427–34.

4. Selvin E, et al. Prevalence of and risk factors for peripheral arterial disease in the United States: results from the National Health and Nutrition Examination Survey, 1999–2000. Circulation. 2004;110(6):738–43.

5. Gerhard-Herman MD, et al. 2016 AHA/ACC guideline on the management of patients with lower extremity peripheral arterial disease: executive summary. Circulation. 2016;135(12):e686–725.

6. Resnick HE, et al. Relationship of high and low ankle brachial index to all-cause and cardiovascular disease mortality. Circulation. 2004;109(6):733–9.

7. Nam SC, et al. Factors affecting the validity of ankle-brachial index in the diagnosis of peripheral arterial obstructive disease. Angiology. 2010;61(4):392–6.

8. Potier L, et al. Use and utility of ankle brachial index in patients with diabetes. Eur J Vasc Endovasc Surg. 2010;41(1):110–6.

9. Klonizakis M, et al. Effect of diabetes on the cutaneous microcirculation of the feet in patients with intermittent claudication. Clin Hemorheol Microcirc. 2015;61(3):439–44.

10. Young MJ, et al. Medial arterial calcification in the feet of diabetic patients and matched non-diabetic control subjects. Diabetologia. 1993;36(7):615–21.

11. Brooks B, et al. TBI or not TBI: that is the question. Is it better to measure toe pressure than ankle pressure in diabetic patients? Diabet Med. 2001;18(7):528–32.

12. Høyer C. The toe-brachial index in the diagnosis of peripheral arterial disease. J Vasc Surg. 2013;58(1):231–8.

13. Sonter JA. The predictive capacity of toe blood pressure and the toe brachial index for foot wound healing and amputation: a systematic review and meta-analysis. Wound Pract Res. 2014;22(4):208–20.

14. Tehan PE, et al. Non-invasive vascular assessment in the foot with diabetes: sensitivity and specificity of the ankle brachial index, toe brachial index and continuous wave Doppler for

detecting peripheral arterial disease. J Diabetes Complications. 2015;30(1):155–60.

15. du Ro H, et al. Photoplethysmography and continuous-wave doppler ultrasound as a complementary test to ankle-brachial index in detection of stenotic peripheral arterial disease. Angiology. 2012;64(4):314–20.

16. Sharafuddin MJ, Marjan AE. Current status of carbon dioxide angiography. J Vasc Surg. 2017;66(2):618–37.

17. Paneni F, et al. Diabetes and vascular disease: pathophysiology, clinical consequences, and medical therapy: part I. Eur Heart J. 2013;34(31):2436–46.

18. Davis WA, et al. Predictors, consequences and cost of diabetes-related lower extremity amputation complicating type 2 diabetes: The fremantle diabetes study. Diabetologia. 2006;49(11):2634–41.

19. Faglia E, et al. Incidence of critical limb ischemia and amputation outcome in contralateral limb in diabetic patients hospitalized for unilateral critical limb ischemia during 1999–2003 and followed-up until 2005. Diabetes Res Clin Pract. 2007;77(3):445–50.

20. Aquino R, et al. Natural history of claudication: long-term serial follow-up study of 1244 claudicants. J Vasc Surg. 2001;34(6):962–70.

21. Jude EB, et al. Peripheral arterial disease in diabetic and nondiabetic patients. A comparison of severity and outcome. Diabetes Care. 2001;24(8):1433–7.

22. Mueller T, Hinterreiter F, Poelz W, Haltmayer M, Dieplinger B. Mortality rates at 10 years are higher in diabetic than in nondiabetic patients with chronic lower extremity peripheral arterial disease. Vasc Med. 2016;21(5):445–52.

23. Icks A, et al. Time-dependent impact of diabetes on mortality in patients after major lower extremity amputation. Diabetes Care. 2011;34(6):1350–4.

24. Zhang Y, et al. Glycosylated hemoglobin in relationship to cardiovascular outcomes and death in patients with type 2 diabetes: a systematic review and meta-analysis. PloS One. 2012;7(8):e42551.

25. Action to control cardiovascular risk in diabetes study group. Effects of intensive glucose lowering in type 2 diabetes. N Engl J Med. 2008;359(24):2545–59.

26. Inzucchi SE, et al. Management of hyperglycemia in type 2 diabetes: a patient-centered approach: position statement of the American Diabetes Association (ADA) and the European Association for the Study of Diabetes (EASD). Diabetes Care. 2012;35(6):1364–79.

27. Society for Vascular Surgery Lower Extremity Guidelines Writing Group. Society for vascular surgery practice guidelines for atherosclerotic occlusive disease of the lower extremities: management of asymptomatic disease and claudication. J Vasc Surg. 2015;61(3 Suppl):2S–41S.

28. Willigendael EM, et al. Influence of smoking on incidence and prevalence of peripheral arterial disease. J Vasc Surg. 2004;40(6):1158–65.

29. Armstrong EJ, et al. Smoking cessation is associated with decreased mortality and improved amputation-free survival among patients with symptomatic peripheral artery disease. J Vasc Surg. 2014;60(6):1565–71.

30. Gabel J, et al. Smoking habits of patients undergoing treatment for intermittent claudication in the vascular quality initiative. Ann Vasc Surg. 2016;44:261–8.

31. Goldberg RJ, et al. Physicians' attitudes and reported practices toward smoking intervention. J Cancer Educ. 1993;8(2):133–9.

32. Newhall K, et al. Impact and duration of brief surgeon-delivered smoking cessation advice on attitudes regarding nicotine dependence and tobacco harms for patients with peripheral arterial disease. Ann Vasc Surg. 2017;38:113–21.

33. Hennrikus D, et al. Effectiveness of a smoking cessation program for peripheral artery disease patients: a randomized controlled trial. J Am Coll Cardiol. 2010;56(25):2105–12.

34. U.S. Department of Health and Human Services. The seventh report of the joint National Committee on prevention, detection, evaluation, and treatment of high blood pressure. Bethesda, MD: National Institutes of Health; 2004.

35. Treatment of Mild Hypertension Research Group. Treatment of mild hypertension study. A randomized, placebo-controlled trial of a nutritional-hygienic regimen along with various drug monotherapies. Arch Intern Med. 1991;151(7):1413–23.

36. Radack K, Deck C. Beta-adrenergic blocker therapy does not worsen intermittent claudication in subjects with peripheral arterial disease. A meta-analysis of randomized controlled trials. Arch Intern Med. 1991;151(9):1769–76.

37. Ahimastos AA, et al. Effect of ramipril on walking times and quality of life among patients with peripheral artery disease and intermittent claudication. A randomized controlled trial. JAMA. 2013;309(5):453–60.

38. Scandinavian Simvastatin Survival Study Group. Randomised trial of cholesterol lowering in 4444 patients with coronary heart disease: the scandinavian simvastatin survival study (4S). Lancet. 2004;344(8934):1383–9.

39. Heart Protection Study Collaborative Group. Randomized trial of the effects of cholesterol-lowering with simvastatin on peripheral vascular and other major vascular outcomes in 20,536 people with peripheral arterial disease and other high-risk conditions. J Vasc Surg. 2007;45(4):645–54.

40. Takemoto M, Liao JK. Pleiotropic effects of 3-hydroxy-3-methylglutaryl coenzyme a reductase inhibitors. Arterioscler Thromb Vasc Biol. 2001;21(11):1712–9.

41. McDermott MM, et al. Statin use and leg functioning in patients with and without lower-extremity peripheral arterial disease. Circulation. 2003;107(5):757–61.

42. Aronow WS, et al. Effect of simvastatin versus placebo on treadmill exercise time until the onset of intermittent claudication in older patients with peripheral arterial disease at six months and at one year after treatment. Am J Cardiol. 2003;92(6):711–2.

43. Nordanstig J, et al. Six-minute walk test closely correlated to "real-life" outdoor walking capacity and quality of life in patients with intermittent claudication. J Vasc Surg. 2014;60(2):404–9.

44. Rooke TW, et al. 2011 ACCF/AHA focused update of the guideline for the management of patients with peripheral artery disease (updating the 2005 guideline): a report of the ACCF/AHA task force on practice guidelines. Circulation. 2011;124(18):2020–45.

45. Masters RK. The impact of obesity on US mortality levels: the importance of age and cohort factors in population estimates. Am J Public Health. 2013;103(10):1895–901.

46. Berrington de Gonzalez A, et al. Body-mass index and mortality among 1.46 million white adults. N Engl J Med. 2010;363(23):2211–9.

47. Farah BQ, et al. Factors associated with sedentary behavior in patients with intermittent claudication. Eur J Vasc Endovasc Surg. 2016;52(6):809–14.

48. Dias RM, et al. Obesity decreases time to claudication and delays post-exercise hemodynamic recovery in elderly peripheral arterial disease patients. Gerontology. 2009;55(1):21–6.

49. Pinto D, et al. The association between sedentary time and quality of life from the osteoarthritis initiative: who might benefit most from treatment? Arch Phys Med Rehabil. 2017;98(12):2485–90.

50. Garg PK, et al. Physical activity during daily life and mortality in patients with peripheral arterial disease. Circulation. 2006;114(3):242–8.

51. Regensteiner JG, et al. Exercise training improves functional status in patients with peripheral arterial disease. J Vasc Surg. 1996;23(1):104–15.

52. Murphy TP, et al. Supervised exercise, stent revascularization, or medical therapy for claudication due to aortoiliac periph-

eral artery disease: the CLEVER study. J Am Coll Cardiol. 2015;65(10):999–1009.

53. Gommans LN, et al. Safety of supervised exercise therapy in patients with intermittent claudication. J Vasc Surg. 2015;61(2):512–518.e2.

54. Antiplatelet Trialists' Collaboration. Collaborative overview of randomised trials of antiplatelet therapy II: maintenance of vascular graft or arterial patency by antiplatelet therapy. BMJ. 1994;308(6922):159–68.

55. Belch J, et al. The prevention of progression of arterial disease and diabetes (POPADAD) trial: factorial randomised placebo controlled trial of aspirin and antioxidants in patients with diabetes and asymptomatic peripheral arterial disease. BMJ. 2008;337:a1840.

56. ASCEND Study Collaborative Group. Effects of Aspirin for primary prevention in persons with diabetes mellitus. N Engl J Med. 2018;379:1529–39

57. Kokoska LA, et al. Aspirin for primary prevention of cardiovascular disease in patients with diabetes: a meta-analysis. Diabetes Res Clin Pract. 2016;120:31–9.

58. Pasala T, et al. Aspirin resistance predicts adverse cardiovascular events in patients with symptomatic peripheral artery disease. Tex Heart Inst J. 2016;43(6):482–7.

59. CAPRIE Steering Committee. A randomised, blinded, trial of clopidogrel versus aspirin in patients at risk of ischaemic events. CAPRIE Steering Committee. Lancet. 1996;348(9038):1329–39.

60. Cacoub PP, et al. Patients with PAD in the charisma trial. Eur Heart J. 2009;30:192–201.

61. Belch JJ, et al. Results of the randomized placebo controlled clopidogrel and ASA in bypass surgery for PAD (CASPAR trial). J Vasc Surg. 2010;52:825–33.

62. Bonaca MP, et al. Vorapaxar in patients with PAD: results of TRA-2 TIMI 50 trial. Circulation. 2013;127:1522–9.

63. Regensteiner JG, et al. Effect of cilostazol on treadmill walking, community-based walking ability, and health-related quality of life in patients with intermittent claudication due to peripheral arterial disease: meta-analysis of six randomized controlled trials. J Am Geriatr Soc. 2002;50(12):1939–46.

64. Feinglass J, et al. Effect of lower extremity blood pressure on physical functioning in patients who have intermittent claudication. The Chicago Claudication Outcomes Research Group. J Vasc Surg. 1996;24(4):503–11.

65. TASC Working Group. Management of peripheral arterial disease. Trans Atlantic Inter-Society Consensus. Eur J Vasc Endovasc Surg. 2000;31:208–90.

66. Toursarkissian. Arterial ulcers: evaluation and treatment.

67. Ruangsetakit C, et al. Transcutaneous oxygen tension: a useful predictor of ulcer healing in critical limb ischaemia. J Wound Care. 2010;19(5):202–6.

68. Capek P, et al. Femoropopliteal angioplasty—factors influencing long-term success. Circulation. 1991;83(2 Suppl):I70–80.

69. Faglia E, et al. Early and five-year amputation and survival rate of diabetic patients with critical limb ischemia: data of a cohort study of 564 patients. Eur J Vasc Endovasc Surg. 2006;32(5):484–90.

70. Hinchliffe RJ, et al. Effectiveness of revascularization of the ulcerated foot in patients with diabetes and peripheral artery disease: a systematic review. Diabetes Metab Res Rev. 2016;32(Suppl 1):136–44.

71. Dick F, et al. Surgical or endovascular revascularization in patients with critical limb ischemia: influence of diabetes mellitus on clinical outcome. J Vasc Surg. 2007;45(4):751–61.

72. Norgren L, et al. Inter-Society consensus for the management of peripheral arterial disease (TASC II). J Vasc Surg. 2007;45(Suppl S):S5–67.

73. Faglia E, et al. Peripheral angioplasty as the first-choice revascularization procedure in diabetic patients with critical limb ischemia: prospective study of 993 consecutive patients hospitalized and followed between 1999 and 2003. Eur J Vasc Endovasc Surg. 2005;29(6):620–7.

74. Bradbury AW, et al. Bypass versus angioplasty in severe ischaemia of the leg (BASIL) trial: an intention-to-treat analysis of amputation-free survival and overall survival in patients randomized to a bypass surgery-first or a balloon angioplasty-first revascularization strat. J Vasc Surg. 2010;51(5 Suppl):5S–17S.

75. Awad S, et al. The impact of diabetes on current revascularisation practice and clinical outcome in patients with critical lower limb ischaemia. Eur J Vasc Endovasc Surg. 2006;32(1):51–9.

76. Wallaert JB, et al. The impact of diabetes on postoperative outcomes following lower-extremity bypass surgery. J Vasc Surg. 2012;56(5):1317–23.

77. Romiti M, et al. Meta-analysis of infrapopliteal angioplasty for chronic critical limb ischemia. J Vasc Surg. 2008;47(5):975–81.

78. Ferraresi R, et al. Long-term outcomes after angioplasty of isolated, below-the-knee arteries in diabetic patients with critical limb ischemia. Eur J Vasc Endovasc Surg. 2009;37(3):336–42.

79. Clark TW, et al. Predictors of long-term patency after femoropopliteal angioplasty: results from the STAR registry. J Vasc Interv Radiol. 2001;12(8):923–33.

80. Markose G, et al. Subintimal angioplasty for femoro-popliteal occlusive disease. J Vasc Surg. 2010;52(5):1410–6.

81. Bargellini I, et al. Primary infrainguinal subintimal angioplasty in diabetic patients. Cardiovasc Intervent Radiol. 2008;31(4):713–22.

82. Zhu YQ, et al. Subintimal angioplasty for below-the-ankle arterial occlusions in diabetic patients with chronic critical limb ischemia. J Endovasc Ther. 2009;16(5):604–12.

83. Tepe G, et al. Management of peripheral arterial interventions with mono or dual antiplatelet therapy -- the MIRROR study: a randomised and double-blinded clinical trial. Eur Radiol. 2012;22(9):1998–2006.

84. Ang H, Koppara TR, Cassese S, et al. Drug coated balloons: technical and clinical progress. Vasc Med. 2020;25(6):577–87.

85. Visonà A, et al. Antithrombotic treatment before and after peripheral artery percutaneous angioplasty. Blood Transfus. 2009;7(1):18–23.

86. Jones CE, et al. Readmission rates after lower extremity bypass vary significantly by surgical indication. J Vasc Surg. 2016;64(2):458–64.

87. Monahan TS, et al. Risk factors for lower-extremity vein graft failure. Semin Vasc Surg. 2009;22(4):216–26.

88. Singh N, et al. Factors associated with early failure of infrainguinal lower extremity arterial bypass. J Vasc Surg. 2008;47(3):556–61.

89. Conte MS, et al. Results of PREVENT III: a multicenter, randomized trial of edifoligide for the prevention of vein graft failure in lower extremity bypass surgery. J Vasc Surg. 2006;43(4):742–51.

90. Toursarkissian B, et al. Early duplex-derived hemodynamic parameters after lower extremity bypass in diabetics: implications for mid-term outcomes. Ann Vasc Surg. 2002;16(5):601–7.

91. Tinder CN, et al. Detection of imminent vein graft occlusion: what is the optimal surveillance program? Semin Vasc Surg. 2009;22(4):252–60.

92. Mattos MA, et al. Does correction of stenoses identified with color duplex scanning improve infrainguinal graft patency? J Vasc Surg. 1993;17:54.

93. Mills JL, et al. The importance of routine surveillance of distal bypass grafts with duplex scanning: a study of 379 reversed vein grafts. J Vasc Surg. 1990;12(4):379–86.

94. Tinder CN, et al. Efficacy of duplex ultrasound surveillance after infrainguinal vein bypass may be enhanced by identification of characteristics predictive of graft stenosis development. J Vasc Surg. 2008;48(3):613–8.

95. Landry GJ, et al. Objective measurement of lower extremity function and quality of life after surgical revascularization for critical lower extremity ischemia. J Vasc Surg. 2014;60(1):136–42.

96. Mills JL, Conte MS, Armstrong DG, et al. The Society for vascular surgery lower extremity threatened limb classification system: risk stratification based on wound, ischemia and foot infection (WIjI). J Vasc Surg. 2014;59:220.

Ophthalmic Disease in Diabetes

53

José Henriques, Sara Vaz-Pereira, João Nascimento,
Marco Medeiros, Susana Henriques,
and Paulo Caldeira Rosa

Abbreviations

Anti-VEGF IV	Anti-VEGF intravitreous injection
BCVA	Best corrected visual acuity
BMI	Body mass index
CRT	Central retinal thickness
DM	Diabetes mellitus
DME	Diabetic macular edema
DR	Diabetic retinopathy
DRS	Diabetic retinopathy study
ESASO	European School for Advanced Studies in Ophthalmology
ESR	Erythrocyte sedimentation rate
ETDRS	Early Treatment Diabetic Retinopathy Study
GADA	Glutamic acid decarboxylase antibodies
HOMA-B	Homoeostasis model assessment estimates of β-cell function
HOMA-IS	Homeostasis model assessment estimate of insulin sensitivity
MA	Microaneurysm
NPDR	Nonproliferative diabetic retinopathy
OCTA	Optical coherence tomography angiography
PDR	Proliferative diabetic retinopathy
PEDF	Pigment epithelium-derived factor
PEVAC	Perifoveal exudative vascular anomalous complex
CRP	C-reactive protein
RDR	Referable diabetic retinopathy
T1DM	Type 1 diabetes mellitus
T2DM	Type 2 diabetes mellitus
VA	Visual acuity
VEGF	Vascular endothelial growth factor
VTDR	Vision-threatening diabetic retinopathy

J. Henriques (✉)
Surgical Retina Unit, Retina Department, Dr. Gama Pinto
Ophthalmology Institute, Lisbon, Portugal

Lisbon Retina Institute, Lisbon, Portugal

S. Vaz-Pereira
Department of Ophthalmology, Hospital de Santa Maria,
Lisbon, Portugal

Department of Ophthalmology, Faculty of Medicine, Universidade
de Lisboa, Lisbon, Portugal

J. Nascimento
Lisbon Retina Institute, Lisbon, Portugal

M. Medeiros
Lisbon Retina Institute, Lisbon, Portugal

Surgical Retina Unit, Retina Department, (CHLC) Centro
Hospitalar Lisboa Central, Lisbon, Portugal

NOVA Medical School, Universidade NOVA de Lisboa,
Lisbon, Portugal

Portuguese Diabetes Association (APDP), Lisbon, Portugal

S. Henriques
Hospital Doutor Fernando da Fonseca, Amadora, Portugal

P. C. Rosa
Lisbon Retina Institute, Lisbon, Portugal

Medical Retina Unit, Retina Department, Dr. Gama Pinto
Ophthalmology Institute, Lisbon, Portugal

© The Author(s), under exclusive license to Springer Nature Switzerland AG 2023
J. Rodriguez-Saldana (ed.), *The Diabetes Textbook*, https://doi.org/10.1007/978-3-031-25519-9_53

Introduction

Diabetes mellitus (DM) is a chronic multisystemic metabolic disease, which is an effect of persistent hyperglycemia and causes deleterious effects in the micro- and macrovasculature [1–4]. It is expected that its incidence and prevalence will continue to increase globally, making it one of the great pandemics of the twenty-first century [5–8].

The eye is one of the main organs affected by this pathology, mainly causing diabetic retinopathy (DR), which is one of the most important microvascular complications of DM [2, 3, 9]. DR has been reported to be one of the leading causes of blindness in the working age population [10–15]. From 1990 to 2010, in England, as a result of the policies of screening and early treatment, DR is no longer considered as the leading cause of blindness and moderate to severe vision loss [16]. Although less known for non-ophthalmologists, there is a spectrum of eye disease related to diabetes that can lead to eye problems or even loss of vision [17–20].

Epidemiology of Diabetes and Diabetic Retinopathy

The diabetic patients are at 25 times more risk of blindness compared to nondiabetic individuals. This was documented by a study that estimated untreated proliferative diabetic retinopathy (PDR) results in an irreversible visual loss in 50% of individuals at five years after diagnosis [21]. The impact of this visual dysfunction is globally recognized [13, 18, 21, 22], involving several countries like the UK that has set up screening programs for early detection and treatment of DR [21]. In the literature, although there is some heterogeneity in the epidemiological data on DR [15, 18], there is an agreement on the fact that this is a current problem with a strong public health impact.

A meta-analysis involving 35 studies carried out worldwide from 1980 to 2008 provided data from 22,896 individuals with diabetes. The estimated global prevalence of DR was 34.6%: 6.96% for PDR, 6.81% for diabetic macular edema (DME), and 10.2% for vision-threatening DR (VTDR) [15].

Studies in the European population showed a prevalence of DR of 36.5–93.6% in type 1 diabetes, 16.3–34.2% in type 2, and 16.3–48.8% in mixed cohorts [13], with VTDR prevalence estimated between 6.7 and 34.9% [13].

In population-based studies, the prevalence of DME among patients with type 1 diabetes was between 4.2 and 7.9%. In patients with type 2 diabetes, it was between 1.4 and 12.8% [13]. Non-stereoscopic fundus photography was used in most of the studies, which affected the accuracy of DME assessment. About half of the studies defined macular edema using the clinically significant macular edema (CSME) criteria, and hence, only the more severe spectrum of DME was captured in these studies [13]. A Cochrane review of the prevalence of DME as assessed by optical coherence tomography (OCT) has found a large range of prevalence rates (19–65%) [13]. This should be considered as a new reference standard for assessment of DME, even in some screening settings [23].

Ling et al. [22] indicated a DR prevalence of 49% in type 1 diabetes and 24.2% in type 2 diabetes in the UK, with a global prevalence of 21.4% for NPDR (nonproliferative diabetic retinopathy), 2.8% for PDR (proliferative diabetic retinopathy), and 6.1% for CSME (clinically significant macular edema).

An important topic in epidemiological DR-related studies is the prevalence of VTDR—either PDR and/or DME. According to a meta-analysis study by Yau et al. (2012), VTDR prevalence was found to be 10.2% globally. These patients need referral and urgent treatment. Some of the studies do a segmentation of the two forms of VTDR [13].

Variability in the Results of Epidemiological Studies

The analysis of the results of multiple studies based on a review of Lee et al. [13] revealed that the prevalence varies depending on the geography and studies reflecting the precociousness DR or its late identification with more advanced disease. Also, there is a difference between diabetes type 1 and type 2. Depending on the epidemiological studies carried out on patients, those who visited hospitals showed a higher prevalence of VTDR compared to those from the community (population-based) who showed lower prevalence of DME and PDR. A wide range of prevalence observed may also be due to the differences in healthcare systems and socioeconomic factors between the studied populations. However, conclusions cannot be drawn as key characteristics, such as known duration of diabetes, vary significantly between the sampled populations [13]. The studies performed in newly diagnosed patients have a lower prevalence of DR since it increases with the duration of the diabetes [13, 24]. It is also higher in Western countries due to urbanization, diet, obesity, and sedentarism [13]. Eastern populations (except in the surrounding regions of Singapore) and the less urbanized and industrialized rural areas have a lower prevalence [13].

Incidence and Progression of DR

In the Wisconsin study, Klein et al. [25] evaluated the progression of DR in individuals with type 1 diabetes over a period of 25 years. The authors have documented a cumulative progression rate of DR of 83%, a progression to PDR of

42%, and improvement of DR in 18%. In addition, the cumulative incidence of macular edema and clinically significant macular edema was 29% and 17%, respectively.

In Portugal, Dutra Medeiros et al. [26] proceeded to assess the incidence and progression of DR in a prospective population-based cohort of type 2 diabetics with five years of follow-up. Referral diabetic retinopathy (RDR) was set to all patients classified with moderate to severe NPDR or PDR, with or without maculopathy or mild NPDR with maculopathy (a little more comprehensive than set to VTDR). The annual incidence of any DR in patients without retinopathy at baseline was 4.60% in the first year, reducing to 3.87% in the fifth year; the cumulative incidence at five years was 14.47%. The risk of any degree of DR, non-referable DR, or RDR was strongly associated with increased duration of diabetes and earlier age at diagnosis.

The Impact of the Nordic (European) Diabetic Classification on Screening of Diabetic Retinopathy

Data-driven algorithms reflect a larger heterogeneity in DM subtypes when compared with the classical division into T1DM and T2DM or glycemic and HbA1c level [27]. Recently, Ahlqvist, E. et al. published a study [28] where six variables were used to carry out a CLUSTER ANALYSIS: age at diagnosis, BMI, HbA1c, GADA, C-peptide, and HOMA-B and HOMA-IS. A Cox and logistic regression was made, and they found 5 clusters [28] (Table 53.1).

The groups 4 and 5 corresponded to 62% of the diabetic patients, who have low complications level; this is the reason why it is advisable to screen these patients only every 2 or 3 years. On the other hand, more attention should be paid to the higher-risk group of eye complications, namely, group 2 and group 1 which correspond to the conventional DM1.

Currently, it is not possible to identify these groups, in our daily practice. However, this screening strategy should be implemented as soon as we can routinely use those tests in diabetic patient care.

OCT as a Current Screening Tool and AI as an Adjunct to Screen Activity

In addition, we should incorporate the new trends toward the use of portable or home OCT and current use of AI in the screening of diabetic retinopathy. Indeed, RetMarkerDR software, a CE-marked Class IIa medical device developed in Portugal, has been used in local DR screening for some years [29]. It has been implemented into a co-existing, human grader-based DR screening program conducted in Portugal. In this case, Retmarker is used to select between "disease" and "no disease" groups. A human grader assessment is only needed for the "disease" subgroup, avoiding the use of this time-consuming practice to analyze normal images. The human resources are directed to those who really need surveillance from an ophthalmologist.

Table 53.1 The Nordic study (European study of Ahlqvist, E. et al. (2018) points to a new diabetic classification: five clusters of recently diagnosed diabetic patients were obtained

Cluster	Name	INITIALS	Prevalence %	Characteristics
1	**Severe autoimmune diabetes**	SAID		**High incidence of retinopathy**
2	**Severe insulin-deficient diabetes**	SIDD		**highest incidence of retinopathy**
3	Severe-insulin resistant diabetes	SIRD		
4	Mild obesity-related diabetes	MOD	22%	Low complictions level if it do.
5	Mild age-related diabetes	MARD	40%	Low complictions level if it do.

The four and five clusters have a low incidence of diabetic complications, namely, eye complications, and correspond at 62% of the diabetic patients. Consequently, the resources should be directed toward the 38% of the patients of the higher risk of developing diabetic retinopathy

OCTA and OCTA as Part of Multimodal Imaging in Diabetic Retinopathy

Structural OCT is a precious tool on assessing DR, showing qualitative and quantitative imaging of macular area and foveal morpho-structure. A multimodal imaging report integrates also IR and color fundus photography, color ultrawide field photography, AF (autofluorescence), en face structural OCT, and OCTA, which can depict the superficial and deep capillary plexus as well as the choroidal plexus. Currently, this multimodal imaging is essential to establish diagnosis and classifying the DR [30].

Diabetic Retinopathy Physiopathology

Several pathophysiological mechanisms are concerned. It is thought that in the retina, there is a change in response to insulin that exists in the peripheral tissues. As a consequence, there is a decrease in the "signaling" PEDG-derived platelet growth factor, which causes a decrease in the survival of pericytes. The capillary walls disappear [31], which has been marked as an early event in the physiopathology of DR. Microstructural and functional changes appear at the vascular and neuronal levels because of the chronic inflammatory state of the retina induced by maintained hyperglycemia. Indeed, it is in the context of the neurovascular retinal unit [32] that the chronic hyperglycemia acts as a key factor in the pathogenesis of DR [2, 3, 9].

This leads to activation of a cascade of events that, without treatment, culminates in the accumulation of fluids in the extravascular space, ischemia, proliferation of abnormal vessels, and blindness [9, 33].

In DR, the first histological changes occur at the level of the retinal capillaries with basement membrane thickening, loss of pericytes, and change of the tight junctions. This leads to loss of the inner blood-retinal barrier incompetence, promoting vascular hyperpermeability, and vaso-occlusive phenomena [9, 33, 34].

At present, the research focuses on the identification of molecular and biochemical mechanisms that contribute to the changes described above [9].

Several potential biochemical mechanisms have been implicated and activated by chronic hyperglycemia, polyols [9, 35–38], the accumulation of advanced glycation products (AGE) [9, 35, 37, 39–42], activation of protein kinase C (PKC) [9, 35, 43], and leukostasis [9, 34, 35]. These channels promote oxidative stress [33, 44], vascu-

lar dysfunction, and the emergence of pro-inflammatory cytokines, such as the vascular endothelial growth factor (VEGF) [9, 33, 34, 45], TNF α [9, 33], nitric oxide (NO) [9], prostacyclin [9], IGF-1 [9, 33], NF-kB [33], PlGF [9], and interleukins 1 and 6 [33]. Of these factors, VEGF has assumed a particular importance, having been identified in the vitreous and retina of individuals with DR [9, 45] and being considered as one of the main stimuli for DME and PDR [46].

VEGF is a potent mitogen of endothelial cells with a molecular weight of about 45 kD [46–48] and is one of the main cytokines expressed as a result of persisting hyperglycemia, resulting in pathologic angiogenesis, vascular permeability, and increased expression of pro-inflammatory cytokines [47, 48]. In this way, VEGF is also been targeted as a therapeutic tool in DR, with anti-VEGF drugs being considered the treatment of choice for DME, alone or in combination with corticosteroids and laser therapy [48].

Another mechanism discussed as responsible for edema in DR is related to the deregulation of the activity carrier of water molecules resulting from the retinal metabolic activity. This was carried out by the Muller cells, in particular, by the change in the activity of water channels (Aquaporin-AQP4) and potassium channels (Kir, Kir 2.1 4.1) with potassium accumulation in the cells of Muller and their hydration and retinal edema [49, 50], which can be reversed by corticosteroids [50].

There is some evidence that in the earliest stages of the disease, VEGF is the main factor implicated in the DME. However, with the evolution of the disease into later phases, DME becomes chronic. Other cytokines [51], in particular IL-1, IL-6, IL-8, IP-10 (protein interferon-inducible protein), and MCP-1 (monocyte chemoattractant protein), related to aggravation and chronicity of the inflammation, are considered responsible for the inadequate response of the anti-VEGF.

DR is the result of complex and multifactorial mechanisms that lead to edema and retinal neovascularization.

Classification of Diabetic Retinopathy and Diabetic Macular Edema

Clinical international classification/disease severity level of diabetic retinopathy (Diabetic Retinopathy GDRPG—Global Project Group 2002) is based on the dilated fundoscopic or color fundus photograph examination [52–54] (Tables 53.2 and 53.3).

Table 53.2 GDRPG—global diabetic retinopathy project group 2002 classification of diabetic retinopathy (DR)

Proposed disease severity level	Findings observable
No apparent retinopathy	No abnormalities
Mild non-proliferative DR	Microaneurysms only
Moderate non-proliferative DR	More than just microaneurysms but less than severe NPDR
Severe non-proliferative DR (if instead of "or" if "and" could be considered very severe non-proliferative DR)	Any of the following: – More than 20 intraretinal hemorrhages in each of the four quadrants – Venous anomalies (venous beading) in two or more quadrants – Intraretinal abnormalities (IRMA) in at least one quadrant No signs of proliferative retinopathy
Proliferative DR	– Neovascularization – Vitreous/preretinal hemorrhage
The Portuguese Retina Study Group believes that any PDR should be subclassified according to gravity as follows [51]:	
Low-risk PDR	Neovascularization in or within 1 DD of the disc (NVD) with area <1/3 of DD or NV beyond 1 DD of the disc (NVE) with an area <0.5 DD
High-risk PDR	Neovascularization in or within 1 DD of the disc (NVD) with area ≥1/3 of DD or NV beyond 1 DD of the disc (NVE) with area ≥0.5DD or any NVD with vitreous hemorrhage
PDR with advanced diabetic eye disease	Any of the following: • Vitreous/preretinal hemorrhage • Rubeosis iridis • Tractional retinal detachment • Fibrovascular proliferation with traction

Table 53.3 GDRPG—diabetic retinopathy global project group 2002 classification of EMD. DD means diameter optic disc

Proposed disease severity level	Findings observable
Macular edema apparently absent	No retinal thickening or hard exudates in the posterior pole
Macular edema apparently present	Retinal thickening or hard exudates in the posterior pole
If macular edema is present, it can be further classified as follows:	
Mild: some retinal thickening or hard exudates in the posterior pole but distant from the center of the macula	
Moderate: retinal thickening or hard exudates approaching the center of the macula but not involving the center	
Severe: retinal thickening or hard exudates involving the center of the macula	

ESASO Classification of Diabetic Maculopathy

An OCT-based classification of diabetic maculopathy has recently been proposed by ESASO (European School of Advanced Studies in Ophthalmology). It includes seven qualitative and quantitative features, scored according to a grading system: central sub-foveal thickness, intraretinal cysts size, status of ellipsoid zone and external limiting membrane, disorganization of the inner retinal layers (DRIL), presence of hyperreflective foci, and presence of subretinal fluid and vitreoretinal relationship. The maculopathy is classified in four different stages, which reflect progressive severity of the disease: early, advanced, severe, and atrophic maculopathy. Some of these OCT parameters could also have prognostic value, such as the DRIL and alteration of ellipsoid zone which are predictors of poor treatment response, and subretinal fluid and hyperreflective foci which are considered inflammation biomarkers [55]. However, this classification based on OCT structural features does not take in consideration the hard exudates and lipoprotein plaques as a signal of chronicity and bad prognosis for visual function nor visual acuity per se, as prognostic and therapeutic biomarkers.

Current Treatment of Diabetic Retinopathy

To address the issue of the treatment, we need to consider both the severity of the disease and the importance of early diagnosis and treatment.

We must take into account that DR can present with different severity levels, depending on the time of evolution of the disease and, as recently shown [28], the subgroup of diabetes. The level of severity is essential to plan the level and complexity of the intervention. In this way, we can adequately plan and allocate human and financial resources according to the level and complexity of each case [56] (Fig. 53.1).

On the other hand, a screening program for early detection and treatment allows an earlier intervention. It has been estimated that only 10% of resource consumption is needed at this time, instead of what would be required in the advanced stages of the disease and with very encouraging results [56]. Preferably, early detection and treatment programs must be carried out with a standard performance of proximity to the diabetic patient, including screening mobile units and use of telemedicine [56].

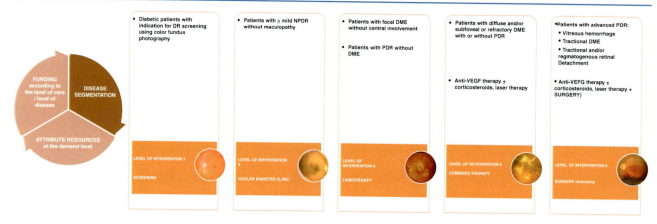

Fig. 53.1 DR levels of intervention and their relevance in health planning. We defined five levels of disease according to the level of severity. Each level of disease corresponds to a level of care. Note that there is an increase in complexity as the level of disease increases

Fig. 53.2 Laser therapy for PDR. Conventional PRP laser should not be avoided in cases of high-risk PDR and PDR in type 1 DM patients. When using a multispot laser, treatment should be more intense so as to be equivalent to conventional PRP laser. Do not wait in severe PDR, particularly in patients with high-risk characteristics

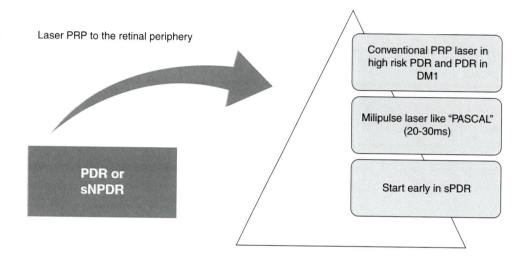

It should be noted that, in each patient, DR can manifest with a predominantly ischemic or exudative component, sometimes mixed. In the first case, we are dealing with an evolution toward very severe NPDR or PDR. In this situation, although there are references to positive results with the use of anti-VEGF [57], the therapy of choice continues to be thermal laser. The treatment is carried out to the periphery of the retina, with the panretinal photocoagulation (PRP) [58] technique or more smoothly, with a technique called targeted retinal photocoagulation (TRP) using a multispot laser [59] (Fig. 53.2). The thermal laser, with a photocoagulation effect, has been a standard therapy of PDR [60] with very long-lasting results. Laser is truly recommended in contexts of low availability of resources, difficulty to follow patients, poor compliance, patients with reduced mobility, PDR in patients with type 1 diabetes, and advanced PDR where it is mostly combined with vitrectomy. In addition to being an effective treatment in the PDR, laser phototherapy has also been used as an efficient eye treatment procedure, thus preventing the onset of blindness due to hyperglycemic

conditions [56, 61–63]. Advanced PDR with vitreous or preretinal hemorrhage and fibrovascular proliferation, particularly associated with retinal or macular detachment, are approached with surgical procedures—vitrectomy associated with intraoperative laser in a PRP pattern [56]. In this setting, a very early vitrectomy, with previous (2–3 days) anti-VEGF IV injection associated with endolaser PRP is an effective long-term treatment for PDR and vitreous hemorrhage.

The exudative component predominates in DME. Early stages of vascular edema, either focal or multifocal, do not imminently threaten fovea. In this case, the laser can still lead to better clinical outcomes [56, 61–63]. It should be emphasized that the laser treatment performed in the macular area follows the softer parameters and small spot diameter to avoid any damage to the microstructure of the macular retina.

It should be emphasized that a clear cut exists between center involving macular edema and other forms of DR with less severe edema [64]. The DRS and ETDRS trials [65, 66] in the 1970s showed that the results of laser photo-

Fig. 53.3 Treatment options for diffuse DME: first line, anti-VEGF; second line, long-acting corticosteroids (eventually as first line in special and chronic cases); third line, which uses laser therapy at macular area for DME (with or without PRP at retinal periphery) as rescue or adjuvant therapy

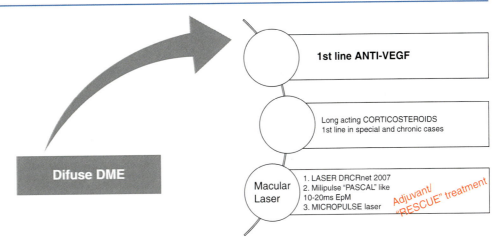

therapy in DME were not encouraging [65, 66]. Only 3% of the treated patients had a gain of 15 ETDRS scale letters at the end of three years, and more than half continued to lose vision despite the laser monotherapy treatment [65]. Many of these patients presented with a diffused or subfoveal exudative component (diffuse DME) and with more advanced levels of disease. We can even say that the treatment paradigm of DR has changed, mainly for diffuse and advanced DME with large lipoprotein exudates, where anti-VEGF (bevacizumab, ranibizumab, aflibercept) [67, 68] therapy is now indicated as the first-line therapy (Fig. 53.3).

Indications for laser use as first line include the vasogenic subform which is clinically characterized by the presence of focally grouped MA and leaking capillaries [69], eyes affected by DME with CRT less than 300 μm [69], PEVAC-like lesions which requires the use of a milipulse low power laser [70], and eyes with persisting vitreomacular adhesion [67]. Subthreshold grid laser treatment can be helpful in eyes with better visual acuity affected by early diffuse DME, in order to avoid the collateral thermal diffusion and the consequent chorioretinal damage [69]. Deferring laser led to superior results, especially in eyes with BCVA at baseline lower than 69 letters [71]. Laser therapy can also be used as rescue after failure of anti-VEGF therapy [72].

Indications for anti-VEGF use as first line include concomitant presence of *neovascularization*, increased *intraocular pressure*, *young age* and the *presence of the lens* because corticosteroids are cataractogenic, *aphakic eye* or *iris-sustained anterior lens* due to possible migration of the device to anterior chamber, and consequent corneal edema. The absence of *inflammation biomarkers* such as subretinal fluid (SRF), hyperreflective retinal spots (HRS), and hard exudates points to the use of anti-VEGF as first line of treatment [64].

Indications for corticosteroids use as first line include *recent cardiovascular disease/recent arterial thromboem-*

bolic events, *pregnancy*/breastfeeding, *noncompliance* or impossibility to return to treatment or follow-up visits, and *vitrectomized eyes.*

Combined therapy: thermal laser with VEGF and prolonged action steroids and surgery. However, the evidence gathered continues to support individualized and multifaceted approach to the patient with DR [73], in which the anti-VEGF agents can be used in combination with the reference treatments, such as corticosteroids [74] and laser phototherapy [68, 75], which act as an adjuvant factor and long-term stabilizer [76] (Fig. 53.4). Currently, the thermal laser with the techniques identified as retinal saving [56, 77, 78] can be combined with an anti-VEGF and/or sub-tenon or intravitreal triamcinolone [79, 80] or extended release devices of dexamethasone [81] or fluocinolone [82]. The last are particularly indicated in patients who have been vitrectomized [83] and as first line in patients with contraindications to anti-VEGF use.

This approach has been rationally demonstrated by enhanced efficacy in clinical trials [72, 84–87] and in better and more efficient management of a healthcare provider system. In about 40% of patients, the response to anti-VEGF monotherapy was not satisfactory [72], and it might make sense to change drug class, shifting for a prolonged action corticosteroid [82], and/or associate the laser treatment (and/or macular periphery) [56].

The combination of drugs appears to be a valid option in order to enhance their global beneficial effects. The different drugs and/or laser therapy act synergistically in the various mechanisms of action that cause edema. The gain in efficacy achieved by combining drugs can reduce the total number of required treatments, decrease the adverse effects of the individual drugs [76], and improve the therapeutic *burden* on the patients [56]. Treatment procedures like vitrectomy and phacoemulsification also go along well with the combination therapy.

The laser therapy, like the vitrectomy, acts as the stabilizing element of the retina in the long term. This has been dem-

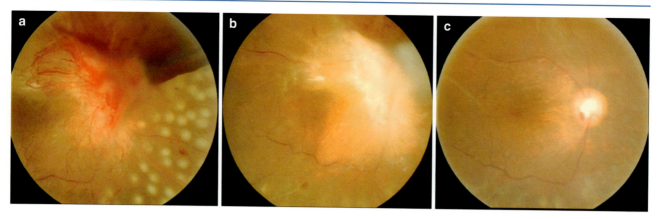

Fig. 53.4 Advanced PDR with vitreous and preretinal hemorrhage in a 35-year-old woman. (**a**) Laser photocoagulation was performed as there was optical transparency. (**b**) Two days after intravitreal ranibizumab injection: there was total regression of neovascularization and a fibrotic "shift" of fibrovascular tissue. (**c**) Two days after vitrectomy with "peeling" of the fibrovascular complex. The result was excellent with the maintenance of visual acuity of 0.8 due to early action in combining therapies. However, this was a highly resource-consuming procedure, which included laser, vitreoretinal surgery, anti-VEGF, and corticosteroids. The treatment could have been simpler by using fewer resources if it was held earlier before reaching advanced PDR

onstrated by the clinical stabilization achieved in laser-treated diabetic patients that lasts for decades.

In the near future, we will continue to use anti-VEGF as well as long-acting steroids in slow-release devices with the features of modulators of neovascularization and edema. The association of genetic therapy opened new frontiers, including the use of viral vectors for transfer of PEDF (pigment epithelium-derived factor) [88–90]. This cytokine has shown to have anti-inflammatory and antioxidant properties [91], as well as the ability to reduce capillary hyperpermeability and edema. The knowledge that laser phototherapy induces retinal environment modeling for production of chemical mediators [92], along with PEDF, either by activation of microglia or the call of medullary stem cells with repair functions, allowed us to further explore this therapy using the laser in earlier phases. Associate methods of improvement of metabolic control [12, 93] and neuroprotection [32] will be the major challenge in treating DM and DR. We anticipate a customized therapy for the individual patient, where the method of treatment will allow to maximize the results and have fewer side effects and fewer visits to the hospital, reducing the burden and treatment cost [93].

Ocular Manifestations of DM Other Than DR

As mentioned above, diabetic eye disease is not limited to DR, even though DR is the best-known microvascular complication (Table 53.4).

Other ocular manifestations of DM can be divided into vitreoretinal, when affecting the vitreous or retina such as the DR, or non-retinal, if they affect other ocular structures [18, 94].

Table 53.4 Ocular manifestations of DM other than DR

Ocular manifestations of DM other than DR	
Blepharitis	Non-arteritic ischemic optic neuropathy
Chalazion	Oculomotor nerve palsy
Dry eye	Asteroid hyalosis
Corneal ulcer	Retinal artery occlusion
Neurotrophic keratitis	Retinal vein occlusion
Loss of accommodation	Ocular ischemic syndrome
Refractive fluctuation of vision	Lipemia retinalis
Cataract	Diabetic papillopathy
Glaucoma	Pupillary abnormalities

Vitreoretinal Manifestations

These include the retinal arterial and venous occlusions and the ocular ischemic syndrome, conditions in which DM is a predisposing factor [18, 94].

The retinal vein occlusions correspond to the second most common vascular retinopathy after DR and are characterized by dilated and tortuous veins associated with intraretinal hemorrhages, cotton-wool spots (localized retinal ischemia), and macular edema. The central retinal vein occlusion involves the whole retina, occurring at the level of the optic disc, and the branch retinal occlusion involves a sector of the retina and is located usually at the level of pathological arteriovenous crossings [18].

The ocular ischemic syndrome (OIS) is a less frequent condition that results from chronic eye hypoperfusion due to significant stenosis/occlusion of the ipsilateral internal carotid or ophthalmic artery. Individuals with this pathology often have multiple systemic risk factors, which include DM, high blood pressure, and dyslipidemia. DM is even considered a major risk factor for carotid disease and consequently the OIS [18, 95].

The appearances of retinal emboli and the retinal arterial occlusions (RAO) are other complications that reflect multiple cardiovascular risk factors of diabetes, especially hypertension and dyslipidemia. The suspicion of an RAO is an ophthalmic emergency, and individuals should be immediately referred to a high-level ophthalmological care center. Symptoms include sudden and painless loss of vision [18]. Changes in the choroidal circulation have also been described [96].

Non-Retinal Manifestations

This group includes disease of eyelids and cornea, crystalline lens, glaucoma, and neuro-ophthalmic disorders.

Eyelids

Blepharitis (inflammation of the eyelids) and chalazion may be the first signs of DM [94].

Cornea

Diabetic patients exhibit reduced corneal sensitivity, resulting in a greater predisposition to infectious keratitis, neurotrophic ulcers, intolerance to contact lenses, erosions, and epithelial defects. There is also a slower healing of the corneal and structural changes in the hemidesmosome of the basal membrane, which leads to persistent epithelial defects even after a minor trauma. Corneal disease symptoms include pain, photophobia, and blurred vision, and the treatment usually consists of lubrication and therapeutic occlusion [18, 94].

Crystalline Lens

Refractive Error

Refractive fluctuation of vision can be a sign of DM and metabolic decompensation due to the change of the power of the lens diopter. This is due to the accumulation of sorbitol by increased activity of the enzyme aldose reductase, which leads to acute lenticular swelling that promotes a hypermetropic shift [94]. It is common when there is a sharp rise in hyperglycemia, often considered an inaugural symptom of DM.

Cataract

Cataracts are also an important cause of impaired vision in diabetic patients, with the risk of cataract increasing with the duration of DM and metabolic control [18]. Patients with type 1 diabetes can sometimes appear with a special type of cataract, a cortical snowflake cataract, which can be rapidly progressive [18]. In individuals with type 2 diabetes, there is worsening of the senile cataract and earlier appearance compared to nondiabetics [18]. Regarding cataract surgery, there are also particularities of DM: (1) preoperative macular edema can compromise visual recovery; (2) DR can rapidly worsen with surgery; (3) there is a prolonged healing time; (4) there is higher risk of postoperative inflammation and infection; and (5) there is higher risk of surgical complications [18, 94].

Glaucoma

Glaucoma is a progressive optic neuropathy, usually associated with increased intraocular pressure and changes in the optic disc and visual field [18].

Case-control trials show a relative risk of primary open-angle glaucoma of 1.6–4.7 in diabetics [18, 94]. DM also disturbs the short posterior ciliary artery self-regulation, exacerbating glaucoma optic neuropathy [18]. Also in DM, there is a greater risk of closed angle glaucoma due to an abnormally large crystalline. Moreover, a crisis of angle closure can also be a complication of an acute hyperglycemia crisis due to the abrupt lenticular edema [94]. Neovascular glaucoma is another type of glaucoma that can arise in diabetics. This type of secondary glaucoma is due to the neovascularization of the iris and angle induced by VEGF, whose production is stimulated by the ischemic retina. In a terminal phase, there is an obstruction of the aqueous humor drainage caused by the fibrovascular tissue in the trabecular meshwork and angle [94].

Neuro-Ophthalmic Disorders

Pupillary Abnormalities

Autonomic neuropathy leading to a denervation of the sphincter and pupillary dilator muscles can contribute to myopic pupils in scotopic conditions and an incomplete response to mydriatic agents [94].

Oculomotor Nerve Palsy

DM has been reported to be a cause of oculomotor palsy in 25–30% of individuals aged over 45 years [18, 94]. These are very common, usually isolated paresis of the III, IV, or VI pairs, and result from microvascular occlusion [18, 94]. Symptoms include binocular diplopia. Usually, there is a spontaneous recovery in 3 months, although recurrence may exist. The presence of other focal neurological signs must lead to the exclusion of compressive injury [18, 94].

Non-Arteritic Ischemic Optic Neuropathy

This condition results in anterior segment ischemia of the optic nerve, and it is estimated that 25% of people with this problem are diabetics [18].

There is an acute and painless decrease in visual acuity, with the presence of a relative afferent pupillary defect and optic disc edema [56]. There is no proven treatment, and the benefit of aspirin remains limited; but even without treatment, this neuropathy usually remains stable [18]. The arteritic variant should be excluded with erythrocyte sedimentation rate (ESR) and C-reactive protein (CRP) and biopsy of the temporal artery due to its reserved prognosis and the need for urgent treatment with intravenous corticosteroids.

Conclusion

This chapter is a review focusing on ocular manifestations of DM, particularly DR, but not neglecting other lesser-known complications. We believe this matter is of particular relevance to the medical doctors who deal with diabetics, sensitizing them on the diabetic eye disease in order to promote a regular ophthalmologic evaluation and enable early detection of these visual debilitating changes.

We live in exciting times, with a constant innovation in prevention, diagnosis, and treatment of DR—the most important ocular complication of DM. However, more evidence with clinical trials on new therapies, clarifying their role, and the use of monotherapy or in combination are required. Other ocular and periocular structures, vessels, and nerves can also be affected by DM. The acquisition of knowledge regarding this issue enables us to diagnose and treat diabetes in a timely manner.Conflicts of InterestJosé Henriques declares having carried out consulting work for Novartis-Alcon, Bausch + Lomb, Bayer, Allergan, and Alimera.

Sara Vaz-Pereira declares having carried out consulting work for Bayer.

João Nascimento declares having carried out consulting work for Novartis, Bausch + Lomb, Alcon, Zeiss, and Bayer.

Marco Dutra Medeiros declares having carried out consulting work for Alcon, Allergan, Zeiss, and Bayer.

Susana Henriques has nothing to disclose.

Paulo Caldeira Rosa declares having carried out consulting work for Novartis, Alcon, and Bayer.

References

1. UK Prospective Diabetes Study (UKPDS) Group. Intensive blood-glucose control with sulphonylureas or insulin compared with conventional treatment and risk of complications in patients with type 2 diabetes (UKPDS 33). Lancet. 1998;352(9131):837–53. http://www.ncbi.nlm.nih.gov/pubmed/9742976. Accessed 3 Sep 2014.
2. Groeneveld Y, Petri H, Hermans J, Springer MP. Relationship between blood glucose level and mortality in type 2 diabetes mellitus: a systematic review. Diabet Med. 1999;16(1):2–13. http://www.ncbi.nlm.nih.gov/pubmed/10229287. Accessed 18 Jul 2017.
3. Stratton IM, Adler AI, Neil HA, et al. Association of glycaemia with macrovascular and microvascular complications of type 2 diabetes (UKPDS 35): prospective observational study. BMJ. 2000;321(7258):405–12. http://www.ncbi.nlm.nih.gov/pubmed/10938048. Accessed 18 Jul 2017.
4. Klein R. Hyperglycemia and microvascular and macrovascular disease in diabetes. Diabetes Care. 1995;18(2):258–68. http://www.ncbi.nlm.nih.gov/pubmed/7729308. Accessed 18 Jul 2017.
5. Harris MI, Flegal KM, Cowie CC, et al. Prevalence of diabetes, impaired fasting glucose, and impaired glucose tolerance in U.S. adults. The third national health and nutrition examination survey, 1988–1994. Diabetes Care. 1998;21(4):518–24. http://www.ncbi.nlm.nih.gov/pubmed/9571335. Accessed 18 Jul 2017.
6. King H, Aubert RE, Herman WH. Global burden of diabetes, 1995-2025: prevalence, numerical estimates, and projections. Diabetes Care. 1998;21(9):1414–31. http://www.ncbi.nlm.nih.gov/pubmed/9727886. Accessed 18 Jul 2017.
7. Wild S, Roglic G, Green A, Sicree R, King H. Global prevalence of diabetes: estimates for the year 2000 and projections for 2030. Diabetes Care. 2004;27(5):1047–53. http://www.ncbi.nlm.nih.gov/pubmed/15111519. Accessed 18 Jul 2017.
8. Shaw JE, Sicree RA, Zimmet PZ. Global estimates of the prevalence of diabetes for 2010 and 2030. Diabetes Res Clin Pract. 2010;87(1):4–14. https://doi.org/10.1016/j.diabres.2009.10.007.
9. Cai J, Boulton M. The pathogenesis of diabetic retinopathy: old concepts and new questions. Eye (Lond). 2002;16(3):242–60. https://doi.org/10.1038/sj.eye/6700133.
10. Kempen JH, O'Colmain BJ, Leske MC, et al. The prevalence of diabetic retinopathy among adults in the United States. Arch Ophthalmol. 2004;122(4):552–63. https://doi.org/10.1001/archopht.122.4.552.
11. Moss SE, Klein R, Klein BE. The 14-year incidence of visual loss in a diabetic population. Ophthalmology. 1998;105(6):998–1003. https://doi.org/10.1016/S0161-6420(98)96025-0.
12. Nabais C, Pereira J, Pereira P, Capote R, Morbeck S, Raposo J. Diabetic retinopathy and associated conditions, what relationship? A study in Portuguese patients with type 2 diabetes. Acta Med Port. 2011;24(Suppl 2):71–8. http://www.ncbi.nlm.nih.gov/pubmed/22849888. Accessed 18 Jul 2017.
13. Lee R, Wong TY, Sabanayagam C. Epidemiology of diabetic retinopathy, diabetic macular edema and related vision loss. Eye Vis (Lond). 2015;2(1):17. https://doi.org/10.1186/s40662-015-0026-2.
14. Bourne RRA, Stevens GA, White RA, et al. Causes of vision loss worldwide, 1990-2010: a systematic analysis. Lancet Glob Health. 2013;1(6):e339–49. https://doi.org/10.1016/S2214-109X(13)70113-X.
15. Yau JWY, Rogers SL, Kawasaki R, et al. Global prevalence and major risk factors of diabetic retinopathy. Diabetes Care. 2012;35(3):556–64. https://doi.org/10.2337/dc11-1909.
16. Liew G, Michaelides M, Bunce C. A comparison of the causes of blindness certifications in England and Wales in working age adults (16–64 years), 1999–2000 with 2009–2010. BMJ Open. 2014;4(2):e004015. https://doi.org/10.1136/bmjopen-2013-004015.
17. Henriques J, Vaz-Pereira S, Nascimento J, Rosa PC. Diabetic eye disease. Acta Med Port. 2015;28(1):107–13. http://www.ncbi.nlm.nih.gov/pubmed/25817504. Accessed 25 Oct 2015.
18. Jeganathan VSE, Wang JJ, Wong TY. Ocular associations of diabetes other than diabetic retinopathy. Diabetes Care. 2008;31(9):1905–12. https://doi.org/10.2337/dc08-0342.
19. Cavallerano JD. A review of non-retinal ocular complications of diabetes mellitus. J Am Optom Assoc. 1990;61(7):533–43. http://www.ncbi.nlm.nih.gov/pubmed/2199552. Accessed 18 Jul 2017.
20. Stanga PE, Boyd SR, Hamilton AM. Ocular manifestations of diabetes mellitus. Curr Opin Ophthalmol. 1999;10(6):483–9. http://www.ncbi.nlm.nih.gov/pubmed/10662255. Accessed 18 Jul 2017.
21. Williams R, Airey M, Baxter H, Forrester J, Kennedy-Martin T, Girach A. Epidemiology of diabetic retinopathy and macular oedema: a systematic review. Eye (Lond). 2004;18(10):963–83. https://doi.org/10.1038/sj.eye.6701476.
22. Ling R, Ramsewak V, Taylor D, Jacob J. Longitudinal study of a cohort of people with diabetes screened by the exeter diabetic

retinopathy screening programme. Eye (Lond). 2002;16(2):140–5. https://doi.org/10.1038/sj/EYE/6700081.

23. Virgili G, Menchini F, Casazza G, et al. Optical coherence tomography (OCT) for detection of macular oedema in patients with diabetic retinopathy. Cochrane Database Syst Rev. 2015;1:CD008081. https://doi.org/10.1002/14651858.CD008081.pub3.

24. Thomas RL, Dunstan FD, Luzio SD, et al. Prevalence of diabetic retinopathy within a national diabetic retinopathy screening service. Br J Ophthalmol. 2015;99(1):64–8. https://doi.org/10.1136/bjophthalmol-2013-304017.

25. Klein R, Knudtson MD, Lee KE, Gangnon R, Klein BEK. The wisconsin epidemiologic study of diabetic retinopathy: XXII the twenty-five-year progression of retinopathy in persons with type 1 diabetes. Ophthalmology. 2008;115(11):1859–68. https://doi.org/10.1016/j.ophtha.2008.08.023.

26. Dutra Medeiros M, Mesquita E, Gardete-Correia L, et al. First incidence and progression study for diabetic retinopathy in Portugal, the RETINODIAB study: evaluation of the screening program for Lisbon region. Ophthalmology. 2015;122:2473. https://doi.org/10.1016/j.ophtha.2015.08.004.

27. Sarría-Santamera A, Orazumbekova B, Maulenkul T, Gaipov A, Atageldiyeva K. The identification of diabetes mellitus subtypes applying cluster analysis techniques: a systematic review. Int J Environ Res Public Health. 2020;17(24):1–27. https://doi.org/10.3390/IJERPH17249523.

28. Ahlqvist E, Storm P, Käräjämäki A, et al. Novel subgroups of adult-onset diabetes and their association with outcomes: a data-driven cluster analysis of six variables. Lancet Diabetes Endocrinol. 2018;6(5):361–9. https://doi.org/10.1016/S2213-8587(18)30051-2.

29. Ribeiro L, Oliveira CM, Neves C, Ramos JD, Ferreira H, Cunha-Vaz J. Screening for diabetic retinopathy in the central region of Portugal. Added value of automated "disease/no disease" grading. Ophthalmologica. 2014;233(2):96–103. https://doi.org/10.1159/000368426.

30. Spaide RF, Fujimoto JG, Waheed NK, Sadda SR, Staurenghi G. Optical coherence tomography angiography. Prog Retin Eye Res. 2018;64:1–55. https://doi.org/10.1016/j.preteyeres.2017.11.003.

31. Enge M, Bjarnegård M, Gerhardt H, et al. Endothelium-specific platelet-derived growth factor-B ablation mimics diabetic retinopathy. EMBO J. 2002;21(16):4307–16. http://www.ncbi.nlm.nih.gov/pubmed/12169633. Accessed 18 Jul 2017.

32. Antonetti DA, Klein R, Gardner TW. Diabetic retinopathy. N Engl J Med. 2012;366(13):1227–39. https://doi.org/10.1056/NEJMra1005073.

33. Kowluru RA, Chan P-S. Oxidative stress and diabetic retinopathy. Exp Diabetes Res. 2007;2007:43603. https://doi.org/10.1155/2007/43603.

34. Patel N. Targeting leukostasis for the treatment of early diabetic retinopathy. Cardiovasc Hematol Disord Drug Targets. 2009;9(3):222–9. http://www.ncbi.nlm.nih.gov/pubmed/19619127. Accessed 18 Jul 2017.

35. El-Asrar AMA. Role of inflammation in the pathogenesis of diabetic retinopathy. Middle East Afr J Ophthalmol. 2012;19(1):70–4. https://doi.org/10.4103/0974-9233.92118.

36. Robison WG, Nagata M, Laver N, Hohman TC, Kinoshita JH. Diabetic-like retinopathy in rats prevented with an aldose reductase inhibitor. Invest Ophthalmol Vis Sci. 1989;30(11):2285–92. http://www.ncbi.nlm.nih.gov/pubmed/2509395. Accessed 18 Jul 2017.

37. Simó-Servat O, Hernández C, Simó R. Genetics in diabetic retinopathy: current concepts and new insights. Curr Genomics. 2013;14(5):289–99. https://doi.org/10.2174/13892029113149990008.

38. Yoshii H, Uchino H, Ohmura C, Watanabe K, Tanaka Y, Kawamori R. Clinical usefulness of measuring urinary polyol excretion by gas-chromatography/mass-spectrometry in type 2 diabetes to assess polyol pathway activity. Diabetes Res Clin Pract. 2001;51(2):115–

23. http://www.ncbi.nlm.nih.gov/pubmed/11165691. Accessed 18 Jul 2017.

39. Chibber R, Molinatti PA, Kohner EM. Intracellular protein glycation in cultured retinal capillary pericytes and endothelial cells exposed to high-glucose concentration. Cell Mol Biol (Noisy-le-Grand). 1999;45(1):47–57. http://www.ncbi.nlm.nih.gov/pubmed/10099839. Accessed 18 Jul 2017.

40. Stitt AW. The role of advanced glycation in the pathogenesis of diabetic retinopathy. Exp Mol Pathol. 2003;75(1):95–108. http://www.ncbi.nlm.nih.gov/pubmed/12834631. Accessed 18 Jul 2017.

41. Goldin A, Beckman JA, Schmidt AM, Creager MA. Advanced glycation end products: sparking the development of diabetic vascular injury. Circulation. 2006;114(6):597–605. https://doi.org/10.1161/CIRCULATIONAHA.106.621854.

42. Schmidt AM, Yan SD, Wautier JL, Stern D. Activation of receptor for advanced glycation end products: a mechanism for chronic vascular dysfunction in diabetic vasculopathy and atherosclerosis. Circ Res. 1999;84(5):489–97. http://www.ncbi.nlm.nih.gov/pubmed/10082470. Accessed 18 Jul 2017.

43. Ways DK, Sheetz MJ. The role of protein kinase C in the development of the complications of diabetes. Vitam Horm. 2000;60:149–93. http://www.ncbi.nlm.nih.gov/pubmed/11037624. Accessed 18 Jul 2017.

44. Gürler B, Vural H, Yilmaz N, Oguz H, Satici A, Aksoy N. The role of oxidative stress in diabetic retinopathy. Eye. 2000;14(5):730–5. https://doi.org/10.1038/eye.2000.193.

45. Wirostko B, Wong T, Simo R. Vascular endothelial growth factor and diabetic complications. Prog Retin Eye Res. 2008;27(6):608–21. https://doi.org/10.1016/j.preteyeres.2008.09.002.

46. Miller JW, Le Couter J, Strauss EC, Ferrara N. Vascular endothelial growth factor A in intraocular vascular disease. Ophthalmology. 2013;120(1):106–14. https://doi.org/10.1016/j.ophtha.2012.07.038.

47. Dugel PU, Hillenkamp J, Sivaprasad S, et al. Baseline visual acuity strongly predicts visual acuity gain in patients with diabetic macular edema following anti-vascular endothelial growth factor treatment across trials. Clin Ophthalmol. 2016;10:1103–10. https://doi.org/10.2147/OPTH.S100764.

48. Stewart MW. Anti-vascular endothelial growth factor drug treatment of diabetic macular edema: the evolution continues. Curr Diabetes Rev. 2012;8(4):237–46. http://www.ncbi.nlm.nih.gov/pubmed/22515701. Accessed 18 Jul 2017.

49. Iandiev I, Pannicke T, Reichel MB, Wiedemann P, Reichenbach A, Bringmann A. Expression of aquaporin-1 immunoreactivity by photoreceptor cells in the mouse retina. Neurosci Lett. 2005;388(2):96–9. https://doi.org/10.1016/j.neulet.2005.06.046.

50. Uckermann O, Kutzera F, Wolf A, et al. The glucocorticoid triamcinolone acetonide inhibits osmotic swelling of retinal glial cells via stimulation of endogenous adenosine signaling. J Pharmacol Exp Ther. 2005;315(3):1036–45. https://doi.org/10.1124/jpet.105.092353.

51. Funatsu H, Noma H, Mimura T, Eguchi S, Hori S. Association of vitreous inflammatory factors with diabetic macular edema. Ophthalmology. 2009;116(1):73–9. https://doi.org/10.1016/j.ophtha.2008.09.037.

52. Wu L. Classification of diabetic retinopathy and diabetic macular edema. World J Diabetes. 2013;4(6):290. https://doi.org/10.4239/wjd.v4.i6.290.

53. Wilkinson CP, Ferris FL, Klein RE, et al. Proposed international clinical diabetic retinopathy and diabetic macular edema disease severity scales. Ophthalmology. 2003;110(9):1677–82. https://doi.org/10.1016/S0161-6420(03)00475-5.

54. International clinical diabetic retinopathy disease severity scale, Detailed Table. 2010. http://www.icoph.org/resources/45/International-Clinical-Diabetic-Retinopathy-Disease-Severity-Scale-Detailed-Table-.html.

55. Panozzo G, Cicinelli MV, Augustin AJ, et al. An optical coherence tomography-based grading of diabetic maculopathy proposed by an international expert panel: the European School for Advanced Studies in ophthalmology classification. Eur J Ophthalmol. 2020;30(1):8–18. https://doi.org/10.1177/1120672119880394.

56. Henriques J, Figueira J, Nascimento J, et al. Retinopatia diabética—orientações clínicas do Grupo de Estudos da Retina de Portugal. Oftalmol Soc Port Oftalmol. 2015;39(4 supl. Out-Dez).

57. Writing Committee for the Diabetic Retinopathy Clinical Research Network. Panretinal photocoagulation vs intravitreous ranibizumab for proliferative diabetic retinopathy: a randomized clinical trial. JAMA. 2015;314(20):2137–46. https://doi.org/10.1001/jama.2015.15217.

58. Figueira J, Silva R, Raimundo M. Laser treatment for proliferative retinopathy. In: Henriques J, Duarte A, Quintão T, editors. Laser manual in ophthalmology—fundamentals and laser clinical practice. 1st ed. Lisbon: SPILM Portuguese Medical Laser Society Publishing; 2017. p. 213–7. https://thea.pt/sites/default/files/documentos/manual_laser_2017_small.pdf.

59. Henriques J, Medeiros MD, Pinto R, Rosa PC. Targeted retinal photocoagulation. PRP with PASCAL. In: Henriques J, Duarte A, Quintão T, editors. Laser manual in ophthalmology-fundamentals and laser clinical practice. 1st ed. Lisbon: SPILM- Portuguese Medical Laser Society; 2017. p. 241–4. https://thea.pt/sites/default/files/documentos/manual_laser_2017_small.pdf.

60. The Diabetic Retinopathy Study Research Group. Photocoagulation treatment of proliferative diabetic retinopathy: the second report of diabetic retinopathy study findings. Ophthalmology. 1978;85(1):82–106.

61. Taylor HR, Binder S, Das T, et al. Updated 2017—ICO guidelines for diabetic eye care. 2017.

62. Hooper P, Boucher M-C, Colleaux K, et al. Contemporary management of diabetic retinopathy in Canada: from guidelines to algorithm guidance. Ophthalmologica. 2014;231(1):2–15. https://doi.org/10.1159/000354548.

63. Photocoagulation for Diabetic Macular Edema. Early treatment diabetic retinopathy study report number 1. Early treatment diabetic retinopathy study research group. Arch Ophthalmol. 1985;103(12):1796–806. http://www.ncbi.nlm.nih.gov/pubmed/2866759. Accessed 10 Aug 2015.

64. Kodjikian L, Bellocq D, Bandello F, et al. First-line treatment algorithm and guidelines in center-involving diabetic macular edema. Eur J Ophthalmol. 2019;29(6):573–84. https://doi.org/10.1177/1120672119857511.

65. Early Photocoagulation for Diabetic Retinopathy. ETDRS report number 9. Early treatment diabetic retinopathy study research group. Ophthalmology. 1991;98(5 Suppl):766–85. http://www.ncbi.nlm.nih.gov/pubmed/2062512. Accessed 18 Jul 2017.

66. Ferris F. Early photocoagulation in patients with either type I or type II diabetes. Trans Am Ophthalmol Soc. 1996;94:505–37. http://www.pubmedcentral.nih.gov/articlerender.fcgi?artid=1312110&tool=pmcentrez&rendertype=abstract. Accessed 14 Apr 2014.

67. Mitchell P, Bandello F, Schmidt-Erfurth U, et al. The RESTORE study: ranibizumab monotherapy or combined with laser versus laser monotherapy for diabetic macular edema. Ophthalmology. 2011;118(4):615–25. https://doi.org/10.1016/j.ophtha.2011.01.031.

68. Stewart MW. Anti-VEGF therapy for diabetic macular edema. Curr Diab Rep. 2014;14(8):510. https://doi.org/10.1007/s11892-014-0510-4.

69. Schmidt-Erfurth U, Garcia-Arumi J, Bandello F, et al. Guidelines for the management of diabetic macular edema by the European Society of Retina Specialists (EURETINA). Ophthalmologica. 2017;237(4):185–222. https://doi.org/10.1159/000458539.

70. Henriques J, Pinto F, Rosa PC, et al. Continuous wave milipulse yellow laser treatment for perifoveal exudative vascular anomalous complex-like lesion: a case report. Eur J Ophthalmol. 2020;32:NP119. https://doi.org/10.1177/1120672120966564.

71. Elman MJ, Ayala A, Bressler NM, et al. Intravitreal Ranibizumab for diabetic macular edema with prompt versus deferred laser treatment: 5-year randomized trial results. Ophthalmology. 2015;122(2):375–81. https://doi.org/10.1016/j.ophtha.2014.08.047.

72. Dugel P, Campbell J, Holecamp N, et al. Long-term response to anti-VEGF therapy for DME can be predicted after 3 injections. An Análises of the protocol I data. In: AAO, ed. AAO Annual Meeting—Sub Specialty Day. AAO; 2015.

73. Pinto R, Henriques J. Retinopatia diabética—tratamento: corticoides, anti-angiogénicos e terapêutica combinada. In: Silva R, Farah ME, editors. Manual de Retina. Neckarsulm: Lidel; 2015. p. 119–23.

74. Zur D, Loewenstein A. Combination therapy for diabetic macular edema. J Ophthalmol. 2012;2012:1–6. https://doi.org/10.1155/2012/484612.

75. Bandello F, Brancato R, Menchini U, et al. Light panretinal photocoagulation (LPRP) versus classic panretinal photocoagulation (CPRP) in proliferative diabetic retinopathy. Semin Ophthalmol. 2001;16(1):12–8. http://www.ncbi.nlm.nih.gov/pubmed/15487693. Accessed 15 Apr 2014.

76. Vaz F, Siva F, Henriques J. O que se entende por terapêutica combinada no tratamento da Retinopatia Diabética? In: Henriques J, Nascimento J, Silva R, eds. 25 Perguntas e Respostas: Retinopatia Diabética—Novo Paradigma de Cuidados. 1ª. GER- Grupo de Estudos da Retina; 2012:123–130. www.ger-portugal.com.

77. Henriques J, Nascimento J, Rosa P, Vaz F, Amaro M. Laser fototérmico e sua interacção com a retina humana. Oftalmol rev SPO. 2013;36:353–64. http://repositorio.hff.min-saude.pt/handle/10400.10/903. Accessed 14 Apr 2014.

78. Gourier H, Pearce E, Chong V. Micropulse technology and concepts. In: Henriques J, Duarte A, Quintão T, editors. LASER manual in ophthalmology—fundamentals and laser clinical practice. 1st ed. Lisbon: SPILM Portuguese Medical Laser Society; 2017. p. 197–201. https://thea.pt/sites/default/files/documentos/manual_laser_2017_small.pdf.

79. Rosa PC, Pinto R, Guitana M. Antiangiogénicos no tratamento da retinopatia diabética. In: Henriques J, Nascimento J, Silva R, editors. 25 Perguntas e respostas: retinopatia diabética—novo paradigma de cuidados. Bogotá: Grupo de E; 2012.

80. Cardillo JA, Melo LAS, Costa RA, et al. Comparison of intravitreal versus posterior sub-tenon's capsule injection of triamcinolone acetonide for diffuse diabetic macular edema. Ophthalmology. 2005;112(9):1557–63. https://doi.org/10.1016/j.ophtha.2005.03.023.

81. Haller JA, Kuppermann BD, Blumenkranz MS, Williams GA, Weinberg DV, Chou CWS. Randomized controlled trial of an intravitreous dexamethasone drug delivery system in patients with diabetic macular edema. Arch Ophthalmol. 2010;128(3):289–96. https://doi.org/10.1001/archophthalmol.2010.21.

82. Calvo P, Abadia B, Ferreras A, Ruiz-Moreno O, Verdes G, Pablo LE. Diabetic macular edema: options for adjunct therapy. Drugs. 2015;75:1461. https://doi.org/10.1007/s40265-015-0447-1.

83. Meireles A, Goldsmith C, El-Ghrably I, et al. Efficacy of 0.2 μg/day fluocinolone acetonide implant (ILUVIEN) in eyes with diabetic macular edema and prior vitrectomy. Eye. 2017;31(5):684–90. https://doi.org/10.1038/eye.2016.303.

84. Wells JA, Glassman AR, Ayala AR, et al. Aflibercept, bevacizumab, or ranibizumab for diabetic macular edema. N Engl J Med. 2015;372(13):1193–203. https://doi.org/10.1056/NEJMoa1414264.

85. Wells JA, Glassman AR, Ayala AR, et al. Aflibercept, bevacizumab, or Ranibizumab for diabetic macular edema: two-year results from a comparative effectiveness randomized clinical trial. Ophthalmology. 2016;123(6):1351–9. https://doi.org/10.1016/j.ophtha.2016.02.022.

86. Jampol LM, Glassman AR, Bressler NM, Wells JA, Ayala AR, Diabetic Retinopathy Clinical Research Network. Anti–vascular endothelial growth factor comparative effectiveness trial for diabetic macular edema. JAMA Ophthalmol. 2016;134(12):1429. https://doi.org/10.1001/jamaophthalmol.2016.3698.

87. Bressler SB, Glassman AR, Almukhtar T, et al. Five-year outcomes of Ranibizumab with prompt or deferred laser versus laser or triamcinolone plus deferred Ranibizumab for diabetic macular edema. Am J Ophthalmol. 2016;164:57–68. https://doi.org/10.1016/j.ajo.2015.12.025.

88. Shen X, Zhong Y, Xie B, Cheng Y, Jiao Q. Pigment epithelium derived factor as an anti-inflammatory factor against decrease of glutamine synthetase expression in retinal Müller cells under high glucose conditions. Graefes Arch Clin Exp Ophthalmol. 2010;248(8):1127–36. https://doi.org/10.1007/s00417-010-1362-5.

89. Tombran-Tink J, Barnstable CJ. Therapeutic prospects for PEDF: more than a promising angiogenesis inhibitor. Trends Mol Med. 2003;9(6):244–50. http://www.ncbi.nlm.nih.gov/pubmed/12829012. Accessed 18 Jul 2017.

90. Vigneswara V, Berry M, Logan A, Ahmed Z. Pigment epithelium-derived factor is retinal ganglion cell neuroprotective and axogenic after optic nerve crush injury. Invest Ophthalmol Vis Sci. 2013;54(4):2624–33. https://doi.org/10.1167/iovs.13-11803.

91. Henriques J, Quintão T, Páris L. Structural and functional changes and possible neuroprotective effects induced by photothermal LASER in the retina. In: Henriques J, Duarte A, Quintão T, editors. LASER manual in ophthalmology—fundamentals and laser clinical practice, vol. 1. 1st ed. Lisbon: SPILM Portuguese Medical Laser Society; 2017. p. 187–92. https://thea.pt/sites/default/files/documentos/manual_laser_2017_small.pdf.

92. Henriques J, Quintão T, Colaço L, Pinto R. Laser action in the human retina: the therapeutic effect of thermal laser. In: Henriques J, Duarte A, Quintão T, editors. Laser manual in ophthalmology—fundamentals and laser clinical practice. 1st ed. Lisbon: SPILM Portuguese Medical Laser Society Publishing; 2017. p. 181–6. https://thea.pt/sites/default/files/documentos/manual_laser_2017_small.pdf.

93. Silva R. Perspetivas futuras no tratamento da retinopatia diabética. In: Henriques J, Nasciment J, Silva R, editors. 25 Perguntas e respostas: retinopatia diabética—novo paradigma de cuidados. Bogotá: Grupo de E; 2012.

94. Negi A, Vernon SA. An overview of the eye in diabetes. J R Soc Med. 2003;96(6):266–72. http://www.ncbi.nlm.nih.gov/pubmed/12782689. Accessed July 18, 2017.

95. Ino-ue M, Azumi A, Kajiura-Tsukahara Y, Yamamoto M. Ocular ischemic syndrome in diabetic patients. Jpn J Ophthalmol. 1999;43(1):31–5. http://www.ncbi.nlm.nih.gov/pubmed/10197740. Accessed July 18, 2017.

96. Lutty GA. Effects of diabetes on the eye. Invest Ophthalmol Vis Sci. 2013;54(14):ORSF81–7. https://doi.org/10.1167/iovs.13-12979.

Diabetes and Oral Health

54

Rosa Maria Díaz-Romero
and Manuel Salvador Robles-Andrade

Objective
- To provide healthcare personnel the necessary elements of the etiology, diagnosis, and treatment of disease in the oral cavity affecting people living with diabetes.
- Analyze systemic interaction models of periodontal disease and poor blood sugar control.

Introduction

For decades, oral health has not been considered among the priorities of government and international organization agendas, perhaps because most of the time poor oral health has affected morbidity and not mortality. Recently, there has been greater awareness from government organizations and even from the population that oral health is part of a person's general well-being. Also, more comprehensive studies have indicated that oral infections constitute a risk factor that generate or increase harmful health events in individuals. This change started in 2000 with the report of the US Surgeon General that was continued in 2002 in the Oral Health Program of the World Health Organization [1] that approved the resolution that urges the inclusion of oral health in chronic disease prevention programs. That is why we are interested in including this work in this chapter. We will provide the main concepts of the dentistry field to the entire multidisciplinary team allowing them to include this component in the comprehensive care of the diabetic patient.

We will start by stating how oral health affects quality of life. We will explain the interaction models of periodontal disease when blood sugar levels are uncontrolled. We will analyze how caries affect the teeth of diabetic people, as well as the repercussions of hyposalivation in the generation of swallowing disorders. We will present how the dentist and/or the periodontist diagnose an oral condition and the different phases that constitute periodontal treatment.

This chapter includes the protocol of diabetic care in the dental office with a clinical guideline followed by the physician, the dietitian, the endocrinologist, the nurse, and the diabetes educator, to detect an oral disease. We will also present the recommendations for the use of antibiotics and antimicrobial prophylaxis useful for the dentist.

> Recently, there has been greater awareness that oral health is part of a person's general well-being with more in-depth studies of how oral infections constitute a risk factor for health in general.

R. M. Díaz-Romero (✉)
Faculty of Dentistry, UNITEC, Mexico City, Mexico
e-mail: rmdiazro@mail.unitec.mx

M. S. Robles-Andrade
Faculty of Dentistry, UNITEC, Mexico City, Mexico

National Institute of Perinatology, Ministry of Health, Mexico City, Mexico

© The Author(s), under exclusive license to Springer Nature Switzerland AG 2023
J. Rodriguez-Saldana (ed.), *The Diabetes Textbook*, https://doi.org/10.1007/978-3-031-25519-9_54

Oral Health and Quality of Life

Oral health is an essential component of good overall health and it is also a basic human right. According to the World Health Organization (WHO) [1], oral diseases have a significant impact in individuals and in society due to the pain these cause, leading to a decreased function and quality of life. The effects of oral diseases are considerable and expensive; it is estimated that treatment represents between 5% and 10% of the health expense in industrialized countries and it is above the resources of many developing countries.

Poor oral health can have severe repercussions in overall health; in the document *Vision 2020 of the International Dental Federation* in 2016 [2], it is stated that pain, dental abscesses, mastication problems, tooth loss, and pigmented or damaged teeth have significant effects in life and in the daily well-being of people. Some of these manifestations can even increase the risk of poor blood sugar control in people living with diabetes. The preservation of oral health is part of the comprehensive well-being of people with diabetes.

> Oral health is a basic human right and its contribution is essential for good quality of life. Oral health is an essential component of good health.

> **Box 54.1**
> It is important for the multidisciplinary team involved in the care of diabetic patients, to be aware of the most important elements the dentist uses to diagnose and provide dental treatment to patients with diabetes.

Periodontal Disease and Systemic Interaction Models

Periodontal Disease and Systemic Interaction Models

The periodontium is a group of tissues that support the tooth, and it is made up of bone, periodontal ligament, radicular cementum, and gingiva. The only visible periodontal tissue is the gingiva that in normal healthy conditions the color is salmon, pink, or coral pink with variations that can be due to the degree of keratinization or to melanic pigmentations; these pigmentations are observed more frequently in Black patients. The external gingival portion is made up of a stratified keratinized epithelium that is firmly attached to a dense base of connective gingival tissue whose main function is to protect the underlying periodontal tissue from external stimuli; this epithelium continues to the gingival groove margin that extends from the crest of the gingival margin to the junctional epithelium; the latter maintains direct attachment to the surface of the tooth [3]. The most frequent periodontal disorders are due to the formation of a bacterial biofilm on the tooth surface; once the biofilm comes into contact with the sulcular epithelium at the level of the gingival margin, an inflammatory response begins in the underlying connective tissue that in 3–4 days becomes powerful enough to begin the destruction of connective tissue, losing up to 70% of the collagen within the inflammatory focus [4]. The clinical manifestation of the interaction between the bacterial biofilm that colonizes the tooth surface and that is in contact with the sulcular epithelium (Fig. 54.1) and the junctional epithelium is called periodontal disease; this term encompasses the two main infections that affect the tooth's supporting tissue: gingivitis and periodontitis.

Gingivitis is an inflammatory process that only affects the gingiva, and it is associated with the accumulation of bacte-

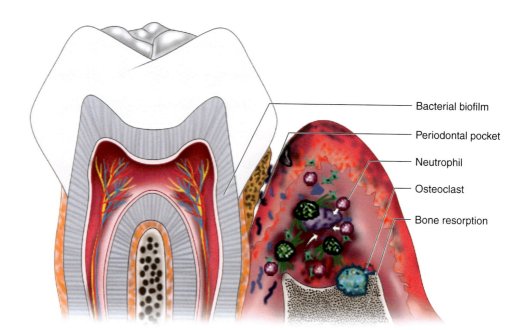

Fig. 54.1 Interaction between the bacterial biofilm and the sulcular and junctional epithelium. The progression of gingivitis to periodontitis involves the proliferation of epithelial cells apically throughout the radicular surface forming periodontal pockets; as these progress, the inflammatory infiltrate increases, starting the bone destruction

Bacterial biofilm

Periodontal pocket

Neutrophil

Osteoclast

Bone resorption

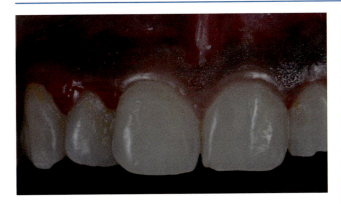

Fig. 54.2 Gingivitis. There is swelling of the gingival margin; it looks erythematous, associated with deposits of bacterial plaque on the teeth

Table 54.1 Strategies suggested to patients for personal plaque control [7]

Strategy	Justification
Teeth brushing at least twice a day	Patients who brush with this frequency keep their teeth for a longer period of time
Use of dental floss once a day	It significantly reduces gingivitis compared to only brushing
Routine use of toothpaste containing triclosan/copolymer	These are more effective in reducing bacterial plaque and gingivitis compared to fluoridated toothpastes
Routine use of mouthwash containing essential oils is suggested	These are effective in reducing bacterial plaque and gingivitis, even in proximal areas

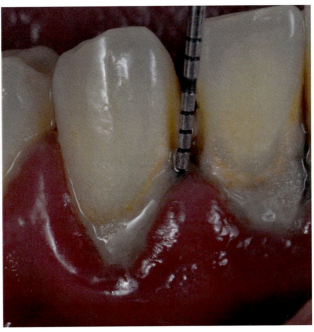

Fig. 54.3 Periodontal probing is a tool used to diagnose periodontitis. Under normal conditions, the probe penetrates the gingival groove 0.5–3 mm; in this case, the probe penetrates 5 mm, reflecting the presence of a periodontal pocket

rial plaque on the dental surface; when the bacteria of the plaque interact with gingival tissue, there is an inflammatory response characterized by an increase in the volume of the gingival margin, a change in the gingival color that looks erythematous and gingival bleeding in the presence of a stimulus (Fig. 54.2) [5]; this infectious process is reversible once the bacterial plaque is removed mechanically with the implementation of personal plaque control (PPC) where patients are instructed to follow an appropriate brushing technique and daily use of dental floss to achieve resolution of the clinical picture a few days after the correct PPC [6] (Table 54.1).

Periodontitis represents the progression of gingivitis to a destructive infectious process associated with the microbiological change of the bacterial biofilm and with a proinflammatory response of the host [8, 9]; this interaction is responsible for the periodontal destruction that causes dental mobility and tooth loss, making this the second cause of tooth loss [10] (Figs. 54.3 and 54.4).

Depending on the individual's susceptibility, the progression of gingivitis to periodontitis may vary; it has been suggested that the progression takes more than 6 months [11, 12]. The main microorganisms associated with periodontitis are *P. gingivalis*, *T. forsythia*, and *T. denticola*; these microorganisms produce enzymes and toxins that damage periodontal tissue and trigger an

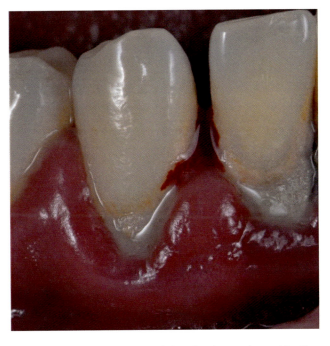

Fig. 54.4 When removing the periodontal probe, we observe bleeding, suggesting an active infection

inflammatory response. Once the inflammatory response is triggered, the red blood cells, fibroblasts, and structural cells of periodontal tissue release proteases, cytokines, and prostaglandins [13]. Proteases degrade collagen fibers giving way to more inflammatory infiltrate. While the connective tissue is destroyed, epithelial cells proliferate apically throughout the radicular surface forming periodontal pockets; as these progress, the inflammatory infiltrate increases, starting the bone destruction mediated by osteocytes [14]. As more plaque accumulates, the microbial density increases, creating a chronic and more destructive response until the tooth is lost at some point [15]. The National Health and Nutrition Examination Survey (NHANES) reported that between 2009 and 2010, 47.2% of the American population over 30 years presented periodontitis [16]. The high prevalence of periodontitis represents a public health issue since it has been associated with a risk factor for the development of cardiovascular diseases [17, 18], to blood glucose control in diabetic patients, where the severity of periodontitis has a negative impact on glucose levels [19], on preterm birth and low birth weight, and on respiratory infections [20], among other chronic inflammatory diseases; furthermore, recently, it was observed that the severity of COVID-19 symptoms significantly increased in patients with poor oral health status and the recovery period was significantly delayed in those with poor oral health, while patients with good oral health had a faster recovery [21]. Among people with diabetes, periodontitis is associated with more diabetes complications. There is evidence that patients with periodontitis and with either type 1 or type 2 diabetes have significantly more renal complications and retinopathy [22].

Periodontal disease is considered as the sixth complication in diabetic patients; in the year 2000 [23], the American Academy of Periodontology stated that "the incidence of periodontitis increases among diabetic patients, increasing the frequency and severity in diabetics with more systemic complications" [24]; the increase in susceptibility is not related to the levels of dental plaque or to dental calculus [25]; collective evidence supports the relationship between both diseases, especially in poorly controlled diabetics [26, 27]. In an epidemiologic study carried out in the United States (NHANES III), individuals with poorly controlled diabetes have 2.9 times higher risk of developing periodontitis, compared to those without diabetes; on the other hand, those who controlled their diabetes properly did not experience any risk increase [28]. It has also been observed that in people with poorly controlled type 2 diabetes, the risk of alveolar bone loss was 11 times greater after 2 years, compared to nondiabetic control individuals [29]. This could be explained by the effect diabetes has in the changing adherence of neutrophils, in chemotaxis, and in phagocytosis that could favor bacterial persistence in the periodontal pocket increasing periodontal destruction significantly. The formation of advanced glycation end products, a key factor in many diabetic complications, is also produced in the peri-

odontium, and its harmful effects over other organ systems may also be reflected in periodontal tissue [30]. Likewise, another study identified a 50% increase in the messenger RNA for the receptor of end products of advanced glycation in subgingival tissue of people with type 2 diabetes, compared to nondiabetic controls [31].

The systemic impact of periodontitis is due to the fact that the extension of the epithelium of periodontal pockets can reach 44–76 cm^2; if we put this into perspective, this represents infected tissue the size of the palm of our hand, having the ability to induce bacteremia and cytokinemia, inducing a low-grade systemic chronic inflammatory process [32]. These bacteremias are the result of mechanical stimulation of the periodontal pocket that became ulcerated during routine activities such as brushing or mastication, where not only do bacteria disseminate but also their products and endotoxins such as lipopolysaccharides [33]. Bacteria and bacterial antigens disseminated from periodontal tissue induce a systemic inflammatory response mediated by white blood cells, endothelial cells, and hepatocytes through the production of IL-1b, IL-6, TNF-a, and PGE2; with continued exposure in the systemic circulation, proinflammatory cytokines induce leukocytosis as well as the production of acute phase proteins such as CRP, fibrinogen, plasminogen, and complement proteins, among others [34, 35]. This bacterial and inflammatory mediator dissemination may have a significant impact on the metabolic condition of a diabetic patient; this is because systemic inflammation can start and disseminate insulin resistance. From an epidemiological standpoint, it has been observed that severe periodontitis is associated with an increase in HbA1C [36] in individuals diagnosed with T2DM [37]. On the other hand, in nondiabetic patients, progression of periodontitis has been associated with an increase in HbA1C and with carbohydrate intolerance; likewise, moderate and severe periodontitis has been linked to a greater risk of triggering diabetic complications like macroalbuminuria, kidney disease, atheroma plaque calcification, and cardio renal mortality [38].

In a systematic review of controlled clinical trials [39], we observed that when periodontal treatment is performed and periodontal infections are eradicated, the average reduction of HbA1C was 0.36%; one of the trials showed that periodontal treatment can even decrease HbA1C levels from 0.4% to 0.5%; this metabolic effect is similar to the one achieved when adding a second glucose-lowering drug to the therapy of diabetic patients [40].

Based on biological plausibility models, epidemiological and therapeutic evidence that link DM to periodontitis in a bidirectional manner (Table 54.2), it is imperative for the attending physician to promote oral health in diabetic patients, by requesting in all cases a consultation with the dentist.

Table 54.2 Evidence in the literature that supports a bidirectional relationship of periodontal disease and diabetes

Author	Key item
Eke PI, dye BA, Wei L, Thornton-Evans GO, Genco RJ	The National Health and Nutrition Survey (NHANES) reported that 47.2% of the American population over 30 years presented periodontitis between 2009 and 2010
Khader YS, Albashaireh ZS, Alomari MA	The high prevalence of periodontitis represents a public health issue. It has been associated with a risk factor for the development of cardiovascular diseases
Mealey BL, Rose LF	To blood glucose control in diabetic patients, where the severity of periodontitis has a negative impact on glucose levels
Haffajee AD. et al.	Periodontitis is a destructive infectious process linked to a microbiological shift in the bacterial biofilm and to a proinflammatory response of the host
Eke PI, et al.	The prevalence of periodontitis in the American population over 30 years is 47.2%
Kinane DF, et al.	Periodontitis has the ability to induce bacteremia and cytokinemia, inducing a low-grade chronic system inflammatory process
Löe H	Periodontitis has been considered the sixth complication of diabetes
Mealey BL, et al.	The severity of periodontitis has a negative impact on glucose levels
Engebretson S, et al.	When periodontal treatment is given and periodontal infections are eradicated, the average HbA1C reduction is 0.36%

The systematic impact periodontitis can have is because the extension of the epithelium of the periodontal pockets can go from 44 to 76 cm^2; in perspective, this represents infected tissue the size of the palm of our hand, having the ability to induce bacteremia and cytokinemia, inducing a low-grade chronic systemic inflammatory process.

Eradicated periodontitis can decrease levels of HbA1 from 0.4% to 0.5%; this metabolic effect is similar to the one achieved when adding a second glucose-lowering drug to the therapy of diabetic patients.

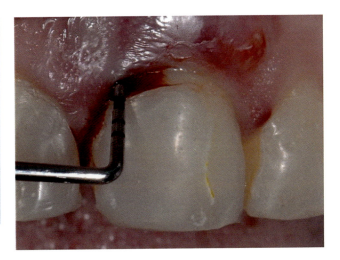

Fig. 54.5 Patient diagnosed with T2DM and periodontitis. We observe that the probe penetrates 9 mm; there is suppuration and bleeding, suggesting an active infection

Based on biological plausibility models, the epidemiologic and therapeutic evidence that link DM bidirectionally to periodontitis, it is essential that the attending physician promotes oral health in diabetic patients, requesting an interconsultation in all cases with the dentist.

Periodontal Diagnosis and Treatment

Diagnosis of periodontitis is clinical and based on the loss of clinical insertion levels, bony loss (Figs. 54.5 and 54.6), periodontal pocket depth, dental mobility, pathological dental migration, and signs of gingival inflammation (change in color, bleeding on probing, volume increase and exudate on probing) [7]. Overall, periodontal treatment is divided into three phases. In phase 1, therapy focuses on eliminating the causal agent (bacterial plaque), defective repairs that contribute to the retention of plaque are removed, and risk factors are controlled (such as smoking, diabetes mellitus, etc.). One of the most important aspects of periodontal phase 1 is providing patients instructions on personal control of bacterial plaque, instructing them on the proper use

of dental floss, an appropriate brushing technique and the items that could facilitate proper oral hygiene [41]. It is absolutely essential to constantly assess the patient's personal plaque control since the long-term therapeutic success depends on it. Treatment of gingivitis consists of eliminating bacterial plaque through mechanical means; as was said before, one of its characteristics is that it is reversible once the bacterial plaque is removed; therefore, patients diagnosed with gingivitis only require periodontal phase 1 (Figs. 54.7 and 54.8).

Unlike gingivitis, periodontitis has an irreversible destructive pattern; in the most recent classification of periodontal diseases, glycemia in diabetic patients is used as an indicator of the rate of periodontitis progression [42]. Periodontitis has to be treated first with nonsurgical means like scaling and root planing, a treatment by means of which bacterial plaque and subgingival calculus are removed using curettes and ultrasonic instruments; on specific clinical scenarios, the use of antibiotics as well as mechanical treatment is necessary

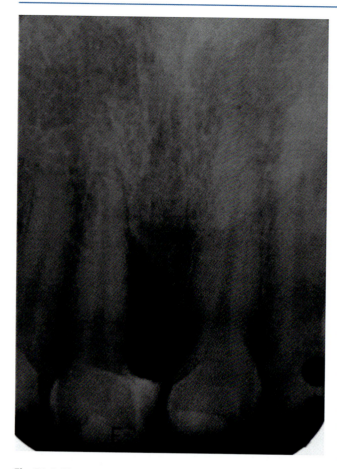

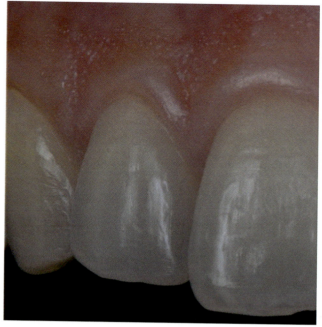

Fig. 54.8 After dental prophylaxis and correct oral hygiene instructions, we observe the resolution of the inflammatory process

Fig. 54.6 X-ray corroborating the presence of vertical bony defect

[43]. If the periodontal pockets persist after the scaling and root planing, periodontal phase 2 is carried out; this is a surgical phase where a flap is lifted in order to perform a deeper periodontal debridement and therefore eliminate the infectious foci. In this phase, the periodontist can place biomaterials that stimulate the periodontal regenerative process [44].

Once the periodontal disease has been controlled, patients start the periodontal phase 3 or maintenance phase. In this phase, patients are reevaluated at 3–6-month intervals to identify if there is any site that has recurred; if so, it is treated at that moment, reinforcing the knowledge so that the patient can follow a good personal plaque control. The maintenance therapy should be carried out for the patient's whole life since the periodontitis can recur.

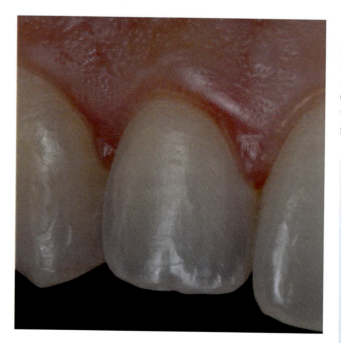

Fig. 54.7 Gingivitis. We observe increased volume of the gingival margin, with an erythematous aspect

Periodontal treatment is divided into three phases. In phase 1 therapy which focuses on eliminating the causal agent (bacterial plaque), the defective repairs that contribute to the retention of plaque are removed, and risk factors are controlled (like smoking, diabetes mellitus, etc.). Periodontal phase 2 is a surgical phase where a flap is raised to perform a deeper periodontal debridement and thus eliminate the infectious foci. In phase 3 or maintenance phase, patients are reassessed in 3–6-month intervals to identify if there is a recurring site; if so, treatment is given at that moment and the knowledge is reinforced so that the patient can perform a proper personal plaque control.

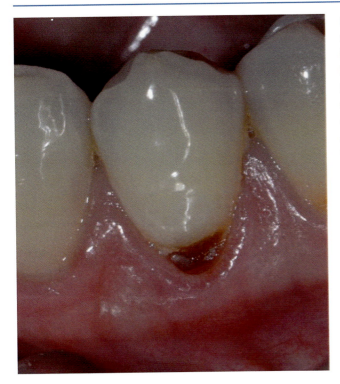

Fig. 54.9 Cervical caries in a diabetic patient

Dental Caries in Diabetics

According to the World Health Organization (WHO), dental caries can be defined as a pathological process characterized by a series of complex chemical and microbiological reactions that end up destroying the tooth. This destruction is the result of the action of acids produced by bacteria in the environment of the dental plaque. Clinically, a caries is characterized by a change in color, loss of transparency, and decalcification of the affected tissue. As the process advances, the tissue is destroyed and cavities are formed.

Throughout the world, around 60%–90% of school-age children and close to 100% of adults have dental caries, often accompanied by pain or a feeling of discomfort.

In diabetics, we observe cervical and atypical caries developed in areas that are not often affected in the rest of nondiabetic patients (Fig. 54.9); however, there is not a unanimous criteria on this theory.

Several reports support the increase in the caries index among diabetics, although there are others who point out a similar risk in nondiabetic patients. These discrepancies have been attributed to the inconsistent characteristics of the clinical evaluations performed, going from the use of several indices like decayed, lost, and filled teeth (CPOD) to bacteriological evaluations; other discrepancies come from the type of populations studied that go from children with type 1 diabetes to elderly patients with type 2 diabetes; however, it is a fact that glucose level in the saliva of nondiabetics is between 0.20 and 2.30 mg/dL, while in diabetics, it goes from 0.45 to 6.30 mg/DI [45]; this condition and the decreased saliva secretion are risk factors for the genesis of decaying processes. These factors alter saliva's buffering capacity that has an effect in the pH of bacterial plaque in teeth, and it affects the rate and the development of caries favoring the growth of microorganisms such as *Streptococcus mutans (Sm)* and *Lactobacillus acidophilus (Lb)* [46]. These are considered bacteriological indicators for their acidogenic and aciduric capacity; in fact, the quantification of these microorganisms has shown a correlation with the decaying process. Scientific evidence indicate that *Streptococcus mutans* is the microorganism associated with the onset of the lesion and *Lactobacillus acidophilus*, with the progression of the lesion; both bacteria are strong producers of acid; therefore, it is considered that the concentration level in saliva, in colony-forming units (CFU) of *Sm* and *Lb* (>105), is associated with intense cariogenic activity, and it is used as an indicator of the high content of fermentable carbohydrates in the oral media, an essential element for greater acidity and thus a greater risk factor. On the other hand, a diabetic patient often develops odontalgias with pulpitis, whose genesis is justified by the microangiopathic processes; the presence of these manifestations is a fact reported in the literature, as well as the repercussions that can cause the dissemination of microorganisms of the oral cavity to the rest of the body (CITA), with the generation of bacteremias that can be the initial factor to trigger generalized bacteremias that have led to death in diabetic patients.

Diabetic patients are more prone to infections; therefore, we have to take the following into account:

– Dental caries is an infection that as it progresses generates the formation of dental abscesses; therefore, this disease should be treated.
– Any dental abscess has to be treated actively to prevent dissemination of bacteria to the blood flow.
– Antibiotic coverage will depend on the type of intervention and the degree of control of diabetes. In some cases, to avoid complications, it is recommended to start preoperative and especially postoperative antibiotic coverage [47].

> In diabetics, we observe cervical and atypical caries developed in areas that we do not often see in nondiabetic patients.

Dental caries is an infection that as it progresses generates the formation of dental abscesses; therefore, this disease should be treated. Any dental abscess has to be treated actively to prevent dissemination of bacteria to the blood flow.

Hyposalivation and Xerostomia

Another anomaly present in diabetics is xerostomia; according to some authors, this disorder is more exacerbated in females. This feeling of "dryness" is caused by the increase in diuresis and a decrease in the volume of extracellular fluid and to changes in the microcirculation of salivary glands that produce hyposialia; xerostomia is often accompanied by glossodynia, taste disorders, burning in the tongue, and halitosis; the decrease of salivary secretion favors the decrease of salivary pH and therefore cariogenic aciduric microorganisms like *Streptococcus mutans* and *Lactobacillus Acidophilus* which proliferate easily. The salivary flow rate is lower in diabetic patients; Screeby in Diabetes Care (1992) states that 63% of patients with T2D refer xerostomia; the authors of this chapter reported 35% [48].

The xerostomia observed in diabetic patients is not only conditioned by poor blood sugar control but also by changes in saliva composition (high protein and potassium content) and autonomic neuropathy that deteriorate glandular secretion.

Xerostomia is the subjective feeling of dryness in the mouth, a symptom reported by the patient. It can be the result of decreased salivary secretion or it can occur in the presence of normal salivary production. Xerostomia is present in 40–60% of diabetic patients who have poor control of the disease with very little salivary production stimulus from the parotid gland compared to patients who are capable of controlling the disease and normal subjects [49].

Hyposalivation in decompensated diabetic patients is explained by the increase in diuresis and polyuria that can affect the production of saliva.

On the other hand, since xerostomia is considered a subjective sensation of dry mouth, it may or may not be attributed to the decrease or interruption of the salivary gland function. Xerostomia not only causes psychological, social, and physical consequences; it also alters food swallowing (Figs. 54.10 and 54.11).

Xerostomia and hyposalivation can be manifestations present in patients with T1D with inappropriate blood glucose control. However, these manifestations can also be related to neuropathy [50].

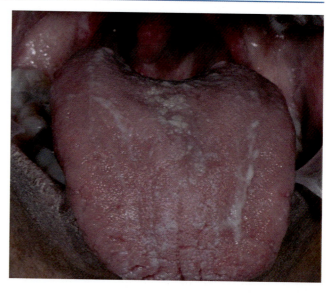

Fig. 54.10 Patient diagnosed with T2DM who presents xerostomia. Clinically, we can see a dehydrated oral mucosa, as well as thick saliva

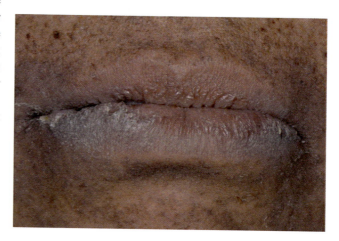

Fig. 54.11 The same patient where we see dehydration of the lip skin

Box 54.2
Xerostomia is a frequent oral condition that can affect oral functions as well as the patient's general well-being.

Box 54.3
Xerostomia in diabetic patients is not only conditioned by poor blood glucose control but also by the changes in saliva composition (high protein and potassium content) and autonomic neuropathy that will deteriorate glandular secretion.

Given its complexity, its treatment requires an interdisciplinary approach that should be focused on improving quality of life, decreasing possible complications, and promoting palliative care. Its etiology has been associated, among other factors, with the presence of systemic diseases including diabetes mellitus. The results of this systematic review and meta-analysis showed a global xerostomia prevalence of 42, 22% (CI of 95%: 33, 97%, and 50, 92%) in people with diabetes and a statistically significant association [51].

Frequent Mucosal Lesions in Diabetics

Candidiasis

Diabetics are prone to fungal infections; this is frequent in our setting. These are produced by the excess growth of *Candida* in the mouth, the digestive tract, the vagina, and other tissues. These are the skin—mucosa disorders that are sometimes systemic and produced by the *Candida* species (the most frequent type is *Candida albicans*). There are local factors such as smoking and the use of total dental prosthesis (Fig. 54.12) that can promote the appearance of candidiasis in the oral cavity as well as by extended periods of hyposalivation in uncontrolled diabetics.

Poor metabolic control is responsible for more fungal infections in diabetic patients than in the rest of the population since the glucose level in saliva acts as a substrate for *Candida*. Taking high doses of antibiotics or prolonged antibiotic use also increases the risk of oral candidiasis. Antibiotics destroy some of the healthy bacteria that prevent candida from proliferating too much.

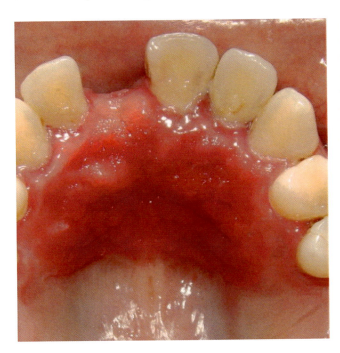

Fig. 54.12 Candidiasis associated with a movable prosthesis in a patient diagnosed with T2DM

Symptoms. Oral candidiasis appears as velvety whitish lesions in the mouth and tongue. Under this whitish material, there is reddish tissue that can bleed easily. Ulcers may increase slowly in number and size.

Exams and Tests. The physician or the dentist can often diagnose oral candidiasis by examining the mouth and tongue since ulcers have a distinctive appearance. If diagnosis is unclear, one of the following tests can be performed to look for candida organisms:
Culture of oral lesions.
Microscopic test of oral scrapings.

Treatment. For oral candidiasis in babies, treatment is often not necessary since it clears on its own after a couple of weeks. If it is a mild case of oral candidiasis after taking antibiotics, eating yoghurt or taking over-the-counter acidophilus capsules may help. The use a soft bristle tooth brush and rinse with a hydrogen peroxide water solution at 3% several times a day can help. Good control of blood sugar levels in people with diabetes can eliminate an oral candidiasis infection. The doctor can prescribe an antifungal mouthwash (nystatin) or chewable tablets (clotrimazole) if the oral candidiasis is severe or if there is a weakened immune system. These products are generally used for 5–10 days. If they do not work, other drugs can be prescribed [52].

Wound Healing and Changes in the Mucosa

Diabetic patients have impaired scarring. There are several theories that try to explain this phenomenon, like poor vascularization, decrease in platelet activity, or disorders in collagen synthesis [53]. Diabetes makes scarring or wounds slower and more difficult than normal. Diabetic patients not only have impaired scarring in acute wounds and slower closure of tissue making them more prone to chronic wounds. This is caused by an early inhibited or impaired inflammatory reaction and by a decrease in the ability to release growth factors and cytokines and the intercellular communication substances with several beneficial functions. When repair cell migration is interrupted, cell repair is hindered, thus decreasing the quality of the granulation status (scarring from the bottom to the top).

There is also diabetic microangiopathy present in the lower limbs, thus reducing the transport and repair capacity of tissue through the blood.

Diabetic patients often develop odontalgia with pulpitis; its genesis is justified by the microangiopathic processes, the frequent appearance of oral ulcers with a delay in wound healing, fissured tongue, and angular cheilitis; one of the most frequent and striking manifestations is reddening and atrophy of the mucosa.

Candidiasis is a frequent disorder in diabetics. Poor metabolic control is responsible for the fungal infections in diabetic patients more than in the rest of the population.

Healthcare Protocol of Diabetics in the Dental Office, Dental Management, Clinical History, and Patient's Level of Control

If we consider the statistics published by the WHO in 2014, the world prevalence of diabetes was 9% among adults over 18 years old. It is calculated that 1.5 million people died as a direct consequence of diabetes in 2012. More than 80% of the diabetes-related deaths were recorded in low- and medium-income countries.

According to WHO forecasts, diabetes will be the seventh cause of mortality in 2030; it is very likely that this type of diabetic patients will seek a dentist's consultation, and these patients may have an asymptomatic disease therefore going undiagnosed.

Clinical Management of Diabetic Patients in the Dental Office

It is very important for the dentist to be prepared to provide dental treatment to the diabetic patient. This includes an appropriate diagnosis of the prediabetic or the diabetic condition, as well as of the oral status of said patient. A full assessment should be performed including a medical and dental history, essential for an accurate diagnosis to create a treatment plan and to manage the patient's condition appropriately. It is important to specify the type of diabetes, the duration, the treatment modality, diet, exercise, oral drugs, or insulin (type and frequency of administration); patients who use insulin with a subcutaneous pump should be properly identified since they are often at risk of developing hypoglycemia since they have tighter control of the blood glucose levels.

Every dental office should have a glucose monitor, and the staff should be familiar with its use in order to measure the patient's capillary blood glucose (whether the patient has a diabetes mellitus diagnosis or not), before any procedure. However, sometimes it is recommended that the patients bring their own glucose monitor to the dental office if they have one at home, to avoid significant variations in the measurements. All the information on the blood glucose levels and HbA_{1C} should be included in the patient's medical record.

Practical recommendations are the following:

1. It is important to highlight the importance of preserving oral health in diabetics. Patients should be instructed on oral self-examination in front of a mirror and if they find an abnormal condition to consult the dentist.
2. What to do before the dental consultation? Blood glucose control should be at appropriate levels. The medication prescribed by the attending physician should not be suspended. When going to the dentist's office, bring a record of the last blood glucose measurements. Medication and therapies are used and information of the attending physician.
3. During the consultation, we must consider that stress causes changes in the body increasing the blood glucose levels. The dentist's consultation generates stress, as dentists are aware of that, so the consult is given early in the day and we recommend the patients no to change their diet or medication.
4. We highlight that the dentist will provide a detailed explanation of the patient's oral condition. He will perform prophylaxis and will instruct the patients on the use of oral hygiene instruments and will provide the next appointment. We recommend diabetic patients to visit the dentist every 4 months for a routine assessment and detection of possible infection foci.
5. If treatment is surgery, what to do before, during, and after the procedure are as follows: Before surgery, work with your dentist to create the safest surgery plan for you. Focus more on your diabetes control weeks before surgery. The dentist will examine and talk to you about your health. It is important to know all the drugs you are taking.
6. During surgery. You will see your dentist before surgery to discuss the control plan for your blood sugar during surgery.
7. After surgery. The dentist or the nursing staff will monitor your blood glucose level frequently. You may have more problems to control it if you have problems to eat, if you are stressed after surgery, or if you have pain or discomfort.
   Be aware of signs of infection such as fever, an incision that is red or warm to the touch, swollen, more pain, or oozing. We recommend being prepared to call the dentist if any questions arise [54].
8. Diabetic patients should be informed that they are at greater risk of developing periodontitis, and if they develop it, blood glucose control will be more complicated having a greater risk of developing diabetes-associated complications like cardiovascular and kidney disease.
9. Patients diagnosed with T1DM, T2DM, or gestational diabetes should have a comprehensive oral examination that includes a periodontal assessment.

10. If periodontitis is diagnosed, it should be managed appropriately; if there is no periodontitis, the patient should follow a preventive program to monitor periodontal changes.

11. Diabetic patients who have extensive tooth loss should be encouraged to have dental rehabilitation in order to have proper mastication and nutrition. When patients loses all their teeth, intake of fibrous food becomes difficult, thus having to change to a softer food diet.

12. Annual oral exams are recommended in children and adolescents diagnosed with diabetes starting at age 6.

13. Patients who are not diagnosed with diabetes but who have obvious risk factors for T2DM and signs of periodontitis should be informed that they are at risk of developing diabetes; we suggest using a HbA1C test and refer them to the doctor for diagnosis.

Antibiotics and Antimicrobial Prophylaxis

The main objective of dental treatment is to eradicate infectious processes and then maintain dental and periodontal health. Controlled diabetic patients are treated the same way nondiabetic patients are; therefore, it is unnecessary to adjust the doses or modify the use of routine drugs in the dentist's consultation. It is important that before the consultation, patients continue their normal diet and their drugs according to the medical prescription. Emergencies and acute infectious processes (with a prior medical interconsultation) should be treated only in uncontrolled diabetic patients; routine treatments should be postponed until blood glucose levels are under control. It is important to consider the presence of organ damage (cardiomyopathy, kidney failure, cirrhosis, emphysema, or alcoholism) since special pharmacological considerations have to be given.

Antibiotics and Antimicrobial Prophylaxis

There is no scientific evidence to support that controlled diabetic patients are prone to postoperative infections when undergoing uncomplicated dentoalveolar surgery; therefore, it is not justified to prescribe antibiotics in these cases; however, if there is a picture of disseminated infection (fever, trismus, lymphadenitis, general discomfort, cellulitis), it is necessary to apply the principles of infection treatment (drainage, elimination of the etiological factor, empirical administration of antibiotics and reassessment).

Antibiotic prophylaxis should not be given routinely to diabetic patients (unless the patient presents another systemic condition that requires it). Routine treatments should be avoided in uncontrolled diabetic patients who have blood glucose levels greater than 250 mg/dL. If an emergency surgical procedure is necessary, appropriate antibiotic prophylaxis is warranted (even though there is no evidence to support it), following the same AHA principles to prevent infectious endocarditis (2 g of amoxicillin 1 h before the procedure). Infections in these patients should be treated aggressively regardless of blood glucose levels.

Guidelines the Physician Should be Aware of to Suspect an Oral Disease

Given that there is a high risk of developing periodontitis and other oral disorders, in a consensus carried out between the American Association of Periodontology and the European Federation of Periodontology on diabetes and periodontitis, the following clinical recommendations were made for physicians and other healthcare professionals:

1. Diabetic patients should be informed that they are at greater risk of developing periodontitis, and if they develop it, blood glucose control will be more complicated, thus making them at risk of developing complications associated with diabetes such as cardiovascular and kidney disease.

2. As part of the initial evaluation, patients diagnosed with T1DM, T2DM, or gestational diabetes should receive an oral and a periodontal examination.

3. Patients diagnosed with T1DM and T2DM should undergo an oral and a periodontal examination annually (even if they do not have an initial diagnosis of periodontitis).

4. Diabetic people who present clinical signs of periodontitis like tooth mobility, dental separation, or gingival oozing should receive immediate dental care.

5. Diabetic patients who present extensive tooth loss should be encouraged to undergo dental rehabilitation for proper mastication and adequate nutrition.

6. All diabetic patients should receive dental education.

7. We recommend oral examinations every year in children and adolescents diagnosed with diabetes starting at age 6.

8. Diabetic patients should be informed that they may present xerostomia and burning mouth and that they are at greater risk of developing candidiasis unlike nondiabetic patients.

Conclusions

Diabetes mellitus has a profound effect on the overall health of patients. Many clinical manifestations are seen in the oral cavity compromising quality of life. When infections are odontogenic, blood sugar control becomes difficult in these patients. That is why there should be a close relationship between the attending physician, the dentist, and other members of the interdisciplinary team who will provide specialized control of any risk factor that may influence the natural history of diabetes.

Concluding Remarks

- Oral health is an essential component of good health and it is a basic human right.
- Poor oral health can have severe repercussions in overall health.
- Periodontal disease is a highly prevalent infection that increases among diabetic patients.
- Periodontal disease increases the frequency and severity in diabetics with more systemic complications.
- Periodontal treatment can help to lower blood glucose levels.
- It is essential that the attending physician promotes oral health in diabetic patients.

Multiple Choice Questions

1. Do oral health and quality of life have any relationship in diabetic people?
    (a) Yes, because treatments constitute 5–10% of the health expense.
    (b) Only if patients do not control their blood glucose levels.
    (c) They do not have any relationship.
    (d) **Yes, because if the mouth is healthy, the person feels well.**
    (e) It depends on the type of diabetes.
2. How is the infectious process that affects support tissue of teeth and characterized by the destruction of teeth called?
    (a) Gingivitis
    (b) **Periodontitis**
    (c) Dental abscess
    (d) Gingival abscess
    (e) Periodontal abscess
3. It is one of the main bacteria associated with periodontitis.
    (a) *S. mutans*
    (b) *S. sanguis*
    (c) *P. gingivalis*
    (d) *S. aureus*
    (e) *L. acidophilus*
4. Dental caries is an infection that as it advances it causes the formation of dental abscesses that should be treated in diabetics only when:
    (a) There is no blood sugar control.
    (b) **They should always be treated to avoid dissemination of bacteria.**
    (c) When purulent abscesses are formed and there is fever.
    (d) When they go to a specialized hospital.
    (e) They should not always be treated; it depends on the depth of the caries.

5. Diabetics are prone to fungal infections such as candidiasis for the following reasons:
    (a) Because the germ is opportunistic
    (b) Because they are immunosuppressed and they have blood glucose that serves as a substrate for candida
    (c) For smoking and having little saliva
    (d) From the effects of the drugs taken by diabetics
    (e) **Due to the poor blood sugar control, the hyposalivation and glucose in the saliva that serves as a substrate for candida**
6. Xerostomia is present in 40–60% of diabetic patients and the causes are:
    (a) The increase in diuresis and the presence of infection foci
    (b) The decreased platelet activity or the changes in the collagen synthesis
    (c) **The increase in diuresis and changes in the microcirculation of salivary glands**
    (d) The periodontal disease and cervical cavities present in the oral cavity
    (e) That diabetics are thirsty constantly
7. What is periodontal phase 1?
    (a) To perform surgical procedures to eradicate infectious foci
    (b) **To eliminate the causal agent in a nonsurgical manner and control risk factors**
    (c) To perform tooth cleaning
    (d) To use antibiotics to eliminate infectious foci
8. What is the effect of periodontal therapy in HbA1c levels?
    (a) They are maintained the same.
    (b) They increase after periodontal treatment.
    (c) They decrease but not significantly.
    (d) **They decrease up to 0.5.**
9. What do we recommended the diabetic patients do before, during, and after the dentist's consultation.
    (a) **Do not suspend medication for going to the dentist and have records of the attending physician and recent blood glucose levels.**
    (b) Have a dental card.
    (c) Have the attending physician's telephone number and all the prescriptions of drugs taken.
    (d) Take the last appointment of the day to avoid any stress.
    (e) Fast before the appointment without brushing their teeth so that the dentist can see the oral condition.
10. Diabetic patients should take prophylactic medication when they present infection in the oral cavity.
    (a) It is always necessary.
    (b) Never.
    (c) Only if they have type 1 diabetes.
    (d) Only elderly patients.

11. An inflammatory process associates to bacterial plaque characterized by an increase in gingival volume and bleeding on probing and is reversible when the bacterial plaque is eliminated.
    (a) Periodontitis
    (b) **Gingivitis**
    (c) Candidiasis
    (d) Linear gingival erythema
    (e) Periodontal abscess

References

1. Organización Mundial de la Salud. The world oral health report 2003. Geneva: OMS; 2003. http://www.who.int/mediacentre/news/releases/2004/pr15/es/.
2. Visión de la FDI 2020. Delinear el futuro de la Salud Bucal. http://www.fdiworldental.org/oral-health/vision-2020/shaping-the-future-of-oral-health.aspx.
3. Hassel TM. Tissues and cells of the periodontium. Periodontol 2000. 1993;3:9–38.
4. Payne WA, Page RC, Olgivie AL, Hall WB. Histopathologic features of the initial and early stages of experimental gingivitis in man. J Periodontal Res. 1975;10:51–64.
5. Löe H, Theilade E, Jensen SB. Experimental gingivitis in man. J Periodontol. 1965;36:177–87.
6. Mariotti A. Dental plaque-induced gingival diseases. Ann Periodontol. 1999;4:7–17.
7. Drisko CL. Periodontal self-care: evidence-based support. Periodontol 2000. 2013;62:243–55.
8. Haffajee AD, Teles RP, Socransky SS. The effect of periodontal therapy on the composition of the subgingival microbiota. Periodontol 2000. 2006;42:219–58.
9. Ledder RG, Gilbert P, Huws SA, Arons L, Ashley MP, Hull PS, McBain AJ. Molecular analysis of the subgingival microbiota in health and disease. Appl Environ Microbiol. 2007;73:516–23.
10. Gemmell E, Yamazaki K, Seymour GJ. Destructive periodontitis lesions are determined by the nature of the lymphocyte response. Crit Rev Oral Biol Med. 2002;13:17–34.
11. Phipps KR, Stevens VJ. Relative contribution of caries and periodontal disease in adult tooth loss for an HMO dental population. J Public Health Dent. 1995;55:250–2.
12. Brecx M, Frohlicher I, Gehr P, Lang NP. Stereological observations on long term experimental gingivitis in man. J Clin Periodontol. 1988;15:621–7.
13. Darveau RP, Tanner A, Page RC. The microbial challenge in periodontitis. Periodontol 2000. 1997;14:12–32.
14. Gemmell E, Marshall RI, Seymour GJ. Cytokines and prostaglandins in immune homeostasis and tissue destruction in periodontal disease. Periodontol 2000. 1997;14:112–43.
15. Schwartz Z, Goulyschin J, Dean DD, Boyan BD. Mechanisms of alveolar bone destruction in periodontitis. Periodontol 2000. 1997;14:158–72.
16. Eke PI, Dye BA, Wei L, Thornton-Evans GO, Genco RJ, on behalf of the participating members of the CDC Periodontal. Disease Surveillance workgroup. Prevalence of periodontitis in adults in the United States: 2009 and 2010. J Dent Res. 2012;91:914–20.
17. Khader YS, Albashaireh ZS, Alomari MA. Periodontal diseases and the risk of coronary heart and cerebrovascular diseases: a meta-analysis. J Periodontol. 2004;75:1046–53.
18. Mealey BL, Rose LF. Diabetes mellitus and inflammatory periodontal disease. Curr Opin Endocrinol Diabetes Obes. 2008;5:135–41.
19. Löe H. Periodontal disease. The sixth complication of diabetes. Diabetes Care. 1993;16:329–34.
20. Scannapieco FA. Role of oral bacteria in respiratory infection. J Periodontol. 1999;70:793–802.
21. Kamel AHM, Basuoni A, Salem ZA, AbuBakr N. The impact of oral health status on COVID-19 severity, recovery period and C-reactive protein values. Br Dent J. 2021;24:1–7.
22. Sanz M, Ceriello A, Buysschaert M, Chapple I, Demmer RT, Graziani F, Herrera D, Jepsen S, Lione L, Madianos P, Mathur M, Montanya E, Shapira L, Tonetti M, Vegh D. Scientific evidence on the links between periodontal diseases and diabetes: consensus report and guidelines of the joint workshop on periodontal diseases and by the International Diabetes Federation and the European Federation of Periodontology. Diabetes Res Clin Pract. 2018;137:231–41.
23. The American Academy of Periodontology. Parameter on periodontitis associated with systemic conditions. J Periodontol. 2000;71:876–8.
24. Taylor GW, Manz MC, Borgnakke WS. Diabetes, periodontal disease, dental caries, and tooth loss: a review of the literature. Comp Cont Edu Dent. 2004;25:179–84.
25. Katz J. Elevates blood glucose levels in patients with severe periodontal disease. J Clin Periodontol. 2001;28:710–2.
26. Castellanos JL, Díaz LM, Gay O. Medicina en odontología en Manejo dental de pacientes con enfermedades sistémicas, vol. 8. México City: El Manual Moderno; 1996. p. 270–83.
27. Tsai C, Hayes C, Taylor GW. Glycemic control of type 2 diabetes and severe periodontal disease in the US adult population. Community Dent Oral Epidemiol. 2002;30:182–92.
28. Taylor GW, Burt BA, Becker MP, Genco RJ, Shlossman M, Knowler WC, Pettitt DJ. Non-insulin dependent diabetes mellitus and alveolar bone loss progression over 2 years. J Periodontol. 1998;69:76–83.
29. Schmidt AM, Weidman E, Lalla E, Yan SD, Hori O, Cao R, Brett JG, Lamster IB. Advanced glycation end products (AGEs) induce oxidant stress in the gingiva: a potential mechanism underlying accelerated periodontal disease associated with diabetes. J Periodontal Res. 1996;31:508–15.
30. Katz J, Bhattacharyya I, Farkhondeh-Kish F, Perez FM, Caudle RM, Heft MW. Expression of the receptor of advanced glycation end products in gingival tissues of type 2 diabetes patients with chronic periodontal disease: a study utilizing immunohistochemistry and RT-PCR. J Clin Periodontol. 2005;32:40–4.
31. Page RC. The pathobiology of periodontal diseases may affect systemic diseases: inversion of a paradigm. Ann Periodontol. 1998;3:108–20.
32. Kinane DF, Riggio MP, Walker KF, MacKenzie D, Shearer B. Bacteraemia following periodontal procedures. J Clin Periodontol. 2005;32:708–13.
33. Li X, Kolltveit KM, Tronstad L, Olsen I. Systemic diseases caused by oral infection. Cain Microbiol Rev. 2000;13:547–58.
34. Elter JR, Hinderliter AL, Offenbacher S, Beck JD, Caughey M, Brodala N, Madianos PN. The effects of periodontal therapy on vascular endothelial function: a pilot trial. Am Heart J. 2006;15:47.
35. Teeuw WJ, Gerdes VE, Loos BG. Effect of periodontal treatment on glycemic control of diabetic patients: a systematic review and meta-analysis. Diabetes Care. 2010;33:421–7.
36. Diaz-Romero RM, Casanova-Roman G, Robles-Andrade MS. Association of uncontrolled glycemia with periodontal, urinary tract and cervical vaginal infections in a group of type 2 diabetic women during pregnancy and during the postnatal period. Int J Diabetes Clin Res. 2016;3:052–7.
37. Borgnakke WS, Ylostalo PV, Taylor GW, Genco RJ. Effect of periodontal disease on diabetes: systematic review of epidemiologic observational evidence. J Clin Periodontol. 2013;40(Suppl 14):135–52.
38. Engebretson S, Kocher T. Evidence that periodontal treatment improves diabetes outcomes: a systematic review and meta-analysis. J Clin Periodontol. 2013;40(Suppl 14):153–63.

39. Engebretson S, Kocher T. Evidence that periodontal treatment improves diabetes outcomes: a systematic review and meta-analysis. J Clin Periodontol. 2013;40(Suppl. 14):S153–63.

40. Armitage GC. Learned and unlearned concepts in periodontal diagnostics: a 50-year perspective. Periodontol 2000. 2013;62:20–36.

41. Lisa JAHM, Lang NP. Surgical and nonsurgical periodontal therapy. Learned and unlearned concepts. Periodontol 2000. 2013;62:218–31.

42. Papapanou PN, Sanz M, et al. Periodontitis: consensus report of workgroup 2 of the 2017 world workshop on the classification of periodontal and peri-implant diseases and conditions. J Clin Periodontol. 2018;45(Suppl 20):S162–70.

43. Cortellini P, Tonetti MS. Clinical and radiographic out- comes of the modified minimally invasive surgical technique with and without regenerative materials: a randomized-controlled trial in intrabony defects. J Clin Periodontol. 2011;38:365–73.

44. Moreira AR, Passos IA, Sampaio FC, Soares MSM, Oliveira RJ. Flow rate, pH and calcium concentration of saliva of children and adolescents with type 1 diabetes mellitus. Braz J Med Biol Res. 2009;42(8):707–11.

45. Malickaa B, Kaczmareka U, Katarzyna S-M. Prevalence of xerostomia and the salivary flow rate in diabetic patients. Adv Clin Exp Med. 2014;23(2):225–33.

46. Sánchez-Pérez L, Sáenz-Martínez L, Luengas-Aguirre I, Irigoyen Camacho E, Álvarez Castro AR, Farmacologia A-GE. Stimulated saliva flow rate analysis and its relation to dental decay. A six years follow-up. Rev ADM. 2015;72(1):33–7.

47. Díaz-Romero RM, Robles-Andrade MS, Ortega-González C. Diabetes mellitus en Farmacología y Terapéutica en Odontología. Espinosa Meléndez 1ª.Edición. México City: Editorial: Medica Panamericana; 2012. p. 251–5.

48. Díaz-Romero RM, Agami Gorinstein C, Ovadia-Rafel R, Villegas-Álvarez F. Xerostomia, hiposalivación y diabetes. Diabetes hoy para el médico y profesional de la salud. 2008;IX(4):2061–4.

49. Sreebny LM, Yu A, Green A, Valdini A. Xerostomia in diabetes mellitus. Diabetes Care. 1992;15:900–4.

50. Edwards JE Jr. Candida species. In: Mandell GL, Bennett JE, Dolin R, editors. Principles and practice of infectious diseases. 7th ed. Philadelphia, PA: Elsevier Churchill Livingstone; 2009: chap 257.

51. Affoo RH, Foley N, Garrick R, Siqueira WL, Martin RE. Meta-analysis of salivary flow rates in young and older adults. J Am Geriatr Soc. 2015;63:2142–51.

52. Sanz-Sánchez I, Bascones-Martínez A. Diabetes mellitus: Su implicación en la patología oral y periodontal. Av Odontoestomatol. 2009;25(5):249–63. http://scielo.isciii.es/scielo.php?script=sci_art text&pid=S021312852009000500003&lng=es.

53. Domek N, Dux K, Pinzur M, Weaver F, Rogers T. J Foot Ankle Surg. 2016;20(16):30064–3.

54. Chapple ILC, Genco R, Working Group 2 of the Joint EFP/AAP Workshop. Diabetes and periodontal diseases: consensus report of the joint EFP/AAP workshop on periodontitis and systemic diseases. J Clin Periodontol. 2013;40(Suppl 14):S106–12.

Renal Disease in Diabetes

55

Carlos A. Garza-García, Virgilia Soto-Abraham, and Magdalena Madero-Rovalo

History

Urinary anomalies in diabetic patients have long been described; many long-standing historical documents refer, for example, to the characteristic sweet taste or smell in the urine of these population. The first description of renal anomalies in diabetic patients goes back to the 1700s, when Domenico Cotugno de Bari described proteinuria in this population [1]. In the next century, Claude Bernard found nephromegaly in diabetic kidneys in 1840 [2], and it was not until 1936 that Kimmelstiel and Wilson described nodular-fibrotic lesions in the glomeruli and diabetic nephropathy, a syndrome characterized by hypertension, proteinuria, and loss of kidney function. Later, in 1969, Harry Keen did a landmark discovery in diabetic nephropathy with the description of albuminuria in diabetic patients and established it as a surrogate for glomerular damage. With all the former discoveries, Mogensen et al. proposed the clinical picture of the natural history for diabetic nephropathy in 1983 [3]. As of today, Mogensen's sequence of diabetic nephropathy continues to be the accepted paradigm with some new features being considered.

Epidemiology of Diabetic Nephropathy

As it is widely known, diabetes has epidemic proportions with a global estimated prevalence of 8.3% in the 2014, corresponding to an approximate of 387 million people worldwide [4], and it is expected to increase to 592 millions of affected individuals by 2035 [5], likely a reflect of worldwide obesity pandemia. Another inherent partner of this world's expected increase in diabetes mellitus is diabetic kidney disease (DKD). For type 1 diabetes, DKD develops in approximately 30% of patients [6] and in about 40% of those with type 2 diabetes. Diabetic population, both types 1 and 2, account for 30–45% of chronic kidney disease (CKD) patients, but since DKD diagnosis is based on the presence of albuminuria as diagnostic criteria, DKD is probably more prevalent when ophthalmologic examination, estimated glomerular filtration rate, and kidney biopsies are included as additional diagnostic criteria.

Pathophysiology

Even though hyperglycemia plays a major role in the development of DKD, other mechanisms have been proposed [7]. Hemodynamic, metabolic, inflammatory pathways, autophagy, and enhanced sodium-glucose transporter-2 (SGLT-2) expression have also been involved in the DKD progression.

Hemodynamic Pathway

Renin-angiotensin-aldosterone system (RAAS) activation, mainly through angiotensin II and endothelin-1, produces a vasoconstriction effect on the efferent arteriole and leads to the widely known hyperfiltration phenomenon. Along with this hemodynamic effect, both molecules enhance mesangial cell hypertrophy and proliferation, extracellular matrix deposition, hypertension, endothelial dysfunction, inflammation, and fibrosis [8].

C. A. Garza-García · V. Soto-Abraham · M. Madero-Rovalo (✉)
Department of Nephrology, Instituto Nacional de Cardiología
Ignacio Chávez, Monterrey, Mexico

© The Author(s), under exclusive license to Springer Nature Switzerland AG 2023
J. Rodriguez-Saldana (ed.), *The Diabetes Textbook*, https://doi.org/10.1007/978-3-031-25519-9_55

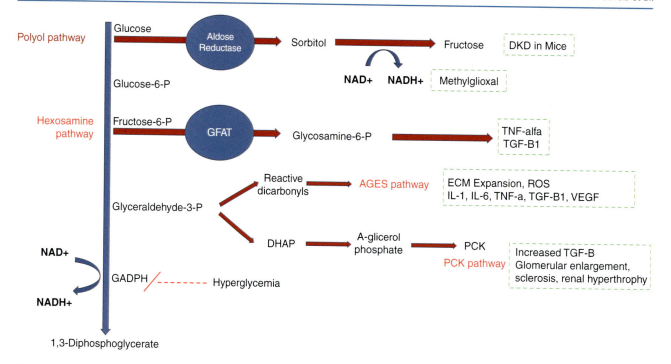

Fi. 55.1 Glycolysis in hyperglycemia. Glycolysis biochemistry is altered by hyperglycemia; it inhibits GADPH and increases upstream pathways, end products of such pathways

Metabolic Pathway

First described in 2001 by Brownlee [9], he showed that hyperglycemia activates superoxide, which inhibits glycolysis last enzymatic step at GADPH (glyceraldehyde-3-phosphate dehydrogenase) preventing formation of 1,3-diphosphoglycerate. The former increases upstream metabolic steps which end up in increased polyol pathway, hexosamine pathway, advanced products of advanced glycation end products (AGEs), and protein kinase C (PKC) (Fig. 55.1).

Polyol Path

Glucose is converted to sorbitol and into fructose afterward. Sorbitol production decreases intracellular NADPH, which ends up in less available glutathione that increases cellular stress and apoptosis. Oxidation of sorbitol leads to fructose generation, which increases NADPH to NAD proportion. This particular change enhances glycolysis inhibition by blockade of GADPH activity. Fructose generated by polyol pathway has shown to be nephrotoxic in mice models [8]; it increases glomerular and tubular damage along with proteinuria and decreases glomerular filtration rate (GFR).

Hexosamine Pathway

This track starts with fructose-6-phosphate which is then converted into glucosamine-6-phosphate, a transcription inducer of inflammatory cytokines such as tumor necrosis factor alpha (TNF-a) and transforming growth factor beta 1 (TGF-

B1). The latter has well-known pathogenic effects such as mesangial matrix expansion and renal cell hypertrophy.

Advanced Glycation End Product (AGE) Pathway

AGE is a generic name for a group of products generated during hyperglycemia due to aberrant glycolysis. The process starts in glyceraldehyde-3-P and ends up in products such as glyoxal and methylglyoxal. These end products damage cells by impairing and/or modifying function of intra- and extracellular proteins, such as laminin and type IV collagen of the glomerular basal membrane (GBM), and increase permeability and thereby proteinuria [10–12]. Also AGEs increase the expression of profibrotic molecules such as fibronectin and collagen types I and IV, leading to extracellular matrix expansion. AGEs by themselves have the property of binding to pro-inflammatory receptors and induce expression of IL-1, IL-6, and TNF-a (tumoral growth factor alpha), TGF-B1 (transforming growth factor beta 1), connective tissue growth factor (CTGF), and vascular endothelial growth factor (VEGF) [11, 13–15].

Protein Kinase C Pathway

Similar to the AGEs, the protein kinase C pathway (PKC) metabolism begins with glyceraldehyde-3-P; hyperglycemia leads to dihydroxyacetone phosphate (DHAP) and ultimately diacylglycerol (DAG). This last element contributes to the activation of PKC, which in turn upregulates prostaglandin E2 and nitric oxide in the afferent arteriole leading to vasodilation and increases angiotensin II over the efferent arteriole ending in vasoconstriction at this point. This vascular phenomenon increases glomerular pressure and corresponds to what is known as glomerular hyperfiltration [16–19]. PKC also mediates VEGF, leading to increased permeability of GBM, and induces CTGF and TFG-B1 which favor thickening of GBM and deposition of extracellular matrix [16].

Inflammatory Pathway

Chronically activated immune system and persistent low-grade inflammation in diabetes have been proposed as contributors to DKD. The latter through an inflammatory transcription factor, NF-kappa-beta (NFKB), is present in human kidney cells along glomerulus and tubule-interstitium. Hyperglycemia induces NFKB, which correlates with interstitial inflammation and proteinuria. Proteinuria by itself further enhances NFKB expression closing a positive feedback loop with hyperglycemia [20–25]. Inflammatory cytokines such as TNF-alpha, IL-1, IL-6, and IL-8 are much more expressed in renal tissue of diabetic models when compared to nondiabetic controls [26, 27]. Inflammatory cytokines correlate positively with the degree of albuminuria in diabetic patients. Also, contribution to GBM thickening, increase in endothelial permeability, apoptosis, and direct toxic effect to renal cells have been proposed as potential pathogenic mechanisms [7].

Autophagy

Autophagy is considered a protective phenomenon that allows cells to maintain homeostasis during starvation or oxidative stress [28, 29]. It allows cells to degradate intracellular proteins and organelles to self-sustain [29, 30]. Podocytes usually have a high level of autophagy. In vitro studies of podocyte exposure to hyperglycemia have shown impairment of this phenomenon and subsequent cellular injury [31–33].

SGLT-2

Hyperglycemia upregulates SGLT-2 in the kidney. This mechanism had been initially considered an evolutionary benefit for glucose claiming and energy storage; however, it has been now shown to have deleterious effects in diabetic patients by further contributing to hyperglycemic state and activation of all the physiopathologic pathways and autophagy impairment [34, 35].

Albuminuria

Emphasis on albuminuria across the scientific literature is explained by its correlation with the loss of glomerular filtration rate and increased cardiovascular risk [1, 2, 36]. Albuminuria is the consequence of a wide, and still not completely understood, interaction within functional (reversible) forces and histopathologic (irreversible) changes [37]. Functional forces are systemic and glomerular hemodynamic disturbances that lead the anatomical structures (glomerular basal membrane, podocyte, and mesangium) to develop irreversible changes. Nonetheless, neither is completely responsible for albuminuria. High hemodynamic pressure over non-damaged structures may not end up in albuminuria, as hemodynamic control over structurally damaged nephrons may not lead to albuminuria either. It has been proposed that the link that regulates interaction between the hemodynamic forces and anatomical structures is the endothelial glicocalix. Endothelial glycocalyx receives sheer stress, hypertension forces, hyperglycemia, and inflammation, among other factors, that ultimately end up in glicocalix degeneration and with it the loose of mechanical and electrical sieving that allows albuminuria.

Albuminuria is also the most sensitive screening tool to diagnose diabetic kidney disease. It is present in up to 55% of patients with DKD regardless of glomerular filtration rate. Only 13% of patients fulfill DKD diagnosis by albuminuria with decreased glomerular filtration rate and as little as 9% have only decreased glomerular filtration rate without albuminuria, as shown in the DEMAND Global [38].

Natural History of Diabetic Nephropathy: The Clinical Picture

From a clinical standpoint, DKD is the dynamic result of multiple risk factors divided as demographic (older age, gender, ethnicity), hereditary (family history for DKD, genetic conditions), systemic conditions (hyperglycemia, obesity, hypertension), kidney injuries (acute kidney injuries, toxins, smoking), and dietary factors (high protein intake). All the former leads to a sequence of susceptibility, initiation, and progression of DKD. The last two stages of this sequence (initiation and progression) correspond to the known and now changing natural history of DKD. Even though the description of DKD natural history involves mainly type 1 diabetics, it is widely accepted for both type 1 and 2 scenarios. A five-stage continuum through time is the result of two main variables, glomerular filtration rate (GFR) and albuminuria (Fig. 55.2).

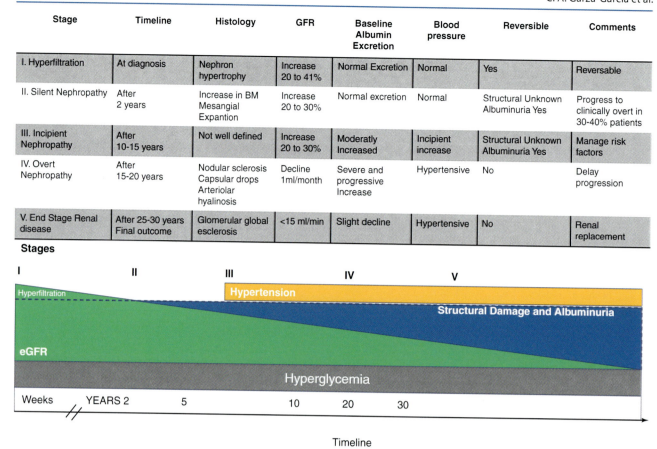

Stage	Timeline	Histology	GFR	Baseline Albumin Excretion	Blood pressure	Reversible		Comments
I. Hyperfiltration	At diagnosis	Nephron hypertrophy	Increase 20 to 41%	Normal Excretion	Normal	Yes		Reversable
II. Silent Nephropathy	After 2 years	Increase in BM Mesangial Expantion	Increase 20 to 30%	Normal excretion	Normal	Structural Unknown Albuminuria Yes		Progress to clinically overt in 30-40% patients
III. Incipient Nephropathy	After 10-15 years	Not well defined	Increase 20 to 30%	Moderatly Increased	Incipient increase	Structural Unknown Albuminuria Yes		Manage risk factors
IV. Overt Nephropathy	After 15-20 years	Nodular sclerosis Capsular drops Arteriolar hyalinosis	Decline 1ml/month	Severe and progressive Increase	Hypertensive	No		Delay progression
V. End Stage Renal disease	After 25-30 years Final outcome	Glomerular global esclerosis	<15 ml/min	Slight decline	Hypertensive	No		Renal replacement

Fig. 55.2 Diabetic nephropathy. (Adapted and modified from Mogensen CE, Christensen CK, and Vittinghus E of the incipient diabetic nephropathy. 1983;32(June))

Early Hypertrophy and Hyperfunction (Hyperfiltration)

Structural, biochemical, and renal function changes are described. Within the structural anomalies, the most remarkable is the increased growth of both kidneys. Such phenomenon is a consequence of tubular hypertrophy and interstitial expansion related to SGLT-2 increased glucose reabsorption along with sodium and water. Hyperglycemia enhances nitric oxide, TFG-B1, CTGF, VEGF, and angiotensin II [1]. Such biochemical environment dilates the afferent arteriole and closes the efferent arteriole, leaving the glomerulus without appropriate autoregulation. The latter allows an elevated intra-glomerular pressure with an enforced 20–40% increase in GFR, a phenomenon known as renal hyperfiltration [2, 3]. Aside from hyperfiltration, dilation of afferent arteriole allows systemic arterial pressure to reflect directly on the glomerulus, further increasing glomerular stress and hyperfiltration effect.

All the abovementioned mechanisms are clinically silent since the main clinical features used to diagnose DKD (GFR and albuminuria) are absent at this stage. Nonetheless, when diabetic patients in this stage of nephropathy exercise with

a ≥ 55% of the maximum expected heart rate (MEHR), they develop albuminuria. This is a lower threshold when compared to nondiabetic healthy individual, where ≥65% of MEHR is needed to start with some degree of albuminuria [3].

Up to this stage of nephropathy, hyperfiltration and exercise-induced albuminuria are reversible by glycemic control within 6 days [3], a fact that further emphasizes that kidney damage from diabetes comes from a long-standing process.

Silent Nephropathy (Glomerular Lesion Without Clinical Disease)

Diabetic patients remain in this stage for many years, without decrease in GFR of development of albuminuria in a steady state. Nonetheless, 30–40% of this group of patients will progress to overt diabetic nephropathy due to multiple histopathologic anomalies established through the glomeruli, tubule-interstitium, and blood vessels. Most remarkable modifications are thickening of the glomerular basal membrane, mesangial expansion, glomerulosclerosis, interstitial inflammation, and fibrosis [2].

Incipient Diabetic Nephropathy

Timeline for this stage corresponds to approximately 10–15 years of diabetic disease, and it is expected in about one-third of diabetic patients. The main characteristic of this phase is the onset and consistency of moderately increased albuminuria in the range between 30 and 300 mg/day. Likewise, steady increase of blood pressure adds on to the development of albuminuria at a rate of about 3 mmHg/year until overt hypertension is detected [2]. Type 1 diabetic patients with mild (<30 mg/day), moderate (30–300 mg/day), and severe (>300 mg/day) albuminuria have a prevalence of hypertension of 42%, 52%, and 79%, respectively. For type 2 diabetic patients, the same categories have a hypertension prevalence of 71%, 90%, and 93% [36].

When albuminuria is found within the first 5 years on new-onset diabetes in the absence of diabetic retinopathy and in the presence of nephrotic syndrome or accelerated loss of kidney function, a biopsy should be considered to rule out other causes of kidney disease other than diabetes.

Evolution of diabetic nephropathy up to this stage is most often accompanied by obesity, hyperuricemia, tobacco use, and noncontrolled hypertension. Treatment of the former entities along with glycemic control may lead to reverse albuminuria and its associated cardiovascular risk.

Overt Diabetic Nephropathy

This phase describes what it is now known as diabetic nephropathy syndrome: decreased GFR, increased proteinuria, and systemic hypertension. This stage's timeline is about 15–20 years after the diagnosis of diabetes mellitus and 30–40% of those who had diabetic renal involvement with progress up to this point. Structural and functional anomalies are irreversible, systemic hypertension is usually present and is the most damaging entity to kidney function, and there is a progressive decline of GFR at an approximate rate of 1 mL/min/month without medical treatment.

End-Stage Renal Failure

Within 25–30 years of diabetes mellitus evolution, end-stage renal disease is expected in those patients who had renal involvement. Clinical picture is not different from any other patient in this stage of kidney disease.

New Findings in the Natural History of Diabetic Nephropathy

The evolution of diabetic nephropathy has now changed. Most patients do not evolve without medical and pharmacological interventions seeking to control progression of disease. The most dramatic change in the natural history described by Mogensen et al. is the possibility to withhold progression of albuminuria from mild to moderate or severe and even when the former and the latter are established and achieve complete remission [39, 40]. Albuminuria evolution has changed since the widespread use of ACE inhibitors and ARBs; further body of knowledge is growing in the field of SGLT-2 receptor antagonists. Different phenotypes of diabetic nephropathy had been postulated, such as the non-albuminuric diabetic nephropathy (Fig. 55.3). However, despite the absence of albuminuria, some patients continue to lose GFR through time. The former evidence has led to new perspectives on the natural history of diabetic nephropathy in the light of comorbidities such as hypertension, obesity, ageing, and pharmacologic treatment. Four different phenotypes have been proposed [41]:

(a) Classical Diabetic Kidney Disease

This group fit into the classical natural history of diabetic kidney disease which resembles Mogensen's work the most, before generalized glucose-lowering and pressure-lowering treatments. Patients develop progressive glomerular hyperfiltration and a linear increment in albuminuria with a linear decline in glomerular filtration rate until kidney failure.

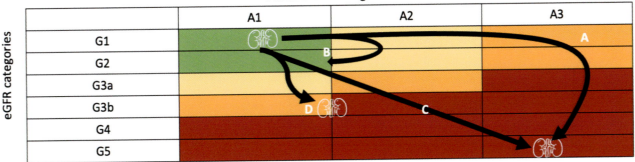

Fig. 55.3 New paradigm of diabetic nephropathy. Diabetic kidney disease trajectories. (**a**) Classic diabetic nephropathy. (**b**) Regression of albuminuria. (**c**) Rapid decliner. (**d**) Non-proteinuria/albuminuric DKD.

(Adapted and modified from Oshima M, Shimizi M, Yamanouchi M. Trajectories of kidney function in diabetes: a clinicopathological update. Nat Rev. Neph. 2021)

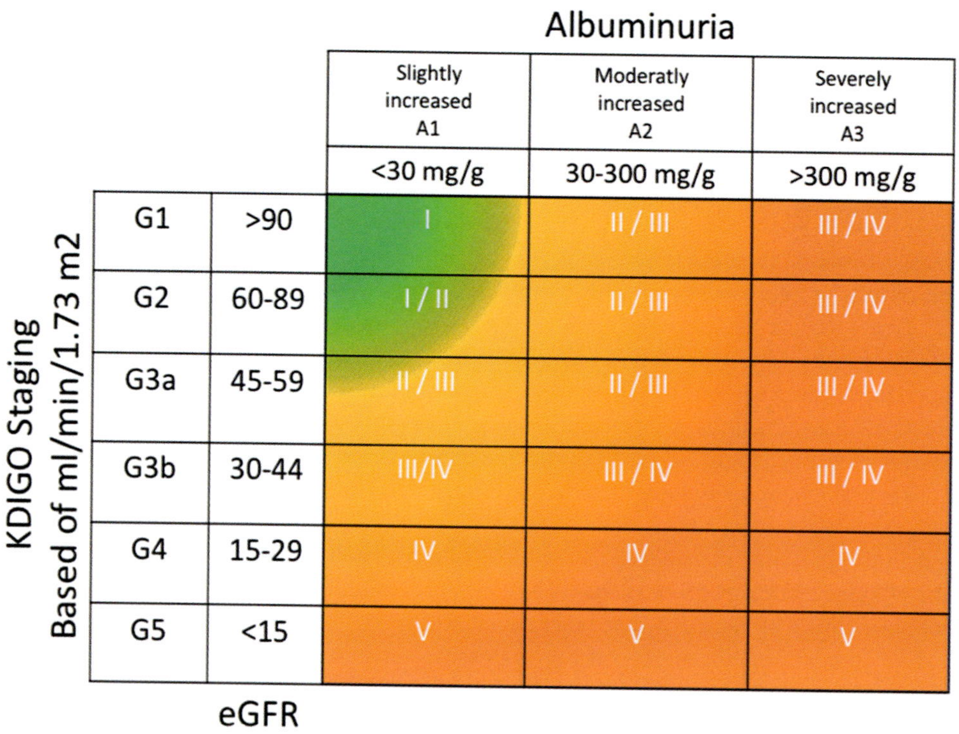

Fig. 55.4 Overlap between KDIGO CKD classification Mogensen's diabetic kidney disease natural history. M = Mogensen's classification stage. G = KDIGO CKD staging. A = Albuminuria. (Adapted and modified: Improving Global Outcomes (KDIGO) CKD Work Group. KDIGO 2012 Clinical practice guideline for the evaluation and management of chronic kidney disease. Kidney inter., Suppl. 2013; 3: 1–150)

Fig. 55.4 Overlap between KDIGO CKD classification Mogensen's diabetic kidney disease natural history. M = Mogensen's classification stage. G = KDIGO CKD staging. A = Albuminuria. (Adapted and modified: Improving Global Outcomes (KDIGO) CKD Work Group. KDIGO 2012 Clinical practice guideline for the evaluation and management of chronic kidney disease. Kidney inter., Suppl. 2013; 3: 1–150)

(b) Regression of Albuminuria

In the current era of generalized metabolic treatment, it has been shown in different populations that a switch and regression from moderate and severe albuminuria to normoalbuminuria may occur, with improvement of blood pressure and glycemia along with renin-angiotensin-aldosterone blockade and inhibition of sodium-glucose cotransporters. Different studies have shown a lower decline in glomerular filtration rate and lower progression to kidney failure and initiation of dialysis.

(c) Rapid Decliner

A rapid GFR decline is defined as a loss of ≥ 5 mL/min/1.73 m^2/year regardless of albuminuria degree. It has been hypothesized that this group may correspond to combined entities that coexist in the patient, such as tubulointerstitial diseases or a formerly damaged kidney on top of which DKD develops. Progression to kidney failure is develop in short period of time.

(d) Non-proteinuric/Non-albuminuric

The prevalence of this phenotype is around 20% for DM1 and up to 40% in DM2. Clinical characteristics for this group are female gender, hypertension, smoking, absence of diabetic retinopathy, and pharmacologic treatment with RAAS blockade. Also, a slower progression of GFR loss and kidney failure had been shown.

Natural History and KDIGO Classification

The KDIGO classification is the most widely used and accepted CKD classification. We propose an overlapping fig-

ure merging Mogensen's described natural history and KDIGO CKD progression (Fig. 55.4).

Nephropathology

Biopsy Adequacy

As for elemental histopathology recommendations, biopsy core should contain at least 12 full glomeruli. For light microscopy, tissue section must be within 2–3 micrometers thick; two slides must be assigned to H&E, two more for PAS stain, one for Masson trichrome, and one for Jone's silver methenamine. As for direct immunofluorescence, non-fixated tissue is recommended to perform frozen sections and incubate with immunoreactants: IgG, IgA, IgM, C1q, C3c, C4c, fibrinogen, albumin, kappa, and lambda. Finally, a small cortex fraction should be fixed in 2.5% glutaraldehyde for electron microscopy. This last technique is quite useful to characterize and differentiate within nondiabetic lesion on top of diabetic damage.

Histology

According to the Renal Pathology Society [40, 42], diabetic nephropathy is described by light microscopy, through four glomerular stages (Table 55.1); interstitial and vascular affections are also described (Table 55.2).

As for the mentioned stages and findings, we consider the following:

Table 55.1 Glomerular classification of diabetic nephropathy based on light microscopy

Class	Description	Criteria
I	Mild or nonspecific changes and EM-proven GBM thickening	Biopsy does not meet criteria for any other class below GMB in EM is >395 nm in females and > 430 nm in males[a]
IIa	Mild mesangial expansion	Biopsy does not meet criteria for classes III and IV Mild mesangial expansion in >25% of the observed mesangium
IIb	Severe mesangial expansion	Biopsy does not meet criteria for classes III and IV Severe mesangial expansion in >25% of the observed mesangium
III	Nodular sclerosis (Kimmelstiel-Wilson lesion)	Biopsy does not meet criteria for class IV At least one convincing Kimmelstiel-Wilson lesion
IV	Advanced diabetic glomerulosclerosis	Global glomerulosclerosis in >50% of glomeruli Lesion from classes I through III to be present

EM electron microscopy, *GBM* glomerular basal membrane
As described by Tervaert TWC, Mooyaart AL, Amann K, Cohen AH, Cook HT, and Drachenberg CB et al. Pathologic classification of diabetic nephropathy. J Am Soc Nephrol. 2010;21 (4):556–63
aIndividuals to be 9 years old of age or older

Table 55.2 Interstitial and vascular lesions of diabetic nephropathy described by light microcopy

Lesion	Criteria	Score
Interstitial lesion	No IFTA	0
	<25% IFTA	1
	25–50% IFTA	2
	>50% IFTA	3
Interstitial inflammation	Absent	0
	Infiltration only in IFTA	1
	Infiltration outside IFTA	2
Vascular lesions		
Arterial hyalinosis	Absent	0
	A least one area of arteriolar hyalinosis	1
	More than one area of arteriolar hyalinosis	2
Presence of large vessel?	*Yes/no*	
Arteriolosclerosis (score by worst artery)	No intimal thickening	0
	Intimal thickening less than thickness of media	1
	Intimal thickening greater than thickness of media	2

As described by Tervaert TWC, Mooyaart AL, Amann K, Cohen AH, Cook HT, and Drachenberg CB et al. Pathologic classification of diabetic nephropathy. J Am Soc Nephrol. 2010;21 (4):556–63

Stage 1. Early morphologic changes develop within the first 5 years of disease and affect glomerular basal membrane but can only be recognized at EM level. These findings correspond to simultaneous thickening and scarring of GBM, tertiary podocyte process effacement, and some focal podocytopenia. As diabetes continue to evolve, GBM accumulate type IV collagen, laminin, and fibronectin leading to double or triple length of its original width. The former thickening damages filtration barrier by direct endothelial damage and fenestral loss. Fibrin and fibrinogen begin to deposit in the subendothelium. At this point, first light microscopy findings are visible through PAS and Jones' methenamine stains, which reveal the important thickening of GBM. Simultaneously, microaneurysms and membrane remodeling as folding and laminated areas even focally duplicated membranes (Fig. 55.5).

Stage 2. After damage has been established at GMB, as a result of direct AGE effect, mesangium begins to accumulate extracellular matrix and leads to mesangiosclerosis. Early mesangiosclerosis is focal and involves only some glomerular segments; progression leads to global and diffuse mesangium replacement which end up in increased size and hyperlobulation.

Stage 3. Most characteristic diabetic kidney disease histologic findings correspond to this stage. Kimmelstiel-Wilson's nodular lesions are appreciated. These lesions are the result of diffuse mesangiosclerosis and microthrombi within the endothelium of dysfunctional microaneurysms. Microthrombi are constantly and chronically produced and reabsorbed, leading to collagen deposits in a laminated manner which finally generates a typical peripheral acellular nodule in the glomerular tuft. It is also common to find in former microaneurysm areas and foam appearance of endothelial and endocapillary cells. Such findings are known as "insudative lesions," a result of intracapillary pressure that manifests as "subcapsular drops," "fibrotic caps," and areas of hyalinosis, all of which share the same physiopathologic nature (Fig. 55.6).

Stage 4. Global sclerosis, nodular structures, and areas of hyalinosis characterize this stage. When more than 90% of the glomeruli present the mentioned findings, advanced interstitial fibrosis and tubular atrophy (IFTA), along with vascular damage, are common (Fig. 55.7). This is the final stage of cumulative damage and results not only of metabolic injury but also from chronic ischemia after vessels develop nodular hyalinosis, sclerosis, tunica media hypertrophy, and tunica intima fibrotic obliteration.

Nowadays, immunofluorescence and immunohistochemistry are considered as part of routine assessment of kidney biopsy (Fig. 55.8). As previously stated, 5 mm of non-fixed renal cortex is desirable for frozen cuts. If the latter is not feasible, the study can be performed from tissue out of the paraffin block, which even though is useful; it must be pointed out that such technique is less sensitive than frozen cuts without fixation.

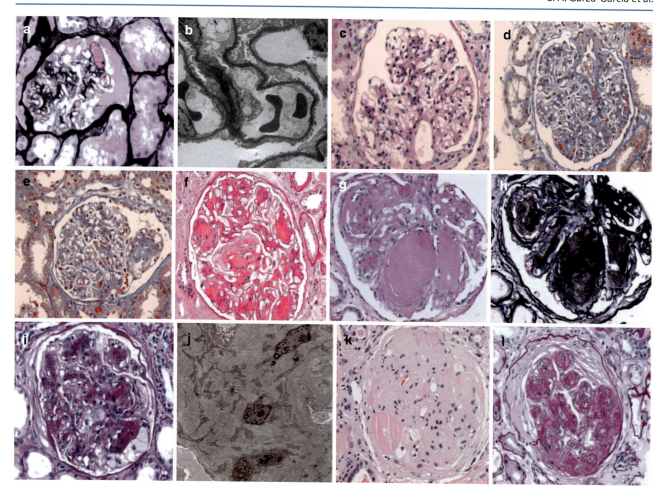

Fig. 55.5 Microphotography showing the different types of diabetic glomerular damage, based on RPS classification. (**a**) Jones Methenamine 40× illustrates a glomeruli with basal membrane irregularities and a microaneurysm. (**b**) Electron microscopy at 2000×, diffuse and homogenous thickening of basal glomerular membrane (RPS Class I). (**c**) PAS 40×, low-moderate expansion of mesangial matrix-generating mesangiosclerosis (Class IIA, RPS). (**d**) Masson's Trichrome 40×, diffuse and homogeneous mesangial thickening, causing glomerular hyperlobulation (Class IIB, RPS). (**e–g**) Microphotography with Masson's Trichrome, PAS [2] and Jones methenamine, respectively. Each at 40×, different stages of acellular collagen forming nodular structures (Class III RPS). (**h**) Residual microaneurysms with endothelial edema within capillary loops, a frequent type of damage in advanced stages of DM. (**i**) Electron microscopy with diffuse collagen deposits within mesangium, characteristic finding in diabetic damage. (**j–l**) H&E and PAS staining, each at 40×, globally sclerosed glomeruli with the presence of hyaline nodules; these findings correspond to DM. When found in most of the glomeruli, it corresponds to Class IV RPS (advanced sclerosis)

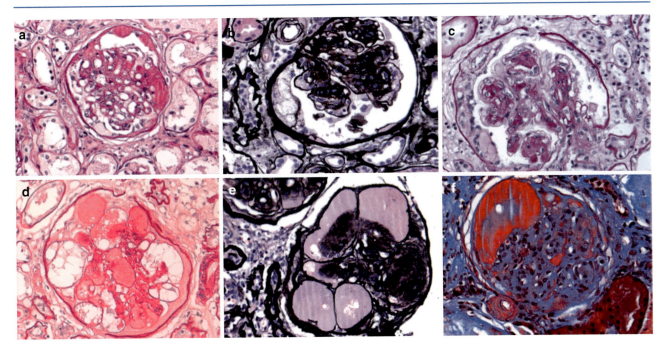

Fig. 55.6 Glomerular insudative lesion. Frequently found in diabetic nephropathy: (**a**) PAS 40×, subcapsular gout, Bowman's capsule-dependent lesion. (**b** and **c**) PAS 40×, fibrous casquet. (**d–f**) PAS, Jones methenamine and Masson's Trichrome, respectively. Each at 40× showing glomerular hyalinosis

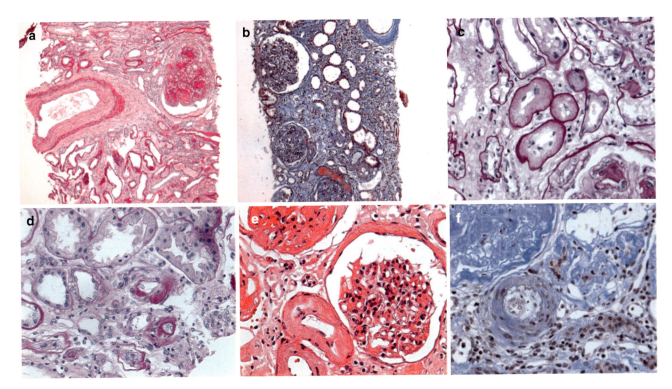

Fig. 55.7 Tubulointerstitial lesions, part of diabetic nephropathy with outmost relevance for renal function prognosis. (**a** and **b**), PAS and Masson's Trichrome 10×, tubulointerstitial fibrosis with loss of tubular "back-to-back" pattern; small caliber arteries present fibrotic damage within arterial intima. (**c**) PAS 40×, lamination and thickening of tubu- lar basal membranes along with atrophic changes. (**d–f**) Microvascular lesions in arterioles, PAS, H&E, and Masson's Trichrome, respectively, each at 40×. Advanced arteriolopathy with complete occlusion of vascular lumen. This finding often leads to chronic ischemic glomerular damage and vessel wall hyalinosis, on top of diabetic damage

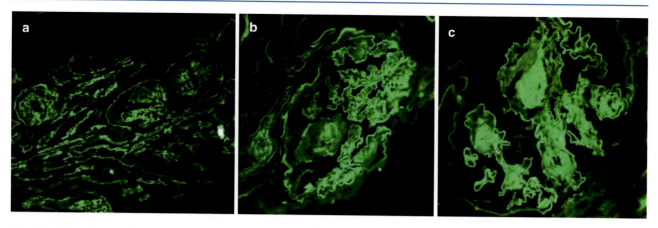

Fig. 55.8 Direct Immunofluorescence in diabetic nephropathy: (**a–c**) Albumin 10× and 40× and IgG 40×, respectively. Hyperfiltration generates linear positivity in glomerular and tubular basal membranes. Albumin shows tubular cytoplasmic reabsorption vacuoles

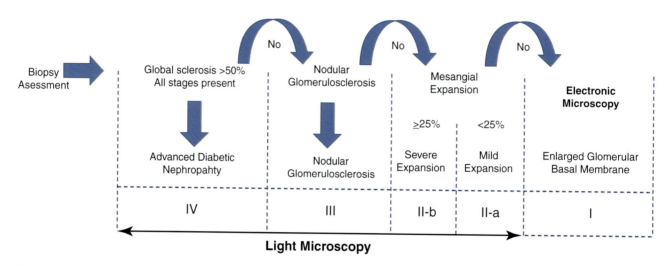

Fig. 55.9 Proposed assessment of kidney biopsy in diabetic nephropathy. (Adapted and modified from as described by Tervaert TWC, Mooyaart AL, Amann K, Cohen AH, Cook HT, and Drachenberg CB et al. Pathologic classification of diabetic nephropathy. J Am Soc Nephrol. 2010;21 (4):556–63)

Tissue out of paraffin block can also be used for indirect immunoperoxidase technique, although with the paramount disadvantage of a less sensitive study.

Diabetic kidney disease continuum implies that histopathologic lesions will not be all at the same stage. A collage of microscopic lesions, from incipient to advanced, will be found. Prevailing histologic findings and the clinical picture ultimately lead to classification, considering an orderly mannered approach by glomerular, interstitial, and vascular findings. It should be emphasized that, being diabetes mellitus such a common entity, it is not uncommon to describe diabetic nephropathy on top of many other nondiabetic entities.

Advanced IFTA is considered the histologic manifestation of end-stage renal disease. As to vessel histology, even though the Renal Pathology Society classification does not make distinction between afferent and efferent arteriolar hyalinosis, it is considered that efferent arteriolar hyalinosis is the most specific vessel finding for diabetic nephropathy, since involvement of the afferent arteriole (afferent arterial hyalinosis) might be present in other entities.

We proposed a flowchart for the evaluation of DKD in kidney biopsy (Fig. 55.9).

It is important to stand out that KDIGO (Kidney Disease: Improving Global Outcomes) 2021 guidelines have proposed the distinction between diabetic nephropathies in which, based on histology, we can affirm such diagnosis. All other cases in which diabetes, albuminuria/proteinuria, and/or diminish glomerular filtration rate are present but without histologic tissue to claim diabetic nephropathy, should be named as diabetic kidney disease (DKD) [43].

Prevention of Diabetic Nephropathy

Avoiding the development of diabetic nephropathy involves treatment of diabetes per se. Glycemic control, antihypertension therapy, and dyslipidemia management are common and comorbid entities that directly impact on the evolution to diabetic nephropathy. However, this is beyond the scope of this chapter, and we will focus specifically on DKD management.

Treatment of Diabetic Nephropathy

Non-pharmacologic Intervention

Salt Intake

Salt intake is associated with increased blood pressure, and therefore, it is considered a risk factor for uncontrolled hypertension and end organ damage with DKD progression. In a systematic review and meta-analysis, by pooling studies with salt reduction in type 1 and type 2 diabetic patients, 13 trials and 254 individuals were included. Mean duration of salt restriction was 1 week for both types of diabetic patients, and median reduction of urinary sodium was 11.9 g/day for type 1 diabetic patients and 7.3 g/day for type 2 diabetic patients. Blood pressure was reduced by −7.11 systolic and −3.13 diastolic mmHg in individuals with type 1 diabetes and −6.90 systolic and −2.87 diastolic mmHg in individuals with type 2 diabetes. The impact of this intervention was considered as effective as the use of one antihypertension medication, and as such, it should be applied to all diabetic patients [44].

Besides salt restriction effect on hypertension, renal and cardiovascular benefits have been described for reduced salt intake in addition to RAAS blockade. The former was described in a pooled analysis of type 2 diabetic patients of RENAAL (Reduction of Endpoints in NIDDM with the Angiotensin II Antagonist Losartan) and IDNT (Irbesartan Diabetic Nephropathy Trial) trials. The former analysis included 1177 participants with established DKD assigned to angiotensin receptor blocker therapy, losartan for RENAAL or irbesartan for IDNT populations, or non-RAAS inhibitors (non-RAASi), further stratified according to urine sodium/creatinine ratio into tertiles of <121 mmol/g (<2.78 g of sodium, <6.05 g of salt), 121–153 mmol/g (2.78–3.51 g of sodium, 6.05–7.65 g of salt), and equal or ≥153 mmol/g. Renal outcomes were defined as a composite of doubling serum creatinine from baseline, serum creatinine ≥6.0 mg/dL, and need for chronic dialysis or transplantation. Cardiovascular outcomes were defined as a composite of death, myocardial infarction, stroke, hospitalization for heart failure, or revascularization procedures. Within ARB and RAASi groups, renal outcomes for ARB therapy in the lower tertile of sodium/creatinine urine ratio had a HR 0.57 (95% CI 0.39–0.84) vs. non RAASi in higher tertile with HR 1.37 (95% CI 0.96–1.96), $P < 0.001$. Same groups for cardiovascular outcomes reported HR 0.65 (95% CI 0.43–0.92) versus HR 1.25 (95% CI 0.89–1.75), $P = 0.021$. Significant difference for renal and cardiovascular endpoints disappeared between groups when comparing high urine sodium/creatinine ratio tertiles [45].

The former illustrates sodium restriction which enhances the renal and cardiovascular benefits of angiotensin receptor antagonism on type 2 diabetic population with DKD.

Protein Restriction

Protein overload hastens renal decline by different mechanisms. Pancreas responds to protein ingestion by increasing glucagon secretion; glucagon generates afferent arteriole vasodilation and increases systemic hemodynamics over the glomerulus. Along with the former, filtrated amino acids are reabsorbed by the proximal convoluted tube with sodium and chloride, which reduces the chloride available to the juxtaglomerular apparatus. The latter leads to the absence of tubuloglomerular feedback, further increasing afferent arteriole dilation. Finally, protein overload to the renal parenchyma, in a low renal mass stage, increases profibrotic cytokines, such as transforming growth factor beta-1 and platelet-derived growth factor [46].

Due to the former mentioned mechanisms of action, low protein diet (LPD, 0.6–0.8 g/kg of body weight/day) was proposed as a therapeutic intervention and proved to be effective in animal models along with nondiabetic kidney disease clinical trials [47]. Therefore, recommendation of LPD was extended to DKD by KDIGO (Kidney Disease Improving Global Outcomes) guidelines [47]. Nonetheless, in diabetic kidney disease, evidence is less clear; there are clinical trials and pooled meta-analysis both pro and against LPD as an effective intervention to slow kidney function decline [46, 47]. A definitive evidence-based recommendation cannot be established.

Interesting proposals are being considered such as starting LPD in eGFR higher than 30 mL/min/1.73 m^2 to preserve eGFR in earlier stages and to avoid malnourishment frequently seen in advanced CKD due to protein energy wasting. In addition, it has been proposed that maintaining or increasing caloric intake and switching carbohydrate, protein, and fat proportions could be of further benefit [46–49].

Pharmacologic Interventions

Renin-Angiotensin-Aldosterone System (RAS)

There is a large body of evidence to back up the use of RAS blockade in DKD being the cornerstone of DKD therapy. ACE inhibitors and ARBs have earned this position due to their positive effect on glomerular filtration preservation, reduction in the development, and progression of proteinuria along with lowering interstitial fibrosis. ACE inhibitors and ARBs are used indistinctly as their effect on the RAS system is directed toward decreasing its activation, even though most of the available evidence for ACE inhibitors is related to type 1 diabetes and for ARBs to type 2 diabetes.

Physiologic explanation of their benefit comes from their effect in systemic and glomerular hemodynamics, by decreasing not only systemic blood pressure but also by decreasing vasoconstriction on efferent arteriole and reducing direct pressure over the glomerulus. The former effect reduces the hyperfiltration phenomenon and clinically translates into GFR preservation and avoidance of proteinuria development, progression, or even regression.

The former was demonstrated in type 1 diabetics in the Collaborative Study Group, where 207 patients received captopril 25 mg three times a day and 202 patients placebo, to a blood pressure goal of ≤140/90 mmHg with a 3-year follow-up. Inclusion criteria corresponded to proteinuria (defined as ≥500 mg per day) and serum creatinine (SCr) of ≤2.5 mg/dL; the primary outcome was doubling of the serum creatinine. By the end of the study, 25 patients in the captopril group and 43 patients in the placebo group had reached the primary outcome, with 48% risk reduction for the captopril group. Subgroup analysis demonstrated that the effect of captopril on outcomes was higher in individuals with increased serum creatinine concentration, 76% for mean SCr 2.0 mg/dL, 55% for mean SCr 1.5 mg/dL, and 17% for 1.0 mg/dL. From the eGFR standpoint, decline in creatinine clearance was 11+/− 21% in captopril group and 17+/−20% in the placebo group ($p = 0.03$) [50].

As for anti-proteinuric effect, a systematic review and meta-analysis that included 646 type 1 diabetic patients (10 clinical trials) with normotensive and moderate increased albuminuria DKD evaluated ACE inhibitor therapy against placebo for this outcome. Reduction in progression to severe albuminuria was reported with an odds ratio of 0.38 (95% CI 0.25–0.57) and regression to low-level albuminuria by 3.07 (95% CI 2.15–4.44). Follow-up at 2 years found 50.5% lower albuminuria in ACE inhibitor-treated patients, compared to placebo ($p < 0.001$) with effect none entirely explained by blood pressure control [51].

In type 2 diabetes, effect of RAS blockade by ARBs also demonstrated reduction in the development and progression of proteinuria along with reduction in GFR decline. The preventing microalbuminuria in type 2 diabetes study (BENEDICT [Bergamo Nephrologic Diabetes Complications Trial]) assessed onset and development of moderately increased albuminuria (primary endpoint) in normoalbuminuric, hypertensive, type 2 diabetic patients. The intervention consisted of a combination of ACEI (trandolapril) and cal-

cium channel blocker (verapamil), either ACEI or calcium channel blocker alone or placebo. Target blood pressure for all participants was 120/80 mmHg, and other antihypertensive medications were allowed to goal. The trial recruited 1204 participants, with a median follow-up of 3.6 years; primary outcome (moderately increased albuminuria) was reached by 5.7% of participants in the combined treatment group, 6.0% in only ACEI group, 11.9% of those receiving calcium channel blocker alone, and in 10% of participant in the placebo group.

In established DKD, a multicentric, randomized, double-blinded, placebo-controlled trial with irbesartan recruited 590 patients with type 2 diabetes and moderately increased albuminuria, assigned groups to placebo, irbesartan 150 mg/day or irbesartan 300 mg/day, with a 2-year follow-up for a primary outcome of severely increased albuminuria or at least 30% increase from baseline. In the intervention arms, 5.2% of patients (10/194) for the 300 mg irbesartan group and 9.7% of patients (9/195) for the 150 mg irbesartan group reached primary outcome, as compared to 14.9% of patients (30/201) in the placebo arm resulting in 70% reduction in albuminuria progression for intervention groups [52]. Regarding GFR, the RENAAL study gathered 1513 patients with type 2 diabetes and randomized to losartan 50 mg, 100 mg, or placebo on top of conventional antihypertensive medication, for a 3.4-year follow-up. Primary outcome was a composite of doubling serum creatinine, and development of end-stage renal disease or death. Secondary outcomes were a composite of morbidity and mortality from cardiovascular causes, proteinuria, and the rate of progression of renal disease. Primary composite was reduced by 16%, double of serum creatinine by 25%, development of end-stage renal disease by 28%, and proteinuria declined by 35% in the losartan groups. There was no effect on mortality [53].

Given the former mentioned data, and many other studies sustaining similar results, double blockade with ACE inhibitor and ARB was explored to obtain more effective results on renal outcomes. The ONTARGET (Ongoing Telmisartan Alone in Combination with Ramipril Global Endpoint Trial) study disregarded the benefit of combined therapy. Such treatment proved increased adverse effects as a composite of need for acute dialysis, double of serum creatinine, and death. The first two endpoints of the composite sustained in individual analysis [54].

Another study to assess the benefit from double blockade in DKD was the Combined Angiotensin Inhibition for the Treatment of Diabetic Nephropathy (VA Nephron-D), which assigned standard baseline therapy of losartan 100 mg per day and randomized participants to lisinopril 10–40 mg per day or placebo. Primary endpoint was eGFR decline, ESRD, and death; secondary endpoint was defined as first occurrence of eGFR decline or ESRD, and safety outcomes were mortality, hyperkalemia, and acute kidney injury. A total of 1448 type 2 diabetic patients with severely increased albuminuria and an eGFR within 30 and 89.9 mL/min/1.73 m² were included and followed for median of 2.2 years. The study was stopped early for significant increased adverse effects in double RAS inhibition groups: hyperkalemia (6.3 events/100 person-years vs. 2.6 events/100 person-years, $p < 0.001$) and acute kidney injury (12.2 vs. 6.7 events/100 person-years, $P < 0.001$) [55].

Aldosterone antagonism has become a valuable tool in the management of chronic kidney disease, for up to 53% of patients on conventional RAS blockade will develop aldosterone escape phenomenon by the end of a 1-year therapy [56]. Compared to ACE inhibitors or ARBs alone, nonselective aldosterone blockade (spironolactone) on top of ACE inhibitors or ARBs significantly reduced 24 h proteinuria [57]. Narrowing to DKD, systematic review and meta-analysis of 7 trials (287 patients) compared ACEI or ARB versus combination therapy of MRA (spironolactone or eplerenone) plus ACEI or ARB. Results showed significantly reduced albuminuria excretion by 69.38% (95% CI -103.53 to −35.22, $p < 0.0001$). As for blood pressure, comparing 296 patients with combined MRA RAS blockade therapy versus 281 patients with RAS blockade alone, significantly decreased systolic and diastolic values were reported, with mean difference − 5.61 (95% CI -9.38 to −1.84, $p = 0.004$) for systolic and − 2.17 (95% CI -4.23 to −0.11, $p = 0.04$) for diastolic blood pressure [57]. In 11 trials pooling within this meta-analysis, GFR did not improve, and as expected, hyperkalemia developed much more (16 studies, 1684 patients) with relative risk of 3.74 (95% CI 2.30–6.09, $p < 00001$) [56].

Summarizing the former evidence, RAS blockade, for which ACEI and ARB have been used interchangeably, is the cornerstone therapy for diabetic kidney disease both in type 1 and 2 diabetes. RAS blocking therapy impacts on the reduction of albuminuria, preservation of GFR, and lowering of fibrotic remodeling. MRA with spironolactone on top of RAS blockade compensates for aldosterone breakthrough, and its major effect is reflected over proteinuria and blood pressure control.

Novel Therapies

Sodium Glucose Transporters

Hyperglycemia induces the proximal convoluted tubule to increase glucose claim, the former is performed in company of sodium, by means of sodium-glucose transporters 1 and 2 (SGLT-1 and SGLT-2, respectively). This leads to a lesser available sodium to be sensed downstream by the macula densa, and as a result, afferent glomerular arteriole is dilated, exposing the glomerulus to direct blood pressure damage while enhancing hyperfiltration phenomenon. Inhibition of sodium-glucose transporters leads to glucosuria and downstream sodium overflow, allowing actual caloric/glucose loss as a desired effect for diabetes treatment in addition to activation of tubule-glomerular feedback.

If we combine RAS blockade with SGLT-2 therapy, we obtain the exact opposite glomerular hemodynamics of diabetic kidney disease pathophysiology. The renal hemodynamics go from dilated afferent and narrowed efferent arterioles, with increased exposure to systemic blood pressure and hyperfiltration on the glomerulus, to a narrow afferent and dilated efferent arteriole, with the opposite effect.

The benefit from the former hypothesis has been tested with positive results in different cardiovascular and renal outcome studies for iSGLT-2. In EMPA-REG OUTCOME trial, type 2 diabetic patients with established cardiovascular disease and eGFR equal or greater than 30 mL/min/1.73 m² of BSA were randomly assigned to receive placebo, empagliflozin 10 mg/day, or 25 mg/day for a median duration of treatment of 2.6 years and median observation time of 3.1 years. RAS blockade, by means of ACEI or ARB, was present in 80.7% of study population at baseline. As for renal outcomes, incident or worsening nephropathy (progression to severely increased albuminuria) occurred in 12.7% in empagliflozin groups versus 18.8% in the placebo group, 0.61 (95% CI 0.53–0.70, $P = <0.001$). Doubling of serum creatinine with a decrease of eGFR to ≤45 mL/min/1.73 m² BSA was 1.5% versus 2.6% in empagliflozin and placebo, respectively, with a relative risk reduction of 44%. Renal replacement therapy was initiated in 13 of 4687 patients in empagliflozin and 14 of 2333 patients in the placebo group, with a relative risk reduction of 55%. Regarding incident albuminuria, there was no difference between medication and placebo groups. The composite of incident or worsening nephropathy or cardiovascular death had a HR for empagliflozin of 0.61 (95% CI 0.55–0.69, $p < 0.001$) [58].

Estimated GFR lowered during the first 4-week period trial in the empagliflozin arms to a mean of −0.82 ± 0.04 mL/min/1.73 m² of BSA for the 25 mg/day and was less evident for the 10 mg/day dose. Estimated GFR remained stable after such period, and mean eGFR annual decline for intervention groups was 0.19 ± 0.11 mL/min/1.73 m² BSA compared to 1.67 ± 0.13 mL/min/1.73 m² BSA in the placebo group, $p < 0.001$. After cessation of trial medication, empagliflozin groups increased eGFR up to 0.55 ± 0.04 mL/min/1.73 m² BSA, making evident the hemodynamic effect of the medication [58].

The Canagliflozin and Cardiovascular Events in Type 2 Diabetes (the CANVAS (Canagliflozin Cardiovascular Assessment Study) Program), another trial for SGLT-2 inhibition, included two sister trials, the CANVAS and CANVAS-R. Both studies were multicentric, double-blinded, randomized, and placebo-controlled. 10,142 DKD participants were assigned to canagliflozin 300 mg/day, 100 mg/day, or placebo for CANVAS and canagliflozin

100 mg/day (with option to increase up to 300 mg/day) or placebo for CANVAS-R. Primary outcome was a composite of death from cardiovascular cause, nonfatal myocardial infarction, and nonfatal stroke. Secondary outcomes were death from any cause, death from cardiovascular cause, progression of albuminuria (30% increase from baseline and category upgrade between normoalbuminuria and moderately or severely increased albuminuria), and another composite of death from cardiovascular cause and hospitalization for heart failure. The mean follow-up was 188.2 weeks. Canagliflozin group had statistically significant less composite of death from cardiovascular cause, nonfatal myocardial infarction, and nonfatal stroke, 26.9 participants per 1000 patient-years versus 31.5 for placebo (HR 0.86, 95% CI 0.75–0.97, $P < 0.001$ non-inferiority and $p = 0.02$ for superiority). Regarding renal outcomes, albuminuria progression was less frequent in intervention groups, 89.4 events per 1000 patient-years versus 128.7 for placebo (HR 0.73, 95% CI 0.67–0.79), along with regression of albuminuria, with 293.4 patients per 1000 patient-year for intervention groups versus 187.5 for placebo (HR 1.70, 95% CI 1.51–1.91). Renal composite of sustained 40% reduction in eGFR, the need for renal replacement therapy, or death from renal causes occurred less in intervention groups, 5.5 in canagliflozin versus 9.0 in placebo per 1000 patient-years (HR 0.60, 95% CI, 0.47–0.77). Death from any cause was not different between canagliflozin and placebo groups [59].

Dapagliflozin and Cardiovascular Outcomes in Type 2 Diabetes (DECLARE-TIMI 58) study randomized patients with type 2 diabetes who have or were at risk for atherosclerotic cardiovascular disease to dapagliflozin or placebo for primary outcomes of major adverse cardiovascular events (MACE) of cardiovascular death, myocardial infarction, or ischemic stroke, and secondary outcomes of renal composite composed of ≥40% decrease in eGFR to less than 60 mL/min/1.73 m^2 of BSA, new end-stage renal disease, death from renal or cardiovascular causes, and death of any cause. A total of 17,160 patients were evaluated, most of which did not have atherosclerotic cardiovascular disease, a primary prevention group of 10,186 patients. Patients were followed for a median of 4.2 years; dapagliflozin was non-inferior to placebo in MACE but did not achieve superiority. Only benefit in a composite of cardiovascular death or hospitalization for heart failure was found, with a 17% relative risk reduction at the expense of lower heart failure events, for there was no difference in cardiovascular events within groups [60].

CREDENCE (Canagliflozin and Renal Events in Diabetes with Established Nephropathy Clinical Evaluation). The goal of the trial was to assess the effect of canagliflozin on renal outcomes among patients with type 2 diabetes mellitus (DM2) and chronic kidney disease (CKD). Patients were randomized in a 1:1 fashion to either canagliflozin 100 mg daily ($n = 2202$) or matching placebo ($n = 2199$). Four thousand four-hundred patients were included with a mean follow-up of 2.62 years. The trial stopped early due to overwhelming benefit. The primary outcome of end-stage renal disease (ESRD), doubling of serum creatinine, and renal or cardiovascular (CV) death, for canagliflozin versus placebo, was 43.2 versus 61.2 per 1000 patient-years (P-Y) ($p = 0.00001$): doubling of serum creatinine, 20.7 versus 33.8/1000 P-Y ($p < 0.001$) for canagliflozin versus placebo, and ESRD, 20.4 versus 29.4/1000 P-Y ($p = 0.002$) for canagliflozin versus placebo [61].

DAPA-CKD (Dapagliflozin and Prevention of Adverse Outcomes in Chronic Kidney Disease). The DAPA-CKD trial was a multinational, multicenter, event-driven, randomized, double-blind, parallel-group, placebo-controlled study involving 4304 patients with CKD and eGFR ≥25 mL/min/1.73 m^2, but ≤75 mL/min/1.73 m^2, and a UACR ≥200 mg/g, but ≤5000 mg/g, with or without type 2 diabetes (T2D). As occurred in the CREDENCE trial, the trial was stopped early due to overwhelming efficacy. Over a median of 2.4 years, a primary outcome event occurred in 197 of 2152 participants (9.2%) in the dapagliflozin group and 312 of 2152 participants (14.5%) in the placebo group (hazard ratio, 0.61; 95% confidence interval [CI], 0.51–0.72; $P < 0.001$). The hazard ratio for the composite of a sustained decline in the estimated GFR of at least 50%, end-stage kidney disease, or death from renal causes was 0.56 (95% CI, 0.45–0.68; $P < 0.001$), and the hazard ratio for the composite of death from cardiovascular causes or hospitalization for heart failure was 0.71 (95% CI, 0.55–0.92; $P = 0.009$). For the first time, this trial demonstrated similar efficacy in subjects with and without diabetes [62].

EMPA-KIDNEY (Empagliflozin in Patients with Chronic Kidney Disease) is an ongoing trial to evaluate renal and cardiovascular outcomes in 6600 patients for the use of empagliflozin on CKD profession; different to other trials, EMPA-KIDNEY would include lower eGFR (CKD-EPI eGFR ≥20–<45 mL/min/1.73 m^2 or) and CKD-EPI eGFR ≥45–<90 mL/min/1.73 m^2 and lower urinary albumin/creatinine ratio ≥ 200 mg/g (or protein/creatinine ratio ≥ 300 mg/g) (Clinical Trial NCT03594110).

Considerations as to adverse effects of SGLT-2 inhibitors as a group include an increased risk for euglycemic ketoacidosis, perineum-necrotizing fasciitis, genitourinary tract infections, hypotension, and acute kidney injury. Medication-specific adverse effects have been described, as in canagliflozin-treated patients, increased incidence for bone fracture, and mid foot/toe amputations. Amputations occur more often in patients with lower-extremity peripheral artery disease and/or diabetic foot.

GLP1 Receptor Agonists (GLP1AR)

Cardiovascular outcome trials for GLP1AR in diabetic population have included chronic kidney disease patients. Data from these trials proved a favorable profile for lixisenatide, exenatide, liraglutide, semaglutide, albiglutide, and dulaglutide for decreasing in albuminuria and may have an effect in lowering eGFR decline rate. Meta-analysis of seven GLP1AR cardiovascular risk outcome trials pooled a 17% risk reduction compared to placebo for a renal composite of severely increased albuminuria, eGFR decline, progression to kidney failure, or death from kidney disease.

As for today, there has not been a completed GLP1RA kidney outcome trial. The Effect of Semaglutide Versus Placebo on the Progression of Renal Impairment in Subjects with Type 2 Diabetes and Chronic Kidney Disease (FLOW) trial started on 2019 and is expected to be completed by 2024 [63].

Finerenone

As previously mentioned, MRAs proved reduction in albuminuria for diabetic and nondiabetic CKD. Finerenone (FRN) is a more selective MRA than spironolactone, with more affinity than eplerenone. Finerenone was evaluated for DKD in the ARTS-DN study, a multicenter, randomized, double-blind, placebo-controlled, parallel group, phase 2B trial in which finerenone at different doses (1.25 mg/day, 2.5 mg/day, 5 mg/day, 7.5 mg/day, 10 mg/day, 15 mg/day, 25 mg/day) or placebo was administered to patients with DKD already on RAS blockade. Eligibility criteria were type 2 diabetic patients already on RAS blockade, with at least moderately increased albuminuria, eGFR ≥30 mL/min/1.73 m^2, first visit serum potassium concentration ≤ 4.8 mmol/L, and 4-week or longer stable non-potassium-sparing diuretic use. Endpoints were evaluation of albuminuria reduction at the end of the 90-day period and adverse effects such as hyperkalemia and eGFR reduction. Effect on albuminuria excretion rate (AER) was noticed in an increasing dose-dependent effect starting on finerenone 7.5 mg/day. Placebo-corrected mean ratios of AER, according to dose, were FRN 7.5 mg/day, 0.79 (90% CI 0.68–0.91, $p = 0.004$), FRN 10 mg/day, 0.76 (90% CI 0.65–0.88, $p = 0.001$), FRN 15 mg/day 0.67 (90% CI 0.58–0.77, $p < 0.001$), and FRN 20 mg/day 0.62 (90% CI 0.54–0.72, $p < 0.001$). Hyperkalemia was reported for the 7.5-, 15-, and 20 mg/day groups in 2.1%, 3.2%, and 1.7%, respectively. There was no difference in eGFR decrease rate of ≥30% [64].

This study suggests the potential benefit from finerenone as another MRA with a lesser adverse effect and dose-dependent effect on reducing albuminuria. Nonetheless, it must be noticed that on the trial, 60% of patients had eGFR of 60 mL/min/1.73 m^2 or more, and serum potassium higher than 4.8 mmol/L was considered an exclusion criteria. Hard endpoints such as cardiovascular events, progression to end-stage renal disease, and dialysis requirement are currently being explored; most recent studies in this regard are FIGARO (Facilitated Immunoglobulin Administration Registry and Outcomes Study) and FIDELIO (Finerenone in Reducing Kidney Failure and Disease Progression).

FIGARO was a double-blind, randomized study that explored cardiovascular outcomes for CKD population with type 2 diabetes treated with finerenone. Eligibility criteria required patients to have ACR of 30 to less than 300 mg/g, eGFR of 25–<90 mL/min per 1.73 m^2 (stage 2–4 CKD) or ACR of 30 to less than 5000 mg/g, and eGFR >60 mL/min per 1.73 m^2 (stage 1 or 2 CKD), both groups on top of maximum tolerated RAAS blockade. Primary outcome was time to event composite of death from cardiovascular causes, nonfatal myocardial infarction, nonfatal stroke, or hospitalization for heart failure. Secondary outcome was kidney failure, sustained decrease of ≥40% in eGFR from baseline, or death from renal causes. Randomization was 7437 patients to finerenone of placebo. Finerenone achieved during a 3.4-year median follow-up, 13% relative risk reduction in primary composite (HR 0.87; 95% CI 0.76–0.98, $P = 0.03$), and 13% relative risk reduction for secondary composite (HR 0.87; 95% CI 0.76–1.01) [65].

FIDELIO was a kidney outcome-driven study for finerenone in chronic kidney disease with type 2 diabetic patients. It was a randomized, double-blind, placebo-controlled trial with 1:1 assignment of 5734 patients to finerenone or placebo. Inclusion criteria were a composite of albumin to creatinine ratio (ACR) of 30 to less than 300 mg/g, eGFR of 25–<60 mL/min per 1.73 m^2 and diabetic retinopathy, or ACR of 300–500 mg/g and eGFR of 25–<75 mL/min per 1.73 m^2. All patients are on maximum tolerated dose of RAAS blockade. The primary outcome was a time-to-event composite of kidney failure, sustained decrease of ≥40% in eGFR from baseline, or death from renal causes. Secondary outcomes were death from cardiovascular causes, nonfatal myocardial infarction, nonfatal stroke, and hospitalization for heart failure. Results for finerenone after a 2.6-year of follow-up were a primary outcome relative risk reduction of 18% (HR 0.82, 95% CI 0.73–0.93; $P = 0.001$) and a secondary outcome relative risk reduction of 14% (HR 0.86, 95% CI 0.75–0.99, $P = 0.03$), lowering risks of progression for CKD and cardiovascular events compared to placebo [66].

Conclusions

Diabetic kidney disease remains the main cause of end-stage kidney failure in the world. Although mechanisms of disease are now better understood, the only accepted medical treatment for DKD is RAS inhibition. Despite this treatment, many patients still progress to kidney failure. Double RAS inhibition is no longer recommended based on two randomized trials. Newer agents such as SGLT-2 inhibitors, GLP1 receptor antagonists, and finerenone are novel and promising therapies that have modified the natural history of the disease. There is still lack of sufficient evidence to combine these agents; however, it is possible that targeting different pathways will result in improved outcomes.

Multiple Choice Questions

1. Which of the following structures must become damaged in order to develop albuminuria:
   (a) Distal collecting duct
   (b) **Glicocalix**
   (c) Juxtaglomerular apparatus
   (d) Urea counter current mechanism
2. The following pathways are responsible for the hyperfiltration mechanism:
   (a) Hexosamine pathway
   (b) Metabolic pathway
   (c) **Hemodynamic pathway**
   (d) Autophagy
3. Hyperfiltration develops in diabetic nephropathy by effect of which of the following:
   (a) Afferent arteriole vasoconstriction
   (b) **Efferent arteriole vasoconstriction**
   (c) Juxtaglomerular apparatus dysfunction
   (d) Glomerular basal membrane thickening
4. Nephropathology description of diabetic nephropathy is based on:
   (a) Electron microscopy description
   (b) Immunofluorescence description
   (c) **Light microscopy description**
   (d) Kimmelstiel-Wilson nodules
5. Earliest nephropathologic findings in diabetic nephropathy.
   (a) Mesangial expansion
   (b) Tubular atrophy
   (c) Interstitial fibrosis
   (d) **Glomerular basal membrane thickening**
6. Most effective treatment for established diabetic nephropathy is based on:
   (a) Endothelin receptor blockade
   (b) Protein restriction
   (c) Diuretic use
   (d) **Renin-angiotensin-aldosterone system blockade**
7. SGLT-2 inhibitor treatment produces which of the following hemodynamic effects in the glomerulus:
   (a) **Vasoconstriction of afferent arteriole**
   (b) Vasodilation of afferent arteriole
   (c) Vasodilation of efferent arteriole
   (d) Vasoconstriction of efferent arteriole
8. Mineralocorticoid antagonist therapy should be considered to compensate for which of the following:
   (a) Hyperfiltration phenomenon
   (b) Albuminuria
   (c) **Aldosterone breakthrough**
   (d) Diuretics hypokalemia effect
9. Overt diabetic nephropathy without treatment leads to glomerular filtration rate loss of.
   (a) **1 mL/min month**
   (b) 1 mL/min week
   (c) 1 mL/min year
   (d) 50% of baseline within first 6 months
10. Which of the following findings must be considered to perform kidney biopsy in diabetic patients
    (a) Development of albuminuria within the first 5 years of diabetes diagnosis
    (b) Development of albuminuria in absence of diabetic retinopathy
    (c) Development of nephrotic syndrome
    (d) **All the above**

References

1. Turner N, Lamiere N, Goldsmith DJ. Oxford textbook of clinical nephrology. 4th ed. Oxford: Oxford University Press; 2016.
2. Mogensen CE. Microalbuminuria, blood pressure and diabetic renal disease: origin and development of ideas. Diabetologia. 1999;42(3):263–85.
3. Mogensen CE, Christensen CK, Vittinghus E. The stages in diabetic renal disease. With emphasis on the stage of incipient diabetic nephropathy. Diabetes. 1983;32(Suppl 2):64–78.
4. Narres M, Claessen H, Droste S, Kvitkina T, Koch M, Kuss O, et al. The incidence of end-stage renal disease in the diabetic (compared to the non-diabetic) population: a systematic review. PLoS One. 2016;11(1):1–28.
5. Harjutsalo V, Groop P-H. Epidemiology and risk factors for diabetic kidney disease. Adv Chronic Kidney Dis. 2014;21(3):260–6.
6. Alicic RZ, Rooney MT, Tuttle KR. Diabetic kidney disease: challenges, progress, and possibilities. Clin J Am Soc Nephrol. 2017;12(12):2032–45.
7. Toth-Manikowski S, Atta MG. Diabetic kidney disease: pathophysiology and therapeutic targets. J Diabetes Res. 2015;2015:697010.
8. Benz K, Amann K. Endothelin in diabetic renal disease. Contrib Nephrol. 2011;172:139–48.
9. Brownlee M. Biochemistry and molecular cell biology of diabetic complications. Nature. 2001;414(6865):813–20.
10. Walton HA, Byrne J, Robinson GB. Studies of the permeation properties of glomerular basement membrane: cross-linking renders glomerular basement membrane permeable to protein. Biochim Biophys Acta. 1992;1138(3):173–83.
11. Forbes JM, Cooper ME, Oldfield MD, Thomas MC. Role of advanced glycation end products in diabetic nephropathy. J Am Soc Nephrol. 2003;14(8 Suppl 3):S254–8.

12. Raabe HM, Höpner JH, Notbohm H, Sinnecker GHG, Kruse K, Müller PK. Biochemical and biophysical alterations of the 7S and NC1 domain of collagen IV from human diabetic kidneys. Diabetologia. 1998;41(9):1073–9.

13. Fukami K, Yamagishi S-I, Ueda S, Okuda S. Role of AGEs in diabetic nephropathy. Curr Pharm Des. 2008;14(10):946–52.

14. Yang CW, Vlassara H, Peten EP, He CJ, Striker GE, Striker LJ. Advanced glycation end products up-regulate gene expression found in diabetic glomerular disease. Proc Natl Acad Sci U S A. 1994;91(20):9436–40.

15. Vlassara H, Striker LJ, Teichberg S, Fuh H, Li YM, Steffes M. Advanced glycation end products induce glomerular sclerosis and albuminuria in normal rats. Proc Natl Acad Sci U S A. 1994;91(24):11704–8.

16. Nagahama T, Hayashi K, Ozawa Y, Takenaka T, Saruta T. Role of protein kinase C in angiotensin II-induced constriction of renal microvessels. Kidney Int. 2000;57(1):215–23.

17. Ruan X, Arendshorst WJ. Role of protein kinase C in angiotensin II-induced renal vasoconstriction in genetically hypertensive rats. Am J Phys. 1996;270(6 Pt 2):F945–52.

18. Williams B, Schrier RW. Glucose-induced protein kinase C activity regulates arachidonic acid release and eicosanoid production by cultured glomerular mesangial cells. J Clin Invest. 1993;92(6):2889–96.

19. Noh H, King GL. The role of protein kinase C activation in diabetic nephropathy. Kidney Int Suppl. 2007;72(106):S49–53.

20. García-García PM, Getino-Melián MA, Domínguez-Pimentel V, Navarro-González JF. Inflammation in diabetic kidney disease. World J Diabetes. 2014;5(4):431–43.

21. Pickup JC. Inflammation and activated innate immunity in the pathogenesis of type 2 diabetes. Diabetes Care. 2004;27(3):813–23.

22. García-García PM. Inflammation in diabetic kidney disease. World J Diabetes. 2014;5(4):431.

23. Sanz AB, Sanchez-Niño MD, Ramos AM, Moreno JA, Santamaria B, Ruiz-Ortega M, et al. NF-kappaB in renal inflammation. J Am Soc Nephrol. 2010;21(8):1254–62.

24. Mezzano S, Aros C, Droguett A, Burgos ME, Ardiles L, Flores C, et al. NF-kappaB activation and overexpression of regulated genes in human diabetic nephropathy. Nephrol Dial Transplant. 2004;19(10):2505–12.

25. Ohga S, Shikata K, Yozai K, Okada S, Ogawa D, Usui H, et al. Thiazolidinedione ameliorates renal injury in experimental diabetic rats through anti-inflammatory effects mediated by inhibition of NF-kappaB activation. Am J Physiol Renal Physiol. 2007;292(4):F1141–50.

26. Navarro JF, Milena FJ, Mora C, León C, García J. Renal proinflammatory cytokine gene expression in diabetic nephropathy: effect of angiotensin-converting enzyme inhibition and pentoxifylline administration. Am J Nephrol. 2006;26(6):562–70.

27. Sekizuka K, Tomino Y, Sei C, Kurusu A, Tashiro K, Yamaguchi Y, et al. Detection of serum IL-6 in patients with diabetic nephropathy. Nephron. 1994;68(2):284–5.

28. Ha H, Hwang I-A, Park JH, Lee HB. Role of reactive oxygen species in the pathogenesis of diabetic nephropathy. Diabetes Res Clin Pract. 2008;82:S42–5.

29. Kroemer G, Mariño G, Levine B. Autophagy and the integrated stress response. Mol Cell. 2010;40(2):280–93.

30. Kume S, Yamahara K, Yasuda M, Maegawa H, Koya D. Autophagy: emerging therapeutic target for diabetic nephropathy. Semin Nephrol. 2014;34(1):9–16.

31. Fang L, Zhou Y, Cao H, Wen P, Jiang L, He W, et al. Autophagy attenuates diabetic glomerular damage through protection of hyperglycemia-induced podocyte injury. PLoS One. 2013;8(4):e60546.

32. Singh R, Kaushik S, Wang Y, Xiang Y, Novak I, Komatsu M, et al. Autophagy regulates lipid metabolism. Nature. 2009;458(7242):1131–5.

33. Yoshizaki T, Kusunoki C, Kondo M, Yasuda M, Kume S, Morino K, et al. Autophagy regulates inflammation in adipocytes. Biochem Biophys Res Commun. 2012;417(1):352–7.

34. Vlotides G, Mertens PR. Sodium-glucose cotransport inhibitors: mechanisms, metabolic effects and implications for the treatment of diabetic patients with chronic kidney disease. Nephrol Dial Transplant. 2015;30(8):1272–6.

35. Kanai Y, Lee WS, You G, Brown D, Hediger MA. The human kidney low affinity Na+/glucose cotransporter SGLT2. Delineation of the major renal reabsorptive mechanism for D-glucose. J Clin Invest. 1994;93(1):397–404.

36. Skorecki K, Chertow GM, Marsden P. Brenner & Rector's the kidney. 10th ed. Filadelfia, PA: Elsevier; 2016.

37. Rabelink TJ, de Zeeuw D. The glycocalyx—linking albuminuria with renal and cardiovascular disease. Nat Rev Nephrol. 2015;11(Box 1):1–10.

38. Thomas MC, Brownlee M, Susztak K, Sharma K, Jandeleit-Dahm KA, Zoungas S, Rossing P, Groop PH, Cooper ME. Diabetic kidney disease. Nat Rev Dis Primers. 2015;1:15018. https://doi.org/10.1038/nrdp.2015.18.

39. Pugliese G. Updating the natural history of diabetic nephropathy. Acta Diabetol. 2014;51(6):905–15.

40. Tervaert TWC, Mooyaart AL, Amann K, Cohen AH, Cook HT, Drachenberg CB, et al. Pathologic classification of diabetic nephropathy. J Am Soc Nephrol. 2010;21(4):556–63.

41. Oshima M, Shimizu M, Yamanouchi M, et al. Trajectories of kidney function in diabetes: a clinicopathological update. Nat Rev Nephrol. 2021;17:740–50. https://doi.org/10.1038/s41581-021-00462-y.

42. Chang A, Gibson IW, Cohen AH, Weening JJ, Jennette JC, Fogo AB. A position paper on standardizing the nonneoplastic kidney biopsy report. Clin J Am Soc Nephrol. 2012;7(8):1365–8.

43. Kidney Disease: Improving Global Outcomes (KDIGO) Blood Pressure Work Group. KDIGO 2021 clinical practice guideline for the management of blood pressure in chronic kidney disease. Kidney Int. 2021;99(3S):S1–S87. https://doi.org/10.1016/j.kint.2020.11.003.

44. Suckling RJ, He FJ, Macgregor GA. Altered dietary salt intake for preventing and treating diabetic kidney disease. Cochrane Database Syst Rev. 2010;12:CD006763.

45. Heerspink HJL, Holtkamp FA, Parving H-H, Navis GJ, Lewis JB, Ritz E, et al. Moderation of dietary sodium potentiates the renal and cardiovascular protective effects of angiotensin receptor blockers. Kidney Int. 2012;82(3):330–7.

46. Otoda T, Kanasaki K, Koya D. Low-protein diet for diabetic nephropathy. Curr Diab Rep. 2014;14(9):523.

47. Klahr S, Levey AS, Beck GJ, Caggiula AW, Hunsicker L, Kusek JW, et al. The effects of dietary protein restriction and blood-pressure control on the progression of chronic renal disease. N Engl J Med. 1994;330(13):877–84.

48. Robertson Lynn M, Waugh N, Robertson A. Protein restriction for diabetic renal disease. Cochrane Database Syst Rev. 2007;4:CD002181.

49. Shah BV, Patel ZM. Role of low protein diet in management of different stages of chronic kidney disease - practical aspects. BMC Nephrol. 2016;17(1):156.

50. Lewis EJ, Hunsicker LG, Bain RP, Rohde RD. The effect of angiotensin-converting-enzyme inhibition on diabetic nephropathy. N Engl J Med. 1993;329(20):1456–62.

51. ACE Inhibitors in Diabetic Nephropathy Trialist Group. Should all patients with type 1 diabetes mellitus and microalbuminuria receive angiotensin-converting enzyme inhibitors? A meta-analysis of individual patient data. Ann Intern Med. 2001;134(5):370–9.

52. Parving HH, Lehnert H, Bröchner-Mortensen J, Gomis R, Andersen S, Arner P, et al. The effect of irbesartan on the development of diabetic nephropathy in patients with type 2 diabetes. N Engl J Med. 2001;345(12):870–8.

53. Brenner BM, Cooper ME, de Zeeuw D, Keane WF, Mitch WE, Parving H-H, et al. Effects of losartan on renal and cardiovascular outcomes in patients with type 2 diabetes and nephropathy. N Engl J Med. 2001;345(12):861–9.

54. Mann JF, Schmieder RE, McQueen M, Dyal L, Schumacher H, Pogue J, et al. Renal outcomes with telmisartan, ramipril, or both, in people at high vascular risk (the ONTARGET study): a multicentre, randomised, double-blind, controlled trial. Lancet. 2008;372(9638):547–53.

55. Fried LF, Emanuele N, Zhang JH, Brophy M, Conner TA, Duckworth W, et al. Combined angiotensin inhibition for the treatment of diabetic nephropathy. N Engl J Med. 2013;369(20):1892–903.

56. Sun L, Sun Y, Shan J, Jiang G. Effects of mineralocorticoid receptor antagonists on the progression of diabetic nephropathy. J Diabetes Investig. 2017;8(4):609–18.

57. Bolignano D, Palmer SC, Navaneethan SD, Strippoli GF. Aldosterone antagonists for preventing the progression of chronic kidney disease. In: Strippoli GF, editor. Cochrane database of systematic reviews. John Wiley & Sons, Ltd: Chichester; 2014. p. 542–51.

58. Wanner C, Inzucchi SE, Lachin JM, Fitchett D, von Eynatten M, Mattheus M, et al. Empagliflozin and progression of kidney disease in type 2 diabetes. N Engl J Med. 2016;375(4):323–34.

59. Neal B, Perkovic V, Mahaffey KW, de Zeeuw D, Fulcher G, Erondu N, et al. Canagliflozin and cardiovascular and renal events in type 2 diabetes. N Engl J Med. 2017;377(7):644–57.

60. Wiviott SD, Raz I, Bonaca MP, Mosenzon O, DECLARE–TIMI 58 Investigators. Dapagliflozin and cardiovascular outcomes in type 2 diabetes. N Engl J Med. 2019;380(4):347–57. https://doi.org/10.1056/NEJMoa1812389.

61. Perkovic V, Jardine MJ, Neal B, CREDENCE Trial Investigators. Canagliflozin and renal outcomes in type 2 diabetes and nephropathy. N Engl J Med. 2019;380(24):2295–306. https://doi.org/10.1056/NEJMoa1811744.

62. Heerspink HJL, Stefánsson BV, Correa-Rotter R, DAPA-CKD Trial Committees and Investigators. Dapagliflozin in patients with chronic kidney disease. N Engl J Med. 2020;383(15):1436–46. https://doi.org/10.1056/NEJMoa2024816. Epub 2020 Sep 24.

63. Michos ED, Tuttle KR. GLP-1 receptor agonists in diabetic kidney disease. Clin J Am Soc Nephrol. 2021;16(10):1578–80. https://doi.org/10.2215/CJN.18771220.

64. Bakris GL, Agarwal R, Chan JC, Cooper ME, Gansevoort RT, Haller H, et al. Effect of finerenone on albuminuria in patients with diabetic nephropathy. JAMA. 2015;314(9):884.

65. Pitt B, Filippatos G, Agarwal R, Anker SD, FIGARO-DKD Investigators. Cardiovascular events with finerenone in kidney disease and type 2 diabetes. N Engl J Med. 2021;385(24):2252–63. https://doi.org/10.1056/NEJMoa2110956.

66. Bakris GL, Agarwal R, Anker SD, Pitt B, Ruilope LM, Rossing P, Kolkhof P, Nowack C, Schloemer P, Joseph A, Filippatos G, FIDELIO-DKD Investigators. Effect of finerenone on chronic kidney disease outcomes in type 2 diabetes. N Engl J Med. 2020;383(23):2219–29. https://doi.org/10.1056/NEJMoa2025845. Epub 2020 Oct 23.

Peripheral Diabetic Neuropathies

Gergely Feher

Introduction

More than 25% of the US population aged ≥65 years has diabetes, and the aging of the overall population is a significant driver of the diabetes epidemic. The epidemic is chiefly of type 2 diabetes and also the associated conditions known as 'diabesity' and 'metabolic syndrome'. In conjunction with genetic susceptibility, particularly in certain ethnic groups, type 2 diabetes is brought on by environmental and behavioural factors such as a sedentary lifestyle, overly rich nutrition and obesity. The prevention of diabetes and control of its micro- and macrovascular complications will require an integrated, international approach if we are to see significant reduction in the huge premature morbidity and mortality it causes [1]. Diabetic neuropathies (DN) encompass a wide range of nerve abnormalities and are common, with prevalence rates reported between 5% and 100% depending on the diagnostic criteria. Diabetic peripheral neuropathy (DPN) is associated with considerable morbidity, increased mortality and diminished quality of life, causing a tremendous economic burden [2]. The duration and severity of hyperglycaemia, presence of dyslipidemia, hypertension and smoking are major risk factors for the development of diabetic polyneuropathy [3]. The different mechanisms involved in different pain sensations are still poorly understood, but there is ample evidence that abnormal discharges from diseased somatosensory neurons are responsible. Spontaneous activity in the peripheral nociceptor system may also trigger central nervous system changes responsible for hyperalgesia and allodynia [1].

Epidemiology

Diabetic peripheral neuropathy (DPN) is a common complication of both type 1 and type 2 diabetes. Despite the different pathophysiologies, there has been a longstanding assumption that the mechanism leading to DPN is shared. Type 2 DM is much more common (90–95%) but has a slightly lower lifetime incidence of neuropathy; the reported prevalence varies between 6 and 51% compared with the 54–59% associated with type 1 DM [4, 5]. The primary risk factor for DPN is hyperglycaemia, but apart from chronic hyperglycaemia, recent studies showed the possible role of large or frequent serum glucose level fluctuations as a possible trigger factor [5]. Whereas treating hyperglycaemia in type 1 DM can significantly reduce the incidence of neuropathy by up to 60–70%, glucose control in type 2 DM has only a marginal 5–7% reduction in the development of neuropathy estimated to affect 30–50% of individuals with diabetes. Many recent studies have implicated cardiovascular risk factors which include age, duration of disease, cigarette smoking, hypertension, elevated triglycerides, higher BMI, alcohol consumption and taller height in the background of DN [1, 4]. Interestingly, between 25% and 62% of patients with idiopathic peripheral neuropathy are reported to have prediabetes, and among individuals with prediabetes, 11–25% are thought to have peripheral neuropathy, and 13–21% have neuropathic pain. Population-based studies suggest a gradient for the prevalence of neuropathy, being highest in patients with manifest diabetes mellitus, followed by individuals with impaired glucose tolerance and then impaired fasting glucose and least in those with normoglycaemia [4].

Pathophysiology

It is generally believed that oxidative stress is the key pathological process inducing nerve damage in diabetes. Oxidative stress, possibly triggered by vascular abnormalities and asso-

G. Feher (✉)
Department of Primary Care, University of Pécs, Pécs, Hungary
e-mail: feher.gergely@pte.hu

© The Author(s), under exclusive license to Springer Nature Switzerland AG 2023
J. Rodriguez-Saldana (ed.), *The Diabetes Textbook*, https://doi.org/10.1007/978-3-031-25519-9_56

ciated microangiopathy in the nerve, is a key pathological process inducing nerve damage in diabetes in humans and experimental models. Diabetes-induced oxidative stress in animal models of in type 1, type 2 and pre-diabetes in sensory neurons and peripheral nerve is demonstrated by increased production of reactive oxygen species (ROS), lipid peroxidation and protein nitrosylation and diminished levels of reduced glutathione and ascorbate. Treatment with antioxidants such as α-lipoic acid, γ-linolenic acid and aldose reductase inhibitors prevents many indices of neuropathy in STZ (streptozotocin)-diabetic rats. The neurons and Schwann cells do initiate protective mechanisms involving upregulation of antioxidant pathways; however, the neurodegenerative outcome is energy failure in the nerve, observed as a decrease in high energy intermediates (e.g. phosphocreatine), impaired axonal transport of proteins and sub-optimal ion pumping [1, 6] (Fig. 56.1).

Polyol pathway hyperactivity: Metabolic disorders are the primary cause of diabetic neuropathy. Hyperglycaemia, induced through decrease of insulin secretion or insulin resistance, is responsible for the enhancement of the polyol pathway activity. The rate-limiting first enzyme of this pathway, aldose reductase, catalyses the formation of sorbitol from glucose, with the oxidation of nicotinamide adenine dinucleotide phosphate (NADPH) to NADP+. Sorbitol is further oxidized to fructose by sorbitol dehydrogenase, which is coupled with the reduction of nicotinamide adenine dinucleotide (NAD+) to NADH. It is described that during hyperglycaemic states, the affinity of aldose reductase for glucose is higher, generating intracellular osmotic stress due to accumulation of sorbitol, since sorbitol does not cross cell membranes. Interesting, the nerve damage following the dia-

betic state seems not to be due to this osmotic stress since it has been reported insignificant sorbitol concentrations in the nerves of diabetic patients [7]. However, the current accepted hypothesis states that polyol pathway hyperactivity is pathogenic primarily by increasing the turnover of cofactors such as NADPH and NAD+, which leads to a decrease in the reduction and regeneration of glutathione, as well as to an increase of advanced glycation end product (AGE) production and activation of diacylglycerol and protein kinase C (PKC) isoforms. Depletion of glutathione could be the primary cause of oxidative stress and be related to the accumulation of toxic species [8]. In fact, aldose reductase inhibitors are effective in preventing the development of diabetic neuropathy in animal models, but they have demonstrated disappointing results and dose-limiting toxicity in human trials [7] (Figs. 56.1 and 56.2).

Oxidative stress and mitochondria: Hyperglycaemia induces activation of classical pathways like AGE, PKC, hexosamine and polyol pathways to mediate cellular damage [7]. Generation of superoxide from mitochondrial electron transport chain is known to contribute towards hyperglycaemia initiated various etiological pathways. Hyperglycaemia enhances the reducing equivalents to electron transport chain (ETC) and the electrochemical potential across the inner mitochondrial membrane and hence increases superoxide production [7]. Superoxide inhibits glyceraldehyde phosphate dehydrogenase (GAPDH) either directly or indirectly through PARP-mediated NADH+ depletion [10]. Inhibition of GAPDH by ROS leads to accumulation of glycolytic intermediates upstream of this enzyme and redirected to initiate cellular pathways like AGE formation. Once the AGEs are formed, they bind to RAGE and activate many other cru-

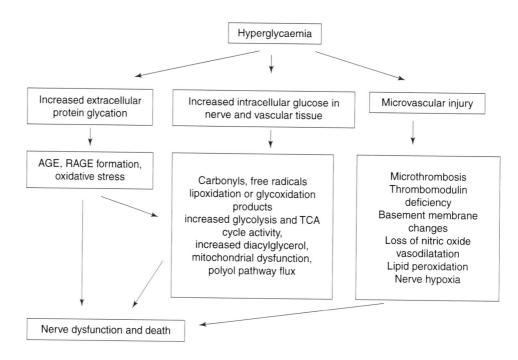

Fig. 56.1 The pathogenesis of diabetic neuropathy (Taken from Deli G et al. Diabetic neuropathies: diagnosis and management. Neuroendocrinology. 2013;98(4):267–80, ref. 1, with permission). *AGE* advanced glycation end product, *RAGE* receptors for AGEs, *TCA* tricarboxylic acid

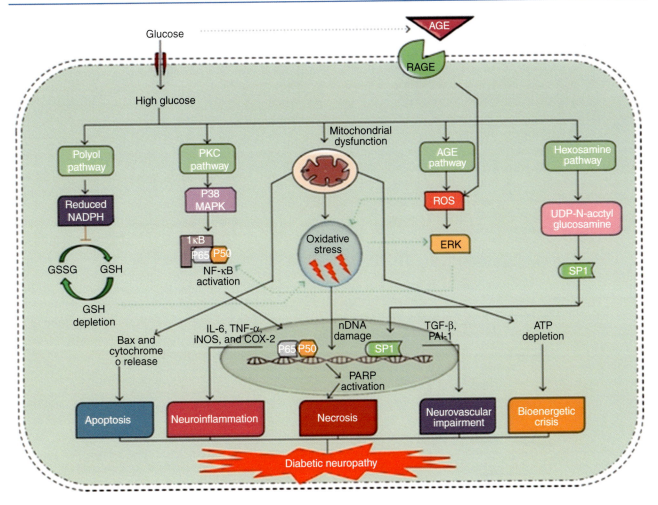

Fig. 56.2 Pathophysiology of diabetic neuropathy. Hyperglycaemia activates numerous metabolic pathways like polyol pathway, protein kinase c (PKC) pathway, advanced glycation end product (AGE) pathway and hexosamine pathway. All these pathways are known to integrate through hyperglycaemia-mediated mitochondrial ROS production. Oxidative stress and these classical pathways in combination activate transcription factors such as nuclear factor kappa enhancer of B cells (NF-κB) and speciality protein-1 (SP-1), resulting in neuroinflammation and vascular impairment. Further, these pathways combined with dysfunctional mitochondria-mediated apoptosis or bioenergetic deple-tion can lead to neuronal damage leading to DN. Poly-ADP ribose polymerase (PARP)-mediated NADH/ATP depletion can lead to neuronal dysfunction due to failure of various energy-dependent processes in neurons. (ERK, extracellular related kinase; IL-6, interleukin-6; iNOS, inducible nitric oxide synthase; COX-2, cyclooxygenase-2; TGF-β, transforming growth factor-β; and PAI-1, plasminogen activator inhibitor-1) (Taken from Sandireddy R et al. Neuroinflammation and oxidative stress in diabetic neuropathy: futuristic strategies based on these targets. Int J Endocrinol. 2014;2014:674987, ref. 9, with permission)

cial pathways like NF-κB and PARP. PKC pathway is activated through dihydroxyacetone phosphate-mediated diacylglycerol (DAG) activation. Hexosamine pathway is activated through enhanced flux of fructose-6-phosphate and polyol pathway by elevated glucose levels. This, in turn, leads to osmotic stress in the cells which further takes the cell towards necrotic cell death. Enhanced activity of Mn-SOD, a mitochondrial form of superoxide dismutase (SOD) or overexpression of uncoupling proteins (UCP-1) in experimental diabetic animals, prevents the development of vascular complications in the animals and also reduced oxidative stress-mediated neuronal damage. The mechanism for this neuroprotective effect can be the reduction of mitochon-drial ROS generation and the clearance of the notorious ROS from the cells. In addition to the above theory, mitochondrial abnormalities and mitochondria-associated oxidative stress stand at a central position in the pathogenesis of diabetic neuropathy. It has been noticed that defects in functioning of ETC chain components compromise ATP production and enhance the generation of free radicals. The free radicals generated causes damage to mitochondrial DNA (mt DNA) and nuclear DNA (nDNA) which in turn aggravates mitochondrial damage. This vicious cycle developed inside mitochondria produces intense oxidative stress and drives the cell towards apoptotic/necrotic death. It is an established fact that diabetes is known to affect the respiratory capacity of ETC functional complexes and thus alters ATP production (Fig. 56.1). Mainly complex I and complex III are known to be affected, which turns out to be electron leakage centres and thus inflates ROS production [7]. Various experimental observations point towards the critical role of mitotoxicity in the pathophysiology of diabetic neuropathy (Figs. 56.1 and 56.2).

Microvascular changes: DNP is frequently associated with microvascular impairment [1, 7]. In clinical and pre-clinical studies, it was found that peripheral perfusion is reduced, not only in the nervous tissue but also in the skin, being an important physiological evidence of microvasculature alteration. As a result, nerve ischaemia occurs, caused by raise in wall thickness and hyalinization of the basal lamina of vessels that nurse peripheral nerves, together with luminal reduction. These alterations are caused by plasma protein scape of capillary membrane to endoneurium, promoting swelling and augmented interstitial pressure in the nerves, accompanied by higher capillary pressure, deposition of fibrin and thrombus development. Hyperglycaemia per se can evoke nerve hypoxia, especially in sensory nerves, altering their electrical stability. Apparently controversial data from clinical studies described that diabetic patients suffering from the DNP presented higher levels of intravascular oxygen and augmented blood flow in the lower limbs than painless patients. As a result of nerve ischaemia, both diabetic patients and animals have shown a progressive nerve loss in proximal and distal segments, resulting in reduction of intraepidermal nerve fibre density. Consequently, axonal degeneration and regeneration also occur but more frequently in patients who do not experience pain. Besides axonal retraction and regeneration, another structural modification related to hyperglycaemia is myelin sheath alteration. The observed demyelinization can be related to Schwann cells' altered capacity to support normal myelin sheath [7] (Figs. 56.1 and 56.2).

Nerve excitability: Sensing ongoing spontaneous pain and paroxysmal shooting pain in the absence of any external stimulus is caused by ectopic impulse generation within the nociceptive pathways [1, 10]. The enhanced excitability can result from altered ion channel function, such as an increase in persistent sodium currents. Persistent sodium currents can be reliably estimated using threshold tracking. In peripheral neuropathy, persistent sodium currents usually increase possibly due to overexpression of sodium channels associated with axonal regeneration and could be responsible for ectopic firings. In diabetic neuropathy, the activation of the polyol pathway mediated by an enzyme, aldose reductase, leads to reduced Na(+)/K(+) pump activity and intra-axonal sodium accumulation; sodium currents are reduced presumably due to decreased trans-axonal sodium gradient [1, 10]. In addition to voltage-gated sodium channels, several other ion channels probably undergo alterations after a nerve lesion, such as voltage-gated potassium channels, which might also contribute to changes in membrane excitability of nociceptive nerves [1, 10] (Fig. 56.3).

Nerve injury also induces upregulation of various receptor proteins such as the transient receptor potential V1 (TRPV1), which is activated by heat at about 41 °C [1]. In neuropathic condition, TRPV1 is downregulated on affected/injured fibres but upregulated on uninjured C-fibres, thereby causing spontaneous nerve activity induced by normal body temperature.

Central sensitization: Central sensitization might develop as a consequence of ectopic activity in primary nociceptive afferent fibres, and structural damage within the CNS itself

Fig. 56.3 Peripheral sensitization changes in the sensitivity of the peripheral terminals of nociceptors to stimuli can contribute to evoked pain. This can occur through inflammatory mediators sensitizing signal transducer proteins, persistent activation of transducer proteins by endogenous agonists, inherited polymorphisms of transducer proteins or an increase in membrane excitability. (Taken from von Hehn CA et al. Deconstructing the neuropathic pain phenotype to reveal neural mechanisms. Neuron. 2012;73(4):638–52, ref. 11 with permission)

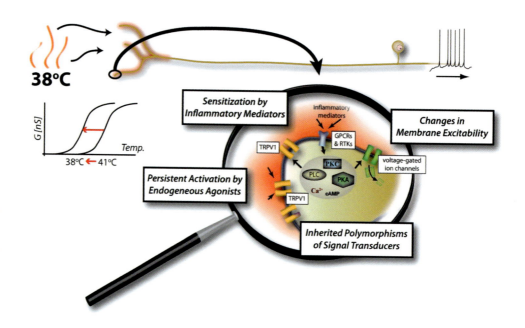

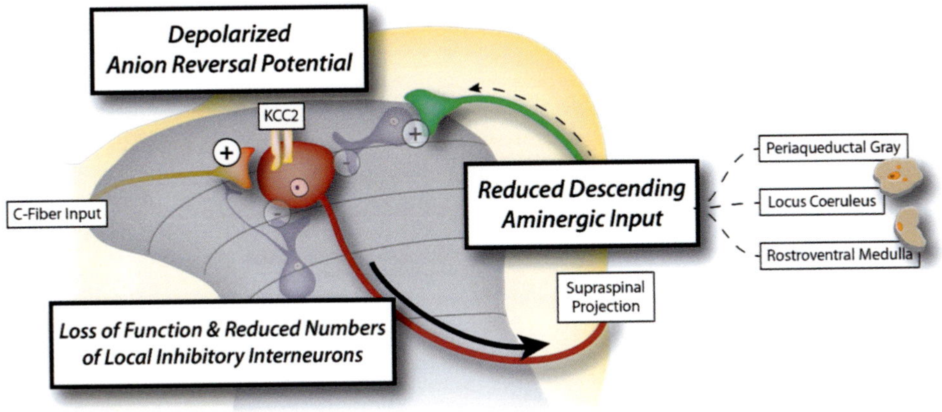

Fig. 56.4 Spinal disinhibition: Excitatory nociceptive signals are enhanced after nerve injury by a reduction in normal inhibitory regulation through a loss of local inhibitory interneurons, a depolarized anion reversal potential and reduced descending inhibition. (Taken from von Hehn CA et al. Deconstructing the neuropathic pain phenotype to reveal neural mechanisms. Neuron. 2012;73(4):638–52, ref. 11 with permission)

might not be necessarily involved. Spinal cord microglia are also strongly activated after nerve injury; the activated microglia not only exhibit increased expression of microglial markers CD 11 b and Iba 1 but also display elevated phosphorylation of p38 mitogen-activated protein kinase. Inhibition of spinal cord p38 has been shown to attenuate neuropathic and postoperative pain, as well as morphine-induced antinociceptive tolerance. Activation of p38 in spinal microglia results in increased synthesis and release of the neurotrophin brain-derived neurotrophic factor and the pro-inflammatory cytokines interleukin-1β, interleukin-6 and tumour necrosis factor-α. Phosphorylation of NMDA and AMPA receptors and expression of voltage-gated sodium channels are also involved both in the spinal cord and supraspinal structures. These mediators can powerfully modulate spinal cord synaptic transmission, leading to increased excitability of dorsal horn neurons, that is, central sensitization, partly via suppressing inhibitory synaptic transmission [1, 7, 10]. Further potent inhibitory neurons, such as descending pathways originating in the brainstem, contribute to modulation of pain processing. Lesions that affect these opioidergic and monoaminergic systems also lead to pain exacerbation via disinhibition [10] (Fig. 56.4).

'Chronic Pain Hurts the Brain'

The pain matrix is composed of several interacting networks. A nociceptive matrix receiving spinothalamic projections (mainly posterior operculoinsular areas) ensures the bodily specificity of pain and is the only one whose destruction entails selective pain deficits. Transition from cortical nociception to conscious pain relies on a second-order network, including posterior parietal, prefrontal and anterior insular areas. Second-order regions are not nociceptive-specific; focal stimulation does not evoke pain, and focal destruction does not produce analgesia, but their joint activation is necessary for conscious perception, attentional modulation and control of vegetative reactions. The ensuing pain experience can still be modified as a function of beliefs, emotions and expectations through activity of third-order areas, including the orbitofrontal and perigenual/limbic networks. The pain we remember results from continuous interaction of these subsystems, and substantial changes in the pain experience can be achieved by acting on each of them. Neuropathic pain (NP) is associated with changes in each of these levels of integration. The most robust abnormality in NP is a functional depression of thalamic activity, reversible with therapeutic manoeuvres and associated with rhythmic neural bursting. Neuropathic allodynia has been associated with enhancement of ipsilateral over contralateral insular activation and lack of reactivity in orbitofrontal/perigenual areas. Although lack of response of perigenual cortices may be an epiphenomenon of chronic pain, the enhancement of ipsilateral activity may reflect disinhibition of ipsilateral spinothalamic pathways due to depression of their contralateral counterpart. This in turn may bias perceptual networks and contribute to the subjective painful experience [12].

In addition to functional changes, morphological alterations at spinal and supraspinal levels have been reported in chronic pain. Neuropathic pain is accompanied by apoptosis of spinal cord cells, sprouting of nerve terminals in somatosensory cortex, grey matter density decrease in PFC associated with reduced cognitive abilities and thalamic atrophy. Morphometric analysis showed that chronic pain particularly in patients with a neuropathic pain component is associated with 5–10% of brain grey matter atrophy in the prefrontal cortex and thalamus. A decrease in grey matter was also

Fig. 56.5 DMN differences between controls and patients. Surface-rendered projection results of a two-sample t-test contrasting the default mode network in the healthy group vs. the pain group. The blue foci indicate the areas that showed significantly less correlational activity in the pain group than in the healthy group. Vice versa the yellow/red foci indicate the areas that showed significantly more correlational activity in the pain group than in the healthy group. (Taken from Cauda F et al. Altered resting state in diabetic neuropathic pain. PLoS One. 2009;4(2):e4542., ref. 13, with permission)

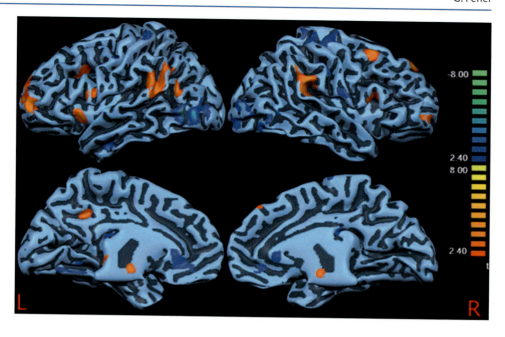

found in brainstem, temporal lobe and somatosensory cortex in addition to PFC in patients with chronic pain; cortical changes were more pronounced in the right hemisphere. It remains to be determined if reduced grey matter density is related exclusively or predominantly to a specific cell population (projection neurons, inhibitory interneurons and microglia) or if different cell types are affected equally. Nerve injury-induced apoptosis in the spinal dorsal horn caused a loss of GABAergic inhibitory interneurons and a decrease in inhibitory synaptic transmission. Microglia was hyperactivated at the spinal level after nerve injury but possibly inhibited in cortical areas in chronic pain [13].

In a revolutionary study by Cauda et al., functional connectivity analyses revealed a cortical network consisting of two anti-correlated patterns: one includes the left fusiform gyrus, the left lingual gyrus, the left inferior temporal gyrus, the right inferior occipital gyrus, the dorsal anterior cingulate cortex bilaterally and the pre- and postcentral gyrus bilaterally, in which its activity is correlated negatively with pain and positively with the controls; the other includes the left precuneus, dorsolateral prefrontal, frontopolar cortex (both bilaterally), right superior frontal gyrus, left inferior frontal gyrus, thalami, both insulae, inferior parietal lobuli, right mammillary body and a small area in the left brainstem, in which its activity is correlated positively with pain and negatively with the controls. Furthermore, a power spectra analysis revealed group differences in the frequency bands wherein the spatial independent component analysis (sICA) signal was decomposed: patients' spectra are shifted towards higher frequencies [14] (Fig. 56.5).

Ever since several studies have confirmed the role of central nervous system impairment. Both somatosensory pathways and cognition-related cerebral areas are involved based

on functional MRI studies, which play a role in the complexity in the development of neuropathic pain and its emotional and mental consequences [15, 16]. Altered functional connectivity can also be detected in patients with type 1 diabetes mellitus [17].

Diagnosis

As it has been previously shown, prediabetes can also be associated with neuropathy. Based on the recent ADA (Americans with Disabilities Act) guidelines, diabetes can be diagnosed on the results of HgBA1C, fasting plasma glucose (FPG) or 2 h postprandial glucose (PG) levels. This statement recommended the use of the A1C test to diagnose diabetes, with a threshold of ≥6.5%. The established glucose criteria for the diagnosis of diabetes (FPG ≥ 7 mmol/l or 2h PG ≥ 11.1 mmol/l) remained valid as well [18].

Prediabetes can be defined as having impaired fasting glucose (IFG) (FPG levels 5.6–6.9 mmol/l) or impaired glucose tolerance (IGT) (2h PG values in the oral glucose tolerance test (OGTT) of 7.8–11.0 mmol/l). It should be noted that the World Health Organization (WHO) and a number of other diabetes organizations define the cutoff for IFG at 110 mg/dl (6.1 mmol/l) [1]. Hence, it is reasonable to consider an A1C range of 5.7–6.4% as identifying individuals with high risk for future diabetes, a state that may be referred to as prediabetes [1, 18]. As with glucose measurements, the continuum of risk is curvilinear—as A1C rises, the risk of diabetes rises disproportionately. Accordingly, interventions should be most intensive follow-up particularly vigilant for those with A1Cs above 6.0%, who should be considered to be at very high risk. Prediabetes is associated with obesity (especially abdominal or visceral obesity), dyslipidemia with high triglycerides and/or low HDL cholesterol and hypertension. The presence of prediabetes should prompt comprehensive screening for cardiovascular risk factors. Standards of lifestyle and medical care can also be found in this guideline [18].

In DPN, sensory deficits usually overshadow motor nerve dysfunction and appear first in the distal portions of the extremities and progress proximally in a 'stocking-glove' distribution with increasing duration or severity of diabetes [1]. In the typical form, the large nerve fibres are damaged later than the small ones [19]. The signs and symptoms of DPN vary depending on fibre type involved, with large fibre disease impairing proprioception and light touch. Small fibre disease impairs pain and temperature perception, leading to paresthesias, dysesthesias and/or neuropathic pain [2] (Table 56.1). Distal weakness occurs only in the most severe cases. Diminished or absent deep tendon reflexes, particularly the Achilles tendon reflex, often indicate mild and otherwise asymptomatic DPN. More advanced asymptomatic neuropathy may first present with late complications such as ulceration or neuroarthropathy (Charcot's joints) of the foot [1, 19].

For diagnosis of DN, bedside examination should include assessment of muscle power, sensations of pinprick, joint position, touch and temperature. Vibration test should be done by tuning fork of a 128 Hz. For touch sensation, mono filament of 1 g is recommended [1]. A number of questionnaires have been developed to help practitioners diagnose neuropathic pain [1, 9, 19]. The DN4 questionnaire is of particular interest, as it can be rapidly completed, is easy to use and has a good diagnostic performance: for a score ≥4/10, it has a sensitivity of 83% and a specificity of 90% for diagnosing neuropathic pain [9, 19]. The main advantage of screening tools is to identify potential patients with NP, particularly by non-specialists. However, these tools fail to identify 10–20% of patients with clinician-diagnosed NP, showing that they cannot replace careful clinical judgement [9] (Table 56.1).

Electrophysiological tests may have no place in the diagnosis of chronic sensorimotor diabetic neuropathy, as they can be normal when only small-diameter fibres are damaged, but are a reliable procedure in the case of mononeuropathies or radiculopathies to exclude any other etiology (demyelinating, toxic polyneuropathies, etc.). Such procedures should be performed only when the clinical presentation is atypical and the diabetic origin uncertain (asymmetrical symptoms or involvement of the upper limbs) [9, 19].

Among laboratory tests, laser-evoked potentials (LEPs) are the best tool for assessing Aδ pathway dysfunction (small-fibre neuropathy) and skin biopsy for assessing neuropathies with distal loss of unmyelinated nerve fibres [1, 9].

Table 56.1 Definition and assessment of negative and positive sensory symptoms and signs in patients with neuropathic pain (Taken from Deli G et al. Diabetic neuropathies: diagnosis and management. Neuroendocrinology. 2013;98(4):267–80, ref. 1, with permission)

Symptom	Sign	Assessment
Negative signs and symptoms		
Hypoesthesia	Reduced sensation	Touch skin with
Pallhypesthesia	To non-painful stimuli	Painter's brush, cotton swab
Hypoalgesia	To vibration	Tuning fork
Thermohypoesthesia	To painful stimuli	Pinprick
	To cold or warm stimuli	Objects of 10 and 45 °C
Spontaneous sensations/pain		
Paraesthesia	Non-painful ongoing sensation	Number per episode
Paroxysmal pain	Painful, shooting electrical attacks for seconds	Grade intensity (0–10)
Superficial pain	Painful ongoing sensation	Threshold for evocation
		Area in cm²
Evoked pain		
Mechanical dynamic allodynia	Normally non-painful stimuli on skin evoke pain	Stroking skin with painter's brush etc.
Mechanical static allodynia		Manual gentle mechanical pressure to the skin
Mechanical punctate or pinprick hyperalgesia	Normally non-painful pressure stimuli on skin evoke pain	Manual gentle pricking of the skin
Temporal summation	Normally stinging-but-not-painful stimuli evoke pain	Pricking the skin with safety pin at <3 s intervals for 30 s
Cold allodynia	Repetitive application of identical single noxious stimuli is perceived as increasing pain sensation	Touch skin with objects of 20 °C
Heat allodynia		Touch skin with objects of 40 °C
Mechanical deep somatic allodynia	Normally non-painful cold stimuli evoke pain	Manual light pressure at joints or muscle
	Normally non-painful heat stimuli evoke pain	
	Normally non-painful pressure on deep somatic tissues evokes pain	

Forms of Diabetic Neuropathy

Several fairly distinct clinical syndromes of diabetic neuropathy have been delineated: the most common as noted is a distal, symmetrical, primarily sensory polyneuropathy affecting feet and legs in a chronic, slowly progressive manner; the others are acute ophthalmoplegia that affects the third and less often the sixth cranial nerve on one side; acute mononeuropathy of limbs or trunk including a painful thoracolumbar radiculopathy; an acute or subacute painful, asymmetrical, predominantly motor multiple neuropathy affecting the upper lumbar roots and the proximal leg muscles ('diabetic amyotrophy'); a more symmetrical, proximal motor weakness and wasting, usually without pain and with variable sensory loss, pursuing a subacute or chronic course; and an autonomic neuropathy involving bowel, bladder, sweating and circulatory reflexes. These forms of neuropathy often coexist or overlap, particularly the autonomic and distal symmetrical types and the subacute proximal neuropathies (Tables 56.2 and 56.3).

Table 56.2 The main features of different patterns of disabling neuropathies in patients with diabetes (Taken from Deli G et al. Diabetic neuropathies: diagnosis and management. Neuroendocrinology. 2013;98(4):267–80, reference 1, with permission)

	Pains	Distal symmetrical sensory loss	Weakness	Sensory ataxia	Autonomic dysfunction	Progression	CSF protein	Electrophysiological test	Nerve biopsy
Length-dependent polyneuropathy	Frequent in distal limbs	Length dependently predominates on pain and temperature sensations	Minor, distal symmetrical	Rare	Common	Years	Variable	Axonal pattern, distal symmetrical	Massive axonal loss
CIDP in diabetic patients	Occasional	Variable predominates on proprioception	Common, often severe proximal and distal	Common	Uncommon	Weeks or months	Increased	Mixed axonal and demyelinative	Variable axon loss and demyelination
Focal/ multifocal diabetic neuropathy	Present in most cases	Variable	Common—asymmetrical—nerve or root territory	Uncommon	Uncommon	Weeks or months	Increased	Axonal pattern, multifocal	Variable

CIDP chronic inflammatory demyelinating polyneuropathy, *CSF* cerebrospinal fluid

Table 56.3 First-line treatment of neuropathic pain (Taken from Deli G et al. Diabetic neuropathies: diagnosis and management. Neuroendocrinology. 2013;98(4):267–80, reference 1, with permission)

Drug	Mode of action	Cautions	Major side effects	Other benefits	NNT	NNH	NNMH
TCA	Inhibition of reuptake of serotonin and/or norepinephrine, block of sodium channels, anticholinergic	Postinfarct states and arrhythmias	Sedation and anticholinergic effects	Improvement of depression and sleep disturbance	1.3–2.4	2.7–6	15–28
SNRI	Inhibition of both serotonin and norepinephrine reuptake	Hepatic dysfunction, renal insufficiency, alcoholism and cardiac disease	Nausea	Improvement of depression	3.1–6	9.6	17–21
Gabapentine	Decreases release of glutamate, norepinephrine and substance P, with ligands on α2-δ subunit of voltage-gated calcium channel	Renal insufficiency	Sedation, dizziness and peripheral oedema	No clinically significant drug interactions	3.3–5.8	2.7–3.7	11–23
Pregabalin	See above	See above	See above	See above plus improvement of sleep disturbance and anxiety	2.9–5	3.7	11–23
Opioids	μ-Receptor agonism, inhibition of norepinephrine and serotonin reuptake	History of substance abuse, suicide risk, driving impairment, concomitant use of SSNRI and tricyclic antidepressant (serotonin syndrome)	Nausea/vomiting, constipation and dizziness	No systemic side effects and rapid onset of analgesic effect	2.6–4.3	3.6	7.8

TCA tricyclic antidepressant, *SNRI* serotonin and norepinephrine reuptake inhibitor, *NNT* number needed to treat, *NNH* number needed to harm, *NNMH* number needed to major harm

Sensorimotor Neuropathy

Distal sensory diabetic polyneuropathy: This is the most common presentation of neuropathy in diabetes, and up to 50% of patients may experience symptoms, most frequently burning pain, electrical or stabbing sensations, paresthesia, hyperesthesia and deep aching pain [1]. These symptoms are generally worse at night and disturb sleep. Together with painful symptoms during the day, this often leads to a reduction in individual's ability to perform daily activities [11].

Examination of the lower limb usually reveals sensory loss of vibration, pressure, pain and temperature perception (mediated by small and large fibres) and absent ankle reflexes [15–17]. Muscle weakness is usually mild, but in some patients, a distal sensory neuropathy is combined with a proximal weakness and wasting [1, 9, 11, 19].

Interestingly, as up to half of the patients may be asymptomatic, a diagnosis may only be made on examination or, in some cases, when the patient presents with a painless foot ulcer [1].

About 10% of diabetic patients experience persistent pain (so-called painful diabetic neuropathy) [11]. Some patients develop predominantly small fibre neuropathy manifesting with pain and paresthesia early in the course of diabetes that may be associated with insulin therapy (insulin neuritis) [8, 20].

Acute diabetic mononeuropathies: Cranial neuropathy in diabetic patients most commonly involve the oculomotor nerve followed by trochlear and facial nerve in order of frequency. Third nerve palsy with pupillary sparing is the hallmark of diabetic oculomotor palsy and is attributed to nerve infarction [8, 9, 11, 19, 21].

Isolated involvement of practically all the major peripheral nerves has been described in diabetes (e.g. carpal tunnel syndrome (CTS) is three times more common in diabetic patients than the normal population and CTS is the second most common neuropathic disease in diabetic patients), but the ones most frequently affected are the femoral, sciatic and peroneal nerves, in that order [22–25]. Rarely is a nerve in the upper extremity affected. In these cases, nerve entrapment seems to be commoner than nerve infarction [8, 9, 11, 19].

The mononeuropathies often emerge during periods of transition in the diabetic illness, for example, after an episode of hyper- or hypoglycaemia, when insulin treatment is initiated or adjusted or when there has been rapid weight loss [1, 8, 9, 11, 19].

Diabetic multiple mononeuropathies and radiculopathies: This category overlaps with the mononeuropathies. A syndrome of painful unilateral or asymmetrical multiple neuropathies tends to occur in older patients with relatively mild or even unrecognized diabetes. Multiple nerves are affected in a random distribution (mononeuritis multiplex).

As in mononeuropathy, the onset is abrupt in one nerve and occurs earlier than the other nerves, which are involved sequentially or irregularly. Nerve infarctions occur because of occlusion of vasa nervosum and should be differentiated from systemic vasculitis [8, 9, 11, 19].

Characteristic diabetic syndromes present subacutely with pain followed by weakness, which affect primarily patients with mild diabetes called radiculoplexus neuropathies (Table 56.3). Three main types can occur, alone or in combination, and include diabetic cervical radiculoplexus neuropathy (DCRPN), diabetic thoracic radiculoneuropathy (DTRN) and diabetic lumbosacral radiculoplexus neuropathy (DLRPN) [8, 9, 11, 19].

Diabetic lumbosacral radiculoplexus neuropathy (DLRPN) occurs in approximately 1% of diabetic patients and probably is the form of diabetic neuropathy that causes the most morbidity [25]. It has been variably known by different names, including diabetic amyotrophy, Bruns-Garland syndrome, diabetic mononeuritis multiplex, diabetic polyradiculopathy, proximal diabetic neuropathy and others [1]. Pain, which can be severe, begins in the low back or hip and spreads to the thigh and knee on one side; the discomfort has a deep, aching character with superimposed lancinating jabs, and there is a propensity for pain to be most severe at night. Although pain is initially the worse symptom, weakness and atrophy become the main problem, which are mainly evident in the pelvic girdle and thigh muscles, although the distal muscles of the leg may also be affected [8, 19].

Diabetic thoracic radiculopathies are a rare but important complication of diabetes mellitus. These typically present with severe pain and dysesthesias along the trunk, chest or abdominal wall and often prompt extensive workups for underlying chest or abdominal pathology [1]. They can be symmetric and can involve multiple dermatomes [8, 9, 11, 19]. While DLRPN is a much more familiar branch of the DRPN spectrum, the cervical segment can also be involved, but it is very rare [8].

Insulin neuritis: In a seemingly paradoxical relationship, both poor glucose control and rapid treatment of hyperglycaemia can be associated with an increased risk of neuropathy. A clinically distinct form of neuropathy that deserves mention is treatment-induced neuropathy in diabetes (TIND). This underdiagnosed iatrogenic small-fibre neuropathy is defined as the acute onset of neuropathic pain and/or autonomic dysfunction within eight weeks of a large improvement in glycaemic control specified as a decrease in glycosylated HbA1c of more than 2% points over 3 months [8]. TIND was first recognized soon after the introduction of insulin and named 'insulin neuritis' [1, 8, 20–22]. For many decades, 'insulin neuritis' was considered a rare cause for acute neuropathy. However, recently published data suggest that it is much more common and clinically relevant. It is most common in type 1 diabetes mellitus (DM) treated with insulin, although rapid glucose correction can occur in both types of diabetes as a result of either insulin or less frequently oral agents. In a study by Gibbons and Freeman, a surprising 10.9% of 954 subjects with diabetes met criteria for TIND, and the risk of developing TIND was associated with the magnitude and rate of HbA1c change [20]. Similar to DPN, the neuropathy of TIND generally follows a length-dependent pattern, but, in contrast, the pain and autonomic symptoms are more extensive and less responsive to opioids. The underlying pathophysiology is poorly understood, although it has been suggested that rapid glycaemic control both with and without insulin leads to hemodynamic changes (arteriovenous shunting) resulting in endoneurial hypoxia of small fibres [8, 20–22].

Diabetes-Associated Chronic Inflammatory Demyelinating Polyneuropathy (CIDP)

Chronic inflammatory demyelinating polyneuropathy (CIDP), as the name implies, is an autoimmune disorder of unknown etiology in two-thirds of the patients; however, in remaining one-third, an etiological cause might be found. Some currently described etiologies include gammopathies including monoclonal gammopathy of undetermined significance (MGUS), multiple myeloma, Castleman's disease and Waldenstrom gammopathy; also, other concurrent disorders like inflammatory bowel disorders, cutaneous melanoma and Hodgkin's lymphoma have been implied [23]. CIDP has typical and atypical phenotypic variants. Only half of CIDP patients have typical CIDP, which exhibits symmetrical sensory and motor symptoms. The remainder has atypical disease, which presents with predominantly focal, sensory, motor, distal or asymmetrical symptoms. Despite increased efforts to identify a biomarker, there is no definitive diagnostic marker for CIDP, and recognition of CIDP is not straightforward in some cases due to its heterogeneous nature [24]. For further details, see the excellent review by Nelligan et al. [25].

Simultaneous occurrence of CIDP and diabetes mellitus (DM) (diabetic CIDP or CIDP-DM) is frequently seen in clinical practice; however, it is ambiguous whether the two disorders are pathogenetically correlated. It is of utmost importance to be familiar with CIDP occurring in diabetics for the reason that contrasting to diabetic polyneuropathy, it may be treatable [23].

There is an increasing body of literature suggesting that the prevalence of CIDP tends to be higher in diabetic patients, especially in those of older age. A recent retrospective health insurance administrative claims database study suggested that the prevalence of CIDP in a nondiabetic population is 6 per 100,000 persons, while the prevalence of CIDP in a patient population with DM is ninefold higher at 54 per 100,000 persons. The association of CIDP with DM remains controversial, as both diseases have increased prevalence in patients over age 50 years. It is a challenge to identify CIDP in a diabetic population due to concomitant axonal damage. Although some patients with CIDP and DM respond to treatment, it is difficult to predict response. Because of the rising prevalence of DM throughout the world, there is a need to differentiate CIDP from DPN accurately [24].

The diagnosis of CIDP relies on a combination of clinical and electrophysiological criteria. A number of criteria have been proposed. The European Federation of Neurological Societies (EFNS)/Peripheral Nerve Society (PNS) guidelines were developed for clinical and research use [26]. The criteria combine clinical features and electrophysiological evidence to define CIDP, with supportive criteria including elevated cerebrospinal fluid (CSF) protein, gadolinium enhancement of nerve roots or plexus on MRI or nerve biopsy findings providing supplemental diagnostic evidence. Electrodiagnostic evidence of peripheral nerve demyelination in motor nerves is required for diagnosis, including distal latency prolongation, reduction of motor conduction velocity, prolongation of F-wave latency and partial motor conduction block, and must be identified in at least two nerves for a diagnosis of 'definite' CIDP. It should be noted that in some cases of pure sensory CIDP where routine motor conduction studies are normal, the EFNS/PNS guidelines may fail to diagnose the condition as CIDP. In these cases, if CIDP is suspected, the proximal region of the peripheral sensory nervous system should be carefully interrogated using sensory-evoked potentials. Although other criteria have been proposed, the EFNS/PNS criteria have good sensitivity and specificity for CIDP diagnosis and are currently the most commonly used [26].

Treatment of Diabetic Neuropathy

In diabetic patients, the risk of DPN and autonomic neuropathy can be reduced with improved blood glucose control, and the improvement of lipid and blood pressure indexes and the avoidance of cigarette smoking and excess alcohol consumption are already recommended for the prevention of other complications of diabetes [1].

Preventive Treatment

Based on the etiology of diabetic neuropathy, several agents have been tested to halt its progression (after the onset of subjective symptoms, only palliative treatments are currently available), thereby improving clinical outcome [23]. A very recent meta-analysis showed that main preventive strategies for DPN are intensive glycaemic control with a target

HbA1c < 6% in patients with type 1 diabetes mellitus and standard control of 7.0–7.9 in patients with type 2 diabetes mellitus, incorporating lifestyle modifications.

An analysis of the literature on experimental peripheral diabetic neuropathy suggests that, to date, all of the pharmacological agents shown to counteract one or several manifestations of painful or insensate neuropathy also have efficacy against nerve conduction velocity deficit [27]. Animal studies using pharmacological and genetic approaches revealed important roles of increased aldose reductase, protein kinase C and poly(ADPribose) polymerase activities, advanced glycation end products and their receptors, oxidative-nitrosative stress, growth factor imbalances and C-peptide deficiency in both painful and insensate neuropathies [27].

Aldose reductase inhibitor treatment was suggested not only improving impaired conduction velocity but also improving a variety of subjective symptoms based on recent studies [24]. These findings may support the hypothesis that the polyol pathway plays a central role in the onset and progress of diabetic neuropathy in human subjects. On the other hand, a Cochrane meta-analysis including 32 trials found no overall significant difference between the treated and control groups (SMD -0.25, 95% CI -0.56 to 0.05), although one subgroup analysis (four trials using tolrestat) is favoured [28]. There was no overall benefit on nerve conduction parameters (27 studies) or foot ulceration (one study). Quality of life was not assessed in any of the studies. While most adverse events were infrequent and minor, three compounds had dose-limiting adverse events that lead to their withdrawal from human use: severe hypersensitivity reactions with sorbinil, elevation of creatinine with zenarestat and alteration of liver function with tolrestat [28]. Interestingly, they may ameliorate cardiac automatic neuropathy especially mild or asymptomatic forms, but it merits further investigations as randomized trials are lacking [29].

Alpha lipoic acid is also a potent antioxidant in experimental models, reported to reduce diabetic microvascular and macrovascular complications in animal models [30]. Four trials (ALADIN I, ALADIN III, SYDNEY, NATHAN II) comprised $n = 1258$ patients (α-lipoic acid $n = 716$; placebo $n = 542$) were included in the first meta-analysis based on the intention-to-treat principle. The results of this meta-analysis provided evidence that treatment with α-lipoic acid (600 mg/day i.v.) over three weeks is safe and significantly improves both positive neuropathic symptoms and neuropathic deficits to a clinically meaningful degree in diabetic patients with symptomatic polyneuropathy [30]. This statement was also included in the ADA guidelines as a Level I, Grade A evidence [1]. On the other hand, this meta-analysis did not fulfil the requirements of the Cochrane Collaboration [30]. In an economical point of view, standard symptomatic treatment seems to be much more cheaper in Europe [1, 30]. The combination of parenteral (600 mg daily for three weeks) and oral therapy (600 mg three times daily for six months) administered over a total of seven months failed to translate into significant improvements [1]. The four-year-follow-up Nathan 1 trial also led to this neutral result [1, 30]. A recent meta-analysis confirmed the abovementioned findings [1, 30]. The current AAN (American Academy of Neurology) and EFNS (European Federation of Neurological Societies) guidelines do not support the use of this drug in neuropathic conditions [1].

Angiotensin-converting enzyme (ACE) or angiotensin receptor blockers (ARB) are widely used in diabetic patient to manage blood pressure and prevent or treat cardiovascular disease and nephropathy. Large-scale studies of the effects of ACE inhibitors or ARBs have not been done, although some small studies and prospective assessments have been performed with positive impact on neuropathy [1].

Symptomatic Treatment: Painful Diabetic Neuropathy

Tricyclic antidepressants (TCA): These are so-called early antidepressant medications. These first-generation medications were effective in the treatment of depression because they enhanced serotonergic or noradrenergic mechanisms or both. They also were the first medication category that proved effective for neuropathic pain in placebo-controlled trials [26]. Unfortunately, the TCAs also blocked histaminic, cholinergic and alpha1-adrenergic receptor sites, and this action brought about unwanted side effects such as weight gain, dry mouth, constipation, drowsiness and dizziness [30]. The cardiovascular effects of TCAs are well characterized and include orthostatic hypotension, slowed cardiac conduction, type 1A antiarrhythmic activity and increased heart rate. Although much of them are temporary and exhibit mild effect, they are generally well tolerated. Based on a Cochrane analysis for diabetic neuropathy, the number needed to treat (NNT) for effectiveness was 1.3 (95% CI 1.2 to 1.5), the number needed to harm (NNH) for minor adverse effects was 6 (95% CI 4.2 to 10.7) and number needed to harm (NNH) for major adverse effects defined as an event leading to withdrawal from a study was 28 (95% CI 17.6–68.9) [31]. Comparison meta-analysis of TCAs and SSRIs showed beneficial safety profiles (but the key effects differed between the drug classes) [1, 31]. On the other hand, their use should be avoided in post-infarct states and in the case of conduction disturbances and cardiac arrhythmias (IA antiarrhythmic effect) [1] (Table 56.3).

Selective serotonin reuptake inhibitors (SSRIs): The SSRIs are increasingly being used to treat a spectrum of depressed patients, including the elderly. As a class, SSRIs have comparable efficacy to TCAs against depression but are generally better tolerated [31]. Despite of their widely use, there is still limited evidence for the role of classical SSRIs in the treatment of painful diabetic neuropathy [31].

The class of serotonin and norepinephrine reuptake inhibitors (SNRIs) now comprises three medications: venlafaxine, milnacipran and duloxetine. These drugs block the reuptake of both serotonin (5-HT) and norepinephrine with differing selectivity. Whereas milnacipran blocks 5-HT and norepinephrine reuptake with equal affinity, duloxetine has a tenfold selectivity for 5-HT and venlafaxine a 30-fold selectivity for 5-HT. All three SNRIs are efficacious in treating a variety of anxiety disorders [32–34].

Venlafaxine (three studies) has an NNT of 3.1 (95% CI 2.2–5.1). The NNH for minor adverse effects 9.6 (95% CI 3.5 to 13) and the number needed to harm (NNH) for major adverse effects defined as an event leading to withdrawal from a study 16.2 (95% CI 8–436) for venlafaxine [1].

Duloxetine at 60 mg daily was also effective in treating painful diabetic peripheral neuropathy in the short term to 12 weeks with a risk ratio (RR) for 50% pain reduction at 12 weeks of 1.65 (95% confidence interval (CI) 1.34–2.03) and number needed to treat (NNT) 6 (95% CI 5–10) [32–34]. In a side effect analysis, it was generally safe and well tolerated, with the three most commonly reported adverse events which were nausea, somnolence and constipation. Modest changes in glycaemia were associated with duloxetine. Aspartate transaminase/alanine transaminase increases were transient and not considered predictive of more severe outcomes [33, 34] (Table 56.3).

Antiepileptic drugs: Antiepileptic drugs (AEDs) have a long history of effectiveness in the treatment of neuropathic pain, dating back to case studies of the treatment of trigeminal neuralgia with phenytoin in 1942 and carbamazepine in 1962 [1, 35–38]. Since 1993, nine new AEDs (felbamate, gabapentin, pregabalin, lamotrigine, topiramate, tiagabine, levetiracetam, oxcarbazepine and zonisamide) have received Food and Drug Administration (FDA) approval for the adjunctive treatment of partial seizures [35–38]. In addition to providing efficacy against epilepsy, these new AEDs may also be effective in neuropathic pain. For example, spontaneous activity in regenerating small caliber primary afferent nerve fibres may be quelled by sodium channel blockade, and hyperexcitability in dorsal horn spinal neurons may be decreased by the inhibition of glutamate release [35–38].

Gabapentin is an effective agent in the treatment of diabetic neuropathy, the NNT for effective pain was 2.9 (95% CI 2.2 to 4.3) and the NNH for minor harm was 3.7 (95% CI 2.4 to 5.4). Persons taking gabapentin can expect to suffer dizziness (21%), somnolence (16%), peripheral oedema (8%) and gait disturbance (9%). Serious adverse events (4%) were no more common than with placebo [35–38] (Table 56.3).

Pregabalin at doses of 300 mg, 450 mg and 600 mg daily was effective in patients with postherpetic neuralgia, painful diabetic neuropathy, central neuropathic pain and fibromyalgia (19 studies, 7003 participants). Pregabalin at 150 mg daily was generally ineffective [1]. The best (lowest) NNT for each condition for at least 50% pain relief over baseline (substantial benefit) for 600 mg pregabalin daily compared with placebo were 5.0 (4.0–6.6) for painful diabetic neuropathy. With 600 mg pregabalin, daily somnolence typically occurred in 15–25% and dizziness occurred in 27–46%. The proportion of participants reporting at least one adverse event was not affected by dose nor was the number with a serious adverse event, which was not more than with placebo [35–38] (Table 56.3).

The efficacy of valproic acid and lamotrigine is doubtful; they are not recommended routinely [32]. Using the Cochrane criteria, carbamazepine seems to be effective; on the other hand, no trial was longer than 4 weeks, of good reporting quality, using outcomes equivalent to at least moderate clinical benefit. In these circumstances, caution is needed in interpretation, and meaningful comparison with other interventions is not possible [1, 35–38]. The efficacy of topiramate is also neutral in this condition [1, 35–38].

Narcotic agents: Short-term studies provide only equivocal evidence regarding the efficacy of opioids in reducing the intensity of neuropathic pain, whereas intermediate-term studies demonstrate significant efficacy of opioids over placebo, which is likely to be clinically important [39]. The opioids studied were classified as weak (tramadol, propoxyphene, codeine) or strong (morphine, oxycodone) [39]. Weak and strong opioids outperformed placebo for pain and function in all types of neuropathic pain based on the result of a recent meta-analysis [39]. Other drugs produced better functional outcomes than opioids, whereas for pain relief, they were outperformed only by strong opioids. Dropout rates averaged 33% in the opioid groups and 38% in the placebo groups [39]. Among the side effects of opioids, only constipation and nausea were clinically and statistically significant.

Benzodiazepines: Agonists at the benzodiazepine binding site of ionotropic gamma-aminobutyric acid (GABA(A)) receptors are in clinical use such as hypnotics, anxiolytics and anticonvulsants since the early 1960s. Analgesic effects of classical benzodiazepines have occasionally been reported in certain subgroups of patients suffering from chronic pain or after spinal delivery through intrathecal catheters. However, these drugs are generally not considered as analgesics. Recent evidence from genetically modified mice now indicates that agents targeting only a subset of benzodiazepine (GABA(A)) receptors should provide pronounced antihyperalgesic activity against inflammatory and neuropathic pain. Several such compounds have been developed recently, which exhibit significant antihyperalgesia in mice and rats and appear to be devoid of the typical side effects of classical benzodiazepines [40].

Other agents: Local lidocaine and capsaicin cream have been shown to be effective in the treatment of neuropathic conditions. They are included as potential therapeutic options in the recent AAN guidelines. Acupuncture, but not traditional Chinese herbal medicine, seems to be slightly effective. Transcutaneous electric nerve stimulation (TENS) should also be considered in the treatment of painful diabetic neuropathy [1].

Comparison: In random effect and fixed effect analyses of duloxetine (DLX), pregabalin (PGB) and gabapentin (GBP), all were superior to placebo for all efficacy parameters, with some tolerability trade-offs. Indirect comparison of DLX with PGB found no differences in 24 h pain severity, but significant differences in subjective global improvement, favouring PGB, and in dizziness, favouring DLX, were apparent. Comparing DLX and GBP, there were no statistically significant differences [41]. In three head-to-head trials, there was no difference between gabapentin and tricyclic antidepressants for achieving pain relief (RR 0.99, 95% CI 0.76 to 1.29) [42]. In a recent network meta-analysis, all interventions remained effective in comparison with placebo (mean difference in change of pain from baseline compared with placebo, amitriptyline, -12.58 [95% CI -16.66 to −8.50]; capsaicin, -9.40 [95% CI -13.92 to −4.88]; gabapentin, -10.22 [95% CI -17.25 to −3.19]; and pregabalin, -10.53 [95% CI -14.74 to −6.32] [35–37]. Based on these results, 5% lidocaine medicated plaster was comparable with the previously mentioned medications [43].

The recent ADA guidelines recommend optimization of glucose control to prevent or delay the development of neuropathy in patients with type 1 diabetes and to slow the progression of neuropathy in patients with type 2 diabetes [44]. Pregabalin, duloxetine are gabapentin are the first line of pharmacological treatments for painful diabetic neuropathy [44]. A very recent narrative in-depth review included pregabalin and duloxetine as first-line treatment options (and gabapentin as a reasonable alternative to pregabalin). Second- and third-line drugs were opioids (they are effective but adverse reactions and addiction concerns should be kept in mind) and topical analgesics. Pathogenesis-oriented treatments such as α-lipoic acid and actovegin should be confirmed in more extensive trials [45].

Combination therapy: Unfortunately there are too few controlled studies (complying with modern requirements for EBM) on combination therapy for neuropathic pain (84). Based on pharmacological, and pharmacokinetical profile, SNRIs and TCAs cannot be combined because of the high possibility of serotonin syndrome. TCAs and gabapentin and pregabalin or SNRI in combination with the abovementioned agents are good possibilities. Opioids can be combined with each of these drugs. Based on the recent AAN guidelines, venlafaxine may be added to gabapentin for a better response, and the EFNS guidelines prefer the combination therapy of TCA-gabapentin and gabapentin-opioids [1].

The recently published COMBO-DN multicentre, double-blind, parallel-group study in diabetic peripheral neuropathic pain addressed whether, in patients not responding to standard doses of duloxetine or pregabalin, combining both medications is superior to increasing each drug to its maximum recommended dose [46]. For initial eight-week therapy, either 60 mg/day duloxetine (groups 1 and 2) or 300 mg/day pregabalin (groups 3 and 4) was given. Thereafter, in the eight-week combination/high-dose therapy period, only nonresponders received 120 mg/day duloxetine (group 1), a combination of 60 mg/day duloxetine and 300 mg/day pregabalin (groups 2 and 3) or 600 mg/day pregabalin (group 4). Eight hundred four patients were evaluated for initial therapy and 339 for combination/high-dose therapy. Fifty percent response rates were 52.1% for combination and 39.3% for high-dose monotherapy (P = 0.068). In exploratory analyses of the initial eight-week therapy uncorrected for multiple comparisons, 60 mg/day duloxetine was found superior to 300 mg/day pregabalin (P < 0.001) [46]. Although not significantly superior to high-dose monotherapy, combination therapy was considered to be effective, safe and well tolerated.

Low-quality evidence raised the possibility of the combination of oxycodone with pregabalin and that of pregabalin with the 5% lidocaine plaster, but future, clear-cut studies are required to drive evidence-based decisions in the clinical setting [47].

Multiple Choice Questions

1. Consequences of peripheral diabetic neuropathy:
   (a) Morbidity
   (b) Discapacity
   (c) Mortality
   (d) Diminished quality of life
   (e) **All of the above**
2. Prevalence of peripheral neuropathy in patients with prediabetes:
   (a) Zero, it is exclusive of patients with diabetes
   (b) 5–10%
   (c) **11–25%**
   (d) 26–40%
   (e) 41–55%
3. Key pathological process inducing nerve damage in diabetes:
   (a) Trauma
   (b) **Oxidative stress**
   (c) Ischaemia
   (d) All of the above
   (e) None of the above
4. Diabetic peripheral neuropathy initially affects:
   (a) One extremity
   (b) Several extremities, asymmetrically
   (c) The proximal portions of the extremities
   (d) **The distal portions of extremities, symmetrically**
   (e) The distal portions of extremities, asymmetrically

5. The percentage of patients with asymptomatic distal sensory diabetic neuropathy is:
   (a) 100%
   (b) 75%
   (c) **50%**
   (d) 25%
   (e) 10%

6. Acute diabetic mononeuropathies are frequently associated:
   (a) With adequate metabolic control
   (b) With viral infections
   (c) With emotional stress
   (d) **With periods of transitions of the disease**
   (e) None of the above

7. Effective doses of pregabalin for the treatment of painful diabetic neuropathy:
   (a) 75 mg/day
   (b) 150 mg/day
   (c) **300 mg/day**
   (d) **450 mg/day**
   (e) **600 mg/day**

8. Traditional benzodiazepines are effective analgesics.
   (a) True
   (b) **False**

9. The evidence regarding the efficacy of opioids in reducing the intensity of neuropathic pain shows that:
   (a) They should be standard therapy.
   (b) They are superior to tricyclic antidepressants.
   (c) They are equally effective to pregabalin.
   (d) **They are only superior to placebo, and the evidence is equivocal**.
   (e) They should not be used.
   (f) They are equally effective to non-steroid anti-inflammatories.

10. In patients with diabetic peripheral pain, the COMBO-DN study showed:
    (a) That combination therapy with duloxetine and pregabalin is superior to high dose monotherapy
    (b) That 300 mg pregabalin is superior to 60 mg duloxetine
    (c) **That 60 mg duloxetine is superior to 300 mg pregabalin**
    (d) That both medications have similar rates of effectiveness and safety
    (e) That doses of duloxetine could be decreased

References

1. Deli G, Bosnyak E, Pusch G, Komoly S, Feher G. Diabetic neuropathies: diagnosis and management. Neuroendocrinology. 2013;98(4):267–80.
2. Yang CP, Lin CC, Li CI, Liu CS, Lin WY, Hwang KL, Yang SY, Chen HJ, Li TC. Cardiovascular risk factors increase the risks of diabetic peripheral neuropathy in patients with type 2 diabetes mellitus: the Taiwan diabetes study. Medicine (Baltimore). 2015;94(42):e1783.
3. Popescu S, Timar B, Baderca F, Simu M, Diaconu L, Velea I, Timar R. Age as an independent factor for the development of neuropathy in diabetic patients. Clin Interv Aging. 2016;11:313–8.
4. Juster-Switlyk K, Smith AG. Updates in diabetic peripheral neuropathy. F1000Res. 2016;5:F1000 Faculty Rev-738.
5. Zhang X, Yang X, Sun B, Zhu C. Perspectives of glycemic variability in diabetic neuropathy: a comprehensive review. Commun Biol. 2021;4(1):1366.
6. Zherebitskaya E, Akude E, Smith DR, Fernyhough P. Development of selective axonopathy in adult sensory neurons isolated from diabetic rats: role of glucose-induced oxidative stress. Diabetes. 2009;58(6):1356–64.
7. Schreiber AK, Nones CF, Reis RC, Chichorro JG, Cunha JM. Diabetic neuropathic pain: physiopathology and treatment. World J Diabetes. 2015;6(3):432–44.
8. Juster-Switlyk K, Smith AG. Updates in diabetic peripheral neuropathy [version 1; referees: 3 approved] 2016. F1000Res. 2016;5:F1000 Faculty Rev.
9. Tesfaye S, Boulton AJ, Dyck PJ, Freeman R, Horowitz M, Kempler P, Lauria G, Malik RA, Spallone V, Vinik A, Bernardi L, Valensi P, Toronto Diabetic Neuropathy Expert Group. Diabetic neuropathies: update on definitions, diagnostic criteria, estimation of severity, and treatments. Diabetes Care. 2010;33(10):2285–93.
10. Baron R, Binder A, Wasner G. Neuropathic pain: diagnosis, pathophysiological mechanisms, and treatment. Lancet Neurol. 2010;9(8):807–19.
11. Tesfaye S, Selvarajah D. Advances in the epidemiology, pathogenesis and management of diabetic peripheral neuropathy. Diabetes Metab Res Rev. 2012;28(Suppl 1):8–14.
12. Garcia-Larrea L, Peyron R. Pain matrices and neuropathic pain matrices: a review. Pain. 2013;154(Suppl 1):S29–43.
13. Neugebauer V, Galhardo V, Maione S, Mackey SC. Forebrain pain mechanisms. Brain Res Rev. 2009;60(1):226–42.
14. Cauda F, Sacco K, Duca S, Cocito D, D'Agata F, Geminiani GC, Canavero S. Altered resting state in diabetic neuropathic pain. PLoS One. 2009;4(2):e4542.
15. Li J, Zhang W, Wang X, Yuan T, Liu P, Wang T, Shen L, Huang Y, Li N, You H, Xiao T, Feng F, Ma C. Functional magnetic resonance imaging reveals differences in brain activation in response to thermal stimuli in diabetic patients with and without diabetic peripheral neuropathy. PLoS One. 2018;13(1):e0190699.
16. Teh K, Wilkinson ID, Heiberg-Gibbons F, Awadh M, Kelsall A, Pallai S, Sloan G, Tesfaye S, Selvarajah D. Somatosensory network functional connectivity differentiates clinical pain phenotypes in diabetic neuropathy. Diabetologia. 2021;64(6):1412–21.
17. Croosu SS, Hansen TM, Brock B, Mohr Drewes A, Brock C, Frøkjær JB. Altered functional connectivity between brain structures in adults with type 1 diabetes and polyneuropathy. Brain Res. 2022;1784:147882.
18. American Diabetes Association Professional Practice Committee, American Diabetes Association Professional Practice Committee, Draznin B, Aroda VR, Bakris G, Benson G, Brown FM, Freeman R, Green J, Huang E, Isaacs D, Kahan S, Leon J, Lyons SK, Peters AL, Prahalad P, Reusch JEB, Young-Hyman D, Das S, Kosiborod M. Classification and diagnosis of diabetes: standards of medical Care in Diabetes-2022. Diabetes Care. 2022;45(Suppl 1):S17–38.
19. Hartemann A, Attal N, Bouhassira D, Dumont I, Gin H, Jeanne S, Said G, Richard JL, Working Group on the Diabetic Foot from the French-speaking Society of Diabetology. Painful diabetic neuropathy: diagnosis and management. Diabetes Metab. 2011;37(5):377–88.
20. Gibbons CH, Freeman R. Treatment-induced diabetic neuropathy: a reversible painful autonomic neuropathy. Ann Neurol. 2010;67(4):534–41.
21. Sandireddy R, Yerra VG, Areti A, Komirishetty P, Kumar A. Neuroinflammation and oxidative stress in diabetic neuropa-

thy: futuristic strategies based on these targets. Int J Endocrinol. 2014;2014:674987.

22. von Hehn CA, Baron R, Woolf CJ. Deconstructing the neuropathic pain phenotype to reveal neural mechanisms. Neuron. 2012;73(4):638–52.

23. Fatehi F, Nafissi S, Basiri K, Amiri M, Soltanzadeh A. Chronic inflammatory demyelinating polyneuropathy associated with diabetes mellitus. J Res Med Sci. 2013;18(5):438–41.

24. Bril V, Blanchette CM, Noone JM, Runken MC, Gelinas D, Russell JW. The dilemma of diabetes in chronic inflammatory demyelinating polyneuropathy. J Diabetes Complicat. 2016;30(7):1401–7.

25. Neligan A, Reilly MM, Lunn MP. CIDP: mimics and chameleons. Pract Neurol. 2014;14(6):399–408.

26. Mathey EK, Park SB, Hughes RA, Pollard JD, Armati PJ, Barnett MH, Taylor BV, Dyck PJ, Kiernan MC, Lin CS. Chronic inflammatory demyelinating polyradiculoneuropathy: from pathology to phenotype. J Neurol Neurosurg Psychiatry. 2015;86(9):973–85.

27. Obrosova IG. Diabetic painful and insensate neuropathy: pathogenesis and potential treatments. Neurotherapeutics. 2009;6(4):638–47.

28. Chalk C, Benstead TJ, Moore F. Aldose reductase inhibitors for the treatment of diabetic polyneuropathy. Cochrane Database Syst Rev. 2007;2007(4):CD004572.

29. Hu X, Li S, Yang G, Liu H, Boden G, Li L. Efficacy and safety of aldose reductase inhibitor for the treatment of diabetic cardiovascular autonomic neuropathy: systematic review and meta-analysis. PLoS One. 2014;9(2):e87096.

30. Mijnhout GS, Alkhalaf A, Kleefstra N, Bilo HJ. Alpha lipoic acid: a new treatment for neuropathic pain in patients with diabetes? Neth J Med. 2010;68(4):158–62.

31. Feighner JP. Mechanism of action of antidepressant medications. J Clin Psychiatry. 1999;60(Suppl 4):4–11.

32. Saarto T, Wiffen PJ. Antidepressants for neuropathic pain: a Cochrane review. J Neurol Neurosurg Psychiatry. 2010;81(12):1372–3.

33. Stahl SM, Grady MM, Moret C, Briley M. SNRIs: their pharmacology, clinical efficacy, and tolerability in comparison with other classes of antidepressants. CNS Spectr. 2005;10(9):732–47.

34. Lunn MP, Hughes RA, Wiffen PJ. Duloxetine for treating painful neuropathy or chronic pain. Cochrane Database Syst Rev. 2009;(4):CD007115.

35. Vinik A. Clinical review: use of antiepileptic drugs in the treatment of chronic painful diabetic neuropathy. J Clin Endocrinol Metab. 2005;90(8):4936–45.

36. Moore RA, Wiffen PJ, Derry S, McQuay HJ. Gabapentin for chronic neuropathic pain and fibromyalgia in adults. Cochrane Database Syst Rev. 2011;(3):CD007938.

37. Moore RA, Straube S, Wiffen PJ, Derry S, McQuay HJ. Pregabalin for acute and chronic pain in adults. Cochrane Database Syst Rev. 2009;(3):CD007076.

38. Smith HS, Argoff CE. Pharmacological treatment of diabetic neuropathic pain. Drugs. 2011;71(5):557–89.

39. Furlan AD, Sandoval JA, Mailis-Gagnon A, Tunks E. Opioids for chronic noncancer pain: a meta-analysis of effectiveness and side effects. CMAJ. 2006;174(11):1589–94.

40. Zeilhofer HU, Witschi R, Hösl K. Subtype-selective GABA(A) receptor mimetics - novel antihyperalgesic agents? Mol Med (Berl). 2009;87(5):465–9.

41. Quilici S, Chancellor J, Löthgren M, Simon D, Said G, Le TK, Garcia-Cebrian A, Monz B. Meta-analysis of duloxetine vs. pregabalin and gabapentin in the treatment of diabetic peripheral neuropathic pain. BMC Neurol. 2009;9:6.

42. Chou R, Carson S, Chan BK. Gabapentin versus tricyclic antidepressants for diabetic neuropathy and post-herpetic neuralgia: discrepancies between direct and indirect meta-analyses of randomized controlled trials. J Gen Intern Med. 2009;24(2):178–88.

43. Wolff RF, Bala MM, Westwood M, Kessels AG, Kleijnen. 5% lidocaine medicated plaster in painful diabetic peripheral neuropathy (DPN): a systematic review. Swiss Med Wkly. 2010;140(21–22):297–306.

44. American Diabetes Association Professional Practice Committee, American Diabetes Association Professional Practice Committee, Draznin B, Aroda VR, Bakris G, Benson G, Brown FM, Freeman R, Green J, Huang E, Isaacs D, Kahan S, Leon J, Lyons SK, Peters AL, Prahalad P, Reusch JEB, Young-Hyman D, Das S, Kosiborod M. 12. Retinopathy, neuropathy, and foot care: standards of medical care in diabetes-2022. Diabetes Care. 2022;45(Suppl 1):S185–94.

45. Ardeleanu V, Toma A, Pafili K, Papanas N, Motofei I, Diaconu CC, Rizzo M, Pantea SA. Current pharmacological treatment of painful diabetic neuropathy: a narrative review. Medicina. 2020;56(1):25.

46. Tesfaye S, Wilhelm S, Lledo A, Schacht A, Tölle T, Bouhassira D, Cruccu G, Skljarevski V, Freynhagen R. Duloxetine and pregabalin: high-dose monotherapy or their combination? The "COMBO-DN study" - a multinational, randomized, double-blind, parallel-group study in patients with diabetic peripheral neuropathic pain. Pain. 2013;154(12):2616–25.

47. Pafili K, Papanas N. Considerations for single- versus multiple-drug pharmacotherapy in the management of painful diabetic neuropathy. Expert Opin Pharmacother. 2021;22(16):2267–80.

Diabetic Cardiac Autonomic Neuropathy

Victoria Serhiyenko and Alexandr Serhiyenko

Abbreviations

ABPM	Ambulatory blood pressure monitoring
BP	Blood pressure
BRS	Baroreflex sensitivity
CAD	Coronary artery disease
CAN	Cardiac autonomic neuropathy
CARTs	Cardiovascular autonomic reflex tests
CHD	Coronary heart disease
CVD	Cardiovascular diseases
DLP	Dyslipidemia
DM	Diabetes mellitus
GLP1-RA	Glucagon-like peptide 1 receptor agonists
HR	Heart rate
HRT	Heart rate turbulence
HRV	Heart rate variability
LV	Left ventricular
MI	Myocardial infarction
MSNA	Muscle sympathetic nerve activity
OH	Orthostatic hypotension
QTi	QT interval
SGLT2i	Sodium glucose transporter 2 inhibitors
SMI	Silent myocardial ischemia
T1DM	Type 1 diabetes mellitus
T2DM	Type 2 diabetes mellitus
α-LA	α-Lipoic acid
ω-3 PUFA	ω-3 Polyunsaturated fatty acids

Core tip: Cardiac autonomic neuropathy (CAN) is a serious complication of diabetes mellitus that is strongly associated with increased risk of cardiovascular mortality. CAN manifests in a spectrum of things, ranging from resting tachycardia, fixed heart rate arrhythmias, intraoperative cardiovascular instability and orthostatic hypotension to development of "silent" myocardial ischemia, "silent" myocardial infarction.

Diabetic patients should be screened for CAN due to the possibility of reversal of cardiovascular denervation in the early stages of the disease. Cardiovascular reflex tests and Holter-derived time and frequency-domain measurements are frequently used for the diagnosis. Therapeutic approaches are promising and may hinder or reverse the progression of the CAN when initiated during the early stages.

Introduction

Diabetes mellitus (DM) is a global epidemic affecting at least 8.3% of the population and 371 million people worldwide with a significant proportion (50%) remaining undiagnosed. It is estimated that almost one of six people are currently at risk of developing diabetes-related complications [1–4].

The majority of patients with long-term course of DM [mainly type 2 diabetes mellitus (T2DM)] are diagnosed

V. Serhiyenko (✉) · A. Serhiyenko
Department of Endocrinology, Danylo Halytsky Lviv National Medical University, Lviv, Ukraine

© The Author(s), under exclusive license to Springer Nature Switzerland AG 2023
J. Rodriguez-Saldana (ed.), *The Diabetes Textbook*, https://doi.org/10.1007/978-3-031-25519-9_57

with coronary heart disease (CHD) due to coronary vessels arterial sclerotic disease. Often the course of CHD is complicated by combination of hypertension, specific kidney arterial involvement, and eyes and lower limbs affection. Metabolic alterations in the myocardium are combined with early coronary atherosclerosis. All these changes in the heart which occur out of prolonged duration of DM among middle age and elderly patients [coronary vessels affection, myocardium changes, diabetic cardiac autonomic neuropathy (CAN), and arterial sclerotic disease] are associated with the term "diabetic heart or diabetic cardiomyopathy" [5, 6].

Cardiac autonomic neuropathy among T2DM patients is characterized by lesion of nerve fibers in the sympathetic and parasympathetic divisions of the autonomic nervous system and is diagnosed unsatisfactorily and may be accompanied by severe orthostatic hypotension (OH), decreased tolerance to the physical loadings, and cause cardiac arrhythmias, ischemia of coronary vessels, *"silent" myocardial infarction (MI)*, "sudden" death syndrome [7–10].

Definition of CAN

Cardiovascular autonomic neuropathy is defined as the impairment of autonomic control of the cardiovascular system in the setting of diabetes after exclusion of other causes [11]. CAN is caused by damage to the autonomic nerve fibers that innervate the heart and blood vessels and leads to abnormalities in cardiovascular dynamics [12]. CAN is usually documented by using several cardiovascular autonomic reflex tests (CARTs) [13–15].

Epidemiology of CAN

CAN is a common chronic complication of type 1 diabetes mellitus (T1DM) and T2DM and is associated with higher morbidity and mortality level among patients with DM. The prevalence of confirmed CAN in unselected people with T1DM and T2DM is around 20%, but figures as high as 65% are reported with increasing age and diabetes duration. Because many studies were hospital based, referral bias cannot be excluded (classes II and III). Clinical correlates or risk markers for CAN are age, diabetes duration, poor glycemic control, microvascular complications (peripheral polyneuropathy, retinopathy, and nephropathy), hypertension, and dyslipoproteinemia (classes I and II). Established risk factors for CAN are glycemic control in T1DM (class I) and a combination of hypertension, dyslipoproteinemia (DLP), obesity, and glycemic control in T2DM (class II) [14, 15].

Screening for CAN should be performed in asymptomatic T2DM at diagnosis and T1DM after 5 years of disease, in particular those at greater risk for CAN due to a history of poor glycemic control [*hemoglobin A$_{1c}$* (HbA$_{1c}$) > 7%], or the presence of one major cardiovascular risk factor (among hypertension, DLP, and smoking), or the presence of macro- or microangiopathic complications (level B). CAN screening may be also required in asymptomatic patients for preoperative risk assessment before major surgical procedures (level C) [14–16].

Risk Factors for the Diabetic Cardiac Autonomic Neuropathy

Current data that differentiate CAN in T1DM and in T2DM in terms of risk factors and natural history are summarized in Table 57.1 [17].

Possible factors associated with high mortality and sudden death due to autonomic neuropathy are [5]:

- Silent myocardial ischemia/infarction.
- Cardiorespiratory arrest/increased perioperative and peri-intubation risk.
- Resting tachycardia.
- Ventricular arrhythmias/prolongation of the QT interval (QTi).
- Hypertension.
- Orthostatic hypotension.

Table 57.1 Cardiac autonomic neuropathy in type 1 and type 2 diabetes mellitus: differences in relation to risk factors and natural history [17]

Diabetes mellitus		
Risk factors	Type 1 diabetes mellitus	Type 2 diabetes mellitus
Age	+	+
Gender (female)	+	−
Obesity	−	+
Hyperinsulinemia	NA	+
Duration of DM	++	++
Smoking	+	+
HbA$_{1c}$	++	++
Hypertension	++	++
Retinopathy	++	+
Hypertriglyceridemia	+	+
Classical diabetic peripheral neuropathy	++	++
Microalbuminuria	++	++
Dyslipoproteinemia (>LDL and <HDL)	+	(+)
Prevalence at diagnosis of DM	7.7%	5%
Prevalence after 10 years	38%	65%
Prevalence (random)	25%	34%

++ strong association; + moderate association; − not found; (+) controversial; NA not applicable

- Flattening of the nocturnal reduction of blood pressure (BP) and heart rate ("non-dipper" phenomenon).
- Exaggerated BP responses with supine position and exercise.
- Abnormal diastolic/systolic left ventricular function.
- Poor exercise tolerance.
- Impaired cardiovascular responsiveness.
- Heat intolerance due to defective sympathetic thermoregulation.
- Susceptibility to foot ulcers and amputations due to arteriovenous shunting and sudomotor dysfunction.
- Hypoglycemia unawareness.
- Increased risk of severe hypoglycemia.
- Obstructive sleep apnea syndrome.

Pathogenesis of CAN

Diabetic CAN is eventually caused by complex interactions among a number of pathogenic pathways. Hyperglycemia is the leading cause of the initiation of this pathogenic process [12, 18–20]. The pathogenesis of diabetic CAN is multifactorial, including increased mitochondrial production of free radicals due to hyperglycemia-induced oxidative/nitrosative stress. Neuronal activity, mitochondrial function, membrane permeability, and endothelial function are impaired by advanced glycosylation end product formation, polyol aldose reductase signaling, protein kinase C and poly(ADP ribose) polymerase activation, and the alteration of the Na^+/K^+-ATPase pump function. Neuronal apoptotic processes are precipitated by endoplasmic reticulum stress induced by hyperglycemia, along with impaired nerve perfusion, DLP, alterations in redox status, low-grade inflammation, and disturbance in Ca^{2+} balance [21–24].

Classification of Diabetic Cardiac Autonomic Neuropathy [25]

Subclinical phase:

- Decreased heart rate variability.
  Early phase:

- Resting tachycardia.
  Advanced stage:

- Exercise intolerance.
- Cardiomyopathy with left ventricular dysfunction.
- Orthostatic hypotension.
- Silent myocardial ischemia.

Clinical Impact of CAN

Clinical Manifestations of CAN

Symptomatic manifestations of CAN include sinus tachycardia, exercise intolerance, and orthostatic hypotension. Orthostatic hypotension (OH) was present in 6–32% of diabetic patients depending on diagnostic cutoffs for fall in systolic blood pressure (20 or 30 mmHg) and the diabetic populations studied [15, 26, 27]. Symptoms of orthostatic intolerance were present in 4–18% of diabetic patients [14, 26, 27]. Orthostatic symptoms, such as light-headedness, dizziness, blurred vision, fainting, or pain in the neck or shoulder when standing, may be worse in the early morning, after meals, during a rise in core temperature, during prolonged standing, or with physical activity [28, 29]. Symptoms may be disabling, are often a barrier to an effective antihypertensive treatment, and may lead to falls in the elderly.

A number of other cardiovascular abnormalities were found in association with CAN [30]. These may play a role in excess mortality and morbidity and contribute to the burden associated with CAN (Table 57.2).

Symptoms and signs associated with diabetic CAN are presented in Table 57.3.

Table 57.2 Abnormalities associated with cardiovascular autonomic neuropathy at the level of cardiovascular system and peripheral vascular function [15]

Cardiovascular system	Peripheral vascular function
Perioperative unstability	↑ peripheral blood flow and warm skin
Resting tachycardia	↑ arteriovenous shunting and swollen veins
Loss of reflex heart rate variations	↑ venous pressure
Hypertension	Leg and foot edema
Exercise intolerance	Loss of protective cutaneous vasomotor reflexes
Orthostatic hypotension	Loss of venoarteriolar reflex with microvascular damage
Postprandial hypotension	↑ transcapillary leakage of macromolecules
Silent myocardial ischaemia	↑ medial arterial calcification
Left ventricular dysfunction and hypertrophy	–
QT interval prolongation	–
Impaired baroreflex sensitivity	–
Non-dipping, reverse dipping	–
Sympathovagal imbalance	–
Dysregulation of cerebral circulation	–
↓ sympathetically mediated vasodilation of coronary vessels	–
↑ arterial stiffness	–

Table 57.3 Symptoms and signs associated with diabetic cardiac autonomic neuropathy [20]

Diabetic cardiac autonomic neuropathy	
Resting tachycardia	
Abnormal blood pressure regulation	Nondipping Reverse dipping
Orthostatic hypotension (all with standing)	Light-headedness Weakness Faintness Visual impairment Syncope
Orthostatic tachycardia or bradycardia and chronotropic incompetence (all with standing)	Light-headedness Weakness Faintness Dizziness Visual impairment Syncope
Exercise intolerance	

Morbidity and Mortality in Cardiac Autonomic Neuropathy

CAN is a significant cause of morbidity and mortality associated with a high risk of cardiac arrhythmias and sudden death, possibly related to "silent" myocardial ischemia (SMI). Cardiovascular disease remains the main cause of excess mortality among patients with T1DM and T2DM. Reduced heart rate variability (HRV) as a marker of autonomic dysfunction has been shown to have dire consequences in terms of morbidity (e.g., progression of coronary atherosclerosis) and mortality independent of cardiovascular risk factors in various populations, including those with prediabetes and DM [12, 31]. In T1DM patients, there is a fourfold increase risk of death [31–33]. CAN is significantly associated with overall mortality [7, 12, 15], and in some but not all studies with morbidity, such as SMI, coronary artery disease (CAD), stroke, diabetic nephropathy progression, and perioperative morbidity. In the Detection of Ischemia in Asymptomatic Diabetic Subjects (DIAD) study, a diminished Valsalva heart rate (HR) ratio (a measure of CAN) was strongly associated with SMI, independent of more traditional risk factors including sex, age, hypertension, and smoking [14, 15, 34]. In the European Epidemiology and Prevention of Diabetes (EURODIAB) study, autonomic dysfunction was present in one-third of T1DM patients and was strongly associated with coexisting cardiovascular disease (CVD) after adjustment to age, HbA$_{1c}$, and duration of diabetes [12]. Results from the Action to Control Cardiovascular Risk in Diabetes (ACCORD) trial again confirmed the association of CAN and mortality. These investigators showed that the individuals in this trial with baseline CAN were 1.55–2.14 times as likely to die as individuals without CAN [35]. Furthermore, CAN in the presence of peripheral neuropathy was the highest predictor of CVD mortality. Indeed, combining indexes of autonomic dysfunction have been shown to be associated with the higher risk

of mortality [7, 33]. There is also strong evidence, based on studies in patients with T1DM and patients with T2DM with a mean follow-up of 9.2 years, that QT interval (QTi) prolongation is an independent predictor of mortality for all-cause and cardiovascular deaths [7, 30, 33, 36]. Thus, CAN assessment can be used for cardiovascular risk stratification in patients with and without established CVD, as a marker for patients requiring more intensive monitoring during the perioperative period and other physiological stresses and as an indicator for more intensive pharmacotherapeutic and lifestyle management of comorbid conditions. There is definitive evidence for a predictive value of CAN on overall mortality (class I). There is some evidence of a predictive value of CAN on morbidity (class II). Orthostatic hypotension, when due to advanced CAN, is associated with an additional increase in mortality risk over that driven by HRV abnormalities (class III). Some cardiovascular abnormalities, closely linked to CAN, are associated with increased mortality: tachycardia (class II), QTi prolongation (class II), and non-dipping status (class III) [15, 37].

CAN is a risk marker of mortality (level A), as well as a risk marker and likely a risk factor for cardiovascular morbidity (level B), and possibly a progression promoter of diabetic nephropathy (level C). Orthostatic hypotension is associated with a worse prognosis than cardiovagal neuropathy (level C). QTi prolongation has prognostic value in diabetes (level B). Non-dipping status is associated with an adverse cardiovascular prognosis in diabetes (level C). Non-dipping status predicts the progression from micro- and macroalbuminuria to renal failure in T2DM (level C) [15].

CAN Assessment

Methods of CAN assessment in clinical practice include assessment of symptoms and signs, *cardiovascular reflex tests* based on HR and blood pressure (BP), and ambulatory blood pressure monitoring (ABPM).

Assessment of Symptoms

Questionnaires have been developed to investigate orthostatic symptoms and their severity in dysautonomic conditions, although they have not been specifically validated for CAN, and validated translations in different languages are lacking. In the Rochester Diabetic Neuropathy Study, the correlation between the autonomic symptoms and the autonomic deficits was weak in T1DM and absent in T2DM patients [28, 29, 38]. Orthostatic symptoms were poorly related to fall in systolic BP on standing. For their clinical impact, orthostatic symptoms should be looked for regularly together with other dysautonomic symptoms in diabetic patients [15].

Assessment of Signs

Resting tachycardia: While abnormalities in HRV are early findings of CAN, resting tachycardia and a fixed HR are characteristic late findings in diabetic patients with vagal impairment. Resting HR of 90–100 b.p.m. and occasional HR increments up to 130 b.p.m. occur. The highest resting HR have been found in patients with parasympathetic damage, occurring earlier in the course of CAN than sympathetic nerve dysfunction; in those with evidence for combined vagal and sympathetic involvement, the rate returns toward normal but remains elevated. A fixed HR that is unresponsive to moderate exercise, stress, or sleep indicates almost complete cardiac denervation. A blunted HR response to adenosine receptor agonists was described in both patients with DM and patients with metabolic syndrome and attributed to earlier stages of CAN [34, 39]. Higher resting HR (>78 b.p.m.) compared with lower resting HR (<58 b.p.m.) and a rise in HR with time have been shown to be powerful, independent risk predictors for all-cause and CVD mortality in several prospective cohorts [9]. The prognostic value of resting HR is a useful tool for cardiovascular risk stratification and as a therapeutic target in high-risk patients [12, 31, 40].

Exercise intolerance: In diabetic patients without evidence of heart disease, but with asymptomatic cardiac vagal neuropathy, exercise capacity and HR, BP, and cardiac stroke volume responses to exercise were diminished. A further decrease in exercise capacity and BP response was seen in patients with both vagal neuropathy and orthostatic hypotension. It is generally recommended that diabetic patients suspected to have CAN should be tested with a cardiac stress test before undertaking an exercise program. The severity of CAN correlated inversely with maximal HR increase during exercise, suggesting CAN contribution to diminished exercise tolerance [14, 15, 41].

Orthostatic hypotension: Orthostatic hypotension is defined as a fall in BP (i.e., > 20 mmHg or more stringent criteria is >30 mmHg for systolic or >10 mmHg for diastolic BP) in response to postural change, from supine to standing [30, 41]. In patients with diabetes, OH is usually a result of damage to the efferent sympathetic vasomotor fibers, particularly in the splanchnic vasculature [12, 28]. Patients with OH are typically represented with light-headedness and presyncopal symptoms. Symptoms, such as dizziness, weakness, fatigue, visual blurring, and neck pain, also might be a result of orthostatic hypotension. Many patients, however, remain asymptomatic despite significant falls in BP. Orthostatic symptoms can also be misjudged as hypoglycemia and can be aggravated by a number of drugs, including vasodilators, diuretics, phenothiazines, and particularly tricyclic antidepressants and insulin [30, 31].

QTi prolongation QTi prolongation has been defined as a QTc (corrected QT for heart rate) ≥460 ms in women and ≥450 ms in men, although in most studies less strict criteria were used. The pathogenesis of QTi prolongation is multifactorial and includes imbalance in cardiac sympathetic innervation, intrinsic metabolic and electrolytic myocardial changes, left ventricular (LV) hypertrophy, and CAD, and genetic factors could lead to QTi prolongation [36, 42]. The day-night modulation of the QT/relative risk relation—on 24-h ECG recordings—was altered in CAN patients free of CAD, LV dysfunction, or hypertrophy, with a reversed day-night pattern and an increased nocturnal QT rate dependence. Reversible QTi prolongation may be induced by hyperinsulinemia in healthy subjects, by hyperglycemia, and by acute hypoglycemia in both healthy and diabetic subjects [36, 43]. In T1DM patients, prolonged QTc was shown to occur frequently during overnight hypoglycemia and was associated with cardiac rate/rhythm disturbances. These findings support an arrhythmic basis for the "dead in bed" syndrome and possibly a provocative role of hypoglycemia-induced sympathetic activation in cardiovascular events [14, 44]. In a meta-analysis of 17 studies including 4584 diabetic patients, QTc prolongation (>441 ms) was a specific (86%) albeit insensitive (28%) index of CAN [38].

Impaired HRV: The earliest clinical indicator of CAN is a decrease in HRV. Variability in the instantaneous beat-to-beat HR intervals is a function of sympathetic and parasympathetic activity that regulates the cardiac functional response to the body's level of metabolic activity. In normal individuals, the HR has a high degree of beat-to-beat variability and HRV fluctuates increasing with inspiration and decreasing with expiration. Initially, clinical relevance of HRV was identified through observations that fetal distress is preceded by alterations in beat-to-beat intervals before any appreciable change occurs in HR itself. The serious implications of abnormal HRV became apparent only in the late 1980s, when it was confirmed that HRV was a strong, independent predictor of mortality after acute myocardial infarction [24, 30, 45, 46]

Non-dipping and reverse dipping: At night, health subjects exhibit a predominance of vagal tone and decreased sympathetic tone, associated with reduction in nocturnal BP. In diabetic CAN this pattern is altered, resulting in sympathetic predominance during sleep and subsequent nocturnal hypertension. This is associated with a higher frequency of LV hypertrophy and both fatal and severe nonfatal cardiovascular events in diabetic CAN subjects [14, 24, 38].

Ambulatory blood pressure monitoring is a standard tool in hypertension research and management with regard to diagnostic, prognostic, and therapeutic issues [47]. It allows the assessment of the diurnal BP pattern, which is mainly regulated by sleep-awake changes in the autonomic cardiovascular function. ABPM may be used for research purposes to:

- Evaluate the circadian BP pattern and its abnormalities (e.g., non-dipping, nocturnal hypertension, extreme dipping, morning surge).
- Study its relationship with autonomic dysfunction, sleep disturbances, and kidney function.
- Assess the 24-h BP response to treatment.
- Evaluate the longer term prognostic implications of circadian BP abnormalities.

Non-dipping and reverse-dipping patterns were associated with CAN, which was the major determinant of the circadian variation in blood pressure. Several observations in both diabetic and nondiabetic patients linked non-dipping to a disruption of the circadian variation in sympathovagal activity, i.e., a diminished increase in vagal activity and a sympathetic predominance during the night. The day-night difference in systolic BP was a moderately accurate diagnostic tool for CAN and reverse dipping as a specific (95%)— albeit insensitive (25%)—marker of CAN [15, 38]. In clinical practice, ABPM in the general population is useful for diagnostic purposes and provides unique and additional information for risk stratification with regard to hypertension-related organ damage and cardiovascular events and for the extent of BP response to treatment [24, 38]. The European Society of Hypertension acknowledges that ABPM may improve predictions of cardiovascular risk in hypertensive patients and recommends that 24-h ABPM should be considered in the presence of either noticeable variability of office BP values or a marked discrepancy between office and home BP values and in case of resistance to drug treatment or suspected hypotensive episodes [24, 38]. Thus, in patients with CAN, ABPM may be particularly useful in detecting non-dipping or reverse-dipping conditions, daytime postural BP changes, and postprandial hypotension and in achieving BP control for the whole 24-h period. Conversely, in clinical practice, the presence of reverse dipping in ABPM may suggest the presence of CAN and thus requires CAN testing [15, 38].

"Silent" myocardial ischemia/cardiac denervation syndrome: The presence of both symptomatic and asymptomatic CAD is increased in diabetic patients, and subclinical neuropathy is an important cause of SMI in patients with diabetes. Five of the 12 studies showed a statistically significant increased frequency of SMI in those with CAN compared with those without CAN [15, 38, 48]. "Silent" ischemia in diabetic patients can either result from CAN, from autonomic dysfunction attributable to CAD itself, or from both. The mechanisms of painless myocardial ischemia are, however, complex and not fully understood. Altered pain thresholds, subthreshold by ischemia not sufficient to induce pain, and dysfunction of the afferent cardiac autonomic nerve fibers have all been suggested as possible mechanisms [12, 38]. Features of a MI in patients with CAN are silence, cough, nausea and vomiting, dyspnea, tiredness, and ECG changes. Reduced appreciation for ischemic pain can impair timely recognition of myocardial ischemia or infarction, thereby delaying appropriate therapy. Thus, patients with CAN warrant more careful attention, and cardiovascular autonomic function testing might be an important component in the risk assessment of diabetic patients with CAD [12].

Intraoperative cardiovascular liability Perioperative cardiovascular morbidity and mortality are increased two- to threefold in patients with diabetes. Compared with nondiabetic subjects, diabetic patients undergoing general anesthesia might experience a greater degree of decline in HR and BP during induction of anesthesia and less of an increase after tracheal intubation and extubation. Vasopressor support is required more often in diabetic individuals with CAN than in those without CAN [30, 49]. The normal autonomic response of vasoconstriction and tachycardia does not completely compensate for the vasodilating effects of anesthesia. There is an association between CAN and more severe intraoperative hypothermia that can result in decreased drug metabolism and impaired wound healing. Reduced hypoxic-induced ventilatory drive [30] requires preoperative CAN screening for loss of HRV. Preoperative cardiovascular autonomic screening might provide useful information for anesthesiologists planning the anesthetic management of diabetic patients and identify those at greater risk of intraoperative complications [12, 30].

Thus, resting HR is not a specific sign of CAN (class IV). After exclusion of other causes, OH suggests an advanced CAN that should be confirmed by CARTs (class I). Orthostatic hypotension (class III), QTi prolongation (class II), and reverse dipping on ABPM are specific but insensitive indices of CAN (class III) [12].

In terms of recommendations, it may be advised that the presence of symptoms and/or signs is not a sufficient criterion for CAN diagnosis but should provide the motivation to perform CAN testing to get a definite diagnosis (level B). Screening of orthostatic symptoms is advisable in any diabetic patient (level B). Regardless of the presence of orthostatic symptoms, the OH test is recommended yearly, in particular in patients over the age of 50 and in hypertensive diabetic patients (level B). CAN testing offers a useful tool to identify patients with potentially poor exercise performance and to prevent adverse outcomes when patients are introduced to exercise training programs (level C). Diabetic patients with unexplained tachycardia should undergo CAN testing (level C). Resting HR may be used in clinical practice for cardiovascular risk stratification (level C). QTi prolongation alone is an insufficient measure of CAN but should prompt further testing (level B). QTc may be used for cardiovascular risk stratification (level B).

ABPM should not be routinely employed for the diagnosis of CAN (level C). However, it is a reliable research tool to explore 24-h BP patterns in different conditions (level B). In the presence of reverse dipping, referral for CAN testing is advisable (level C). ABPM may be useful in patients with CAN to detect non-dipping, to determine risk stratification for cardiovascular mortality and nephropathy progression, and to adjust antihypertensive treatment (level C) [12].

Cardiovascular Autonomic Reflex Tests

Autonomic balance involves complex interactions with several physiological mechanisms that act to maintain heart rate and BP within normal limits. Recent investigations have suggested that autonomic dysfunction (e.g., heightened activity of the sympathetic nervous system and suppressed activity of the parasympathetic nervous system) impairs the ability of the *autonomic nervous system* to regulate the cardiovascular system. Thus, autonomic imbalance might be a key component involved in both the etiology and the clinical course of CVD. What is also emerging is that one needs to distinguish the difference between autonomic imbalance and clear evidence of autonomic neuropathy. Autonomic imbalance produces a number of interesting and trying clinical situations, such as orthostatic tachycardia, orthostatic bradycardia, and OH, and can be responsible for predisposition to arrhythmias and "sudden" death [12, 40]. CARTs assess cardiovascular autonomic function through time-domain HR response to deep breathing, Valsalva maneuver, and postural change, and by measuring the end-organ response, that is, HR and BP changes, although indirect autonomic measures are considered the gold standard in autonomic testing. Heart rate variations during deep breathing, Valsalva maneuver, and lying-to-standing (HR tests) are indices mainly of parasympathetic function, whereas the OH, the BP response to a Valsalva maneuver, and sustained isometric muscular strain provide indices of sympathetic function. These tests are noninvasive, safe, clinically relevant (they correlate with tests of peripheral nervous system function), easy to carry out, sensitive, specific, reproducible, and standardized, and therefore they are considered consolidated, gold standard measures of autonomic function [12].

Diagnostic tests of CAN are summarized in Table 57.4.

Normal, borderline and abnormal values in tests of cardiovascular autonomic function are summarized in Table 57.5.

The Toronto Consensus [38] has concluded the following regarding diagnosis of CAN:

- The following CARTs are the gold standard for clinical autonomic testing: HR response to deep breathing, standing and Valsalva maneuver, and BP response to standing (class II evidence).
- These CARTs are sensitive, specific, reproducible, easy to carry out, safe, and standardized (classes II and III).
- The Valsalva maneuver is not advisable in the presence of proliferative retinopathy and when there is an increased risk of retinal hemorrhage (class IV).
- CARTs are subject to a number of confounding or interfering factors (class III).
- Age is the most relevant factor affecting HR tests (class I).
- A definite diagnosis of CAN and CAN staging requires more than one HR test and the OH test (class III).

The main clinical indications of the autonomic reflex tests are the following [15, 17, 38]:

- Diagnosis and staging of CAN in T2DM patients (at diagnosis and annually thereafter).

Table 57.4 Cardiovascular autonomic reflex tests [12]

Test	Technique	Normal response and values
Beat-to-beat HRV	With the patient at rest and supine, heart rate is monitored by ECG while the patient breathes in and out at six breaths per minute, paced by a metronome or similar device	A difference in HR of >15 beats per minute is normal and < 10 beats per minute is abnormal. The lowest normal value for the expiration-to-inspiration ratio of the R-R interval decreases with age: Age 20–24 years, 1.17; 25–29, 1.15; 30–34, 1.13; 35–39, 1.12; 40–44, 1.10; 45–49, 1.08; 50–54, 1.07; 55–59, 1.06; 60–64, 1.04; 65–69, 1.03; and 70–75, 1.02
Heart rate response to standing	During continuous ECG monitoring, the R-R interval is measured at beats 15 and 30 after standing	Normally, a tachycardia is followed by reflex bradycardia. The 30:15 ratio should be >1.03, borderline 1.01–1.03
Heart rate response to the Valsalva maneuver	The subject forcibly exhales into the mouthpiece of a manometer to 40 mmHg for 15 s during ECG monitoring	Healthy subjects develop tachycardia and peripheral vasoconstriction during strain and an overshoot bradycardia and rise in BP with release. The normal ratio of longest R-R to shortest R-R is >1.2, borderline 1.11–1.2
Systolic blood pressure response to standing	Systolic BP is measured in the supine subject. The patient stands, and the systolic BP is measured after 2 min	Normal response is a fall of <10 mmHg, borderline fall is a fall of 10–29 mmHg, and abnormal fall is a decrease of >30 mmHg
Diastolic blood pressure response to isometric exercise	The subject squeezes a handgrip dynamometer to establish a maximum. Grip is then squeezed at 30% maximum for 5 min	The normal response for diastolic BP is a rise of >16 mmHg in the other arm, borderline 11–15 mmHg

Table 57.5 Normal, borderline, and abnormal values in tests of cardiovascular autonomic function [5]

	Normal	Borderline	Abnormal
Tests reflecting mainly parasympathetic function			
Heart rate response to Valsalva maneuvre (Valsalva ratio)	≥1.21	1.11–1.20	≤1.10
Heart rate (R-R interval) variation	≥15 beats/min	11–14 beats/min	≤10 beats/min
During deep breathing (maximum-minimum heart rate) immediate heart rate response to standing (30:15 ratio)	≥1.04	1.01–1.03	≤1.00
Tests reflecting mainly sympathetic function			
Blood pressure response to standing (fall in systolic blood pressure in mmHg)	≤10	11–29	≥30
Blood pressure response to sustained handgrip (increase in diastolic blood pressure	≥16 mmHg	11–15 mmHg	≤10 mmHg

- Diagnosis and staging of CAN in T1DM patients (5 years after diagnosis and annually thereafter).
- Stratification of cardiovascular risk: in pre-operatory testing, pre-physical activity, indication of selective beta-blocker, and suspected silent ischemia.
- Differential diagnosis of other manifestations of CAN (regardless of DM duration): assess whether gastroparesis, erectile dysfunction, OH, dizziness, syncope, or tachycardia in diabetic persons are due to dysautonomia.
- Evaluate the progression of autonomic failure and monitor response to therapy (e.g., continuous infusion of insulin, post-transplants, and use of antioxidants).
- Differential diagnosis of other causes of neuropathy such as autoimmune autonomic neuropathy (chronic inflammatory demyelinating polyneuropathy, celiac disease, amyotrophy) or toxic-infectious neuropathy (alcohol, primary neuritic *Hansen's* disease, human immunodeficiency virus) as well as in cases where the presence of autonomic neuropathy is disproportionate to the sensorimotor neuropathy.

The most sensitive and specific diagnostic tests currently available to evaluate CAN in clinical research are (1) HRV, (2) baroreflex sensitivity (BRS), (3) muscle sympathetic nerve activity (MSNA), (4) plasma catecholamines, and (5) heart sympathetic imaging [50].

Heart Rate Variability

Heart rate is never completely stable. Continuous tonic, phasic, and transient external and internal stimuli of multiple origins affect HR to a variable but measurable extent. Five different mechanisms have been described: (1) sympathetic and para-sympathetic efferences to the sinus node; (2) neurohumoral influences (e.g., catecholamines, thyroid hormones), (3) stretch of the sinus node, (4) changes in local temperature; and (5) ionic changes in the sinus node. Under resting conditions, it can be assumed that the short-term HRV is essentially determined by the first and third factors. The sympathetic and parasympathetic stimuli directly influence HR and are responsible for a physiologic variation in the heart rate, or HRV. The HRV can be evaluated in the time and frequency domains [38, 45, 50].

Time-domain measures of the normal R-R intervals include the difference between the longest and shortest R-R intervals, the standard deviation of 5-min average of normal R-R intervals (SDANN), and the root-mean-square of the difference of successive R-R intervals (rMSSD). Longer recordings (e.g., 24-h) allow the calculation of additional indices, as the number of instances per hour in which two consecutive R-R intervals differ by more than 50 ms over 24 h (pNN50). Essentially, all these indices explore the parasympathetic activity.

In the frequency domain, the use of spectral analysis of R-R interval (and other cardiovascular and respiratory signals) allows a precise description of the different fluctuations. The components of the HRV obtained by spectral analysis provide information about both the sympathetic and parasympathetic influences on the heart [38, 50]. Based on studies using acceptable techniques, there is evidence of reduced parasympathetic modulation of HR in diabetes and also reduced modulation of systolic BP in the low-frequency region [38, 51] particularly after sympathetic stimulation in response to tilting or in the microcirculation. As most of the CARTs essentially explore the parasympathetic activity, there is no other simple test of sympathetic activity capable of identifying early (functional or anatomic) autonomic sympathetic abnormality [50]. CARTs are considered the gold standard for CAN testing. Impaired HRV time- and frequency-domain indices have been reported in diabetic patients before CARTs abnormalities arise. However, the few studies that assessed the diagnostic accuracy against the reference standard of CARTs found only fair results. Time- and frequency-domain analysis of 24-h ECG recordings has documented an abnormal nocturnal sympathetic predominance in diabetic patients that was linked to BP non-dipping. In obese patients, weight loss was associated with an improvement in global HRV and in parasympathetic HRV indices [7, 50].

In this way, HRV testing is a clinically relevant measure in addition to CARTs and provides key information about autonomic-parasympathetic and sympathetic-modulation of the cardiovascular system. Analysis of HRV can be done using statistical indices in the time and frequency domains. Time-domain indices of global HRV and total spectral power of HRV represent the index of parasympathetic activity, as well as the HRV spectral power in the high-frequency region, while the relative proportion (not the absolute power) in the low frequencies of HRV provides a relative measure of sympathetic modulation. This interpretation should be made with cautions if respiratory artifacts (slow breaths) cannot be excluded. Application of the technique is critically dependent upon understanding of the underlying physiology, the mathematical analyses used, and the many confounders and possible technical artifacts [46, 50].

In this way, misinterpretation of power spectrum takes place due to irregular respiratory pattern and verbalization during breathing, creating artifactual low frequencies and false "sympathetic overactivity."

Use of the absolute power of R-R interval low-frequency spectral data as evidence of sympathetic activity. In case of very low HRV (2–4% of total variability found in healthy subjects), the interpretation of spectral components is affected by the presence of non-autonomic components in the respiratory range. Other confounding factors (such as drugs) similar as those reported for CARTs [50, 52].

Recommendations [50]

- The best approach to HRV testing involves the analysis of ECG recordings in conjunction with respiration and beat-to-beat BP recordings (level C). When respiration cannot be recorded, breathing rate should be controlled (15 breaths/min) and hyperventilation or slow deep breathing avoided (level B). The subjects must not speak during recordings (level C). The optimal recording time is 4–5 min during well-controlled rest. Longer times (7 min) may be preferable if fast Fourier transform methods are used and if frequent ectopics are to be edited. Long uncontrolled recording times should be avoided (level C). When testing is done under stable conditions, autoregressive or fast Fourier transform methods can be used. When fast changes are to be expected (e.g., during interventions), autoregressive algorithms are preferred or alternatively special time-varying techniques.
- Age-related reference curve should be obtained for the healthy population in the same environment, and using the methodology adopted, construct 95% confidence limits (level B).
- Other recommendations on confounding factors are similar as those reported for CARTs.
- Used with the appropriate methodology, HRV has an increasingly important role in clinical research and therapeutic trials.

During 24-h Recordings

- If the goal is to define the circadian pattern of autonomic activity, long-duration spectra (e.g., 1 h) and autoregressive algorithms are preferable.

- If the goal is to define relatively faster modifications, shorter time windows (e.g., 5 min) are preferable. Special time-varying techniques can provide beat-to-beat autonomic changes.

Heart Rate Turbulence

Another Holter-based technique for evaluating CAN is the HR turbulence (HRT). HRT refers to sinus rhythm cycle length fluctuations following isolated premature ventricular beats. After an initial acceleration, the sinus rate decelerates after a premature ventricular beat. There are two components of HRT, turbulence onset and turbulence slope. A transient vagal inhibition triggers the mentioned initial acceleration in HR as a response to the missed baroreflex afferent input due to hemodynamically ineffective ventricular contraction. The successive deceleration in heart rate is caused by a sympathetically mediated overshoot of arterial pressure through vagal recruitment. HRT evaluation can be used in the risk assessment after acute MI and in the monitoring of disease progression in heart failure and CAN [22, 53]. A turbulence slope of below 3.32 ms/R-R is 97% sensitive and 71% specific for the diagnosis of CAN as detected by the CART in patients with T2DM [22, 54].

Baroreflex Sensitivity

The BRS is an interesting approach as it combines information derived from both HR and blood pressure. The measurement of the cardiac vagal arm BRS can be done with several methods: drugs or physical maneuvers can be applied to modify BP; alternatively, spontaneous blood pressure variations can be used. In all cases, the response in heart rate to the changes in BP is quantified. None of the BRS tests available today—based on drug-induced or physically induced changes in BP, spontaneous BP fluctuations with the sequences technique, or spectral analysis—have shown so far a definite advantage over the others or a clinically relevant difference [50, 55].

Longitudinal studies have demonstrated that BRS has important independent prognostic value in cardiac patients [50, 55] and in diabetic patients. Although some observations in diabetic patients support an early impairment of BRS before CARTs abnormalities, very few studies have evaluated so far the diagnostic accuracy of BRS measures as compared with the reference standard of CARTs with inconsistent results. Thus, no definite conclusion is possible on the diagnostic characteristics for CAN of BRS assessment, in particular on its sensitivity. In patients without CAN, an early stage of functional BRS abnormalities [17, 50] still responsive to lifestyle intervention—physical training or dietary improvement and weight reduction—has been documented.

BRS assessment may warrant use for identifying subjects at risk for CAN and also in clinical trials [50, 56].

In this way, cardiac vagal BRS assessment is an important component of autonomic testing as it combines information derived from both HR and blood pressure. Cardiac vagal BRS is a widely recognized independent prognostic index for cardiovascular mortality and morbidity in the general—mainly cardiac and the diabetic—population (class II). No definite conclusion is possible on the diagnostic characteristics of BRS assessment (classes III–IV). The presence of early abnormalities with respect to CARTs and their reversibility with appropriate treatments warrant the clinical use of BRS in identifying subjects at risk for CAN and to test potential therapeutic approaches (classes II–III). Pharmacological methods allow assessment of BRS across a range of physiologically relevant BP and when used with microneurography measurement of the sympathetic baroreflex. But this invasive technique is limited to research purposes. The methodology of BRS (in particular spontaneous BRS) is simple and fast. All BRS techniques require a dedicated beat-to-beat noninvasive blood pressure monitor. None of the BRS tests today available have shown a definite advantage over the other or a clinically relevant difference (class II) [50].

Fluctuations induced by drifts of the noninvasive blood pressure monitors. Most methods need a large number of arbitrary constraints imposed by the calculations that may affect the results. Respiratory pattern: although BRS measures in general do not need a strict control of respiratory pattern, slow breathing increases BRS and reduces sympathetic efferent drive; therefore, some feedback from respiration is necessary to correctly interpret the results. Age-related reduction in BRS. Other confounding factors (e.g., drugs) are similar as those for CARTs [50].

If the spontaneous approach is adopted, it is suggested to use a battery of methods based on the simplest single 5-min recording procedure (spontaneous BRS) and present the results in terms of a central measure (average or median) (level C) [50]:

- Recording should be performed during spontaneous breathing for 4–5 min, under monitored respiration or during controlled breathing at 15 breaths/min (level C).
- Pre-filtering of the data improves the agreement between methods and provides a more robust estimate of BRS (level C).
- The recording time should be kept between 4 and 5 min of well-controlled rest. Avoid long uncontrolled recording times (level C).
- The subjects must not speak during recordings (level C).
- Age-related reference curves should be obtained from the healthy population of the same environment and for the methodology adopted and construct 95% confidence limits (level B).

- Other recommendations on confounding factors are similar as those reported for CARTs.

Muscle Sympathetic Nerve Activity

Increased resting MSNA and blunted responsiveness to physiological hyperinsulinaemia or glucose ingestion have been described in T2DM having neuroadrenergic autonomic dysfunction and resembles insulin-resistant states and obesity. MSNA abnormalities in these conditions reverse with weight loss [50]. In contrast, T1DM is associated with a significant decrease in the number of bursts by about half [57]. Although reproducibility is similar to nondiabetic subjects, obtaining good-quality recordings is much more difficult in patients with diabetic polyneuropathy than in nondiabetic subjects [50], presumably as a result of a reduction in the conducting sympathetic nerve fibers.

In this way, the MSNA is the only method allowing direct and continuous measurement of sympathetic nerve traffic (class I). MSNA is the only method that can directly assess the sympathetic vascular arm of the arterial or cardiopulmonary baroreflex (class I). Type 1 diabetes appears to be associated with a reduction of MSNA (class IV). In early T2DM, resting MSNA might be increased, possibly due to hyperinsulinemia (class IV). The technique is difficult, invasive, and time-consuming, requires specialized trained operator, and cannot be repeated often in the same subject (class II) [50].

Confounders. BP variation, large inter-individual variations, food intake, age, posture, hypoxia, hydration, exercise, female reproductive hormones, arousal, sleep, mental stress, and ethnicity [50].

Recommendations. MSNA should not be routinely employed for the diagnosis of CAN (level C). MSNA should be employed with standard CARTs or for specific tests aimed at measuring vascular sympathetic modifications (e.g., glycemic clamps) (level C) [50].

Catecholamine Assessment and Cardiovascular Sympathetic Tests

Norepinephrine plasma appearance rate is in principle the biochemical equivalent of MSNA. Norepinephrine plasma appearance rate and clearance have been determined in idiopathic autonomic neuropathy as well as in diabetic CAN. While norepinephrine clearance is low in idiopathic autonomic neuropathy, this was not the case in CAN, and accordingly in diabetic CAN no additional diagnostic power was added by the inclusion of [³H]-norepinephrine kinetic studies [50, 58]. Thus, catecholamine kinetics is an interesting technique which may give more information about catecholamine production and clearance across different regions but is unsuitable to be used as a diagnostic tool yet. Plasma dihydroxyphenylalanine (DOPA) is not related to sympathetic neuropathy and has a mixed neuronal and non-neuronal origin. Plasma 3,4-dihydroxyphenylglycol (DHPG) may be a more sensitive marker of overall sympathetic innervation than supine plasma norepinephrine [50], and simultaneous measurement of norepinephrine and DHPG yields more information than measurement of either alone. Catecholamine assessment in diabetes showed in general lower than normal responses to postural changes, exercise, hypoglycemia, and CARTs. A subnormal orthostatic increment in plasma norepinephrine is a specific but not sensitive index of baroreflex-sympathoneural failure or sympathetic noradrenergic denervation [50].

Highlights. Clinical investigations including catecholamine determinations have contributed significantly to the understanding of the pathophysiology of CAN (class III). In the diagnostic context, the significance has been less prominent, partly due to the limited inclusion of the essays in clinical evaluations. Plasma catecholamine concentrations can indicate sympathetic noradrenergic and adrenomedullary hormonal system activity. Because levels of catecholamines are extremely responsive to lifestyle factors such as posture, temperature, dietary intake, medications, distress, and comorbidities, the clinical diagnostic value of plasma levels of catecholamines depends importantly on controlling or monitoring these factors (class III). Whole-body plasma norepinephrine and epinephrine respond rather slowly (minutes) to different physiological maneuvres. During turnover studies, different regional norepinephrine and epinephrine activities are "diluted" into a large plasma pool, contributing to blunted responses. Standardization of experimental conditions is to a large extent prohibitive for clinical routine purposes. In general, there is no neurochemical index that specifically assesses cardiac sympathetic innervation or function. This requires measurement of rates of entry of norepinephrine into the venous drainage of the heart, in turn requiring right heart catheterization, measurement of coronary sinus blood flow, and infusion of tracer-labeled norepinephrine [50]

Confounders. Plasma norepinephrine concentrations increase with age. Thus, age matching is mandatory for comparisons. Smoking increases sympathetic nervous activity and catecholamine concentrations; 24 h tobacco abstention is required for comparisons. Posture, emotional stress, and ambient temperature all affect catecholamine concentrations and should thus be standardized [50].

Recommendations. In a number of experimental conditions, plasma catecholamine measurements are mandatory. For clinical routine diagnosis and staging of CAN, the usefulness of plasma catecholamine concentrations is less obvious (level C). Plasma norepinephrine, epinephrine, and DHPG concentrations should be measured when whole-body sympathetic activity is assessed together with other relevant physiological parameters (HR, BP, cardiac output, hormonal and metabolic events) [50].

Heart Sympathetic Imaging and Heart Function Tests

Direct assessment of cardiac sympathetic innervation is possible using radiolabeled catecholamines or sympathomimetic amines that are actively taken up by sympathetic nerve terminals. Although in principle, it is possible to directly assess the integrity of both the parasympathetic as well as the sympathetic nervous system, there has been a paucity of research on parasympathetic imaging of the heart. Cardiac sympathetic neuroimaging, before and after administration of particular pharmacologic probes, can assess specific aspects of neuronal function. This combination has rarely been used [50].

Four tracers have been utilized to visualize the sympathetic nervous innervation of the heart: [123I]-*meta*-iodobenzylguanidine (MIBG), [11C]-*meta*-hydroxyephedrine (HED), 6-[18F] dopamine, and [11C]-epinephrine [32, 50, 59, 60].

The washout rates from the myocardium of [11C]-epinephrine or 6-[18F]-dopamine can give information on vesicular integrity. In subjects with T1DM and CAN, the washout rates of [11C]-epinephrine parallels those of [11C]-HED, suggesting regional differences in vesicular uptake or retention. Causes of defective tracer uptake or increased washout from the heart are a matter of current research [50, 61].

The interpretation of findings using sympathetic neurotransmitter analogues is complicated by the fact that alterations in sympathetic nervous system tone may also affect the retention of these tracers, and this fact is often not considered as an explanation for the clinical findings. In the isolated rat heart model, elevated norepinephrine concentrations in the perfusion increased neuronal HED clearance rates consistent with the concept that neuronal "recycling" of HED can be disrupted by increased synaptic norepinephrine levels. Alternatively at high norepinephrine concentrations, non-neuronal uptake of HED into myocardial cells and impaired retention may be an interfering factor [50].

Additionally, interpretation of early myocardial [123I]-MIBG retention is complicated by increased body mass index and diastolic BP which have been reported to reduce myocardial MIBG uptake. Moreover, difficulties and delays in acquisition of utilizable images can complicate the interpretation of the measurement obtained. The delivery of tracers is critically influenced by myocardial perfusion, so myocardial retention of tracers should be performed with a quantitative analysis of myocardial blood flow. This can be performed using positron emission tomography in order to derive a myocardial retention index [50, 62]. However, although regional perfusion deficiencies can be excluded using single-photon emission computed tomography, quantitative analysis of regional myocardial perfusion cannot be performed. Additionally, myocardial ischemia or damage is also known to result in cardiac denervation which may occur in the absence of alterations in CARTs [32, 63], whereas CAN is associated with impaired vasodilatory capacity in response to adenosine. Anoxic ischemia severely decreases the efficiency of vesicular sequestration and thus accelerates the loss of radioactivity, giving the false impression of denervation. Left ventricular dysfunction in DM has also been reported to reduce [123I]-MIBG retention and increased washout rate [50].

Highlights. Scintigraphic tracers directly assess the structural integrity of the sympathetic nervous system supply to the heart (class III). [123I]-MIBG scanning and single-photon emission computed tomography are widely used and available at most secondary care institutions; however, MIBG scanning is approved and reimbursed for evaluation of pheochromocytoma and so far not for evaluation of cardiac sympathetic innervation. Most data relate to the evaluation of cardiac sympathetic integrity; few studies evaluate the respiratory system. The relationships of deficits in tracer uptake/washout to sympathetic neuronal integrity and function are poorly understood: current tracers may not be the most optimum. Combined neuroimaging-pharmacologic approaches are required. Scintigraphic data correlates with HRV testing but have greater sensitivity to detect changes in sympathetic neuronal structure and/or function [50, 64] (class III). Scintigraphic data correlate with indices of myocardial perfusion and LV dysfunction in T1DM (class III). Limited studies demonstrate that decreased "uptake" and excessive "washout" of MIBG-derived radioactivity is an adverse prognostic finding in a spectrum of conditions including DM and that scintigraphic data are affected by the quality of glucose control (class III). Cost of scintigraphic studies is considerable [32, 50, 65]

Confounders. Parasympathetic tracers are not yet generally available. [11C]-HED and 6-[18F]-dopamine positron emission tomography have limited availability and are not reimbursed. Damage to the myocardium and LV dysfunction interferes with tracer uptake and washout independently of changes in CARTs. Regional myocardial [123I]-MIBG "uptake" is semi-quantitative and not a clean index of neuronal uptake, which occurs extremely rapidly. [123I]-MIBG retention is affected by body mass index, diastolic BP, and local factors which influence the tracer uptake and retention. Delivery of tracers is critically influenced by myocardial perfusion (myocardial retention of tracers should be performed with quantitative analysis of myocardial blood flow) [50].

The effects of the following on the kinetics of myocardial tracer retention are poorly understood: age (except for 6-[18F]-dopamine), gender, glucose, insulin, DLP, hypertension, and vasoactive agents. Methodology for the assessment of sympathetic integrity is not standardized. Normative values have not been developed [50].

Recommendations [50]

- Scintigraphic studies should not be routinely employed for the diagnosis of CAN and should be utilized in concert with standard CARTs (level C).
- Scintigraphic studies are extremely valuable in the identification of sympathetic noradrenergic denervation as a mechanism of neurogenic orthostatic hypotension (level B).
- [123I]-MIBG single-photon emission computed tomography offers semiquantitative assessment, and [11C]-HED, 6-[18F]-dopamine, and [11C]-epinephrine positron emission tomography offer quantitative assessment of cardiac sympathetic integrity (level B).
- There is no standardized methodology for scintigraphic assessment of cardiac sympathetic integrity, and only limited data on the reproducibility exist (level C).
- Scintigraphic tracer uptake is affected by myocardial perfusion, and tracer retention is affected by available energy for the active neuronal and vesicular uptake transporters (level C).
- The results of scintigraphy should be compared with an appropriate control population (level C).
- Scintigraphic studies offer good sensitivity to detect sympathetic neuronal loss in the heart (level C).
- Scintigraphy is appropriate to explore the effects of sympathetic denervation on cardiac physiology, metabolism, and function (level C).
- Scintigraphy is useful as a marker of cardiac sympathetic denervation in cross-sectional and longitudinal research studies (level C).

Diagnostic Criteria for CAN

No unanimous criteria for diagnosis of CAN have been adapted to date. A single abnormal result among the two or three heart rate tests actually performed was considered a sufficient criterion for early CAN diagnosis. However, the presence of abnormalities in more than one test on several occasions was indicated as preferable for diagnosis [38, 66]. In addition, the presence of two or three abnormal results (two for borderline, three for definite) among the seven autonomic cardiovascular indices (including the five standard CARTs and other time and frequency domain indices of HRV) was recommended as a criterion for CAN diagnosis [67].

The Toronto Consensus established four reasons why the diagnosis of CAN is relevant to clinical practice [38]:

- For diagnosing and staging the different clinical forms of CAN: initial, definite, and advanced or severe.
- For the differential diagnosis of clinical manifestations (e.g., resting tachycardia, OH, and dyspnea upon exercise) and their respective treatment.
- For stratifying the degree of cardiovascular risk and the risk of other diabetic complications (nephropathy, retinopathy, and "silent" myocardial ischemia).
- To adapt the goal of glycated hemoglobin (HbA_{1c}) in each patient: for example, those with severe CAN should have a less aggressive glycemic control due to the risk of asymptomatic hypoglycemia in these patients, while patients with initial stages of CAN should have a more intensive glycemic control.

CARTs are the gold standard clinical tests for cardiovascular autonomic neuropathy [38]. Following the eighth International Symposium on Diabetic Neuropathy in 2010, criteria for diagnosis and staging of CAN are defined in the CAN Subcommittee of the Toronto Consensus Panel statement [23, 38, 68]. Accordingly, only one abnormal CARTs result is sufficient to diagnose possible or early CAN among the seven autonomic function analysis (five CARTs, time-domain and frequency-domain HRV tests), two or three abnormal tests indicate definite or confirmed CAN; and severe/advanced CAN can be indicated by concurrent orthostatic hypotension [23, 38, 68].

Staging of CAN

Ewing et al. proposed a classification based on "early involvement" (one abnormal result on HR test or two borderline results), "definite involvement" (two or more abnormal results on HR tests), and "severe involvement" (presence of OH) [26]. An "autonomic neuropathy score"—obtained by scoring the results of CARTs—has been used with the dual advantage of quantifying the progression of CAN and providing an overall quantitative result [38]. While an abnormal OH test, result generally occurs late in diabetes and subsequent to abnormalities in the HR tests; no chronological order or a markedly different prevalence of abnormalities among the HR tests has been found [38, 67]. Considering progression from an early to an advanced involvement, instead of from parasympathetic to sympathetic neuropathy, would appear to be the most appropriate approach to CAN staging, although OH may on rare occasions precede abnormalities in HR tests [26, 38]. The available information regarding the duration required to progress from an earlier to a later stage of CART impairment is scant, and it is not documented that a progression to OH and symptomatic forms

invariably occur in all patients. The combination of CARTs with tests for sudomotor function may provide a more accurate diagnosis of diabetic autonomic neuropathy [38].

Conclusions [38]

- The following CARTs are the gold standard for clinical autonomic testing: HR response to deep breathing, standing, and Valsalva maneuver, and BP response to standing (class II).
- These CARTs are sensitive, specific, reproducible, easy to perform, safe, and standardized (classes II and III).
- The Valsalva maneuver is not advisable in the presence of proliferative retinopathy and when there is an increased risk of retinal hemorrhage (class IV).
- CARTs are subject to a number of confounding or interfering factors (class III). Age is the most relevant factor affecting heart rate tests (class I).
- A definite diagnosis of CAN and CAN staging requires more than one HR test and the OH test (class III).

Recommendations [38]

- Diagnosis of CAN is based on the use of CARTs for HR response to deep breathing, standing, Valsalva maneuver, and for BP response to standing (level A).
- For the diagnosis and monitoring of CAN, more than one HR test and the OH test are required (level B).
- Performance of CARTs should be standardized and the influence of confounding variables minimized (level A).
- Age-related normal ranges of HR tests are strictly required (level A).
- CAN diagnosis and staging: (1) the presence of one abnormal cardiovagal test result identifies the condition of possible or early CAN, to be confirmed over time; (2) at least two abnormal cardiovagal results are required for a definite or confirmed diagnosis of CAN; and (3) the presence of OH in addition to HR test abnormalities identifies severe or advanced CAN (level B).
- CARTs allow CAN staging from early to advanced involvement (level C).
- Progressive stages of CAN are associated with increasingly worse prognosis (level B).

Management of CAN

Clinical effectiveness of CAN diagnosis in clinical forms of CAN and the awareness of CAN for the therapeutic strategy in asymptomatic forms of CAN are presented in Fig. 57.1.

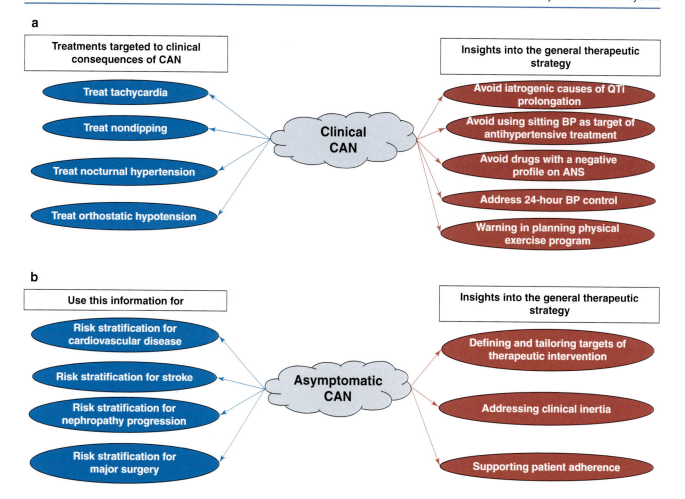

Fig. 57.1 (**a**) Clinical effectiveness of cardiac autonomic neuropathy (CAN) diagnosis in clinical forms of CAN and (**b**) the awareness of CAN for the therapeutic strategy in asymptomatic forms of CAN. *QTi* QT interval, *BP* blood pressure, *ANS* autonomic nervous system.

(Adapted from Spallone V [14], with permission from Publisher. Copyright ©2019 Korean Diabetes Association From Diabetes Metab J. 2019 43:1:16. Reprinted with permission from The Korean Diabetes Association)

Intensive Glycemic Control and Multifactorial Risk Intervention

Compensation state of T2DM is recognized as a primary goal in the prevention of development and/or progression of CVD [2, 3, 18, 35, 69]. Insulin resistance (IR) is a defining feature in most cases of T2DM and plays a key role in the pathogenesis of myocardial alternations. Obviously, pharmacological agents that are used in the treatment of diabetes should have positive qualities for correction of functional and structural disorders of the cardiovascular system [10, 70]. Theoretically, pharmacological agents that improve insulin sensitivity [metformin, thiazolidinediones (TZD)] appear to be the most appropriate in this regard. It is established that metformin has a positive effect on glucose metabolism; Ca^{2+} concentration in cardiomyocytes, but metformin,

unlike TZD, does not show any positive effect on optimization of glucose metabolism in the myocardium [6, 54]. TZD stimulates receptor transcription factors, activated by peroxisome proliferator-activated receptor-γ (PPAR-γ), which improves insulin sensitivity and reduces the level of circulating free fatty acids (FFA). It is likely that TZD, despite the absence of the myocardium PPAR-γ type receptors, improves the functional state of the myocardium by reducing the content of FFA. However, the use of TZD among patients with CVD is limited due to the possibility of fluid retention and/or development of edema [71].

In the Steno 2 study, an intensive multifactorial cardiovascular risk intervention reduced the progression or the development of CAN among T2DM patients with microalbuminuria [72]. However, the beneficial effect of intensive glycemic control on CAN in T2DM has not been specifically proven [14, 19, 73].

Lifestyle Modification

Nutrition and physical activity. Correction of obesity. Limit salt intake to 2–4 g/day. Limit smoking, alcohol, and foods that contain caffeine. It has been established that compliance with recommended lifestyle modifications (exercise, weight loss, etc.) helps improve insulin sensitivity level. Sedentary lifestyle (less than 1000 kcal/week) is accompanied by the risk of mortality three times higher than when living an active lifestyle. Dosed physical activity reduces hyperinsulinemia and encourages the tendency to normalize lipid metabolism in addition to body weight decrease. Physical activity is associated with higher HRV and lower HR, therefore may be a predictor of positive changes in HRV indices [46, 74]. Obtaining the necessary amount of energy combined with physiologic food ration forms the dietary principles. The traditional Mediterranean diet (Greece and Southern Italy) is associated with longevity and/or low mortality due to CVD complications, decrease incidence of T2DM, and low frequency of wide range of chronic diseases, including rheumatoid arthritis, Parkinson's disease, and others [25, 75, 76].

Treatment of Dyslipoproteinemia

For DLP pharmacotherapy using statins, fibrates, bile acid sequestrants, nicotinic acid and its derivatives, products of long-chain ω-3 and ω-6 polyunsaturated fatty acids (PUFA), or as an alternative, their combination with cholesterol absorption inhibitors [54, 77–79].

Statins Statins (along with lifestyle changes) should be prescribed to patients with T2DM aged over 40 where there is at least one of the risk factors for CVD (regardless of basic lipid levels); prescription of statins among patients with T2DM aged under 40 years without diagnosed CVD should be considered when low-density lipoprotein (LDL) cholesterol level exceeds 2.6 mmol/L [78, 80, 81]. Achievement of LDL level in the blood <1.8 mmol/L or reduction by 30–40% compared with initial level (in case of failure to achieve value targets in the course of the prescription of the maximum tolerable dose statin) is suitable for patients at high risk of CVD, particularly patients with T2DM. However, statins are often ineffective when used for treatment of atherogenic DLP as pharmacological agents to achieve reduction in triglycerides (TG) and increase high-density lipoprotein (HDL) cholesterol; statin use (even at high doses) only partially solves the problem of the risk of CVD [80, 82].

Fibrates Fibrates limit the availability of substrates for the synthesis of TG in the liver, encourage lipoprotein lipase effects, increase LDL receptor/ligand interaction, stimulate cholesterol secretion with bile, stimulate reverse cholesterol transport, that is accompanied by reduction of TG and very LDL (VLDL) cholesterol levels, and improve insulin sensitivity. Possible mechanisms that help fibrates improve insulin sensitivity are fibrate binding to receptors that activate PPAR-β enhances fatty acids oxidation in the liver and, consequently, causes increase of insulin sensitivity; fibrates are involved in the regulation of adipokine expression [adiponectin, leptin, tumor necrosis-α (TNF-α), resistin, etc.], accompanied by the increase of insulin sensitivity [83].

Bile acid sequestrants Bile acid sequestrants are safe lipid-lowering medicaments, however often causing gastrointestinal adverse reactions. The second-generation bile acid sequestrants, including colesevelam, bind bile acids with higher affinity and better tolerance. It is used as a supplement to diet therapy and physical activity to reduce the concentration of LDL cholesterol among patients with primary DLP, during monotherapy and/or in combination therapy with statins, and to improve glycemic control among patients with T2DM. In addition, it is important that the bile acid sequestrants reduce the concentration of glucose and HbA_{1c} in the blood (approximately 0.9%) [38, 84] and thus may be useful in the treatment of hypercholesterolemia among patients with T2DM.

Niacin Niacin is the most efficient pharmacological agent for raising HDL cholesterol level and, to a lesser extent, to reduce the concentration of TG and LDL cholesterol. It is reported that the therapeutic effect of prolonged forms of niacin on lipid profile occurs with the medicament intake in the dose range 0.5–2.0 g. A common reason for not using niacin, which significantly affects patient's susception and accurate application, is the problem of "flushing." Current approach to this issue is the use of combined prolonged form of niacin with laropiprant, an inhibitor of prostaglandin D_2 [77].

Long-chain ω-3 PUFAs The use of long-chain ω-3 PUFAs due to their effects on glucose homeostasis and IR (IR reduction in muscle > adipose tissue >> liver) presumably inhibits insulin secretion and delays the development of T2DM) influences the state of lipid metabolism (decrease TG concentrations, presumably increase the concentration of HDL, cholesterol, improve lipid profile among patients with T2DM and DLP), moderately reduces BP, improves endothelial function, reduces the inflammation, and improves antioxidant protection [79, 85–89].

Ezetimibe Ezetimibe is used as a nutrition and exercise supplement to reduce the concentration of LDL cholesterol, total cholesterol (TC), and treatment of homozygous familial hypercholesterolemia. Despite some reservations, ezetimibe remains the medicine of first choice among other pharmacological agents in the absence of target specific level of LDL cholesterol using statin monotherapy [81].

Combined treatment Therapy of first choice for T2DM in case of lipid profile correction is usage of statins to achieve specific target of LDL cholesterol level <2.6 mmol/L for primary prevention and <1.8 mmol/L for secondary prevention of CVD. Failure to get this target is the indication to combine statins with other lipid-lowering agents of other pharmacological groups. A number of international guidelines as a compulsory component of CVD risk monitoring recommend to control apolipoprotein B level on the first-priority basis [81, 90].

Correction of Metabolic Abnormalities in the Myocardium

Correction of metabolic abnormalities in the myocardium is the basis of pharmacotherapy that aims at optimization of the energy metabolism of the myocardium. Pharmacological impact system includes the following main aspects: use of metabolism regulators; energy-saving solutions; activators of endogenic high-energy compounds and O_2 transportation; inhibitors of metabolic acidosis; membrane's protection (inhibition of lipid peroxidation membranes of cardiomyocytes); and stabilization of lysosomal membranes, neutralization of membranotropic action of humoral agents of lysosomal proteases, and others. Medicaments that enhance cell energy state (means of potential energy supply survival of ischemic myocardium). Deterioration of intracellular reserves of carbohydrates needs to be replenished by use of glycolysis activation measures. The use of macroergic phosphates (ATP, etc.) as a direct energy source is problematic, as the therapeutic effect of ATP in case of ischemia probably has less to do with disposing of its macroergic bonds but more with involving products of catabolism of ATP into energy metabolism of cardiomyocytes [6, 54].

Modulators of metabolism. Insulin resistance affects myocardial function by reducing glucose transportation and oxidation of carbohydrates, enhancing the use of free fatty acids, inhibition of Ca^{2+} transportation in the sarcolemma, violation of the structure, and function of regulatory contractile proteins of myofibrils. In case of DM, the reduction of myocardial energy formation leads to inhibition of glucose oxidation and preferential oxidation of fatty acids in the myocardium and skeletal muscle, which increases sensitivity to myocardial ischemia and leads to significant disturbances of Ca^{2+} homeostasis and deterioration of diastolic and systolic myocardial function. The presence of CAD among patients with diabetes worsens the disease and significantly increases cardiovascular mortality. It is considered that even the initial stages of glycemic profile violations may influence the myocardial metabolism and contribute to the development of cardiomyopathy [91]. It is important that myocardial dysfunction is a suppositive stage of chronic hyperglycemia elaboration. Thus, dysfunction of cells metabolism, rather than systemic hyperglycemia, is the reason for elaboration of cardiac malfunction [54, 76].

Metabolic medicaments. Optimization of myocardial energy metabolism is based on increased myocardial glucose oxidation, which enhances cardiac function and protects myocardial fibers from ischemic and reperfusion injuries. Myocardial use of glucose in case of chronic disease may be improved due to intake of the medicines that can improve fatty acids metabolism and inhibit their oxidation. New therapeutic approach has been implemented after advent of trimetazidine—the first representative of a new class of metabolic agents—inhibitors of 3-ketoacyl coenzyme A thiolase. *Trimetazidine* reduces oxidation of fatty acids; stimulates glucose intake; restores the link between glycolysis and carbohydrate oxidation, which leads to the formation of ATP, reducing O_2 consumption; redirects fatty acids toward phospholipids; and increases cell tolerance to ischemic and reperfusion injuries; increases the oxidation of glucose and the activity of Na^+, K^+-ATPase, and Ca^{2+}-pumps in the sarcoplasmic reticulum. Anti-ischemic properties of trimetazidine do not depend on changes in hemodynamics and are associated with a distinct recovery of mechanical function after ischemia, which makes it recognized as cardyo-cytoprotective agent. Trimetazidine prescription improves glucose metabolism, reduces endothelin-1 among patients with diabetic cardiomyopathy, is accompanied by a significant positive changes in ejection fraction parameters among patients with heart failure, and improves quality of life parameters and NYHA functional class [92]. Another pharmacological agent that facilitates the inhibition of metabolism of fatty acids is *perhexiline*. Perhexiline prescription to patients with heart failure significantly contributes to the improvement of EF, VO_2max, and quality of life. Unfortunately, the clinical use of this medicament is limited because of the risk of hepatotoxicity and peripheral neuropathy [93]. *Ranolazine* is the third antianginal pharmacological agent with a potential of metabolism modificator. However, the following factors do not allow to implement its use: the degree of inhibition of fatty acids metabolism is limited by physiological indicators; ranolazine prescription associates with the possibility of QTi interval prolongation [94].

Limitation of extracellular Ca^{2+} into the cell. Blockers of Ca^{2+}-channels show a protective effect on myocardium in case of ischemia. In terms of correction of cell power, the most pathogenetically efficient option is the use of Ca^{2+} blockers; however they only eliminate secondary dysfunction links of oxidative phosphorylation in mitochondria. Prescription of β-adrenergic receptor blockers for T2DM with CAD and CAN has significant pathogenetic grounds as high sympathetic activity that is followed by CAN, accelerates the development of CVD, and significantly affects prognosis. In addition, several studies demonstrated the ability of β-blockers to reduce the incidence of SMI episodes and improve prognosis among these patients. However, adrenergic receptors and β-blockers negatively affect the performance of glycemic profile; increase the risk of hypoglycemia, showing a negative effect on blood lipid profile and can provoke acute heart failure. The above-described events occur with prescription of non-selective β-blockers. Selective β-adrenergic receptor blockers, including metoprolol, are free of side effects, including the effectiveness of metoprolol in the treatment of CVD demonstrated in numerous controlled studies. *Metoprolol* has cardioprotective properties; improves prognosis among patients with CAD; and has a fair tolerance in case of prolonged use. Cardioselective β-blockers can also balance the effects of autonomic dysfunction; in particular, by resisting sympathetic stimulation, they can restore parasympathetic–sympathetic balance. However, traditional antianginal agents that affect hemodynamic parameters (β-blockers, Ca^{2+} antagonists, etc.) have lower tolerance among elderly due to the high risk of the interaction of pharmacological agents with a significant incidence of side effects [6, 54].

Total HRV has been shown to be increased and parasympathetic/sympathetic balance improved by angiotensin-converting enzyme (ACE) inhibition in patients with mild autonomic neuropathy through increases in nerve blood flow [52, 66]. Prostaglandin analogs have been shown to be effective through the same mechanism [66, 74]. Cardioselective beta-blockers are considered to have positive effects on autonomic dysfunction. For example, the addition of metoprolol to ramipril therapy in patients with type 1 diabetes resulted in recovery of HRV parameters [11, 95]. Furthermore, bisoprolol improved HRV in heart failure [91]. In a study including individuals with long-term diabetes and diabetic neuropathy, the combination of ACE inhibition and angiotensin-receptor blockade improved autonomic neuropathy [12]. In addition, it was showed that losartan therapy significantly improved HRV in patients with ischemic cardiomyopathy [96]. Similarly, sympathovagal imbalance in heart failure patients was improved following the administration of spironolactone along with enalapril, furosemide, and digoxin [97]. Such evidence reveals that combination therapies appear to provide better results than monotherapies [22, 23].

Medicaments contain micro- and macro-elements, primarily Mg^{2+}. One of the risk factors that can decrease insulin sensitivity is hypomagnesaemia. It is suggested that Mg^{2+} deficiency plays a significant role in increasing the risk of diabetic macro- and microvascular complications and, especially, the risk of CAD [6, 76].

Thrombosis Prevention and Treatment

Platelets obtained from patients with T2DM and tested in vitro are characterized by a real ability to aggregate under the influence of ADP, adrenaline, collagen, arachidonic acid,

and thrombin. Aggregation of platelets is significantly increased in the second, irreversible phase, which depends on the transformation of arachidonic acid into labile prostacyclin and thromboxane. Thus, the possibility of ADP receptors of platelet membranes blocking is a pathogenetically justified measure. Prescription of antiplatelet agents, namely acetylsalicylic acid (ASA), clopidogrel, and others, can help prevent blood clots, stenocardia, and development of MI. The active clopidogrel metabolite irreversibly binds to ADP receptor on the platelet membrane, which leads to inhibition of adenylate cyclase, inhibition of ADP-dependent secretion of platelet granules, and inhibition of ADP-dependent process of binding fibrinogen receptor to the platelet membrane, does not affect the expression of receptors directly, blocks myointymal proliferation in case of vascular damage, and unlike ASA does not affect the activity of cyclooxygenase. Effect of clopidogrel and ASA synergy is demonstrated in the study of platelet ex vivo. However, clopidogrel is a more effective pharmacological agent within the frames of the combined risk of MI, stroke, and the syndrome of "sudden death" reduction [54, 98].

Aldose Reductase Inhibitors

Aldose reductase inhibitors (ARI) inhibit the *polyol* pathway for *glucose metabolism*, preventing the reduction of the redox potentials. Analysis of the double-blind, placebo-controlled study established that tolrestat contributes to the improvement of independent tests results and vibration sensitivity among patients with symmetric diabetic peripheral neuropathy (DPN). *Zenarestat* prescription for 12 months was accompanied by a dose-dependent change in the spissitude of nerve tissue, increased the velocity of nerve impulses, and improved myocardial systolic function. *Zoporestat and ranirestat*—medicaments of a new generation of ARI group—showed sufficient efficacy in experimental studies [60].

While the use of aldose reductase inhibitors (epalrestat, fidarestat, and AS-3201), which reduce nerve sorbitol, had a positive influence on HRV in patients with mild abnormalities, they were ineffective in advanced CAN patients [54, 66].

Replacement Therapy with the Help of Myoinositol

Several individual clinical trials were conducted for the study of myoinositol efficacy in the treatment of diabetic neuropathy. The results are quite positive; but in the future, clinical double-blind, placebo-controlled trials are needed [99].

Aminoguanidine

Aminoguanidine improves capacity of nerve velocity, increases blood flow, inhibits the formation of advanced glycation end products, and delays the emergence and development of albuminuria. Analysis of controlled trials confirmed quite aminoguanidine high efficiency among patients with diabetic neuropathy, but the development of a number of side effects terminated their application. The use of aminoguanidine derivatives is accompanied by clinical efficacy and lack of adverse side effects [7, 73]. The results are promising, but need further clinical double-blind, placebo-controlled studies.

Neurotrophic Therapy

Inhibition of nerve growth factor (NGF) expression and its receptors suppresses NGF axonal retrograding transport and reduces the activity of small unmyelinated neurons and their neuropeptides, including substance P and gene-linked calcitonin peptide. The use of recombinant human NGF normalizes neuropeptide concentration and prevents the development of sensory neuropathy in the experiment. However, the results of clinical placebo-controlled studies deny the positive impact of recombinant human NGF among patients with diabetic neuropathy [7, 73].

Antineural Autoimmunity Human Immunoglobulin for Intravenous Use

Intravenous human immunoglobulin prescription is recommended for patients with diabetic peripheral neuropathy (DPN), which have signs of antineural autoimmunity symptomes. The side effects include headache, and the main danger could be the development of an anaphylactic reaction; however, it affects mainly patients with deficiency of immunoglobulin A [7, 73].

Endoneural Perfusion Inhibition with the Development of Hypoxia

Experimental and clinical studies have shown benefit in the efficiency of vasodilators when used for improvement of nerve flow velocity, but there is not enough information about the impact of vasodilators on the course of DPN during clinical double-blind placebo-controlled studies. The research results of characteristics that impact the angiotensin-converting enzyme inhibitors on heart rate variability parameters among diabetic patients with CAN appeared to show diametrically opposed results. In particular, prescription of *quinapril* for 3 months was accompanied by statistically sig-

nificant increased parasympathetic activity, and the use of trandolapril for 12 months did not affect the performance of autonomic myocardial function. However, most of these pharmacological agents have no proven clinical and electrophysiological positive effects and have certain limitations and contraindications [30, 73].

Activation of Free Radical Stress

Considering that one of the major pathogenetic mechanisms of neuropathy is oxidative stress, the need for antioxidants prescription is obvious [100, 101]. Great therapeutic potential is observed in α-lipoic acid (α-LA) and creates pathogenic evidence for the use of this pharmacological agent [100, 101]. Mechanism of α-LA action is not fully developed, but specific attention should be paid to two hypotheses. First, α-LA phenomenon causes dose-dependent proliferation of neuroblastoma cultured cells. Changes in the membrane fluidity that are mediated through sulfhydryl groups α-LA are considered to cause this effect. This is confirmed by the following results of several studies, including experimental neuropathy induced by acrylamide, followed by a significant inhibition of proliferation of the above phenomenon; overlay and/or progression of experimental distal neuropathy, mainly caused by a decrease of content of substances in axons containing sulfhydryl groups (e.g., glutathione); α-LA in vivo and in vitro enhances spontaneous processes of expansion and improvement of the structural and functional nerve terminals membranes state; and prescription of α-LA stimulates the regeneration of nerve terminals in case of the partial denervation, as well as experimental hexacarbon neuropathy. Second, and the most probable mechanism, is the ability of α-LA to function as a radical binder (cleaner) [54, 67, 102].

Vitamins with Antioxidant Properties [a Liposoluble Vitamin B₁ (Benfotiamine)], Combined Medications

There are enough experimental and clinical results of studies that suggest that the hyperinsulinemia, IR, and chronic hyperglycemia in T2DM have a negative impact on the metabolism of thiamine particularly due to the inhibition of the functional state of the thiamine transporter-1 and thiamine transporter-2, responsible for the reabsorption of vitamin in the proximal tubules of the kidneys; and transketolase (TK) activity, which can lead to the congestion of intermediates in the initial stages of glycolysis [glyceraldehyde-3-phosphate (GA3P), fructose-6-phosphate (F6P), and dihydroxyacetone-phosphate]. Congestion of intermediates in case of chronic hyperglycemia increases the production of free radicals in the mitochondria, followed by inhibition of glyceraldehyde-3-phosphate dehydrogenase (GAPDH). Increased concentrations of GA3P, F6P, and GAPDH can initiate induced hyperglycemia, metabolic fates that favor the overlay of vascular injury, including activation of proteinkinase-C, accumulation of advanced glycation end products (AGEs), hexosamine biosynthetic fates activation, and dicarbonyl compounds. Activation with dicarbonyl compounds is followed by further stimulation of the AGEs formation, which is also associated with functional impaired and structural state of cardiomyocytes [59, 103, 104].

It is clear that the correction of thiamin deficiency must be performed using exogenous vitamin B_1 or benfotiamine (monophosphate S-benzoyl-thiamine, high-bioavailable liposoluble vitamin B_1 derivatives). Results of experimental and clinical studies suggest a positive effect of benfotiamine prescription on prevention of diabetic vascular disease progression. Benfotiamine broad therapeutic potential has a good efficiency on medications containing soluble thiamine derivatives for the purpose of regulating the activity of free radical processes, correction of endothelial dysfunction in case of CVD, and stabilization of clinical and antioxidant effects [105].

Benfotiamine can promote neuronal and vascular deficiency correction through the participation of nitrogen oxide processes, which have a significant therapeutic potential for the treatment of CVD. The use of thiamine and α-LA combination has a great significance in the treatment of diabetic angio-neuropathy. In particular, it demonstrated that prescription of benfotiamine and α-LA to patients with T1DM was followed by normalization of hyperglycemia and for 4 weeks it promoted the normalization of prostacyclin synthase suppressed by diabetes and increase of TK activity in monocytes in two to three times [105–107].

Fatty Acids Metabolism Disorders (γ-Linolenic Acid, Acetyl L-Carnitine)

Vasoactive prostanoids, metabolites and dihomo-γ-linolenic acid (DGLA), including prostaglandins and other eicosanoids, are necessary for the physiological behavior of nerve conductivity and blood flow. The results of double-blind, placebo-controlled studies showed that prescription of DGLA to patients with DPN is followed by positive dynamics in clinical course, as well as increase in the speed of nerve conductivity. L-carnitine's main function is to strengthen the metabolism of fatty acids, but there is experimental evidence of L-carnitine's ability to activate glucose metabolism. It is believed that T2DM is characterized by malfunction of L-carnitine exchange in the mitochondria. The results of several studies showed that prescription of L-carnitine helps to improve energy supplies and LV function. It is established

that propionyl-L-carnitine improves the functional status, used as glucose energy oxidation in the rat's affected myocardium (despite the increased level of fatty acids). Nutrition of diabetic mice with obesity with L-carnitine addition increases the level of acyl-carnitine in the blood, muscle, liver, and adipose tissue and increases levels of pyruvate dehydrogenase activity in the muscles; prescription of zinc–carnitine mixture reduces hyperglycemia and improves glucose tolerance. L-carnitine infusion with the help of hyperinsulinemic-euglycemic clamp improves glucose profile control and reduces the concentration of circulating lipids. L-carnitine prescription for 3 or 6 months for newly diagnosed patients with T2DM with lipid metabolism disorders is followed by a statistically significant decrease in lipoprotein(a) [Lp(a)] levels. The results of double-blind, placebo-controlled studies among patients with verified hyperLP(a) established that L-carnitine (2 g/day) encouraged a significant decrease in the concentration of Lp(a) levels; L-carnitine incorporation into nutrition of patients with newly diagnosed T2DM is followed by similar changes; and combined L-carnitine with simvastatin (20 mg/day) treatment is much more efficient in decreasing the concentration of lipids, including TG and Lp(a) than statin monotherapy. Thus, L-carnitine can be used as one of the components for lipid-modifying therapy among patients with T2DM [108, 109].

ω-3 PUFAs Medications

A fundamentally new approach to assessing the biological role of eicosapentaenoic (EPA) and docosahexaenoic acid (DHA) is associated with long-term epidemiological studies results among Inuits, which established a small percentage of CVD. The Greenlandic Inuits were observed to have an increased bleeding duration, lower levels of TC, TG, and VLDL-cholesterol; and a significant increase in TC lipid membranes of EPA and DHA contents, arachidonic acid concentration reduction, and linoleic acid. For the first time, these results allowed to express a reasonable assumption about the protective effect of DHA and especially EPA from the damaging effects on the internal vessel wall capable of inducing experiment CAD—a phenomenon of TC activation—and high blood viscosity, enhanced the cyclic endoperoxide synthase, including prostaglandin H_2, thromboxane A_2 (TXA$_2$) activation of endothelial cell proliferation, hypercholesterolemia, and hypertriglyceridemia. Prescription of EPA and DHA is followed by a decrease in the "rigidity" of red blood cells, which is obviously associated with labilization of erythrocyte plasmalemma based on rapid and intensive incorporation of long-chain ω-3 PUFAs phospholipids into membrane and decreased synthesis of vasoconstrictor active ingredients [79].

The ability of exogenous EPA and DHA to incorporate phospholipid blood cell membranes and membrane phospholipids of endothelial cells blood vessels affects the fundamental plasmalemma properties and receptor function for the perception and processing of extracellular information. Accumulating long-chain polyenes acids labilizes plasmalemma, changing the microviscosity of its lipid matrix, which causes the transformation of the basic plasmalemma properties: permeability, generation of biopotentials, and ions transit. Changes in the lipid environment of receptor structures affects their functional activity and enzyme systems control in the cell, which primarily relates to the corpuscular adenylate cyclase, whose function is related to the metabolism of phospholipids [87, 110].

Analysis of experimental and clinical studies proves that ω-3 PUFA inhibit the absorption of cholesterol in the intestine and its synthesis in the liver, lead to increased clearance of lipoproteins in the blood, prevent the development of IR in experimental diabetes, decrease level of BP, dose-dependently prevent the development of diabetes, improve the sensitivity of platelets to ADP and collagen, contribute to positive changes in the parameters of coagulation and endothelial cells migration, and inhibit the proliferation of smooth muscle cells. However, the studies aimed to investigate the features of ω-3 PUFA in T2DM are numerically small, and obtained results do not always testify to their effectiveness [88, 89, 111]. In particular, the results of the ORIGIN trial demonstrated that administration of 1 g ω-3 PUFAs did not reduce the rate of death caused by cardiovascular reasons or their outcomes during a period of 6 years among patients with dysglycemia and additional cardiovascular risk factors. In this trial, the dose of ω-3 PUFA was not chosen on the basis of any estimate of its effect on TG levels; nevertheless, a significant reduction in the TG level was shown. However, this study did not apply to treatment of CAN, and it was decided to continue the study for a few more years [85]. In the same time, American Diabetes Association (ADA, 2005) recommended the prescription of α-LA and ω-3 PUFAs in algorithms of DPN treatment [66] and in ADA recommendations (2014) and results of some trials: prescription of ω-3 PUFAs in DLP treatment among patients with T2DM and cardiovascular diseases [1, 88].

Symptomatic Treatment of Orthostatic Hypotension

Orthostatic hypotension syndrome is manifested by dizziness and possibility of loss of consciousness. Hypovolemia and sympathoadrenal disorders are the most common char-

acteristic features among patients with DM and orthostatic hypotension. Orthostatic hypotension among most diabetic patients progresses asymptomatically and, therefore, does not require correction. However, in severe cases, it is key traumatic factor [38, 112].

Treatment of OH is required only when symptomatic with the therapeutic goal to minimize postural symptoms rather than to restore normotension. The first step encompasses non-pharmacological measures with the attempt to (1) identify other causes of OH, e.g., volume depletion, and avoid, when possible, drugs exacerbating postural symptoms, such as psychotropic drugs, diuretics, and α-adrenoreceptor antagonists; (2) educate patients regarding behavioral strategies such as gradual staged movements with postural change, mild isotonic exercise, head-up bed position during sleep, physical counter-maneuvres (e.g., leg-crossing, stooping, squatting, and tensing muscles), use of portable folding chairs, increased fluid and salt intake if not contraindicated, drinking water rapidly, and avoidance of large meals rich in carbohydrates; and (3) use of elastic garment over the legs and abdomen. If symptoms persist despite these measures, a pharmacological treatment should be considered [38].

Treatment of symptomatic postural hypotension among patients with CAN is very complicated because of the need to achieve a balance between changes in BP in the vertical and horizontal position. The increase of peripheral venous inflow is achieved through the use of elastic tightening body linen. It is inappropriate to prescribe psychotropic and diuretic drugs and eliminate the possibility of electrolyte disorders and/or reduce the fluid volume [38].

The peripheral selective α1-adrenergic agonist *midodrine* is a first-line drug that exerts a pressor effect through both arteriolar constriction and venoconstriction of the capacitance vessels. The dosing should be individually tailored (up to two to four times 10 mg/day, with the first dose taken before arising and use avoided several hours before planned recumbency particularly in patients with documented supine hypertension). Adverse events are pilomotor reactions, pruritus, supine hypertension, bradycardia, gastrointestinal symptoms, and urinary retention. *Midodrine* is the only medication approved by the Food and Drug Administration for the treatment of symptomatic orthostatic hypotension [38].

The *9-α-fluorohydrocortisone* is first-choice drug that acts through sodium retention, a direct constricting effect on partially denervated vessels, and an increase in the water content of the vessel wall leading to a reduced distensibility. Possible adverse effects include supine hypertension, hypokalemia, congestive heart failure, and peripheral edema. The initial dose should be 0.05–0.1 mg daily with individual titration to 0.1–0.3 mg daily [38, 112].

Erythropoietin was proposed to increase standing blood pressure via several mechanisms: (1) increasing red cell mass and central blood volume, (2) correcting the anemia frequently associated with severe CAN, and (3) neurohumoral effects on the vascular wall and vascular tone regulation. It can be administered in diabetic patients with hemoglobin levels under 11 g/dL subcutaneously or intravenously at doses between 25 and 75 U/kg three times/week with an hemoglobin target of 12 g/dL followed by lower maintenance doses [38, 112].

Other possible treatments include (1) *desmopressin acetate*, a vasopressin analogue useful to correct nocturnal polyuria and morning orthostatic hypotension; (2) *somatostatin analogues* aimed at inhibiting the release of vasoactive gastrointestinal peptides, enhancing cardiac output, and increasing forearm and splanchnic vascular resistance, with severe cases of hypertension as possible adverse events in diabetic patients; (3) *caffeine* and (4) *acarbose*, both useful in attenuating postprandial hypotension in autonomic failure [38, 112, 113].

While pharmacological treatments, such as midodrine, clonidine, octreotide, fludrocortisone acetate, erythropoietin, nonselective beta-blockers and pyridostigmine bromide appear promising, all have mild to severe side effects, including hypertension [22, 35].

New Glucose-Lowering Medications and Autonomic Nervous System

Sodium Glucose Transporter 2 Inhibitors (SGLT2i)

It would be of interest to understand whether some of the positive effects on the cardiovascular system of these drugs are mediated by interaction with the autonomic nervous system in the kidney or directly in the central nervous system. However, clinical trials with SGLT2i using ABPM do not confirm to a preferential lowering effect on nocturnal versus daytime systolic BP, despite the diuretic and natriuretic effect of these drugs and the dipping restoration found with SGLT2i in rat models of obesity and metabolic syndrome [14, 114].

Glucagon-like Peptide 1 Receptor Agonists (GLP1-RA)

Experimental findings in mice and rats document that the central and peripheral administration of a glucagon-like peptide 1 receptor agonist (GLP1-RA) increased heart rate, reduced frequency-domain indices of HRV, and increased sympathetic activity [14, 115].

However, it should be noted that the GLP1-RA effects on heart rate and the autonomic nervous system need to be reconciled with the favorable cardiovascular outcomes in clinical trials of at least some GLP1-RAs (liraglutide, semaglutide, exenatide ER) [14].

The Toronto Consensus Panel on Diabetic Neuropathy concluded the following in relation to CAN treatment [38]:

- Intensive diabetes therapy retards the development of CAN in T1DM (level A).
- Intensive multifactorial cardiovascular risk intervention retards the development and progression of CAN in T2DM (level B).
- Lifestyle intervention might improve HRV in prediabetes (level B) and diabetes (level B).
- Symptomatic orthostatic hypotension might be improved by non-pharmacological measures (level B) and by midodrine (level A) and/or fludrocortisone (level B).

The recommendations from the Toronto Consensus Panel on Diabetic Neuropathy are as follows:

Diabetes therapy in patients with type 1 and type 2 diabetes should consider the individual risk profile and comorbidities (class I).

Lifestyle intervention should be offered as a basic preventive measure (class I).

Given the limited evidence from very few large-scale randomized clinical trials, recommendations cannot be given for pharmacological and non-pharmacological treatments of CAN.

Drugs that might reduce HRV should be avoided in patients with CAN (class III).

Resting tachycardia associated with CAN can be treated with cardioselective beta-blockers (class I).

The first therapeutic approach in symptomatic orthostatic hypotension should consider the exclusion of drugs exacerbating orthostatic hypotension, correction of volume depletion (class I), and other non-pharmacological measures (class IIa).

Pharmacotherapy of symptomatic orthostatic hypotension should include midodrine (class I) or fludrocortisones or a combination of both in non responders to monotherapy (class IIa).

Because of the limited evidence, the potential risk of any pharmacological treatment should be thoroughly weighed against its possible benefit (class I).

CARTs should be used as end points in prospective observational and clinical trials.

Concluding Remarks

Cardiac autonomic neuropathy is a serious complication of diabetes mellitus that is strongly associated with increased risk of cardiovascular mortality.

Screening for CAN must be performed to asymptomatic patients with type 2 diabetes at diagnosis and type 1 diabetic patients after 5 years of disease, in particular those (but not only) at greater risk for CAN.

Diagnosis of CAN is based on the use of CARTs, which are considered as the gold standard for clinical autonomic testing: the presence of one abnormal cardiovagal test result identifies the condition of possible or early CAN, to be confirmed over time; (2) at least two abnormal cardiovagal results are required for a definite or confirmed diagnosis of CAN; and (3) the presence of OH in addition to HR test abnormalities identifies severe or advanced CAN.

Lifestyle intervention is a basic preventive measure and may improve HRV. Intensive diabetes therapy retards the development of CAN in type 1 diabetes and intensive multifactorial cardiovascular risk intervention retards the development and progression of CAN in type 2 diabetes. Resting tachycardia by CAN can be treated with cardioselective β-blockers. Pharmacotherapy of symptomatic orthostatic hypotension should include midodrine or fludrocortisone or a combination of both in nonresponders to monotherapy.

The promising methods include research and use of tools that increase blood flow through the vasa vasorum, including butaprost (prostacyclin analogue), TXA_2 blockers, and drugs that contribute into strengthening and/or normalization of Na^+, K^+-ATPase (cilostazol, a potential phosphodiesterase inhibitor), α-LA, DGLA, and ω-3 PUFAs and the simultaneous prescription of α-LA, ω-3 PUFAs, and DGLA [8, 20, 30, 67, 95]. In addition, the combination of α-LA, ω-3 PUFAs, DGLA, and ARI is the most rational pathogenetically justified use.

Multiple Choice Questions

1. At what timepoint screening for CAN must be performed?
   (a) Asymptomatic patients with T2DM at diagnosis and patient with T1DM after 5 years of disease.
   (b) Asymptomatic patients with T2DM after 5 years of disease and type 1 diabetic patients at diagnosis.
   (c) Only patients with clinical signs of CAN.
   (d) Only patients with the history of poor glycemic control.
   (e) Screening for CAN shouldn't be performed.

2. Which risk factors are known for the development of CAN?
   (a) Diabetes duration.
   (b) Poor glycemic control.
   (c) Microvascular complications.
   (d) Combination of hypertension, dyslipidemia and obesity.
   (e) All listed above.

3. What method is considered as a gold standard for CAN diagnosis?
   (a) CARTs.
   (b) Orthostatic hypotension.
   (c) QTc prolongation on ECG.
   (d) Reverse dipping on ABPM.
   (e) Resting tachycardia by physical assessment.

4. What result based on the use of CARTs could confirm definite CAN?
   (a) At least two abnormal results of cardiovascular tests/or two for borderline, and three for definite.
   (b) At least three abnormal results of cardiovascular tests/or three for borderline, and four for definite.
   (c) At least one abnormal result of cardiovascular tests/or two for borderline.
   (d) At least four abnormal results of cardiovascular tests.
   (e) Orthostatic hypotension.

5. What signs are needed to undergo CAN testing?
   (a) Orthostatic hypotension.
   (b) Resting tachycardia.
   (c) QTc prolongation.
   (d) Reverse dipping by ABPMA.
   (e) All of above.

6. List a definition that is true for CAN management and prevention.
   (a) Lifestyle intervention is a basic preventive measure.
   (b) Resting tachycardia can be treated with cardioselective β-blockers.
   (c) Intensive diabetes therapy retards the development of CAN in type 1 diabetes mellitus, and intensive multifactorial cardiovascular risk intervention retards the development and progression of CAN in type 2 diabetes.
   (d) Symptomatic orthostatic hypotension should be treated with midodrine or fludrocortisone or a combination of both in nonresponders to monotherapy.
   (e) All answers are correct.

7. Patient complains (suffers) from tachycardia and exercise intolerance. After examination anemia was diagnosed. Despite this, patient was directed to CAN testing, and CARTs were performed. Results: the deep breathing test-borderline, all others normal. Check the correct answer.

(a) Possible early CAN.

(b) Definite confirmed CAN.

(c) Severe advanced CAN.

(d) Symptomatic CAN.

(e) Insufficient information for CAN diagnosis.

8. By performing the screening of orthostatic symptoms to asymptomatic type 2 diabetic patient, a fall in systolic blood pressure of 30 mmHg and diastolic of 11 mmHg was found. The patient didn't have any other specific conditions that could lead to orthostatic hypotension. Patient was referred for CAN screening and CARTs were performed: three heart rate test abnormalities were found. What stage of CAN patient suffers from?

(a) Possible early CAN.

(b) Definite confirmed CAN.

(c) Severe advanced CAN.

(d) Symptomatic CAN.

(e) CAN is excluded.

9. Patient with newly diagnosed type 2 diabetes mellitus and arterial hypertension had undergone ABPM test. It is also known that patient suffers from obesity and dyslipidemia. The results had shown the presence of reverse dipping. Should this patient be referred for CAN testing?

(a) Of course patient should be referred.

(b) CAN testing is inappropriate.

(c) Yes, he should but in 5 years.

(d) Just if he has clinical signs of CAN.

(e) Yes, but after the normalization of blood pressure profile.

10. Which drugs should include pharmacotherapy of symptomatic orthostatic hypotension by CAN?

(a) Midodrine and/or fludrocortisone.

(b) Erythropoetin.

(c) Desmopressin acetate.

(d) Somatostatin analogues.

(e) Nonselective β-blockers.

Correct Answers

1. (a) Asymptomatic patients with T2DM at diagnosis and patient with T1DM after 5 years of disease

   According to the Consensus of the CAN Subcommittee of the Toronto Consensus Panel on Diabetic Neuropathy, screening for CAN must be performed to asymptomatic patients with type 2 diabetes at diagnosis and type 1 diabetic patients after 5 years of disease, in particular those (but not only) at greater risk for CAN (level B). Screening for CAN may be also required for preoperative risk assessment before major surgical procedure (level C).

2. (e) All listed above

   Risk markers for CAN are age, diabetes duration, poor glycemic control, microvascular complications (nephropathy, peripheral polyneuropathy, retinopathy), hypertension, and dyslipidemia (classes I and II). For type 1 diabetic patients, the established risk factors for CAN development is poor glycemic control (class I), and for type 2 is the combination of hypertension, dyslipidemia, obesity, and poor glycemic control (class II).

3. (a) CARTs

   Resting tachycardia may reflect diabetic autonomic dysfunction, but it also can reflect sympathetic hyperactivity and/or vagal impairment by some cardiovascular diseases, low physical activity, anemia, and other conditions. Orthostatic hypotension suggests advanced CAN that should be confirmed by CARTs (class I) but after exclusion of other pathophysiological conditions (hypovolemia, deconditioning, influence of some drugs). QTc could be prolonged due to imbalance in cardiac sympathetic innervation, intrinsic metabolic and electrolytic changes, CAD, and genetic factors. Non-dipping and reverse dipping patterns are associated with CAN, as by this conditions, vagal activity is impaired with sympathetic predominance during the night and disrupted circadian variation. So resting heart rate is not a specific sign of CAN (class IV), orthostatic hypotension (class III), QTc prolongation (class II), and reverse dipping on ABPM (class III) are specific but insensitive indices for CAN and requires CAN testing. Diagnosis of CAN is based on the use of CARTs, which are considered as the gold standard for clinical autonomic testing: heart rate response to deep breathing (standing), Valsalva maneuver, blood pressure response to standing (class II, level A).

4. (a) At least two abnormal results of cardiovascular tests/ or two for borderline and three for definite

   According to the Consensus of the CAN Subcommittee of the Toronto Consensus Panel on Diabetic Neuropathy, for the definite or confirmed diagnosis of CAN is required the presence of at least two abnormal cardiovagal test results/or two for borderline, three for definite.

5. (e) All above

   According to the Consensus of the CAN Subcommittee of the Toronto Consensus Panel on Diabetic Neuropathy, all of the listened above clinical findings can alert on the presence of CAN. Especially, orthostatic hypotension suggests an advanced CAN that should be confirmed by CARTs (class I); resting tachycardia is not a specific sign of CAN (class IV), but patients with unexplained tachycardia should undergo CAN testing (level C). Qtc prolongation (class II) alone, as a reverse dipping on ABPM (class III) are an insufficient measure of CAN, but should be sign to referral for CAN testing (level B and C accordingly).

6. (e) All answers are correct

   According to the existing data, all definitions are correct. Lifestyle intervention is a basic preventive measure (class I) and may improve HRV (level B). Resting tachycardia by CAN can be treated with cardioselective β-blockers (class I). Intensive diabetes therapy retards the development of CAN in type 1 diabetes (level A) and intensive multifactorial cardiovascular risk intervention retards the development and progression of CAN in type 2 diabetes (level B). Pharmacotherapy of symptomatic orthostatic hypotension should include midodrine (class I, level A) or fludrocortisone (level B) or a combination of both in non-responders to monotherapy (class II A).

7. (e) Insufficient information for CAN diagnosis

Patient complaints could be explained by anemia. The presence of one abnormal cardiovagal test result identifies the condition of possible or early CAN that should be confirmed over time (level B). As the result was on borderline it is insufficient for CAN diagnosis. So, patient should undergo CAN testing after treatment of anemia.

8. (c) Severe advances CAN

According to the Consensus of the CAN Subcommittee of the Toronto Consensus Panel on Diabetic Neuropathy, after exclusion of other causes, orthostatic hypotension suggests an advanced CAN that should be confirmed by CARTs (class I); the presence of orthostatic hypotension in addition to abnormal heart rate test (two or more) identifies severe or advanced CAN.

9. (a) Of course patient should be referred

This patient should be referred to CAN diagnostic tests. There are several reasons to perform screening for CAN: (1) he has established risk factors for CAN development, combination of hypertension, dyslipidemia, and obesity in type 2 diabetes mellitus (class II); (2) diabetes mellitus type 2 is newly diagnosed (level B); and (3) In the presence of reverse dipping referral for CAN testing is advisable (level C).

10. (a) Midodrine and/or fludrocortisone.

Pharmacotherapy of symptomatic orthostatic hypotension should include midodrine (class I) or fludrocortisones or a combination of both in nonresponders to monotherapy (class IIa).

The first-line medication by orthostatic hypotension is the peripheral selective α_1-adrenergetic agonist midodrine (class I, level A). The dosing regimen should be individually tailored (the usual starting dose is 2.5 mg three times daily, most patients are controlled at or below 30 mg per day given in three or four (up to six) divided doses, but a total daily dose of 30 mg should not be exceeded. Fludrocortisone could be the first-choice drug that acts through sodium retention, a direct constricting effect on partially denervated vessels and an increase in the water content of the vessel wall leading to a reduced distensibility. In nonresponders to monotherapy, the combination of midodrine and fludrocortisone should be prescribed.

Glossary

Cardiac autonomic neuropathy Cardiac autonomic neuropathy chronic complication of diabetes mellitus is defined as the impairment of autonomic control of the cardiovascular system in the setting of diabetes after exclusion of other causes and is usually documented by using several cardiovascular autonomic reflex tests.

Cardiovascular autonomic reflex tests Cardiovascular autonomic reflex tests these tests are considered the gold standard in autonomic testing. Heart rate variations during deep breathing, Valsalva maneuver, and lying-to-standing (HR tests) are indices mainly of parasympathetic function; whereas the orthostatic hypotension, the blood pressure response to a Valsalva maneuver, and sustained isometric muscular strain provide indices of sympathetic function.

Orthostatic hypotension Orthostatic hypotension is defined as a fall in BP (i.e., >20 mmHg or more stringent criteria is >30 mmHg for systolic or >10 mmHg for diastolic BP) in response to postural change, from supine to standing.

Non-dipping status Non-dipping status a fall in average sleeping blood pressure <10% from baseline.

Reverse dipping Reverse dipping nocturnal hypertension.

References

1. American Diabetes Association. Standards of medical care in diabetes-2014. Diabetes Care. 2014;37(Suppl 1):14–80. https://doi.org/10.2337/dc14-S014.

2. American Diabetes Association. Standards of medical care in diabetes-2016. Diabetes Care. 2016;39(Suppl 1):1–2. https://doi.org/10.2337/dc16-S001.

3. International Diabetes Federation. IDF Diabetes Atlas. 7th ed. Brussels: International Diabetes Federation; 2015.

4. Rodriguez-Saldaña J. Preface: a new disease? In: Rodriguez-Saldaña J, editor. Diabetes textbook: clinical principles, patient management and public health issues. Basel: Springer; 2019; p. 1–8. https://link.springer.com/book/10.1007/978-3-030-11815-0.

5. Kempler P, Tesfaye S, Chaturvedi N, Stevens LK, Webb DJ, Eaton S, et al. EURODIAB IDDM Complications Study Group. Autonomic neuropathy is associated with increased cardiovascular risk factors: the EURODIAB IDDM complications study. Diabet Med. 2002;19:900–9. https://doi.org/10.1046/j.1464-5491.2002.00821.x.

6. Wanders D, Plaisance EP, Judd RL. Pharmacological effects of lipid-lowering drugs on circulating adipokines. World J Diabetes. 2010;1:116–28. https://doi.org/10.4239/wjd.v1.i4.116.

7. Maser RE, Lenhard MJ. Cardiovascular autonomic neuropathy due to diabetes mellitus: clinical manifestations, consequences, and treatment. J Clin Endocrinol Metab. 2005;90:5896–903. https://doi.org/10.1210/jc.2005-0754.

8. Prince CT, Secrest AM, Mackey RH, Arena VC, Kingsley LA, Orchard TJ. Cardiovascular autonomic neuropathy, HDL cholesterol, and smoking correlate with arterial stiffness markers determined 18 years later in type 1 diabetes. Diabetes Care. 2010;33:652–7. https://doi.org/10.2337/dc09-1936.

9. Vinik AI, Casellini C, Parson HK, Colberg SR, Nevoret ML. Cardiac autonomic neuropathy in diabetes: a predictor of

cardiometabolic events. Front Neurosci. 2018;12:591. https://doi.org/10.3389/fnins.2018.00591.

10. Ziegler D, Zentai CP, Perz S, Rathmann W, Haastert B, Döring A, Meisinger C. Prediction of mortality using measures of cardiac autonomic dysfunction in the diabetic and nondiabetic population: the MONICA/KORA Augsburg cohort study. Diabetes Care. 2008;31:556–61. https://doi.org/10.2337/dc07-1615.

11. Tandon N, Ali MK, Narayan KM. Pharmacologic prevention of microvascular and macrovascular complications in diabetes mellitus: implications of the results of recent clinical trials in type 2 diabetes. Am J Cardiovasc Drugs. 2012;12:7–22. https://doi.org/10.2165/11594650-000000000-00000.

12. Vinik AI, Maser RE, Ziegler D. Autonomic imbalance: prophet of doom or scope for hope. Diabet Med. 2011;28:643–51. https://doi.org/10.1111/j.1464-5491.2010.03184.x.

13. Anonymous. Assessment: clinical autonomic testing report of the therapeutics and technology assessment Subcommittee of the American Academy of Neurology. Neurology. 1996;46:873–80.

14. Spallone V. Update on the impact, diagnosis and management of cardiovascular autonomic neuropathy in diabetes: what is defined, what is new, and what is unmet. Diabetes Metab J. 2019;43:3–30. https://doi.org/10.4093/dmj.2018.0259.

15. Spallone V, Bellavere F, Scionti L, Maule S, Quadri R, Bax G, et al. Recommendations for the use of cardiovascular tests in diagnosing diabetic autonomic neuropathy. Nutr Metab Cardiovasc Dis. 2011;21:69–78. https://doi.org/10.1016/j.numecd.2010.07.005.

16. Ko SH, Park SA, Cho JH, Song KH, Yoon KH, Cha BY, et al. Progression of cardiovascular autonomic dysfunction in patients with type 2 diabetes: a 7-year follow-up study. Diabetes Care. 2008;31:1832–6. https://doi.org/10.2337/dc08-0682.

17. Rolim LC, de Souza JST, Dib SA. Tests for early diagnosis of cardiovascular autonomic neuropathy: critical analysis and relevance. Front Endocrinol (Lausanne). 2014;4:173. https://doi.org/10.3389/fendo.2013.00173.

18. Bakkar NZ, Dwaib HS, Fares S, Eid AH, Al-Dhaheri Y, El-Yazbi AF. Cardiac autonomic neuropathy: a progressive consequence of chronic low-grade inflammation in type 2 diabetes and related metabolic disorders. Int J Mol Sci. 2020;21:9005. https://doi.org/10.3390/ijms21239005.

19. Frontoni S, Di Bartolo P, Avogaro A, Bosi E, Paolisso G, Ceriello A. Glucose variability: an emerging target for the treatment of diabetes mellitus. Diabetes Res Clin Pract. 2013;102:86–95. https://doi.org/10.1016/j.diabres.2013.09.007.

20. Pop-Busui R. Cardiac autonomic neuropathy in diabetes. A clinical perspective. Diabetes Care. 2010;33:434–41. https://doi.org/10.2337/dc09-1294.

21. Albers JW, Pop-Busui R. Diabetic neuropathy: mechanisms, emerging treatments, and subtypes. Curr Neurol Neurosci Rep. 2014;14:473. https://doi.org/10.1007/s11910-014-0473-5.

22. Balcıoğlu AS, Müderrisoğlu H. Diabetes and cardiac autonomic neuropathy: clinical manifestations, cardiovascular consequences, diagnosis and treatment. World J Diabetes. 2015;6:80–91. https://doi.org/10.4239/wjd.v6.i1.80.

23. Fisher VL, Tahrani AA. Cardiac autonomic neuropathy in patients with diabetes mellitus: current perspectives. Diabetes Metab Syndr Obes. 2017;10:419–34. https://doi.org/10.2147/DMSO.S129797.

24. Ozdemir M, Arslan U, Türkoğlu S, Balcıoğlu S, Cengel A. Losartan improves heart rate variability and heart rate turbulence in heart failure due to ischemic cardiomyopathy. J Card Fail. 2007;13:812–7. https://doi.org/10.1016/j.cardfail.2007.08.002.

25. Kempler P, editor. Neuropathies. Nerve dysfunction of diabetic and other origin. Budapest: Springer; 1997.

26. Ewing DJ, Martyn CN, Young RJ, Clarke BF. The value of cardiovascular autonomic function tests: 10 years experience in diabetes. Diabetes Care. 1985;8:491–8. https://doi.org/10.2337/diacare.8.5.491.

27. Valensi P, Johnson NB, Maison-Blanche P, Extramania F, Motte G, Coumel P. Influence of cardiac autonomic neuropathy on heart rate dependence of ventricular repolarization in diabetic patients. Diabetes Care. 2002;25:918–23. https://doi.org/10.2337/diacare.25.5.918.

28. Low PA, Walsh JC, Huang CY, McLeod JC. The sympathetic nervous system in diabetic neuropathy. A clinical and pathological study. Brain. 1975;98:341–56. https://doi.org/10.1093/brain/98.3.341.

29. Low PA. Prevalence of orthostatic hypotension. Clin Auton Res. 2008;18:8–13. https://doi.org/10.1007/s10286-007-1001-3.

30. Vinik AI, Erbas T. Diabetic autonomic neuropathy. In: Buijs RM, Swaab DF, editors. Handbook of clinical neurology, vol. 117. Edinburgh: Elsevier; 2013. p. 279–94. https://doi.org/10.1016/B978-0-444-53491-0.00022-5.

31. Vinik AI, Maser RE, Ziegler D. Neuropathy: the crystal ball for cardiovascular disease? Diabetes Care. 2010;33:1688–90. https://doi.org/10.2337/dc10-0745.

32. Nagamachi S, Jinnouchi S, Kurose T, Ohnishi T, Flores LG 2nd, Nakahara H, et al. 123I-MIBG myocardial scintigraphy in diabetic patients: relationship with 201Tl uptake and cardiac autonomic function. Ann Nucl Med. 1998;12:323–31. https://doi.org/10.1007/BF03164921.

33. Ziegler D, Schatz H, Conrad F, Gries FA, Ulrich H, Reichel G. Effects of treatment with the antioxidant alpha-lipoic acid on cardiac autonomic neuropathy in NIDDM patients. A 4-month randomized controlled multicenter trial (DEKAN study). Diabetes Care. 1997;20:369–73. https://doi.org/10.2337/diacare.20.3.369.

34. Vinik AI, Erbas T, Casellini CM. Diabetic cardiac autonomic neuropathy, inflammation and cardiovascular disease. J Diabetes Investig. 2013;4:4–18. https://doi.org/10.1111/jdi.12042.

35. Pop-Busui R, Boulton AJ, Feldman EL, Bril V, Freeman R, Malik RA, et al. Diabetic neuropathy: a position statement by the American Diabetes Association. Diabetes Care. 2017;40:136–54. https://doi.org/10.2337/dc16-2042.

36. Valensi P, Extramiana F, Lange C, Cailleau M, Haggui A, Maison Blanche P, et al. Influence of blood glucose on heart rate and cardiac autonomic function. The DESIR study. Diabet Med. 2011;28:440–9. https://doi.org/10.1111/j.1464-5491.2010.03222.x.

37. Veglio M, Chinaglia A, Cavallo-Perin P. QT interval, cardiovascular risk factors and risk of death in diabetes. J Endocrinol Investig. 2004;27:175–81. https://doi.org/10.1007/BF03346265.

38. Spallone V, Ziegler D, Freeman R, Bernardi L, Frontoni S, Pop-Busui R, et al. Cardiovascular autonomic neuropathy in diabetes: clinical impact, assessment, diagnosis, and management. Diabetes Metab Res Rev. 2011;27:639–53. https://doi.org/10.1002/dmrr.1239.

39. Hage FG, Iskandrian AE. Cardiovascular imaging in diabetes mellitus. J Nucl Cardiol. 2011;18:959–65. https://doi.org/10.1007/s12350-011-9431-7.

40. Vinik AI, Ziegler D. Diabetic cardiovascular autonomic neuropathy. Circulation. 2007;115:387–97. https://doi.org/10.1161/CIRCULATIONAHA.106.634949.

41. Vinik AI, Camacho PM, Davidson JA, Handelsman Y, Lando HM, Leddy AL, et al. Task force to develop an AACE position statement on autonomic testing. American Association of Clinical Endocrinologists and American College of endocrinology position statement on testing for autonomic and somatic nerve dysfunction. Endocr Pract. 2017;23:1472–8. https://doi.org/10.4158/EP-2017-0053.

42. Santini V, Ciampittiello G, Gigli F, Bracaglia D, Baroni A, Cocconetti E, et al. QTc and autonomic neuropathy in diabetes: effects of acute hyperglycaemia and n-3 PUFA. Nutr Metab Cardiovasc Dis. 2007;17:712–8. https://doi.org/10.1016/j.numecd.2006.09.006.

43. Rosengård-Bärlund M, Bernardi L, Fagerudd J, Mäntysaari M, Af Björkesten CG, Lindholm H, et al. FinnDiane Study Group. Early

autonomic dysfunction in type 1 diabetes: a reversible disorder? Diabetologia. 2009;52:1164–72. https://doi.org/10.1007/s00125-009-1340-9.

44. Desouza CV, Bolli GB, Fonseca V. Hypoglycemia, diabetes, and cardiovascular events. Diabetes Care. 2010;33:1389–94. https://doi.org/10.2337/dc09-2082.

45. Benichou T, Pereira B, Mermillod M, Tauveron I, Pfabigan D, Maqdasy S, et al. Heart rate variability in type 2 diabetes mellitus: a systematic review and meta-analysis. PLoS One. 2018;13:e0195166. https://doi.org/10.1371/journal.pone.0195166.

46. Sessa F, Anna V, Messina G, Cibelli G, Monda V, Marsala G, et al. Heart rate variability as predictive factor for sudden cardiac death. Aging (Albany NY). 2018;10:166–77. https://doi.org/10.18632/aging.101386.

47. Mancia G, De Backer G, Dominiczak A, Cifkova R, Fagard R, Germano G, et al. 2007 ESH-ESC guidelines for the management of arterial hypertension: the task force for the management of arterial hypertension of the European Society of Hypertension (ESH) and of the European Society of Cardiology (ESC). J Hypertens. 2007;25:1105–87. https://doi.org/10.1097/HJH.0b013e3281fc975a.

48. Wackers FJ, Young LH, Inzucchi SE, Chyun DA, Davey JA, Barrett EJ, et al. Detection of silent myocardial ischemia in asymptomatic diabetic subjects: the DIAD study. Diabetes Care. 2004;27:1954–61. https://doi.org/10.2337/diacare.27.8.1954.

49. Burgos LG, Ebert TJ, Assiddao C, Turner LA, Pattison CZ, Wang-Cheng R, et al. Increased intraoperative cardiovascular morbidity in diabetics with autonomic neuropathy. Anesthesiology. 1989;70:591–7. https://doi.org/10.1097/00000542-198904000-00006.

50. Bernardi L, Spallone V, Stevens M, Hilsted J, Frontoni S, Pop-Busui R, et al. Methods of investigation for cardiac autonomic dysfunction in human research studies. Diabetes Metab Res Rev. 2011;27:654–64. https://doi.org/10.1002/dmrr.1224.

51. Mogensen UM, Jensen T, Kober L, Kelbaek H, Mathiesen AS, Dixen P, et al. Cardiovascular autonomic neuropathy and subclinical cardiovascular disease in normoalbuminuric Type 1 diabetic patients. Diabetes. 2012;61:1822–30. https://doi.org/10.2337/db11-1235.

52. Shakespeare CF, Katritsis D, Crowther A, Cooper IC, Coltart JD, Webb-Peploe MV. Differences in autonomic nerve function in patients with silent and symptomatic myocardial ischaemia. Br Heart J. 1994;71:22–9. https://doi.org/10.1136/hrt.71.1.22.

53. Bauer A, Malik M, Schmidt G, Barthel P, Bonnemeier H, Cygankiewicz I, et al. Heart rate turbulence: standards of measurement, physiological interpretation, and clinical use: International Society for Holter and Noninvasive Electrophysiology Consensus. J Am Coll Cardiol. 2008;52:1353–65. https://doi.org/10.1016/j.jacc.2008.07.041.

54. Serhiyenko VA, Serhiyenko AA. Cardiac autonomic neuropathy: risk factors, diagnosis and treatment. World J Diabetes. 2018;9:1–24. https://doi.org/10.4239/wjd.v9.i1.1.

55. La Rovere MT, Pinna GD, Maestri R, Robbi E, Caporotondi A, Guazzotti G, et al. Prognostic implications of baroreflex sensitivity in heart failure patients in the beta-blocking era. J Am Coll Cardiol. 2009;53:193–9. https://doi.org/10.1016/j.jacc.2008.09.034.

56. Cseh D, Climie RE, Offredo L, Guibout C, Thomas F, Zanoli L, et al. Type 2 diabetes mellitus is independently associated with decreased neural baroreflex sensitivity: the Paris prospective study III. Arterioscler Thromb Vasc Biol. 2020;40:1420–8. https://doi.org/10.1161/ATVBAHA.120.314102.

57. Hoffman RP, Sinkey CA, Anderson EA. Microneurographically determined muscle sympathetic nerve activity levels are reproducible in insulin-dependent diabetes mellitus. J Diabetes Complicat. 1998;12:307–10. https://doi.org/10.1016/S1056-8727(98)00010-5.

58. Hilsted J. Catecholamines and diabetic autonomic neuropathy. Diabet Med. 1995;12:296–7. https://doi.org/10.1111/j.1464-5491.1995.tb00479.x.

59. González-Ortiz M, Martínez-Abundis E, Robles-Cervantes JA, Ramírez-Ramírez V, Ramos-Zavala MG. Effect of thiamine administration on metabolic profile, cytokines and inflammatory markers in drug-naïve patients with type 2 diabetes. Eur J Nutr. 2011;50:145–9. https://doi.org/10.1007/s00394-010-0123-x.

60. Schemmel KE, Padiyara RS, D'Souza JJ. Aldose reductase inhibitors in the treatment of diabetic peripheral neuropathy: a review. J Diabetes Complicat. 2010;24:354–60. https://doi.org/10.1016/j.jdiacomp.2009.07.005.

61. DeGrado TR, Hutchins GD, Toorongian SA, Wieland DM, Schwaiger M. Myocardial kinetics of carbon-11-meta-hydroxyephedrine (HED): retention mechanisms and effects of norepinephrine. J Nucl Med. 1993;34:1287–93.

62. Allman KC, Stevens MJ, Wieland DM, Hutchins GD, Wolfe ER Jr, Greene DA, Schwaiger M. Noninvasive assessment of cardiac diabetic neuropathy by C-11 hydroxyephedrine and positron emission tomography. J Am Coll Cardiol. 1993;22:1425–32. https://doi.org/10.1016/0735-1097(93)90553-D.

63. Stevens MJ, Dayanikli F, Raffel DM, Allman KC, Sandford T, Feldman EL, et al. Scintigraphic assessment of regionalized defects in myocardial sympathetic innervation and blood flow regulation in diabetic patients with autonomic neuropathy. J Am Coll Cardiol. 1998;31:1575–84. https://doi.org/10.1016/S0735-1097(98)00128-4.

64. Freeman MR, Newman D, Dorian P, Barr A, Langer A. Relation of direct assessment of cardiac autonomic function with metaiodobenzylguanidine imaging to heart rate variability in diabetes mellitus. Am J Cardiol. 1987;80:247–50. https://doi.org/10.1016/S0002-9149(97)00337-8.

65. Schnell O, Muhr D, Weiss M, Dresel S, Haslbeck M, Standl E. Reduced myocardial 123I-metaiodobenzylguanidine uptake in newly diagnosed IDDM patients. Diabetes. 1996;45:801–5. https://doi.org/10.2337/diab.45.6.801.

66. Boulton AJ, Vinik AI, Arezzo JC, Bril V, Feldman EL, Freeman R, et al. Diabetic neuropathies: a statement by the American Diabetes Association. Diabetes Care. 2005;28:956–62. https://doi.org/10.2337/diacare.28.4.956.

67. Ziegler D. Can diabetic polyneuropathy be successfully treated? MMW Fortschr Med. 2010;152:64–8. https://doi.org/10.1007/BF03366224.

68. Dimitropoulos G, Tahrani AA, Stevens MJ. Cardiac autonomic neuropathy in patients with diabetes mellitus. World J Diabetes. 2014;6:245–58. https://doi.org/10.4239/wjd.v5.i1.17.

69. Soares-Miranda L, Sandercock G, Vale S, Santos R, Abreu S, Moreira C, Mota J. Metabolic syndrome, physical activity and cardiac autonomic function. Diabetes Metab Res Rev. 2012;28:363–9. https://doi.org/10.1002/dmrr.2281.

70. Vincent AM, Calabek B, Roberts L, Feldman EL. Biology of diabetic neuropathy. Handb Clin Neurol. 2013;115:591–606. https://doi.org/10.1016/B978-0-444-52902-2.00034-5.

71. Valensi P, Pariès J, Attali JR. French Group for Research and Study of diabetic neuropathy. Cardiac autonomic neuropathy in diabetic patients: influence of diabetes duration, obesity, and microangiopathic complications—the French multicenter study. Metabolism. 2003;52:815–20. https://doi.org/10.1016/S0026-0495(03)00095-7.

72. Gaede P, Lund-Andersen H, Parving HH, Pedersen O. Effect of a multifactorial intervention on mortality in type 2 diabetes. N Engl J Med. 2008;358:580–91. https://doi.org/10.1056/NEJMoa0706245.

73. Callaghan BC, Cheng HT, Stables CL, Smith AL, Feldman EL. Diabetic neuropathy: clinical manifestations and current treatments. Lancet Neurol. 2012;11:521–34. https://doi.org/10.1016/S1474-4422(12)70065-0.

74. Shin S, Kim KJ, Chang HJ, Lee BW, Yang WI, Cha BS, et al. The effect of oral prostaglandin analogue on painful diabetic neuropathy: a double-blind, randomized, controlled trial. Diabetes Obes Metab. 2013;15:185–8. https://doi.org/10.1111/dom.12010.

75. Derosa G, Limas CP, Macías PC, Estrella A, Maffioli P. Dietary and nutraceutical approach to type 2 diabetes. Arch Med Sci. 2014;10:336–44. https://doi.org/10.5114/aoms.2014.42587.

76. Sytze Van Dam P, Cotter MA, Bravenboer B, Cameron NE. Pathogenesis of diabetic neuropathy: focus on neurovascular mechanisms. Eur J Pharmacol. 2013;719:180–6. https://doi.org/10.1016/j.ejphar.2013.07.017.

77. AIM-HIGH Investigators. The role of niacin in raising high-density lipoprotein cholesterol to reduce cardiovascular events in patients with atherosclerotic cardiovascular disease and optimally treated low-density lipoprotein cholesterol: baseline characteristics of study participants. The Atherothrombosis Intervention in Metabolic syndrome with low HDL/high triglycerides: impact on Global Health outcomes (AIM-HIGH) trial. Am Heart J. 2011;161:538–43. https://doi.org/10.1016/j.ahj.2010.12.007.

78. Ascaso JF. Advances in cholesterol-lowering interventions. Endocrinol Nutr. 2010;57:210–9. https://doi.org/10.1016/j.endonu.2010.03.008.

79. Serhiyenko VA, Serhiyenko LM, Serhiyenko AA. Omega-3 polyunsaturated fatty acids in the treatment of diabetic cardiovascular autonomic neuropathy: a review. In: Moore SJ, editor. Omega-3: dietary sources, biochemistry and impact on human health. New York: Nova Science Publishers; 2017. p. 79–154.

80. Blum A, Shamburek R. The pleiotropic effects of statins on endothelial function, vascular inflammation, immunomodulation and thrombogenesis. Atherosclerosis. 2009;203:325–30. https://doi.org/10.1016/j.atherosclerosis.2008.08.022.

81. Fleg JL, Mete M, Howard BV, Umans JG, Roman MJ, Ratner RE, et al. Effect of statins alone versus statins plus ezetimibe on carotid atherosclerosis in type 2 diabetes: the SANDS (Stop Atherosclerosis in Native Diabetics Study) trial. J Am Coll Cardiol. 2008;52:2198–205. https://doi.org/10.1016/j.jacc.2008.10.031.

82. Tesfaye S, Selvarajah D. Advances in the epidemiology, pathogenesis and management of diabetic peripheral neuropathy. Diabetes Metab Res Rev. 2012;28:8–14. https://doi.org/10.1002/dmrr.2239.

83. Belfort R, Berria R, Cornell J, Cusi K. Fenofibrate reduces systemic inflammation markers independent of its effects on lipid and glucose metabolism in patients with the metabolic syndrome. J Clin Endocrinol Metab. 2010;95:829–36. https://doi.org/10.1210/jc.2009-1487.

84. Staels B. A review of bile acid sequestrants: potential mechanism(s) for glucose-lowering effects in type 2 diabetes mellitus. Postgrad Med. 2009;121:25–30. https://doi.org/10.3810/pgm.2009.05.suppl53.290.

85. Bosch J, Gerstein HC, Dagenais GR, Díaz R, Dyal L, Jung H, et al. n-3 fatty acids and cardiovascular outcomes in patients with dysglycemia. N Engl J Med. 2012;367:309–18. https://doi.org/10.1056/NEJMoa1203859.

86. De Roos B, Mavrommatis Y, Brouwer IA. Long-chain n-3 polyunsaturated fatty acids: new insights into mechanisms relating to inflammation and coronary heart disease. Br J Pharmacol. 2009;158:413–28. https://doi.org/10.1111/j.1476-5381.2009.00189.x.

87. Ebbesson SO, Devereux RB, Cole S, Ebbesson LO, Fabsitz RR, Haack K, et al. Heart rate is associated with red blood cell fatty acid concentration: the Genetics of Coronary Artery Disease in Alaska Natives (GOCADAN) study. Am Heart J. 2010;159:1020–5. https://doi.org/10.1016/j.ahj.2010.03.001.

88. Jeppesen C, Schiller K, Schulze MB. Omega-3 and omega-6 fatty acids and type 2 diabetes. Curr Diab Rep. 2013;13:279–88. https://doi.org/10.1007/s11892-012-0362-8.

89. Kandasamy N, Joseph F, Goenka N. The role of omega-3 fatty acids in cardiovascular disease, hypertriglyceridaemia and diabetes mellitus. Br J Diabetes Vasc Dis. 2008;8:121–8. https://doi.org/10.1177/14746514080080030301.

90. Tomassini JE, Mazzone T, Goldberg RB, Guyton JR, Weinstock RS, Polis A, et al. Effect of ezetimibe/simvastatin compared with atorvastatin on lipoprotein subclasses in patients with type 2 diabetes and hypercholesterolaemia. Diabetes Obes Metab. 2009;11:855–64. https://doi.org/10.1111/j.1463-1326.2009.01061.x.

91. Witteles RM, Fowler MB. Insulin-resistant cardiomyopathy clinical evidence, mechanisms, and treatment options. J Am Coll Cardiol. 2008;51:93–102. https://doi.org/10.1016/j.jacc.2007.10.021.

92. Fragasso G, Palloshi A, Puccetti P, Silipigni C, Rossodivita A, Pala M, et al. A randomized clinical trial of trimetazidine, a partial free fatty acid oxidation inhibitor, in patients with heart failure. J Am Coll Cardiol. 2006;48:992–8. https://doi.org/10.1016/j.jacc.2006.03.060.

93. Lee L, Campbell R, Scheuermann-Freestone M, Taylor R, Gunaruwan P, Williams L, et al. Metabolic modulation with perhexiline in chronic heart failure: a randomized, controlled trial of short-term use of a novel treatment. Circulation. 2005;112:3280–8. https://doi.org/10.1161/CIRCULATIONAHA.105.551457.

94. Morrow DA, Scirica BM, Karwatowska-Prokopczuk E, Murphy SA, Budaj A, Varshavsky S, et al. Effects of ranolazine on recurrent cardiovascular events in patients with non-ST-elevation acute coronary syndromes: the MERLIN-TIMI 36 randomized trial. JAMA. 2007;297:1775–83. https://doi.org/10.1001/jama.297.16.1775.

95. Tesfaye S, Boulton AJM, Dyck PJ, Freeman R, Horowitz M, Kempler P, et al. Diabetic neuropathies: update on definitions, diagnostic criteria, estimation of severity, and treatments. Diabetes Care. 2010;33:2285–93. https://doi.org/10.2337/dc10-1303.

96. Orchard TJ, LLoyd CE, Maser RE, Kuller LH. Why does diabetic autonomic neuropathy predict IDDM mortality? An analysis from the Pittsburgh epidemiology of diabetes complications study. Diabetes Res Clin Pract. 1996;34:165–71. https://doi.org/10.1016/S0168-8227(96)90025-X.

97. Rhee SY, Kim YS, Chon S, Oh S, Woo JT, Kim SW, et al. Long-term effects of cilostazol on the prevention of macrovascular disease in patients with type 2 diabetes mellitus. Diabetes Res Clin Pract. 2011;91:11–4. https://doi.org/10.1016/j.diabres.2010.09.009.

98. Dhule SS, Gawali SR. Platelet aggregation and clotting time in type II diabetic males. Natl J Physiol Pharm Pharmacol. 2014;4:121–3. https://doi.org/10.5455/njppp.2014.4.290920131.

99. Pop-Busui R, Evans GW, Gerstein HC, Fonseca V, Fleg JL, Hoogwerf BJ, et al. Effects of cardiac autonomic dysfunction on mortality risk in the action to control cardiovascular risk in diabetes (ACCORD) trial. Diabetes Care. 2010;33:1578–84. https://doi.org/10.2337/dc10-0125.

100. Csányi G, Miller FJ. Oxidative stress in cardiovascular disease. Int J Mol Sci. 2014;15:6002–8. https://doi.org/10.3390/ijms15046002.

101. Mallet ML, Hadjivassiliou M, Sarrigiannis PG, Zis P. The role of oxidative stress in peripheral neuropathy. J Mol Neurosci. 2020;70:1009–17. https://doi.org/10.1007/s12031-020-01495-x.

102. Ibrahimpasic K. Alpha lipoic acid and glycaemic control in diabetic neuropathies at type 2 diabetes treatment. Med Arch. 2013;67:7–9. https://doi.org/10.5455/medarh.2013.67.7-9.

103. Adaikalakoteswari A, Rabbani N, Waspadji S, Tjokroprawiro A, Kariadi SH, Adam JM, Thornalley PJ. Disturbance of B-vitamin

status in people with type 2 diabetes in Indonesia-link to renal status, glycemic control and vascular inflammation. Diabetes Res Clin Pract. 2012;95:415–24. https://doi.org/10.1016/j.diabres.2011.10.042.

104. Stracke H, Gaus W, Achenbach U, Federlin K, Bretzel RG. Benfotiamine in diabetic polyneuropathy (BENDIP): results of a randomised, double blind, placebo-controlled clinical study. Exp Clin Endocrinol Diabetes. 2008;116:600–5. https://doi.org/10.1055/s-2008-1065351.

105. Serhiyenko VA, Serhiyenko LM, Serhiyenko AA. Recent advances in the treatment of neuropathies in type 2 diabetes mellitus patients: focus on benfotiamine (review and own data). In: Berhardt LV, editor. Advances in medicine and biology (numbered series), vol. 166. New York: Nova Science Publishers; 2020. p. 1–80.

106. Haupt E, Ledermann H, Köpcke W. Benfotiamine in the treatment of diabetic polyneuropathy-a three-week randomized, controlled pilot study (BEDIP study). Int J Clin Pharmacol Ther. 2005;43:71–7. https://doi.org/10.5414/CPP43071.

107. Moss CJ, Mathews ST. Thiamin status and supplementation in the management of diabetes mellitus and its vascular comorbidities. Vitam Miner. 2013;2:111. https://doi.org/10.4172/vms.1000111.

108. Power RA, Hulver MW, Zhang JY, Dubois J, Marchand RM, Ilkayeva O, et al. Carnitine revisited: potential use as adjunctive treatment in diabetes. Diabetologia. 2007;50:824–32. https://doi.org/10.1007/s00125-007-0605-4.

109. Solfrizzi V, Capurso C, Colacicco AM, D'Introno A, Fontana C, Capurso SA, et al. Efficacy and tolerability of combined treatment with L-carnitine and simvastatin in lowering lipoprotein(a) serum levels in patients with type 2 diabetes mellitus. Atherosclerosis. 2006;188:455–61. https://doi.org/10.1016/j.atherosclerosis.2005.11.024.

110. Bang HO, Dyerberg J. The bleeding tendency in Greenland Eskimos. Dan Med Bull. 1980;27:202–5.

111. Harris WS. Omega-3 fatty acids and cardiovascular disease: a case for omega-3 index as a new risk factor. Pharmacol Res. 2007;55:217–23. https://doi.org/10.1016/j.phrs.2007.01.013.

112. Freeman R. Clinical practice. Neurogenic orthostatic hypotension. N Engl J Med. 2008;358:615–24. https://doi.org/10.1056/NEJMcp074189.

113. Lahrmann H, Cortelli P, Hilz M, Mathias CJ, Struhal W, Tassinari M. EFNS guidelines on the diagnosis and management of orthostatic hypotension. Eur J Neurol. 2006;13:930–6. https://doi.org/10.1111/j.1468-1331.2006.01512.x.

114. Rahman A, Fujisawa Y, Nakano D, Hitomi H, Nishiyama A. Effect of a selective SGLT2 inhibitor, luseogliflozin, on circadian rhythm of sympathetic nervous function and locomotor activities in metabolic syndrome rats. Clin Exp Pharmacol Physiol. 2017;44:522–5. https://doi.org/10.1111/1440-1681.12725.

115. Valensi P, Chiheb S, Fysekidis M. Insulin- and glucagon-like peptide-1-induced changes in heart rate and vagosympathetic activity: why they matter. Diabetologia. 2013;56:1196–200. https://doi.org/10.1007/s00125-013-2909-x.

Autonomic Visceral Neuropathy and Gastrointestinal Disorders

58

Anne Mohr Drewes, Christina Brock, and Asbjørn Mohr Drewes

Chapter Objectives

- The autonomic nervous system consists of the enteric, parasympathetic, and sympathetic nerve systems. In the early stages of autonomic neuropathy, the vagal nerve seems to be the most vulnerable consequently compromising its function.
- Autonomic neuropathy is one of the most burdensome symptoms in patients with diabetes mellitus. It is, however, frequently under-diagnosed.
- In patients with longstanding diabetes, up to 40% suffer from gastrointestinal symptoms.
- Symptoms induced by visceral neuropathy cover the entire gastrointestinal tract and includes nausea and vomiting, bloating, early satiety, diarrhoea, and constipation.
- Both hyperglycaemic and hypoglycaemic episodes coalesce to form a cumulative indirect cascade which initiates and maintains neuro-inflammation in diabetic autonomic neuropathy.

Introduction

The brain–gut axis is a bidirectional nexus of the sensory input from the gastrointestinal (GI) tract and efferent pathways, which is involved in secretion of digestive hormones, homeostatic regulation, and gut motility. This axis comprises among other the autonomic nervous system (ANS), comprising the enteric nervous system (ENS), parasympathetic and sympathetic branches, which have a delicate regulatory interaction. Therefore, the ANS has an essential role, and any dysfunction leads to impaired mediation of visceral regulation. Consequently, damage to the ANS such as development of diabetic autonomic neuropathy (DAN) is one of the most burdensome complications to diabetes, yet frequently under-diagnosed. These complications cause symptoms in the GI tract such as nausea, vomiting, diarrhoea, and constipation, see Fig. 58.1. It is difficult to diagnose DAN, but it may be defined as impaired functions of the involved nerves controlling the involuntary body functions such as the cardiovascular, urinary, pulmonary, and digestive systems [1]. Cardiac autonomic neuropathy is a measureable impaired regulation of the heart function, leading to dysrhythmias, such as atrial fibrillation, tachycardia, and even cardiac arrest [2]. Patients with cardiac autonomic neuropathy develop an impaired adaptability of the heart rate, assessed as reduced heart rate variability [3], see Chap. 59 for further elaboration. In this chapter, we focus on autonomic gastrointestinal neuropathy in patients with diabetes, explaining the underlying pathophysiology and the symptomatology in the GI tract.

Diabetic autonomic neuropathy could be defined as impaired functions of nerves controlling involuntary body functions.

A. M. Drewes (✉)
Department of Medicine, Regional Hospital Horsens, Horsens, Denmark
e-mail: anne@drewes.dk

C. Brock · A. M. Drewes
Mech-Sense, Department of Gastroenterology and Hepatology, Clinical Institute, Aalborg University Hospital, Aalborg, Denmark

© The Author(s), under exclusive license to Springer Nature Switzerland AG 2023
J. Rodriguez-Saldana (ed.), *The Diabetes Textbook*, https://doi.org/10.1007/978-3-031-25519-9_58

Fig. 58.1 Gastro intestinal
disorders related to autonomic
neuropathy

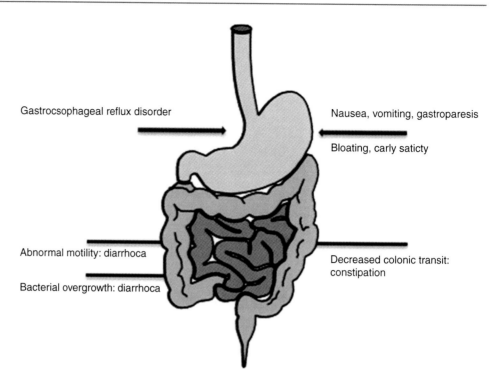

Fig. 58.1 Gastro intestinal disorders related to autonomic neuropathy

Neuropathy in Diabetes Mellitus

Neuropathy can objectively be demonstrated in 40–50% of who are diagnosed with diabetes for >20 years [4]. Recent research found evidence that in patients with long-term type 1 diabetes and polyneuropathies, there was prolonged neuronal transmission and altered neuronal brain responses at all levels of the neuraxis. The increased central conduction time was associated with diminished parasympathetic tone. This confirms that diabetes induced neuronal impairment at all levels, involving autonomic, central, and peripheral nerves [5]. It has been shown that structural changes in endoneuronal capillary morphology and vascular reactivity exist prior to neuropathy in patients with type 2 diabetes [6]. Furthermore, such endoneuronal hypoxia was associated with reductions in nerve conduction velocities. The pathophysiology underlying these findings is however complex and multifactorial and includes neuronal changes within Schwann cells, axons, and the microvascular compartment [7]. In addition, several biochemical mechanisms triggered by hyperglycaemia or hypoglycaemia also leads to neuropathy, which will be elaborated in this chapter, see Fig. 58.2.

The ENS innervates the gastrointestinal tract, gallbladder, and pancreas with motorneurons, sensory neurons, and interneurons. ENS controls the fluid transport between the gut and its lumen, local blood flow, as well as the gut motility. These functions are maintained as the ENS receive and integrate the incoming information leading to efferent transmission, which regulate the digestive system from the brainstem.

Thus, there is a close connection to the central nervous system (CNS) in order to balance physiological demands. Due to the enormous amount of neurones that correspond closely to the number in CNS, the ENS is recognized as the second brain [8, 9]. All these neurones and their interconnections are vulnerable to DAN [10].

The neuronal tissue in the brain might undergo changes as well [11, 12]. Animals where diabetes has been induced showed changes in the CNS. Furthermore, functional brain imaging and electroencephalographic recordings in patients with diabetes confirm functional and structural brain changes [3]. The imaging studies demonstrated mainly microstructural changes in brain areas involved in visceral sensory processing in patients with diabetes and GI symptoms. The encephalographic studies indicated that altered insular processing of sensory stimuli could be the key player in symptom generation. In particular, one study found that the deeper the insular electrical source was located, the more GI symptoms the patients experienced [13]. Another study found that GI symptoms and beat-to-beat interval (as a proxi of autonomic tone) were correlated to reorganization in the opercular cortex. Furthermore, the shift in operculo-cingulate networks was related to decreased quality of life in the patients [14]. These studies with electroencephalography were often conducted in combination with quantitative sensory testing and mostly it was found that stimulation of the GI organs induced hyposensitivity. This is in line with patients suffering from somatic diabetic neuropathy where pain and other sensations typically are associated with hypo-

Fig. 58.2 Structural changes and biochemical mechanism triggered by hyperglycaemia or hypoglycaemia may induce visceral neuropathy

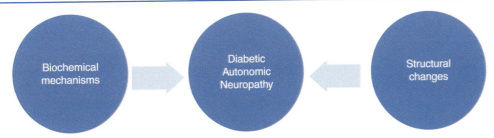

algesia to stimulation of the skin. The imaging findings and electrophysiological changes within the brain were associated with GI symptoms in patients with diabetes, therefore they might represent a biomarker for disease severity and hence be a new therapeutic target for neuromodulation or pharmacological therapy [3]. In Fig. 58.3, a conceptual model illustrating the different nerve pathways that may contribute to the GI symptoms in DM is shown.

In the early stages of DAN, alterations in the ENS are masked and difficult to detect. However, the vagal nerve due to its length and widespread appearance is most vulnerable to impaired function, and thus most work regarding DAN characterizes the vagal function [15]. The vagal nerve is the longest of the cranial nerves, and among other functions, it transmits signals from the gut wall receptors, sensitive to chemical and mechanical stimuli, controlling gut motility, secretion, and feeding behaviour [16]. Patients with diabetes and GI symptoms experience gastric retention and a delay in transit with segmentation of barium column within the small intestine, which was similar to changes found in patients with vagotomy [17, 18]. It has been shown in animal studies that the presence of glucose-responsive neurons have been identified in the CNS which may alter the vagal efferent activity [18]. Therefore, the systemic changes in blood glucose experienced in both hyper- and hypoglycaemic episodes might have a direct effect on the parasympathetic tone. Increased blood glucose level increases the level of oxidative stress and pro-inflammatory cytokines involved in neuroinflammation. Recent studies have shown that both electrical and pharmacological stimulation of the vagal nerve reduces the level of pro-inflammatory cytokines in both healthy, experimental inflammatory and auto-immune diseases [19, 20]. Hence, enhanced vagal tone might activate the cholinergic anti-inflammatory reflex and may have the potential to modulate the immune system [21, 22]. Therefore, it is plausible that enhanced vagal activity might have a protective function on diabetes-induced neuroinflammation. Taken together, the multifaceted mechanisms linked to ENS and ANS explain the variety of symptoms underlying DAN [23].

In experimental models of diabetes, reduced levels of neurotrophic support, including insulin-like growth factor and nerve growth factor, have been found. These findings have implicated reduced endoneuronal blood flow and thereby causing neuronal damage. The consequence of such

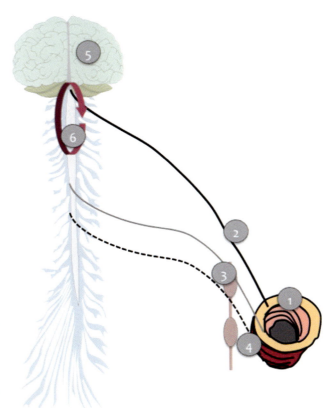

Fig. 58.3 Nerve pathways and mechanisms that may contribute to gastrointestinal symptoms in patients with diabetes mellitus: (1) Biochemical, vascular and degenerative changes in the enteric nervous system; Autonomic neuropathy that may affect (2) the vagal nerve (black line) and (3) sympathetic pathways (grey line) and indirectly modulate sensations from the gut; (4) Affection of visceral (and somatic in case the peritoneum is involved) afferents (dotted line) mediating sensations such as pain; (5) Structural and functional changes in the brain (and spinal cord), together with (6) affection of spino-bulbo-spinal loops

impairment in blood flow also leads to alteration of the nitric oxide metabolism and the Na+/K+ ATP-ase activity [24]. Furthermore, animal studies indicated that a changed Na+/K+ pump function may occur as a result of C-peptide deficiency. This may cause shunting glucose through the polyol pathway leading to increased levels of sorbitol and alteration of nerve excitability recovery cycle, which ultimately leads to neuronal damage [25, 26]. A last mechanism to mention is nerve damage through complement activation, as it has been reported in several peripheral neuropathies [27, 28]. A study on chronic peripheral neuropathy in children found a cell surface deficiency of the protein CD59, which is a complement regulatory protein. Furthermore, sural nerve biopsies from patients with diabetes have shown presence of activated complement proteins and membrane attack complex neoantigen [27]. Complement activation might be a potential new area to investigate when explaining autonomic neuropathy.

The Hyperglycaemia Hypothesis

Consequences of hyperglycaemia are increased intracellular glucose level and cellular toxicity. This glucotoxicity alters cell function in different ways causing increased level of diacylglycerol (which in turn activates protein kinase C) and synthesis of polyols and hexosamines that accumulate intracellularly [29–31]. These metabolic pathways are summarized in Fig. 58.4 and is shortly explained in the following:

A minor branch of glycolysis is the hexosamine biosynthesis pathway, where fructose-6-phosphate converts to glucosamine-6-phosphate, which is a rate-limited enzyme. Hexosamine accumulate intracellular causing oxidative stress. Second, another intracellular metabolic pathway is the polyol. When the polyol pathway is activated, it may cause reduction of Na^+/K^+ -ATPase activity and osmotic damage and intracellular oxidative stress [32]. Third, increase in diacylglycerol and protein kinase C pathways is believed to increase the activity of cytosolic phospholipase A2 and produce prostaglandin E_2, as well as other pro-inflammatory mediators, which inhibit cellular (Na^+/K^+) ATPase [33, 34].

The exact mechanism by which these pathways lead to altered cell function is not fully understood, but taken together they coalesce to induce oxidative stress [35]. In the mitochondria, levels of free radicals, such as nitrogen species and superoxide rise. However, the ability to gather free radicals is reduced because of a reduction of the proton donor nicotinamide-adenine-dinucleotide [30]. Additionally, this mechanism may activate an enzyme, poly(ADP-ribose) polymerase, of great importance to deoxyribonucleic acid repair, and this activation may cause break-up of the deoxyribonucleic acid strands. The consequence of this mechanism is critically level of adenosine triphosphate in, e.g. Schwann cells, possibly leading to neuronal death [34].

When superoxide level rises, an inhibition of the key enzyme in glycolysis (glyceraldehyde-3-phosphate dehydrogenase) is manifest, resulting in enhanced activity in the involved biochemical pathways including further production of polyols, hexosamines, poly(ADP-ribose) polymerase, and advanced glycation end products, and thereby closing the loop of a vicious cycle [35]. For further reading, the following references are recommended: [36–38].

It has been found that the hyperglycaemia theory may be more valid for patients with type 1 than type 2 diabetes. Additionally, a Cochrane review found that improved glucose control prolongs the onset of peripheral sensorimotor neuropathy in type 1 DM, whereas it only had a modest, non-significant relative risk reduction in patients with type 2 DM after a follow-up period of 4 years. Contrarily, when the follow-up period was 15 years for the same cohort, the effect of increased glucose control showed significant risk reduction [39–41]. Even though these studies were conducted on peripheral axons, similar mechanisms are likely present in other nerve tissues, such as the ANS.

Finally the formation of advanced glycation end-products contribute to the intracellular non-enzymatic glycation of proteins, in which the extracellular matrix interacts with various receptors and possibly leads to pro-inflammatory gene expression that further amplifies the process [38].

The Influence of Severe Hypoglycaemia

Prolonged and severe hypoglycaemia may result in increased release of excitatory amino acids, which may cause uncontrolled triggering calcium influx. This again activates proteolytic enzymes that are known to cause neuronal damage [41]. Furthermore, hypoglycaemic levels of glucose may be counter-regulated through hormones inducing an acute rise in blood viscosity and haematocrit levels, which influences capillary blood flow especially when structural changes of the metabolic pathways and vessel of the neurons are already present [42].

Taken together, the biochemical pathways induced by hyperglycaemia and consequences of hypoglycaemia coalesce to form a cumulative indirect cascade that can initiate and summate neuro-inflammation, as is observed in DAN.

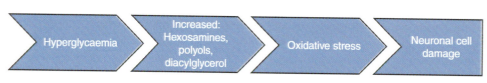

Fig. 58.4 Hyperglycaemia induces an increased level of hexosamines, polyols, and diacylglycerol within the cell, which may cause oxidative stress inducing cell damage

Gastrointestinal Disorders in Patients with Diabetes

Diabetic neuropathy may induce gastrointestinal symptoms, which will be elaborated in the following section (see Table 58.1). In several studies, patients with diabetes have reported more symptoms originating from the GI tract in comparison to people without diabetes [43–45]. Up to 20% of patients with diabetes have diarrhoea and up to 60% suffered from constipation [17, 44]. One study reported that long-term type 1 DM was accompanied by increased frequency of upper GI symptoms [46, 47]. On the other hand, another study found the prevalence of upper gastrointestinal symptoms, abdominal pain, and constipation was not significantly increased [48]. The prevalence of these symptoms varied which could have different explanations. However, due to lack of consensus, the assessment of GI symptoms varies, and thus to ensure consistency between study sites, it has been suggested to use the Diabetes Bowel Symptom Questionnaire in future epidemiological and clinical studies [49]. These disorders are difficult to treat which is why a multidisciplinary team including gastroenterologists, diabetologists, nurses, dieticians, surgeons, psychologist, and other health professionals should work together to help the patient. One main goal should be to prevent further progression by tight glycaemic control and then to ease symptoms which will be elaborated briefly in the following sections [50].

Gastrointestinal Reflux Disease

Patients with diabetes often suffer from nausea and vomiting [51]. One reason may be autonomic neuropathy-induced gastro-oesophageal reflux disease (GORD), where gastric content into the oesophagus causing complications or symptoms. Symptoms include heartburn and regurgitation. Clinical findings in GORD may also include laryngitis, chronic cough, and bronchospasm [52]. GORD could be seen in patients with DAN due to a hyperglycaemia-induced lower oesophageal sphincter pressure and increased amount of transient lower oesophageal sphincter relaxations.

Table 58.1 Possible diabetic neuropathy-induced gastrointestinal symptoms

Diabetic neuropathy-induced symptoms
Nausea
Vomiting
Reflux
Gastroparesis
Bloating
Constipation
Diarrhoea

Furthermore, studies report that impaired relaxation of the gastric fundus might cause early satiety and dyspeptic symptoms that also influence the symptom pattern in GORD [53].

Patients experiencing reflux should in many cases undergo endoscopy possibly accompanied by biopsy. Acidic and non-acidic content in the oesophagus can be assessed with pH impedance monitoring, and the swallowing and sphincter functions can be investigated with oesophageal high-resolution manometry, which is especially relevant in diabetic patients where neuropathy is suspected.

Reflux treatment is individual and determined by severity and progress. First, it is important to avoid provoking factors such as large meals, coffee, and alcohol. Symptoms caused by reflux can be treated with proton-pump inhibitors, but occasionally antacids, H_2 blockers, or foaming agents are used. However, symptoms such as nausea and vomiting are mainly controlled from the brain; therefore, it is mandatory to consider dysfunction of the CNS when other causes are ruled out [3]. It is expected that the alterations in the CNS system persist even long after the primary cause (if any) is ruled out.

Gastroparesis

The most common cause of gastroparesis is diabetes, and of all cases of gastroparesis, about one-third originates from diabetes-induced gastroparesis [54, 55]. The cumulative incidence for gastroparesis is approximately 5% for patients with type 1 DM and 1% for type 2 DM [56]. Even though gastroparesis proceeds the presence of delayed gastric emptying, most research have focused on this topic, as it is present in 30–50% with long-lasting diabetes [57]. The typical patient experiencing symptomatic gastroparesis has a long history of insulin-dependent diabetes and poor glycaemic control lasting for several years. In some cases, recent onset of gastroparesis is the only diabetic complication experienced by the patient. Other symptoms may include nausea, vomiting, bloating, early satiety, and epigastric pain [58]. Furthermore, gastroparesis predisposes for small intestinal dysfunction in up to 80% of those presented with clinical symptoms, which may lead to small intestinal bacterial overgrowth or interaction between host and gut microbiota [59]. One study investigating the microbiome in patients with type 1 diabetes even indicated that the patients had a decreased diversity, reduced stability, and more classified members in their microbiome compared with healthy controls [60]. Bacterial overgrowth as well as transit problems and constipation can secondarily cause abdominal pain [61].

The detailed anamnesis is crucial when diagnosing a patient with gastroparesis, and the use of validated questionnaires, such as the PAGI-SYM, are used to assess the patient reported symptoms from which the Gastroparesis Cardinal

Symptom Index can be calculated [62]. To investigate a gastroparetic patient, gastroscopy is often needed to rule out differential diagnosis such as celiac disease, ulcers, and cancer. If symptoms resemble those seen after truncal vagotomy (mild gastric dilation, poor to no peristalsis, residual gastric secretions despite a prolonged fast, atonic duodenal bulb, and open pylorus), then the diagnosis is straightforward. However, a proportion of these patients have no gastroscopic abnormalities [17, 63]. In such cases, motility investigations such as scintigraphy or radiopague markers are needed [64]. Scintigraphy is in most laboratories the "gold standard" to assess gastric emptying time, where retention of a meal labelled with ^{99m}Tc sulfur colloid is compared to normal reference values [57]. Recently, the wireless motility capsule (such as the SmartPill), which consist of a portable receiver, a wireless transmitting capsule, and displaying software has been taken into use. Following consumption of a standard meal, the participant swallows the capsule, which samples and transmits pressure, pH, and temperature data, from which segmental transit times (including gastric emptying time) can be derived [65, 66]. Alternative tests to asses gastric emptying include breath tests which measures the non-radioactive isotope ^{13}C labelled digestible substance and measure the metabolized isotope in the breath, emptying of radiopaque markers from the stomach by use of fluoroscopy, ultrasonography, ultrasound, and the paracetamol absorption test which is valid for gastric emptying of liquid meals [57, 64, 67–70].

The treatment of gastroparesis is challenging, but patients should be encouraged to focus on glycaemic control. The antiemetic drug metoclopramide has shown control of symptoms in 30–60% of patients and domperidone has shown effective in up to 60% of cases [71]. However, it must be underlined that there is no association between symptom improvement and changes in gastric motility following treatment with prokinetics [72]. Furthermore, most prokinetics are limited to short-term use due to the risk of irreversible tardive dyskinesia and cardiovascular side effects. Furthermore, symptoms can be diminished by use of pharmacological agent that increases motility such as erythromycin or (off label) prucalopride. New molecular targets are currently identified, and relamorelin, a synthetic ghrelin analogue, has shown promising results accelerating gastric emptying [73]. Endoscopic procedures such as botulinum toxin injections and myomectomy of the pylorus are also promising [61]. Constipation—if present—should also be adequately treated as it may give "upstream" motility disorders.

Another important aspect is nonpharmacological treatment with dietary consulting to improve glycaemic control [61]. In theory, patients with concomitant functional disorders or bloating may benefit from Low Fermentable Oligo-, Di-, and Mono-saccharides and Polyols diet (low-FODMAP) [74]. It is a dietary intervention under investigation in dys-

motility disorders, which is why it might benefit selected diabetic patients with neuropathy-induced dysmotility [75]. Avoidance of these carbohydrates should be global, and it is important to recognize that ingestions of FODMAPs are not the cause of the disease, but limited intake may represent an opportunity to reduce the patient symptoms [74]. Another dietary intervention has been studied by Olausson EA et al. [76]. In this study, patients with diabetes mellitus and gastroparesis were to eat a small particle diet. They found that patients on this diet improved in key symptoms such as nausea and vomiting. Furthermore, gastric electrical stimulation has been approved by the US Food and Drug Administration to alleviate symptoms in gastroparesis. The underlying mechanisms are debated and a growing body of evidence points toward alteration of the sympatico–vagal balance rather than enhancing gastric motility [77]. Nonetheless, the procedure has shown to decrease both symptom frequency and severity [78]. A potentially new method is stimulation of the vagal nerve during the skin together with deep breathing. This has been shown to increase gastric contractions in healthy volunteers [79], and currently a study is undergoing to explore this method in patients with diabetes [80].

Diarrhoea

Diarrhoea is observed in up to 20% of patients. The diarrhoea can be present as episodic, loose stool consistency, and periods with normal bowel function alternating with constipation [17, 59]. The cause of idiopathic diabetic diarrhoea is not known; however, the most recognized explanation is shifted sympatico–vagal balance as both sympathectomy and truncal vagotomy can cause diarrhoea. It may be caused by rapid transit or slow transit together with bacterial overgrowth [59, 81]. Even though autonomic neuropathy often induce prolonged transit times, it may also indirectly cause diabetic diarrhoea [17]. Furthermore, a study found that long-standing diabetes was associated with a decrease in number of interstitial cells of Cajac as well as decreased inhibitory innervation and an increase in excitatory innervation causing diarrhoea [82].

Abnormal and dis-coordinated motility of the small bowel may also lead to small intestinal bacterial overgrowth, which potentially also causes diarrhoea [83]. Third, faecal incontinence due to *anorectal dysfunction* can be present due to a weakened internal anal sphincter and lowered rectal sensory threshold [84]. Finally, as insulin is a trophic hormone for the acinar and ductal cells in pancreas, *pancreatic exocrine insufficiency* must be considered, especially when steatorrhoea is found, and as a parallel, patients with pancreatitis may have demolished the visceral nerves [85]. Appropriate test with pancreatic enzyme therapy or pancreatic function test is recommended.

Diagnosis of neuropathy-induced diarrhoea serves to exclude differential diagnosis that can lead to chronic watery diarrhoea, for example microscopic colitis or irritable bowel syndrome. If differential diagnosis can be excluded, the diagnosis idiopathic diabetic diarrhoea can be made (non-specific radiological findings and clinical symptoms) [17].

In order to treat patients with severe and long-lasting diabetic neuropathy-induced diarrhoea, there are six important targets: (1) hydration, nutrient deficiency, and correction of electrolyte deficiencies, (2) fibre supplementation which might be helpful in some cases, however it may also worsen gastroparesis, (3) symptomatic treatment with, e.g. codeine or loperamide as antidiarrheal medication by prolonging transit time and reduction of peristalsis, (4) treatment of underlying causes such as bacterial overgrowth with probiotics/antibiotics, (5) enzyme supplementation in case of exocrine pancreas insufficiency [71], and (6) glycaemic control in order to reverse underlying mechanisms [86].

Constipation

Motility disorders, more specifically reduced colonic transit time due to dysfunction of the ENS and ANS leads to constipation [53, 87]. A study investigating the prevalence of constipation in diabetics showed that 60% reported constipation and thus it is the most commonly reported symptom. Furthermore, the same study reported that 76% of the patients suffered from at least one GI symptom [17]. Furthermore, reduced bowel motility may result in specific constipation that occasionally leads to overflow incontinence that influences the clinical picture [71]. Of note, 80% of patients with diabetic diarrhoea also suffered from periods with constipation.

Constipation can be evaluated with radiopaque markers, scintigraphy, or different capsules as mentioned above and recently reviewed in [65]. In patients with functional gastrointestinal disorders, a reduction in caecal and colonic contractility, as well as bloating and distension was associated with excessive fermentation in the caecum assessed as a higher pH-drop across the iliocaecal junction [88]. A recent study found that patients with type 1 diabetes had prolonged small bowel transit, colonic transit, gastric emptying, and whole-gut transit time compared with healthy controls. Furthermore, prolonged colonic transit time in association with an increased fall in pH across the ileocecal junction was found [66]. Similar findings were shown in a recent paper where the wireless motility capsule was used to show pan-enteric prolongation of gastrointestinal transit times and a more acidic caecal pH, which may represent heightened caecal fermentation in diabetics [66].

Constipation could be due to alterations in the microbiota—or vice versa—however the exact mechanism on how alterations in microbiota influences the colonic motility. One study indicates that the breakdown of short chain fatty acids induces acidic milieu and thus modifies motility rhythm in the hindgut [89]. In support of this, animals who received antibiotics were shown to modulate their gut microbiota, which consequently improved their glucose tolerance and sensitivity to insulin [90]. Similar mechanisms are plausible in humans but need to be investigated in further detail.

Constipation may be treated conservatively with regular exercise, increased intake of dietary fibres, and focus on hydration. A non-pharmacological vibrating capsule has reduced constipation by improving peristaltic waves in the large intestine, however further studies are needed. Medical interventions may include bulk fibres or laxatives. In patients with slow-transit constipation, it is preferred to use osmotic laxatives compared to fibre supplementation and bulking agents. As the latter stimulates the intestines to absorb excessive amounts of fluid from the body. Frequently, osmotic active drugs are also used in combination with enemas. The reader is referred to [50, 61, 91].

In chronic constipation due to autonomic neuropathy and slow transit newer drugs such as prucalopride, a selective 5-HT receptor agonist may prove to be useful as it enhances colonic transit. Furthermore, lubiprostone stimulates secretion of electrolyte secretion and colonic water through activating of type 2 chloride channels in enterocytes. Another plausible target in the future is altering the composition of the microbiota through dietary alterations or faecal transplantation.

Diagnosis of Diabetic Autonomous Neuropathy

The clinician should ideally investigate the GI symptoms as described in section "Gastrointestinal Disorders in Patients with Diabetes" of this chapter. Additionally when gut symptoms arise in patients with diabetes, autonomic neuropathy should always be suspected, especially if the patient also suffers from distal symmetric polyneuropathy. Conventional measures of the autonomic function are indirect methods that rely on cardiovascular reflexes. However, the detection of early and subtle abnormalities in the parasympathetic system remains controversial, as the methods are relatively insensitive to sympathetic deficits [1, 92]. Classically, the ANS function has been correlated to recordings of the peroneal nerve [1, 93]. However, these methods are unspecific, invasive, and time consuming, which could explain why the most popular and the most utilised is time domain derived parameters of Heart Rate Variability or sudomotor reflex testing. One way to measure real-time brainstem vagal efferent activity known as cardiac vagal tone is with the neuroscope. A non-invasive measurement using ECG electrodes to detect phase shift in the beat-to-beat RR interval, which is described in detail elsewhere [94]. Another method in the future may be to measure potential biomarkers such as N-acetylaspartate with magnetic resonance imaging, which have been found to be reduced in patients with type 1 diabetes and central neuronal dysfunction or loss [95]. However, diagnosing DAN remains complicated as there is poor association between autonomic function testing and experienced GI symptoms [1].

There is no consensus regarding the optimal test parameters [96–98], and the shortcomings of each methods and their interpretation is responsible for the lack of formal diagnosing of DAN. Thus, such diagnosis is frequently delayed, the causes of which are most certainly multifactorial but arguably includes the non-specificity of presenting symptoms, the lack of clinician appreciation, and the limited availability of specialised diagnostic services. Nevertheless, diagnosis of DAN is important as it has a pivotal role in the pathophysiology of a number of diabetes-induced complications.

Concluding Remarks

Manifest DAN is one of the most burdensome symptoms, yet frequently under-diagnosed. The autonomic neuropathy induces symptoms such as nausea, vomiting, bloating, early satiety, diarrhoea, and constipation, which undoubtedly compromise the quality of life in these patients. The frequently presence of GI symptoms in patients with diabetes should make the clinician focus on DAN. Conservative and symptomatic treatment should accompany the suspicion of DAN, and if possible, the underlying cause should be treated. Ideally, treatment should be individualised as the symptom complex differs between patients. New emerging therapies are in pipeline and future research will undoubtedly result in improvement of the armamentarium clinicians have available for treatment of the severe complications associated with DAN.

Multiple Choice Questions

1. The autonomic nervous system comprises.
   - (a) The sympathetic, parasympathetic branch.
   - (b) **The enteric nervous system, parasympathetic, and sympathetic branches.**
   - (c) The sympathetic branch.
   - (d) The parasympathetic and enteric nervous system.
   - (e) The brain, the so-called second brain "the enteric nervous system" and the sympathetic branch.

2. In patients with longstanding diabetes up to how many percentage of the patients suffer from GI symptoms such as nausea and vomiting.
   - (a) 10%
   - (b) 12%
   - (c) 20%
   - (d) 25%
   - (e) **40%**

3. Which part of the gastrointestinal tract can be affected by visceral neuropathy?
   - (a) The upper GI tract.
   - (b) The lower GI tract.
   - (c) The bowel.
   - (d) Only the anorectal part of the GI tract.
   - (e) **It is possible that the neuropathy cover the entire gastrointestinal tract causing symptoms such as nausea and vomiting, bloating, early satiety, diarrhoea, and constipation.**

4. In order to treat patients with reflux which statement is most correct?
   - (a) The only treatment is avoiding provoking factors such as large meals.
   - (b) The only treatment is medical including combinations of antacids and proton pump inhibitors.
   - (c) **First, it is important to avoid provoking factors such as large meals, coffee, and alcohol. Symptoms caused by reflux can be treated with antacids, H_2 blockers, proton pump inhibitors, or foaming agents.**
   - (d) Constipation treatment should be the first option.
   - (e) Currently no treatment exists.

5. The typical patient experiencing symptomatic gastroparesis is?
   - (a) A newly diagnosed type 1 diabetic.
   - (b) **A patient with a long history of insulin-dependent diabetes and poor glycaemic control lasting for several years.**
   - (c) A diabetic with extreme alcohol abuse.
   - (d) A newly diagnosed type 2 diabetic.
   - (e) A patient with a long history of well-controlled diabetes.

6. Hypoglycaemia has been shown to cause cell damage, but how?
   - (a) It increases levels of NO in the entire body.
   - (b) Unhealthy levels of calcium leaves the cell.
   - (c) Reduction in release of excitatory amino acids protecting the cell.
   - (d) **Increased release of excitatory amino acids, which may cause uncontrolled triggering calcium influx. This again activates proteolytic enzymes that are known to cause neuronal damage.**
   - (e) The production of reactive oxygen species is limited.

7. In order to treat patients with diabetes and diarrhoea, which statement is most correct?

   (a) **Hydration, nutrient deficiency and correction of electrolyte, antidiarrheal medication to prolonging transit time and reduce peristalsis, as well as reducing faecal volume in order to control symptoms, treatment of the underlying cause.**

   (b) Antidiarrheal medication for 1 week.

   (c) Hydration, nutrient deficiency and correction of electrolyte, and treatment of underlying cause such as bacterial overgrowth which should be treated with antibiotics.

   (d) Hydration, nutrient deficiency and correction of electrolyte, and treatment of underlying cause such as anorectal dysfunction.

   (e) Surgery of the intestines.

8. Which of the following statements about the pathophysiological explanation behind visceral neuropathy is most correct?

   (a) Hyperglycaemia is the only main player in inducing oxidative stress.

   (b) Hypoglycaemia is the only main player in pro-inflammatory mechanism.

   (c) Hyperglycaemia and hypoglycaemia are the only main players in inducing neuronal damage.

   (d) **Peripheral and autonomic neurons, as well as their interconnections, are particularly vulnerable to hyperglycaemia. It is obvious that any increase in glucose is associated with increased risk of injury to the organ including neuropathy.**

   (e) Hyperlipidaemia is main player alone to induce oxidative stress and pro-inflammatory mechanisms.

9. The measurements of GI symptoms have varied in many studies. What should researcher be aware of in future studies?

   (a) Every patient with gut symptoms should be offered an upper endoscopy locating symptoms.

   (b) Every patient with gut symptoms should be offered an upper endoscopy as well as a colonoscopy to investigate the entire gastrointestinal tract.

   (c) **In future epidemiological and clinical studies, the Diabetes Bowel Symptom Questionnaire is suggested as a consistent method to measure GI symptoms.**

   (d) A computed tomography scan of the body should be conducted in order to cover every symptom in patients with diabetes.

   (e) The variation is unavoidable and must be accepted.

10. When should autonomic neuropathy be suspected in patient with diabetes?

    (a) When newly diagnosed.

    (b) When the patients asks about it without symptoms.

    (c) **When gut symptoms arise, especially if the patient also suffers from distal symmetric polyneuropathy.**

    (d) When changing medicine.

    (e) Always.

Further Reading

1. Feldman M, Schiller LR. Disorders of gastrointestinal motility associated with diabetes mellitus. Ann Intern Med. 1983 Mar;98(3):378-84

   – Provides an overview of gastrointestinal symptoms in patients with diabetes

2. Rayner CK, Samsom S, Jones KL, Horowitz M. Relationships of Upper Gastrointestinal Motor and Sensory Function With Glycemic Control. Diabetes Care. 2001 Feb;24(2):371-81

   – A great article to read if you wish to know more about the effect of acute change in blood glucose toward the upper gastrointestinal tract.

3. Sangnes DA, Søfteland E, Biermann M, Gilja OH, Thordarson H, Dimcevski G. Gastroparesis- causes, diagnosis and treatment. Tidsskr Nor Laegeforen. 2016 May 24; 136(9):822-6. Doi: 10.4045/tidsskr.15.0503. eCollection 2016

   – This article provides a thorough knowledge about gastroparesis in relation to diabetes.

4. Brock C, Brock B, Pedersen AG, Drewes AM, Jessen N, Farmer AD. Assessment of the cardiovascular and gastrointestinal autonomic complications of diabetes. World J Diabetes 2016 Aug 25;7(16):321-32. doi:

   – This article is recommended as further reading if one is interested in knowing more about the cardiovascular system and the gastrointestinal tract in relation to DAN.

References

1. Brock C, Brock B, Pedersen AG, Drewes AM, Jessen N, Farmer AD. Assessment of the cardiovascular and gastrointestinal autonomic complications of diabetes. World J Diabetes. 2016;7(16):321–32.

2. Dimitropoulos G, Tahrani AA, Stevens MJ. Cardiac autonomic neuropathy in patients with diabetes mellitus. World J Diabetes. 2014;5(1):17–39.

3. Drewes AM, Søfteland E, Dimcevski G, Farmer AD, Brock C, Frøkjær JB, et al. Brain changes in diabetes mellitus patients with gastrointestinal symptoms. World J Diabetes. 2016;7(2):14–26. http://www.pubmedcentral.nih.gov/articlerender.fcgi?artid=4724575&tool=pmcentrez&rendertype=abstract

4. Sandireddy R, Yerra VG, Areti A, Komirishetty P, Kumar A. Neuroinflammation and oxidative stress in diabetic neuropa-

thy: futuristic strategies based on these targets. Int J Endocrinol. 2014;2014:674987.

5. Nissen TD, Meldgaard T, Nedergaard RW, Juhl AH, Jakobsen PE, Karmisholt J, Drewes AM, Brock B, Brock C. Peripheral, synaptic and central neuronal transmission is affected in type 1 diabetes. J Diabetes Complicat. 2020;34:107614.

6. Ostergaard L, Finnerup NB, Terkelsen AJ, Olesen RA, Drasbek KR, Knudsen L, et al. The effects of capillary dysfunction on oxygen and glucose extraction in diabetic neuropathy. Diabetologia. 2015;58(4):666–77.

7. Vinik AI, Park TS, Stansberry KB, Pittenger GL. Diabetic neuropathies. Diabetologia. 2000;43(8):957–73.

8. Grundy D, Schemann M. Enteric nervous system. Curr Opin Gastroenterol. 2005;21(2):176–82.

9. Powley TL. Vagal input to the enteric nervous system. Gut. 2000;47 Suppl 4:iv30–2; discussion iv36.

10. Rudchenko A, Akude E, Cooper E. Synapses on sympathetic neurons and parasympathetic neurons differ in their vulnerability to diabetes. J Neurosci. 2014;34(26):8865–74.

11. Lelic D, Brock C, Softeland E, Frokjaer JB, Andresen T, Simren M, et al. Brain networks encoding rectal sensation in type 1 diabetes. Neuroscience. 2013;237:96–105.

12. Brock C, Softeland E, Gunterberg V, Frokjaer JB, Lelic D, Brock B, et al. Diabetic autonomic neuropathy affects symptom generation and brain-gut axis. Diabetes Care. 2013;36(11):3698–705.

13. Brock C, Graversen C, Frokjaer JB, Softeland E, Valeriani M, Drewes AM. Peripheral and central nervous contribution to gastrointestinal symptoms in diabetic patients with autonomic neuropathy. Eur J Pain. 2013;17(6):820–31.

14. Lelic D, Brock C, Simrén M, Froekjaer JB, Søfteland E, Dimcevski G, Gregersen H, Drewes AM. The brain networks encoding visceral sensation in patients with gastrointestinal symptoms due to diabetic neuropathy. Neurogastroenterol Motil. 2014;26(1):46–58. https://doi.org/10.1111/nmo.12222.

15. Schönauer M, Thomas A, Morbach S, Niebauer J, Schönauer U, Thiele H. Cardiac autonomic diabetic neuropathy. Diab Vasc Dis Res. 2008;5(4):336–44.

16. Yuan H, Silberstein SD. Vagus nerve and Vagus nerve stimulation, a comprehensive review: part III. Headache. 2016;56(3):479–90.

17. Feldman M, Schiller LR. Disorders of gastrointestinal motility associated with diabetes mellitus. Ann Intern Med. 1983;98(3):378–84. https://doi.org/10.7326/0003-4819-98-3-378.

18. Mizuno Y, Oomura Y. Glucose responding neurons in the nucleus tractus solitarius of the rat: in vitro study. Brain Res. 1984;307(1–2):109–16.

19. Brock C, Brock B, Aziz Q, Moller HJ, Pfeiffer Jensen M, Drewes AM, et al. Transcutaneous cervical vagal nerve stimulation modulates cardiac vagal tone and tumor necrosis factor-alpha. Neurogastroenterol Motil. 2016;29(5).

20. Olofsson PS, Rosas-Ballina M, Levine YA, Tracey KJ. Rethinking inflammation: neural circuits in the regulation of immunity. Immunol Rev. 2012;248(1):188–204.

21. Koopman FA, Chavan SS, Miljko S, Grazio S, Sokolovic S, Schuurman PR, et al. Vagus nerve stimulation inhibits cytokine production and attenuates disease severity in rheumatoid arthritis. Proc Natl Acad Sci U S A. 2016;113(29):8284–9. https://doi.org/10.1073/pnas.1605635113.

22. Bonaz B, Sinniger V, Pellissier S. Anti-inflammatory properties of the vagus nerve: potential therapeutic implications of vagus nerve stimulation. J Physiol. 2016;594:5781–90.

23. Bird SJ, Brown MJ. Diabetic neuropathies. Neuromuscul Disord Clin Pract. 2014;9781461465(October):647–73.

24. Ekberg K, Johansson B-L. Effect of C-peptide on diabetic neuropathy in patients with type 1 diabetes. Exp Diabetes Res. 2008;2008:457912.

25. Krishnan AV, Kiernan MC. Altered nerve excitability properties in established diabetic neuropathy. Brain. 2005;128(Pt 5):1178–87.

26. Wahren J, Ekberg K, Johansson J, Henriksson M, Pramanik A, Johansson BL, et al. Role of C-peptide in human physiology. Am J Physiol Endocrinol Metab. 2000;278(5):E759–68.

27. Ghosh P, Sahoo R, Vaidya A, Chorev M, Halperin JA. Role of complement and complement regulatory proteins in the complications of diabetes. Endocr Rev. 2015;36(3):272–88. https://doi.org/10.1210/er.2014-1099.

28. Flyvbjerg A. Diabetic angiopathy, the complement system and the tumor necrosis factor superfamily. Nat Rev Endocrinol. 2010;6(2):94–101.

29. Chowdhury SKR, Smith DR, Fernyhough P. The role of aberrant mitochondrial bioenergetics in diabetic neuropathy. Neurobiol Dis. 2013;51:56–65.

30. Tomlinson DR, Gardiner NJ. Glucose neurotoxicity. Nat Rev Neurosci. 2008;9(1):36–45.

31. Hosseini A, Abdollahi M. Diabetic neuropathy and oxidative stress: therapeutic perspectives. Oxid Med Cell Longev. 2013;2013:168039.

32. Williamson JR, Chang K, Frangos M, Hasan KS, Ido Y, Kawamura T, et al. Hyperglycemic pseudohypoxia and diabetic complications. Diabetes. 1993;42(6):801–13.

33. Cameron NE, Cotter MA, Jack AM, Basso MD, Hohman TC. Protein kinase C effects on nerve function, perfusion, Na(+), K(+)-ATPase activity and glutathione content in diabetic rats. Diabetologia. 1999 Sep;42(9):1120–30.

34. Koya D, King GL. Protein kinase C activation and the development of diabetic complications. Diabetes. 1998;47(6):859–66.

35. Koppen B, Stanton B. Berne & levy physiology. 6th ed. Mosby; 2010.

36. Obrosova IG, Drel VR, Pacher P, Ilnytska O, Wang ZQ, Stevens MJ, et al. Oxidative-nitrosative stress and poly(ADP-ribose) polymerase (PARP) activation in experimental diabetic neuropathy: the relation is revisited. Diabetes. 2005;54(12):3435–41.

37. Edwards JL, Vincent AM, Cheng HT, Feldman EL. Diabetic neuropathy: mechanisms to management. Pharmacol Ther. 2008;120(1):1–34.

38. Sytze Van Dam P, Cotter MA, Bravenboer B, Cameron NE. Pathogenesis of diabetic neuropathy: focus on neurovascular mechanisms. Eur J Pharmacol. 2013;719(1–3):180–6.

39. Callaghan BC, Little AA, Feldman EL, Hughes RAC. Enhanced glucose control for preventing and treating diabetic neuropathy. Cochrane database Syst Rev. 2012;6:CD007543.

40. The Diabetes Control and Complications Trial Research Group, Nathan DM, Genuth S, Lachin J, Cleary P, Crofford O, Davis M, Rand L, Siebert C. The effect of intensive treatment of diabetes on the development and progression of long-term complications in insulin-dependent diabetes mellitus. N Engl J Med. 1993;329(14):977–86.

41. Linn T, Ortac K, Laube H, Federlin K. Intensive therapy in adult insulin-dependent diabetes mellitus is associated with improved insulin sensitivity and reserve: a randomized, controlled, prospective study over 5 years in newly diagnosed patients. Metabolism. 1996;45(12):1508–13.

42. Brands AMA, Kessels RPC, de Haan EHF, Kappelle LJ, Biessels GJ. Cerebral dysfunction in type 1 diabetes: effects of insulin, vascular risk factors and blood-glucose levels. Eur J Pharmacol. 2004;490(1–3):159–68.

43. Ricci JA, Siddique R, Stewart WF, Sandler RS, Sloan S, Farup CE. Upper gastrointestinal symptoms in a U.S. national sample of adults with diabetes. Scand J Gastroenterol. 2000;35(2):152–9.

44. Spangeus A, El-Salhy M, Suhr O, Eriksson J, Lithner F. Prevalence of gastrointestinal symptoms in young and middle-aged diabetic patients. Scand J Gastroenterol. 1999;34(12):1196–202.

45. Bytzer P, Talley NJ, Hammer J, Young LJ, Jones MP, Horowitz M. GI symptoms in diabetes mellitus are associated with both poor glycemic control and diabetic complications. Am J Gastroenterol. 2002;97(3):604–11.

46. Schvarcz E, Palmer M, Ingberg CM, Aman J, Berne C. Increased prevalence of upper gastrointestinal symptoms in long-term type 1 diabetes mellitus. Diabet Med. 1996;13(5):478–81.

47. Mjornheim A-C, Finizia C, Blohme G, Attvall S, Lundell L, Ruth M. Gastrointestinal symptoms in type 1 diabetic patients, as compared to a general population. A questionnaire-based study. Digestion. 2003;68(2–3):102–8.

48. Janatuinen E, Pikkarainen P, Laakso M, Pyorala K. Gastrointestinal symptoms in middle-aged diabetic patients. Scand J Gastroenterol. 1993;28(5):427–32.

49. Quan C, Talley NJ, Cross S, Jones M, Hammer J, Giles N, et al. Development and validation of the diabetes bowel symptom questionnaire. Aliment Pharmacol Ther. 2003;17(9):1179–87.

50. Meldgaard T, Keller J, Olesen AE, Olesen SS, Krogh K, Borre M, Farmer A, Brock B, Brock C, Drewes AM. Pathophysiology and management of diabetic gastroenteropathy. Ther Adv Gastroenterol. 2019;12:1–17. https://doi.org/10.1177/1756284819852047.

51. Quigley EM, Hasler WL, Parkman HP. AGA technical review on nausea and vomiting. Gastroenterology. 2001;120(1):263–86.

52. Patti MG. An evidence-based approach to the treatment of gastroesophageal reflux disease. JAMA Surg. 2016;151(1):73–8.

53. Yarandi SS, Srinivasan S. Diabetic gastrointestinal motility disorders and the role of enteric nervous system: current status and future directions. Neurogastroenterol Motil. 2014;26(5):611–24.

54. Camilleri M, Parkman HP, Shafi MA, Abell TL, Gerson L. Clinical guideline: management of gastroparesis. Am J Gastroenterol. 2013;108(1):18–37. quiz 38

55. Parkman HP, Hasler WL, Fisher RS. American Gastroenterological Association technical review on the diagnosis and treatment of gastroparesis. Gastroenterology. 2004;127(5):1592–622.

56. Jung H-K, Choung RS, Locke GR 3rd, Schleck CD, Zinsmeister AR, Szarka LA, et al. The incidence, prevalence, and outcomes of patients with gastroparesis in Olmsted County, Minnesota, from 1996 to 2006. Gastroenterology. 2009;136(4):1225–33.

57. Ma J, Rayner CK, Jones KL, Horowitz M. Diabetic gastroparesis: diagnosis and management. Drugs. 2009;69(8):971–86.

58. Waseem S, Moshiree B, Draganov PV. Gastroparesis: current diagnostic challenges and management considerations. World J Gastroenterol. 2009;15(1):25–37.

59. Phillips LK, Rayner CK, Jones KL, Horowitz M. An update on autonomic neuropathy affecting the gastrointestinal tract. Curr Diab Rep. 2006;6(6):417–23.

60. Giongo A, Gano KA, Crabb DB, Mukherjee N, Novelo LL, Casella G, et al. Toward defining the autoimmune microbiome for type 1 diabetes. ISME J. 2011;5:82–91.

61. Meldgaard T, Olesen SS, Farmer AD, Krogh K, Wendel AA, Brock B, Drewes AM, Brock C. Diabetic enteropathy: from molecule to mechanism-based treatment. J Diabetes Res. 2018;2018:3827301. https://doi.org/10.1155/2018/3827301.

62. Revicki DA, Rentz AM, Dubois D, Kahrilas P, Stanghellini V, Talley NJ, et al. Development and validation of a patient-assessed gastroparesis symptom severity measure: the gastroparesis cardinal symptom index. Ailment Pharmacol Ther. 2003;18(1):141–50.

63. Zitomer BR, Gramm HF, Kozak GP. Gastric neuropathy in diabetes mellitus: clinical and radiologic observations. Metabolism. 1968;17(3):199–211.

64. Olausson EA, Brock C, Drewes AM, Grundin H, Isaksson M, Stotzer P, et al. Measurement of gastric emptying by radiopaque markers in patients with diabetes: correlation with scintigraphy and upper gastrointestinal symptoms. Neurogastroenterol Motil. 2013;25(3):e224–32.

65. Gronlund D, Poulsen JL, Sandberg TH, Olesen AE, Madzak A, Krogh K, et al. Established and emerging methods for assessment of small and large intestinal motility. Neurogastroenterol Motil. 2017;29(7).

66. Farmer AD, Pedersen AG, Brock B, Jakobsen PE, Karmisholt J, Mohammed SD, et al. Type 1 diabetic patients with peripheral neuropathy have pan-enteric prolongation of gastrointestinal transit times and an altered caecal pH profile. Diabetologia. 2017;60:709–18.

67. Saad RJ, Hasler WL. A technical review and clinical assessment of the wireless motility capsule. Gastroenterol Hepatol (N Y). 2011;7(12):795–804.

68. Lee JS, Camilleri M, Zinsmeister AR, Burton DD, Kost LJ, Klein PD. A valid, accurate, office based non-radioactive test for gastric emptying of solids. Gut. 2000;46(6):768–73.

69. Medhus AW, Lofthus CM, Bredesen J, Husebye E. Gastric emptying: the validity of the paracetamol absorption test adjusted for individual pharmacokinetics. Neurogastroenterol Motil. 2001;13(3):179–85.

70. Sangnes DA, Søfteland E, Biermann M, Gilja OH, Thordarson H, Dimcevski G. Gastroparesis - causes, diagnosis and treatment. Tidsskr Nor Lægeforen. 2016;136(9):822–6. https://doi.org/10.4045/tidsskr.15.0503.

71. Krishnan B, Babu S, Walker J, Walker AB, Pappachan JM. Gastrointestinal complications of diabetes mellitus. World J Diabetes. 2013;4:51. https://doi.org/10.4239/wjd.v4.i3.51.

72. Janssen P, Scott Harris M, Jones M, et al. The relation between symptom improvement and gastric emptying in the treatment of diabetic and idiopathic gastroparesis. Am J Gastroenterol. 2013;108(9):1382–91.

73. Chedid V, Camilleri M. Relamorelin for the treatment of gastrointestinal motility disorders. Expert Opin Investig Drugs. 2017;26(10):1189–97.

74. Gibson PR, Shepherd SJ. Evidence-based dietary management of functional gastrointestinal symptoms: the FODMAP approach. J Gastroenterol Hepatol. 2010;25(2):252–8.

75. Parrish CR. Nutritional considerations in the patient with gastroparesis. Gastroenterol Clin North Am. 2015;44(1):83–95. https://doi.org/10.1016/j.gtc.2014.11.007.

76. Olausson EA, Storsrud S, Grundin H, Isaksson M, Attvall S, Simren M. A small particle size diet reduces upper gastrointestinal symptoms in patients with diabetic gastroparesis: a randomized controlled trial. Am J Gastroenterol. 2014 Mar;109(3):375–85.

77. Frokjaer JB, Ejskjaer N, Rask P, Andersen SD, Gregersen H, Drewes AM, et al. Central neuronal mechanisms of gastric electrical stimulation in diabetic gastroparesis. Scand J Gastroenterol. 2008;43(9):1066–75.

78. Buckles DC, Forster J, McCallum RW. The treatment of gastroparesis in the age of the gastric pacemaker: a review. MedGenMed. 2003;5(4):5.

79. Frokjaer JB, Bergmann S, Brock C, Madzak A, Farmer AD, Ellrich J, et al. Modulation of vagal tone enhances gastroduodenal motility and reduces somatic pain sensitivity. Neurogastroenterol Motil. 2016;28(4):592–8.

80. Okdahl T, Bertoli D, Brock B, Krogh K, Knop FK, Brock C, Drewes AN. Study protocol for a multicentre, randomised, parallel group, sham-controlled clinical trial investigating the effect of transcutaneous vagal nerve stimulation on gastrointestinal symptoms in people with diabetes complicated with diabetic autonomic neuropathy: the DAN-VNS study. BMJ Open. 2021;11(1):e038677. https://doi.org/10.1136/bmjopen-2020-038677.

81. Drewes VM. Mechanical and electrical activity in the duodenum of diabetics with and without diarrhea. Pressures, differential pressures and action potentials. Am J Dig Dis. 1971;16(7):628–34.

82. He CL, Soffer EE, Ferris CD, Walsh RM, Szurszewski JH, Farrugia G. Loss of interstitial cells of cajal and inhibitory

innervation in insulin-dependent diabetes. Gastroenterology. 2001;121(2):427–34.

83. Rezaie A, Pimentel M, Rao SS. How to test and treat small intestinal bacterial overgrowth: an evidence-based approach. Curr Gastroenterol Rep. 2016;18(2):8.

84. Wald A. Incontinence and anorectal dysfunction in patients with diabetes mellitus. Eur J Gastroenterol Hepatol. 1995;7(8):737–9.

85. Poulsen JL, Olesen SS, Malver LP, Frokjaer JB, Drewes AM. Pain and chronic pancreatitis: a complex interplay of multiple mechanisms. World J Gastroenterol. 2013;19(42):7282–91.

86. Selby A, Friendenberg FK. Pathophysiology, differential diagnosis, and treatment of diabetic diarrhea. Springer Science; 2019.

87. Camilleri M, Malagelada JR. Abnormal intestinal motility in diabetics with the gastroparesis syndrome. Eur J Clin Invest. 1984;14(6):420–7.

88. Arora Z, Parungao JM, Lopez R, Heinlein C, Santisi J, Birgisson S. Clinical utility of wireless motility capsule in patients with suspected multiregional gastrointestinal dysmotility. Dig Dis Sci. 2015;60(5):1350–7.

89. Jones KL, Russo A, Stevens JE, Wishart JM, Berry MK, Horowitz M. Predictors of delayed gastric emptying in diabetes. Diabetes Care. 2001;24(7):1264–9.

90. Carvalho BM, Guadagnini D, Tsukumo DML, Schenka AA, Latuf-Filho P, Vassallo J, et al. Modulation of gut microbiota by antibiotics improves insulin signalling in high-fat fed mice. Diabetologia. 2012;55(10):2823–34.

91. Rao SSC. Constipation: evaluation and treatment of colonic and anorectal motility disorders. Gastrointest Endosc Clin N Am. 2009;19(1):117–39.

92. Wieling W, Borst C, van Dongen Torman MA, van der Hofstede JW, van Brederode JF, Endert E, et al. Relationship between impaired parasympathetic and sympathetic cardiovascular control in diabetes mellitus. Diabetologia. 1983;24(6):422–7.

93. Ewing DJ, Burt AA, Williams IR, Campbell IW, Clarke BF. Peripheral motor nerve function in diabetic autonomic neuropathy. J Neurol Neurosurg Psychiatry. 1976;39(5):453–60.

94. Farmer AD, Coen SJ, Kano M, Naqvi H, Paine PA, Scott SM, et al. Psychophysiological responses to visceral and somatic pain in functional chest pain identify clinically relevant pain clusters. Neurogastroenterol Motil. 2014;26(1):139–48.

95. Hansen TM, Brock B, Juhl A, Drewes AM, Vorum H, Andersen CU, Jakobsen PE, Karmisholt J, Froekjaer JB, Brock C. Brain spectroscopy reveals that N-acetylaspartate is associated to peripheral sensorimotor neuropathy in type 1 diabetes. J Diabetes Complicat. 2019;33(4):323–8. https://doi.org/10.1016/j.jdiacomp.2018.12.016.

96. Spallone V, Ziegler D, Freeman R, Bernardi L, Frontoni S, Pop-Busui R, et al. Cardiovascular autonomic neuropathy in diabetes: clinical impact, assessment, diagnosis, and management. Diabetes Metab Res Rev. 2011;27(7):639–53.

97. Tesfaye S, Boulton AJM, Dyck PJ, Freeman R, Horowitz M, Kempler P, et al. Diabetic neuropathies: update on definitions, diagnostic criteria, estimation of severity, and treatments. Diabetes Care. 2010;33(10):2285–93.

98. Bernardi L, Spallone V, Stevens M, Hilsted J, Frontoni S, Pop-Busui R, et al. Methods of investigation for cardiac autonomic dysfunction in human research studies. Diabetes Metab Res Rev. 2011;27(7):654–64.

Urologic Complications in Patients with Diabetes

59

Ivan Mauricio Schroeder-Ugalde,
Karen Yhadira Sanchez-Lastra, and Angel Enrique Garcia-Cortes

Introduction

Diabetes Mellitus (DM) is a group of metabolic diseases associated with high glucose levels that cause systemic long-term damage, dysfunction, and failure of several tissues [1]. Among the consequences of this chronic hyperglycemic state, patients with DM suffer several urologic complications that involve endothelial and neural damage all along the genitourinary tract with significant economical and quality-of-life costs.

The worldwide incidence of urologic complications associated with DM is increasing because of the high incidence of obesity in the entire world [2]. The effect of obesity in our society is growing at a worrying rate, and it is associated with an increasing risk of noninsulin-dependent diabetes. Clinicians have the opportunity to prevent, diagnose, and change the evolution of these urologic complications among patients with diabetes by maintaining a proper weight [3].

Diabetes has been associated with an earlier presentation and increased severity of urologic complications [4]. DM leads to nerve function disturbance, loss of innervation of neuromuscular nerve terminals, abnormal immune response, and altered sympathetic/parasympathetic innervation [5]. Therefore, peripheral accumulations of fat in the abdominal region of patients with diabetes has been associated to an increased risk of urologic complications such as urinary incontinence, erectile dysfunction, benign prostatic hyperplasia, urinary tract infections, and possibly with cancer [3].

Bladder Dysfunction (BD) and Cystopathy

Generally, the beginning of bladder lesions of diabetes is not very evident, and they are not recognized until the disease is in the most advanced stages. Between 20 and 50% of all diabetic patients are affected, although some studies raise this figure to 88% of cases. No correlation has been observed between the type and duration of diabetes or the age of the patients, although it was shown that 80% of cases with a neurogenic diabetic bladder have lesions in other organs (kidney, eye, penis, arteries, etc.). (Campbell-Walsh 12 ed).

Bladder dysfunction or dysfunction in the bladder outflow tract attributed to any alteration of the nervous system. Some bladder symptoms that occur in patients with diabetes mellitus are known as diabetic bladder dysfunction or diabetic cystopathy, which include lower urinary tract symptoms (LUTS) characterized by increased postvoid residual volume due to inadequate emptying of the bladder, resulting in increased bladder capacity, worsened by reduced sensation and contraction of the bladder [6].

The cornerstone for evaluation is the questioning of urologic history, sexuality, bowel behavior, and neurologic history. Within the specific urological history, we must take into account the onset of symptoms, relief after urination, the beginning and end of urination, if there is presence of interruption of urination, mode and type of urination, enuresis and a strict record is essential in a urination diary.

Almost half of patients with DM suffer from different degrees of bladder dysfunction (74% men and 59.26% women), which causes an increase in postvoid residual urine and urinary incontinence, causing infections, bladder stones, or eventually kidney damage [7]. In men, bladder disorders are made worse by the enlargement of the prostate associated with age.

In Mexico, approximately 12% of the population suffers from type 2 diabetes mellitus, so the prevalence of bladder dysfunction due to this cause is common in the urological delivery, it is important to know how to detect it and refer it in time to the urology specialist to its timely treatment.

I. M. Schroeder-Ugalde (✉)
Hospital Angeles Universidad and UROMED,
Ciudad de México, CDMX, Mexico

K. Y. Sanchez-Lastra · A. E. Garcia-Cortes
Hospital Regional Lic. Adolfo Lopez Mateos ISSSTE,
Mexico City, Mexico

© The Author(s), under exclusive license to Springer Nature Switzerland AG 2023
J. Rodriguez-Saldana (ed.), *The Diabetes Textbook*, https://doi.org/10.1007/978-3-031-25519-9_59

Obese and diabetic women are expected to have more pelvic floor disorders, such as stress urinary incontinence and overactive bladder [4] that could be related to increased abdominal pressure from the abdominal panniculus that exerts pressure unwanted over the pelvic organs, uterus, bladder, urethral sphincters and vagina [3], peripheral neuropathy, and loss of bladder support. Insulin treatment in women with diabetes mellitus increases the risk of urge incontinence, compared to women treated with metformin, which has no effect on incontinence [8, 9].

Bladder hypersensitivity is reported as the most common finding, ranging from 39% to 61% in patients with diabetes mellitus, in numerous clinical studies [6]. Furthermore, an important predictor of bladder dysfunction is the presence of peripheral neuropathy, renal disease, and the association of metabolic syndrome [4].

Pathophysiology

During the early stages of diabetic cystopathy, there is an increase in the storage capacity of the bladder, which affects its compliance or ability to adapt to pressure as the bladder fills [10]. Several mechanisms have been described that induce abnormalities in bladder function at the detrusor muscle level, including changes in intracellular connections and excitability, muscarinic receptor density, genetic traits, and changes in intracellular signaling. All of these contributing factors result in decreased contractility and increased postvoid residual volume. Compensatory bladder hypertrophy results in increased bladder instability that decreases its contraction force due to collagen deposits, rendering detrusor muscle tension ineffective [10]. Another theory is the associated increase in diuresis due to the hyperglycemic state resulting in neural and endothelial damage, which collectively can lead to detrusor muscle hypertrophy in an attempt to adapt to these changes. On the other hand, abnormalities in calcium and potassium cell wall channels increase detrusor muscle activity and increase hyperactivity [11]. Furthermore, rabbit models have shown that overexpression of aldose reductase and increased lipid peroxidation products result in decreased detrusor contractility [12].

Another problem that influences bladder hypertrophy could be an increase in oxidative stress, associated with greater damage to the bladder muscles [13] or induced by a deficiency in axonal transport of neural growth factor (NGF). Bladder tissue remodeling is also associated with downregulation of tissue growth factor (TGF) and collagen mRNA levels, which induce an increase in elastin synthesis. These factors can result in an increase in bladder compliance in patients with diabetes associated with a reduction in collagen synthesis [14].

Neuronal control of bladder function consists of an interaction between autonomic sympathetic and parasympathetic, somatic afferent and efferent pathways. Patients with diabetic cystopathy have somatic and autonomic neuropathy. In addition, cells subjected to long periods of exposure to hyperglycemia suffer an accumulation of oxidative stress products, which cause axonal degeneration and nerve damage, decrease nerve conduction, trigger diabetic cystophaty, and erectile dysfunction [15]. In addition, decreased bladder filling sensation, caused by nerve damage, can cause excessive distention and increased hypocontractility of the bladder wall in diabetic patients. Diabetic cystopathy also involves neuropathic changes, produced by hyperexcitability of the urethral afferent reflex, leading to external urethral sphincter dysfunction and reduced urethral smooth muscle relaxation with obstruction to urine outflow.

Long-standing diabetes also affects the peristaltic function of the ureters by interfering with ureteral muscle cells and nerve function, causing upper urinary tract dysfunction, urine stasis, and eventually kidney stone formation [5]. The voiding reflex is a neural stimulus controlled by the M2 and M3 receptors. Patients with diabetes have a greater number of muscarinic receptors in the urothelium that increase sensory nerve activity and modify detrusor contraction, causing greater bladder dysfunction and urinary stasis [11].

Clinical Manifestations

In the early stages of the diabetic bladder, compensatory changes maintain the ability to maintain a normal diuresis. In later stages, decreased voiding pressure and increased urethral obstruction lead to larger volumes of postvoid residual urine, producing a wide variety of symptoms ranging from urgency to urinate and incontinence (a sensation urinary leakage) (40% to 80% risk) to the most severe expression of overflow incontinence (in which the bladder empties due to excess residual urine without patient control) [16].

Diabetic patients can complain of lower urinary tract symptoms, including urgency, difficulty in initiating, maintaining and ending urination, inadequate voiding or sensation of residual urine, frequent urination during the day and night, slow or decreased urinary flow of different severity levels. Consequently, voiding reflexes appear to be diminished or inactive, causing a progressive asymptomatic increase in bladder capacity, which can eventually cause urinary retention, bladder stone formation, diverticula, infection, upper urinary tract dilation, and kidney damage. . In contrast, diabetic bladder dysfunction can also present as overactive bladder syndrome with corresponding frequent day and night bladder emptying, urgency, and lower urinary tract symptoms. Hypersensitivity and hypercontractility of the bladder are more common than hypocontractility [6].

Diabetic cystopathy and bladder dysfunction are common in long-standing diabetic patients. They can be asymptomatic or manifest a wide spectrum of clinical symptoms, ranging from voiding discomfort due to overactive bladder and urge incontinence due to decreased bladder sensation, to overflow incontinence and acute urinary retention [4]. Bladder symptoms can be divided into irritating and obstructive. Irritant symptoms involve the overexcited detrusor muscle, causing urgency, polyakiuria, nocturia, and urge incontinence, known as overactive bladder syndrome. Obstructive symptoms include decreased size and strength of voiding flow, terminal dribbling, decreased sensation of a full bladder, and high postvoid residual urine. Obstructive symptoms are related to a pseudo-obstructive bladder, represent the last phase of visceral diabetic neuropathy, and are associated with a low urine flow that can be demonstrated with uroflowmetry, high postvoid residual and urodynamic studies, which show a hypotonic bladder in cystometry caused by a myogenic alteration of the microvasculature and neuronal cells. [10, 17].

Diagnosis

The approach to the study of diabetic cystopathy depends on the individual patients symptoms, severity, renal function, and impact on quality of life. In patients with symptoms of bladder dysfunction, physicians should take a detailed history including the International Male Prostate Symptom Score, physical examination with neurological reflex and rectal examination, presence of pelvic organ prolapse, followed by tests of laboratory to evaluate kidney function (serum creatinine), infections (urine test), and clinical chemistry. Similarly, a sexual history, the presence of genital or sexual dysfunction, the sensation in the genital area, specific to the man (erection, orgasm and ejaculation) and specific to the woman (dyspareunia and orgasm), within the habits bowel movements, presence of fecal incontinence, urgency, rectal sensation, stool pattern, and the onset of this complication. In the neurological history, if you have a congenital or acquired condition, mental status, neurological symptoms, spasticity, or autonomic dysreflexia.

The diagnosis of diabetic neurogenic bladder is based on the performance of a complete urodynamic study (flowmetry, cystometry, electromgraphy, and urethral pressure profiles). The most common findings of the final stages of the disease are the loss of voiding sensation with significant increase of bladder capacity and decreased detrusor contraction (areflexia) with low voiding flow and presence of residual postvoiding urine. The picture must be differentiated from infravesical urinary obstruction, which is achieved with a pressure/flow study. Urodynamic evaluation is an essential component of the examination, although it is not indicated in all cases. It includes cystometrogram, simultaneous flow and pressure studies, sphincter electromyography, and postvoid residue measurement [6]. It is recommended that the patient has to carry out a voiding diary prior to the urodynamic study. Diabetic women have significantly higher nocturia scores on lower urinary tract symptom questionnaires, with weaker urinary flows, reduced voiding volumes, increased residual urine volumes, and lower peak flow rates by uroflowmetry [4].

Treatment

The first step in managing any type of diabetes complications is blood glucose control. The treatment of diabetic cystopathy depends on the severity of the symptoms, but in the early stages, it is basically conservative and, in case of complications, they should be treated accordingly [18]. The treatment of diabetic neurogenic bladder resides in the treatment of symptoms, the prevention of urinary infection, the maintenance of renal function, and continence with an adequate bladder emptying. However, there is no cure for the disease. When there is an unstable bladder, the use of anticholinergics is of great help to improve symptoms (Campbell-Walsh 12 ed). In patients who complain of urgency, different types of first-line therapy are available to control detrusor overactivity, including oral muscarinic drugs, and more uroselective anticholinergics with fewer adverse effects (oxybutynin, tolterodine, darifenacin, or solifenacin). A recently approved β3 adrenergic agonist (mirabegron) that increases urine storage capacity, by direct relaxation of detrusor smooth muscle, can be used to provide rapid relief of symptoms [19, 20]. Infiltration of the detrusor muscle with botulinum toxin has been shown to decrease urge incontinence. A surgical approach could be offered in severe cases of unresolved urge incontinence with selective muscarinic anticholinergics, including bladder denervation, myomectomy, and bladder augmentation with ileal cystoplasty. All of them are associated with the risk of increased postvoid volume, urinary tract infection, kidney damage, and stone formation [18].

In men with additional bladder outlet obstruction associated with an enlarged prostate, initial treatment includes the use of alpha blockers such as terazosin, tamsulosin, and alfuzosin. In advanced stages, transurethral resection of the prostate could be considered.

In cases of failure to empty the bladder, frequent clean intermittent catheterization is the best option to avoid permanent use of indwelling catheters, due to the risk of increased infection rate, lower urinary tract lithiasis, and squamous cell carcinoma of the bladder [21].

All these measures are always carried out to protect kidney function, since, by increasing bladder pressure, due to the increase in urinary volume and the lack of accommodation of the bladder, they can cause a deterioration in kidney function and worsen the damage per se. That is what diabetes mellitus does to the kidneys (Campbell-Walsh 12ed.). Similarly, within the objectives of treatment, they are to avoid urinary tract infection, achieve or maintain urinary continence, preserve the ability to urinate, and improve the quality of life of the patient.

Benign Prostatic Hyperplasia (BPH) and Urethral Obstruction

Benign prostatic hyperplasia (BPH) is an age-related phenomenon that affects up to 50% of men aged 60–69 years and almost 90% at age 90 [22]. DM is frequently associated with BPH due to the same age of incidence [23]. BPH has been largely associated to metabolic disorders including diabetes, metabolic syndrome, obesity, and hypertension. Preclinical and clinical studies have shown that increased plasma insulin levels are positive independent predictors of BPH, as well as high fasting glucose level and hyperlipidemia; all of them have shown a positive correlation to the progression of BPH [24–26].

Pathophysiology

Several theories have been proposed in the pathogenesis of BPH. The most convincing however is that prolonged chronic ischemia and repeated ischemia-reperfusion injury in the bladder could generate oxidative stress, which increases sympathetic nerve activity and vascular damage, further hypoxia of the bladder and prostate, abnormal cell proliferation, in addition to an increase of lower urinary tract symptoms [22]. Endothelial dysfunction and nitric oxide (NO) deficiency are among the most important factors in the development of diabetic complications, affecting the lower urinary tract as well. Relaxation of the urethral sphincter is partially affected by NO, which in turn causes outflow obstruction and hyper-excitability of afferent neurons associated with progression of diabetes [27]. All these factors, in addition to the increased risk of overactive bladder in diabetic patients are closely related to peripheral nerve irritation [28]. Another possible explanation for the presence of BPH in diabetic patients involves insulin-like growth factor (IGF). Beta cells of patients with Type 2 diabetes secrete higher concentrations of insulin; the resulting hyperinsulinemia stimulates IGF synthesis. Activation of the prostate IGF receptors may also cause prostate growth [29, 30] which could be explained because of homology of insulin and IGF receptors [31] and cross-activity to insulin action [32].

The pathogenesis of BPH is multi-factorial and characterized by basal cell hypertrophy, secretory alterations of lami-

nal cells, infiltration of lymphocytes with production of pro-inflammatory cytokines, stromal proliferation, diminished apoptosis, trans-differentiation and extracellular matrix production, abnormal autonomous innervation, and modification of the neuroendocrine cell function among others [22]. Disturbances in fatty acid metabolism are also influential in the progression of BPH, including inflammation, oxidative stress, peroxidation of lipids and accumulation of 8-hydroxy-2′-deoxyguanosine, and increased androgen synthesis [33].

Clinical Manifestations

Initially, patients with BPH complain of symptoms of LUTS (which already mentioned includes nocturia, frequency, urgency, weakened stream, hesitancy, intermittency, straining, and a sense of incomplete emptying) [34]. Progressive evolution toward complications in the urinary tract is more important than symptoms related to micturition. They are significant and include bleeding, lithiasis, renal insufficiency, and infections [35], but the most serious and painful manifestation is acute urinary retention, the inability to urinate, characterized by intense pain in the pelvis [36].

Diagnosis

Evaluation of BPH in diabetic patients includes a detailed medical history, including LUTS questions, severity, and influence in their quality of life. The American Urological Association Symptoms Index (AUA-SI) is a questionnaire that allows physicians to quantify symptoms at diagnosis and over time in response to treatment. Digital rectal examination should be included in the physical examination. PSA (Prostate-specific antigen), urinalysis, and frequency/volume chart may be filled, as well as uroflowmetry, post void residual ultrasound, and renal ultrasound in order to diagnose complications [34].

Treatment

To avoid complications, effective and conservative drug treatment for BPH is currently available. Patients with a small prostate are routinely treated with alpha-1 blocker monotherapy as first-line therapy, either with nonselective blockers such as doxazosin and terazosin or uroselective blockers such as tamsulosin, alfuzosin, and silodosin. All of them have similar effectiveness but diverse side-effect profiles. Characteristic side effects include postural hypotension, dizziness, rhinitis, asthenia, sexual dysfunction, and abnormal ejaculation. Storage and voiding symptoms improve briefly after initiation of treatment. Alpha-1 blockers do not prevent BPH progression. For that reason, prostate volume and symptom progression should be monitored during the follow-up of the patient [34, 37].

Patients with a small prostate associated to voiding symptoms, the diagnosis of overactive bladder should be considered and treated as previously mentioned with anticholinergics, keeping in mind the need to monitor by dynamic bladder ultrasound the possibility of urinary retention, even though the risk is low.

In patients with enlarged prostate (over 30–40gr), the use alpha-1 blockers in combination with an alpha 5 reductase inhibitor (finasteride or dutasteride) that block the conversion of dehidrotestosterone from testosterone is highly recommended, in order to diminishing the prostate volume at long term with a faster effect on the relaxation of the bladder neck. In case of failure with all these therapies, the surgical approach is the next option. Transurethral resection of the prostate is the gold standard, but newer techniques such as bipolar resection, and the use of laser vaporization, botox infiltration, cryotherapy and high intensity focused ultrasound among others, represent less invasive approaches than open adenomectomy [36, 37].

Sexual Dysfunction

Men and women with diabetes are affected by sexual dysfunctions, which are defined as the inability to achieve or maintain an adequate sexual response to complete a sexual encounter or intercourse resulting in a satisfactory orgasmic sensation. Sexual dysfunctions include disorders of libido, ejaculatory problems, orgasmic abnormalities, and erectile dysfunction. The reported prevalence of sexual dysfunction in men with type 2 diabetes is up to 46%. Sexual dysfunction in women is harder to diagnose but it has been proposed that its prevalence in type 1 diabetes is 71% and 42% in females with type 2 diabetes [38, 39].

Almost half of nonsexually active men and women with type 2 diabetes report that their sexual life do not fulfills their sexual needs, suggesting that they are more concerned and even more distressed than sexually active patients. Commonly, women argue that lack of sexual activity is related to a number of reasons, including lack of interest, physical problems that make it difficult or unpleasant, absence of partner, or having a partner with physical limitations [40].

Sexual dysfunctions involve a group of alterations that affect significantly the quality of life of these patients and include reduced desire, decreased arousal, orgasmic abnormalities, and painful intercourse [41].

Leading risk factors that further affect diabetic men and women include age, length of diabetes [40] co-medications, obstetric history, neurogenic and vascular complications, and infections among others.

Erectile Dysfunction (ED)

It is defined as a long term, consistent, or recurrent inability to attain and/or maintain penile erection sufficient for sexual satisfaction. It is the third most frequent complication of diabetes and considered as one of the most significant complaints affecting quality of life [42]. Manifestations usually appear after 10 to 12 years after the onset of diabetes, because of diabetic endothelial and neural damage associated with persistent high serum glucose levels [43].

The WHO Global Report on Diabetes states that the number of people with diabetes has risen from 108 million in 1980 to 422 million in 2014 and that the global prevalence among adults has risen from 4.7% to 8.5% over the same period. The overall prevalence of erectile dysfunction in diabetes is 59.1%, but significantly different across countries, South America 74.6%, Oceania and Africa 71.3%, and lowest amongst North American studies with 34.5% . Diabetic male patients generally have a greater prevalence and an earlier onset of erectile dysfunction than men without diabetes and it appears 10–15 years earlier in diabetic than in nondiabetic men. Erectile dysfunction in diabetics is directly associated with poor glycemic control as well as greater duration and severity of diabetes [44]. Moreover, it has been demonstrated that ED is an early sign of cardiovascular events, particularly coronary heart disease. Prevention of cardiovascular disease through screening and management of cardiovascular risk factors in men with ED is very important [45].

Pathophysiology

The aetiology of ED in diabetes is considered to be multifactorial, pathophysiologic changes associated with diabetes can broadly be classified as vasculopathy, neuropathy, hypogonadism, and local pathological factors.

Men with erectile dysfunction that have macrovascular disease have diminished vasodilating responses causing less relaxation of the vascular smooth muscle tissue because of changes in the vessel that predispose to subsequent atherosclerosis, plaque formation, thrombosis leading to occlusive macrovascular disease, and microvascular disease due to deficient production of nitrate oxide in nonadrenergic noncholinergic neurons and in the endothelium [46]. These abnormalities are associated with important accumulation of advanced glycation products, altered expression of arginase, a competitor of the NO synthase for its substrate L-arginine [47, 48]. All of these abnormalities cause a tendency toward vasoconstriction, such as that caused by phenilephrine and endothelin-1, resulting in lack of vasodilatation and inadequate penile erection.

Numerous mechanisms play important roles in the pathophysiology of erectile dysfunction in diabetic males, one of them is the polyol pathway, which forms sorbitol by action of the enzyme aldose reductase. Sorbitol accumulates inside the cells, causing diminished myo-inositol levels (a precursor of the phosphatidylinositol), required for the adequate functioning of the Na-K ATPase pump. Increased sorbitol concentrations additionally produce progressive peripheral nerve damage [49].

Regarding vascular component, endothelial damage is a central issue in ED, because in comparison with healthy males, diabetic male patients have a diminished arterial inflow, which has been observed microscopically with reduced diameter and deficient morphology of the vascular wall [50]. Contraction of cavernosal smooth muscle cells is also affected by hyperglycemia, which results in an increased forced response to vasoconstrictors. This could be partially explained because of sensitization in protein kinase C and Rho A-Rho kinase Ca^{2+} pathways, which may cause a tendency toward a flaccid stage and modify the responses to NO [51]. All of these mechanisms are further compromised by other factors that impact erectile function including apoptosis or atrophy of the cavernous smooth muscle, due to diminished expression of blc2, intracellular release of Ca^{2+}, increased connective tissue proliferation due to tumor growth factor beta causing fibrosis, and a deficient response to NO in the cavernous and sinusoidal artery, with a decrease in neuronal and endothelial levels of NO synthetase. In brief, there are several components that take place in the endothelial and neural damage in the periphery and central nervous system, which globally impact on ED in patients with DM.

Diabetes is associated with peripheral and autonomic neuropathy and both of these can contribute to ED. The mechanism for ED is due to the reduced or absent parasympathetic activity needed for relaxation of the smooth muscle of the corpus cavernosum, which is produced by the decrease of norepinephrine levels as well as an increase in acectylcholine, resulting in increased NO synthase (NOS) activity, which releases NO.

Other factor is Hypogonadism, associated with type 2 diabetes. One study reported that 20% of diabetic men with ED had frank hypogonadism with a total testosterone level below 8 nmol/L and 31% had borderline low total testosterone levels between 8 and 12 nmol/L. The mechanism of hypogonadism in diabetes is incompletely understood. Hypogonadism is also associated with obesity and advancing age, common factors in type 2 diabetes.

Diagnosis

The International Questionnaire for Erectile Function helps to determine the degree of erectile dysfunction and evaluate the progression or response to medical treatment, one of the questionnaires is the International Index of Erectile Function (IIEF) and its short form, IIEF5 (also known as SHIM: Sexual Health Inventory for Men). The erectile function domain of IIEF and SHIM has been validated to assess the presence and the severity grade of ED. In the erectile function domain of IIEF, men scoring ≤25 are classified as having ED and those scoring >25 are considered not to have ED, with a sensitivity of 97% and specificity of 88%. The SHIM scale, those who score ≤ 21 are considered to have ED and those scoring >21 are considered not to have ED and sensitivity 98% and specificity of 88%.

In certain cases, in which a more precise evaluation of vascular flows is needed, an echo Doppler could be performed to determine cavernous artery flux and morphology. In selected cases, other studies to determine the degree of damage of myelinated pudendal somatosensory fibers and unmyelinated fibers can be done. Additional studies include assessment of nocturnal penile tumescence and electrostimulation. Most of these studies, however, are more commonly used in research protocols than in everyday clinical practice [52].

Treatment

Approximately 20% of patients with ED received pharmacological treatment, for that reason, clinicians should broadly evaluate sexuality among DM patients, trying to improve the sexual activity of patients and consequently their quality of life [40]. Glycemic control is an important factor, a decrease in or maintenance of hemoglobin A1c below 7.0% were significantly associated with a change on IIEF-5.

The first line of treatment are oral medications (phosphodiesterase 5 inhibitors), followed by intracavernosal injection (alprostadil), and finally penile prosthesis.

The daily use of phosphodiesterase 5 inhibitors can improve not only sexual function but also diminishes urinary tract symptoms associated with prostate enlargement. Meta-analysis has confirmed that phosphodiesterase 5 inhibitors are effective treatments of ED in patients with diabetes [53].

Sildenafil citrate, tadalafil, udenafil, and vardenafil hydrochloride are the oral agents for the treatment of erectile dysfunction. All PDE5 inhibitors are less efficacious in diabetic men. They all share the same mechanism of action, which involves the hydrolysis of guanosine monophosphate to guanosine 5′-monophosphate, diminishing it, causing an increase in the relaxation of the cavernosal smooth muscle mediated by NO, increasing the blood flow into the corpus cavernosum, and causing penile erection [54]. Vardenafil and sildenafil are more effective on an empty stomach and start working after 30 min, with peak action at 1 h and a window of action of 4–6 h. Tadalafil has a long half life with a therapeutic window of 36–48 h, which may aid spontaneity.

Common side effects of phosphodiesterase 5 inhibitors are headache, dyspepsia, bluish eye sight, and facial flushing; lumbar musculoskeletal pain has been found in patients receiving tadalafil and mirodenafil [53]. Phosphodiesterase type 5 inhibitors are contraindicated in those who are on nitrates, because of the potential for a dramatic fall in blood pressure.

Vacuum erection devices cause blood flow to be directed into the penis, and when a satisfactory erection is obtained, a compressive device is applied at the base of the penis in order to prevent blood return and lose the erection. Side effects include cold penis due to noncirculating blood, loss or diminished sensation due to nerve compression, and the uncomfortable process to obtain the erection using the device [55]. External support devices that hold the flaccid penis to allow penetration have been designed, but the use of these instruments has not gained acceptance among patients and their partners.

Another medical option is intraurethral suppositories of prostaglandin E-1 which are injected into the urethra. In men with diabetes, their reported efficiency rate to achieve satisfactory intercourse is 60%, although in clinical practice, they have not proved to be as effective [56, 57]. Injections of prostaglandin E-1 directly into the corpus cavernosum have a direct effect on blood vessels, causing immediate penile erections, with a reported response rate above 83% [58]. Main limitations include the need of injection prior to the sexual encounter, its impact on the spontaneity of sexual intercourse, and adverse effects including penile pain, hematomas, infection, fibrosis and priapism, prolonged and painful erections [59].

Patients not responding to medical therapy, unsatisfied with side effects or patients who prefer a permanent solution should consider a penile prosthesis implant (PPI). PPI improves flaccidity and rigidity, male satisfaction and correlates positively with satisfaction of the sexual partner. The rate of complications related to penile implantation is lower than 5%; they may be catastrophic however and include misplacement, migration, perforation, and a low risk of infection (less than 1.8%) using antibiotic prophylaxis, antibiotic impregnation, or hydrophobic-coated prosthesis [60].

Urinary Tract Infections

Urinary tract infection (UTI) is the most common infection among patients with diabetes mellitus [7, 8], with estimates of diabetics suffering from UTI reaching 10% of patients visiting hospitals [61].

The worldwide prevalence of urinary tract infections (UTI) is around 150 million persons per year [62]. DM patients have a higher incidence of infections in general, and UTI are not the exception. In a cohort of over 6000 patients with diabetes mellitus enrolled into 10 clinical trials of diabetes therapies, the incidence of urinary infection was 91.5/1000 person/years for women and 28.2/11,000 for men. [63]. In the Dutch National Survey of General Practice, patients with Type 1 diabetes mellitus were1.96 times more likely to experience urinary infection and with Type 2 diabetes 1.24 times more likely. [64]. In a recent study of a cohort of 460 hospitalized participants, the overall prevalence of UTI was 27.39% among diabetic patients and 17.83% among nondiabetic participants, with a higher prevalence in ages between 40 and 49 and a higher prevalence between women (43%) in comparison with men (13.8%) [61]. The high prevalence of UTI recorded among the age group 40–49 years could be due to increased rate of sexual activity in this age group. Metabolic abnormalities and long-term complications including neuropathy and nephropathy are presumed to be determinants of increased infectious morbidity [65].

The variety of UTI patients with diabetes ranges from asymptomatic bacteriuria to cystitis, pyelonephritis, renal abscess, xantogranulomatouse pyelonephritis to severe urosepsis [66]. DM is also associated with severe cutaneous infections of the genitals such as Fournier's gangrene.

Asymptomatic bacteriuria is more prevalent in women, due to the anatomical length of the urethra, and it is closer to the warm, moist, vulvar, and perianal areas that are commonly colonized by enteric bacteria [66]. Asymptomatic bacteriuria occurs in 8–26% of diabetic women, a prevalence estimated to be 2–3 times higher than nondiabetic women [67].

DM female patients frequently suffer bacterial cystitis with higher prevalence of both asymptomatic bacteriuria and symptomatic UTI added to recurrent complications, compared to healthy women [62]. Bacterial cystitis is frequently suffered by diabetic patients; it is more common in women than in men, especially in those with type 2 DM. Diabetic women have a higher prevalence of asymptomatic bacteriuria than healthy women, and they have a greater tendency for developing symptomatic UTI and recurrent complications with higher incidence of more serious complications [68, 69]. For women with diabetes and asymptomatic bacteriuria, those with type 2 diabetes have an increased risk for pyelonephritis and subsequent impairment of renal function [68, 69].

Type 2 DM is more than a risk factor for community acquired UTI and is a high predisposition for healthcare associated UTI, such as catheter-associated UTI, postrenal transplant recurrent UTI, and catheter-associated UTI [66]. Hospitalization due to pyelonephritis occurs more frequently in diabetic patients, and they are at higher risk of developing acute pyelonephritis, which could progress to renal abscess, pyelitis or emphysematous cystitis or pyelonephritis, and bacteriemia [66, 70]. In a Canadian report, diabetic women were 6–15 times more frequently hospitalized for acute pyelonephritis and diabetic men 3.4–17 times [71].

A retrospective analysis found that diabetes mellitus was one of four variables independently associated with a poor outcome (clinical or bacteriological failure or relapse) of therapy for acute pyelonephritis. Other evidence supporting increased severity of infection is an increased frequency of bacteremia, more prolonged duration of fever, and increased mortality (12.5% with diabetes and 2.5% without) in older patients with diabetes. Over 90% of episodes of emphysematous pyelonephritis cases occur in persons with diabetes and 67% of episodes of emphysematous csystitis [72]. Other clinical manifestations that are unique or strongly associated with diabetes include abscess formation and renal papillary necrosis.

Pathophysiology

The development of UTI in women is preceded by colonization of the vaginal and periurethral epithelium by the infecting organism. Ascension to the bladder may then ensue E. coli causes the overwhelming majority of UTIs. Normal host defense mechanisms usually prevent entry to or persistence of bacteria within the urinary tract. The growth rate of bacteria and fungi in urine is stimulated by glycosuria [73]. In addition, higher renal parenchymal glucose levels create a favorable atmosphere for multiplication of many microorganisms [66]. A reduction of urinary Tamm Horsfall glycoprotein (THP) excretion which correlates with reduction of renal mass is consistently observed in diabetic nephropathy. Glycation of THP in patients with diabetes or renal diseases also reduces the capacity of THP to inhibit bacterial adherence to human uroepithelium [74].

Bacterial attachment to the uroepithelium is the necessary initiating event permitting bacterial persistence. Uropathogenic E. coli are specialized for success in the urinary tract, elaborating virulence determinants such as adhesins (type 1, P and S fimbriae, and afimbrial adhesin), which bind to specific molecules in the uroepithelium, such as glycosphingolipids and uroplakins [75]. A recent study examined the ability of three representative clinical isolates of uropathogenic E. coli to adhere to uroepithelial cells collected from urine of women with and without diabetes.

Uropathogenic E. coli expressing type 1 fimbriae were twice as adherent to cells from women with diabetes as compared with cells collected from the women without diabetes.

Local urinary cytokines regulate host defence against urinary tract infections. DM results in abnormalities in the host immune defense system that may result in higher risk of developing infection. Immunologic impairments such as defective migration and phagocytes alterations of chemotaxis in polymorphonuclear leukocytes are common in DM patients [76]. A potential risk factor for urinary tract infection is polymorphonuclear leukocyte dysfunction in a high-glucose state. Significantly lower urinary IL-8- and Il-6-concentrations are found in diabetic women compared with nondiabetic controls, and these lower levels correlate with lower urinary leukocyte counts [68, 69]. One recent study shows that monocytes from women with type 1 diabetes produced lower amounts of proinflammatory cytokines upon stimulation with lipolysaccharide, women with diabetes who developed bacteriuria also produced lower urinary IL-6 concentrations, as compared with specimens from bacteriuric control subjects without diabetes [68, 69]. Diminished neutrophil responses, lower levels of cytokines and leukocytes facilitate adhesion of microorganisms to uroepithelial cells and the development of infections [77].

General host factors associated with risk of infection in patients with diabetes include age, metabolic control, duration of diabetes mellitus, microvascular complications, urinary incontinence, and cerebrovascular disease or dementia. The only risk factor associated with acute cistitis in premenopausal women with Type 1 diabetes was sexual activity. Previously suggested as possible risk factors, duration of diabetes or elevated HBA1c levels have not been shown to increase the risk of urinary tract infections in recent studies [68, 69].

The increased frequency of UTI in patients with diabetes might be associated to nerve damage caused by hyperglycemia, affecting the capacity of bladder to sense the presence of urine and leading to stagnation of urine for a long time, or inadequate bladder emptying due to ineffective detrusor contraction, increasing the probability of infections [62]. Over 50% of men and women with diabetes have bladder dysfunction which may impair voiding and facilitate infection. Urinary incontinence is consistently associated with urinary tract infection in diabetic women, but this association is not likely causative. Bladder dysfunction occurs in 26–86% of diabetic women depending on age, extent of neuropathy, and duration of diabetic disease. The possibility that voiding disorders are contributing to UTI should be considered in all diabetic patients.

Also of importance is the fact that many diabetic patients are infected with non-Escherichia coli species, in particular Klebsiella, other gram-negative rods, enterococci, and group B streptococci. Additionally, urinary infections with Candida

Albicans occur commonly in diabetic women but infrequently in other women.

Clinical Manifestations

UTI in DM patients can be the origin of severe complications that can end up in sepsis, organ failure, and death. Therefore, it is important to be vigilant of the usual clinical manifestations such as urinary urgency, frequency, bad urine odor, pain, dysuria, tenesmus, incomplete emptying and incontinence for lower UTI; and costovertebral angle pain or tenderness, fever, chills for upper UTI [66]. Diabetic patients generally present with symptoms similar to nondiabetic patients, but clinical signs may be altered in some patients with peripheral or autonomic neuropathy. Patients with diabetes are more likely to have more severe presentations of pyelonephritis including fever bacteremia and bilateral renal involvement. Less frequent presentations of urinary infection which occur most often in patients with diabetes include emphysematous cystitis or pyelonephritis, ureteral obstruction secondary to papillary necrosis, and renal or perinephric abscesses.

Diagnosis

Frequent and early screening for UTI should be performed in DM patients with suggestive symptoms, in order to establish the appropriate early treatment and to avoid complications.

As soon as the clinical diagnosis of UTI is suspected, a midstream urine sample must be examined, looking for the presence of leukocytes (more than 10 leukocytes/mm^3) or a positive dipstick leukocyte esterase test to detect pyuria. Microscopic or macroscopic hematuria is sometimes observed [66] associated to positive nitrites and the presence of bacteriuria. A urine specimen for culture should be obtained prior to initiating antimicrobial therapy for every diabetic patient presenting with pyelonephritis or complicated urinary tract infection. Women with symptoms consistent with acute cystitis and who do not have diabetic nephropathy or other long-term complications, particularly if they have a prior history of recurrent acute cystitis, do not usually require a urine culture. However, these women should also have a urine specimen for culture if this is a recurrent episode within 1 month of treatment, if empiric therapy has failed, or if there has been recent antimicrobial treatment so resistant organisms are more likely.

Pyuria is a universal accompaniment of symptomatic urinary tract infection. Thus, the presence of pyuria, by itself, is not useful for diagnosis of urinary tract infection or to differentiate asymptomatic and symptomatic infection. The absence of pyuria, however, is useful to exclude urinary tract infection in patients with questionable symptoms.

A diagnosis of bacteriuria is made when >105 cfu/ml of an organism is isolated from a voided urine specimen. Despite the fact that Escherichia coli is the most frequent bacteria in patients with urinary tract infections, unusual, multidrug resistant and aggressive pathogens are more prevalent in DM patients, including Klebsiella, gram negative rods, enterococci, group B streptococci, Pseudomonas and Proteus mirabilis [78]. Type 2 DM is a risk factor for fungal UTI, such as candida, these patients are more predisposed to be infected by resistant pathogens, including extended-spectrum β-lactamase-positive Enterobacteriaceae, fluoroquinolone-resistant Uropathogens, carbapenem-resistant Enterobacteriaceae, and vancomycin-resistant Enterococci [66].

The increased frequency of serious complications of urinary tract infection in patients with diabetes requires a low threshold for obtaining diagnostic imaging. Ultrasound scanning is safer, less costly, and easier to perform. These methods allowed detection of calculi, obstruction, and incomplete bladder emptying. Computerized tomography (CT) is now accepted as the most sensitive imaging modality for diagnosis and follow-up of abnormalities potentially associated with urinary tract infections. An enhanced CT scan is preferred, but contrast media should be used with caution in patients with diabetes mellitus or with renal disease.

Treatment

Treatment of urinary tract infection in patients with diabetes is generally similar to nondiabetic patients. Key factors to consider include whether the patient is asymptomatic or symptomatic, whether infection is localized to the bladder or kidney, and renal function. Glycemic control is helpful in the control of (UTI) [62].

Assuming that asymptomatic bacteriuria is more common and that the consequences more deleterious among women with diabetes, the question as to whether to attempt to eradicate it is of considerable relevance. In a randomized controlled trial of type 1 and type 2 diabetic women with asymptomatic bacteriuria, women were randomized to treatment with antimicrobials or no treatment for episodes of asymptomatic bacteriuria >3 years. Importantly, the study demonstrated that screening and treatment episodes of asymptomatic bacteriuria had no impact on overall occurrence of symptomatic urinary tract infections or hospitalizations [79]. Therefore there are no short- or long-term benefits for treatment of asymptomatic bacteriuria in women with diabetes mellitus. Asymptomatic bacteriuria by itself is not associated with an increased rate of progression to renal impairment or other long-term complications in patients with diabetes [80].

Acute cystitis in women with good glucose control and without long-term complications should be managed as uncomplicated urinary infection, usually with short-term antimicrobial therapy [81]. However, patients with pyelonephritis and severe systemic symptoms including nausea and vomiting or hemodynamic instability should be hospitalized for initial parenteral antibiotic therapy.

The choice of initial empiric antimicrobial therapy should consider current treatment guidelines, the patient's metabolic status and tolerance, the clinical presentation, and known or suspected local or institutional susceptibility of uropathogens (Table 59.1). The use of trimethoprim, cotrimoxazole, or nitrofurantoin is considered as the standard regimen of antibiotic therapy [82]. Broad spectrum cephalosporins and fluoroquinolones are the drugs of choice for pyelonephritis. However, alternate regimens such as the carbapenems meropenem, ertapenem or doripenem or betalactam/beta lactamase inhibitors such as piperacillin/tazobactam or ampicillin/sulbactam may be appropriate if antimicrobial resistance is a concern. For patients who present with severe sepsis or septic shock, broad spectrum antimicrobial therapy to provide maximal coverage for resistant organisms should be initiated pending urine culture results. Antimicrobials with nephrotoxic side effects, e.g., aminoglycosides should be used with caution in patients with renal insufficiency. Nitrofurantoin should be avoided in renal failure as drug metabolites accumulate and may cause peripheral neuropathy [83]. There are studies reporting higher frequency of extended spectrum beta-lactamase producing E. coli and Klebsiella pneumonia in diabetic patients. However, these studies didn't report whether diabetes was an independent risk factor for increased resistance [84].

Among women with type 1 diabetes, sexual activity has been identified as the most important risk factor for the development of urinary tract infections, similar to women without diabetes. Continuous or postcoital prophylaxis with low-dose antimicrobial agents and intermittent self-treatment with antimicrobials are the recommended strategies to prevent recurrent urinary tract infections in women without diabetes which also could be useful in women with diabetes [85].

Recurrent infection in young women without long-term complications of diabetes is managed as acute uncomplicated cystitis, including antimicrobial therapy given as long-term low dose or post intercourse prophylaxis for women with very frequent recurrence. For patients with complicated infection, it is essential to identify and correct any known urologic abnormalities and to optimize voiding, including use of intermittent catheterization where appropriate.

Conclusions

Patients with diabetes are highly susceptible to urologic complications. They may be serious, life threatening, and affect quality of life. The underlying mechanisms determining the increased risk and severity of infection are not fully described, but alterations in specific components of the host response, metabolic abnormalities, and long-term complications of diabetes likely contribute. It is important to take into account these comorbidities in the management of diabetes and to understand their pathogenesis to prevent systemic dissemination. Many patients with diabetes accept these comorbidities are part of their disease but clinicians should be aware, interrogate, and screen for these complications in order to indicate the adequate treatment. Controlled clinical trials of therapy comparing patients with and without diabetes mellitus or diabetic patients stratified by adequacy of control and complications will be necessary to improve management of this common and important problem.

Table 59.1 Recommendations for antimicrobial therapy in uncomplicated cystitis in patients with diabetes mellitus

Antimicrobial	Regimen	Duration
First-line		
Fosfoycin trometamol	3000 mg	Single dose
Nitrofurantoin	50–100 mg orally 3–4 times a day	5 days
Nitrofurantoin monohydrate/ macrocrystals	100 mg twice a day	5 days
Trimethoprim/ sulfamethoxasole	800/160 mg orally every 12 h	3 days
Alternatives		
Ciprofloxacin	250–500 mg orally every 12 h	3 days
Levofloxacin	250–500 mg every 12 h	3 days
Norfloxacin	400 mg orally every 12 h	3 days
Ofloxacin	200 mg orally every 12 h	3 days
Cephalexin	500 mg 4 times daily	7 days
Axetil cefuroxime	500 mg twice daily	7 days
Cefpodoxime proxetil	100 mg orally every 12 h	3 days
Cefixime	400 mg daily	3 days

Multiple Choice Questions

1. Urologic complications in people with diabetes are associated to:
   (a) Nerve function disturbances
   (b) Loss of innervations of neuromuscular terminals
   (c) Abnormal immune responses
   (d) Altered sympathetic/parasympathetic innervations
   (e) **All of the above**
2. Peripheral accumulations of fat in the abdominal region of DM patients have been associated to an increased risk of urologic complications including:

(a) **Urinary incontinence**
(b) **Erectile dysfunction**
(c) **Benign prostatic hyperplasia**
(d) **Urinary tract infections**
(e) **Cancer**

3. Diabetic cystopathy is characterized by:
(a) **Urinary incontinence**
(b) **Increased post voiding residual volume**
(c) **Urinary tract infection**
(d) All of the above
(e) None of the above

4. Bladder symptoms of diabetic cystopathy include:
(a) **Polyakiuria**
(b) Decreasing caliber and strength of the voiding flow
(c) Terminal dribbling
(d) **Urgency incontinence**
(e) High postvoid residual urine

5. Infiltration of the detrusor muscle can be achieved with:
(a) Oxybutynin
(b) Solifenacin
(c) **Botulinum toxin**
(d) Darifenacin
(e) Tolterodine

6. Positive predictive predictors of benign prostatic hyperplasia:
(a) Urinary tract infection
(b) Plasma insulin levels
(c) Dysuria
(d) **Urinary urgency**
(e) Fasting blood glucose

7. Patients with benign prostatic hypertrophy and enlarged prostate should be treated with:
(a) Nonselective alpha-1 blockers
(b) Selective alpha-1 blockers
(c) Alpha reductase inhibitors
(d) **Alpha-1 blockers combined with 5 alpha reductase inhibitors**
(e) Surgical management is the only option

8. The reported prevalence of sexual dysfunction in men with type 2 diabetes:
(a) 18%
(b) 37%
(c) **46%**
(d) 53%
(e) 71%

9. The reported prevalence of sexual dysfunction in women with type 1 diabetes:
(a) 18%
(b) 37%
(c) 46%
(d) 53%
(e) **71%**

10. Erectile dysfunction:
(a) is a minor complaint of men with diabetes
(b) has not been quantified
(c) is usually present at diagnosis
(d) **is the third most common chronic complication and the most significantly affecting quality of life**
(e) is common but less relevant regarding quality of life

References

1. American Diabetes Association. Diagnosis and classification of diabetes mellitus. Diabetes Care. 2011;34(1):S62–9.
2. Rull JA, Aguilar-Salinas CA, Rojas R, Rios-Torres JM, Gómez-Pérez FJ, Olaiz G. Epidemiology of type 2 diabetes in Mexico. Arch Med Res. 2005;36(3):188–96.
3. Mobley D, Baum N. The obesity epidemic and its impact on urologic care. Rev Urol. 2015;17(3):165.
4. Karoli R, Bhat S, Fatima J, Priya S. A study of bladder dysfunction in women with type 2 diabetes mellitus. Indian J Endocrinol Metab. 2014;18(4):552.
5. Canda AE, Dogan H, Kandemir O, Atmaca AF, Akbulut Z, Balbay MD. Does diabetes affect the distribution and number of interstitial cells and neuronal tissue in the ureter, bladder, prostate, and urethra of humans? Cent European J Urol. 2014;67(4):366.
6. Golbidi S, Laher I. Bladder dysfunction in diabetes mellitus. Front Pharmacol. 2010;1:136.
7. Kebapci N, Yenilmez A, Efe B, Entok E, Demirustu C. Bladder dysfunction in type 2 diabetic patients. Neurourol Urodyn. 2007;26(6):814–9.
8. Brown JS, Nyberg LM, Kusek JW, Diokno AC, Foldspang FNH, Herzog AR, Hunskarr S, Milsom I, Nygaard I, Subak LL, Thom DH. Proceedings of the National Institute of Diabetes and Digestive and Kidney Diseases international symposium on epidemiologic issues in urinary incontinence in women. Am J Obstet Gynecol. 2003;188:S77–88.
9. Jackson RA, Vittinghoff E, Kanaya AM, Resnick HE, Kritchevsky S, Miles T, Simonsick E, Brown JS. Aging and body composition. Obstet Gynecol. 2004;104:301–7.
10. Liu G, Daneshgari F. Temporal diabetes- and diuresis-induced remodeling of the urinary bladder in the rat. Am J Physiol Regul Integr Comp Physiol. 2006;291:R837.
11. Cheng JT, Yu BC, Tong YC. Changes of M3-muscarinic receptor protein and mRNA expressions in the bladder urothelium and muscle layer of streptozotocin-induced diabetic rats. Neurosci Lett. 2007;423:1–5.
12. Changolkar AK, Hypolite JA, Disanto M, Oates PJ, Wein AJ, Chacko S. Diabetes induced decrease in detrusor smooth muscle force is associated with oxidative stress and overactivity of aldose reductase. J Urol. 2005;173:309–13.
13. Satriano J. Kidney growth, hypertrophy and the unifying mechanism of diabetic complications. Amino Acids. 2007;33:331–9.
14. Gray MA, Wang CC, Sacks MS, Yoshimura N, Chancellor M, Nagatomi J. Time dependent alterations of select genes in streptozotocin-induced diabetic rat bladder. Urology. 2008;71:1214–9.
15. Beshay E, Carrier S. Oxidative stress plays a role in diabetes-induced bladder dysfunction in a rat model. Urology. 2004;64:1062.
16. Brown JS, Barrett-Connor E, Nyberg LM, Kusek JW, Orchard TJ, Ma Y. Incontinence in women with impaired glucose tolerance: results of the diabetes prevention program. J Urol. 2004;171:325–6.

17. Daneshgari F, Liu G, Birder L, Hanna-Mitchell AT, Chacko S. Diabetic bladder dysfunction: current translational knowledge. J Urol. 2009;182:S18–26.

18. Liu G, Daneshgari F. Diabetic bladder dysfunction. Chin Med J. 2014;127(7):1357.

19. Aizawa N, Homma Y, Igawa Y. Effects of mirabegron, a novel b3-adrenoceptor agonist, on primary bladder afferent activity and bladder microcontractions in rats compared with the effects of oxybutynin. Eur Urol. 2012;62:1165–73.

20. Chapple C, Nitti V, Khullar V, Wyndaele J, Herschom S, Van Kerrebroeck P, Beth M, Siddiqui E. Onset of action of the b3-adrenoceptor agonist, mirabegron, in phase II and III clinical trials in patients with overactive bladder. World J Urol. 2014;32(6):1565–72. https://doi.org/10.1007/s00345-014-1244-2.

21. Deli G, Bonsbyak E, Pusch G, Komoly S, Feher G. Diabetic neuropathies: diagnosis and management. Neuroendocrinology. 2013;98(4):267–80.

22. Shimizu S, Tsounapi P, Shimizu T, Honda M, Inoue K, Dimitriadis F, Saito M. Lower urinary tract symptoms, benign prostatic hyperplasia/benign prostatic enlargement and erectile dysfunction: are these conditions related to vascular dysfunction? Int J Urol. 2014;21(9):856–64.

23. Berger P, Deibl M, Halpern EJ, Lechleitner M, Bektic J, Horninger W, Fritsche G, Steiner H, Pelzer A, Bartsch G, Frauscher F. Vascular damage induced by type 2 diabetes mellitus as a risk factor for benign prostatic hyperplasia. Diabetologia. 2005;48:784–9.

24. Chen KC, Sung SY, Lin YT, Hsieh CL, Shen KH, Peng CC, Peng RY. Benign prostatic hyperplasia complicated with T1DM can be alleviated by treadmill exercise—evidences revealed by the rat model. BMC Urol. 2015a;15(1):113.

25. Chen Z, Miao L, Gao X, Wang G, Xu Y. Effect of obesity and hyperglycemia on benign prostatic hyperplasia in elderly patients with newly diagnosed type 2 diabetes. Int J Clin Exp Med. 2015b;8(7):11289.

26. Gacci M, Corona G, Vignozzi L, Salvi M, Serni S, De Nunzio C, Maggi M. Metabolic syndrome and benign prostatic enlargement: a systematic review and meta-analysis. BJU Int. 2015;115(1):24–31.

27. Torimoto K, Fraser MO, Hirao Y, De Groat WC, Chancellor MB, Yoshimura N. Urethral dysfunction in diabetic rats. J Urol. 2004;171:1959–64.

28. Wei-Chia L. The impact of diabetes on the lower urinary tract dysfunction. JTUA. 2009;20:155–61.

29. Ikeda K, Wada Y, Foster HE, Wang Z, Weiss RM, Latifpour J. Experimental diabetes-induced regression of the rat prostate is associated with an increased expression of transforming growth factor-beta. J Urol. 2000;164(1):180–5.

30. Vikram A, Jena GB, Ramarao P. Increased cell proliferation and contractility of prostate in insulin resistant rats: linking hyperinsulinemia with benign prostate hiperplasia. Prostate. 2010;70(1):79–89.

31. Ullrich A, Gray A, Tam AW, Yang-Feng T, Tsubokawa M, Collins C, Henzel W, Le Bon T, Kathuria S, Chen E. Insulin-like growth factor I receptor primary structure: comparison with insulin receptor suggests structural determinants that define functional specificity. EMBO J. 1986;5(10):2503–12.

32. Liu JL. Does IGF-I stimulate pancreatic islet cell growth? Cell Biochem Biophys. 2007;48(2–3):115–25.

33. Shankar E, Bhaskaran N, MacLennan GT, Liu G, Daneshgari F, Gupta S. Inflammatory signaling involved in high-fat diet induced prostate diseases. J Urol Res. 2015;2(1):1018.

34. Elterman DS, Barkin J, Kaplan SA. Optimizing the management of benign prostatic hyperplasia. Ther Adv Urol. 2012;4(2):77–83.

35. Marks LS, Roehrborn CG, Andriole GL. Prevention of benign prostatic hyperplasia disease. J Urol. 2006;176(4):1299–306.

36. He LY, Zhang YC, He JL, Li LX, Wang Y, Tang J, et al. The effect of immediate surgical bipolar plasmakinetic transurethral resection of the prostate on prostatic hyperplasia with acute urinary retention. Asian J Androl. 2016;18(1):134.

37. Mcvary KT, Roehrborn CG, Avins AL, Barry MJ, Bruskewitz RC, Donell RF, Foster HE Jr, Gonzalez CM, Kaplan SA, Penson DF, Ulchaker JC, Wei JT. Update on AUA guideline on the management of benign prostatic hyperplasia. J Urol. 2011;185(5):1793–803.

38. Enzlin P, Mathieu C, Van den Bruel A, Bosteels J, Vanderschueren D, Demyttenaere K. Sexual dysfunction in women with type 1 diabetes: a controlled study. Diabetes Care. 2002;25:672–7.

39. Owiredu WK, Amidu N, Alidu H, Sarpong C, Gyasi-Sarpong CK. Determinants of sexual dysfunction among clinically diagnosed diabetic patients. Reprod Biol Endocrinol. 2011;25(9):70.

40. Bjerggaard M, Charles M, Kristensen E, Lauritzen T, Sandbæk A, Giraldi A. Prevalence of sexual concerns and sexual dysfunction among sexually active and inactive men and women with screen-detected type 2 diabetes. Sex Med. 2015;3(4):302–10.

41. Doruk H, Akbay E, Çayan S, Akbay E, Bozlu M, Acar D. Effect of diabetes mellitus on female sexual function and risk factors. Arch Androl. 2005;51(1):1–6.

42. Latini DM, Penson DF, Lubeck DP, Wallace KL, Henning JM, Lue TF. Longitudinal differences in disease specific quality of life in men with erectile dysfunction: results from the exploratory comprehensive evaluation of erectile dysfunction study. J Urol. 2003;169:1437–42.

43. Sun P, Cameron A, Seftel A, Shabsigh R, Niederberger C, Guay A. Erectile dysfunction-an observable marker of diabetes mellitus? A large national epidemiological study. J Urol. 2007;117(4):1588.

44. Goldstein I, Jones LA, Belkoff LH, Karlin GS, Bowden CH, Peterson CA, Day WW. Avanafil for the treatment of erectile dysfunction: a multicenter, randomized, double-blind study in men with diabetes mellitus. Mayo Clin Proc. 2012;87(9):843–52.

45. Malavige LS, Wijesekara P, Ranasinghe P, Levy JC. The association between physical activity and sexual dysfunction in patients with diabetes mellitus of European and south Asian origin: the Oxford sexual dysfunction study. Eur J Med Res. 2015;20(1):1–7.

46. Morano S. Pathophysiology of diabetic sexual dysfunction. J Endocrinol Invest. 2003;26(3 Suppl):65–9.

47. Bivalacqua TJ, Hellstrom WJ, Kadowitz PJ, Champion HC. Increased expression of arginase II in human diabetic corpus cavernosum: in diabetic-associated erectile dysfunction. Biochem Biophys Res Commun. 2001;283:923–7.

48. Seftel AD, Vaziri ND, Ni Z, Razmjouei K, Fogarty J, Hampel N, Polak J, Wang RZ, Ferguson K, Block C, Haas C. Advanced glycation end products in human penis: elevation in diabetic tissue, site of deposition, and possible effect through iNOS or eNOS. Urology. 1997;50(6):1016–26.

49. Neves D. Advanced glycation end-products: a common pathway in diabetes and age-related erectile dysfunction. Free Radic Res. 2013;47(Suppl 1):49–69.

50. Grant P, Jackson G, Baig I, Quin J. Erectile dysfunction in general medicine. Clin Med. 2013;13(2):136–40.

51. Chitaley K, Wingard CJ, Clinton Webb R, Branam H, Stopper VS, Lewis RW, Mills TM. Antagonism of rho-kinase stimulates rat penile erection via a nitric oxide-independent pathway. Nat Med. 2001;7:119–22.

52. Dean RC, Lue TF. Physiology of penile erection and pathophysiology of erectile dysfunction. Urol Clin North Am. 2005;32(4):379–v.

53. Balhara YPS, Sarkar S, Gupta R. Phosphodiesterase-5 inhibitors for erectile dysfunction in patients with diabetes mellitus: a systematic review and meta-analysis of randomized controlled trials. Indian J Endocrinol Metab. 2015;19(4):451.

54. Boulton AJ, Selam JL, Sweeney M, Ziegler D. Sildenafil citrate for the treatment of erectile dysfunction in men with type II diabetes mellitus. Diabetologia. 2001;44:1296–301.

55. Levine LA, Dimitriou RJ. Vacuum constriction and external erection devices in erectile dysfunction. Urol Clin North Am. 2001;28:335–41.

56. Fulgham PF, Cochran JS, Denman JL, Feagins BA, Gross MB, Kadesky KT, Adesky MC, Clark AR, Roehrborn CG. Disappointing initial results with transurethral alprostadil for erectile dysfunction in a urology practice setting. J Urol. 1998;160:2041–6.

57. Huang SA, Lie JD. Phosphodiesterase-5 (PDE5) inhibitors in the management of erectile dysfunction. PT. 2013;38:407–19.

58. Heaton JP, Lording D, Liu SN, Litonjua AD, Guangwei L, Kim SC, Kim JJ, Zhi-Zhou S, Israr D, Niazi D, Rajatanavin R, Suyono S, Benard F, Casey R, Brock G, Belanger A. Intracavernosal alprostadil is effective for the treatment of erectile dysfunction in diabetic men. Int J Impot Res. 2001;13:317–21.

59. Perimenis P, Gyftopoulos K, Athanasopoulos A, Barbalias G. Diabetic impotence treated by intracavernosal injections: high treatment compliance and increasing dosage of vaso-active drugs. Eur Urol. 2001;40:398–402.

60. Antonini G, Busetto GM, De Berardinis E, Giovannone R, Vicini P, Del Giudice F, Perito PE. Minimally invasive infrapubic inflatable penile prosthesis implant for erectile dysfunction: evaluation of efficacy, satisfaction profile and complications. Int J Impot Res. 2016;28(1):4–8.

61. Flores-Mireles AL, Walker JN, Caparon M, Hultgren SJ. Urinary tract infections: epidemiology, mechanisms of infection and treatment options. Nat Rev Microbiol. 2015;13(5):269–84.

62. Sewify M, Nair S, Warsame S, Murad M, Alhubail A, Behbehani K, Tiss A. Prevalence of Urinary Tract Infection and Antimicrobial Susceptibility among Diabetic Patients with Controlled and Uncontrolled Glycemia in Kuwait. J Diabetes Res. 2015;2016:6573215.

63. Hammar N, Farahmand B, Gran M, Joelson S, Andersson SW. Incidence of urinary tract infection in patients with type 2 diabetes. Experience from adverse event reporting in clinical trials. Pharmacoepidemiol Drug Saf. 2010;19:1287–92.

64. Muller LM, Gorter KJ, Hak E, Goudzwaard WL, Schellevis FG, Hoepelma AL, Rutten GE. Increased risk of common infections in patients with type 1 and type 2 diabetes mellitus. Clin Infect Dis. 2005;142:20–7.

65. McMahon MM, Bristrian BR. Host defenses and susceptibility to infection in patients with diabetes mellitus. Infect Dis Clin N Am. 1995;9:1–9.

66. Nitzan O, Elias M, Chazan B, Saliba W. Urinary tract infections in patients with type 2 diabetes mellitus: review of prevalence, diagnosis, and management. Diabetes Metab Syndr Obes. 2015;8:129.

67. Zhanel GC, Harding GK, Nicolle LE. Asymptomatic bacteriuria in patients with diabetes mellitus. Rev Infet Dis. 1991;13:150–4.

68. Geerlings SE, Stolk RP, Camps MJ, Netten PM, Collet TJ, Hoepelman AI. Risk factors for symptomatic urinary tract infection in women with diabetes. Diabetes Care. 2000a;23:1737–41.

69. Geerlings SE, Stolk RP, Camps MJ, Netten PM, Hoekstra JB, Bouter PK, Braveboer B, Collet TJ, Jansz AR, Hoepelman AM. Asymptomatic bacteriuria can be considered a diabetic complication in women with diabetes mellitus. Adv Exp Med Biol. 2000b;485:309–14.

70. Stapleton A. Urinary tract infections in patients with diabetes. Am J Med. 2002;113(suppl 1A):80S–4S.

71. Nicolle LE, Friesen D, Harding GKM, Roos LL. Hospitalization for acute pyelonephritis in Manitoba, Canada, during the period from 1989 to 1992; impact of diabetes, pregnancy, and aboriginal origin. Clin Infect Dis. 1996;22:1051–6.

72. Thomas AA, Lane BR, Thomas AZ, Remer EM, Campbell SC, Shoskes DA. Emphysemathous cystitis: a review of 135 cases. BJU Int. 2007;100:17–20.

73. Werner T Geno-und phänotypische Charakter- isierung von E.coli bei Patienten mit Diabetes mellitus Typ 2 und einer asymptomatischen Bak- teriurie und Patientennach Nierentransplantation. Promotionsschrift (Theses to M.D.-Qualifuing), University of Jena:2008.

74. Serafini-Cessi F, Malagolini N, Cavallone D. Tamm-Horsfall glycoprotein: biology and clinical relevance. Am J Kidney Dis. 2003;42:658–16.

75. Johnson JR. Microbial virulence determinants and the pathogenesis of urinary tract infection. Infect Dis Clin N Am. 2003;17:261–278, viii.

76. Dalal S, Nicolle L, Marrs CF, Zhang L, Harding G, Foxman B. Long-term escherichia coli asymptomatic bacteriuria among women with diabetes mellitus. Clin Infect Dis. 2009;49(4):491–7.

77. Hamdan HZ, Kubbara E, Adam AM, Hassan OS, Suliman SO, Adam I. Urinary tract infections and antimicrobial sensitivity among diabetic patients at Khartoum, Sudan. Ann Clin Microbiol Antimicrob. 2015;14(1):1.

78. Ronald A. The etiology of urinary tract infection: traditional and emerging pathogens. Am J Med. 2002;113:14–9.

79. Harding GK, Zhanel GC, Nicolle LE, Cheang M. Antimicrobial treatment in diabetic women with asymptomatic bacteriuria. N Engl J Med. 2002;347:1576–83.

80. Meiland R, Geerlings SE, Stolk RP, Netten PM, Schneeberger PM, Hoepelman AIM. Asymptomatic bacteriuria in women with diabetes mellitus: effect on renal function after 6 years of follow-up. Arch Intern Med. 2006;166:2222–7.

81. Gupta K, Hooton TM, Naber KG, et al. International clinical practice guidelines for the treatment of acute uncomplicated cystitis and pyelonephritis in women: a 2010 update of the IDSA and ESCMID guidelines. Clin Infect Dis. 2011;52(5):e103–20.

82. Grabe M, Bishop MC, Bjerklund-Johansen TE, Botto H, Cek M, Lobel B, Naber KG, Palou J, Tenke P, Wagenlehner F. Guidelines on urological infections. Eur Assoc Urol. 2009:1–108. http://www.uroweb.org/online-guidelines/

83. Munar MY. Singh 1L drug dosing adjustments in patients with chronic kidney disease. Am Fam Physician. 2007;75:1487–149.

84. Colodner R, Rock W, Chazan B, Keller N, Guy N, Sakran W, Raz R. Risk factors for the development of extended-spectrum beta-lactamase-producing bacteria in nonhospitalized patients. Eur J Clin Microbiol Infect Dis. 2004;23:163–7.

85. Fihn SD. Clinical practice: acute uncomplicated urinary tract infection in women. N Engl J Med. 2003;349:259–66.

Musculoskeletal Complications of Diabetes Mellitus

Deep Dutta, Rajiv Singla, Meha Sharma, Aarti Sharma, and Sanjay Kalra

Introduction

Musculoskeletal complications of diabetes are a diverse set of disorders which are associated with significant impairment of the quality of life in affected patients. Lack of awareness amongst patients and also perhaps amongst the caregivers contributes to increased morbidity due to this complications amongst patient with diabetes.

In contrast to the extensively studied microvascular and macrovascular complications of DM, data and evidence on the musculoskeletal complications of Diabetes Mellitus (DM) is largely derived from observational studies. Pathogenic mechanisms for many of these conditions are yet to be fully elucidated. An important aspect of the musculo-skeletal complication of DM is that their occurrence is not limited to individuals with diabetes. Such conditions are also known to occur in a diverse set of non-diabetes disorders. The only exception to this rule is perhaps the diabetic muscle infarction (DMI)/ myonecrosis, which is believed to occur exclusively amongst patients with DM [1].

In a study from Kerala, the prevalence of rheumatologic and musculoskeletal disorders was observed to be very common in patients with diabetes having a prevalence of 42.58% in a cohort of 310 individuals. With the exponential increase in the burden of diabetes, especially in India, the burden of patients with musculoskeletal complication of diabetes is also going to increase manifold. Some of the unique challenges with type-2 diabetes in India is the nearly two decade earlier onset in Indians as compared to rest of the globe, a greater insulin resistance, systemic inflammation, a more severe beta cell impairment, greater central adiposity, increased body fat percentage, and a more rapid progression from prediabetes to diabetes [2]. Duration as well as severity of diabetes has been often linked with increased occurrence and severity of the musculo-skeletal complication of diabetes. In this chapter, a review of the major musculoskeletal complications of diabetes has been done, highlighting their pathophysiology, treatment modalities, and outcomes (Table 60.1).

Musculoskeletal manifestations can be divided largely into three categories:

- Bone effects of diabetes
- Muscle effects of diabetes
- Joint and connective tissue effects of diabetes

D. Dutta
Department of Endocrinology, CEDAR Superspeciality Healthcare, New Delhi, India

R. Singla
Department of Endocrinology, Kalpavriksh Healthcare, New Delhi, India

M. Sharma
Department of Rheumatology, CEDAR Superspeciality Healthcare, New Delhi, India

A. Sharma
Department of Rheumatology, Maharaj Agrasen Hospital, New Delhi, India

S. Kalra (✉)
Department of Endocrinology, Bharti Hospital, Karnal, India

Table 60.1 Musculoskeletal involvement in diabetes mellitus

Conditions occurring more frequently in DM
- Shoulder capsulitis
- Limited joint mobility
- Dupuytren's disease
- Stenosing flexor tenosynovitis (trigger finger)
- Neuropathic charcot arthropathy
- Calcific shoulder periarthritis
- Carpal tunnel syndrome

Conditions unique to DM
- Diabetic muscle infarction

Condition sharing risk factors of DM and metabolic syndrome
- Diffuse idiopathic skeletal hyperostosis
- Crystal-induced arthritis
- Osteoarthritis

Miscellaneous
- Bone health and osteoporosis

© The Author(s), under exclusive license to Springer Nature Switzerland AG 2023
J. Rodriguez-Saldana (ed.), *The Diabetes Textbook*, https://doi.org/10.1007/978-3-031-25519-9_60

Bone Effects of Diabetes: Bone Density and Fracture Risk

Effect of diabetes on bone health is quite complex and interesting. Effect varies with type of diabetes and with site of skeletal system. Both type 1 and type 2 diabetes are associated with poor bone health and increased fracture rate, but their effect on bone mineral density varies. Type 1 diabetes is associated with decreased bone density in majority of studies done. Uncontrolled type 1 diabetes may, in fact, prevent an adolescent from acquiring peak bone mass. When assessed in midlife, most of the studies show, bone mineral density to be decreased. Low body mass index, lower lean mass contributes to lower BMD in patients with T1DM. Different studies have consistently shown that fracture risk is increased by around two times, at lumber spine, hip, and distal radius in patients with type-1 diabetes. Major pathophysiologic factor responsible for decreased bone density in type 1 diabetes is lack of insulin that, otherwise, acts as an anabolic agent for bone. Raised blood glucose in uncontrolled diabetes also deteriorates bone quality by formation of non-enzymic glycated collagen cross-links which are much weaker than, usually formed, enzymic pyrilodine cross-links. Another important factor predisposing to poor bone health in this population is low body mass index. Only measure, which is effective, for prevention and recovery is adequate glycaemic control as that would signify normal blood glucose levels with optimum insulin therapy [3].

Situation in type 2 diabetes is much more complex as these patients often have associated hyperinsulinism. Bone mineral density in type 2 diabetes can vary from low to normal to some patients even increased, depending on the disease state and the clinical scenario. Raised BMI in obese type-2 DM patients has a trophic effect on BMD. However, it must be highlighted that even in patients with normal to increased BMI in T2DM, the fracture rates has been consistently demonstrated to be increased in T2DM. This can be attributed to the poor bone quality in such patients, secondary to glycation of bone matrix secondary to persistent hyperglycaemia in patients with T2DM. The authors have observed in a cohort of type-2 diabetes patients that is the lean mass, which has the maximum impact on bone health in diabetes. A greater lean mass leads to a greater dynamic loading of the bones, which has a trophic effect on bone health and density. Sarcopenia due to any cause is associated with low bone density in diabetes.

Apart from weakening the bone, accumulation of advanced glycosylation end-products (AGEs) in the organic bone matrix by nonenzymatic glycation interfere with normal osteoblast development, function, and attachment to the collagen matrix. In type 2 diabetes, differential effect at trabecular and cortical sites has also been noted with preservation of trabecular bone and loss of cortical bone mass. There are clinical studies which show that in T2DM, most of the fractures occur at sites that are rich in cortical bone. Risk factors other than bone density also need to be kept in mind in patients with diabetes, most notable being microvascular complication (esp. neuropathy and retinopathy), macrovascular complications, and muscle weakness.

Smoking, use of glucocorticoids, associated inflammatory diseases like inflammatory arthropathy all are associated with poorer bone mineral density and bone health in diabetes. Bone health is often a neglected aspect of diabetes management. It would a good clinical practice from the clinician's point of view to avoid medications which are associated with impaired bone health in patients of diabetes with established low bone mineral density. Pioglitazone and SGLT2 inhibitors have been linked to adverse bone mineral outcomes in diabetes. Pioglitazone (thiazolidinediones) inhibits bone formation directly, by diverting mesenchymal stem cell precursors from the osteoblast to the adipocyte lineage. SGLT2 inhibitors use has been linked to increased phosphate reabsorption from the kidneys. Increased phosphate reabsorption and increased circulating phosphorous leads to secondary hyperparathyroidism, increased circulating levels of phosphatonins, all of which have an adverse impact on bone mineral density. The high prevalence of vitamin-D deficiency also contributes to impaired bone mineral health and peak bone mass in adulthood.

Muscle Effects of Diabetes

Muscles are a major user of insulin-mediated glucose uptake. In face of insulin resistance in type 2, proteomics studies have revealed weakened metabolic flexibility, i.e. difficulty in switching between glucose metabolism and fatty acid utilization with preferential oxidative-to-glycolytic shift. There is altered mitochondrial function, reduced lipid oxidation, increased cellular stress response, and enhanced detoxification mechanisms. All these metabolic change result in changes in contractile proteins and altered cytoskeletal proteins and also fatigue and tiredness.

Acute and chronic neuropathies associated with diabetes can lead to muscle atrophy and weakness. For example, carpal tunnel syndrome (discussed in sections ahead) can lead to atrophy of hand muscles, and distal polyneuropathy can lead to loss of small muscles of foot. Primary diseases of muscles seen in diabetics include diabetic myonecrosis and amyotrophy.

Diabetic Myonecrosis

Spontaneous infarction of muscle in diabetic patients is a rare but well-known entity. Approximately 200 cases have been reported in literature so far. The pathophysiology for diabetic myonecrosis has not been fully elucidated, but it is proposed to be ischemic in nature without any obvious athero-embolism or vascular occlusion of any major artery. It is more commonly seen in patients who are dependent on insulin and already have underlying microvascular complications.

Clinically, the disease has slight male preponderance and patient usually present with a disabling and constant pain involving quadriceps muscles. Other areas which can be involved in minority of cases include calf muscles, upper limb, and neck muscles. There may be an apparent swelling at site of involvement. Asymmetry is a hallmark of this disease. Bilateral involvement occurs in one-third of patients. Blood investigation reveals raised levels of ESR and CRP, while creatine kinase may be raised or normal during early or late stage of presentation, respectively. Leucocyte count and temperature are normal and helps in differentiation from infective pathology. Sonography reveals diffuse or focal muscle edema and is invaluable in ruling out deep vein thrombosis or major arterial thrombosis. Magnetic resonance imaging is investigation of choice in such cases and the involved muscle shows hyperintensity on T2-weighted sequences and addition of contrast differentiates non-enhancing infarcted muscle from surrounding inflammation or edema. Additional findings on MRI can be subcutaneous edema, subfascial fluid, and loss of the normal fatty intramuscular septa. Biopsy is not generally indicated, but reveals muscle edema and infarction along with evidence of microangiopathy.

Disease generally resolves on its own by 6–12 weeks. Rest and pain relief are mainstay of therapy. But as there is evidence of microangiopathy and association with other microvascular complications, antiplatelets are generally advised. Constant vigil, however, is required as some of the cases can be complicated by compartment syndrome. Moreover, recurrence rate is very high and half of the cases would have recurrence. The mean mortality rate associated with DMI is 10% within 2 years of initial diagnosis, predominantly as a result of macrovascular complications.

Diabetic Amyotrophy

Amyotrophy or diabetic lumbosacral plexopathy has overlapping clinical presentation with diabetic myonecrosis. But, amyotrophy occurs predominantly in type 2 patients who are fairly controlled or has recently been diagnosed. It also pres-

ent with acute onset proximal leg pain followed by muscle weakness. Disease is usually unilateral at onset, but bilateral involvement eventually occurs in majority of patients. About one-third of patients may have distal onset of disease. This condition is also associated with distal and proximal sensory loss. New onset autonomic symptoms may occur in up to half of the patients and more than 80% patients would report loss of at least 10% body weight. Rarely, muscles of upper limb and thorax can be involved.

Underlying pathophysiology is not clear (e.g., ischemic, metabolic and/or inflammatory), though there is general consensus that ischemic injury due to non-systemic microvasculitis is most likely cause. Electrodiagnostic studies, in presence of typical features, are sufficient to clinch the diagnosis. Abnormalities are localized to lumbosacral plexus and peripheral nerves of lower limb. HIV and cytomegalovirus can cause similar disease with same electrodiagnostic findings. Inflammatory myopathies such as polymyositis and dermatomyositis should always be ruled out. Associated classical cutaneous manifestations makes easy for dermatomyositis to be ruled out. Polymyositis is classically associated with elevated levels of creatine-phosphokinase (CPK) in the blood which is not seen in amyotrophy.

Disease usually runs a self-limited course with spontaneous resolution but some residual problem remains in large majority in form of either weakness or persistent pain. Course of disease can run over months. Treatment is only symptomatic. No evidence exists to favour treatment with steroids, immunosuppressants, or immunoglobulins.

Joint and Connective Tissue Effects of Diabetes

Joint and connective tissue diseases are more common in people with diabetes (Table 60.2). There is no single mechanism that has been shown to account for the development of joint and connective tissue effects of diabetes, viz. limited joint mobility (LJM), shoulder adhesive capsulitis, stenosing flexor tenosynovitis, and Dupuytren's contracture amongst

Table 60.2 Prevalence of joint and connective tissue diseases in people with and without diabetes

Musculoskeletal disorder	With diabetes (%)	Without diabetes (%)
Shoulder capsulitis	11–30	2–10
Limited joint mobility	8–50	0–26
Dupuytren's disease	20–63	5–10
Carpal tunnel syndrome	11–16	2–5
Stenosing flexor tenosynovitis	10–12	<1
Diffuse idiopathic skeletal hyperostosis	13–50	2–15

others. However, the shared cause of these conditions seems to involve abnormal connective tissue deposition around joints, in tendon sheaths, and in the palmar fascia, respectively.

Accumulation of advanced glycation end products (AGEs) with cross-linking of collagen and other macromolecules has been proposed as a potential pathogenetic mechanism. It is likely that poorer glycaemic control over time with resulting AGE formation influences the development of hand and shoulder problems amongst patients with DM.

Adhesive Capsulitis of the Shoulder (Frozen Shoulder Syndrome, Shoulder Periarthritis) Enter Box 60.1

Box 60.1 Adhesive Capsulitis of Shoulder

Painful progressive restriction of shoulder motion
30 months: Average duration of symptoms
10–29% prevalence amongst diabetics
Treatment: Analgesics, physiotherapy, intra-articular corticosteroid injection, arthroscopic capsular release

The prevalence of adhesive capsulitis is 11–29% in patients with T2DM, as compared to only 2–3% in healthy euglycaemic individuals. Risk factors for adhesive capsulitis include older age, increased duration of diabetes, history of myocardial infarction, presence of peripheral neuropathy and nephropathy. Adhesive capsulitis usually presents as painful progressive restriction of range of shoulder movement, especially on abduction and external rotation. Its natural history can be divided into three phases: pain, stiffness, and recovery. The length of the recovery phase depends on the duration of the stiffness phase, with symptoms lasting for an average of 30 months. Adhesive capsulitis can involve any of the large joints in diabetes. Frozen shoulder syndrome is perhaps the most common type of adhesive capsulitis (Table 60.2). Shoulder adhesive capsulitis is more likely to develop in older individuals with either type of DM and in those with longer duration of disease amongst patients with type 1 DM, history of myocardial infarction, associated nephropathy, and/or neuropathy [4].

Analgesics physical therapy and intra-articular corticosteroid injection are first-line therapy during the initial painful phase of shoulder adhesive capsulitis. Intra-articular injection, early in the course of the disease, has been linked to improved outcomes and better mobility in the long run. It must be highlighted that oral corticosteroids have limited role and should be routinely used in patients with adhesive capsulitis. Oral glucocorticoids are not associated with improved mobility outcomes in the long run and additionally

they adversely affect glycaemic control. Intensive physiotherapy including stretching and mobilization also has a key role in improving clinical outcomes. Arthroscopic capsular release has been an effective treatment modality for refractory shoulder adhesive capsulitis in a few patients. Radiographic-guided hydro-dilation and manipulation under anesthesia have been tried in refractory patients with mixed long-term outcomes.

Limited Joint Mobility (Diabetic Cheiro-Arthropathy) Enter Box 60.2

Box 60.2 Limited Joint Mobility

Collagen disease seen only in diabetes
Prevalence 8–50%
Stiff hands with thick, tight, and waxy skin
Asymptomatic
Harbinger of microvascular disease

Limited joint mobility (LJM) also known as 'diabetic cheiro-arthropathy' is characterized by stiff hands. The skin is markedly thick, tight, and waxy especially on the dorsal aspects of the hands which are usually, symmetrically affected: mimicking scleroderma.

Patients with LJM have limited extension of the metacarpophalangeal, proximal interphalangeal, and distal interphalangeal joints, usually beginning in the ulnar digits and spreading radially. Screening for LJM can be done by physical examination. The prayer (preachers) sign involves the patient holding the hands opposed to one another vertically with elbows flexed and wrists extended. A positive sign is observed by an inability of the patient to completely approximate the palmar surface of the digits.

In the table top sign, the patient places the palms flat on a hard surface with the digits spread. Normally, the entire palmar surface of the digits should contact the table. If the test is positive, the digits and palm will not lie flat. Both these tests can also be positive with Dupuytren's contracture. The prayer sign is also useful for staging of LJM as follows:

Stage 0: normal findings on prayer sign examination.
Stage 1: involvement of one or two interphalangeal joints bilaterally.
Stage 2: Inability to approximate three or more interphalangeal joints bilaterally.
Stage 3: Hand deformity at rest.

The prevalence of LJM in diabetes varies from 8% to 50%. The frequency of LJM in diabetics increases with increasing diabetes duration. The importance of LJM can be highlighted by the fact that its presence is an indicator for other associated more grave microvascular and macrovascular complications of diabetes. An association with microvascular complications (retinopathy, microalbuminuria) has been shown, both in Type 1 and in Type 2 diabetes. LJM increases the risk for microvascular disease in Type 1 diabetes. There is an 83% risk for microvascular complications after 16 years of diabetes in the presence of LJM, compared with a 25% risk in the absence of LJM. Patients with LJM may be at higher risk for foot ulceration because of concomitant limited joint mobility at the hallux.

Treatment of LJM is not very satisfactory. Physiotherapy to increase the range of motion in the hand joints is fundamental. This involves active and passive mobilization and use of corrective splints. Glucocorticoids injection of flexor tendon sheaths leads to resolution of finger contractures in every two out of three patients with LJM. At a more practical level, optimization of glycaemic control is believed to be vital for the management of LJM.

Dupuytren Contracture (DD)

DD is a progressive fibro-proliferative disorder resulting in abnormal scar-like tissue in the palmar fascia leading to irreversible, permanent, painless, and progressive contracture of the involved digits. DD is commonly bilateral, and 'Dupuytren-like' fibrotic tissue can occur on the dorsum of the hand over the knuckles (Garrod's pads), feet (Lederhose's disease), and penis (Peyronie's disease). The ring finger is the most frequently involved, followed by the little finger, and then middle finger; the index finger and thumb are rarely involved.

The incidence of DD also increases with concurrent patient clinical conditions or factors such as diabetes, smoking, chronic alcoholism, seizures, and infection. Microvascular changes in smokers may play a role. Hand examination also reveals palpable palmar nodule or nodules.

The prevalence of DC in diabetes ranges between 20% and 63%, considerably higher than amongst nondiabetic subjects (13%). DC in diabetic subjects is associated with diabetes duration, long-term poor metabolic control, and presence of microvascular complications. LJM and DC may coexist in the same patient [5].

DD must be distinguished from several other conditions that affect the hand, including trigger finger, stenosing tenosynovitis, a ganglion cyst, or a soft-tissue mass. Unlike DC, trigger finger typically involves pain with flexion followed by the inability to extend the affected digit. Stenosing tenosynovitis may be distinguished from DD by pain and a history of overuse or trauma. A small, movable nodule that is tender to palpation at the metacarpophalangeal joint is likely a ganglion cyst. Treatment of DC involves optimized glycaemic control and physiotherapy. Topical steroid injection and surgery are reserved for the more severe cases. Surgery yields satisfactory results.

Calciphylaxis

Calciphylaxis is a form of small vessel vasculitis. It has been reported in patients with renal failure as well as diabetes. Clinically, they present as small tender areas on the skin, initially red in color, which then become subcutaneous nodules, leading to poorly healing necrotizing skin ulcers. Key to treatment is to ensure a good glycaemic control and analgesics for pain relief.

Stenosing Flexor Tenosynovitis (Trigger Finger)

Stenosing flexor tenosynovitis typically presents with locking (or 'triggering') of fingers in flexion, extension, or both, most commonly involving the thumb, middle, and ring fingers. At clinical examination, locking is reproducible on active or passive finger flexion. Moreover, a nodule is palpable at the base of affected finger. The prevalence of stenosing flexor tenosynovitis ranges between 5% and 36% amongst patients with type 1 and 2 DM, as compared with 2% in the general population. Compared with nondiabetics, patients with DM are more likely to have multiple fingers involved simultaneously by stenosing flexor tenosynovitis [6].

In diabetic subjects, it is associated with diabetes duration, long-term poor metabolic control, and presence of microvascular complications. Additionally, it has been suggested as an indicator of glucose dysmetabolism that should prompt glucose measurement and oral glucose tolerance test in the general population. Treatment of stenosing flexor tenosynovitis includes modification of activities to avoid triggering of digits, nonsteroidal anti-inflammatory drug therapy, splinting, corticosteroid injection into the tendon sheath, and surgical release. Corticosteroid injections into the tendon sheath has been especially found to be beneficial in patients with disease duration of less than 6 months and having nodular type of disease. In these patients, the success rate of a single injection is as high as 96%.

Calcific Shoulder Periarthritis (Tendinitis)

Calcific tendinitis is a painful condition most commonly affecting the shoulder in which calcium hydroxyapatite crystals deposit predominantly in periarticular areas. In the shoulder, these crystals may also deposit within the tendons of the rotator cuff. The incidence of calcific shoulder periarthritis is increased amongst patients with DM. Calcific tendinitis may coexist with adhesive capsulitis in the shoulder.

Carpal Tunnel Syndrome (CTS)

Carpal Tunnel Syndrome is a common compression neuropathy of the median nerve associated with many conditions including diabetes. Classically, these patients present with the wasting of the muscles of the thenar eminence (abductor pollicis brevis, extensor pollicis longus, and extensor policis brevis). The typical presentation is hand paresthesia involving the median nerve distribution. Paresthesia and pains are usually exacerbated in the night. Apart from diabetes, CTS is also associated with rheumatoid arthritis, pregnancy, and obesity. Diabetes may induce structural alterations of tendon, increase obesity, and produce metabolic abnormalities that result in proliferation or fibrosis of the connective tissues surrounding the nerve. Transforming growth factor-beta has a key role in the pathogenesis of CTS. Increased TGFb is seen in TGF which is associated with increased localized inflammation and collagen deposition. The prevalence of CTS in diabetes has been reported at 11–25%, and it is more common in women. Conversely, 5–8% of patients with carpal tunnel syndrome may have diabetes. Two classic signs, Tinel's sign and Palen's test, are very helpful in establishing the diagnosis. A positive Tinel's sign refers to the elicitation of paresthesia and/or pain in the hand (mainly thenar and thumb area) by tapping over the median nerve on the volar aspect of the wrist. Palen's test is positive if similar symptoms are produced when the patient flexes both wrists completely and opposes the dorsal surfaces of the hands to each other.

Management focuses on analgesics and splints, while topical steroid injection and surgery may be indicated in more severe cases. Endoscopic tendon release procedures are increasingly being used in CTS to relieve the median nerve from compression, with good clinical outcomes. Recent studies have suggested that a single dose of ultrasound-guided perineural platelet-rich plasma (PRP) injection can provide therapeutic effect for at least 1 year post injection [7].

Reflex Sympathetic Dystrophy

Also known as algodystrophy, Sudeck's atrophy, and chronic regional pain syndrome type 1, this disorder is characterized by pain, swelling, trophic changes, and vasomotor disturbances with impaired mobility of the body part involved. The development of the condition is usually preceded by a trauma, which may range from trivial injury to a surgery or a fracture. Apart from diabetes, reflex sympathetic dystrophy is also seen in hyperthyroidism, hyperparathyroidism, and type IV hyperlipidemia. A large variety of treatment options have been used in reflex sympathetic dystrophy ranging from analgesics, physiotherapy, intravenous bisphosphonates, calcitonin, oral corticosteroids, and sympathetic ganglion blocks. Clinical outcomes are usually good. In rare patients, it may lead to contractures.

Diffuse Idiopathic Skeletal Hyperostosis (DISH), Forestier's Disease

Diffuse idiopathic skeletal hyperostosis (DISH) is a condition characterized by ossification of spinal ligaments associated with large bridging osteophytes between vertebral bodies. Obesity, hyperlipidemia, hyperuricemia, hypertension, hyperinsulinemia, and diabetes are thought to be associated with DISH.

The diagnosis of DISH is based on radiologic features. Radiographic criteria for the diagnosis of DISH include the presence of 'flowing' osteophytes along the anterolateral aspects of at least four contiguous vertebral bodies, the preservation of intervertebral disk spaces, and the absence of changes of degenerative spondylosis or spondyloarthropathy. Analgesics, heat application, exercise, and local corticosteroid injections have been used to treat patients with DISH. Targeted spine strengthening exercise and posture training program reduced kyphometer measured, but not radiographic-measured kyphosis in people with DISH [8].

Crystal-Induced Arthritis and Gout

Calcific tendinitis is clearly associated with diabetes. Similar calcific processes certainly occur in blood vessels of diabetic patients as well as in spinal ligaments in DISH. Metabolic changes, consequent to chronic high glucose and insulin levels, may produce important changes in connective tissues that might predispose to pathologic calcification.

Gout is an inflammatory arthropathy characterized by increased deposition of mono-sodium urate crystals in the joint. Gout is more common in Caucasians where it effects 1–2% of the population. Risk factors for gout include hyperuricemia, male sex, renal impairment, alcohol use, and increased consumption of meat. Insulin resistance, which is very common is type-2 diabetes, is associated with decreased uric acid excretion and hence is associated with hyperuricemia. Serum urate concentration and gout is strongly associated with central adiposity and insulin resistance. Few meta-analysis have showed that the prevalence of gout in type-2 diabetes may be as high as 25%. It must be highlighted that amongst the anti-hypertension medicines and anti-lipid medication, losartan and fenofibrate have urate-lowering effects. Hence, special consideration should be given to these drugs when type-2 diabetes patients with hyperuricemia/gout is planned to be put on hypertension or lipid medications. Mycophenolate mofetil therapy with pegloticase and anakinra are new upcoming therapies for refractory gout [9, 10].

Osteoarthritis

Osteoarthritis is the most common form of arthritis in adults and as such would frequently co-occur with diabetes by chance alone. Clear clinical evidence that diabetes predisposes to premature or severe osteoarthritis is lacking. The fact that obesity is a common risk factor for both osteoarthritis and diabetes makes epidemiologic studies difficult. Peripheral neuropathy may also adversely affect joints and increase the risk of advanced, aggressive forms of osteoarthritis. There seems to be propensity for diabetic patients to have more severe pain and radiographic changes both preoperatively and postoperatively, an increased risk of deep tissue infection as well as an increased revision rate compared with nondiabetic controls. Whether insulin resistance worsens or not when therapeutic doses of oral glucosamine are used to treat osteoarthritis remains controversial. Intra-articular injections of autologous fat with or without platelet rich plasma is a new upcoming therapy for severe osteoarthritis [11].

Charcot Arthritis

Charcot's arthropathy is a form of destrictive arthritis. It is seen in diabetes usually as an association with peripheral neuropathy. It is a debilitating condition observed in 0.4% of patients with diabetes and is associated with limb deformity, gait instability, ulcers and may lead to limb amputation also. Four different stages of Charcot arthropathy have been described. In the earliest stage (Stage 0), the patient usually complains of pain in the joint. The join may or may not have swelling. X-rays of the joint are normal at this stage. MRI is the most sensitive tool for diagnosis at this stage where it can pick up marrow edema, subchondral cysts, and microfractures. In Stage 1, the X-rays of the joint now start showing varying degrees of osteolysis, bone fragmentation, and architectural destruction. Stages 0 and 1 are the clinically active stages of the disease characterized by joint pain swelling, redness, and localized increase in skin temperature. In stage 2, the clinical signs of local inflammation usually resolves, coalescence starts which may be visible on joint X-rays. Stage 3 is known as the reconstructive stage, where fusion or ankylosis of the bones occur. Stages 0 and 1 usually last up to 6 months whereas stages 2 and 3 last up to 24 months.

Charcot's arthropathy most commonly involves the foot. Altered architecture of the foot as a result of the deformity leads to abnormal foot pressure distributions, leading to increased risk of foot ulcers at the high pressure points. Tarsometatarsal followed by the mid-tarsal joint involvements are the two most common types of Charcot arthropathy. After foot, knees, elbows, and the shoulder joints are most commonly affected by Charcot's arthropathy.

The pathogenesis of Charcot's arthropathy is yet to be fully elucidated. Localized joint inflammation and osteoclast activation is central to the pathogenesis of Charcot arthropathy. Increased local levels of tumor necrosis factor alpha, interleukins (IL-1, IL6), RANK ligand have been documented in Charcot arthropathies. Abnormal weight bearing due to diabetic neuropathy leads to small microtrauma to the foot, which leads to foot inflammation and hyperemia which sets up a vicious cycle of joint inflammation and damage resulting to Charcot arthropathy.

The most important aspect of managing Charcot arthropathy, especially in the acute stage is joint immobilization, and absolute cessation of weight bearing. Nonweight bearing total contact cast (TCC) is the treatment of choice for managing Charcot foot. This leads to significant reduction in joint inflammation and reduces the risk of deformity also. Bisphosphonates (pamidronate, alendronate, zoledronate) have been demonstrated to be useful in reducing joint inflammation and hastening recovery in patients with Charcot arthropathy, both in observational studies as well as randomized controlled trials. Small studies have also showed the beneficial effects of RANK ligand inhibitors (denosumab) in the management of Charcot arthropathy. Surgery has no role in the management of Charcot arthropathy in the active stage. Surgery has a role in inactive or burnt out stage of the disease, where it helps in joint stabilization, and helps improving the pressure distribution of the joint, which would help in preventing ulcers. Therapeutic footwears have an important role in improving foot pressure distribution in patients with Charcot's foot, help in healing of foot ulcers, and also providing limited mobility to the patients.

Diabetic Foot

One of the most devastating complications of diabetes is diabetic foot. Foot problems in diabetes occur due to combination of abnormalities affecting vascularity, peripheral nerves, skin and musculoskeletal system.

Foot problems in diabetes can be largely divided into infective and noninfective complications.

Charcot's foot is characterized by destruction of small foot joints and complete disorganization of anatomy of foot. Neuropathy is the main contributor in this condition with both peripheral and autonomic neuropathy playing significant roles. Peripheral neuropathy makes the insensate foot take repeated trauma and also to transmit pressure in not-so-optimal way. This creates false pressure points and puts undue stress on small joints of foot. Autonomic neuropathy, on the other hand, impairs regulation of blood flow to foot and thus exposing bones of foot to excessive bone loss during periods of increased blood flow. Charcot foot is great danger to health of any diabetic as this condition cannot be reversed and puts patient at grave risk of foot ulcer and infections. It can present early on, as an acute inflammatory process which is frequently mistaken for gout, osteomyelitis or injury, and then develops into chronic arthritis with severe deformities. It is always a clinical challenge to differentiate between Charcot foot and osteomyelitis. Systemic signs of infection (fever, leucocytosis), breach in skin of foot, positive probe test and positive labeled leucocyte scan favor a diagnosis of osteomyelitis. MRI and Tc bone scan have also been used to differentiate between them.

Proper foot care education to patient to avoid further deterioration and to prevent ulcers is of paramount importance. Non-weight bearing and immobilization of the affected limb have been the mainstays of therapy. Bisphosphonates have also been reported to be useful for the acute phase of Charcot arthropathy.

A detailed discussion of ulceration and infective complications of foot in diabetes is beyond the scope of this chapter. However, general principles for wound care remain the same. There are two ways in which diabetic foot is at disadvantage. One, diabetic foot is more predisposed to trauma. Any skeletal abnormality in foot in patient with diabetes predisposes them to increased risk of trauma because of sensory loss. Diabetic patients with minor trauma to foot are more likely to ignore because of lack of pain. Insensate foot also alters proprioception and thus makes these patients more prone to falls and major trauma while walking. Moreover, neuropathy further contributes to deformity of foot, e.g. atrophy of mid-foot muscles causes clawing. Associated autonomic neuropathy results in dry skin and more risk of fissures. Second, altered blood supply to foot, due to vasculopathy, makes these trauma and infection difficult to heal. Moreover, delivery of antibiotics is also hampered. And because of this reason, patient vasculature is a must for a normal foot in diabetics. In the presence of vascular adequacy, even if minor wounds are sustained they would heal with basic care.

The main goal should be prevention of diabetic foot ulcers. In this regard, at-home foot skin temperature monitoring is a great way to predict sites of increased risk of foot ulcer. At-home foot temperature monitoring significantly reduces incidence of diabetic foot ulcer recurrence at or adjacent to measurement sites over usual care, only if the participants reduce ambulatory activity when hotspots are found or when aiming to prevent ulcers at any foot site [12].

Conclusion

Musculoskeletal complications of diabetes hence are a large number of diverse set of disorders. In contrast to other complications of diabetes, a good clinical eye has a key role in the diagnosis of these disorders. Many a times, these complications are missed in a busy clinic practice, as most of these complications are not severe and life threatening, although lack of their diagnosis and timely treatment may lead to significant morbidity in the patients.

Multiple Choice Questions

1. Anti-diabetic medications linked with adverse impact on bone health include:
   (a) Sulfonylureas
   (b) Insulin
   (c) **SGLT-2 inhibitors**
   (d) DPP-4 inhibitors
   (e) **Glitazones**
2. All of the following are true regarding diabetic myonecrosis except:
   (a) Painful
   (b) ESR is raised
   (c) Spontaneously resolving.
   (d) **Recurrence rates are low**
   (e) Asymmetrical
3. All of the following are true regarding diabetic amyotrophy except:
   (a) Asymmetrical
   (b) Predominantly motor involvement and muscle wasting.
   (c) Spontaneously resolving.
   (d) **Definitive role of immunosuppresive and glucocorticoids in management**
   (e) **Sensory involvement is absent**
4. Most commonly involved joints in adhesive capsulitis in patients with diabetes:
   (a) Knee
   (b) **Shoulder**
   (c) Hips
   (d) Elbow
   (e) Metacarpophalangeal
5. Carpel tunnel syndrome leads to wasting of the following small muscles of the hand except:
   (a) abductor pollicis brevis
   (b) **abductor policis longus**
   (c) extensor pollicis brevis
   (d) extensor pollicis longus
   (e) **Opponens pollicis**
6. Carpel tunnel syndrome is due to the involvement of the following nerve:
   (a) Ulnar nerve
   (b) **Median nerve**

    (c) Radial nerve

    (d) Cutaneous nerve of the forearm

    (e) Superficial peroneal nerve

7. Antihypertensive medications with uric acid lowering effects include.

    (a) amlodipine

    (b) ramipril

    (c) lisinopril

    (d) olmesartan

    (e) **losartan**

8. Anti-lipid medication with uric acid lowering properties

    (a) **Fibrates**

    (b) statins

    (c) bile acid binding resins

    (d) PCSK9 inhibitors

    (e) Ezetimibe

9. Medications acting on bone metabolism found to be beneficial in Charcot's arthropathy include:

    (a) teriparatide

    (b) **bisphosphonates**

    (c) calcitonin

    (d) **denosumab**

    (e) saracatanib

10. The pathogenesis of Charcot's arthropathy involves all except:

    (a) increased inflammatory cytokines

    (b) increased osteoclast activation

    (c) **decreased RANK-L expression**

    (d) **increased osteoblast activation**

    (e) increased local hyperemia.

References

1. SerbanAL UGF. Rheumatic manifestations in diabetic patients. J Med Life. 2012;5(3):252–7.
2. Maisnam I, Dutta D, Mukhopadhyay S, Chowdhury S. Lean mass is the strongest predictor of bone mineral content in type-2 diabetes and normal individuals: an eastern India perspective. J Diabetes Metab Disord. 2014;13(1):90.
3. Silva MBG, Skare TL. Musculoskeletal disorders in diabetes mellitus. Rev Bras Reumatol. 2012;52(4):594–609.
4. Lebiedz-Odrobina D, Kay J. Rheumatic manifestations of diabetes mellitus. Rheum Dis Clin N Am. 2010;36:681–99.
5. Mathew AJ, Nair JB, Pillai SS. Rheumatic-musculoskeletal manifestations in type 2 diabetes mellitus in South India. Int J Rheum Dis. 2011;14:55–60.
6. Papana N, Maltezos E. The diabetic hand: a forgotten complication? J Diabetes Complicat. 2010;24:154–62.
7. Chen SR, Shen YP, Ho TY, Li TY, Su YC, Chou YC, Chen LC, Wu YT. One-year efficacy of platelet-rich plasma for moderate-to-severe carpal tunnel syndrome: a prospective, randomized, double-blind, Controlled Trial. Arch Phys Med Rehabil. 2021;102(5):951–8.
8. Katzman WB, Parimi N, Gladin A, Poltavskiy EA, Schafer AL, Long RK, Fan B, Wong SS, Lane NE. Sex differences in response to targeted kyphosis specific exercise and posture training in community-dwelling older adults: a randomized controlled trial. BMC Musculoskelet Disord. 2017;18(1):509. https://doi.org/10.1186/s12891-017-1862-0.
9. Khanna PP, Khanna D, Cutter G, Foster J, Melnick J, Jaafar S, Biggers S, Rahman AKMF, Kuo HC, Feese M, Kivitz A, King C, Shergy W, Kent J, Peloso PM, Danila MI, Saag KG. Reducing immunogenicity of Pegloticase with concomitant use of mycophenolate mofetil in patients with refractory gout: a phase II, randomized, double-blind, Placebo-Controlled Trial. Arthritis Rheumatol. 2021;73(8):1523–32.
10. Saag KG, Khanna PP, Keenan RT, Ohlman S, Osterling Koskinen L, Sparve E, Åkerblad AC, Wikén M, So A, Pillinger MH, Terkeltaub R. A randomized, phase II study evaluating the efficacy and safety of anakinra in the treatment of gout flares. Arthritis Rheumatol. 2021;73(8):1533–42.
11. Louis ML, Dumonceau RG, Jouve E, Cohen M, Djouri R, Richardet N, Jourdan E, Giraudo L, Dumoulin C, Grimaud F, George FD, Veran J, Sabatier F, Magalon J. Intra-articular injection of autologous microfat and platelet-rich plasma in the treatment of knee osteoarthritis: a double-blind randomized comparative study. Arthroscopy. 2021;37(10):3125–3137.e3. https://doi.org/10.1016/j.arthro.2021.03.074.
12. Bus SA, Aan de Stegge WB, van Baal JG, Busch-Westbroek TE, Nollet F, van Netten JJ. Effectiveness of at-home skin temperature monitoring in reducing the incidence of foot ulcer recurrence in people with diabetes: a multicenter randomized controlled trial (DIATEMP). BMJ Open Diabetes Res Care. 2021;9(1):e002392. https://doi.org/10.1136/bmjdrc-2021-002392.

Diabetes and the Skin

61

Justine Mestdagh, Sterre Blanche Laura Koster, Jeffrey Damman, and Hok Bing Thio

Chapter Objectives/Key Features

- There are several skin manifestations in diabetes mellitus, some of them occur frequently.
- Some of these are specific for Type 1 diabetes mellitus, others for Type 2 and some occur in both.
- Medications used to treat diabetes mellitus may also cause skin adverse effects.

Introduction

Many diabetes mellitus patients develop skin manifestations during the course of the disease and children are no exception [1, 2]. Prevalence rates range from 30 to 80% [2, 3]. However, we should keep in mind that diabetes is a highly prevalent disease and therefore should remain critical toward studies trying to determine a direct relationship without being aware of possible confounding factors. The skin is a large organ of the human body and is directly visible to the outside world. Because of this, patients tend to care a lot about their skin, sometimes more than clinicians realize [4].

Skin manifestations of diabetes mellitus are diverse and range from cosmetic concerns to severe conditions more frequently seen in long-standing disease. Recognizing these is a rewarding clinical skill to master, since some of them may be important diagnostic clues as well as markers of advanced disease [5]. Some diabetes-related skin defects can be a port of entry for later infections. Several medications can affect the skin shortly after intake. Some skin manifestations are more specific for diabetes than others. Besides evaluating the skin for establishing a diagnosis of diabetes, it can also be a help for evaluating treatment success, study results, and glucose levels.

Pathogenesis

Pathogenesis of skin involvement in diabetes mellitus can be seen as a collaborative, cumulative phenomenon of biochemical, vascular, neurological, immune-mediated and metabolic changes with longstanding hyperglycemia as its key pathogenic player. Diabetics with hemoglobin A1c values <8 mmol/ml tend to have less cutaneous involvement than those with hemoglobin A1c values >8 mmol/ml [2].

Increased oxidative stress and chronic high levels of circulating glucose lead to a non enzymatical chemical reaction between glucose and proteins, lipids and nucleic acids. The chemical reactions between amino acids and the carbonyl group of glucose are called Maillard reaction. First reversible Schiff's bases are formed followed by the conversion to stable products. Finishing transforming chemical reaction leads to the formation of advanced glycation end products (AGE) which bind to specific receptor on many cell surfaces initiating numerous intracellular signaling cascades leading to diabetic complications [6]. Due to formation of AGE and oxidative stress, vascular damages appear [7]. Neuropathy leads to hypo- or even anhidrosis, vascular dilation causing erythema and hyposensation. Vascular and neurological changes are responsible for loss of sensation, impaired blood supply, and failure of homeostatic regulatory mechanism in end organs such as the skin.

Today, skin autofluorescence (SAF) can be measured easily by a quick, non-invasive method. The SAF serves then as

J. Mestdagh
Department of Dermatology, University Hospital Gent, Ghent, Belgium

S. B. L. Koster · H. B. Thio (✉)
Department of Dermatology, Erasmus University Medical Center, Rotterdam, The Netherlands
e-mail: h.thio@erasmusmc.nl

J. Damman
Department of Pathology, Erasmus University Medical Center, Rotterdam, The Netherlands
e-mail: j.damman@erasmusmc.nl

© The Author(s), under exclusive license to Springer Nature Switzerland AG 2023
J. Rodriguez-Saldana (ed.), *The Diabetes Textbook*, https://doi.org/10.1007/978-3-031-25519-9_61

a quantitative parameter of the cutaneous AGE which in turn can be used to predict and early detection of diabetic vascular complications [8].

Hyperglycemia increases the flux through to pyolol- and hexosamine pathways with activation of protein kinase C, NFkappa b, mitogen-activated protein kinase (MAPK), and others [9]. Consequently, this leads to endothelial proliferation and basement membrane thickening with deposition of periodic acid-Schiff stain positive (PAS+) material with narrowing of arterioles, capillaries, and venules.

Keratinocyte function is frequently altered which leads to an impaired epidermal barrier function and delayed wound healing. [10–12] Decreased hydration might play a role. pH values of the skin are higher than in non-diabetic patients leading to an increase in bacterial colonization.

Skin Manifestations of Diabetes Mellitus

Certain skin manifestations are specific for Type 1 diabetes mellitus, others for Type 2 and some occur in both. In the following text, diseases appear in alphabetical order. Whether they occur predominantly in Type 1 diabetes mellitus, 2, or both will be mentioned.

Acanthosis Nigricans

Acanthosis nigricans (Fig. 61.1) consists of velvety hyperpigmented plaques in the intertriginous areas of the skin. Frequently skin tags are found within these lesions. Most patients are asymptomatic although maceration, malodor, and discomfort have been reported. It is the most frequent skin condition in diabetes, almost all Type 2 diabetic patients develop acanthosis nigricans to a certain extent. It is more frequently seen in Hispanics and native as well as African Americans; men and women are equally affected. Besides diabetes, acanthosis nigricans can also appear in obese individuals, patients with insulin resistance (both independently associated) and less frequently in patients with acromegaly, Cushing syndrome, and leprechaunism. It is sometimes observed in malignancies (especially those of the stomach) and associated with certain medications, for example, nicotinic acid, corticosteroids, and rarely repetitive insulin injections. Lastly, it can appear in healthy individuals as well [13, 14].

Histopathology of the affected skin (Fig. 61.2) reveals hyperkeratosis, papillomatosis, mild acanthosis, and sometimes hyperpigmentation of the basal layer. There is usually no dermal inflammation. The hyperkeratosis causes the darkened aspect and papillomatosis causes accentuation of skin markings. High levels of circulating insulin bind the tyrosine

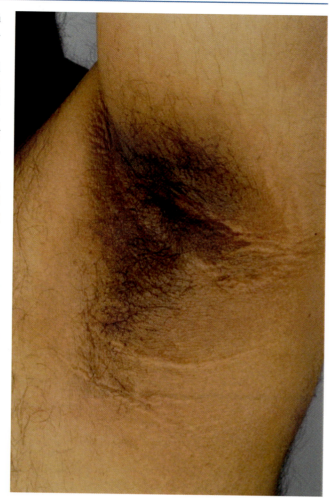

Fig. 61.1 Acanthosis nigricans

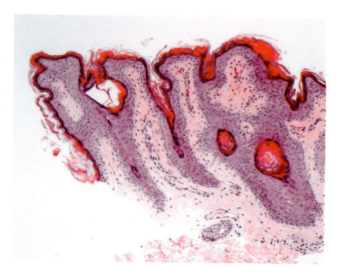

Fig. 61.2 Acanthosis nigricans. Acanthosis nigricans: the lesion shows hyperkeratosis and papillomatosis usually without dermal inflammation.

kinase growth factor receptors (e.g., insulin-like growth factor 1receptor) on fibroblasts and keratinocytes. This stimulates these cells to grow, causing the typical skin manifestations.

People with extensive acanthosis nigricans seem to have higher fasting plasma insulin levels [15, 16].

Weight reduction, exercise, and if necessary, glucose lowering treatment in combination with lipid lowering drugs may reduce insulin resistance and improve acanthosis nigricans. If patients experience discomfort, ointments containing salicylic acid, urea, lactic acid, or retinoids may reduce the hyperkeratotic lesions. Systemic retinoids have been used in severe cases. Recurrence is often seen after discontinuation of therapy.

Acrochordon

Acrochordon (Figs. 61.3 and 61.4), also called fibroma molle, fibroepithelial polyp, or skin tag is a soft pedunculated flesh colored papule in the axillae, neck, eyelids, and in the inframammary region. Patients are asymptomatic apart from possible cosmetic concerns and rarely experience pain or irritation when the fibroma contains nerve endings.

There is a slight female predisposition and its prevalence increases with age. The association between acrochordon and obesity is well established, but they are also an independent marker for diabetes, especially Type 2 [17]. Skin tags have been detected in 23% of diabetic patients compared to 8% in a healthy control group. Though there is some controversy regarding the total amount of skin tags per individual and the associated risk of diabetes, current literature seems to show that the higher the number, the higher the risk for diabetes mellitus. Patients with over 30 skin tags are especially at risk. A positive correlation has also been found between the total

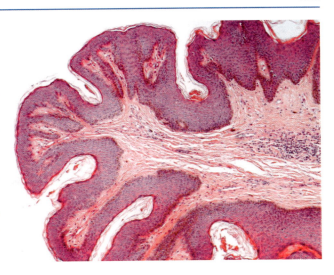

Fig. 61.4 Acrochordon. Acrochordon or fibroepithelial polyp: the papules show a fibrovascular core covered by epidermis showing hyperplasia sometimes resembling seborrheic keratosis. The stroma often shows loosely arranged collagen, an increased number of blood vessel and (in larger lesions) fat cells

number of skin tags and mean fasting plasma glucose [18, 19] making skin tags an even more sensitive cutaneous marker for diabetes than acanthosis nigricans. Clinicians should be aware of this association when taking note of multiple acrochordons. As mentioned earlier, high levels of circulating insulin stimulate keratinocytes to grow, which could help explain the higher prevalence of skin tags in diabetics. Treatment is not necessary, but if patients want them to be removed, they can be excised. Electrodessication and cryotherapy are two valid alternatives.

Acquired Perforating Dermatosis

Acquired perforating dermatosis (Fig. 61.5) presents with scaly highly pruritic follicular hyperkeratotic dome-shaped papules and nodules, often with central umbilication or a central keratotic plug on the extensor surfaces of the lower extremities and in some cases also on the face, trunk, and dorsal area of the hands.

This chronic disease is rare but more frequently seen in Afro-Americans with diabetes (both Type 1 and 2) and chronic kidney disease or hemodialysis (as high as 10%). However, it can also occur in diabetics with normal kidney function [20–22].

Skin conditions to be included in the differential diagnosis are prurigo nodularis, folliculitis, arthropod bites, multiple keratoacanthomas, psoriasis vulgaris, and lichen planus. Pathologic examination (Figs. 61.6 and 61.7) shows a hyperplastic invaginating epidermis containing parakeratosis, degenerated connective tissue and cellular debris, following the transepidermal elimination of dermal collagen and elastin.

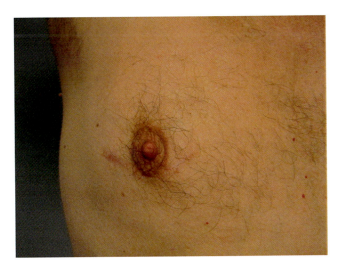

Fig. 61.3 Acrochordon in the right axilla

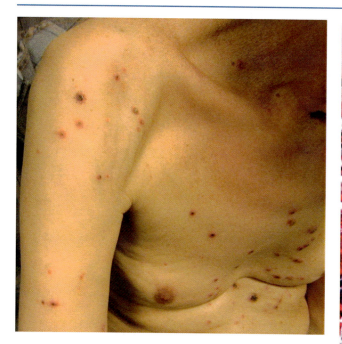

Fig. 61.5 Acquired perforating dermatosis

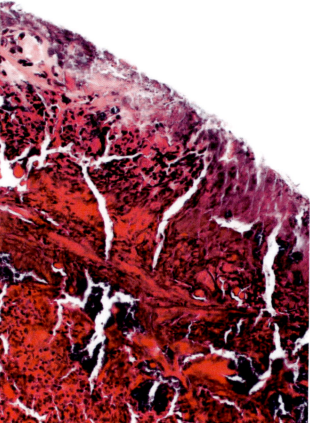

Fig. 61.7 Acquired perforating dermatosis. The lesion shows an invaginating epidermis containing a parakeratotic plug with degenerated connective tissue fibers and cellular debris

first in the dermis or epidermis, pruritus is probably rather the cause of these changes than the effect. Acquired perforating dermatosis is difficult to treat. Treating the pruritus is the main goal. Coexisting disease should be treated according to current standards though dialysis does not improve the disease course. Topical glucocorticoids, antihistamines, topical and systemic retinoids, doxycycline, allopurinol, cryotherapy, and phototherapy are all used for symptom relief.

Bullosis Diabeticorum

Patients suffering from bullosis diabeticorum present with uni- to bilateral spontaneous tense non-inflammatory bullae on normal appearing skin of the dorsolateral sides of the lower extremities and sometimes of the hands. Though it is thought to be a distinct marker for diabetes, it is the rarest skin manifestation in diabetes occurring in 0.5% of all diabetic patients. No large population studies have confirmed this so its frequency might be higher. It does occur more in men with longstanding poorly controlled Type 1 diabetes mellitus with peripheral neuropathy [23, 24].

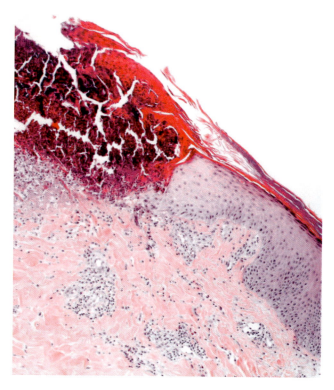

Fig. 61.6 Acquired perforating dermatosis. The lesion shows an invaginating epidermis containing a parakeratotic plug with degenerated connective tissue fibers and cellular debris

The cause is probably a multifactorial interplay between glycation of collagen, Koebner phenomenon, microvasculopathy, and inflammatory reaction to altered dermal collagen or deposition of substances which are not removed by dialysis. It is unclear whether the abnormality appears

There are three known subtypes. In the first, "classic" type, the cleavage level of the bullae is intraepidermal [25], the fluid in these bullae is clear and sterile and the surrounding epidermis shows spongiosis. There is no pain. These bullae resolve spontaneously without scars in a few weeks but recurrence is possible. Histopathological examination shows a subepidermal blister with early re-epithelialization. The second type consists of bullae filled with hemorrhagic fluid. The cleavage level lies below the dermoepidermal junction. Healing comes with scarring and atrophy. The third type appears on tanned skin, and its cleavage level lies within the lamina lucida of the dermoepidermal junction. Healing leaves no scars. The differential diagnosis of bullosis diabeticorum includes primary autoimmune blistering such as pemphigus, bullous pemphigoid, erythema multiforme, epidermolysis bullosa acquisita, and porphyria cutanea tarda. Immunofluorescence tests are negative. Bullosis diabeticorum is associated with high blood glucose levels but venous pressure elevation may also play a role. Microangiopathic vessels offer less blood to the skin which then becomes more prone to acantholysis, and thus blister formation. Other possible causes are autoimmune phenomena, exposure to UV light, and alterations in calcium and magnesium levels [23, 26, 27]. Spontaneous resolution is seen within 2 to 5 weeks [28]. No treatment is needed besides the prevention of complications, e.g., chronic ulcers and bacterial infections. In cases of major discomfort, aspiration can be considered. Nevertheless, recurrence of bullae is frequent.

Diabetic Cheiroarthropathy (Diabetic Stiff Hand or Limited Joint Mobility Syndrome)

People with diabetic cheiroarthropathy have a thickened waxy skin and bilateral limited joint mobility of the hands and fingers leading to flexion contractures (e.g., Dupuytren's disease). This process starts at the fifth digit and progresses radially. It can extend to the wrists, elbows, ankles, knees, toes, and cervicothoracic spine. Clinical examination can reveal a prayer sign, which is the inability to approximate the palmar surfaces of the hands and fingers. Some patients have Huntley papules, which are multiple tiny papules grouped on the dorsal sides of the fingers or periungally. On histologic examination, a hyperkeratotic epidermis and dermal papillary hypertrophy is noticed. Up to 30% of diabetics have diabetic cheiroarthropahty. Incidence increases with disease duration but not with diabetes control. Although it is more common in patients with Type 1 and Type 2 diabetes mellitus than in other individuals, the disease can occur in people without diabetes. If presenting in diabetic patients, it is a predictor of other complications (especially retinopathy and nephropathy). In children with Type 1 diabetes, it is the earliest clinically apparent long-term complication [1].

Differences in the collagen household of the skin such as increased glycosylation of collagen lead to irreversible crosslinking of collagen and other proteins and decreased collagen degradation. Other possible contributing factors are microangiopathy, neuropathy [29, 30], and accumulation of AGE which, after binding their receptors, would stimulate inflammatory and fibrogenic growth factor receptors and cytokines via protein kinase C.

Diabetic cheiroarthropathy is not yet treatable but control of diabetes and physiotherapy are likely to be helpful. Phototherapy, radiotherapy, prostacyclin, penicillin, ciclosporin, factor XIII, and sorbinol have been applied without spectacular results. Research in animals is currently underway, investigating drugs blocking the protein crosslinking or blocking interactions between AGE and their receptors in the early stages of the disease.

Diabetic Dermopathy

Lesions of diabetic dermopathy or so-called shin spots are dynamic, various stages can present in the same patient at the same time. They are usually asymmetrical, 0.5 to 1 cm large red to brown hyperpigmentated spots ranging from atrophic macules to plaques. Plaques are more frequently recognized. These appear bilateral on the extensor parts of the legs but can rarely occur elsewhere and are usually asymptomatic. It is one of the most common skin manifestations in diabetes (Type 1 and 2) with a prevalence of up to 70%, although it is rare in children [1]. It is more frequent in men aged 50 and over and patients with poorly controlled diabetes. Although the association is strong, it is not entirely specific for diabetes mellitus since 20% on nondiabetic people have similar lesions [3]. Patients presenting with this dermopathy should be screened for diabetes especially if they present with four or more shin spots because they are thought to represent postinflammatory hyperpigmentation and cutaneous atrophy in the setting of poor vascular supply and microtrauma [31].

Shin spots may precede abnormal glucose metabolism but may also be a marker for microangiopathic complications such as retinopathy, nephropathy, and neuropathy, as well as macroangiopathic complications, especially coronary artery disease [32, 33]. Differential diagnosis with dermatophytosis should be made. Diabetic dermopathy should be a clinical diagnosis, and there is no need for skin biopsy. If performed, a specific histopathologic findings are seen such as hyperpigmentation of the epidermal basal layer, hemosiderin and melanin in the dermis, and thickening of the arteriolar basement membrane. There is no effective treatment but some lesions resolve spontaneously in 18–24 months on average though atrophic hypopigmented scars are seen afterward. Infection prevention can be indicated and new lesions may always arise.

Disseminated Granuloma Annulare

Granuloma annulare (Fig. 61.8) is a rare benign inflammatory disease. The main efflorescences are erythematous papules which slowly expand centrifugally and resolve centrally to reveal annular plaques with superficial scaling. The back of the hands and arms are usually affected. Patients are usually asymptomatic but can experience pruritus. The disease can occur at any age but is mostly seen in children and adolescents. Multiple subtypes exist. Its relation to diabetes has been the subject of many discussions over the years and now only the disseminated form is believed to be associated with diabetes and even this correlation is only based on retrospective studies and currently no case control studies are available [34, 35]. Generalized granuloma annulare can also be seen in malignancies, thyroid dysfunction, hepatitis B, C and HIV infections [36–40]. Histology reveals a granulomatous reaction pattern showing palisading of histiocytes (and sometimes giant cells) and lymphocytes surrounding an area of necrobiotic/collagenolytic collagen (complete type) (Fig. 61.9). The necrobiotic areas show deposition of mucin. The incomplete type shows interstitial inflammation with histiocytes (sometimes admixed with giant cells) and lymphocytes and also mucin deposition can be found (incomplete/interstitial form). Pathologists sometimes have difficulties differentiating this disease from necrobiosis lipoidica because both present with infiltrating palisaded histiocytes and collagen degeneration in the dermis. In the disseminated form, inflammation may be mild and the areas of inflammation are often found in the papillary dermis as seen in lichen nitidus. Also, necrobiosis and mucin deposition might be less profound. Not only pathologists have a hard time differentiating these diseases, they are also clinically resembling and might even coexist. Some authors suggest that generalized granuloma annulare is an early phase of nec-

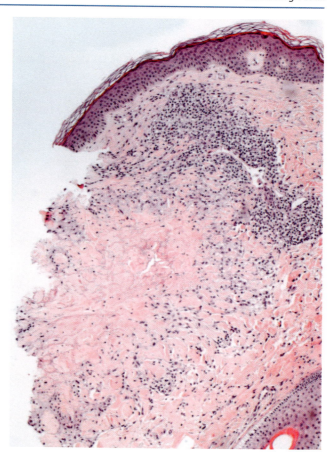

Fig. 61.9 Disseminated granuloma annulare. Areas of necrobiosis are surrounded by palisading histiocytes and lymphocytic inflammation. Although the histopathological features can be identical to classical granuloma annulare, disseminated granuloma annulare often shows a mild infiltrate located in the papillary dermis.

robiosis lipoidica, [41] although in the former no epidermal atrophy or yellow discoloration is seen.

In contrast to localized forms, generalized granuloma annulare only rarely resolves spontaneously. A protracted and relapsing course is usually seen with often therapy-resistant lesions. Many different types of treatment have been used including cryotherapy, topical, intralesional or systemic corticosteroids, phototherapy (UVA1 and PUVA), chlorambucil, pentoxifylline, cyclosporine, fumaric acid ester derivatives, potassium iodide, niacinamide, etanercept, infliximab, adalimumab, efalizumab, hydroxychloroquine, and dapsone.

Eruptive Xanthomas

Eruptive xanthomas are small (1–2 mm) yellow papules with erythematous border appearing in weeks to months, mostly asymptomatic but sometimes tender. They appear most frequently on the extensor surfaces of the limbs and the buttocks. Lesions often occur as a result of Koebner phenomenon on pressure sites. The yellow discoloration is due to foamy

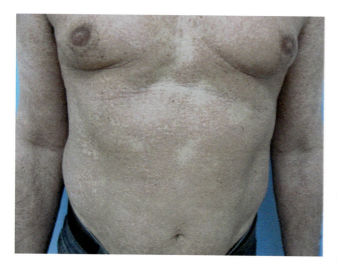

Fig. 61.8 Disseminated granuloma annulare

macrophages in the dermal inflammatory infiltrate of lymphocytes and neutrophils. They are associated with elevated eruptive triglycerides in the blood of patients with poorly controlled diabetes (especially Type 2), in familial hypertriglyceridemia and in patients using excessive amounts of alcohol. Insulin stimulates the activity of lipoprotein lipase and plays a role in the metabolism of triglycerides. This leads to a decreased clearance of very low density lipoproteins and chylomicrons. This can be aggravated further by polyphagia caused by glycosuria [42, 43]. Clinicians should be aware of a significantly elevated risk of pancreatitis [44]. Only 0.1% of patients with diabetes will develop eruptive xanthomas. The main treatment objective is controlling the hypertriglyceridemia and to be aware of other problems related to this condition. Control of diabetes and hyperlipidemia leads to swift disappearance of the xanthomas. Local therapeutic options are application of trichloroacetic acid, excision, curettage, and CO_2 laser therapy.

Infections

Recurrent skin infections may be the presenting feature of diabetes. Bacterial and fungal infections appear more frequently, more severe, and atypical. Skin infections occur in 20–50% of diabetic patients, more frequently in Type 2 and are associated with poor glycemic control. Patients with well-controlled diabetes are not at higher risk of infections. Viral infection on the contrary are not more frequent. For further details, we refer to Chap. 66 on infections.

Lichen Planus

Lichen planus (Fig. 61.10) is a chronic inflammatory disease of the skin, mucous membranes, scalp, and nails. Lesions are pruritic and present as flat-topped polygonal violaceous papules. Wickham striae can be visible on oral mucosa only and consist of a fine reticular network of white arborizing lines but lichen planus can also affect genital mucosa. Four Ps (pruritic, purple, polygonal, and papules or plaques) can be used as a mnemonic. The exact pathogenesis of lichen planus is not clear but it has been postulated to be a T-cell-mediated autoimmune process, resulting in damage of keratinocytes [45–47]. Microscopic examination of a skin specimen reveals specific changes consisting of a lichenoid lymphocytic infiltrate with liquefactive degeneration (Fig. 61.11). Half of the patients with lichen planus have impaired glucose metabolism and approximately 25% suffer from diabetes. The reverse relationship has been examined much less, and the association is still controversial. Prevalence ranges from 0.9 to 1.4% in the general population vs. 2 to 4% in patients with either Type 1 or 2 diabetes [48–50]. Although the dis-

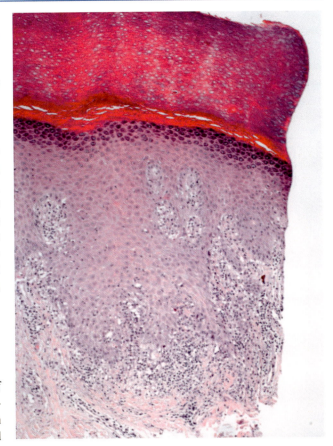

Fig. 61.10 Lichen planus. The lesion shows hyperkeratosis, acanthosis, and a lichenoid interface dermatitis with scattered apoptotic cells along the basement membrane

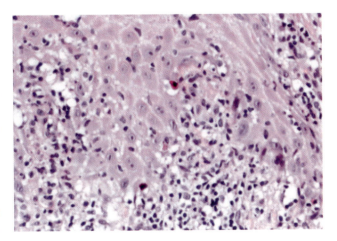

Fig. 61.11 Lichen planus. An interface dermatitis is noted with scattered apoptotic keratinocytes along the basal layer

ease is usually self-limiting, patients are frequently treated. Topical corticosteroids should be tried first. If necessary other options include oral corticosteroids, oral retinoids, cyclosporine, and phototherapy which have all shown efficacy.

Necrobiosis Lipoidica

Necrobiosis lipoidica (Fig. 61.12) is a chronic inflammatory skin disorder of collagen degeneration with a granulomatous response, thickening of the blood vessel walls and fat deposition [51]. A small clinical study determined that patients with necrobiosis lipoidica had a higher proportion of natural antibodies against such as actin, myosin, keratin, desmin when compared to patients with Type 1 diabetes mellitus and healthy control subjects [52, 53]. The disease is typically seen in patients in the third to fourth decade. Normally patients are asymptomatic though pain and pruritus can occur. Necrobiosis lipoidica starts with bilateral non-scaling red papules mostly seen on the pretibial regions though other regions can be involved. Red-brown rims may indicate disease activity. There is a centrifugal spreading pattern. Red papules slowly turn into atrophic lesions with central yellow discoloration possibly due to underlying dermal fibrosis and lipid excess in the dermis or due to the formation of advanced glycation end products, especially 2-(2-furoyl)-4[5]-(2-furanyl)-1H-imidazole which has a yellow hue. Telangiectasia can be seen through the translucent plaque. In advanced disease, large plaques can be seen and 35% of the lesions show ulceration. It should be known that chronic ulceration is a risk factor for the development of squamous cell carcinomas. Necrobiosis lipoidica is generally recognized in association with diabetes mellitus, however, the precise biological association remains unclear. In addition, quite recently necreobiosis lipoidica also has been associated with obesity, hypertension, dyslipidemia, and thyroidal disorder [54, 55]. The prevalence of necrobiosis lipoidica ranges from 0.3 to 1.2% in all diabetics to 2 to 3% in the insulin-dependent subtype. Even higher percentages in female patients have been reported. Necrobiosis lipoidica is thought to be the best recognized skin-associated disease of diabetes although it is rare. Prevalence ranges from 0.3 to 1.2% of all diabetics to 2 to 3% in the insulin-dependent subtype and even higher rates in female patients. Patients with Type 1 diabetes develop the disease earlier than those with Type 2 diabetes. Diabetes usually proceeds with the onset of necrobiosis lipoidica by 10 years although simultaneous and reverse patterns can be seen [56]. The association is less strong if the skin disease presents on other body parts than the legs. Whether the severity of diabetes and the activity of necrobiosis lipoidica are correlated is still uncertain. Its presence is worth mentioning given the higher prevalence of retino- and nephropathy. Histology shows a dermal infiltrate which usually affects the entire thickness of the dermis. The infiltrate tends to be horizontally orientated showing intervening layers of granulomatous inflammation and horizontal layers of necrobiosis (sandwich), in areas showing palisading of histiocytes surrounding necrobiosis. The deep dermis often shows admixture with lymphocytes and plasmacells (Fig. 61.13). Whether microangiopathy, neuropathy, trauma, immunoglobulin deposition causing vasculitis or a combination of these forms the origin of the collagen matrix destruction is still under discussion. Necrobiosis lipoidica is very

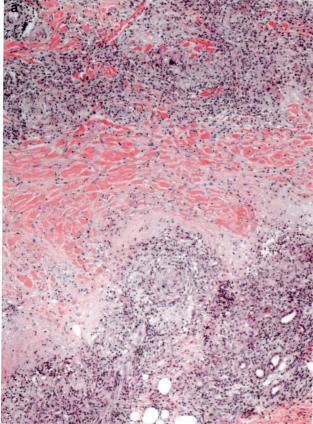

Fig. 61.13 Necrobios lipoidica. The infiltrate shows horizontal "sandwich" layering of (**a**) granulomatous inflammation and necrobiosis (**b**) and fibrosis. The deep dermis often shows a surrounding lymphocytic infiltrate admixed with plasmacells (**c**).

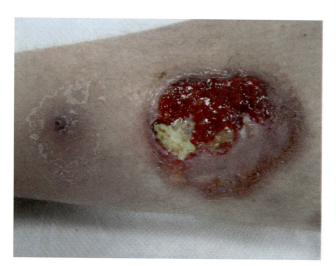

Fig. 61.12 Necrobiosis lipoidica

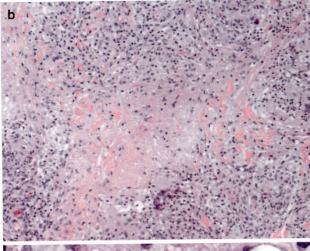

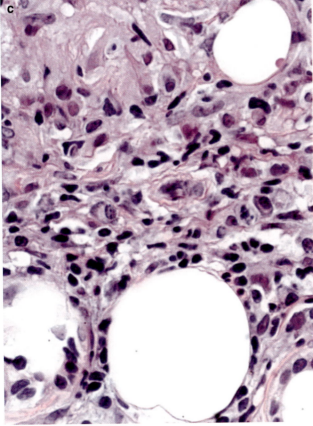

Fig. 61.13 (continued)

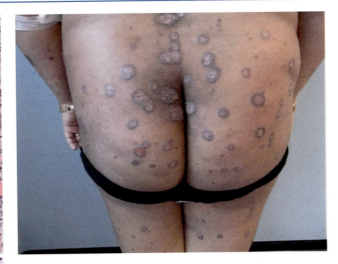

Fig. 61.14 Psoriasis vulgaris

ation (PUVA). Lesions tend to relapse with therapy cessation. Spontaneous resolution is seen in 13–19% of patients after 6 to 12 years [42].

Psoriasis Vulgaris

Psoriasis (Fig. 61.14) is a chronic immune-mediated inflammatory disease of the skin. Patients present with erythematous scaly papules and plaques occurring most frequently in areas of friction [53]. It is common; the prevalence worldwide is estimated to be 1–3% [59]. Association between these two diseases has been made but up until now no consensus was made. Patients with diabetes may present with a more edematous inflammatory course of psoriasis as well as more therapy-resistant psoriasis [60]. Treatment consists of topical (e.g., calcipotriol, corticosteroids, and tacrolimus) or systemic immunomodelators, as well as UV light [53].

Pruritus, Xerosis Cutis, and Keratosis Pilaris

Xerosis cutis, xeroderma, or dry skin is one of the earliest and most frequent skin signs in diabetes, found in almost half the diabetic population. Dry mucous membranes, for example laryngitis scleroticans sicca can be observed as well. Xerosis can be demonstrated in diabetics by measuring transipedermal water loss and high frequency conductance of the forearm [54]. We should keep in mind that both xerosis cutis and diabetes mellitus are very common. The presence of xerosis cutis increases the risk of complications, including infection and ulceration [53]. Pruritus is the main complaint patients present with. In atopic patients, the prevalence of xerosis cutis is higher.

hard to treat, but sometimes slow healing occurs. No positive effect of glycemic control has been demonstrated so far [57, 58]. Topical steroids (if necessary under occlusion) are a therapeutic option but can also worsen the atrophy. If an active border is seen, intralesional steroids may be of help. Topical calcineurin inhibitors and compression therapy might be effective. Systemic treatment is possible with chloroquine, fumaric acid ester derivatives, mycophenolate mofetil, cyclosporine, anti-TNF alpha, and psoralen with ultraviolet A radi-

Xerosis cutis is believed to result from sympathetic and sensory neuropathy and also vasculopathy. Sweat gland dysfunction starts with thermoregulatory dysfunction of the extremities and later on the entire body (global anhidrosis), although the reverse can occur (e.g., postprandial gustatory sweating on the face, neck, and chest). Chronic generalized pruritus can be a sign of undiagnosed diabetes as well as truncal pruritus, burning feet syndrome, pruritus vulvae, and anogenital pruritus although the latter may be secondary to candidiasis or streptococci infection. Clinicians should keep in mind that underlying illness and drug reactions also cause pruritus. Regular use of emollients helps to prevent this skin problem.

Keratosis pilaris consists of rough follicular papules and variable erythema on the extensor surfaces of the extremities and sometimes on the face, buttocks, and trunk. It flares up in wintertime. 11.7% of children with Type 1 diabetes have keratosis pilaris but it is very common in non-diabetic patients as well. Xerosis cutis certainly plays a role in this disease. Treatment is difficult and not strictly necessary but emollients as well as keratolytic agents, retinoids, and topical corticosteroids of low potency can be helpful.

Rubeosis Faciei—Palmar Erythema and Periungual Telangiectasia

Acral erythema is an erysipelas-like erythema of the hands (especially the thenar and hypothenar region) and feet and has a mostly patchy distribution due to microangiopathy [61]. It differs from physiological erythema caused by warmth, emotional state, hand elevation, and external pressure in its distribution and aspect of the erythema.

Rubeosis faciei is a relatively common chronic flushed appearance of the face, neck, and upper extremities. It is more easily to notice in Fitzpatrick skin types one and two.

These two asymptomatic skin signs both result from small vessel occlusive disease with compensatory hyperemia of superficial blood vessels or from decreased vascular tone. Described prevalence in patients with Type 1 and 2 diabetes range from less than 10% to over 60% [62–65]. This might be due to confounding factors such as Fitzpatrick skin type [66], severity of disease, and inpatient status. It is associated with vessel engorgement which contributes to visual impairment in diabetics. The erythema (Fig. 61.15) is directly related to disease duration. Improvement is seen with adequate control of blood sugar levels but these phenomena flare up with concomitant use of vasodilating therapies or vasodilators such as caffeine and alcohol.

Periungual telangiectasia are clinically visible dilated capillary veins due to loss of capillary loops and dilation of other surrounding capillaries. It is seen in 40–50% of all patients with diabetes. It can also be seen in connective tis-

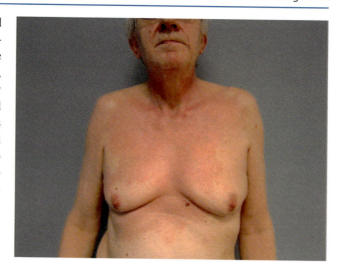

Fig. 61.15 Erythema

sue diseases such as scleredema and dermatomyositis. It is highly likely that nail folds show erythema and that cuticles are ragged (this should not be confused with paronychia caused by infection). Some patients are asymptomatic while others experience discomfort in their fingertips. No treatment is necessary [53].

Different skin types are divided based on skin color and response to ultraviolet irradiation.

Skin Thickening and Scleredema Diabeticorum

Skin thickening and scleredema diabeticorum are associated with long-term disease progression and diabetic neuropathy ($P < 0.05$) [67] and is a cutaneous marker for other microvascular complications.

There are three subtypes of skin thickening. In the first subtype, there is a benign asymptomatic thickening which is only measurable with ultrasonography. This type is seen in nearly 25% of all diabetic patients. The second type of skin thickening is clinically noticeable. Phenotypes range from Huntley papules to diabetic hand syndrome in 8 to 50% of diabetic patients [68, 69]. The initial complaints in diabetic hand syndrome consist of stiffness and progresses to limited joint mobility and possibly Dupuytren contracture (caused by shortening of skin anchoring ligaments).

Scleredema diabeticorum is a rare asymptomatic diffuse ill-defined erythematous induration of the upper back and neck possibly extending to the deltoid and lumbar region. Acral regions are spared. The skin can have a peau d'orange aspect. Reduced elasticity of the skin can result in reduced joint mobility, and thus stiffness frequently coexists. Two-and-a-half to 14% of patients with diabetes suffer from this condition. Men and obese patients with long lasting Type 2 diabetes are at higher risk. Pathology reports show an unaffected epidermis and a homogenous thickened dermis with activated fibroblasts and enlarged collagen bundles separated by mucin deposition. It is important to take a full thickness excisional biopsy. An excess of blood glucose leads to collagen synthesis by fibroblasts and retarded collagen degradation and glycosaminoglycan depositions. Scleredema is also seen in rheumatoid arthritis, hyperparathyroidism, Sjögren's syndrome, and seldom in IgG paraproteinemia or malignancy.

Scleredema diabeticorum and classic scleredema are clinically difficult to distinguish but appear to have distinct light and electron microscopic features [70]. Scleredema diabeticorum does not improve with glycemic control although this measure is believed to be an important preventive tool. Treatment is often difficult and includes UVA (psoralen UVA as well as UVA1) and systemic therapy such as oral corticosteroids, cyclosporine, cyclophosphamide. In severe cases, radiotherapy could give some relief [71–74].

Ulcers

see Chap. 65, foot complications.

Vitiligo

In vitiligo (Fig. 61.16), depigmented maculae are seen which are slowly progressive. The extent of affected skin ranges from localized to generalized and even universal and is mostly seen on the face, hands, and genitals. Histopathology shows the absence of melanocytes in the basal layer after Melan A staining (Figs. 61.17 and 61.18). It is possible that some melanocytes are seen around the hair follicles. The depigmentation is the result of immune mediated melanocyte loss or function loss, and tyrosinase is the main antigen

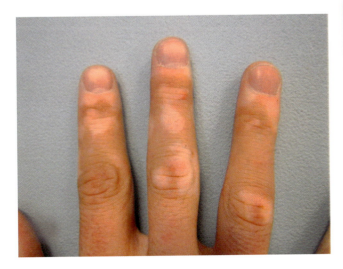

Fig. 61.16 Vitiligo

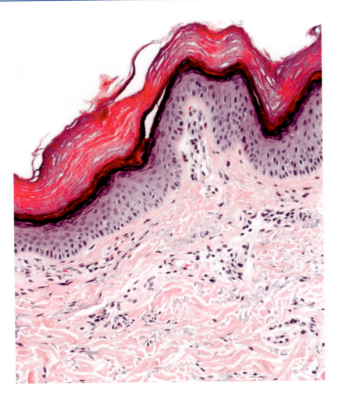

Fig. 61.17 Vitiligo. Absence of melanocytes (HE stain)

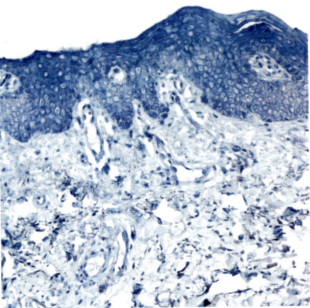

Fig. 61.18 Vitiligo. Absence of melanocytes (Melan A stain)

recognized. One in three patients has a positive family history of vitiligo. One to 7% of insulin-dependent diabetics suffers from vitiligo [2] compared to a 0.2 to 1% prevalence in the global population making it the most common depigmenting disorder [5]. Due to the high number of Type 2 diabetics, these patients will be seen more often with vitiligo, though it is relatively more prevalent in Type 1 diabetes. The combination of Type 1 diabetes and vitiligo is suggestive for polyglandular autoimmune syndrome. This is a rare immune-mediated endocrinopathy with at least two affected endocrine glands. In these cases, vitiligo is often more difficult to treat. Patients should avoid sun exposure. Topical corticosteroids of high potency can give satisfying results if applied early on (with or without narrow-band ultraviolet B). Topical calcineurin inhibitors have shown some benefit. PUVA and 8-methoxypsoralen lotion can be used as well. In generalized vitiligo, treatment with ultraviolet B light may be an option as well. Camouflage therapy is an option if patients have cosmetic concerns.

Yellow Skin

The yellow skin of some diabetic patients consists of an orange to yellow discoloration of the skin, most obvious on the palms and soles. The sclerae are spared in contrast to patients suffering from jaundice. Yellow nails (Fig. 61.19) affects up to 40% of diabetic patients, especially the elderly. The yellow color is best visible at the distal part of the nails, and these discolored nails have a slower growth rate and appear more curved due to poor vascularization of the nail matrix. Differential diagnosis includes physiological processes in the elderly, onychomycosis, yellow nail syndrome, yellow nails due to lymphedema or respiratory tract disease [75].

The relationship of both discolorations to diabetes mellitus is questionable. Some believe that diabetic patients are exposed to higher levels of carotene in their diet rich of fruits and vegetables, which together with an impaired hepatic conversion leads to carotenemia and thus yellow discoloration of skin and nails. Differential diagnosis of carotenemia includes jaundice hypothyroidism, hypogonadism, hypopituitarism, bulimia and anorexia nervosa [13].

Another possibility is the formation of advanced glycation end products, especially 2-(2-furoyl)-4[5]-(2-furanyl)-1H-imidazole, which has a yellow hue as mentioned earlier. There is currently no treatment available.

Mucormycosis

Mucormycosis is a rare opportunistic fungal infection, with a high mortality rate, caused by fungal species belonging to the order Mucorales (class Zygomycetes). Mucormycosis occurs in immunocompromised patients. Risk factors include poorly controlled diabetes mellitus, end-stage renal disease, hematologic malignancies, and solid organ transplantation. It can affect various organs, including sinuses, nose, eyes, brain, intestine, lungs, and skin. Clinical presentation depends on the anatomical site of involvement, which is associated with the predisposing medical condition. Diabetes mellitus, for example, was found to be correlated with rhino-cerebral mucormycosis [76]. In the skin, it presents as an indurated plaque which rapidly evolves into a necrotic ulcer. The diagnosis can be confirmed by histological evalution; broad non-septate hyphae can be observed in blood vessels (Fig. 61.20).

Whilst mucormycosis is prevalent globally, the disease is most common in India [77]. Lately, higher infection rates have been reported worldwide in COVID-19 patients [78, 79]. The exact incidence and prevalence remain unknown. Treatment of mucormycosis is difficult, as mucorales are naturally resistant to most antifungals. Amphotericin B and surgical debridement or excision are the most effective options [78].

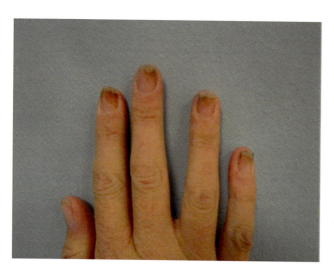

Fig. 61.19 Yellow nails

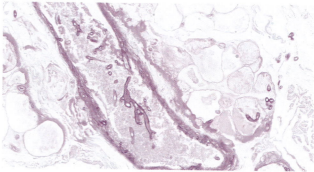

Fig. 61.20 Mucormycosis: Broad non-septate hyphae in a vascular lumen and wall. PAS+ stain

Necrotising Fasciitis

Necrotising fasciitis is a bacterial infection, localised in any of the layers within the soft tissue compartment (dermis, subcutaneous fat tissue, superficial fascia, deep fascia, or muscle). It is a rapidly progressive disease with a high mortality rate. Early recognition, surgical treatment (amputation, fasciotomy, and debridement of necrotic tissue), plus intravenous antibiotic therapy, and hemodynamic support are the most important factors effecting survival rate [80, 81]. Patients usually present with pain disproportionate to clinical signs, which may include erythema with poorly defined edges, oedema, and bullae. At a later stage, purpura and necrotic tissue may be present. Furthermore, patients can present with signs of sepsis, such as hypotension, tachycardia, and fever [81, 82]. Microscopically an extensive diffuse neutrophilic infiltrate can be seen in the subcutaneous fat tissue (Fig. 61.21a, b). However, necrotising fasciitis is a clinical diagnosis.

Necrotising fasciitis may result from any skin damage (i.e., minor trauma, skin biopsy, laceration, insect bite, needle puncture [particularly intravenous drug use], chronic ulcer, herpes zoster, surgical wound, skin abscess). Diabetes mellitus is the most common co-morbidity associated with necrotising fasciitis. A possible explanation why patients with diabetes are more prone to necrotizing fasciitis is that peripheral sensory polyneuropathy increases susceptibility to minor trauma. Next to this, tissue hypoxia caused by vasculopathy and the underlying immunodeficiency in diabetic patients may ease out bacterial colonization [83]. Other predisposing factors include use of immunosuppressants, malnutrition, and peripheral arterial disease [3]. COVID-19 can be an aggravating factor [84].

COVID-19, the Skin, and Diabetes

COVID-19, caused by the novel coronavirus SARS-CoV-2, is most notorious for causing respiratory pathology. However, multiple extrapulmonary manifestations have been described, among which is skin manifestations. Erythematous rash, chil-

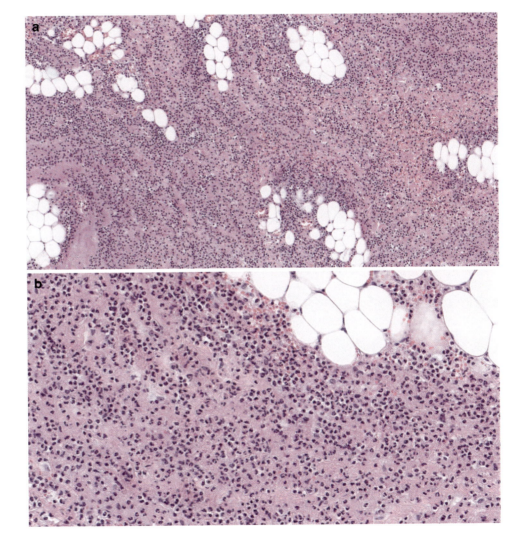

Fig. 61.21 (a) (Magnification 10×)—necrotising fasciitis: An extensive and almost pure diffuse neutrophilic infiltrate in the subcutaneous fat. (b) (Magnification 40×)—necrotising fasciitis: An extensive and almost pure diffuse neutrophilic infiltrate in the subcutaneous fat

blain-like lesions, and urticarial lesions were most commonly reported [85, 86]. Other manifestations include exanthema in various forms (morbilliform/maculopapular/papulovesicular), livedoid/necrotic lesions, and purpura/petechiae. The skin lesions were often accompanied by pruritus and were mostly self-resolving [83–87]. SARS-CoV-2 enters the human cells via the angiotensin-converting enzyme 2 (ACE2) receptor, which is expressed in various organs, including the skin. Especially, keratinocytes in the epidermis show a high expression of ACE2, which can explain the presence of cutaneous manifestations in COVID-19 patients [85, 88].

Diabetes mellitus is one of the comorbidities associated with COVID-19, and diabetic patients are at risk of developing a more severe disease manifestation. Hyperglycemia and ketosis, as a result of deterioration in pancreatic β-cell function and apoptosis, caused by elevated cytokine levels, are mechanisms that may account for the more severe disease course. Next to this, the presence of ACE2 receptors in the pancreas might contribute to insulin deficiency and hyperglycemia. Consequently, COVID-19 can be associated with deterioration of skin manifestations of diabetes mellitus [88, 89].

Side Effects of Medication

Side Effects of Insulin

Insulin Lipodystrophy.
Atrophy and hypertrophy of the skin might both occur although they are less frequently seen since the use of more pure insulins and synthetic analogues. Hypertrophy used to be present in two-thirds of insulin-dependent patients, but this number has been reduced to 1 to 2 %. It is characterized by a localized hypertrophy of subcutaneous fat. In these hypertrophic areas, insulin absorption is delayed; therefore, patients should rotate the injection site. Hypertrophy resolves spontaneously.

Atrophy at the insulin injection sites is due to an immunological reaction including IgM, IgE, and C3 in dermal blood vessels initiating a signal cascade that inhibits adipocyte differentiation [90]. Duration of exposure and depot formation play a role in the onset of atrophy. Substitution with fast acting insulin has been suggested as therapy [3]. It is unknown why women are more likely to develop atrophy and why men suffer from lipohypertrophy more often.

Continuous subcutaneous insulin infusion with the latest types of infusion materials does not frequently induce local infections, although allergy to tape and certain tubing constituents can be seen.

Allergic reactions to insulin are seen in approximately 2.4% of insulin-dependent diabetics. They can be classified into four categories (immediate local, generalized, delayed, and biphasic). Immediate local reactions range from erythema to urticaria and are assumed to be IgE mediated. Peak intensity is reached in 15–30 min and resolves within an hour. The immediate local reaction may progress to generalized erythema and urticaria. Anaphylaxis is rare. Delayed forms (4–24 h after injection appearing 2 weeks after the start with insulin therapy [3, 11]) present most frequently with itchy nodules at the injection site. Biphasic reactions are rare and consist of a combination of an immediate and a delayed local reaction in patients with symptoms resembling serum sickness. Treatment with topical corticosteroids is almost always successful.

Oral Hypoglycemic Medication

A wide range of quit frequently appearing cutaneous drug reactions to oral antidiabetic agents have been described ranging from pruritus, photosensitivity, allergic reactions, erythema multiforme, erythema nodosum, urticarial and pruritus to lichenoid, and morbilliform eruptions.

- Sulphonylurea has the most skin-related side effects, as approximately 1 to 5% of patients develop cutaneous reactions within 2 months of treatment. Maculopapular eruptions are the most common. Other cutaneous side effects include erythema, urticaria, erythema multiforme, exfoliative dermatitis, erythema nodosum, pemphigus vulgaris, psoriasiform, and lichenoid drug eruptions. Most sulfonylureas can induce photosensitivity. Even with a negative patch test, oral antidiabetic therapies should be switched.
- Approximately 20 % develop an alcohol flush with symptoms of redness, warmth, headache, tachycardia, and seldom dyspnea within 15 min after alcohol consumption and disappearing within the hour. Second- generation sulphonylureas present with less cutaneous side effects.
- Meglinitinides or glinides rarely cause cutaneous reactions (<0.01%). If present, they usually consist of pruritus, rash, urticarial, or generalized reactions such as anaphylaxic shock.
- Biguanides such as metformin cause cutaneous side effects ranging from psoriasiform drug eruptions and leucocytoclastic vasculitis to phototoxic reactions and erythema multiforme.
- Thiazolidinediones glitazones can seldom cause edema.
- Dipeptidyl peptidase IV inhibitors give dose-dependent necrotic skin lesions in monkeys. Increased rates of angioedema are noted only if they are used together with ace inhibitors due to inhibition of the degradation of bradykinin and substance P. Case reports show severe skin reactions such as bullous pemphigoid, Stevens–Johnson syndrome and toxic epidermal necrosis.

– Alpha glucosidase inhibitors-like acarbose have been responsible for acute generalized exanthematous pustulosis and erythema multiforme.
– Injection of Glucagon-like-peptide-1 receptor agonist (or incretinomimetics) can cause local granulomatous reactions (e.g., eosinophilic sclerosing lipogranulomas).

Concluding Remarks

The skin is often involved in diabetes mellitus as well as in side effects of medications used to treat diabetes. Some of those skin diseases are more specific for diabetes than others and some are more frequent in Type 1, others in Type 2 or both types of diabetes mellitus.

The intensity ranges from mild to severe. Recognizing these skin conditions may be of great value since they can be the presenting symptom in diabetes mellitus, port of entry for infection, or sign of advanced disease.

Multiple Choice Questions

1. Which statement is false?
   A. **A Circa 10% of all patients with diabetes mellitus develop skin manifestations.**
      False, 30–80% of all patients with diabetes mellitus develop skin manifestations.
   B. Patients care a lot about the appearance of their skin.
   C. Disseminated granuloma annulare can be observed in diabetes mellitus patients, malignancies, thyroid dysfunction, hepatitis B, C, and HIV infections.
   D. Skin manifestations of diabetes mellitus can be present before the diagnosis of diabetes mellitus.
   E. Some of the skin manifestations of diabetes mellitus are linked to neuropathy and angiopathy.
2. What is true about acanthosis nigricans?
   A. Acanthosis nigricans can only occur in patients with diabetes mellitus.
   B. Acanthosis nigricans is highly disabling.
   C. **Acanthosis nigricans occurs in the intertriginous areas.**
      Correct, especially in the neck, armpits, and groins.
   D. After treatment no recurrence is possible.
   E. It occurs more often in the Caucasian race.
3. Acquired perforating dermatosis is (Fig. 60.22).
   A. easy to treat.
   B. a frequently appearing dermatosis.
   C. is most frequently seen on the flexor areas of the lower extremities.
   D. **a highly pruritic skin disease.**
Correct. It presents with scaly highly pruritic follicular hyperkeratotic papules and nodules.

E. more frequently seen in Caucasian people.
4. Which statement about bullosis diabeticorum is false?
   A. There are three known subtypes.
   B. **all subtypes heal without scarring.**
      False, the cleavage level of the second subtype lies below the dermoepidermal junction so healing leaves scars.
   C. It occurs more frequently in men with longstanding poorly controlled Type 1 diabetes.
   D. No treatment is needed.
   E. Primary autoimmune blistering should be excluded.
5. Diabetic dermopathy is.
   A. **a synonym for shin spots.**
      Correct, these are asymmetric red to brown hyperpigmentated spots.
   B. a synonym for diabetic stiff hands.
   C. no reason to screen for diabetes mellitus.
   D. a skin manifestation that never preceeds to diabetes mellitus.
   E. a unilateral appearing dermatosis.
6. Which statement concerning eruptive xanthomas is false?
   A. A Patients with eruptive xanthomas are usually asymptomatic.
   B. There is a correlation with elevated blood triglycerides.
   C. There is an elevated risk of pancreatitis.
   D. **Systemic treatment is indicated.**
      False, the main treatment objective is controlling the hypertriglyceridemia. Local therapeutics can be used.
   E. 10% of all diabetes mellitus patients develop eruptive xanthomas.
7. Which statement on granuloma annulare is false?
   A. Granuloma annulare is a rare benign inflammatory disease.
   B. This disease usually occurs on the hands and arms.
   C. **All forms occur more frequently in patients with diabetes mellitus.**
      False, only the disseminated form occurs more frequently in diabetes mellitus patients.
   D. It is sometimes histopathologically difficult to distinguish from necrobiosis lipoidica.
   E. Multiple subtypes exist.
8. Which statement on lichen planus is true?
   A. Lichen planus is a chronic inflammatory disease due to overactivity of the B cells.
   B. Lichen planus only occurs on the oral mucous membrane.
   C. The relationship to diabetes mellitus is completely clear.
   D. Lichen planus only occurs on the skin.
   E. **Four Ps can be used as a mnemonic.**

Correct, it stands for pruritic, purple, polygonal, papules, or plaques.

9. What is true about necrobiosis lipoidica?
   A. **A It is important to diagnose.**
      Correct, prevalence of retinopathy and nephropathy is higher in this subgroup of patients.
   B. Never preceeds to diabetes mellitus.
   C. Occurs in the first and second decade.
   D. This skin condition never heals.
   E. This skin condition is easy to treat.

10. Which statement on vitiligo is false?
   A. Patients with vitiligo should avoid sun exposure.
   B. After melan A staining, no melanocytes are observed on histopathological examination.
   C. **It occurs more often in Type 2 diabetes.**
      False, vitiligo occurs more frequently in Type 1 diabetes. Both are auto-immune diseases.
   D. Ultraviolet B light may be of help in the treatment of this disease.
   E. Topical corticosteroids and calcineurin inhibitors are used in the treatment of vitiligo.

Glossary

Atrophy A loss of tissue from the epidermis, dermis, or subcutaneous tissues. There may be fine wrinkling and increased translucency if the process is superficial.

Erythema Redness of the skin produced by vascular congestion or increased perfusion.

Koebner phenomenon The onset of new inflammatory skin lesions after minor trauma such as scratching.

Macula A circumscribed alteration in the color of the skin.

Nodule A solid mass in the skin, which can be observed as an elevation or can be palpated. It is more than 0.5 cm in diameter. It may involve epidermis and dermis, dermis and subcutis, or subcutis alone. It may consist of fluid, other extracellular material (e.g., amyloid), inflammatory, or neoplastic cells.

Papule A circumscribed palpable elevation, less than 0.5 cm in diameter. By careful examination it is often possible to determine whether the thickening involves predominantly the epidermis or the dermis and what type of pathological process is concerned. The only distinction between a papule and a nodule is the size, and this is artificial; some lesions characteristically occur at the smaller size of a papule, whereas others typically enlarge from a papule to become a nodule. Recording a finite size is more useful.

Plaque An elevated area of skin, usually defined as 2 cm or more in diameter. It may be formed by the extension or coalescence of either papules or nodules as in psoriasis and granuloma annulare, respectively. Small plaque is sometimes used for such lesions 0.5–2 cm in diameter.

Sclerosis Diffuse or circumscribed induration of the subcutaneous tissues. It may also involve the dermis, when the overlying epidermis may be atrophic. It is characteristically seen in scleroderma, but may occur as a sequel to or in association with many different processes.

Ulcer A loss of dermis and epidermis, often with loss of the underlying tissues.

Vesicles and bullae Visible accumulation of fluid within or beneath the epidermis. Vesicles are small (less than 0.5 cm in diameter) and often grouped. Bullae, which may be of any size over 0.5 cm, should be subdivided as multilocular (due to coalesced vesicles, typically in eczema) or unilocular [91]

References

1. Baselga Torres E, Torres-Pradilla M. Manifestaciones cutáneas en ninos con diabetes mellitus y obesidad. Actas Dermosifiliogr. 2014;105:546–57.
2. Van Hattem S, Bootsma AH, Thio HB. Skin manifestations of diabetes. Cleve Clin J Med. 2008;75(11):772–87.
3. Demirseren DD, Emre S, Akoglu G, et al. Relationship between skin diseases and extracutaneous complications of diabetes mellitus : clinical analysis of 750 patients. Am J Clin Dermatolo. 2014;15:65–70.
4. Han G. A new appraisal of dermatologic manifestations of diabetes mellitus. Cutis. 2014;94(1):E21–6.
5. Duff M, Demidova O, Blackburn S, et al. Cutaneous manifestations of diabetes mellitus. Clin Diabetes. 2015;33:40–8.
6. Halban PA, Polonsky KS, Bowden DW, Hawkins MA, Ling C, Mather KJ, et al. Beta-cell failure in type 2 diabetes: postulated mechanisms and prospects for prevention and treatment. Diabetes Care. 2014;37(6):1751–8.
7. Brownlee M. The pathobiology of diabetic complications: a unifying mechanism. Diabetes. 2005;54:1615–25.
8. Hosseini MS, Razavi Z, Ehsani AH, Firooz A, Afazeli S. Clinical significance of Non-invasive skin autofluorescence measurement in patients with diabetes: a systematic review and meta-analysis. EClinicalMedicine. 2021;16(42):101194.
9. Barlovic DP, Soro-Paavonen A, Jandeleit-Dahm KA. RAGE biology, atherosclerosis and diabetes. Clin Sci (Lond). 2011;121(2):43–55.
10. Wertheimer E, Trebicz M, Eldar T, et al. Differential roles of insulin receptor and insulin-like growth factor-1 receptor in differentiation of murine skin keratinocytes. J Invest Dermatol. 2000;115:24–9.
11. Benoliel AM, Kahn-Perles B, Imbert J, et al. Insulin stimulates haptotactic migration of human epidermal keratinocytes through activation of NF-kappa B transcription factor. J Cell Sci. 1997;110:2089–97.
12. Tsao MC, Walthall BJ, Ham RG. Clonal growth of normal human epidermal keratinocytes in a defined medium. J Cell Physiol. 1982;110:219–29.
13. Ahmed I, Goldstein B. Diabetes mellitus. Clin Dermatol. 2006;24(4):237–46.
14. Murphy-Chutorian B, Han G, Cohen SR. Dermatologic manifestations of diabetes mellitus: a review. Endocrinol Metab Clin N Am. 2013;42(4):869–98.
15. Brockow K, Steinkraus V, Rinninger F, Abeck D, Ring J. Acanthosis nigricans: a marker for hyperinsulinemia. Pediatr Dermatol. 1995;12:323–6.
16. Stuart CA, Gilkison CR, Smith MM, Bosma AM, Keenan BS, Nagamani M. Acanthosis nigricans as a risk factor for non-insulin-dependent diabetes mellitus. Clin Pediatr. 1998;37:73–9.
17. Kahana M, Grossman E, Feinstein A, et al. Skin tags: a cutaneous marker for diabetes mellitus. Acta Derm Venereol Suppl (Stockh). 1986;67:175–7.

18. Rasi A, Soltani-Arabshahi R, Shahbazi N. Skin tag as a cutaneous marker for impaired carbohydrate metabolism: a case-control study. Int J Dermatol. 2007;46:1155–9.

19. Sudy E, Urbina F, Maliqueo M, Sir T. Screening of glucose/insulin metabolic alterations in men with multiple skin tags on the neck. JDDG. 2008;6(10):852–6.

20. Levy L, Zeichner JA. Dermatologic manifestations of diabetes. J. Diabetes. 2012;4:68–76.

21. Ferringer T, Miller F. Cutaneous manifestations of diabetes mellitus. Dermatol Clin. 2002;20:483–92.

22. Farrel AM. Acquired perforating dermatosis in renal and diabetic patients. Lancet. 1997;349:895–6.

23. Lipsky BA, Baker PD, Ahroni JH. Diabetic bullae: 12 cases of a purportedly rare cutaneous disorder. Int J Dermatol. 2000;39:196–200.

24. Oursler JR, Goldblum OM. Blistering eruption in a diabetic. Bullosis diabeticorum. Arch Dermatol. 1991;127:247–50.

25. Perez MI, Kohn SR. Cutaneous manifestations of diabetes mellitus. J Am Acad Dermatol. 1994;30:519–31.

26. James WD, Odom RB, Goette DK. Bullous eruption of diabetes mellitus. A case with positive immunofluorescence microscopy findings. Arch Dermatol. 1980;116:1119–92.

27. Derighetti M, Hohl D, Krayenbuhl BH, Panizzon RG. Bullosis diabeticorum in a newly discovered type 2 diabetes mellitus. Dermatology. 2000;200:366–7.

28. Martinez DP, Diaz JO, Bobes CM. Eruptive xanthomas and acute pancreatitis in a patient with hypertriglyceridemia. Int Arch Med. 2008;1:6.

29. Hollister DS, Brodell RT. Finger 'pebbles'. A dermatologic sign of diabetes mellitus. Postgrad Med. 2000;107:209–10.

30. Quondamatteo F. Skin and diabetes mellitus: what do we know? Cell Tissue Res. 2014;355(1):1–21.

31. Morgan AJ, Schwartz RA. Diabetic dermopathy: a subtle sign with grave implications. J Am Acad Dermatol. 2008;58(3):447–51.

32. Romano G, Moretti G, Di Benedetto A, et al. Skin lesions in diabetes mellitus: prevalence and clinical correlations. Diabetes Res Clin Pract. 1998;39:101–6.

33. Morgan AJ, Schwartz RA. Diabetic dermopathy: a subtle sign with grave implications. J Am Acad Dermatol. 2008;58:447–51.

34. Yun JH, Lee JY, Kim MK, et al. Clinical and pathological features of generalized granuloma annulare with their correlation: a retrospective multicenter study in Korea. Ann Dermatol. 2009;21(2):113–9.

35. Dabski K, Winkelmann RK. Generalized granuloma annulare: clinical and laboratory findings in 100 patients. J Am Acad Dermatol. 1989;20:39–47.

36. Toro JR, Chu P, Yen TS, et al. Granuloma annulare and human immunodeficiency virus infection. Arch Dermatol. 1999;135:1341–6.

37. Goucha S, Khaled A, Kharfi M, et al. Granuloma annulare. G Ital Dermatol Venereol. 2008;143:359–63.

38. Granel B, Serratrice J, Rey J, et al. Chronic hepatitis C virus infection associated with a generalized granuloma annulare. J Eur Acad Dermatol Venereol. 2006;20:186–9.

39. Ma HJ, Zhu WY, Yue XZ. Generalized granuloma annulare and malignant neoplasms. Am J Dermapathol. 2003;25:113–6.

40. Li A, Hogan DJ, Sanusi ID, et al. Granuloma annulare and malignant neoplasms. Am J Dermapathol. 2003;25:113–6.

41. Marchetti F, Geraduzzi T, Longo F, Faleschini E, Ventura A, Tonini G. Maturity-onset diabetes of the young with necrobiosis lipoidica and granuloma annulare. Pediatr Dermatol. 2006;23:247–50.

42. Ferringer T, Miller F 3rd. Cutaneous manifestations of diabetes mellitus. Dermatol Clin. 2002;20:483–92.

43. Parker F. Xanthomas and hyperlipidemias. J Am Acad Dermatol. 1985;13:1–30.

44. Kala J, Mostow EN. Images in clinical medicine. Eruptive xanthoma. N Engl J Med. 2012;366(9):835.

45. Gorouhi F, Davari P, Fazel N. Cutaneous and mucosal lichen planus: a comprehensive review of clinical subtypes, risk factors, diagnosis and prognosis. Sci World J. 2014;2014:742826.

46. Iijima W, Ohtani H, Nakayama T, et al. Infiltrating CD8+ T cells in oral lichen planus predominantly express CCR5 and CXCR3 and carry respective chemokine ligands RANTES/CCL5 and IP-10/CXCL10 in their cytolytic granules: a potential self-recruiting mechanism. Am J Pathol. 2003;163:261–8.

47. Usatine RP, Tinitigan M. Diagnosis and treatment of lichen planus. Am Fam Physician. 2011;84:53–60.

48. Seyhan M, Ozcan H, Sahin I, et al. High prevalence of glucose metabolism disturbance in patients with lichen planus. Diabetes Res Clin Pract. 2007;77:198–202.

49. Puri N. A study on cutaneous manifestations of diabetes mellitus. Our Dermatol Online. 2012;3:83–6.

50. Mahajan S, Koranne RV, Sharma SK. Cutaneous manifestations of diabetes mellitus. Indian J Dermatol Venereol Leprol. 2003;69:105–8.

51. Wake N, Fang JC. Images in clinical medicine. Necrobiosis lipoidica diabeticorum. N Engl J Med. 2006;355:e20.

52. Haralambous S, Blackwell C, Mappouras DG, et al. Increased natural autoantibody activity to cytoskeleton proteins in sera from patients with necrobiosis lipoidica, with or without insulin-dependent diabetes mellitus. Autoimmunity. 1995;20:267–75.

53. Horton B, Boler L, Subauste AR. Diabetes mellitus and the skin: recognition and Management of Cutaneous Manifestations. South Med J. 2016;109(10):636–46.

54. Hashemi DA, Brown-Joel ZO, Tkachenko E, Nelson CA, Noe MH, Imadojemu S, Vleugels RA, Mostaghimi A, Wanat KA, Rosenbach M. Clinical features and comorbidities of patients with necrobiosis Lipoidica with or without diabetes. JAMA Dermatol. 2019;155(4):455–9.

55. Erfurt-Berge C, Heusinger V, Reinboldt-Jockenhöfer F, Dissemond J, Renner R. Comorbidity and therapeutic approaches in patients with necrobiosis Lipoidica. Dermatology. 2022;238(1):148–55.

56. Den Hollander JC, Hajdarbegovic E, Thio B, van der Leest RJT. Cutaneous manifestations of diabetes mellitus. In: Hall JC, Hall BJ, editors. Hall's manual of skin as a marker of underlying disease. Shelton: PMPH-USA; 2011. p. 245–59.

57. O'Toole EA, Kennedy U, Nolan JJ, et al. Necrobiosis lipoidica: only a minority of patients have diabetes mellitus. Br J Dermatol. 1999;140(2):283–6.

58. Cohen O, Yaniv R, Karasik A, Trau H. Necrobiosis lipoidica and diabetic control revisited. Med Hypotheses. 1996;46:348–50.

59. Non Arunachalam M, Dragoni F, Colucci R, et al. Non-segmental vitiligo and psoriasis comorbidity: a case-control study in Italian patients. J Eur Acad Dermatol Venereol. 2014;28(4):433–7.

60. Köstler E, Porst H, Wollina U. Cutaneous manifestations of metabolic diseases: uncommon presentations. Clinic Dermatol. 2005;23:457–64.

61. Yamaoka H, Sasaki H, Yamasaki H, et al. Truncal pruritus of unknown origin may be a symptom of diabetic polyneuropathy. Diabetes Care. 2010;33:150–5.

62. Singh R, Barden A, Mori T, et al. Advanced glycation end-products: a review. Diabetogia. 2001;44:129–46.

63. Young RJ, Hannan WJ, Frier BM, et al. Diabetic lipohypertrophy delays insulin absorption. Diabetes Care. 1984;7(5):479–80.

64. Naf S, Esmatjes E, Recasens M, et al. Continuous subcutaneous insulin infusion to resolve an allergy to human insulin. Diabetes Care. 2002;25:634–5.

65. Huntley A. Diabetes mellitus: review. Dermatol Online J. 1995;1:2. http://dermatology.cdlib.org/DOJvol1num2/diabetes/dmreview.html. Accessed July 30 2008

66. Lieverman LS, Rosenbloom AL, Riley WJ, et al. Reduced skin thickness with pump administration of insulin. N Engl J Med. 1980;303:940–1.

67. High AH, Tomasini CF, Argenziano G, Zalaudek I. Basic Principles of dermatology. In: Bolognia JL, Jorizzo JL, Schaffer JV, editors. Dermatology third edition. Philadelphia: Elsevier Saunders; 2012. p. 1–42.

68. Brik R, Berant M, Vardi P. The scleroderma-like syndrome of insulin-dependent diabetes mellitus. Diabetes Metab Rev. 1991;7:121–8.

69. Collier A, Matthews DM, Kellett HA, et al. Change in skin thickness associated with cheiroarthropathy in insulin dependent diabetes mellitus. Br Med J (Clin Res Ed). 1986;292:936.

70. Krasagakis K, Hettmannsperger U, Trautmann C, et al. Persistent scleredema of Buschke in a diabetic: improvement with high-dose penicillin. Br J Dermatol. 1996;134:597–8.

71. Eberlein-Konig B, Vogel M, Katzer K, et al. Succesfull UVA1 phototherapy in a patient with scleredema adultorum. J Eur Acad Dermatol Venereol. 2005;19:203–4.

72. Hager CM, Sobhi HA, Hunzelmann N, et al. Bath-PUVA therapy in three patients with scleredema adultorum. J Am Acad Dermatol. 1998;38:240–2.

73. Bowen AR, Smith L, Zone JJ. Scleredema adultorum of Buschke treatment with radiation. Arch Dermatol. 2003;139:780–4.

74. Konemann S, Hesselmann S, Bolling T, et al. Radiotherapy of benign diseases-scleredema adultorum Buschke. Strahlenther Onkol. 2004;180:811–4.

75. de Berker D, Richert B, Baran R. Acquired disorders of the nails and nail unit. In: Griffiths C, Barker J, Bleiker T, Chalmers R, Creamer D, editors. Rook's textbook of dermatology. 9th ed. Chichester, West Sussex: John Wiley & Sons Inc; 2016. p. 95.1–95.65.

76. Jeong W, Keighley C, Wolfe R, Lee WL, Slavin MA, Kong DCM, Chen SC. The epidemiology and clinical manifestations of mucormycosis: a systematic review and meta-analysis of case reports. Clin Microbiol Infect. 2019;25(1):26–34.

77. Prakash H, Chakrabarti A. Epidemiology of Mucormycosis in India. Microorganisms. 2021;9(3):523.

78. Garre V. Recent advances and future directions in the understanding of Mucormycosis. Front Cell Infect Microbiol. 2022;24(12):850581.

79. Stone N, Gupta N, Schwartz I. Mucormycosis: time to address this deadly fungal infection. Lancet Microbe. 2021;2(8):e343–4.

80. Nawijn F, Smeeing DPJ, Houwert RM, Leenen LPH, Hietbrink F. Time is of the essence when treating necrotizing soft tissue infections: a systematic review and meta-analysis. World J Emerg Surg. 2020;8(15):4.

81. Stevens DL, Bryant AE. Necrotizing soft-tissue infections. N Engl J Med. 2017;377(23):2253–65.

82. Goh T, Goh LG, Ang CH, Wong CH. Early diagnosis of necrotizing fasciitis. Br J Surg. 2014;101(1):e119–25.

83. McArdle P, Gallen I. Necrotising fasciitis in diabetics. Lancet. 1996;348(9026):552.

84. McGee SA, Barnum M, Nesbit RD. The epidemiology of necrotizing fasciitis at a rural level 1 trauma center during the COVID-19 pandemic. Am Surg. 2022;5:31348221074251.

85. Zhao Q, Fang X, Pang Z, Zhang B, Liu H, Zhang F. COVID-19 and cutaneous manifestations: a systematic review. J Eur Acad Dermatol Venereol. 2020;34(11):2505–10.

86. Jia JL, Kamceva M, Rao SA, Linos E. Cutaneous manifestations of COVID-19: a preliminary review. J Am Acad Dermatol. 2020;83(2):687–90.

87. Genovese G, Moltrasio C, Berti E, Marzano AV. Skin manifestations associated with COVID-19: current knowledge and future perspectives. Dermatology. 2021;237(1):1–12.

88. Gupta A, Madhavan MV, Sehgal K, Nair N, Mahajan S, Sehrawat TS, Bikdeli B, Ahluwalia N, Ausiello JC, Wan EY, Freedberg DE, Kirtane AJ, Parikh SA, Maurer MS, Nordvig AS, Accili D, Bathon JM, Mohan S, Bauer KA, Leon MB, Krumholz HM, Uriel N, Mehra MR, Elkind MSV, Stone GW, Schwartz A, Ho DD, Bilezikian JP, Landry DW. Extrapulmonary manifestations of COVID-19. Nat Med. 2020;26(7):1017–32.

89. Albulescu R, Dima SO, Florea IR, Lixandru D, Serban AM, Aspritoiu VM, Tanase C, Popescu I, Ferber S. COVID-19 and diabetes mellitus: unraveling the hypotheses that worsen the prognosis (review). Exp Ther Med. 2020;20(6):194.

90. Blanco M, Hernández MT, Strauss KW, Amaya M. Prevalence and risk factors of lipohypertrophy in insulin-injecting patients with diabetes. Diabetes Metab. 2013;39(5):445–53.

91. Coulson IH, Benton EC, Ogden S. Diagnosis of skin disease. In: Griffiths C, Barker J, Bleiker T, Chalmers R, Creamer D, editors. Rook's textbook of dermatology. 9th ed. Chichester, West Sussex: John Wiley & Sons Inc; 2016. p. 4.1–4.26.

Further Reading

Behm B, Schreml S, Landthaler M, Babilas P. Skin signs in diabetes mellitus. J Eur Acad Dermatol Venereol. 2012;26(10):1203–11.

Makrantonaki E, Jiang D, Hossini AM, et al. Diabetes mellitus and the skin. Rev Endocr Metab Disord. 2016;17(3):269–82.

Foot Complications

62

Lawrence B. Harkless, Jarrod Shapiro,
and Joel Rodriguez-Saldana

Introduction

Patient C was a 50-year-old diabetic male truck driver. He presented to the emergency department with a red, hot, painful, swollen right foot and lower leg. There were no open lesions with unilateral edema and diffuse erythema. A venous duplex ultrasound was negative for deep venous thrombosis. Laboratory data showed no leukocytosis. The patient was admitted, placed on broad spectrum I.V. antibiotics, and discharged three days later. He returned to the emergency department 3 days after discharge with the same complaint of persistent redness and swelling. A second venous ultrasound was negative for thrombosis, and he was discharged home with a new oral antibiotic and a referral to the podiatry clinic. After a 2 week delay in obtaining an appointment, the patient noted his right foot had changed shape and was flatter in the arch than the contralateral foot. The deformity progressed to ulceration requiring surgical intervention. This unfortunate outcome in which the correct diagnosis of acute Charcot neuroarthropathy was missed resulted in considerable patient morbidity and increased healthcare utilization.

Diabetic foot complications are serious events in the lives of patients with diabetes. Historically, pedal complications were underappreciated by the general medical community; however, international efforts have improved the recognition of this very serious problem. All health professionals involved with diabetic patients should be well informed about the potential complications of diabetic foot syndrome. This chapter will discuss diabetic foot complications with an emphasis on a conceptual framework of the epidemiology,

risk, and wound-healing concepts underlying these complications. A detailed discussion of diabetic foot ulcerations, infections (including skin and soft tissue structure infections and osteomyelitis), Charcot neuroarthropathy, and the role of targeted partial foot amputations will provide healthcare professionals with an understanding of this detrimental disease.

Diabetes is highly common with an estimated 194 million diabetics worldwide [1]. It has also been estimated that 344 million people will be diabetic by 2030 [1]. Of this number of affected people, 15% will develop a diabetic foot ulcer at some time [2], which corresponds to 2% to 6% of diabetics yearly with an estimated 6.9 million that will be affected in 2030 [2]. Diabetes has a significant and often catastrophic effect on patients' lives with global health implications. It is estimated that diabetic patients overall have a 15% risk of lower limb amputation [3]. Of this number, 85% are preceded by an ulcer [2]. Patients who develop an ulcer have a 34% risk of developing another wound within 1 year of healing the index ulcer and a 70% chance at 5 years [4].

Patients often fair poorly with the onset of foot ulceration. Diabetic foot ulcers that progress to lower limb amputation set off a catastrophic chain of events with a 50% risk of contralateral foot ulceration and a 50% rate of contralateral limb amputation within 2 to 5 years [5]. Mortality rates are significantly worsened when considering diabetic foot complications. Five-year mortality rates are 45%, 18%, and 55% for patients with neuropathic, neuroischemic, and ischemic ulcerations, respectively [6]. Limb amputations have similarly dismal survival outcomes. Mayfield et al. reviewed Veterans Affairs discharge documents of 5180 patients who underwent some type of lower limb amputation. They found a 56% 5-year mortality rate after transtibial and 70% mortality after transfemoral amputation [7]. Hoffman et al. found similar poor prognoses after major limb amputation with 1,3,5, and 10-year survival rates of 78%, 61%, 44%, and 19%, respectively [8].

The addition of Charcot neuroarthropathy worsens yet the prognosis of these patients. Sohn et al. found a 59% incidence of foot ulceration in those with Charcot foot (538 of

L. B. Harkless
School of Podiatric Medicine, Department of Surgery, UTRGV
School of Podiatric Medicine, Edinburgh, TX, USA
e-mail: lawrence.harkless@utrgv.edu

J. Shapiro
Western University of Health Sciences College of Podiatric
Medicine, Chino Valley Medical Center, Chino, CA, USA

J. Rodriguez-Saldana (✉)
Multidisciplinary Diabetes Center Mexico, Mexico City, Mexico

© The Author(s), under exclusive license to Springer Nature Switzerland AG 2023
J. Rodriguez-Saldana (ed.), *The Diabetes Textbook*, https://doi.org/10.1007/978-3-031-25519-9_62

911 patients). Of these, 66% were treated for foot ulcer at the time of Charcot diagnosis [9]. They also found the relative risk of amputation for patients with foot ulcer and Charcot was 12 times higher than those with Charcot alone [9].

The cost of diabetic foot complications may also be catastrophic. Ramsey et al. retrospectively reviewed 8905 patients from a health maintenance organization and found the cost for a 40- to 65-year-old diabetic male with a new foot ulcer in 1999 was $27,987 over a 2-year period [2]. With inflation, this corresponds in 2016 to $40,003 [10].

These figures demand a specific set of conclusions. The first is that the majority of diabetic foot ulcers and major limb amputations are preventable. When they occur, a foot ulcer greatly increases the risk of further complications such as soft tissue and bone infection and must be treated aggressively. Third, limb amputation is preceded by foot ulceration that becomes secondarily infected with limb amputation as the end result. Finally, the costs associated with diabetic foot complications are extraordinary and place a very large burden on the world's healthcare system.

This has led some to consider how diabetic foot complications compare with other diseases. Armstrong, et al. compared the 5-year mortality rates of neuropathic ulcers and amputations with various types of cancer [6]. They found 5-year mortality rates of neuropathic ulcers and amputations to be equivalent to colon cancer and worse than Hodgkin's disease, breast cancer, and prostate cancer (Fig. 62.1). This has prompted the concept of *malignant diabetes* in which diabetic foot complications are markers for a diabetic process that has advanced to a severity equivalent to (and some-times worse than) cancer (courtesy Jeff Robbins, DPM, personal communication).

With this background in mind, it is possible to consider a conceptual pathological framework for diabetic foot complications with an emphasis on healing concepts, risk assessment, and psychosocial aspects that play an important role in this process.

At a macroscopic level, the continuum of diabetic foot ulceration to infection to amputation is clearly understood. The hyperglycemic process leads to peripheral neuropathy (discussed below) and loss of large and small sensory fibers. This loss of protective sensation reduces or eliminates the capacity to sense low-grade repetitive or single high-grade traumatic pressures to specific aspects of the foot. Low-grade microtrauma is mediated by the presence of structural deformity or limited joint motion [11, 12] (Fig. 62.2). As pressures continue to wear away epidermis, deeper layers become exposed creating the neuropathic ulcer. If the ulcer remains exposed, the likelihood to become colonized with opportunistic skin flora with contamination cellulitis and infection is high. Chronic or acute infection may lead to osteomyelitis of the nearby bone with possible amputation.

Treating pedal complications successfully requires an understanding of the normal wound-healing process. Aberrant healing associated with diabetic foot complications is discussed later in this chapter. Initial wound healing begins with the hemostatic inflammatory phase, mediated by neutrophils, which diminish in number after the first 24 h and replaced with macrophages and lymphocytes. The proliferative repair phase occurs between several days after injury to the first few weeks,

Fig. 62.1 Five-year mortality percentages comparing neuropathic ulceration and amputation with other common malignant diseases (Armstrong et al. with permission)

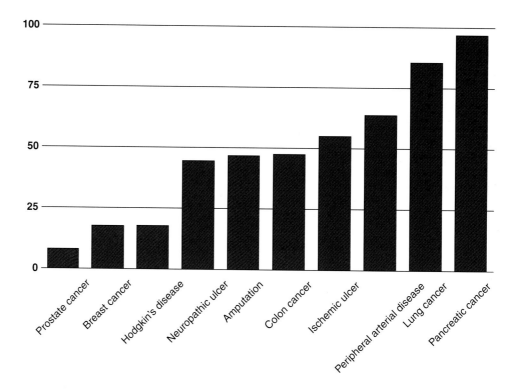

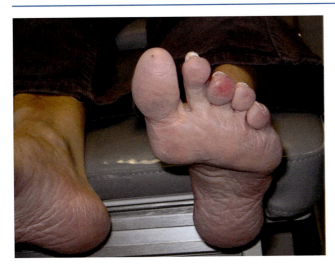

Fig. 62.2 Preulcerative digital erythema due to chronic repetitive low-grade pressures caused by hammertoe deformity

Table 62.1 Vascular risk spectrum

Risk Type	Historical Component
Macrovascular disease	CAD, CVA/TIA, intermittent claudication
Microvascular disease	Retinopathy, nephropathy, neuropathy
Functional microvascular disease	Gastroparesis, impotence
Metabolic syndrome	Impaired glucose tolerance(IGT) pre diabetes, insulin resistance(IR), HTN, hyperlipidemia, obesity smoking
Family history	History of DM and complications

with steadily increasing fibroblasts and endothelial cells. It is at this stage that the typical diabetic foot ulcer healing process stalls. The final phase, remodeling, occurs after several weeks with type 1 collagen replacing the prior epidermal type III collagen, leaving a healed skin surface with approximately 80% of its original tensile strength [13]. During the proliferative phase, three mechanisms occur: connective tissue deposition (described above), contraction (mediated by myofibroblasts), and epithelialization [13]. Each of these phases is mediated by various cytokines and cell signaling pathways. Successfully, healing diabetic foot ulcers will heal by a variable combination of these three methods.

Peripheral vascular disease has a profound effect on the assessment, treatment, and prognosis of diabetic foot complications. Diabetics with peripheral arterial disease (PAD) are at significantly greater risk for poor outcomes. Jude et al. examined the relationship between diabetes and PAD severity and outcomes by examining the lower-extremity angiograms and medical records of 58 patients with diabetes and 78 without. The results of their analysis depicted that patients with diabetes had greater PAD severity in the profunda femoris and all arterial segments below the knee ($P \leq 0.02$). Furthermore, diabetes was associated with a risk for amputation that was five times greater than that for nondiabetic patients (41.4% vs 11.5%, odds ratio [OR] 5.4, $P < 0.0001$) and mortality that was double for nondiabetic patients (51.7% vs. 25.6%, OR 3.1, $P = 0.002$) [14].

When considering the risk spectrum of peripheral arterial disease in the diabetic patient, it is efficacious to consider an organized approach using the patient's medical history. Harkless and Holmes created a vascular risk spectrum from patient historical data [15]. Table 62.1 lists the pertinent components of this risk spectrum. The clinician obtains the appropriate history, including the listed components, and determines a low, medium, or high risk for the presence of peripheral arterial disease. This system has not been validated but provides the clinician with a basis in which to understand the presence of PAD and order further testing.

Each of the risk components described above cumulatively increases the risk for peripheral arterial disease and an increased chance of poor outcomes when combined with other complications such as neuropathic ulceration, Charcot arthropathy, or infection. The UKPDS trial found for each 1% increase in glycosylated hemoglobin, there was a 28% increase in peripheral arterial disease at 6 years after diagnosis. Additionally, each 10-mmHg increase in systolic blood pressure increased the risk by 25%, and smoking, prior diagnosis of coronary artery disease, and dyslipidemia were also independent risk factors for PAD [16].

The significance of this vascular risk spectrum is compounded by the concept of metabolic memory in which diabetes complications persist and progress after glycemic control is established. The converse of this, in which intensive glycemic control has a prolonged protective effect despite later reversion to conventional therapy, was termed the "legacy effect" after the UKPDS trial [17]. Increasing research evidence demonstrates that microvascular complications such as retinopathy and nephropathy in diabetics may be mediated by epigenetic DNA methylation, thus modifying gene expression [18]. The presence of advanced glycation end products (via cross-linking and irreversibly altering protein function) and oxidative stress (through creation of reactive oxygen species and subsequent tissue damage) have also been implicated [19, 20]. Experimental evidence for this process was noted during the Diabetes Control and Complications Trial (DCCT) [21] in which a continued retinopathy effect was noted in the conventional treatment group despite later enrollment and intensive glycemic treatment during the EDIC trial [22]. This process may be logically extrapolated from retinopathy and nephropathy to peripheral neuropathy since these three complications are intimately linked. Further research needs to delineate the mechanisms and biological effects of metabolic memory as they pertain to peripheral neuropathy and diabetic foot complications.

Diabetic pedal complications are made more challenging by patient psychosocial aspects. Nonadherence to medical instruction is highly common in this population with significant lower extremity effects. Armstrong et al. performed a prospective study of 20 diabetic patients with plantar ulcers. They placed a pedometer on the hip and in a removable cast boot and tracked ambulatory activity. Only 28% of walking activities at home were performed while wearing the removable cast boot, and the highest utilizers were the boot only 60% of the time [23]. In a similar study, patients were prescribed prescription shoes with a pedometer to track usage to prevent ulceration. Eighty-five percent of patients wore the shoes outside the home, but only 15% wore them when inside the home, which correlated with more steps per day out of the shoes [24]. Additionally, other studies have demonstrated improved ulcer healing outcomes when protocols were utilized that eliminated the chance of noncompliance [25–28].

Charcot Neuroarthropathy

Charcot neuroarthropathy is a well-documented but poorly understood catastrophic imbalanced inflammatory reaction that occurs most often in the diabetic population in developed countries. This disorder was originally described in patients with tertiary neurosyphilis and knee joint destruction and has generally poor outcomes if not recognized early and treated properly [29–31].

Charcot arthopathy appears clinically as a mild to moderately painful joint destructive disease, but at the molecular level, it has been hypothesized as due to an imbalance in pro-inflammatory cytokines responsible for bone growth regulation [32]. Jeffcoate et al. offer the most current description of this disorder as being initiated by an insult to the foot or ankle which then stimulates osteoclast formation by activating nuclear transcription factor κB (NF-κB) which leads to a significant osteoclastic and lytic process with subsequent bone destruction. This molecule is itself activated by receptor activator of NF-κB ligand (RANKL) and has been implicated as an etiologic factor of blood vessel tunica media calcification [33]. Further research will help elucidate this process and will likely lead to medications that will reduce the effects of this devastating disease.

Clinically, Charcot arthropathy presents in two forms [32] acute and [33] chronic. In the acute phase, the affected foot or ankle presents most commonly with moderate to severe edema, erythema, calor, and variable pain. Patients will present a variable history with or without a known traumatic episode. Due to peripheral neuropathy with loss of sensation, diabetic patients may feel limited pain in comparison to a fully sensate person and may have no recollection of trauma. A low-grade chronic trauma or a more significant injury may be the inciting event.

Charcot arthropathy in which no ulcerations are present create a diagnostic dilemma. One must consider the broad differential diagnosis of an erythematous, edematous foot, including acute gouty arthropathy, cellulitis, osteomyelitis, occult or overt trauma, and deep venous thrombosis. This clinical dilemma may be difficult for the physician to sort out and is best handled with emergent referral of a lower extremity specialist. The index of suspicion for each of these differentials may be lowered with appropriate laboratory and imaging studies. However, one must maintain a high index of suspicion for osteomyelitis in a patient with this presentation. Cellulitis and osteomyelitis may be ruled out based on the understanding that the vast majority of foot infections occur via contiguous spread infection (skin surface bacteria entering the deeper tissues through a breach in the skin) rather than hematogenously. Hematogenous spread osteomyelitis in the diabetic foot is an extremely rare occurrence. However, we have seen several patients with bacteremia seed a Charcot joint. A search of the literature demonstrates no case studies of hematogenous spread osteomyelitis to the diabetic foot. This may be due in part to the smaller number of long bones in the foot and lack of open growth plates as is found in the more common pediatric hematogenous osteomyelitis of the tibia and femur. In cases where there is ulceration with Charcot changes, ruling out osteomyelitis becomes much more difficult.

A careful physical examination should be undertaken, looking for any open lesions in the typically edematous, erythematous foot with warmth and variable pain to palpation [30]. Early stages may show no morphological changes to foot structure, however later in the disease, after joint destruction has occurred, the classic rocker-bottom foot is easily witnessed (Figs. 62.3, 62.4, and 62.5). Charcot arthropathy may occur at any joint of the foot and ankle;

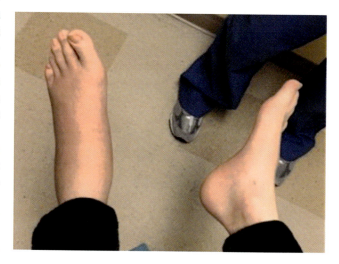

Fig. 62.3 Acute Charcot left foot. Note the edema and subtle erythema. The left foot was warmer than the right. Radiographs at this stage were negative for joint destruction or dislocation

Fig. 62.4 Classic rocker bottom foot deformity secondary to Charcot midfoot collapse. Radiograph of same patient demonstrating Lisfranc and naviculocuneiform collapse

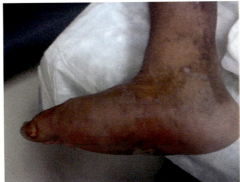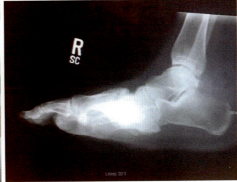

however, the tarsometatarsal joint is most commonly involved. Though slightly less common, ankle Charcot is potentially devastating in its poor outcomes [29].

Temperature differences have been shown to assist with diagnosis of Charcot arthropathy and monitor resolution of the acute phase. A greater than 2 °C temperature difference using an infrared dermal thermometer is helpful in diagnosing acute Charcot and in monitoring progression out of the acute and into the coalescence phase [34, 35]. Thermometry should be used 15 min after cast and dressings are removed, and the thermometer should be accurate to ±0.1 °C [36].

Laboratory studies are often inconclusive with either a demonstrable leukocytosis and elevated nonspecific inflammatory markers, such as erythrocyte sedimentary rate (ESR) and C-reactive protein (CRP), or these values may also be found to be in the normal reference range [34, 37]. It has been shown that the acute local inflammation is dissociated from the systemic inflammatory response in these patients [34], and this lack of a systemic response may help providers in differentiating this disorder from infection. Other laboratory values may demonstrate elevations in glycemic indicators and renal dysfunction. No definitive validated laboratory markers for the specific diagnosis of Charcot neuroarthropathy exist outside of limited research studies.

Typical imaging studies begin with foot and/or ankle radiographs depending on the suspected joint involvement. During the earliest stages of Charcot, radiographs may demonstrate no abnormal findings other than increased soft tissue density and volume. Later stages will be clearly evident on plain film radiographs with joint destruction, fragmentation, dislocation (during the development phase) and progressive sclerosis, ankylosis, and rounding of bone fragments (during the coalescence and remodeling phases) (Figs. 62.6 and 62.7).

Charcot neuroarthopathy of the foot progresses through four primary stages that blend intimately making it difficult to determine if a patient has progressed to the next stage. The modified Eichenholtz classification [38, 39] is most commonly used to stage the disorder. Stage 0 is the most acute (inflammatory) stage with the classic "red, hot, and swollen"

appearance. Radiographs are the most often utilized initial imaging modality [40] and commonly show no joint destructive changes in the earliest stage. Stage 1 is the development phase, which also appears as a foot with warmth, erythema, and variable edema. Radiographs may show early mild destruction and joint diastasis. Stage 2 is the coalescence phase in which the inflammatory process subsides with clinical normalization and radiographic changes that appear more chronic in nature with sclerosis of prior lucent bone and a blunting or smoothed appearance to bony fragments. The final third stage is termed remodeling which demonstrates a more chronic appearance similar to stage 2. The timeline of each of these stages vary.

An anatomic classification has also been proposed by Sanders and Frykberg [41]. They defined the location of the Charcot destruction coupled with the frequency of complications as follows:

Pattern I: Forefoot = 15%.
Pattern II: Tarsometatarsal joint = 40%.
Pattern III: Naviculo-cuneiform, Talo-navicular, Calcaneo-cuboid joints = 30%.
Pattern IV: Ankle and/or subtalar joint = 10%.
Pattern V: Calcaneus = 5%.

Other imaging modalities, though useful for other pathologic entities, do not provide significant diagnostic assistance. Computed tomography may assist with diagnosing early nondisplaced fractures [40]. Magnetic resonance imaging (MRI) in most cases is not necessary and may in fact create a diagnostic dilemma. Joint fragmentation, fracture, and bone marrow edema involving multiple joints, the typical Charcot appearance on MRI, may be difficult to differentiate from osteomyelitis, acute exacerbations of chronic osteoarthritis, or gouty arthropathy. In situations where ulceration is present, radiologists will be unable to rule out osteomyelitis. Bone scintigraphy should be avoided due to its lack of specificity [42]. Any inflammatory condition may appear as increased radiotracer uptake, even on delayed phases and white blood cell labeled studies. The reader is cautioned to take careful

Fig. 62.5 Chronic Charcot of the right midfoot with collapse and rocker bottom appearance. Note the medial arch ulceration due to increased focal plantar pressures

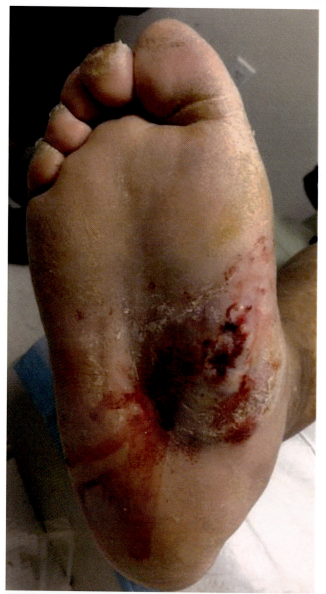

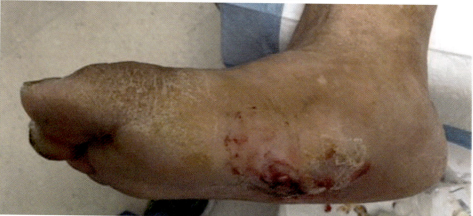

consideration of the results for all advanced imaging studies for the diagnosis of Charcot neuroarthropathy.

Treatment of the Charcot foot varies based on the acuity of the presentation. Acute Charcot arthropathy management consists of stabilization of any comorbid disorders such as establishing appropriate glycemic control, hydration, and intravenous antimicrobials if infection is suspected. Additionally, local wound care is important if ulceration is identified concurrently with arthropathy. Sharp debridement removes bacterial contamination, while most wound care must

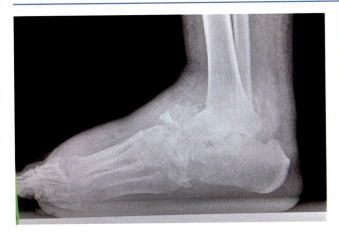

Fig. 62.6 Acute Charcot arthropathy involving the midtarsal and subtalar joints

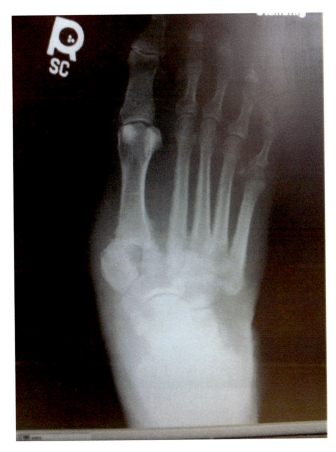

Fig. 62.7 Late development early coalescent Charcot arthropathy involving the Lisfranc and intercuneiform joints

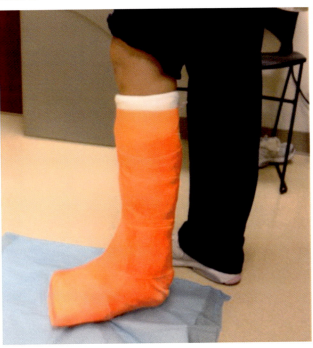

Fig. 62.8 Total contact cast for treatment of acute Charcot neuroarthropathy

Clinicians should be aware of the protracted time frame for the acute phase to transition into the coalescent phase where protected weightbearing is possible. Sinacore studied 30 subjects with 35 acute onset presentations of Charcot of the foot and ankle. The midfoot was most commonly involved (46 patients), followed by the hindfoot (23 patients), forefoot (20 patients), and ankle (11 patients). All patients were treated with total contact casting, and the healing endpoint was defined as discontinuation of the necessity for TCC as determined by the treating physician. In 100% of cases, the average healing time was 86 ± 45 days [43]. Providers may take from this a rule-of-thumb of 1 to 2 months for transitioning out of the acute Charcot phase.

Total contact casting (TCC) (Fig. 62.8) is a modified method of below the knee cast that involves applying minimal under-cast padding to the extremity and using a cast that conforms to the shape of the leg and foot. This device attempts to maintain the shape of the foot during the acute destructive process of Charcot. The patient should be maintained in the TCC until the acute phase of destruction has resolved with cast changes weekly at first until the initial edema resolves. The TCC requires considerable training to appropriately apply, and if placed incorrectly may result in abrasions, ulcerations, and an increased potential for limb amputation. This device should be applied only by trained specialists. Pinzur et al. found patients were able to safely bear weight in a TCC with biweekly changes lasting an average of 5.8 weeks. Patients were considered safe for transition into prescription shoes at an average of 12 weeks [44]. In the emergency department, an appropriate alternative is to apply a removable cast walker to the patient with instructions not to remove (Fig. 62.9).

be established. In cases of abscess formation, operative incision and drainage, and, rarely, amputation may be necessary.

The cornerstone of treatment for acute Charcot neuroarthropathy is protected offweighting with total contact casting. The patient must remain completely nonweightbearing on the affected limb using any manner that will guarantee patient adherence. This may be accomplished via crutches, roller cart, or wheelchair depending on patient psychosocial capabilities and available resources.

Charcot arthropathy involving the ankle joint is somewhat different in outcomes compared with pedal joints and often involves a surgical approach. Schon et al. found an improved overall outcome of this disorder when treated surgically as opposed to nonsurgically with casting and bracing. They found a greater loss of correction with nonsurgical care and improved success rates with surgical intervention [45].

The effect of bisphosphonate therapy for the treatment of acute Charcot arthropathy has revealed conflicting and controversial results. Jude et al. in 2001 randomized 39 patients with acute Charcot to either a single intravenous dose of pamidronate 90 mg or placebo (saline) in a double blind manner. Patients were then followed for 12 months during

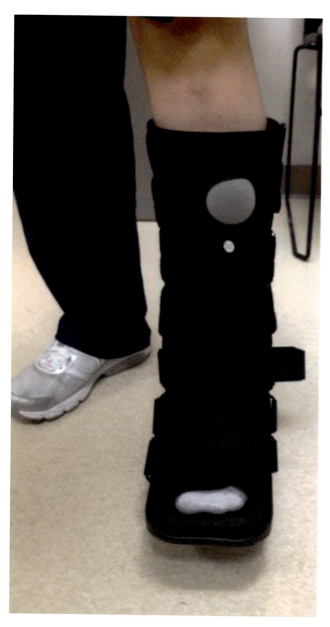

Fig. 62.9 Removable cast walker as an alternative to total contact casting

which skin temperature, bone-specific alkaline phosphatase, and deoxypyridinoline crosslinks were measured. Patients given the pamidronate were observed to have an initial reduction in bone turnover as compared with placebo with similar levels at the end of the study [46]. This was the first study to examine a potentially definitive treatment for Charcot arthropathy. Subsequently, several studies examined the outcomes of bisphosphonate therapy on acute Charcot with one study finding increased time to clinical resolution with zoledronic acid and possibly extending the time to resolution [47].

Significant methodological flaws in this body of research demonstrate low experimental numbers, various treatment methods (e.g., intravenous versus oral formulations and different experimental drugs), and lack of long-term follow-up [48, 49]. Two systematic reviews have stated that skin temperature and inflammatory markers decrease with bisphosphonate therapy, but studies have failed to demonstrate improved clinical outcomes and might even prolong the resolution phase [50, 51]. Due to the lack of long-term outcomes and questionable results, we currently recommend against the use of bisphosphonates for acute Charcot neuroarthropathy.

Currently, the joint destruction and subsequent deformity of Charcot are irreversible. Thus, long-term care consists of shoe gear modifications, sometimes requiring custom shoes, custom foot orthoses, and regular serial observation by a foot specialist. Some physicians prefer to place these patients into a Charcot Restraint Orthotic Walker (CROW), which is a custom molded below knee brace that attempts to redistribute plantar pressures (Fig. 62.10). The primary goal is prevention of ulceration and amputation.

In certain situations, surgical intervention may be necessary, including demonstrated instability, preulcerative callus formation, and ulceration. Surgical options are beyond the scope of this chapter but generally include tendoachilles lengthening to reduce forefoot pressures, ostectomy procedures to reduce bony prominence, realignment arthrodesis to create a more functionally stable and plantigrade foot, and limb amputation. Each of these reconstructive procedures should be considered salvage methods in an attempt to avoid amputation.

Outcomes for patients with Charcot arthropathy of the foot vary. When considering the risk of amputation, it is clear that patients with mild joint destruction and minimal to no subsequent deformity are at relatively low risk. Sohn et al. retrospectively reviewed a Veterans' Affairs national cohort of 911 patients with incident Charcot arthropathy and 15,117 patients with diabetic foot ulcers (without amputations). They found the overall amputation rate for patients with Charcot was not significantly different from the overall diabetic population with foot ulcers. However, patients with both Charcot and the

Fig. 62.10 Custom-made Charcot Restraint Orthotic Walker (CROW) for offweighting the Charcot foot

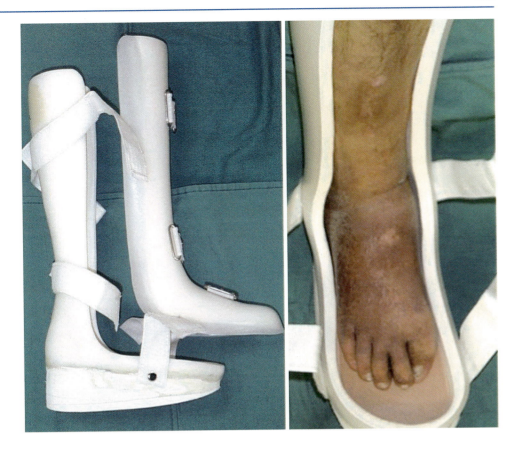

presence of a foot ulcer were 12 times more likely to undergo a limb amputation, and patients with ulcer alone were 7 times more likely to undergo a limb amputation than those with Charcot alone [9]. This demonstrates that Charcot alone does not increase the risk of amputation, but when coupled with a foot ulcer, the risks are much higher.

When considering mortality, the risk profile is different. Sohn et al. examined a cohort of 1050 patients with Charcot arthropathy and compared them to diabetic patients with foot ulcer and those with diabetes alone. During a 5-year follow-up, they found 18.8% of patients with diabetes alone died, 37.0% with foot ulcer died, and 28.3% of the Charcot patients died. These researchers found the presence of Charcot independently and significantly increased the mortality rate of these patients [52].

These findings show that Charcot arthropathy is a complex and serious disease with a high rate of complications and potential morbidity and mortality. Physicians should maintain a very high index of suspicion in any diabetic patient with an acute presentation of erythema, edema, warmth, and new onset pain, despite the presence or absence of ulceration. A low threshold for acute splinting or casting with strict nonweightbearing protocols is the best current treatment to prevent long-term deformity and complications. Further research will be necessary to better elucidate the etiology and treatment of Charcot arthropathy.

Foot Amputation

Amputation is often the final stage of a long process, and in the diabetic this may often be considered a failure of prior care. However, a modified view of this concept may be appropriate to better understand the role of amputations in the foot. As discussed in the introduction to this chapter, major limb amputation (transtibial and transfemoral levels) has significant associated morbidity and mortality in the diabetic population. This may be observed through several lenses. First, these patients already have significant comorbidities, including advanced cardiovascular disease, among others.

Additionally, major limb amputation leads to a greater energy expenditure during walking. Waters et al. performed a seminal study in 1976 in which they compared several gait parameters in patients with above knee, below knee, and Symes ankle disarticulation amputations to a control group of normal subjects. They found improved gait velocity, cadence, stride length, oxygen uptake, maximum aerobic activity, and heart rate in patients with the more distal amputations [53]. Similarly, Gailey et al. compared transtibial amputee oxygen consumption, heart rate, and self-selected walking speed with a non-amputee control group. They also found increased metabolic costs in the amputee group. However, when stratifying the amputee group by length of amputation, they found a significant improvement in these parameters with increased amputation stump length [54].

However, it has been shown that length of the residual limb also correlates with mortality. There are no studies that show amputation itself leads directly to increased mortality. This correlation is likely complex and may be hypothesized as a population with significant comorbidities, especially cardiovascular, with the additional physiologic stressor of the amputation (increased energy expenditure and decreased ambulatory capability) accelerating the rate of development of the already present comorbidities.

Several research studies although have demonstrated improved mortality when comparing partial foot amputations to major limb amputations [55–57]. Table 62.2 shows a synthesis of studies that compared mortality by level of amputation: digital, below knee, and above knee levels. As shown, the 1 and 5 year mortality trends are decreased in favor of those that involve only the forefoot as compared with the leg.

With this general trend toward improved outcomes with more distal amputations, it is important to strongly consider partial foot amputations as significant tools to help patients maintain an active life and potentially improved life expectancy.

It is the intention of this section to provide clinicians with general information about the options available for pedal amputations. Interested surgeons should refer to other textbooks for procedure specifics. A variety of pedal amputations exist, all of which spare the remaining portions of the foot with variable success, most of which prevent major limb amputation.

The choice of which amputation to perform is highly patient-specific and depends on therapy goals, reason for amputation (cellulitis, abscess, gas gangrene, osteomyelitis, malignancy, or gangrene secondary to peripheral arterial disease). A detailed work-up must be performed including obtaining an appropriate history, physical, and laboratory and imaging data. Additionally, the preoperative functional status and psychosocial history must be evaluated to appreciate the anticipated postoperative level of function.

Table 62.2 Mortality percentages by level of lower limb amputation demonstrating improvements with increasingly distal amputations [55–57]

Amputation level	30 day mortality %	1 year mortality %	5 year mortality %
Toe	1.7	6.6	46
TMA	2.7	8.5	45
BKA	7.0	25.5	56
AKA	11.1	49.4	70

Peripheral arterial disease is a major risk factor for failure of partial foot amputations [58]. Patients with peripheral arterial disease should undergo a comprehensive evaluation with noninvasive vascular testing, angiography, and consultation with a vascular surgeon. Revascularization should be performed before amputation unless an acute infection necessitates incision and drainage with debridement. It is sometimes necessary to stage the definitive amputation after emergent debridement and subsequent revascularization. Very little evidence is available to assist caregivers in determining the best timing of amputation after revascularization.

Caselli et al. attempted to answer this question by retrospectively reviewing 23 diabetic patients with ischemic foot ulcers who underwent successful transluminal percutaneous angioplasty (PTA) and 20 patients who underwent unsuccessful PTA. They used transcutaneous oxygen pressure measurement ($TcPO_2$) on the dorsal surface of the foot before and after PTA at 1, 7, 14, 21, and 28 days postoperative as a marker of improved perfusion. In the successful revascularization group, $TcPO_2$ measurements progressively improved and peaked at 4 weeks while the unsuccessful group saw no significant rise in $TcPO_2$. These researchers suggested waiting 3 to 4 weeks for the definitive amputation when delay is possible [59]. Currently, timing of amputation after revascularization is determined anecdotally based on clinician experience rather than via sound research-based evidence. Clearly, further research with well-designed prospective methodology is necessary.

Digital Amputation (Fig. 62.11)

Indications for digital amputation in the diabetic foot most commonly include isolated gangrene of a toe, osteomyelitis, and severe soft tissue infection. Amputation of a single digit may be performed along any portion of the length of the digit including the distal or proximal interphalangeal joint or at the metatarsophalangeal joint. When possible, it is preferable to leave as much of the digit as possible. The remaining stump acts as to prevent the contiguous digits from falling into the space previously occupied by the amputated digit. Hammertoe contractures though must be taken into consideration as this may cause the remaining post-amputation portion of the toe to be plantar flexed with increased distal pressures and future ulceration.

Ray Amputation

Amputation of a toe (Fig. 62.12) and part or all of the associated metatarsal is another common procedure that is

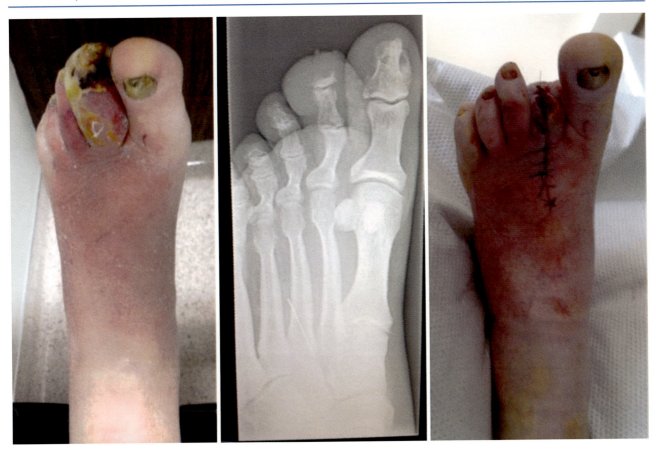

Fig. 62.11 Digital amputation with disarticulation at the metatarsophalangeal joint on patient with second toe distal phalangeal osteomyelitis and necrotizing abscess formation. Partial closure immediately with delayed primary closure 3 days later

Fig. 62.12 Partial toe amputations. Left: 2 weeks postoperative with uneventful healing. Note buttressing effect the residual toe provides. Right: dislocation of first metatarsophalangeal joint with almost 90° hallux abduction due to prior lesser toe amputations and loss of lateral buttress

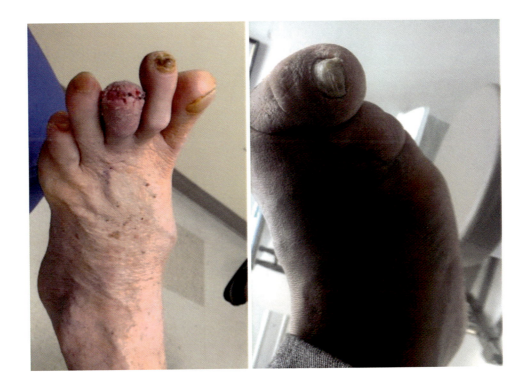

commonly performed on patients with osteomyelitis of a digit that extends into the metatarsophalangeal joint or abscess of the affected ray. Due to firm fascial septae that separate the individual rays, it is often possible to resect a ray in an isolated manner. This procedure is easily performed with a racket-type incision that extends proximally along the metatarsal to the necessary amputation level (Fig. 62.13).

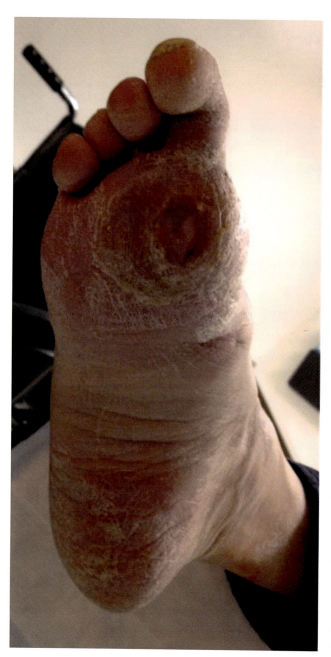

Fig. 62.13 Recurrent neuropathic ulcer status post partial first ray amputation. Note the lesser hammertoe contractures and ulceration secondary to transfer pressure

Transmetatarsal Amputation

Amputation of all toes and a portion of their associated metatarsals, the transmetatarsal amputation, is a powerful and highly useful procedure in the diabetic foot. This procedure is indicated in forefoot gangrene, osteomyelitis, abscess, or forefoot tumor (Figs. 62.14 and 62.15). Due to increased plantar pressures and altered gait kinematics [60] percutaneous Achilles tendon lengthening is commonly performed with this procedure to prevent postoperative plantar stump ulceration. This procedure has a high success rate, allowing patients to ambulate with minimal shoe modifications.

Isolated and Panmetatarsal Head Resection

Although not considered true amputations, removal of an isolated metatarsal head or removal of all of the metatarsal heads (panmetatarsal head resection) may be important alternative tissue-sparing procedures useful in specific situations. These include neuropathic plantar ulcers and isolated or multiple metatarsal head osteomyelitis without extended bone or soft tissue involvement. A retrospective review of 34 panmetatarsal head resection procedures with average follow-up of 20.9 months revealed an overall success rate of 97% with 1 ulcer recurrence and no amputations [61].

Figure 62.16 demonstrates the utility of this procedure. Patient SR was a 48-year-old long-term diabetic male with a chronic right foot plantar neuropathic ulcer that did not respond to several offweighting modalities. The patient had previously undergone second and third metatarsal head resections with resultant rigid deformity. Due to peripheral arterial disease, the patient underwent a femoral to posterior tibial bypass and 1 month later panmetatarsal head resection. At 5-year follow-up, the patient remained ulcer free. Internally, offweighting the forefoot successfully resolved this patient's ulcer.

Tarsometatarsal (Lisfranc) Midtarsal (Chopart) Amputations (Figs. 62.17 and 62.18)

These more proximal foot amputations have historically been less utilized due to increased long-term complications, especially plantar reulceration [62]. Previously, this was due to a less biomechanically stable foot with focal plantar pressures and the absence of adequate prosthetic devices. When possible, a more distal amputation such as the transmetatarsal level is preferable. However, in cases of more significant tissue loss where limb

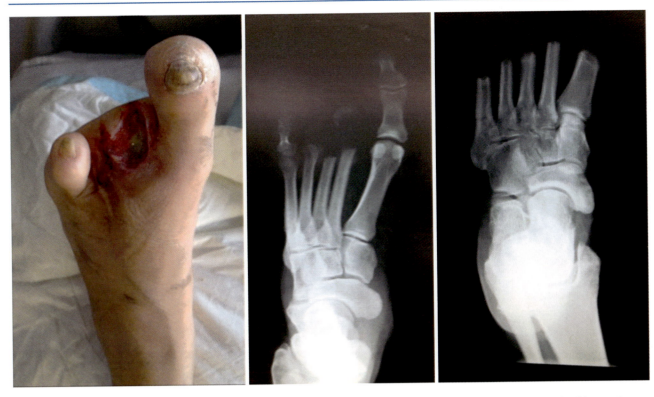

Fig. 62.14 Series of a patient who underwent transmetatarsal amputation after multiple prior digital and partial ray amputations with osteomyelitis of the second metatarsal head and a nonfunctional forefoot. Left: preoperative clinical appearance with visible second metatarsal head. Middle: preoperative dorsoplantar radiograph with second metatarsal head fracture and osteomyelitis. Right: postoperative dorsoplantar radiograph after successful transmetatarsal amputation

Fig. 62.15 Diabetic male with severe peripheral arterial disease and critical limb ischemia (top image). Patient underwent endovascular intervention and staged transmetatarsal amputation with Achilles tendon lengthening. Dorsal weightbearing view (bottom left) with plantar view (bottom right) demonstrating successful healing without recurrent ulceration

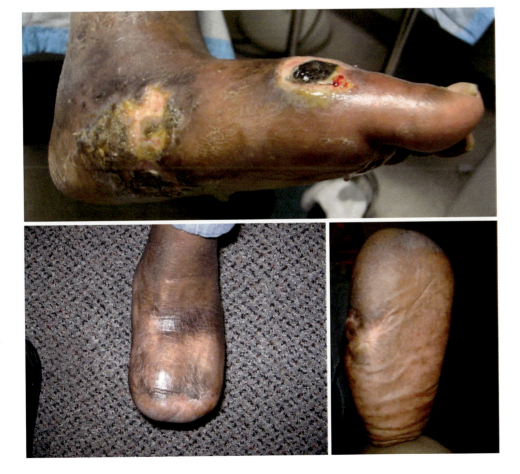

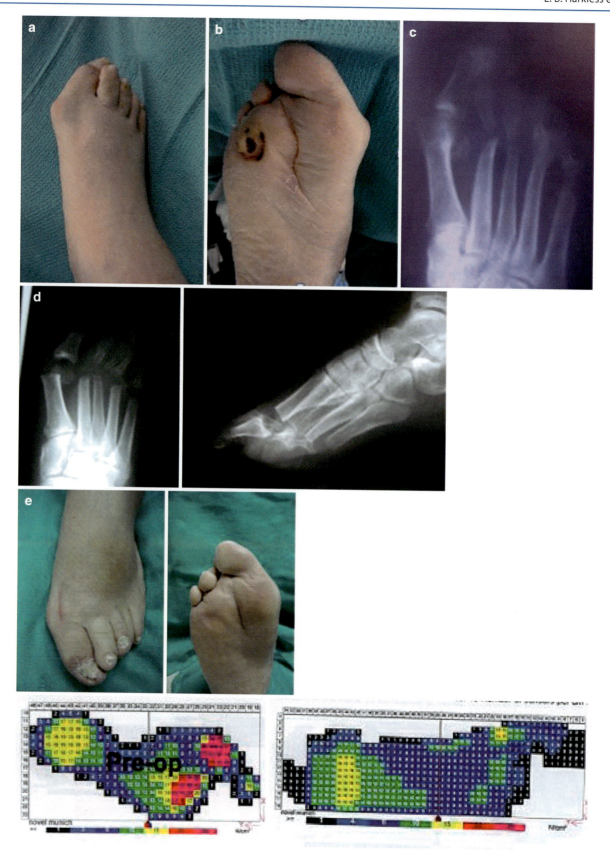

Fig. 62.16 Clinical and radiographic image series of patient SR who underwent panmetatarsal head resection after revascularization for non-healing plantar neuropathic ulceration. Images **A, B, C** = preoperative clinical and radiographic appearance. **D** = Postoperative radiographic appearance. **E** = 5-year follow-up clinical appearance. Note ulcer-free appearance. Bottom row shows E-med pressure sensing system with preoperative (left) and postoperative (right) pressures (red = highest pressures, black = lowest). Note the significant long-term pressure reductions

Fig. 62.17 Right foot Lisfranc amputation with removal of fifth metatarsal base and peroneus brevis attachment. Altered biomechanics led to varus foot position with lateral overload and recurrent plantar ulceration

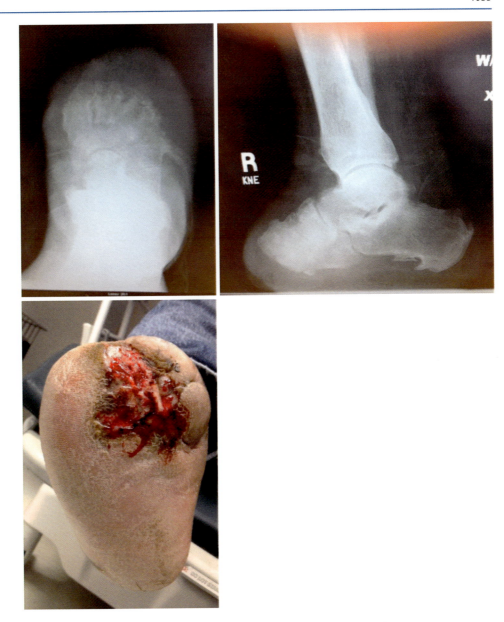

salvage is attempted, these procedures have an important role. Preservation of the bases of the first and fifth metatarsals when possible retains their respective tendon insertions with improved outcomes. Accessary soft tissue balancing techniques improve the mechanical function of the residual foot. These include gastrocnemius recession, Achilles tendon lengthening, Achilles tenotomy or tenectomy, tibialis anterior transfer, peroneus brevis transfer, and posterior tibial tenotomy [62, 63].

The partial foot amputations outlined above have variable outcomes. The majority of clinical studies are retrospective in nature, and further well-designed prospective comparative studies are necessary. Given this limitation, there is a relative consensus that isolated partial or total digital amputations generally have positive results. However, amputation of the hallux or first ray is a unique situation that may have variably poor outcomes. In 1997, Murdoch et al. retrospectively

reported on a 10-year cohort of diabetic patients who underwent either great toe or partial first ray amputations. Sixty percent of these patients eventually underwent a second amputation, 17% underwent a later below knee amputation, and 11% had a transmetatarsal amputation on the same extremity. The mean time to second amputation was 10 months from the index procedure [64]. Kadukammakal et al. retrospectively reviewed 48 patients who underwent 50 partial first-ray amputations between 2003 and 2009 and found 24 cases required further surgical intervention with 12 of those converted to a transmetatarsal amputation with a mean time of 9 months to definitive amputation [65]().

Similarly, Izumi et al. in 2006 retrospectively analyzed a population of 277 diabetic patients who underwent a first-time amputation. They looked at repeat amputation after first amputation at 1, 3, and 5 years [66]. They found the reampu-

Fig. 62.18 Chopart amputation for lesser tarsal osteomyelitis after failed Lisfranc amputation. Preoperative radiograph (left). Postoperative radiograph (right) and clinical appearance (bottom) after successful Chopart amputation and Achilles tendon lengthening

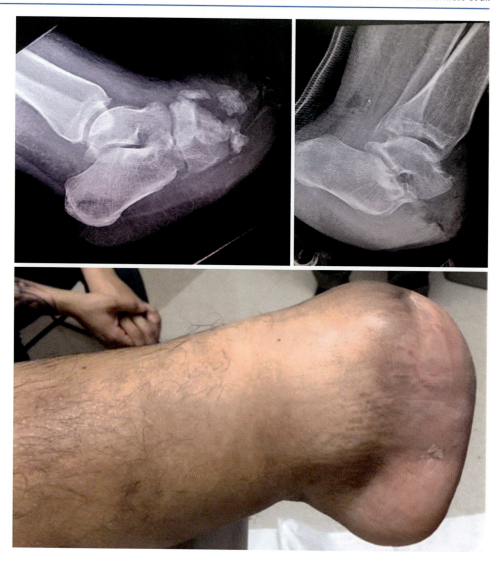

Table 62.3 Ipsilateral limb amputation rates by level of original amputation level [67]

Level of index amputation	1-year (%)	3-years (%)	5-years (%)
Toe	22.8	39.6	52.3
Ray	28.7	41.2	50
Transmetatarsal	18.8	33.3	42.9
Major limb	4.7	11.8	13.3

tation rates noted in Table 62.3. As indicated in the table these researchers found an increasing trend in future amputations over time. However, the rate of change decreased when comparing toe and ray amputations to the transmetatarsal level, indicating the inherent problematic long-term success of the more minor pedal amputations. This increased complication rate is due to the altered biomechanics of the residual foot in otherwise ambulatory patients. For example, after partial first ray amputation, it is highly predictable to see hammertoe contractures of the remaining toes and altered weightbearing plantar pressures. These deformities then predispose the neuropathic patient to further ulceration, infection, and subsequent amputation.

The transmetatarsal amputation has gained popularity as an increasingly successful forefoot amputation. The aforementioned studies demonstrate the decreased reamputation rates versus hallux and partial first ray amputation. This was shown early in a retrospective cohort study of 53 patients undergoing first-time amputation with a success rate of 37.1% in patients undergoing partial first ray amputations and 93.3% in patients undergoing transmetatarsal amputation [67]().

Conclusion

All interventions discussed herein rely fully on involvement of the patient and adherence to treatment regimens. Unfortunately, this may be difficult in practice. Nonadherence in patients with diabetic foot complications is high.

Depression has a significant effect on the diabetic patient and has been shown to decrease health-related quality of life, decrease self footcare, and increase number and severity of diabetes-related complications [68, 69]. Major depression has been linked with a two-fold increased risk of incident ulcers [70] and a five-fold increased risk of ulcer recurrence [71]. Depression also increases the amputation risk with a 33% increased risk of major amputation and 12% increased risk of any amputation (major or minor) [72].

Specialists caring for patients with diabetic foot complications must be cognizant of the home and social environment as well as any individual factors that may involuntarily increase nonadherence to medical therapy. Time should be taken to educate the patient about his or her situation and the steps necessary for care, and it must be determined if the patient is cognitively able to understand the various needs to effect positive outcomes.

The complications associated with the diabetic foot are highly significant and require greater focus to improve patient outcomes. Due to the complexity of the diabetic patient, no single medical provider can successfully perform all of the necessary interventions. Thus, a team approach is integral to appropriate care. The team approach, in which all providers involved with limb preservation participate in the joint care of patients, has become increasingly common with designated amputation prevention centers to focus on all aspects of the diabetic foot. Table 62.4 lists the possible members of the amputation prevention service [73], but it must be understood that at the center of this team is the patient.

Several recent studies have demonstrated both improved outcomes and decreased healthcare costs with this team approach. VanGils et al. reported on the outcomes of a collaborative approach between podiatry and vascular surgery services in a Veterans' Affairs population. During a 55-month follow-up, they found an 86.5% limb loss avoidance rate at 3 years which remained 83% at 5 years [74]. Similarly, a collaborative approach including vascular surgery, orthopedics, endocrinology, plastic surgery, and nursing in a Turkish limb preservation service found an overall amputation rate of 39.4% with 30% below knee amputations [75], an improvement in the rate of major amputations. Driver et al. reporting on the outcomes of a multispecialty limb preservation service, found an 82% decrease in any lower limb amputations over a 4-year period despite a rising number of diabetic patients [76].

In conclusion, diabetic foot complications were a previously poorly understood phenomenon that today has demonstrated significant improvements in outcomes. When understood properly and treated with a comprehensive interprofessional care model diabetic foot ulcers, Charcot neuroarthropathy, and infections such as osteomyelitis may be successfully treated with improved patient ambulatory activity and quality of life.

Table 62.4 Potential members of an amputation prevention service

Certified diabetes educator
Endocrinologist
General surgeon
Infectious disease specialist
Internist
Nephrologist
Nurse
Nutritionist
Podiatrist/orthopedist
Pedorthotist/orthotist/prosthetist
Psychologist/psychiatrist
Vascular surgeon

Multiple Choice Questions

1. Five year mortality rate for patients with neuropathic foot ulcers:
   (a) 30%
   (b) 35%
   (c) 40%
   (d) **45%**
   (e) 50%
2. Diabetic foot ulcers:
   (a) Are not preventable
   (b) Are mostly not preventable
   (c) **Are mostly preventable**
   (d) Are unavoidable
   (e) None of the above
3. Compared with some types of cancer, 5-year mortality rates from neuropathic ulcers and amputations:
   (a) **Are higher**
   (b) Are lower
   (c) Are equal
   (d) Have not been compared
   (e) Are not comparable
4. A crucial initial event on the development of diabetic foot ulcers:
   (a) Low grade microtrauma
   (b) **Loss of protective sensation**
   (c) Lower limb ischemia
   (d) Infection
   (e) Structural deformities
5. The stage at which the typical foot ulcer healing process stalls:
   (a) The hemostatic inflammatory phase
   (b) **The proliferative phase**
   (c) The remodeling phase
6. Compared to patients without diabetes, the risk of amputation in patients with diabetes and peripheral artery disease is:
   (a) Two times higher
   (b) Three times higher

(c) Four times higher

(d) **Five times higher**

(e) Six times higher

7. Historical components of the vascular risk spectrum include:

(a) Macrovascular disease

(b) Microvascular disease

(c) Functional microvascular disease

(d) A and B are correct

(e) **A, B, and C are correct**

8. According to the UKPDS trial, each 1% increase in glycosylated hemoglobin increases the risk of peripheral artery disease:

(a) 12%

(b) **28%**

(c) 34%

(d) 43%

(e) 51%

9. Independent risk factors for peripheral artery disease include all of the following, except:

(a) Hyperglycemia

(b) Smoking

(c) Systolic blood pressure

(d) **Diastolic blood pressure**

(e) Dyslipidemia

10. Different studies have shown that a team approach reduces the risk of lower limb amputations approximately:

(a) 30%

(b) 40%

(c) 50%

(d) **80%**

(e) Compared to traditional management, no reduction have been demonstrated.

References

1. Wild S, et al. Global prevalence of diabetes: estimates for the year 2000 and projections for 2030. Diabetes Care. 2004;27(5):1047–53.

2. Ramsey S, et al. Incidence, outcomes, and cost of foot ulcers in patients with diabetes. Diabetes Care. 1999;22(3):382–7.

3. Reiber GE, Boyko EJ, Smith DG. Lower extremity foot ulcers and amputation in diabetes. In: Harris MI, Cowie CC, Stern MP, et al., editors. Diabetes in America. 2nd ed. Washington: DC, US Government Printing Office; 1995.

4. Apelqvist J, Larsson J, Agardh CD. Long-term prognosis for diabetic patients with foot ulcers. J Intern Med. 1993;233(6):485–91.

5. Larsson J, Agardh CD, Apelqvist J, Stenström A. Long term prognosis after healed amputation in patients with diabetes. Clin Orthop Relat Res. 1998;350:149–58.

6. Moulik P, et al. Amputation and mortality in new-onset diabetic foot ulcers stratified by etiology. Diabetes Care. 2003;26(2):491–4.

7. Mayfield J, et al. Survival following lower-limb amputation in a veteran population. J Rehabil Res Dev. 2001;38(3):341–5.

8. Hoffman M, et al. Survival of diabetes patients with major amputation is comparable to malignant disease. Diab Vasc Dis Res. 2015;12(4):265–71.

9. Sohn M, et al. Lower-extremity amputation risk after Charcot arthropathy and diabetic foot ulcer. Diabetes Care. 2010;33(1):98–100.

10. US Inflation Calculator. Coinnews Media Group. http://www.usinflationcalculator.com/. Last accessed April 2016.

11. Young MJ, et al. The effect of callus removal on dynamic plantar foot pressures in diabetic patients. Diabet Med. 1992;9:55–7.

12. Ledoux W, et al. Relationship between foot type, foot deformity, and ulcer occurrence in the high-risk diabetic foot. J Rehabil Res Dev. 2005;42(5):665–72.

13. Cho CY, Lo JS. Dressing the part. Dermatol Clin. 1998;16(1):25–47.

14. Jude EB, Oyibo SO, Chalmers N, Boulton AJM. Peripheral arterial disease in diabetic and nondiabetic patients. A comparison of severity and outcome. Diabetes Care. 2001;24:1433–7.

15. Holmes C, Harkless L. Linking risk factors: the role of history in predicting outcome. Diabetic Foot. 2004;7(3):116–22.

16. Adler A, et al. UKPDS 59: hyperglycemia and other potentially modifiable risk factors for peripheral vascular disease in type 2 diabetes Adler et al. Diabetes Care. 2002;25(1):894–9.

17. White NH, Sun W, Cleary PA, Danis RP, Davis MD, Hainsworth DP, et al. Prolonged effect of intensive therapy on the risk of retinopathy complications in patients with type 1 diabetes mellitus: 10 years after the diabetes control and complications trial. Arch Ophthalmol. 2008;126:1707–15.

18. El-Osta A, Brasacchio D, Yao D, Pocai A, Jones PL, Roeder RG, et al. Transient high glucose causes persistent epigenetic changes and altered gene expression during subsequent normoglycemia. Exp Med. 2008;205:2409–17.

19. Zong H, Ward M, Stitt AW. AGEs, RAGE, and diabetic retinopathy. Curr Diab Rep. 2011;11:244–52.

20. Kowluru RA, Chan PS. Oxidative stress and diabetic retinopathy. Exp Diabetes Res. 2007;2007:43603.

21. The diabetes control and complications trial research group. The effect of intensive treatment of diabetes on the development and progression of long-term complications in insulin-dependent diabetes mellitus. N Engl J Med. 1993;329:977–86.

22. Epidemiology of diabetes interventions and complications (EDIC). Design, implementation, and preliminary results of a long-term follow-up of the diabetes control and complications trial cohort. Diabetes Care. 1999;22:99–111.

23. Armstrong DG, Lavery LA, Kimbriel HR, Nixon BP, Boulton AJM. Activity patterns of patients with diabetic foot ulceration. Diabetes Care. 2003;26(9):2595–7.

24. Armstrong DG, Abu-Rumman PL, Nixon BP, Boulton AJ. Continuous activity monitoring in persons at high risk for diabetes-related lower-extremity amputation. J Am Podiatr Med Assoc. 2001;91(9):451–5.

25. Armstrong DG, Rosales MA, Gashi A. Efficacy of Fifth Metatarsal Head Resection for Treatment of Chronic Diabetic Foot Ulceration. J Am Podiatr Med Assoc. 2005;95(4):353–6.

26. Armstrong DG, Nguyen HC, Lavery LA, van Schie CH, Boulton AJ, Harkless LB. Off-loading the diabetic foot wound: a randomized clinical trial. Diabetes Care. 2001;24(6):1019–22.

27. Piaggesi A, Schipani E, Campi F, Romanelli M, Baccetti F, Arvia C, Navalesi R. Conservative surgical approach versus non-surgical Management for Diabetic Neuropathic Foot Ulcers: a randomized trial. Diabet Med. 1998;15:412–7.

28. Waaijmann R, et al. Adherence to wearing prescription custom-made footwear in patients with diabetes at high risk for plantar foot ulceration. Diabetes Care. 2013;36:1613–8.

29. Pakarinen TK, et al. Long-term outcome and quality of life in patients with Charcot foot. Foot Ankle Surg. 2009;15(4):187–91.

30. Milne T, et al. Developing an evidence-based clinical pathway for the assessment, diagnosis and Management of Acute Charcot Neuro-Arthropathy: a systematic review. J Foot Ankle Res. 2013;6(30):1–12.

31. Sochocki M, et al. Health related quality of life in patients with Charcot arthropathy of the foot and ankle. Foot Ankle Surg. 2008;14:11–5.

32. Jeffocoate W, et al. The role of proinflammatory cytokines in the cause of neuropathic osteoarthropathy (acute Charcot foot) in diabetes. Lancet. 2005;366:2058–61.

33. Hofbauer L, Schoppet M. Clinical implications of the Osteoprotegrin/RANK/RANKL system for bone and vascular diseases. J Am Med Assoc. 2004;292(4):490–5.

34. Petrova N, et al. Is there a systemic inflammatory response in the acute Charcot foot? Diabetes Care. 2007;30(4):997–8.

35. Armstrong D, Lavery L. Monitoring healing of acute Charcot's arthropathy with infrared dermal thermometry. J Rehabil Res Dev. 1997;34(3):317–21.

36. Bharara M, et al. Thermography and thermometry in the assessment of diabetic neuropathic foot: a case for furthering the role of thermal techniques. Int J Low Extrem Wounds. 2006;5(4):250–60.

37. Judge M. Infection and neuroarthropathy: the utility of C-reactive protein as a screening tool in the Charcot foot. J Am Podiatr Med Assoc. 1998;98(1):1–6.

38. Rosenbaum A. Classifications in brief: Eichenholtz classification of Charcot arthropathy. Clin Orthop Relat Res. 2015;473(3):1168–71.

39. Shibata T, et al. The results of arthrodesis of the ankle for leprotic neuroarthropathy. J Bone Joint Surg. 1990;72:749–56.

40. Aliabadi P, et al. Imaging of neuropathic arthropathy. Semin Musculoskelet Radiol. 2003;7(3):217–25.

41. Sanders LJ, Frykberg RG. Diabetic neuropathic osteoarthropathy: the Charcot foot. In: Frykberg RG, editor. The high risk foot in diabetes mellitus. New York: Churchill Livingston; 1991. p. 297–338.

42. Fosbøl M, et al. Three-phase bone scintigraphy for diagnosis of Charcot neuropathic osteoarthropathy in the diabetic foot – does quantitative data improve diagnostic value? Clin Physiol Funct Imaging. 2017;37(1):30–6.

43. Sinacore D. Acute Charcot arthropathy in patients with diabetes mellitus: healing times by foot location. J Diabetes Complicat. 1998;12:287–93.

44. Pinzur M, et al. Treatment of Eichenholz stage I Charcot foot arthropathy with a weight-bearing Total contact cast. Foot Ankle Int. 2006;27(56):324–9.

45. Schon LC, et al. Charcot neuroarthropathy of the foot and ankle. Clin Orthop Relat Res. 1998;349:116–31.

46. Jude EB, et al. Bisphosphonates in the treatment of Charcot neuroarthropathy: a double-blind randomized controlled trial. Diabetalogia. 2001;44(11):2032–7.

47. Pakarinen TK, et al. The effect of zoledronic acid on the clinical resolution of Charcot neuroarthropathy. Diabetes Care. 2011;34:1514–6.

48. Pitocco D, et al. Six-month treatment with Aledronate in acute Charcot neuroarthropathy. Diabetes Care. 2005;28(5):1214–5.

49. Anderson J, et al. Bisphosphonates fort he treatment of Charcot neuroarthropathy. J Foot Ankle Surg. 2004;43(5):285–9.

50. Richard JL, et al. Treatment of acute Charcot foot with bisphosphonates: a systematic review of the literature. Diabetalogia. 2012;55(5):1258–64.

51. Al-Nammari SS, et al. A Surgeon's guide to advances in the pharmacological management of acute Charcot neuroarthropathy. Foot Ankle Surg. 2013;19(4):212–7.

52. Sohn MW, et al. Mortality risk of Charcot arthropathy compared with that of diabetic foot ulcer and diabetes alone. Diabetes Care. 2009;32(5):816–21.

53. Waters R, et al. Energy cost of walking of amputees: the influence of level of amputation. J Bone Joint Surg. 1976;58:42–6.

54. Gailey S, et al. Energy expenditure of trans-tibial amputees during ambulation at self-selected pace. Prosthetics Orthot Int. 1994;18(2):84–91.

55. Mayfield J, et al. Survival following lower-limb amputation in a veteran population. J Rehab Res Develop. 2001;38(3):341–5.

56. Izumi Y, et al. Mortality of first-time amputees in diabetics: a 10 year observation. Diab Res Clin Pract. 2009;83:126–31.

57. Brown M, et al. Partial foot amputations in patients with diabetic foot ulcers. Foot Ankle Int. 2012;33(9):707–16.

58. Nerone V, et al. Reamputation after minor foot amputation in diabetic patients: factors leading to limb loss. J Foot Ankle Surg. 2013;52(2):184–7.

59. Caselli A, et al. Transcutaneous oxygen tension monitoring after successful revascularization in diabetic patients with Ischaemic foot ulcers. Diabet Med. 2005;22(4):460–5.

60. Garbalosa JB, et al. Foot function in diabetic patients after partial amputation. Foot Ankle Int. 1996;17(1):43–8.

61. Giurini J, et al. Panmetatarsal head resection. A viable alternative to the transmetataral amputation. J Am Podiatr Med Assoc. 1993;83(2):101–7.

62. Garwood C, Steinberg G. Soft tissue balancing after partial foot amputations. Clin Podiatr Med Surg. 2016;33(1):99–111.

63. Schweinberger M, Roukis T. Soft-tissue and osseous techniques to balance forefoot and midfoot amputations. Clin Podiatr Med Surg. 2008;25(4):623–39.

64. Murdoch D, et al. The natural history of great toe amputations. J Foot Ankle Surg. 1997;36(3):204–8.

65. Kadukammakal J, et al. Assessment of partial first-ray resections and their tendency to Progress to Transmetatarsal amputations. J Am Podiatr Med Assoc. 2012;102(5):412–6.

66. Izimi Y, et al. Risk of Reamputation in diabetic patients stratified by limb and level of amputation: a 10 year observation. Diabetes Care. 2006;29(3):566–70.

67. Cohen M, et al. Panmetatarsal head resection and Transmetatarsal amputation versus solitary partial first ray resection in the neuropathic foot. J Foot Surg. 1991;30(1):29–33.

68. Simon G, et al. Diabetes complications and depression as predictors of health service costs. Gen Hosp Psychiatry. 2005;27:344–51.

69. Egede L, et al. The effect of depression on self-care behaviors and quality of Care in a National Sample of adults with diabetes. Gen Hosp Psychiatry. 2009;31:422–7.

70. Williams LH. Depression and incident diabetic foot ulcers: a prospective cohort study. Am J Med. 2010;123(8):748–54.

71. Monami M, et al. The diabetic person beyond a foot ulcer: healing, recurrence, and depressive symptoms. J Am Podiatr Med Assoc. 2008;98(2):130–6.

72. Williams LH, et al. Depression and incident lower limb amputations in veterans with diabetes. J Diabetes Complications. 2011;25(3):175–82.

73. Rogers L, et al. Toe and flow: essential components and structure of the amputation prevention team. J Am Podiatr Med Assoc. 2010;100(5):342–8.

74. Van Gils CC, et al. Amputation prevention by vascular surgery and podiatry collaboration in high-risk diabetic and nondiabetic patients. The operation desert foot experience. Diabetes Care. 1998;22(5):678–83.

75. Aksoy DY, et al. Change in the amputation profile in diabetic foot in a tertiary reference center: efficacy of team working. Exp Clin Endocrinol Diabetes. 2004;112(9):526–30.

76. Driver VR, et al. Reducing amputation rates in patients with diabetes at a military medicalcenter: the limb preservation service model. Diabetes Care. 2005;28(2):248–53.

Diabetes and Cancer

63

Joanna Wojciechowska, Wojciech Krajewski,
Tomasz Zatoński, and Joel Rodriguez-Saldana

Chapter Objectives

- The prevalence of diabetes mellitus type 2 and cancers of various sites is dramatically increasing nowadays. It was established that diabetes mellitus (mainly type 2 diabetes mellitus) predisposes do oncogenesis in various human organs.
- The main factors leading to neoplastic transformation in diabetics are hyperinsulinaemia, hyperglycaemia and chronic inflammation induced by excessive adipose tissue.
- Anti-diabetic medications interfere with the risk of neoplastic transformation—some of them elevate the risk, some reduce the risk and some express inconsistent activity.
- Certain anti-diabetic medications express potential usefulness in improving effectiveness of conventional chemotherapy.
- Diabetics with T2DM and coexisting neoplasm have worse disease-free and overall survival than patients with neoplasm but without T2DM.

J. Wojciechowska (✉) · T. Zatoński
Department and Clinic of Otolaryngology, Head and Neck Surgery, Wrocław Medical University Hospital, Wrocław, Poland

W. Krajewski
Department and Clinic of Otolaryngology, Head and Neck Surgery, Wrocław Medical University Hospital, Wrocław, Poland

Department and Clinic of Urology, Wrocław Medical University Hospital, Wrocław, Poland
e-mail: wk@sofstar.pl

J. Rodriguez-Saldana
Multidisciplinary Diabetes Center Mexico,
Ciudad de México, Mexico

Introduction

Diabetes mellitus (DM), one of the most common diseases all around the world, comprises a large group of metabolic disorders. DM is characterized by persistent hyperglycaemia caused by inaccurate function of insulin or its reduced excretion from pancreatic beta cells. Long-lasting hyperglycaemia results in damage and improper function of various organs. The morbidity of T2DM is rapidly increasing especially in middle-aged people (45–65 years). Interestingly, recent evidence implies that there is a significant correlation between DM and neoplastic transformation [1–9]. The association was observed both for type 1 diabetes mellitus (T1DM) and type 2 diabetes mellitus (T2DM) [10]; nevertheless the majority of studies concern T2DM [11, 12]. It has been shown that DM (especially T2DM) increases the risk of various cancers in men and women [10, 11]. Up to now, little is known about the links between T1DM and carcinogenesis. Nevertheless, it was observed that T1DM enhances the overall risk of pancreas, liver, oesophagus, colon and rectum, and stomach, thyroid, brain, lung, endometrium, ovary, cervix, squamous cell skin cancers and acute lymphatic leukaemia in women [10–13]. The strongest association between DM and carcinogenesis is observed for pancreatic and liver cancers in patients with T2DM [14]. Additionally, according to the current knowledge there is also a relationship between neoplastic transformation and anti-diabetic medications [6]. However, the exact mechanisms leading to this connection need further investigation [1, 15].

Historical Facts

The first description of diabetes (a state of polyuria) was found in the Ebers Papyrus in 1552 BC by Egyptian physician Hesy-Ra. This description was found in Thebes (Egypt) in 1862 AD by Egyptologist Georg Ebers. The term "diabetes" comes from Greek meaning "siphone" and was introduced by Areteus from Cappadocia (81-138 AD) who described main symptoms of this disease [16, 17]. The main differences between the two most common types of DM (type 1 and type 2) were observed and described by Himsworth in 1936 [18].

Epidemiology

The number of persons with diabetes mellitus in 2021 estimated by the International Diabetes Federation (IDF) among adults (aged 20–79 years) reached 537 million of people [19]. Nevertheless, approximately 50% of DM cases remain undiagnosed. The IDF estimates that in 2040 the number of persons with diabetes will amount 785 million people [19].

The World Health Organization (WHO) has declared that cancer is the leading cause of death worldwide, accounting for nearly ten million deaths in 2020 [20]. The most common new causes of cancer in 2020 were breast (2.26 million cases), lung (2.21 million cases), colon and rectum (1.93 million cases), prostate (1.41 million cases), skin (non-melanoma) (1.20 million cases) and stomach (1.09 million cases) [20]. The most common causes of cancer death in 2020 were lung, colon and rectum, liver, stomach and breast, and according to the WHO, the annual incidence of new cancer cases will reach 22 million in the next two decades [20]. Normal cells transform into malignant cancer cells through a complex process, including initiation, promotion and progression involving more aggressive growth, angiogenesis and metastases [21].

Types of Diabetes Mellitus

Diabetes is a group of disease entities that can be classified as follows:

T1DM (previously known as "insulin-dependent diabetes mellitus") is caused by autoimmune or idiopathic process of self-aggression leading to rapid destruction of pancreatic β-cells. As a result, the level of insulin, the pancreatic hormone responsible for maintaining glycaemic control, is minimal or undetectable. T1DM usually appears as ketoacidosis with its main symptoms including polyuria, polydipsia, nausea, vomiting, stomachache, weakness, acetone breath and Kussmaul breathing. T1DM concerns 5–10% of all cases of diabetes. The autoimmune process is characterized by the presence of four types of antibodies: ICA (islet cell antibodies), IAA (insulin autoantibodies), anti-GAD (anti-glutamid acid decarboxylase), IA-2 and IA-2B (tyrosine phosphatase-related islet antibodies). These antibodies can be detected months of even years before first symptoms of the disease. Generally, T1DM is not an inherited disease; however, there is a proven genetic predisposition determined by HLA (human leukocyte anti-

gens). The highest susceptibility to T1DM occurs in patients with haplotype HLA-DRB1*03 (DR3) or HLA-DRB1*04 (DR4) with DQB1*03:02 (DQ8) [22]. Conversely, the HLA-DQ6 haplotype is considered to protect against developing T1DM. T1DM may appear at any age but is usually diagnosed during childhood (before 30 years). The exception is LADA (Latent Autoimmune Diabetes of Adults) that occurs in adults. T1DM treatment is based on multiple doses of exogenous insulin preparations for the lifetime.

T2DM (previously known as "non-insulin-dependent diabetes mellitus") is the most common form of diabetes (up to 95% of all cases). T2DM is generally characterized by insulin resistance of insulin-dependent tissues (adipose tissue, liver and muscle cells) leading to improper, excessive secretion of insulin and hyperinsulinaemia [23]. Insulin insensitivity causes a decreased glucose uptake of target tissues and increased serum glucose level [18]. Other pathologies in T2DM comprise increased amount of circulating inflammatory cytokines, adipokines, lipotoxic free fatty acids or amyloid deposits in pancreatic islet cells [24]. Risk factors of T2DM include genetic, inherited predisposition, sedentary lifestyle, obesity, ageing, cigarettes smoking and/or excessive alcohol consumption. This type of diabetes commonly affects middle-aged or older people albeit during the last two decades an increasing trend has occurred in adolescents. The genetic susceptibility to T2DM is more significant than observed in T1DM. Confirmed positive family history is associated with a 2–4 times increased risk of T2DM [24]. Recently discovered genes connected with high risk of developing T2DM are insulin receptor, potassium channels, proteases or transcription factors genes [16, 24]. The onset and early stages of T2DM are usually asymptomatic and progressive, and the slow development of the disease leads to delayed diagnosis. Being asymptomatic years before diagnosis, patients with T2DM are more prone to develop macrovascular or microvascular complications [24]. Management in T2DM is based on lifestyle changes, medical nutrition therapy, physical activity, diabetes education and support, and anti-diabetics [25–27]. Reducing body weight and physical activity are the firsts steps of therapy and essential in every stage of the disease. Pharmacotherapy must be patient-adjusted and includes a variety of glucose-lowering drugs such as biguanides (metformin), sulfonylureas, meglitinides, α-glucosidase inhibitors, thiazolidinediones (TZD), dipeptidyl peptidase four inhibitors (DPP-4-i), glucagon-like peptide-1 agonists (GLP-1) and sodium-glucose co-transporter 2 inhibitors (SGLT2 inhibitors). If all mentioned methods are insufficient to achieve glycaemic control, insulin injections are required. Insulin may be used as monotherapy or in combination with other anti-diabetic drugs.

Additional etiological classes of diabetes include monogenic types, including MODY (maturity onset diabetes of the young), an inherited form caused by an autosomal dominant gene. The pathophysiology of this type of diabetes is based on improper beta cells secretion of insulin with preserved insulin function [23]. Monogenic-type diabetes usually manifests in childhood (younger than 25) and is characterized by hyperglycaemia, insulin deficiency and mild clinical symptoms. Insulin resistance is not observed in MODY. Therapy in this type is of diabetes based on medical nutrition and oral anti-diabetics. Secondary causes of known aetiology include genetic defects of beta cells and insulin function, diabetes caused by drugs or other chemicals, infections, endocrinopathies, diseases of the exocrine pancreas or genetic syndromes.

Gestational diabetes (GDM) is a state of glucose intolerance that begins or is diagnosed during pregnancy. GDM is caused by insulin resistance during gestation and affects up to 7% of pregnant women. Insulin resistance in women with GDM is higher than in healthy ones, probably because of chronic insulin resistance observed in the first group [28]. During pregnancy, levels of hormones opposing insulin action (placental lactogen, oestrogen, progesterone and prolactin) are elevated, leading to excessive insulin secretion. Risk factors of GDM include obesity, GDM in previous pregnancies, positive family history of diabetes, current glucosuria and history of macrosomia in previous pregnancies. The management in GDM is based on medical nutrition, exercise and if this management is insufficient, insulin injections. Gestational diabetes is a risk factor for T2DM after childbirth T2DM [29]. Most of the studies about the association of diabetes are focused on Type 2 diabetes and cancer are focused on probably because of a higher prevalence of T2DM than T1DM.

Diabetes Mellitus and Oncogenesis—The Main Correlation

The association between DM and carcinogenesis was described for the first time in 1910 by Maynard and Pearson [30–31]. One hundred years afterwards, a consensus report presented by the American Diabetes Association (ADA) and the American Cancer Society (ACS) in 2010 described possible factors linking diabetes and cancer which could be divided into three main groups including modifiable risk factors, non-modifiable risk factors and biological links between DM and cancer [1, 32].

Links between DM and oncogenesis according to the ADA and the ACS:

- Modifiable risk factors:
  - overweight (BMI >25 and <30) and obesity (BMI >30)
  - physical activity (at least 5 days a week for 30 min a day reduces the probability of T2DM development)
  - smoking
  - alcohol abuse

- Non-modifiable risk factors:
  - sex (men are more prone than women)
  - age (adults aged between 55 and 60 years and older are more prone)
  - race (African Americans are more prone than Caucasians)
- Biological links:
  - hyperinsulinaemia (the effect of resistance to endogenous insulin or by exogenous insulin used as a medication).
  - hyperglycaemia
  - fat-induced chronic inflammation

Biological Linking Factors

(hyperinsulinaemia, hyperglycaemia, fat-induced chronic inflammation)

Role of Hyperinsulinaemia in Cancer Biology

Epidemiological studies have shown that high levels of insulin or C-peptide predict an increased risk for colorectal, breast, pancreas, bladder and endometrial cancer [21]. Insulin resistance and hyperinsulinaemia are important factors in the development of type 2 diabetes and additionally, insulin stimulates cell proliferation and promotes carcinogenesis in experimental animals [33]. Insulin resistance blocks signalling in the metabolic pathway involved in glucose metabolism, but does not inhibit activation of the cell signalling pathway involving cell differentiation [21]. The pro-neoplastic features of insulin are induced by activation of its receptors, Insulin Receptor [IR] and Insulin-like Growth Factor-1 is a polypeptide synthesized by almost all cells, although primarily by the liver [21]. Insulin resistance is able to activate the IGF-R receptor (IGF-R) because of approximately 60% structural homology of IGF-R and IR [33]. Similarly, IR may be stimulated by insulin and by both Insulin-like growth factors, IGF-1 and IGF-2 [34]. Ligand-induced IR autophosphorylation triggers intracellular mechanisms. The most important is activation of PI3K/Akt/mTOR (phosphoinositide 3-kinase/protein kinase B/mammalian target of rapamycin) signalling pathway. Stimulation of PI3K/Akt/mTOR signalling pathway plays a critical role in oncogenesis [35]. Interestingly, activation of IGF-R (by both insulin and IGF) results in more significant pro-neoplastic effects than activation of IR. IR and IGF-R are critical in tumourigenesis also because of the fact that their concentration in various cancer cells is higher than in normal cells; thus the effect of insulin and IGF on neoplastic cells is enhanced [36, 37].

Indirect Effects of Hyperinsulinaemia on Cancer Biology

– Up-regulation of bioavailable IGF-1 by hyperinsulinaemia-induced down-regulation of IGF-binding protein 1,2 and IGF-binding protein-3. IGF-binding proteins are crucial in IGF serum transfer and activity. IGF binding to specific proteins does not exert its biological effects (biological inactivity) [36, 38].
– Up-regulation of IGF-1 in growth hormone (GH)-dependent manner (*Explanation:* Insulin stimulates growth hormone receptors (GHR) located in the liver leading to elevated release of GH. Subsequently, GH promotes IGF-1 synthesis) [39].
– Up-regulation of leptin, a pro-neoplastic adipokine [40].
– Reduced synthesis of sex hormone binding protein (SHBG) in the liver (*Explanation:* SHBG plays an important role in transfer and activity of sex hormones (testosterone, oestrogen). Reduced amount of SHBG leads to high bioavailability of sex hormones that presumably results in development of hormone-related cancers (e.g. endometrial, breast cancer) [41].

The Role of Hyperglycaemia in Cancer Biology

It was established that cancer cells require high glucose levels to grow and survive. Cancer cells are more sensitive to high serum glucose levels than normal cells because of their elevated concentration of glucose receptors (GLUT-1, GLUT-3). These cells are characterized by rapid development and metabolism, and therefore they require high glucose resources [42]. The link between glucose and cancer dates back to the Warburg effect, described by Otto Warburg in 1924, which states that "the prime cause of cancer is the replacement of the respiration of oxygen (oxidation of glucose) in normal body cells by fermentation of sugar [43]. Hyperglycaemia enables neoplastic transformation via stimulation of cells' quick growth and development, suppression of apoptosis and metastasis promotion [44]. Increased blood glucose levels affect the normal cellular system at three steps contributing to dysregulated growth: (1) DNA (genetic), (2) RNA transcription, (3) Protein (translation) [45].

Mechanisms Leading to Proliferative Activity of Hyperglycaemia [21, 44, 45]

– Elevated expression of PPAR α and γ (*peroxisome proliferator-activated receptor*) (*Explanation:* PPAR α

and γ interfere with lipid metabolic pathways and speed up neoplastic cells development).
– *Elevated expression of* glucose receptors (GLUT-1, GLUT-3) leading to increased cellular glucose intake.
– Elevated expression of EFG (epithelial growth factor) that activates neoplastic pathways via binding to its receptor EGFR (epithelial growth factor receptor).
– Increased amounts of ROS (reactive oxygen species) and SOD (superoxide dismutase) leading to free radicals and other reactive molecules which could produce oxidative damage to DNA, mutations in oncogenes and tumour suppressor genes (*Explanation:* Oxidative stress is a critical triggering factor of insulin resistance, a tumour-promoting factor. In addition, it induces glucose-mediated inflammation and increased synthesis of transcriptional factors including NF-κB, activating protein-1 and early growth response-1. These mechanisms lead to tumour growth and metastasis).

Mechanisms Leading to Anti-apoptotic Activity of Hyperglycaemia [44]

– Reduced amount of PDH (prolyl hydroxylase) resulting in increased levels of HIF-α (hypoxia-inducible factor α) (*Explanation:* The majority of energy in tumour cells is produced in a hypoxic environment, via aerobic glycolysis. HIF-α is a critical factor involved in cancer cell existence in hypoxic milieu; thus hyperglycaemia-induced high amount of HIF-α promotes tumour cells growth and survival).

Mechanisms Leading to Hyperglycaemia-Mediated Metastasis [44–47]

– Increased zinc intake resulting in cancer cells dislocation (*Explanation:* Increased zinc intake is caused by hyperglycaemia-induced high expression of zinc receptors. Zinc is an intracellular signalling molecule, able to convert extracellular impulses to intracellular processes and to mediate interaction between cells).
– Up-regulation of urokinase plasminogen activator (uPA), a critical mediator in cancer cells displacement.
– Stimulation of ETM (epithelial to mesenchymal transition) process, a mechanism that enables cancer cells to metastasise.

Moreover, hyperglycaemia induces epigenetic changes resulting in constant activation of oncogenic pathways, a phenomenon called "hyperglycaemic memory". Activation of oncogenic pathways is regulated by overexpression of well-known neoplastic mediators, nuclear factor-κB (NF-κB) and neuregulin-1 (Nrg1) [44].

Role of Obesity and Fat-Induced Chronic Inflammation in Cancer Biology

Adipose tissue consists of adipocytes, endothelial, immune cells like and cytokines, associated with cancer risk and progression [21]. The vast majority of patients with T2DM are obese or overweight. Besides being a risk factor for T2DM and various cardiovascular disorders, obesity reveals pro-neoplastic activity [48–52]. Nowadays, the correlation between obesity and carcinogenesis has been widely discussed. It was reported that adiposity promotes the development of breast, endometrial, pancreatic, colorectal and oesophageal cancer [48–49]. Meta-analysis of case-control and prospective cohort studies has confirmed that T2DM is an independent risk factor for the development of non-Hodgkin lymphoma, and cancer of the bladder, breast, colon and rectum, endometrium, liver and pancreas [48], and some studies report that nearly 40% of all cancers can be attributed to overweight and obesity [49]. Obesity presumably exerts its pro-neoplastic activities in various ways. It interferes with sex hormones physiology, induces chronic inflammation and changes profile of adipose tissue polypeptide hormones (adipokines) [41, 49]. Adipose tissue is a crucial endocrine organ and in condition of abundance leads to dysregulation of endocrine mechanisms. Excessive adipose tissue expresses high amounts of aromatase, an enzyme critical in converting androgens to oestrogens, leading to high levels of oestrogens, which accompanied by low concentration of progesterone increases the risk of oestrogen-related breast and endometrial cancers [21, 41, 49]. Obesity-induced chronic inflammation is characterized by increased production of proinflammatory cytokines including interleukin-6, resistin and TNF-alpha (Tumour Necrosis Factor-alpha), which in turn lead to an increase in insulin levels, further increasing the inflammatory response [41]. Moreover, excessive adipose tissue secretes high amount of VEGF (Vascular Endothelial Growth Factor) and MMP (matrix metalloproteinases) leading to tumour growth and metastasis, respectively [41]. Adiponectin and leptin are two antagonist adipokines with significant impact on carcinogenesis [49, 50]. The level of adiponectin is decreased and the level of leptin is increased in patients with excessive adipose tissue. Adiponectin sensitizes cells to insulin, suppresses cells growth and metabolism, and exerts pro-apoptotic mechanisms, whereas leptin stimulates proliferation of cancer cells [49, 50]. In clinical studies, adiponectin inhibited tumour development in in vitro breast cancer cell lines and in animals afflicted by sarcomas [51, 52]. Conversely, leptin exacerbates insulin resistance and induces tumour-promoting processes, stimulates angiogenesis and tumour proliferation, and prevents apoptosis [49].

Diabetes and the Correlation with Oncogenesis in Particular Organs

Various studies emphasize that DM may induce neoplastic transformation [6]. Nevertheless, the exact influence of DM on carcinogenesis in particular organs has not been fully elucidated and the results of different studies remain conflicting. The positive correlation between DM and tumourigenesis was observed for organs of digestive system (pancreas, colon and liver), genitourinary system (bladder, kidney, endometrium), head and neck region and breast [53, 54]. On the other hand, a negative, inverse correlation was found only for prostate cancer which increases with increasing duration of diabetes [48]. The majority of the recent studies concern pancreatic and liver cancers; thus these two entities would be discussed more precisely than others. The current knowledge of the association between DM and cancers of particular organs is discussed below.

Pancreatic Cancer

The correlation between DM and increased risk of pancreatic cancer (PaC) was confirmed by various studies [55]. However, the association between diabetes and PaC remains unclear, because of a two-way relationship. PaC may lead to increased glucose and insulin levels followed by abnormal glucose metabolism, and abnormal glucose metabolism may cause neoplastic transformation in pancreatic cells. Huxley et al. reported a 50% increased risk of PaC in patients with T2DM history shorter than 5 years [56] and Elena et al. suggested that persons with diabetes have a 40% higher risk of PaC than people without diabetes [57]. In this study, the highest level of risk was observed in patients with DM lasting for 2–8 years; DM of 9 or more years was not associated with increased risk of PaC and may be possibly caused by hypoinsulinaemia that develops along with diabetes duration [57]. Conversely, an elevated risk of PaC in patients with long-lasting DM was reported in another study [58]. It has also been shown that patients with obesity and T2DM have a 54% higher risk of PaC [57]. On the other hand, Grote et al. observed a statistically significant increased risk of PaC in patients with HbA (1c) ≥6,5% compared with ≤5,4%, independently of obesity or insulin resistance [59]. It was found that patients with diabetes and T2DM have a higher propensity to suffer from PaC because of high serum concentration of insulin and its precursors. The authors did not find a significant association between T1DM and PaC [59, 214]. On the other hand, another study reported a two-times higher risk of PaC in patients with

T1DM or MODY than in people without diabetes [60]. There are also studies implying genetic predisposition to PaC in individuals with diabetes [61, 62]. Interestingly, Prizment et al. checked 10 different SNPs (Single Nucleotide Polymorphisms) related to DM and found a positive association between PaC incidence and DM only for one of the examined SNPs—GCKR rs780094 (glucokinase gene which rises plasma fasting glucose level) [61]. Additionally, it has been shown that GCKR rs780094 is associated with a higher risk of T2DM and PSA-detected prostate cancer [63]. Another research examining the genetic susceptibility to PaC in diabetics found a higher PaC risk in patients with glucose-rising allele of MADD rs11039149, FTO rs8050136 and MTNR1B rs1387153 variants. The inverse association was observed for BCL11A rs243021 [62].

Liver Cancer: it was established that T2DM as well as T2DM-related metabolic disorders stimulate tumourigenesis in hepatic cells. Hepatocellular carcinoma (HCC) is the most frequently observed primary malignant cancer in the liver and is also commonly present in diabetics [64]. In 1986 Lawson reported for the first time the positive association between higher prevalence of HCC in diabetics [65] and other authors confirmed this finding [66, 67]. Besides being observed in diabetics, HCC frequently occurs in patients with non-alcoholic fatty liver disease (NAFLD) and in those with obesity and insulin resistance [67]. NAFLD is a condition commonly seen in individuals with T2DM and is critically correlated with adiposity. NAFLD as well as T2DM and obesity stimulates tumourigenesis in liver cells via various mechanisms including modified adipokines profile (increased leptin level and decreased adiponectin level), oxidative stress (imbalance between antioxidant and prooxidant factors) and lipotoxicity (malfunction or death of non-adipose tissue cells caused by accumulation of excess lipids). Through the portal circulation, the liver is exposed to high amounts of circulating insulin. Constantly high insulin levels, via elevated production of IGF-1, lead to multiplication and apoptotic suppression in hepatic cells [68]. According to a meta-analysis of 25 cohort studies, the incidence of HCC is significantly increased in both men and women with DM [66], and other authors reached to consistent conclusions [64, 65, 68]. It is difficult to establish whether T2DM is an independent risk factor for HCC or whether T2DM leads to HCC via induction of other liver disorders including NAFLD, steatosis, alcohol abuse, cirrhosis and HCV/HBV infections [63, 69]. Beyond these contributing factors, the association between DM and HCC remains unclear [1].

Colon/Colorectal Cancer: a variety of studies established that T2DM predisposes to colon and colorectal cancers (CRC). A meta-analysis conducted by Larsson et al. revealed that DM is a significant risk factor for CRC [70]. The relative risk among diabetics was approximately 30% higher than in non-diabetics and was similar in both genders and the overall mortality of CRC is approximately 1.5 times higher in diabetics than in non-diabetics [70]. The positive association between T2DM and colon/colorectal cancer was also described in another study which found that the incidence of cancer was similar in colon and in rectum, with no statistically significant difference between genders [71]. Another meta-analysis revealed a 1.22-fold higher relative risk of CRC in people with diabetes [54]. Similar results were reported in other studies [53, 72].

Bladder Cancer: according to current knowledge there is also a positive association between T2DM and oncogenesis in bladder cells [73, 74]. The association was observed for both female and male diabetics. Woolcott et al. found an increased risk of bladder cancer in patients with diabetes with higher levels of risk in females [75]. Conversely, Zhu et al. reported a statistically significant increased risk for bladder cancer in men with T2DM [76].

Kidney Cancer: the clear association between renal cell cancer (RCC) and DM has not been fully elucidated. Various studies reported conflicting results. A prospective study of women with T2DM conducted by Hee-Kyung et al. revealed increased risk of renal cell cancer (RCC) in this group [77]. Similar associations were described in Japanese men and in Czech diabetics [78, 79]. No such correlation was found in another study [80]. Qayyum et al. suggested that DM is not an independent risk factor of RCC, but when combined with obesity or hypertension, it increased the risk of RCC [81]. Another study did not confirm that DM is a risk factor for RCC; however it revealed an increased risk of death from RCC in diabetics [82].

Endometrial Cancer: a significant role of DM in endometrial carcinogenesis was emphasized by a number of authors and it was also strongly implied that DM is an independent risk factor of endometrial carcinogenesis [83]. Lindemann et al. established a three times increased risk of endometrial cancer (EC) in diabetic women [84]. Interestingly, the risk of EC is more than six times higher in obese diabetics in comparison with non-obese non-diabetics [38]. An investigation on the influence of elevated serum glucose level on EC development revealed that both elevated serum glucose level caused by impaired glucose metabolism and DM increased the risk of EC [85]. It was suggested that DM might predispose to EC via hyperinsulinaemia-dependent reduced levels of adiponectin and through obesity-related decreased concentration of SHBG. The reduced levels of SHBG lead to elevated bioavailable oestrogen and testosterone amounts and eventually stimulate endometrial oncogenesis [49–86].

Breast Cancer: the significant correlation between DM and the high risk of oncogenesis in breast tissues has been widely discussed in the literature and is now well established [87, 88].

The revealed causes of breast carcinogenesis in DM include [87–89]:

- activation of IR or IGF-R through IGF
- overexpression of IR in breast tissue
- activation of insulin-dependent IP3-K/AKT/mTOR pathway
- hyperglycaemia
- insulin-induced increased level of bioavailable IGF-1
- insulin-induced increased concentration of leptin
- insulin-induced reduced level of adiponectin
- insulin-induced reduced level of SHBG resulting in increased amount of bioavailable oestradiol

The correlation between DM and breast cancer is mainly observed in postmenopausal women [87]. Nondiabetic postmenopausal obese women with hyperinsulinaemia are at higher risk of BC incidence in comparison to normoinsulinemic ones [90]. The presumed inequalities in the prevalence of BC in post- and premenopausal diabetic females may be induced by different oestrogen concentrations (modified indirectly by insulin) observed in these populations [32].

The correlation between T2DM and BC incidence was also studied in MKR (MKR is a mouse model of T2DM, which has a genetically modified IGF-1 receptor) [91]. The authors of this study documented a positive relationship between BC and high insulin concentrations in MKR female mice with hyperinsulinaemia. The hyperinsulinaemic milieu in MKR led to proliferation and oncogenesis in breast cells. Subsequently, specimens of tumour and breast tissues from examined mice were taken for further research. The obtained tissues presented elevated level of IR and increased IR/IGF-1R activation that resulted in insulin-dependent metabolic effects and proliferation of mammary glands [91]. Overexpression of IGF-1R in breast tissue in transgenic mice and its influence on BC incidence was also emphasized in another study [92].

Head and Neck Cancers: studies investigating the association between DM and head and neck cancers (HNCs) are sparse with conflicting results. Some authors reported positive association, some reported negative inverse association and some found no correlation. The majority of precise studies focus on particular organs of the head and neck area. In general, the incidence of HNC was weakly associated with T2DM or no significant relationship was revealed [93, 94]. On the other hand, there is also the presumption that head and neck squamous cell carcinoma (HNSCC) is slightly inversely associated with T2DM [95].

Laryngeal Cancer

Japanese men with diabetes present a significantly higher risk of laryngeal cancer independently of smoking status [96]. Other studies on Japanese population of diabetics found an increased risk of laryngeal cancer in both genders [78, 97]. Conversely, the risk of laryngeal cancer incidence was decreased in a large group of U.S. veterans with T2DM [98]. No significant association between these two diseases was observed in another study [99].

Pharyngeal Cancer

A significantly higher risk of oropharyngeal and nasopharyngeal cancers was reported in Taiwanese individuals with T2DM [3]. The risk of pharyngeal cancer is higher in those with long-lasting T2DM in comparison to those with a short history of T2DM [99].

Oral Cancer

The increased risk of oral cancer incidence in diabetics has also been described [3, 99].

Prostate Cancer: according to the current knowledge, prostate cancer (PC) is the only neoplasm that is inversely related to DM [100], and a number of research documented a significant protective influence of DM on PC incidence [100–102]. This association is presumably a result of hyperglycaemia-induced low concentrations of testosterone and hypoinsulinaemia in patients with T1DM or long-lasting T2DM. Physiologically, insulin inhibits the hepatic synthesis of IGF-1-binding protein leading to increased bioavailability of IGF-1, which subsequently may induce prostate cells' proliferation. Hypoinsulinaemia in T1DM or long-lasting T2D consequently results in low circulating IGF-1 and suppresses prostate cells' multiplication.

Opposite results implying that DM promotes the development of advanced PC were found in a Japanese population where it was shown that people with diabetes aged 40–64 years had a significantly increased relative risk of PC incidence [103]. Men older than 40–64 years had also elevated PC risk, but the risk was lower than in younger patients [104].

Anti-diabetic Medications and Their Influence on Neoplastic Transformation

It was widely discussed that via intervening in mechanisms of cell cycle and cellular survival, anti-diabetic medications have a potential impact on carcinogenesis [6]. Presumably, the main linking factor between oncogenesis and anti-diabetic medications is in their capacity to stimulate insulin secretion or from exogenous administration. T2DM can be controlled by either oral or injectable medications, whereas T1DM is based on multiple insulin doses. A number of studies have examined the role of anti-diabetics to increase or decrease the risk of cancer development or mortality and the effects of cancer therapy on insulin resistance and hyperglycaemia [105].

- Anti-diabetic medications decreasing insulin levels include:
  - metformin
  - thiazolidinediones (TZD)
- Anti-diabetic medications increasing insulin levels:
  - sulfonylureas
  - exogenous insulin
- Anti-diabetic medications decreasing insulin resistance include:
  - metformin
  - TZD

Hyperglycaemia and hyperinsulinaemia are well-known carcinogenesis-promoting factors; normalizing serum glucose and insulin concentrations may presumably prevent neoplastic transformation. Conversely, other studies have shown that glucose-lowering therapies do not increase the risk of cancer in patients with T2DM [106, 107]. The majority of studies on the association between anti-diabetic medications and oncogenesis concern metformin; thus, this drug will be discussed in detail.

Metformin: Mechanism of Action and Its Influence on Carcinogenesis

Metformin is a member of the biguanide family with activity as insulin sensitizer. Current recommendations consider metformin as a first-line medication for T2DM therapy [26, 108–110]. It is established that metformin suppresses oncogenesis through systemic (indirect, interfering in serum levels of glucose and insulin) and cellular (direct, targeted at tumour cells) mechanisms [32, 36, 111–121]. By comparison to normal cells, cancer cells tend to synthesize more ATP through glycolysis than normal cells [114]. This metabolic shift is a hallmark of cancer and facilitates the uptake and incorporation of more nutrients into nucleotides, amino acids and lipids required for highly proliferating cells [114].

Indirect Impact of Metformin on Neoplastic Transformation [6, 105, 113–120]

- Reduction of the serum glucose concentration via:
  - inhibition of hepatic gluconeogenesis (in LKB1/ AMPK-dependent and/or -independent way).

  - inhibition of hepatic glycogenolysis by promoting hepatic adenosine monophosphate kinase phosphorylation
  - prevention of glucagon-dependent release of glucose from liver cells by accumulating AMP
  - suppression of gastrointestinal absorption of glucose
- Reduction of the serum insulin concentration.
- Suppression of inflammatory response by inhibiting the activation of NF-κB (*Explanation:* NF-κB is a critical factor in inflammatory response. Chronic inflammation stimulates oncogenesis [122–124]).
- Inhibition of metastatic progression by interfering in cancer stem cells biology (*Explanation:* Cancer stem cells are capable of undergoing epithelial to mesenchymal transition (EMT), a crucial process in metastasis, and a marker of unfavourable prognosis and cancer aggressiveness. Metformin is able to inhibit metastasis by damaging cancer stem cells [125–127]).
- Stimulation of the immune system, leading to CD8 T-cells production, by modifying fatty acid metabolism [128].
- Suppression of UPR (unfolded protein response) leading to activation of apoptosis [36].
- High local concentration of metformin after oral intake reduces the risk of oncogenesis (observed for colon cancer) [129].

Direct Impact of metformin on Neoplastic Transformation

- Reduction of ATP synthesis leading to inhibition of the formation of factors crucial for cancer cell survival.
- (*Explanation:*
- *Metformin → modifications in respiratory complex I → energetic stress → reduced production of ATP → activation of AMPK → inhibition of mTOR pathway → antiproliferative and energy saving mechanisms, inhibition of growth factor formation (insulin, IGF-1, glucose, leptin), inhibition of proteins and fatty acids formation)*
- Inhibition of mTOR pathway in AMPK-independent manner by decreasing insulin and IGF-1 concentrations.
- Activation of LKB1-dependent signalling resulting in suppression of oncogenesis (LKB1, *liver kinase B1*, is a well-known neoplastic suppressor).
- Reduction of the reactive oxygen species (ROS) formation.
- Suppression of VEGF, a critical factor of tumour vascularity formation.

- Suppression of HIF-1, a critical factor of tumour cells perseverance in hypoxic milieu.
- Cell cycle arrest and apoptosis induction via activation of cell cycle inhibitory components (p53, p21, cyclin D1).
- Modification of multidrug resistance 1 gene (MDR1 gene) and microRNA encoding P-glycoprotein (*Explanation*: Tumour cells are characterized by high expression of P-lycoprotein. Because of the fact that P-glycoprotein has the ability to eliminate hydrophobic chemotherapeutics from cancer cell, high concentration of P-glycoprotein in tumour cells reduces the effectiveness of chemotherapy).

Effects of Metformin on Neoplasms of the Digestive System

1. *Pancreatic cancer:* it has been shown that patients taking metformin have significantly decreased risk of pancreatic cancer by comparison to non-users and in those on insulin administration [130, 131].
2. *Liver cancer:* the risk of liver cancer is also significantly reduced in diabetics on metformin therapy [132, 133].
3. *Colorectal cancer:* researches examining the effect of metformin on colorectal cancer presented conflicting results. Whereas some of them observed a protective activity of metformin on CRC, others reported opposite outcomes [133–135].

Effects of Metformin on Neoplasms of the Genitourinary System

1. *Prostate cancer:* It was established that anti-diabetic therapy based on metformin reduces the risk of prostate cancer (up to 44% reduction in Caucasians) [136]. Other studies consistently reported a decreased risk of prostate cancer in metformin users [137, 138]. Interestingly, metformin users had also significantly a lower risk of advanced prostate cancer. The anti-neoplastic effect of metformin increased with the duration on metformin therapy [139].
2. *Kidney cancer:* In vitro studies on human kidney cancer cell lines 786-O revealed that metformin-mediated increased expression of microRNA-26a, a regulatory RNA critical in cell diversification, led to suppression of 786-O cells proliferation and oncogenesis [140].
3. *Ovarian cancer:* Various authors described that metformin reduced the risk of ovarian cancer incidence in women with T2DM undergoing metformin therapy.

Metformin also improved overall survival and extended disease-free period in females with ovarian cancer [141, 142]. An in vitro study conducted on epithelial ovarian cancer cell lines OVCAR-3 and OVCAR-4 documented metformin-mediated anti-oncogenic results. Moreover, chemotherapy for ovarian cancer revealed better anti-neoplastic effects of cisplatin when enriched with metformin usage [143].

4. *Breast cancer:* Besides being helpful in chemotherapy for ovarian cancer, metformin revealed its usefulness in chemotherapy for breast cancer. Metformin was able to damage BC stem cells refractory to chemotherapy based on doxorubicin. Such treatment schedule enabled destruction of BC stem cells (using metformin) and BC non-stem cells (using doxorubicin) [98]. Metformin also improved anti-neoplastic effects of chemotherapy for BC based on trastuzumab and on taxane [144, 145].

Effects of Metformin on Lung Cancer

It has been shown that the use of metformin may lead up to a 45% decrease in the incidence of lung cancer [146]. Metformin enhanced the effectiveness and final outcomes of chemotherapy for advanced non-small cell lung cancer (NSCLC) in individuals with T2DM [147].

Effects of Metformin on Head and Neck Cancers

According to sparse studies on the association between metformin and HNSCC in individuals with T2DM, metformin may presumably reduce the risk of HNSCC incidence. A statistically significant decrease was observed for nasopharyngeal and oropharyngeal cancers [148]. This anti-diabetic drug was also able to suppress the proliferation of HNSCC cells, and to decrease the probability of HNSCC recurrence and metastasis [149, 150]. It led to better overall condition in diabetics with HNSCC, especially in those with laryngeal cancer [151]. On the other hand, there is also a report of no substantial interference of metformin on the HNSCC risk in diabetics [95].

Sulfonylureas: Mechanism of Action and Influence on Carcinogenesis

The most important sulfonylureas used as anti-diabetic medications are Glyburide, Glimepiride and Glipizide. Their main mechanism of action is regulation of insulin secretion by closing the potassium channel located in pancreatic β cells. Sulfonylureas-induced potassium channels closure results in elevated insulin efflux and increased postprandial and fasting insulin levels. Whereas potassium channels closure presumably induce anti-tumourigenic mechanisms, sulfonylureas-stimulated hyperinsulinaemia promotes tumourigenesis [152]. Nevertheless, the exact effect of sulfonylureas on oncogenesis and cancer biology has not been fully elucidated [153]. The results of various studies on this issue remain conflicting. In addition, particular sulfonylureas presumably have different influence on carcinogenesis. Significantly elevated risk of cancer incidence in individuals with T2DM undergoing sulfonylureas therapy was reported by a variety of authors [135, 154, 155]. Diabetics on sulfonylureas had an increased risk of liver and colon cancer and decreased risk of prostate cancer [155, 156]. According to clinical reports, gliclazide was able to reduce the risk of neoplasm development in diabetics, whereas glyburide reduced the risk in some studies, and increased in others [157–159]. Until today, the relationship between glimepiride, glipizide and oncogenesis has not been established [158].

Exogenous Insulin: Influence on Carcinogenesis

The group of exogenous insulins comprise human insulin and insulin analogues. The vast majority of studies investigating the association between exogenous insulin and oncogenesis imply tumour-promoting effects of exogenous insulin [154, 160]. Patients on long-acting insulin analogues (glargine and detemir) are more prone to undergo carcinogenesis in comparison to non-insulin users [113, 161]. Nevertheless, the risk is lesser than observed in human insulin users [162]. Diabetics on insulin revealed increased risk of liver, pancreatic, renal, stomach, liver and respiratory tumours, and reduced risk of prostate cancer [156, 163]. Studies focusing on glargine effect on cancer biology present conflicting results. Diabetics on glargine had increased risk of breast, prostate and pancreatic cancers incidence and reduced risk of colon and colorectal cancers [164–166]. Glargine investigations in vitro have shown suppressed apoptosis and tumour-promoting activity in human endometrioid endometrial carcinoma, breast adenocarcinoma and CRC cells [167–169]. No significant correlation between glargine and oncogenesis was observed in another study [170].

Thiazolidinediones: Mechanism of Action and Influence on Carcinogenesis

Thiazolidinediones are a group of PPARγ agonists currently used in T2DM treatment. The main components of this group are Pioglitazone, Rosiglitazone, Troglitazone, Netoglitazone, Ciglitazone and Efatutazone. TZD-induced stimulation of PPARγ sensitizes insulin-dependent tissues to insulin that leads to better glycaemic regulation. The speculation that TZD may presumably have an impact on cancer biology was made after finding that a variety of neoplasms are characterized by elevated expression of PPARγ. Nevertheless, the possible influence of TZDs on oncogenesis may be induced in PPARγ-dependent and PPARγ-independent manner. TZD-mediated activation of PPARγ in cancer cells interfered with cell cycle and led to cell cycle arrest and apoptosis [171].

PPARγ-independent anti-neoplastic activity of TZD [171, 172]:

- Suppression of antiapoptotic Bcl-2 (B-cell leukaemia/lymphoma)/Bcl-xL function resulting in apoptosis of cancer cells
- Inhibition of androgen activation by interfering in gene encoding androgen receptor
- Degradation of specificity protein 1 (Sp1) resulting in reduction of survivin (an apoptosis inhibitor), EGFR (epidermal growth factor), and intercellular and vascular cell adhesion molecules ICAM-1 and VCAM-1
- (*Explanation*: Specificity protein 1 is a critical protein in cell cycle. This protein is able to modify genes encoding cell cycle and vascular endothelial growth factor. Such ability enables Sp1 to interfere with development, metabolism and metastasis of cancer cells.)
- Down-regulation of various well-established cancer-promoting molecules including β-catenin, cyclin D1 and FLIP (FLICE-like inhibitory protein)

The majority of studies suggested that TZDs have anti-neoplastic activity and reduces the risk of various cancers incidence [155, 173, 174]. On the other hand, there are reports indicating that these drugs may also reveal tumour-promoting features. It was observed that TZDs as a group decreased the risk of breast, lung and colorectal cancers [175]. Pioglitazone and rosiglitazone were able to reduce the risk of liver cancer, pioglitazone but not rosiglitazone reduced the risk of breast cancer and rosiglitazone reduced the risk of colorectal cancer [174, 176]. Netoglitazone revealed anti-neoplastic activity against human pancreatic cancer cells, colorectal cancer cells, multiple myeloma and prostate cancer cells (mainly androgen-irrespective prostate cancer cells) [177–179]. Efatutazone suppressed colon cancer development in mice and suppressed in vitro anaplastic thyroid carcinoma cell lines [180]. Suppressed proliferation of ovarian, prostate and lung cancer cells was observed after Troglitazone administration [180]. Possibly, TZDs may also improve the efficacy of chemotherapy. Chemotherapy for breast and pancreatic cancer cells was improved after rosiglitazone administration. Rosiglitazone presumably reduced chemoresistance in neoplastic cells [181]. Additionally, TZDs enhanced the effectiveness of anti-neoplastic therapy for soft tissue sarcoma and thyroid cancer [182].

On the other hand, there are also studies implying that TZDs as a group may induce pro-neoplastic effects. Such significant correlation was found in diabetic women undergoing rosiglitazone treatment [183]. Several studies suggested that diabetics on Pioglitazone therapy had increased risk of bladder cancer, NHL and melanoma [22, 184–187].

Incretin-Based Medications: Mechanisms of Action and Influence on Carcinogenesis

Dipeptidyl peptidase-4 inhibitors (DDP-4-i) and Glucagon-like peptide 1 agonists (GLP-1 agonists) are anti-diabetic medications used in T2DM that interact with the incretin system.

Dipeptidyl Peptidase-4 Inhibitors (DDP-4-i) include Sitagliptin, Saxagliptin, Vildagliptin, Alogliptin and Linagliptin. Dipeptidyl peptidase-4 inhibitors' main function is based on inhibiting the enzyme Dipeptidyl peptidase-4 (DDP-4) that is critical in destruction of Glucagon-like peptide-1 (GLP-1). Consequently, suppression of DDP-4 leads to increased serum concentration of GLP-1. Unlike GLP-1 agonists, DDP-4-i do not delay the gastric emptying rate and do not promote the sensation of satiety. A variety of studies found that DDP-4-i users were at higher risk to suffer from pancreatic cancer. However, the risk was significantly lesser than observed in diabetics on sulfonylureas and comparable in individuals on TZDs [188–191]. No pro-neoplastic activity of DDP-4-i was found in mice and in human individuals with T2DM [106, 192]. On the other hand, laboratory studies on rats revealed diminished colon tumourigenesis and reduced reactive oxygen species in long-term administration of Sitagliptin [193]. In addition, sitagliptin enhanced engraftment of Umbilical Cord Blood transplantation in adults with haematological neoplasms [194].

Glucagon-like Peptide 1 Agonists (GLP-1 agonists) include Liraglutide, Exenatide and Semaglutide. GLP-1 agonists elevate glucose-mediated insulin synthesis and its efflux in pancreatic β *cells in a precise and controlled way. They reduce glycogenolysis and glucagon secretion. GLP-1 agonists slow down the* gastrointestinal motility leading to delayed absorption of carbohydrates and lesser increase in serum glucose level [27]. Additionally, they promote satiety via interfering in the central nervous system. Whereas several studies found decreased risk of oncogenesis in GLP-1 agonist users, other research reported opposite results. Exenatide was able to suppress the development of human prostate cancer cells and murine CT26 colon cancer cells [195–196]. Moreover, it presented anti-neoplastic activity against breast cancer cells [197]. Liraglutide-induced stimulation of GLP-1R (GLP-1 receptors) suppressed neoplastic transformation and metastasis in human pancreatic cancer cells in in vitro and in vivo investigation. The anti-neoplastic activity was a result of suppression of PI3K/Akt pathway [198]. On the other hand, GLP-1 agonists elicited tumourigenesis in rodent thyroid C-cells, but not in human thyroid C-cells nor in thyroid gland in diabetics [199–200]. The proliferation observed in rodent C-cells might be caused by GLP-1-receptors–mediated excretion of calcitonin [201]. Presumably, mainly various levels of GLP-1 receptors in humans and in rodents caused this difference. There are also reports implying elevated risk of pancreatic cancer incidence in GLP-1 agonist users [189, 191].

Alpha-Glucosidase Inhibitors (AGIs)

Mechanisms of Action and Influence on Carcinogenesis: the main components of this group are Acarbose, Voglibose and Miglitol. AGIs slow down digestion and absorption of polysaccharides in the gastrointestinal tract by inhibiting enzymes sucrose (invertase) and maltase in the proximal small intestine, leading to delayed increase in postprandial serum glucose level and better glycaemic control. AGIs elevated intestinal hormones activity and enhanced intestinal microbiota [202]. Reports of the influence of AGIs on oncogenesis are scarce. According to current knowledge AGIs may reduce the risk of colorectal, lung and gastric cancers [203, 204]. The risk of kidney cancer is presumably elevated in diabetics undergoing AGIs therapy [205]. Conversely, no significant influence of AGIs on both carcinogenesis and cancer-related mortality was revealed in another study [206].

Sodium-Glucose Co-transporter 2 Inhibitors (SGLT2 Inhibitors)

Mechanism of Action and Influence on Carcinogenesis: SGLT2 inhibitors are a new class of anti-diabetic medications used in T2DM treatment. The main components of this group are Empagliflozin, Canagliflozin, Dapagliflozin and Ertugliflozin. SGLT2 is a glucose transporter located in the proximal renal tubules; their main role is glucose reabsorption of approximately 90% of the renal glucose filtrate. Consequently, SGLT2 inhibitors are able to significantly lower serum glucose levels via enhancing glucose excretion by the kidneys. Additionally, SGLT2 inhibitors elevate insulin sensitivity, improve insulin secretion from pancreatic beta cells and decrease gluconeogenesis [207]. As SGLT2 inhibitors are quite novel drugs the precise association between them and oncogenesis has not been completely established. Correlation between these two entities has already been observed, but it is still based on sparse research. Studies assessing the correlation between Dapagliflozin and bladder cancer have shown that Dapagliflozin might elevate the risk of oncogenesis in bladder cells, albeit without statistical significance. No increase in neoplastic transformation in bladder tissue was found in mice and rats receiving Dapagliflozin, and for in vitro human bladder transitional cell carcinoma (TCC) cell lines [208]. Moreover, Dapagliflozin presumably did not increased the risk of breast cancer [208]. Studies about Canagliflozin have not documented an increased risk of neoplastic transformation in bladder, breast and kidneys [208]. Another study on SGLT2-expressing neoplasms (pancreatic and prostate cancers) found that Dapagliflozin and Canagliflozin significantly reduced tumour growth and enhanced death of tumour cells [209]. This finding should draw attention to the potential anti-neoplastic role of SGLT2 inhibitors in SGLT2-expressing tumours. Tumour-suppressing activity of Canagliflozin was also observed for prostate and lung cancer cells. The anti-neoplastic role in this study was presumably induced by inhibiting mitochondrial complex-I supported respiration that resulted in limitation of cellular proliferation [210]. Nevertheless, observations about the potential anti-neoplastic activities of SGLT2 inhibitors require further investigation.

Summary

The prevalence of diabetes mellitus type 2 and cancers of various sites is dramatically increasing nowadays. Both entities are important causes of death all over the world. A number of studies proved that DM increases the risk of oncogenesis in various organs. The association was predominantly observed in T2DM possibly because of potential T2DM-induced tumour-promoting factors. The mechanisms linking DM and neoplastic transformation in various types of organs are probably different and have not been clearly explained yet. The vast majority of attention is put on three groups of linking factors, including modifiable, non-modifiable and biological. Modifiable risk factors include overweight and obesity, physical inactivity, smoking and alcohol abuse. Non-modifiable risk factors comprise age between 55 and 60 years or more, male gender and African American race. Biological risk factors include hyperinsulinaemia, insulin resistance, hyperglycaemia and chronic inflammation induced by excessive adipose tissue. According to current knowledge the most significant factor linking T2DM and oncogenesis is obesity. Moreover, several studies suggest that there is also correlation between DM duration and the risk of carcinogenesis albeit the results of these investigations are inconsistent. It was established that many tumours overexpress receptors for insulin leading to higher susceptibility to both metabolic and mitogenic activity of insulin in tumour cells. Furthermore, diabetics with T2DM and coexisting neoplasm have worse disease-free and overall survival than patients with neoplasm but without T2DM. In accordance with collected data, individuals with DM are more prone to suffer from cancers of digestive tract system (liver, pancreatic, colon/colorectal cancers) and genitourinary system (bladder and endometrial cancers). Breast cancer is also more commonly observed in diabetic women than in non-diabetic ones. Correlation between DM and renal cancer and HNC is not clear. Data investigating the association between DM and HNC are lacking. Current knowledge implies that DM increases the risk of both oral cavity and pharyngeal neoplasms. It was also established that DM predisposes to perineural invasion in patients with oral squamous cell cancer. In addition, the prognosis in patients with oral cavity cancer and DM is worse than in those without DM. The relationship between DM and laryngeal cancer is inconsistent; some authors suggest an increased risk, some authors report a lower risk and some have not found a relationship between these diseases. Conversely, several studies have reported a protective, anti-neoplastic effect of DM on the risk of prostate cancer, with a significantly inverse association between PC and DM. This protective association is presumably a result of hyperglycaemia-induced low concentration of testosterone and hypoinsulinaemia in patients with T1DM or long-lasting T2DM. Nevertheless, other reports indicate an increased risk of prostate carcinogenesis. The potentially protective effect of DM on prostate cancer requires further investigation.

Recent analyses have shown that anti-diabetic drugs may modify the risk of oncogenesis in persons with diabetes, albeit with inconsistent results. Some drugs presumably increase the risk, whereas others reduce the risk of tumourigenesis. The majority of studies on this matter concern metformin, a drug of first choice in T2DM. It was been shown that metformin reduces the risk of cancer and improves the overall survival in diabetics. Favourable outcomes with the use of metformin have been observed in a wide variety of cancers including breast, pancreas, liver, colon, prostate, lungs and ovaries. Several authors have also revealed an inhibitory effect of metformin on human renal cancer cell lines 786-O. According to studies examining the influence of metformin on HNC, metformin decreased the risk of HNC (the most significant reduction was found for oro- and nasopharyngeal cancers) and improved overall survival in patients with laryngeal squamous cell carcinoma. It has also been suggested that SGLT2 inhibitors express potential anti-neoplastic activity, albeit the evidence is still sparse. The influence of other anti-diabetic medications including sulfonylureas, exogenous insulin, TZDs, alpha-glucosidase inhibitors, incretin-based drugs (GLP-1 agonists and DDP-4-i) on cancer incidence and prognosis remains inconsistent.

Based on the above information, it can be assumed that diabetes mellitus and oncogenesis are presumably combined entities. It is increasingly recognized that diabetes increases the risk of developing cancer [211]. Diabetes and cancer commonly coexist and outcomes in people with both conditions are poorer than in those who have cancer but no diabetes [211]. Greater attention should be devoted to screen patients with diabetes mellitus for the main causes of cancer, especially those with T2DM. These patients require precise, regular follow-up in order not to omit any neoplastic transformation [211]. Careful screening should also be performed in individuals on anti-diabetic drugs [212].

The correlation between DM/anti-diabetic medications and carcinogenesis requires further investigation to establish exact, general and cell-intrinsic mechanisms linking these entities. Attention should also be drawn to potential anti-neoplastic activities of particular anti-diabetic drugs. Therapeutic nihilism should be avoided and a personalized approach to managing hyperglycaemia in people with cancer is required [211].

Concluding Remarks

- Diabetics (mainly with T2DM) are more prone to suffer from cancers of digestive tract system (liver, pancreatic, colon/colorectal cancers) and genitourinary system (bladder and endometrial cancers). Breast cancer is also more commonly observed in diabetic women than in non-diabetic ones.
- Prostate cancer risk is presumably inversely associated with diabetes mellitus.
- Metformin may reduce the risk of cancer incidence and improve overall survival in diabetics. Favourable effect of metformin was observed in a wide variety of cancers including breast, pancreatic, liver, colon, prostate, lungs and ovaries. Its potential usefulness in chemotherapy is promising and still studied.
- SGLT2 inhibitors express potential anti-neoplastic activity. The influence of sulfonylureas, exogenous insulin, TZDs, alpha-glucosidase inhibitors, incretin-based drugs (GLP-1 agonists and DDP-4-i) on cancer incidence and prognosis remains inconsistent.

Multiple-Choice Questions

1. The linking factors between diabetes mellitus and oncogenesis are:
   (a) Hyperglycaemia
   (b) Hypoinsulinaemia
   (c) Hyperinsulinaemia
   (d) **a, c.** (The biological factors linking DM and oncogenesis include hyperinsulinaemia, insulin resistance, hyperglycaemia and chronic inflammation induced by excessive adipose tissue. According to current knowledge the most significant factor linking T2DM and oncogenesis is obesity.)
   (e) a, b, c

2. Fat-induced chronic inflammation leading to oncogenesis is characterized by:
   (a) Increased level of adiponectin and decreased level of leptin
   (b) Increased level of leptin and decreased level of adiponectin
   (c) Increased production of proinflammatory cytokines including IL-6, resistin and TNF-alpha
   (d) **b, c.** (Excessive adipose tissue interferes with sex hormones physiology (high amounts of aromatase converting oestrogens to androgens), induces chronic inflammation and changes profile of adipose tissue polypeptide hormones (adipokines). Obesity-induced chronic inflammation is characterized by increased production of proinflammatory cytokines including interleukin-6, resistin and TNF-alpha (Tumour Necrosis Factor-alpha). The level of adiponectin is reduced and the level of leptin is increased in patients with excessive adipose tissue. Adiponectin sensitizes cells to insulin, suppresses cells growth and metabolism, and exerts pro-apoptotic mechanisms, whereas leptin stimulates proliferation of cancer cells.)
   (e) All answers are false

3. Pro-neoplastic features of insulin are induced by activation of:
   (a) Insulin Receptor
   (b) Insulin-like Growth Factor Receptor
   (c) Growth Hormone Receptor
   (d) a, b, c
   (e) **a, b.** (The pro-neoplastic features of insulin are induced by activation of its receptors (Insulin Receptor and Insulin-like Growth Factor Receptor), as well as via Insulin-like Growth Factor. Ligand-induced IR autophosphorylation triggers intracellular mechanisms. The most important one is activation of PI3K/Akt/mTOR (phosphoinositide 3-kinase/protein kinase B/mammalian target of rapamycin) signalling pathway. Stimulation of PI3K/Akt/mTOR signalling pathway plays a critical role in oncogenesis. Activation of IGF-R results in more significant pro-neoplastic effects than activation of IR.)

4. Indirect effects of hyperinsulinaemia on cancer biology:
   (a) **Increased level of Growth Hormone (GH) leading to elevated concentration of Insulin Like Growth Factor-1 (IGF-1).** (Insulin stimulates growth hormone receptors (GHR) located in the liver leading to elevated release of GH. Subsequently,

GH promotes IGF-1 synthesis. IGF-1 is a mitogenic factor.)

   (b) Increased concentration of pro-neoplastic adipose tissue hormone—adiponectin

   (c) Increased concentration of anti-neoplastic adipose tissue hormone—leptin

   (d) a, b, c

   (e) All answers are false

5. Tumour-promoting mechanism of hyperglycaemia:

   (a) Reduced expression of glucose transporters (GLUT-1 and GLUT-3)

   (b) Reduced level of hypoxia-inducible factor α (HIF-α), a critical anti-neoplastic factor

   (c) **Increased expression of PPAR α and γ (peroxisome proliferator-activated receptor)** (PPAR α and γ interfere with lipid metabolic pathways and speed up neoplastic cells development)

   (d) a, b, c

   (e) b, c

6. Which statements are correct:

   (a) Diabetes mellitus type 2 elevates the risk of endometrial cancer

   (b) Diabetes mellitus type 2 elevates the risk of prostate cancer via reducing testosterone levels

   (c) The risk of hepatocellular carcinoma is increased in patients with type 2 diabetes mellitus

   (d) a, b, c

   (e) **a, c.** (It is suggested that DM might predispose to EC via hyperinsulinaemia-dependent reduced level of adiponectin and via obesity-related decreased concentration of SHBG. Reduced level of SHBG leads to elevated bioavailable oestrogen and testosterone amounts and eventually stimulates endometrial oncogenesis

     Liver is exposed to circulation of high amounts of insulin because of its portal vessels. Constantly high insulin levels, via elevated production of IGF-1, lead to multiplication and apoptosis suppression in hepatic cells.

     According to current knowledge prostate cancer (PC) is the only neoplasm that is conversely related to DM. This association is presumably a result of hyperglycaemia-induced low concentration of testosterone and hypoinsulinaemia detected in T1DM or long-lasting T2DM.)

7. Anti-neoplastic features of metformin comprise:

   (a) Reduction of the serum insulin concentration

   (b) Reduction of the serum glucose concentration via inhibition of gluconeogenesis and glycogenolysis in the liver

   (c) Stimulation of mTOR pathway, a critical anti-neoplastic pathway

   (d) a, b, c

   (e) **a, b (answer c is false because metformin** inhibits mTOR pathway in AMPK-independent manner by decreasing insulin and IGF-1 concentrations. mTOR pathway plays a critical role in oncogenesis).

8. Choose the correct statement:

   (a) Metformin reduces the risk of liver cancer

   (b) Metformin reduces the risk of pancreatic cancer

   (c) Metformin reduces the risk of ovarian cancer

   (d) **All answers are correct**

   (e) All answers are false

9. Anti-diabetic medications that influence the risk of neoplastic transformation are:

   (a) Metformin

   (b) Thiazolidinediones

   (c) Sulfonylureas

   (d) Dipeptidyl peptidase-4 inhibitors

   (e) **a, b, c, d.** (A majority of studies present that metformin reduces the risk of neoplastic transformation. The influence of sulfonylureas, thiazolidinediones and dipeptidyl peptidase-4 inhibitors on cancer incidence and prognosis remains inconsistent.)

10. Diabetes mellitus type 2 promotes oncogenesis via:

   (a) Activation of insulin-dependent IP3-K/AKT/mTOR pathway

   (b) Insulin-induced increased level of bioavailable IGF-1

   (c) Insulin-induced increased concentration of leptin

   (d) Insulin-induced reduced level of SHBG resulting in increased amount of bioavailable oestradiol

   (e) **a, b, c, d**

Glossary

Hyperinsulinaemia Increased serum insulin level.

Hyperglycaemia Increased serum glucose level.

Pro-neoplastic Promoting neoplastic transformation.

PI3K/Akt/mTOR signalling pathway (phosphoinositide 3-kinase/protein kinase B/mammalian target of rapamycin signalling pathway)— Critical pathway in oncogenesis.

IGF-binding proteins Proteins crucial in IGF serum transfer and bioavailability.

Urokinase plasminogen activator (uPA) A critical mediator in cancer cell displacement.

ETM (Epithelial to Mesenchymal Transition process) A mechanism that enables cancer cells to metastasise.

Adipokines Adipose tissue polypeptide hormones, e.g. leptin, adiponectin.

SNPs (Single Nucleotide Polymorphisms) A sequence in a single nucleotide that is observed at a specific position in the genome.

NAFLD (non-alcoholic fatty liver disease) A condition of fat deposits accumulation not induced by alcohol abuse. NAFLD is associated with metabolic syndrome and insulin resistance.

Lipotoxicity Malfunction or death of non-adipose tissue cells caused by accumulation of excessive lipids.

Oxidative stress Imbalance between antioxidant and pro-oxidant factors.

Oncogenesis, tumourigenesis, carcinogenesis A group of mechanisms leading to transformation of normal cells to cancer cells.

Milieu A setting in which something happens (environment, surrounding).

Gluconeogenesis A process of glucose biosynthesis.

Glycogenolysis A process of biochemical degradation of glycogen to glucose.

NF-κB A factor controlling transcription of DNA and cells survival.

OVCAR Epithelial ovarian cancer cell lines.

Stem cell Undifferentiated cells which have the ability to differentiate into specialized cells, and to divide to synthesize more stem cells.

References

1. Giovannucci E, Harlan DM, Archer MC, Bergenstal RM, Gapstur SM, Habel LA, et al. Diabetes and cancer: a consensus report. Diabetes Care. 2010;33:1674–85.
2. Jee SH, Ohrr H, Sull JW, Yun JE, Ji M, Samet JM. Fasting serum glucose level and cancer risk in Korean men and women. JAMA. 2005;293:194–202.
3. Tseng KS, Lin C, Lin YS, Weng SF. Risk of head and neck cancer in patients with diabetes mellitus: a retrospective cohort study in Taiwan. JAMA Otolaryngol Head Neck Surg. 2014;140:746–53.
4. Noto H, Tsujimoto T, Sasazuki T, Noda M. Significantly increased risk of cancer in patients with diabetes mellitus: a systematic review and meta-analysis. Endocr Pract. 2011;17:616–28.
5. Joost H-G. Diabetes and cancer: Epidemiology and potential mechanisms. Diab Vasc Dis Res. 2014;11:390–4.
6. Wojciechowska J, Krajewski W, Bolanowski M, Krecicki T, Zatonski T. Diabetes and cancer: a review of current knowledge. Exp Clin Endocrinol Diabetes. 2016;124:263–75.
7. Bonagiri PR, Shubrook JH. Review of associations between type 2 Diabetes and cancer. Clin Diabetes. 2020;38:256–65.
8. Wang M, Yang Y, Liao Z. Diabetes and cancer: epidemiological and biological links. World J Diabetes. 2020;15:227–38.
9. Zhang C, Le A. Diabetes and Cancer: The Epidemiological and Metabolic Associations. In: Le A, editor. The Heterogeneity of Cancer Metabolism. Advances in Experimental Medicine and Biology. New York: Springer. p. 1311.
10. Harding JL, Shaw JE, Peters A, Carstensen B, Magliano DJ. Cancer risk among people with type 1 and type 2 Diabetes: disentangling true associations, detection bias and reverse causation. Diabetes Care. 2015;38:264–70.
11. Ling L, Brown K, Miksza JK, Howells L, Morrison A, Issa E, et al. Association of Type 2 Diabetes with cancer: a meta-analysis with bias analysis for unmeasured confounding in 151 cohorts comprising 32 million people. Diabetes Care. 2020;43:2313–22.
12. Zendehdel K, Nyren O, Ostenson CG, Adami HO, Ekbom A, Ye W. Cancer incidence in patients with type 1 diabetes mellitus: a population-based cohort study in Sweden. J Natl Cancer Inst. 2003;95:1797–800.
13. Shu X, Ji J, Li X, Sundquist J, Sundquist K, Hemminki K. Cancer risk among patients hospitalized for type 1 diabetes mellitus: a population-based cohort study in Sweden. Diabet Med. 2010;27:791–7.
14. Vigneri P, Frasca F, Sciacca L, Pandini G, Vigneri R. Diabetes and cancer. Endocr Relat Cancer. 2009;16:1103–23.
15. Decensi A, Puntoni M, Goodwin P, Cazzaniga M, Gennari A, Bonanni B, et al. Metformin and cancer risk in diabetic patients: a systematic review and meta-analysis. Cancer Prev Res. 2010;3:1451–61.
16. Ahmed AM. History of diabetes mellitus. Saudi Med J. 2002;23:373–8.
17. Loriaux DL. Diabetes and the Ebers papyrus: 1552 B.C. Endocrinologist. 2006;16:55–6.
18. Olokoba AB, Obateru OA, Olokoba LB. Type 2 diabetes mellitus: a review of current trends. Oman Med J. 2012;27:269–73.
19. International Diabetes federation. IDF Atlas 10th ed 2021.
20. World Health Organization. Cancer. Accessed December 7 2021. https://www.who.int/news-room/fact-sheets/detail/cancer
21. Collins KK. The Diabetes-Cancer Link. Diabetes Spectrum. 2014;27:276–80.
22. Nguyen C, Varney MD, Harrison LC, Morahan G. Definition of high-risk type 1 diabetes HLA-DR and HLA-DQ types using only three single nucleotide polymorphisms. Diabetes. 2013;62:2135–40.
23. American Diabetes Association. Classification and diagnosis of Diabetes. Standards of medical Care in Diabetes 2021. Diabetes Care. 2021;44(Suppl 1):S15–33.
24. Stumvoll M, Goldstein BJ, van Haeften TW. Type 2 diabetes: principles of pathogenesis and therapy. Lancet. 2005;365:1333–46.
25. Moore H, Summerbell C, Hooper L, Cruickshank K, Vyas A, Johnstone P, et al. Dietary advice for treatment of type 2 diabetes mellitus in adults. Cochrane Database Syst Rev. 2004;2004:CD004097.
26. Brunetti L, Kalabalik J. Management of type-2 diabetes mellitus in adults: focus on individualizing non-insulin therapies. P T. 2012;37:687–96.
27. Nathan DM, Buse JB, Davidson MB, Ferrannini E, Holman RR, Sherwin R, et al. Medical management of hyperglycemia in type 2 diabetes: a consensus algorithm for the initiation and adjustment of therapy: a consensus statement of the American Diabetes Association and the European Association for the Study of Diabetes. Diabetes Care. 2009;32:193–203.
28. Buchanan TA, Xiang AH. Gestational diabetes mellitus. J Clin Invest. 2005;115:485–91.
29. Perkins JM, Dunn JP, Jagasia SM. Perspectives in gestational Diabetes mellitus: a review of screening, diagnosis, and treatment. Clinical Diabetes. 2007;25:57–62.
30. Maynard G. A statistical study in cancer death-rates. Biometrika. 1910;7:276–304.
31. Pearson K, Elderton LA, EM. On the correlation of death rates. J R Stat Soc. 1910;73:534–9.
32. Gallagher EJ, LeRoith D. Diabetes, cancer, and metformin: connections of metabolism and cell proliferation. Ann N Y Acad Sci. 2011;1243:54–68.
33. Del Barco S, Vazquez-Martin A, Cufi S, Oliveras-Ferraros C, Bosch-Barrera J, Joven J, et al. Metformin: multi-faceted protection against cancer. Oncotarget. 2011;2:896–917.
34. Kiselyov VV, Versteyhe S, Gauguin L, De Meyts P. Harmonic oscillator model of the insulin and IGF1 receptors' allosteric binding and activation. Mol Syst Biol. 2009;5:243.

35. Cui Y, Andersen DK. Diabetes and pancreatic cancer. Endocr Relat Cancer. 2012;19:F9–F26.

36. Kourelis TV, Siegel RD. Metformin and cancer: new applications for an old drug. Med Oncol. 2012;29:1314–27.

37. Belfiore A. The role of insulin receptor isoforms and hybrid insulin/IGF-I receptors in human cancer. Curr Pharm Des. 2007;13:671–86.

38. Friberg E, Mantzoros CS, Wolk A. Diabetes and risk of endometrial cancer: a population-based prospective cohort study. Cancer Epidemiol Biomark Prev. 2007;16:276–80.

39. Baxter RC, Brown AS, Turtle JR. Association between serum insulin, serum somatomedin and liver receptors for human growth hormone in streptozotocin diabetes. Horm Metab Res. 1980;12:377–81.

40. Somasundar P, Yu AK, Vona-Davis L, McFadden DW. Differential effects of leptin on cancer in vitro. J Surg Res. 2003;113:50–5.

41. van Kruijsdijk RC, van der Wall E, Visseren FL. Obesity and cancer: the role of dysfunctional adipose tissue. Cancer Epidemiol Biomark Prev. 2009;18:2569–78.

42. Vander Heiden MG, Cantley LC, Thompson CB. Understanding the Warburg effect: the metabolic requirements of cell proliferation. Science. 2009;324:1029–33.

43. Menendez JA, Joven J, Cominas-Faja B, Oliveras-Ferraros C, Cuyás E, Martin-Castillo B, et al. The Warburg effect version 2.0. Metabolic reprogramming of cancer stem cells. Cell Cycle. 2013;128:1166–79.

44. Ryu TY, Park J, Scherer PE. Hyperglycemia as a risk factor for cancer progression. Diabetes Metab J. 2014;38:330–6.

45. Ramteke P, Deb A, Shepal V, Kumar BM. Hyperglycemia associated metabolic and molecular alterations in cancer risk, Progression, treatment, and mortality. Cancers. 2019;11:1402.

46. Li D. Diabetes and pancreatic cancer. Mol Carcinog. 2012;51:64–74.

47. Fukada T, Yamasaki S, Nishida K, Murakami M, Hirano T. Zinc homeostasis and signaling in health and diseases: zinc signaling. J Biol Inorg Chem. 2011;16:1123–34.

48. Garg SK, Maurer H, Reed K, Selagamsetty R. Diabetes and cancer: two diseases with obesity as a common risk factor. Diabetes Obes Met. 2014;16:97–110.

49. Renehan AG, Zwahlen M, Egger M. Adiposity and cancer risk: new mechanistic insights from epidemiology. Nat Rev Cancer. 2015;15:484–98.

50. Doerstling SS, O'Flanagan CH, Hursting S. Obesity and cancer metabolism: a perspective on interacting tumor-intrinsic and extrinsic factors. Front Oncol. 2017;7:1–11.

51. Lega IC, Lipscombe LL. Diabetes, obesity and cancer - pathophysiology and clinical implications. Endocr Rev. 2020;41:33–52.

52. Brown JC, Carson TL, Thompson HJ, Agurs-Collins. The triple health threat of Diabetes, obesity, and cancer - epidemiology, disparities, mechanisms and interventions. Obesity. 2021;29:954–9.

53. Grossmann ME, Nkhata KJ, Mizuno NK, Ray A, Cleary MP. Effects of adiponectin on breast cancer cell growth and signaling. Br J Cancer. 2008;98:370–9.

54. O'Rourke RW. Obesity and cancer: at the crossroads of cellular metabolism and proliferation. Surg Obes Relat Dis. 2014;10:1208–19.

55. Sun L, Yu S. Diabetes mellitus is an independent risk factor for colorectal cancer. Dig Dis Sci. 2012;57:1586–97.

56. Wu L, Yu C, Jiang H, Tang J, Huang HL, Gao J, et al. Diabetes mellitus and the occurrence of colorectal cancer: an updated meta-analysis of cohort studies. Diabetes Technol Ther. 2013;15:419–27.

57. Balasubramanyam M. Diabetic oncopathy--one more yet another deadly diabetic complication! Indian J Med Res. 2014;140:15–8.

58. Huxley R, Ansary-Moghaddam A, Berrington de Gonzalez A, Barzi F, Woodward M. Type-II diabetes and pancreatic cancer: a meta-analysis of 36 studies. Br J Cancer. 2005;92:2076–83.

59. Elena JW, Steplowski E, Yu K, Hartge P, Tobias GS, Brotzman MJ, et al. Diabetes and risk of pancreatic cancer: a pooled analysis from the pancreatic cancer cohort consortium. Cancer Causes Control. 2013;24:13.

60. Grote VA, Rohrmann S, Nieters A, Dossus L, Tjonneland A, Halkjaer J, et al. Diabetes mellitus, glycated haemoglobin and C-peptide levels in relation to pancreatic cancer risk: a study within the European prospective investigation into cancer and nutrition (EPIC) cohort. Diabetologia. 2011;54:3037–46.

61. Stevens RJ, Roddam AW, Beral V. Pancreatic cancer in type 1 and young-onset diabetes: systematic review and meta-analysis. Br J Cancer. 2007;96:507–9.

62. Prizment AE, Gross M, Rasmussen-Torvik L, Peacock JM, Anderson KE. Genes related to diabetes may be associated with pancreatic cancer in a population-based case-control study in Minnesota. Pancreas. 2012;41:50–3.

63. Pierce BL, Austin MA, Ahsan H. Association study of type 2 diabetes genetic susceptibility variants and risk of pancreatic cancer: an analysis of PanScan-I data. Cancer Causes Control. 2011;22:877–83.

64. Murad AS, Smith GD, Lewis SJ, Cox A, Donovan JL, Neal DE, et al. A polymorphism in the glucokinase gene that raises plasma fasting glucose, rs1799884, is associated with diabetes mellitus and prostate cancer: findings from a population-based, case-control study (the ProtecT study). Int J Mol Epidemiol Genet. 2010;1:175–83.

65. Davila JA, Morgan RO, Shaib Y, McGlynn KA, El-Serag HB. Diabetes increases the risk of hepatocellular carcinoma in the United States: a population based case control study. Gut. 2005;54:533–9.

66. Lawson DH, Gray JM, McKillop C, Clarke J, Lee FD, Patrick RS. Diabetes mellitus and primary hepatocellular carcinoma. Q J Med. 1986;61:945–55.

67. Dyson J, Jaques B, Chattopadyhay D, Lochan R, Graham J, Das D, et al. Hepatocellular cancer: the impact of obesity, type 2 diabetes and a multidisciplinary team. J Hepatol. 2014;60:110–7.

68. Wang C, Wang X, Gong G, Ben Q, Qiu W, Chen Y, et al. Increased risk of hepatocellular carcinoma in patients with diabetes mellitus: a systematic review and meta-analysis of cohort studies. Int J Cancer. 2012;130:1639–48.

69. Noureddin M, Rinella ME. Nonalcoholic fatty liver disease, diabetes, obesity, and hepatocellular carcinoma. Clin Liver Dis. 2015;19:361–7.

70. El-Serag HB, Hampel H, Javadi F. The association between diabetes and hepatocellular carcinoma: a systematic review of epidemiologic evidence. Clin Gastroenterol Hepatol. 2006;4:369–80.

71. Gao C, Yao SK. Diabetes mellitus: a "true" independent risk factor for hepatocellular carcinoma? Hepatobiliary Pancreat Dis Int. 2009;8:465–73.

72. Larsson SC, Orsini N, Wolk A. Diabetes mellitus and risk of colorectal cancer: a meta-analysis. J Natl Cancer Inst. 2005;97:1679–87.

73. Yang YX, Hennessy S, Lewis JD. Type 2 diabetes mellitus and the risk of colorectal cancer. Clin Gastroenterol Hepatol. 2005;3:587–94.

74. Jiang Y, Ben Q, Shen H, Lu W, Zhang Y, Zhu J. Diabetes mellitus and incidence and mortality of colorectal cancer: a systematic review and meta-analysis of cohort studies. Eur J Epidemiol. 2011;26:863–76.

75. Xu X, Wu J, Mao Y, Zhu Y, Hu Z, Xu X, et al. Diabetes mellitus and risk of bladder cancer: a meta-analysis of cohort studies. PLoS One. 2013;8:e58079.

76. Larsson SC, Orsini N, Brismar K, Wolk A. Diabetes mellitus and risk of bladder cancer: a meta-analysis. Diabetologia. 2006;49:2819–23.

77. Woolcott CG, Maskarinec G, Haiman CA, Henderson BE, Kolonel LN. Diabetes and urothelial cancer risk: the multiethnic cohort study. Cancer Epidemiol. 2011;35:551–4.

78. Zhu Z, Wang X, Shen Z, Lu Y, Zhong S, Xu C. Risk of bladder cancer in patients with diabetes mellitus: an updated meta-analysis of 36 observational studies. BMC Cancer. 2013;13:310.

79. Hee-Kyung J, Willett WC, Cho E. Type 2 diabetes and the risk of renal cell cancer in women. Diabetes Care. 2011;34:1552–6.

80. Inoue M, Iwasaki M, Otani T, Sasazuki S, Noda M, Tsugane S. Diabetes mellitus and the risk of cancer: results from a large-scale population-based cohort study in Japan. Arch Intern Med. 2006;166:1871–7.

81. Svacina S. Tumours of kidneys, urinary bladder and prostate in obesity and diabetes. Vnitrni lekarstvi. 2008;54:464–7.

82. Zucchetto A, Dal Maso L, Tavani A, Montella M, Ramazzotti V, Talamini R, et al. History of treated hypertension and diabetes mellitus and risk of renal cell cancer. Ann Oncol. 2007;18:596–600.

83. Qayyum T, Oades G, Horgan P, Aitchison M, Edwards J. The epidemiology and risk factors for renal cancer. Current Urology. 2013;6:169–74.

84. Washio M, Mori M, Khan M, Sakauchi F, Watanabe Y, Ozasa K, et al. Diabetes mellitus and kidney cancer risk: the results of Japan collaborative cohort study for evaluation of cancer risk (JACC study). Int J Urol. 2007;14:393–7.

85. Lucenteforte E, Bosetti C, Talamini R, Montella M, Zucchetto A, Pelucchi C, et al. Diabetes and endometrial cancer: effect modification by body weight, physical activity and hypertension. Br J Cancer. 2007;97:995–8.

86. Lindemann K, Vatten LJ, Ellstrom-Engh M, Eskild A. Body mass, diabetes and smoking, and endometrial cancer risk: a follow-up study. Br J Cancer. 2008;98:1582–5.

87. Lambe M, Wigertz A, Garmo H, Walldius G, Jungner I, Hammar N. Impaired glucose metabolism and diabetes and the risk of breast, endometrial, and ovarian cancer. Cancer Causes Control. 2011;22:1163–71.

88. Soliman PT, Wu D, Tortolero-Luna G, Schmeler KM, Slomovitz BM, Bray MS, et al. Association between adiponectin, insulin resistance, and endometrial cancer. Cancer. 2006;106:2376–81.

89. Liao S, Li J, Wei W, Wang L, Zhang Y, Li J, et al. Association between diabetes mellitus and breast cancer risk: a meta-analysis of the literature. Asian Pac J Cancer Prev. 2011;12:1061–5.

90. Larsson SC, Mantzoros CS, Wolk A. Diabetes mellitus and risk of breast cancer: a meta-analysis. Int J Cancer. 2007;121:856–62.

91. Schernhammer ES, Holly JM, Pollak MN, Hankinson SE. Circulating levels of insulin-like growth factors, their binding proteins, and breast cancer risk. Cancer Epidemiol Biomark Prev. 2005;14:699–704.

92. Gunter MJ, Hoover DR, Yu H, Wassertheil-Smoller S, Rohan TE, Manson JE, et al. Insulin, insulin-like growth factor-I, and risk of breast cancer in postmenopausal women. J Natl Cancer Inst. 2009;101:48–60.

93. Novosyadlyy R, Lann DE, Vijayakumar A, Rowzee A, Lazzarino DA, Fierz Y, et al. Insulin-mediated acceleration of breast cancer development and progression in a nonobese model of type 2 diabetes. Cancer Res. 2010;70:741–51.

94. Jones RA, Moorehead RA. The impact of transgenic IGF-IR overexpression on mammary development and tumorigenesis. J Mammary Gland Biol Neoplasia. 2008;13:407–13.

95. Stott-Miller M, Chen C, Chuang SC, Lee YC, Boccia S, Brenner H, et al. History of diabetes and risk of head and neck cancer: a pooled analysis from the international head and neck cancer epidemiology consortium. Cancer Epidemiol Biomark Prev. 2012;21:294–304.

96. Becker C, Jick SS, Meier CR, Bodmer M. Metformin and the risk of head and neck cancer: a case-control analysis. Diabetes, Obes Met. 2014;16:1148–54.

97. Stott-Miller M, Chen C, Schwartz SM. Type II diabetes and metabolic syndrome in relation to head and neck squamous cell carcinoma risk: a SEER-Medicare database study. Cancer Epidemiol. 2013;37:428–33.

98. Nakamura K, Wada K, Tamai Y, Tsuji M, Kawachi T, Hori A, et al. Diabetes mellitus and risk of cancer in Takayama: a population-based prospective cohort study in Japan. Cancer Sci. 2013;104:1362–7.

99. Kuriki K, Hirose K, Tajima K. Diabetes and cancer risk for all and specific sites among Japanese men and women. Eur J Cancer Prev. 2007;16:83–9.

100. Atchison EA, Gridley G, Carreon JD, Leitzmann MF, McGlynn KA. Risk of cancer in a large cohort of U.S. veterans with diabetes. Int J Cancer. 2011;128:635–43.

101. Bosetti C, Rosato V, Polesel J, Levi F, Talamini R, Montella M, et al. Diabetes mellitus and cancer risk in a network of case-control studies. Nutr Cancer. 2012;64:643–51.

102. Kasper JS, Giovannucci E. A meta-analysis of diabetes mellitus and the risk of prostate cancer. Cancer Epidemiol Biomark Prev. 2006;15:2056–62.

103. Waters KM, Henderson BE, Stram DO, Wan P, Kolonel LN, Haiman CA. Association of diabetes with prostate cancer risk in the multiethnic cohort. Am J Epidemiol. 2009;169:937–45.

104. Bansal D, Bhansali A, Kapil G, Undela K, Tiwari P. Type 2 diabetes and risk of prostate cancer: a meta-analysis of observational studies. Prostate Cancer Prostatic Dis. 2013;16(151–8):S1.

105. Li Q, Kuriyama S, Kakizaki M, Yan H, Sone T, Nagai M, et al. History of diabetes mellitus and the risk of prostate cancer: the Ohsaki cohort study. Cancer Causes Control. 2010;21:1025–32.

106. Tseng CH. Diabetes and risk of prostate cancer: a study using the National Health Insurance. Diabetes Care. 2011;34:616–21.

107. Shlomai G, Neel B, LeRoith D, Gallagher J. Type 2 Diabetes mellitus and cancer: the role of pharmacotherapy. J Clin Oncol. 2016;35:4261–70.

108. Simo R, Plana-Ripoll O, Puente D, Morros R, Mundet X, Vilca LM, et al. Impact of glucose-lowering agents on the risk of cancer in type 2 diabetic patients. The Barcelona case-control study. PLOS One. 2013;8:e79968.

109. Franchi M, Asciutto R, Nicontra F, Merlino L, La Vecchia C, Corrao G, et al. Metformin, other antidiabetic drugs, and endometrial cancer risk: a nested case-control study within Italian healthcare utilization databases. Eur J Cancer Prev. 2017;26:225–31.

110. American Diabetes Association. Pharmacologic approaches to glycemic treatment standards of medical Care in Diabetes – 2021. Diabetes Care. 2021;44(Suppl 1):S111–24.

111. Garber AJ, Handelsman Y, Grunberger G, Einhorn D, Abrahamson MJ, Barzilay JI, et al. Consensus statement by the American Association of Clinical Endocrinologists and American College of endocrinology on the comprehensive type 2 diabetes management algorithm - 2020 executive summary. Endocr Pract. 2020;26:107–39.

112. National Institute for Health and Care Excellence (NICE) (2017) Type 2 diabetes in adults: management. NICE guideline. Available from nice.org.uk/guidance/ng28.

113. Rattan R, Ali Fehmi R, Munkarah A. Metformin: an emerging new therapeutic option for targeting cancer stem cells and metastasis. J Oncol. 2012;2012:928127.

114. Evans JM, Donnelly LA, Emslie-Smith AM, Alessi DR, Morris AD. Metformin and reduced risk of cancer in diabetic patients. BMJ. 2005;330:1304–5.

115. Rosta A. Diabetes and cancer risk: oncologic considerations. Orv Etil. 2011;152:1144–55.

116. Song I-S. Metformin as an anticancer drug: a commentary on the metabolic determinants of cancer cell sensitivity to glucose limitation and biguanides. Journal of Diabetes Investigation. 2015;6:516–8.

117. Hanly EK, Darzynkiewicz Z, Tiwari RK. Biguanides and targeted anti-cancer treatments. Genes Cancer. 2015;6:3–4.

118. Podhoerecka M, Ibanez B, Dmoszynska A. Metformin- its potential anti-cancer and anti-aging effects. Postepy Hig Med Dosw. 2017;71:170–5.

119. Romero R, Erez O, Hütteman M, Maymon E, Panaitescu B, Conde-Agudelo A, et al. Metformin, the aspirin of the 21st century: its role in gestational diabetes mellitus, prevention of pre-eclampsia and cancer, and the promotion of longevity. Am J Obstet Gynecol. 2018;217:282–302.

120. Abdelgadir E, Ali R, Rashid F, Bashier A. Effect of metformin on different non-Diabetes related conditions, a special focus on malignant conditions: review of literature. J Clin Med Res. 2017;9:388–95.

121. Lv Z, Guo Y. Metformin and its benefits for various diseases. Front Endocrinol. 2020;11:1–10.

122. Ahmad E, Sargeant JA, Zaccardi F, Khunti K, Webb DR, Davies MJ. Where does Metformin stand in modern day Management of Type 2 Diabetes? Pharmaceuticals. 2020;13:427.

123. Drzewoski J, Hanefeld M. The current and potential therapeutic use of metformin - the good old drug. Pharmaceuticals. 2021;14:122.

124. Hirsch HA, Iliopoulos D, Struhl K. Metformin inhibits the inflammatory response associated with cellular transformation and cancer stem cell growth. Proc Natl Acad Sci U S A. 2013;110:972–7.

125. Mani SA, Guo W, Liao MJ, Eaton EN, Ayyanan A, Zhou AY, et al. The epithelial-mesenchymal transition generates cells with properties of stem cells. Cell. 2008;133:704–15.

126. Hirsch HA, Iliopoulos D, Tsichlis PN, Struhl K. Metformin selectively targets cancer stem cells, and acts together with chemotherapy to block tumor growth and prolong remission. Cancer Res. 2009;69:7507–11.

127. Hollier BG, Evans K, Mani SA. The epithelial-to-mesenchymal transition and cancer stem cells: a coalition against cancer therapies. J Mammary Gland Biol Neoplasia. 2009;14:29–43.

128. Pearce EL, Walsh MC, Cejas PJ, Harms GM, Shen H, Wang LS, et al. Enhancing CD8 T-cell memory by modulating fatty acid metabolism. Nature. 2009;460:103–7.

129. Pollak M. Potential applications for biguanides in oncology. J Clin Invest. 2013;123:3693–700.

130. Bodmer M, Becker C, Meier C, Jick SS, Meier CR. Use of anti-diabetic agents and the risk of pancreatic cancer: a case-control analysis. Am J Gastroenterol. 2012;107:620–6.

131. Li D, Yeung SC, Hassan MM, Konopleva M, Abbruzzese JL. Antidiabetic therapies affect risk of pancreatic cancer. Gastroenterology. 2009;137:482–8.

132. Zhang ZJ, Zheng ZJ, Shi R, Su Q, Jiang Q, Kip KE. Metformin for liver cancer prevention in patients with type 2 diabetes: a systematic review and meta-analysis. J Clin Endocrinol Metab. 2012;97:2347–53.

133. Lee MS, Hsu CC, Wahlqvist ML, Tsai HN, Chang YH, Huang YC. Type 2 diabetes increases and metformin reduces total, colorectal, liver and pancreatic cancer incidences in Taiwanese: a representative population prospective cohort study of 800,000 individuals. BMC Cancer. 2011;11:20.

134. Singh S, Singh H, Singh PP, Murad MH, Limburg PJ. Antidiabetic medications and the risk of colorectal cancer in patients with diabetes mellitus: a systematic review and meta-analysis. Cancer Epidemiol Biomark Prev. 2013;22:2258–68.

135. Bodmer M, Becker C, Meier C, Jick SS, Meier CR. Use of metformin is not associated with a decreased risk of colorectal cancer: a case-control analysis. Cancer Epidemiol Biomark Prev. 2012;21:280–6.

136. Wright JL, Stanford JL. Metformin use and prostate cancer in Caucasian men: results from a population-based case-control study. Cancer Causes Control. 2009;20:1617–22.

137. Preston MA, Riis AH, Ehrenstein V, Breau RH, Batista JL, Olumi AF, et al. Metformin use and prostate cancer risk. Eur Urol. 2014;66:1012–20.

138. Kato H, Sekine Y, Furuya Y, Miyazawa Y, Koike H, Suzuki K. Metformin inhibits the proliferation of human prostate cancer PC-3 cells via the downregulation of insulin-like growth factor 1 receptor. Biochem Biophys Res Commun. 2015;461:115–21.

139. Murtola TJ, Tammela TL, Lahtela J, Auvinen A. Antidiabetic medication and prostate cancer risk: a population-based case-control study. Am J Epidemiol. 2008;168:925–31.

140. Yang FQ, Wang JJ, Yan JS, Huang JH, Li W, Che JP, et al. Metformin inhibits cell growth by upregulating microRNA-26a in renal cancer cells. Int J Clin Exp Med. 2014;7:3289–96.

141. Febbraro T, Lengyel E, Romero IL. Old drug, new trick: repurposing metformin for gynecologic cancers? Gynecol Oncol. 2014;135:614–21.

142. Dilokthornsakul P, Chaiyakunapruk N, Termrungruanglert W, Pratoomsoot C, Saokeaw S, Sruamsiri R. The effects of metformin on ovarian cancer: a systematic review. Int J Gynecol Cancer. 2013;23:1544–51.

143. Gotlieb WH, Saumet J, Beauchamp MC, Gu J, Lau S, Pollak MN, et al. In vitro metformin anti-neoplastic activity in epithelial ovarian cancer. Gynecol Oncol. 2008;110:246–50.

144. Vazquez-Martin A, Oliveras-Ferraros C, Del Barco S, Martin-Castillo B, Menendez JA. The anti-diabetic drug metformin suppresses self-renewal and proliferation of trastuzumab-resistant tumor-initiating breast cancer stem cells. Breast Cancer Res Treat. 2011;126:355–64.

145. Jiralerspong S, Palla SL, Giordano SH, Meric-Bernstam F, Liedtke C, Barnett CM, et al. Metformin and pathologic complete responses to neoadjuvant chemotherapy in diabetic patients with breast cancer. J Clin Oncol. 2009;27:3297–302.

146. Lai SW, Liao KF, Chen PC, Tsai PY, Hsieh DP, Chen CC. Antidiabetes drugs correlate with decreased risk of lung cancer: a population-based observation in Taiwan. Clin Lung Cancer. 2012;13:143–8.

147. Tan BX, Yao WX, Ge J, Peng XC, Du XB, Zhang R, et al. Prognostic influence of metformin as first-line chemotherapy for advanced nonsmall cell lung cancer in patients with type 2 diabetes. Cancer. 2011;117:5103–11.

148. Yen YC, Lin C, Lin SW, Lin YS, Weng SF. Effect of metformin on the incidence of head and neck cancer in diabetics. Head Neck. 2015;37(9):1268–73.

149. Sikka A, Kaur M, Agarwal C, Deep G, Agarwal R. Metformin suppresses growth of human head and neck squamous cell carcinoma via global inhibition of protein translation. Cell Cycle. 2012;11:1374–82.

150. Rego DF, Pavan LM, Elias ST, De Luca CG, Guerra EN. Effects of metformin on head and neck cancer: a systematic review. Oral Oncol. 2015;51:416–22.

151. Sandulache VC, Hamblin JS, Skinner HD, Kubik MW, Myers JN, Zevallos JP. Association between metformin use and improved survival in patients with laryngeal squamous cell carcinoma. Head Neck. 2014;36:1039–43.

152. Yasukagawa T, Niwa Y, Simizu S, Umezawa K. Suppression of cellular invasion by glybenclamide through inhibited secretion of platelet-derived growth factor in ovarian clear cell carcinoma ES-2 cells. FEBS Lett. 2012;586:1504–9.

153. Noto H, Goto A, Tsujimoto T, Osame K, Noda M. Latest insights into the risk of cancer in diabetes. Journal of Diabetes Investigation. 2013;4:225–32.

154. Chang CH, Lin JW, Wu LC, Lai MS, Chuang LM. Oral insulin secretagogues, insulin, and cancer risk in type 2 diabetes mellitus. J Clin Endocrinol Metab. 2012;97:E1170–5.

155. Onitilo AA, Engel JM, Glurich I, Stankowski RV, Williams GM, Doi SA. Diabetes and cancer II: role of diabetes medica-

tions and influence of shared risk factors. Cancer Causes Control. 2012;23:991–1008.

156. Hsieh MC, Lee TC, Cheng SM, Tu ST, Yen MH, Tseng CH. The influence of type 2 diabetes and glucose-lowering therapies on cancer risk in the Taiwanese. Exp Diabetes Res. 2012;2012:413782.

157. Gonzalez-Perez A, Garcia Rodriguez LA. Prostate cancer risk among men with diabetes mellitus (Spain). Cancer Causes Control. 2005;16:1055–8.

158. Yang X, So WY, Ma RC, Yu LW, Ko GT, Kong AP, et al. Use of sulphonylurea and cancer in type 2 diabetes-the Hong Kong Diabetes registry. Diabetes Res Clin Pract. 2010;90:343–51.

159. Pasello G, Urso L, Conte P, Favaretto A. Effects of sulfonyl-ureas on tumor growth: a review of the literature. Oncologist. 2013;18:1118–25.

160. Monami M, Lamanna C, Balzi D, Marchionni N, Mannucci E. Sulphonylureas and cancer: a case-control study. Acta Diabetol. 2009;46:279–84.

161. Blin P, Lassalle R, Dureau-Pournin C, Ambrosino B, Bernard MA, Abouelfath A, et al. Insulin glargine and risk of cancer: a cohort study in the French National Healthcare Insurance Database. Diabetologia. 2012;55:644–53.

162. Buchs AE, Silverman BG. Incidence of malignancies in patients with diabetes mellitus and correlation with treatment modalities in a large Israeli health maintenance organization: a historical cohort study. Metab Clin Exp. 2011;60:1379–85.

163. Dejgaard A, Lynggaard H, Rastam J, Krogsgaard TM. No evidence of increased risk of malignancies in patients with diabetes treated with insulin detemir: a meta-analysis. Diabetologia. 2009;52:2507–12.

164. Karlstad O, Starup-Linde J, Vestergaard P, Hjellvik V, Bazelier MT, Schmidt MK, et al. Use of insulin and insulin analogs and risk of cancer - systematic review and meta-analysis of observational studies current. Drug Saf. 2013;8:333–48.

165. Colmers IN, Bowker SL, Tjosvold LA, Johnson JA. Insulin use and cancer risk in patients with type 2 diabetes: a systematic review and meta-analysis of observational studies. Diabetes Metab. 2012;38:485–506.

166. Stammberger I, Essermeant L. Insulin glargine: a reevaluation of rodent carcinogenicity findings. Int J Toxicol. 2012;31:137–42.

167. Lim S, Stember KG, He W, Bianca PC, Yelibi C, Marquis A, et al. Electronic medical record cancer incidence over six years comparing new users of glargine with new users of NPH insulin. PLoS One. 2014;9:e109433.

168. Teng JA, Hou RL, Li DL, Yang RP, Qin J. Glargine promotes proliferation of breast adenocarcinoma cell line MCF-7 via AKT activation. Horm Metab Res. 2011;43:519–23.

169. Aizen D, Sarfstein R, Bruchim I, Weinstein D, Laron Z, Werner H. Proliferative and signaling activities of insulin analogues in endometrial cancer cells. Mol Cell Endocrinol. 2015;406:27–39.

170. Qin J, Teng JA, Zhu Z, Chen JX, Wu YY. Glargine promotes human colorectal cancer cell proliferation via upregulation of miR-95. Horm Metab Res. 2015;47:861–5.

171. Bordeleau L, Yakubovich N, Dagenais GR, Rosenstock J, Probstfield J, Chang YP, et al. The association of basal insulin glargine and/or n-3 fatty acids with incident cancers in patients with dysglycemia. Diabetes Care. 2014;37:1360–6.

172. Wei S, Yang J, Lee SL, Kulp SK, Chen CS. PPARgamma-independent antitumor effects of thiazolidinediones. Cancer Lett. 2009;276:119–24.

173. Weng JR, Chen CY, Pinzone JJ, Ringel MD, Chen CS. Beyond peroxisome proliferator-activated receptor gamma signaling: the multi-facets of the antitumor effect of thiazolidinediones. Endocr Relat Cancer. 2006;13:401–13.

174. Govindarajan R, Ratnasinghe L, Simmons DL, Siegel ER, Midathada MV, Kim L, et al. Thiazolidinediones and the risk of lung, prostate, and colon cancer in patients with diabetes. J Clin Oncol. 2007;25:1476–81.

175. Monami M, Dicembrini I, Mannucci E. Thiazolidinediones and cancer: results of a meta-analysis of randomized clinical trials. Acta Diabetol. 2014;51:91–101.

176. Colmers IN, Bowker SL, Johnson JA. Thiazolidinedione use and cancer incidence in type 2 diabetes: a systematic review and meta-analysis. Diabetes Metab. 2012;38:475–84.

177. Chang CH, Lin JW, Wu LC, Lai MS, Chuang LM, Chan KA. Association of thiazolidinediones with liver cancer and colorectal cancer in type 2 diabetes mellitus. Hepatology. 2012;55:1462–72.

178. Kumagai T, Ikezoe T, Gui D, O'Kelly J, Tong XJ, Cohen FJ, et al. RWJ-241947 (MCC-555), a unique peroxisome proliferator-activated receptor-gamma ligand with antitumor activity against human prostate cancer in vitro and in beige/nude/ X-linked immunodeficient mice and enhancement of apoptosis in myeloma cells induced by arsenic trioxide. Clin Cancer Res. 2004;10:1508–20.

179. Yamaguchi K, Lee SH, Eling TE, Baek SJ. A novel peroxisome proliferator-activated receptor gamma ligand, MCC-555, induces apoptosis via posttranscriptional regulation of NAG-1 in colorectal cancer cells. Mol Cancer Ther. 2006;5:1352–61.

180. Min KW, Zhang X, Imchen T, Baek SJ. A peroxisome proliferator-activated receptor ligand MCC-555 imparts antiproliferative response in pancreatic cancer cells by PPARgamma-independent up-regulation of KLF4. Toxicol Appl Pharmacol. 2012;263:225–32.

181. Joshi H, Pal T, Ramaa CS. A new dawn for the use of thiazolidinediones in cancer therapy. Expert Opin Investig Drugs. 2014;23:501–10.

182. Feng YH, Velazquez-Torres G, Gully C, Chen J, Lee MH, Yeung SC. The impact of type 2 diabetes and antidiabetic drugs on cancer cell growth. J Cell Mol Med. 2011;15:825–36.

183. Frohlich E, Wahl R. Chemotherapy and chemoprevention by thiazolidinediones. Biomed Res Int. 2015;2015:845340.

184. Ramos-Nino ME, MacLean CD, Littenberg B. Association between cancer prevalence and use of thiazolidinediones: results from the Vermont Diabetes information system. BMC Med. 2007;5:17.

185. Ferwana M, Firwana B, Hasan R, Al-Mallah MH, Kim S, Montori VM, et al. Pioglitazone and risk of bladder cancer: a meta-analysis of controlled studies. Diabet Med. 2013;30:1026–32.

186. Jin SM, Song SO, Jung CH, Chang JS, Suh S, Kang SM, et al. Risk of bladder cancer among patients with diabetes treated with a 15 mg pioglitazone dose in Korea: a multi-center retrospective cohort study. J Korean Med Sci. 2014;29:238–42.

187. Turner RM, Kwok CS, Chen-Turner C, Maduakor CA, Singh S, Loke YK. Thiazolidinediones and associated risk of bladder cancer: a systematic review and meta-analysis. Br J Clin Pharmacol. 2014;78:258–73.

188. Ferrara A, Lewis JD, Quesenberry CP Jr, Peng T, Strom BL, Van Den Eeden SK, et al. Cohort study of pioglitazone and cancer incidence in patients with diabetes. Diabetes Care. 2011;34:923–9.

189. Gokhale M, Buse JB, Gray CL, Pate V, Marquis MA, Sturmer T. Dipeptidyl-peptidase-4 inhibitors and pancreatic cancer: a cohort study. Diabetes Obes Met. 2014;16:1247–56.

190. Butler AE, Galasso R, Matveyenko A, Rizza RA, Dry S, Butler PC. Pancreatic duct replication is increased with obesity and type 2 diabetes in humans. Diabetologia. 2010;53:21–6.

191. Tella SH, Rendell MS. DPP-4 inhibitors: focus on safety. Expert Opin Drug Saf. 2015;14:127–40.

192. Tseng CH, Lee KY, Tseng FH. An updated review on cancer risk associated with incretin mimetics and enhancers. J Environ Sci Health C Environ Carcinog Ecotoxicol Rev. 2015;33:67–124.

193. Kissow H, Hartmann B, Holst JJ, Viby NE, Hansen LS, Rosenkilde MM, et al. Glucagon-like peptide-1 (GLP-1) receptor agonism

or DPP-4 inhibition does not accelerate neoplasia in carcinogen treated mice. Regul Pept. 2012;179:91–100.

194. Femia AP, Raimondi L, Maglieri G, Lodovici M, Mannucci E, Caderni G. Long-term treatment with sitagliptin, a dipeptidyl peptidase-4 inhibitor, reduces colon carcinogenesis and reactive oxygen species in 1,2-dimethylhydrazine-induced rats. Int J Cancer. 2013;133:2498–503.

195. Farag SS, Srivastava S, Messina-Graham S, Schwartz J, Robertson MJ, Abonour R, et al. In vivo DPP-4 inhibition to enhance engraftment of single-unit cord blood transplants in adults with hematological malignancies. Stem Cells Dev. 2013;22:1007–15.

196. Nomiyama T, Kawanami T, Irie S, Hamaguchi Y, Terawaki Y, Murase K, et al. Exendin-4, a GLP-1 receptor agonist, attenuates prostate cancer growth. Diabetes. 2014;63:3891–905.

197. Koehler JA, Kain T, Drucker DJ. Glucagon-like peptide-1 receptor activation inhibits growth and augments apoptosis in murine CT26 colon cancer cells. Endocrinology. 2011;152:3362–72.

198. Ligumsky H, Wolf I, Israeli S, Haimsohn M, Ferber S, Karasik A, et al. The peptide-hormone glucagon-like peptide-1 activates cAMP and inhibits growth of breast cancer cells. Breast Cancer Res Treat. 2012;132:449–61.

199. Zhao H, Wang L, Wei R, Xiu D, Tao M, Ke J, et al. Activation of glucagon-like peptide-1 receptor inhibits tumourigenicity and metastasis of human pancreatic cancer cells via PI3K/Akt pathway. Diabetes Obes Met. 2014;16:850–60.

200. Samson SL, Garber A. GLP-1R agonist therapy for diabetes: benefits and potential risks. Curr Opin Endocrinol Diabetes Obes. 2013;20:87–97.

201. Nauck MA, Friedrich N. Do GLP-1-based therapies increase cancer risk? Diabetes Care. 2013;36(Suppl 2):S245–52.

202. Hegedus L, Moses AC, Zdravkovic M, Le Thi T, Daniels GH. GLP-1 and calcitonin concentration in humans: lack of evidence of calcitonin release from sequential screening in over 5000 subjects with type 2 diabetes or nondiabetic obese subjects treated with the human GLP-1 analog, liraglutide. J Clin Endocrinol Metab. 2011;96:853–60.

203. Joshi SR, Standl E, Tong N, Shah P, Kalra S, Rathod R. Therapeutic potential of alpha-glucosidase inhibitors in type 2 diabetes mellitus: an evidence-based review. Expert Opin Pharmacother. 2015;1:1959–81.

204. Tseng YH, Tsan YT, Chan WC, Sheu WH, Chen PC. Use of an alpha-glucosidase inhibitor and the risk of colorectal cancer in patients with Diabetes: a Nationwide. Population-Based Cohort Study Diabetes Care. 2015;38:2068–74.

205. Chen YL, Cheng KC, Lai SW, Tsai IJ, Lin CC, Sung FC, et al. Diabetes and risk of subsequent gastric cancer: a population-based cohort study in Taiwan. Gastric Cancer. 2013;16:389–96.

206. Lai SW, Liao KF, Lai HC, Tsai PY, Sung FC, Chen PC. Kidney cancer and diabetes mellitus: a population-based case-control study in Taiwan. Ann Acad Med Singap. 2013;42:120–4.

207. Wu L, Zhu J, Prokop LJ, Murad MH. Pharmacologic therapy of Diabetes and overall cancer risk and mortality: a meta-analysis of 265 studies. Sci Rep. 2015;5:10147.

208. Malhotra A, Kudyar S, Gupta AK, Kudyar RP, Malhotra P. Sodium glucose co-transporter inhibitors - a new class of old drugs. Int J Appl Basic Med Res. 2015;5:161–3.

209. Lin HW, Tseng CH. A review on the relationship between SGLT2 inhibitors and cancer. Int J Endocrinol. 2014;2014:719578.

210. Scafoglio C, Hirayama BA, Kepe V, Liu J, Ghezzi C, Satyamurthy N, et al. Functional expression of sodium-glucose transporters in cancer. Proc Natl Acad Sci U S A. 2015;112:E4111–9.

211. Villani LA, Smith BK, Marcinko K, Ford RJ, Broadfield LA, Green AE, et al. The diabetes medication canagliflozin reduces cancer cell proliferation by inhibiting mitochondrial complex-I supported respiration. Mol Metab. 2016;5:1048–56.

212. Chowdhury TA, Jacob P. Challenges in the management of people with diabetes and cancer. Diabet Med. 2019;36:795–802.

Further Reading

Decensi A, Puntoni M, Goodwin P, Cazzaniga M, Gennari A, Bonanni B, et al. Metformin and cancer risk in diabetic patients: a systematic review and meta-analysis. Cancer Prevent Res. 2010;3:1451–61. *A systemic review with meta-analysis presenting the inverse association between metformin and cancer risk*

Feng YH, Velazquez-Torres G, Gully C, Chen J, Lee MH, Yeung SC. The impact of type 2 diabetes and antidiabetic drugs on cancer cell growth. J Cell Mol Med. 2011;15:825–36. *Another study assessing the influence of anti-diabetic medications on cancer biology*

Giovannucci E, Harlan DM, Archer MC, Bergenstal RM, Gapstur SM, Habel LA, et al. Diabetes and cancer: a consensus report. Diabetes Care. 2010;33:1674–85. *A clear and comprehensive consensus report on the correlation between diabetes mellitus and oncogenesis*

Pollak M. Potential applications for biguanides in oncology. J Clin Invest. 2013;123:3693–700. *A study on potential usefulness of biguanides (metformin with its antineoplastic activities) in oncology*

Renehan AG, Zwahlen M, Egger M. Adiposity and cancer risk: new mechanistic insights from epidemiology. Nat Rev Cancer. 2015;15:484–98. *A study presenting increased risk of cancer incidence in patients with adiposity (adiposity is significantly correlated with type 2 diabetes mellitus)*

Ryu TY, Park J, Scherer PE. Hyperglycemia as a risk factor for cancer progression. Diabetes Metab J. 2014;38:330–6. *A study explaining the tumor-promoting activity of hyperglycemia*

Tsilidis KK, Kasimis JC, Lopez DS, Ntzani EE, Ioannidis JP. Type 2 diabetes and cancer: umbrella review of meta-analyses of observational studies. BMJ. 2015;350:g7607. *A comprehensive meta-analysis on the correlation between type 2 diabetes mellitus and cancer*

Wojciechowska J, Krajewski W, Bolanowski M, Krecicki T, Zatonski T. Diabetes and Cancer: a Review of Current Knowledge. Exp Clin Endocrinol Diabetes. 2016;124(5):263–75. *A review article written by the authors of this chapter. The chapter is based on this article. The article, similarly to this chapter, analyse the association between diabetes mellitus (mainly type 2 diabetes mellitus) and cancer risk and cancer biology. The article also present the association between diabetes mellitus and antidiabetic medications*

Wu L, Zhu J, Prokop LJ, Murad MH. Pharmacologic therapy of diabetes and overall cancer risk and mortality: a meta-analysis of 265 studies. Sci Rep. 2015;5:10147. *A meta-analysis assessing the association between anti-diabetic pharmacotherapy and cancer risk and mortality*

Diabetes in Children and Adolescents

64

América Liliana Miranda Lora,
Montserrat Espinosa Espíndola, Martha Beauregard Paz,
Jorge Mario Molina Díaz, and Miguel Klünder Klünder

Objectives
- To identify the types of diabetes mellitus that can affect children and adolescents.
- To provide information about diagnostic tests for identifying the etiology of diabetes mellitus in children and adolescents.
- To describe the epidemiology, risk factors, clinical presentation, treatment, and follow-up for comorbidities in pediatric patients with type 1 and 2 diabetes.

type of diabetes is important for the choice of treatment, educational approach, nutritional program, and prevention of complications.

The care and management of children and adolescents with diabetes have unique aspects such as the following: (1) changes in insulin sensitivity related to growth and sexual development; (2) dependency care; and (3) neurological susceptibility to changes in glucose levels. A multidisciplinary team of specialists in pediatric diabetes should provide care to these patients. Family and individual management education are important for achieving a balance between adult supervision and independent self-care [2].

Introduction

Diabetes mellitus is one of the most common chronic diseases in pediatric patients. The prevalence of diabetes in adolescents from 12 to 19 years of age in the United States during 2005–2014 was 0.8%, of which 28.5% was undiagnosed, and the prevalence of prediabetes was 17.7% [1].

Several decades ago, type 1 diabetes was considered to occur only in children; and T2D, only in adults. However, the proportion of adult patients with type 1 diabetes and the incidence of T2D in children and young adults have been increasing. Given the current obesity epidemic, distinguishing between type 1 and 2 diabetes in children can be difficult. Currently, excessive weight is common in children with type 1 diabetes, whereas autoantibodies and ketosis may be present in patients with T2D. However, the identification of the

Definition and Diagnostic Tests for Diabetes in Children

The term *diabetes mellitus in children* describes a group of disorders of abnormal carbohydrate metabolism that result in hyperglycemia in patients ≥10 and <18 years of age [3]. The diagnostic criteria for diabetes mellitus and increased risk of diabetes (prediabetes) of the Expert Committee of the American Diabetes Association are essentially the same in children and adults [4].

Diagnostic Tests for Diabetes

- Measurement of fasting plasma glucose levels ≥126 mg/dL with no caloric intake for at least 8 h.[1]
- Measurement of 2-h plasma glucose levels ≥200 mg/dL during an oral glucose tolerance test using a glucose load containing 1.75 g of anhydrous glucose per kilogram of body weight dissolved in water, with a maximum of 75 g of anhydrous glucose (footnote 1).

A. L. M. Lora · M. E. Espíndola · M. B. Paz
Epidemiological Research Unit in Endocrinology and Nutrition,
Hospital Infantil de México Federico Gómez,
Ciudad de México, Mexico

J. M. M. Díaz
Department of Pediatric Endocrinology, Hospital Infantil de
México Federico Gómez, Ciudad de México, Mexico

M. K. Klünder (✉)
Hospital Infantil de México Federico Gómez,
Ciudad de México, Mexico

---

[1] In the absence of unequivocal hyperglycemia, results should be confirmed by repeat testing.

© The Author(s), under exclusive license to Springer Nature Switzerland AG 2023
J. Rodriguez-Saldana (ed.), *The Diabetes Textbook*, https://doi.org/10.1007/978-3-031-25519-9_64

- Measurement of HbA1c levels ≥6.5% using a method certified and standardized to the Diabetes Control and Complications Trial assay.* Marked discordance between the measured HbA1c and plasma glucose levels should raise the possibility of assay interference. In conditions such as hemoglobinopathies, pregnancy, glucose-6-phosphate dehydrogenase deficiency, HIV, hemodialysis, recent blood loss, or transfusion or erythropoietin therapy, HbA1c should not be used to diagnose diabetes. However, the studies that formed the basis for this recommendation included only adults, and whether the same HbA1c cutoff point should be used to diagnose diabetes in children and adolescents remains unclear. The American Diabetes Association has suggested that this criterion underestimates the prevalence of prediabetes and diabetes in obese children and adolescents [4–6].
- Measurement of random plasma glucose levels ≥200 mg/dL in a patient with classic symptoms of hyperglycemia or hyperglycemia crisis.

Diagnostic Tests for Increased Risk of Diabetes (Prediabetes)

- Impaired fasting glucose test: fasting plasma glucose levels of 100–125 mg/dL
- Impaired glucose tolerance test: 2-h plasma glucose levels of 140–199 mg/dL during an oral glucose tolerance test
- HbA1c analysis: 5.7–6.4% [4]

Etiological Classification

Distinguishing among the types of diabetes in all groups at onset has difficulties, and the true diagnosis becomes more obvious over time. The diabetes mellitus classification of the American Diabetes Association, which depends on causation, distinguishes the following types [4]:

- **Type 1 diabetes mellitus.** This is characterized by an absolute insulin deficiency, usually as a result of the autoimmune destruction of pancreatic beta cells (type 1A) or secondary to defects in insulin secretion from inherited defects in pancreatic beta cell glucose sensing (type 1B).
- **T2D mellitus.** This is characterized by insulin resistance resulting from defects in the action of insulin on its target tissues and is associated with varying and usually progressive failure of beta cell secretion.

- **Genetic defects of beta cell function (monogenic diabetes).** This type of diabetes is characterized by impaired insulin secretion by pancreatic beta cells caused by a single gene mutation. This genetically heterogeneous group includes the following: neonatal diabetes, mitochondrial diabetes, and maturity-onset diabetes of the young (MODY). These forms of diabetes represent <5% of patients with diabetes and are generally characterized by onset before the age of 25 years. The diagnosis of monogenic diabetes should be considered in children with the following conditions [7–10]:
  - Diabetes in the first 6 months of life
  - A family history of diabetes in first-degree relatives who lack the characteristics of type 1 diabetes (no islet autoantibodies, low or no insulin requirements >5 years after diagnosis [stimulated C-peptide level >200 pmol/L]) [9]
  - Strong family history of diabetes but without typical features of T2D (nonobese and low-risk ethnic group)
  - Mild fasting hyperglycemia (100–150 mg/dL), especially if young and nonobese
  - Children with diabetes not characteristic of type 1 or 2 diabetes that occurs in successive generations (suggestive of an autosomal dominant pattern of inheritance)
  - A prolonged honeymoon period of >1 year or an unusually low requirement of insulin (<0.5 U/kg/day) after 1 year of diabetes

    Neonatal diabetes. This rare disorder has an incidence of 1:300,000–1:400,000 live births [11]. It presents in the first 6 months of life and can be either transient or permanent. All children diagnosed with diabetes in the first 6 months of life should undergo immediate genetic testing for neonatal diabetes [4]. In patients diagnosed between 6 and 12 months of age, testing for neonatal diabetes mellitus should be limited to those without islet antibodies, as most patients in this age group have type 1 diabetes [9]. Almost 50% of cases are permanent, and the most common cause is an autosomal dominant defect in *KNJ11* or *ABCC8*, which encode the Kir6.2 and SUR1 subunits of the ATP-sensitive potassium channel, respectively. However, other genetic defects include the following [4, 12]:

    KCNJ11. Autosomal dominant inheritance. It causes a permanent or transient form. Clinical features include intrauterine growth restriction, possible developmental delay, and seizures and response to sulfonylureas.

    INS. Autosomal dominant inheritance. This is a permanent form of neonatal diabetes associated with intrauterine growth restriction and controlled with insulin.

ABCC8. Autosomal dominant inheritance. It causes a permanent or transient form. Patients usually have intrauterine growth restriction, rare developmental delay, and response to sulfonylureas.

6q24 (PLAG1, HYMA1). The inheritance is autosomal dominant. Mechanisms include uniparental disomy of chromosome 6, paternal duplication, or maternal methylation defect. It is a transient form. The clinical features are intrauterine growth restriction, macroglossia, and umbilical hernia. It may be treatable with medications other than insulin therapy.

GATA6. Autosomal dominant inheritance. It is a permanent form with pancreatic hypoplasia, cardiac malformations, pancreatic exocrine insufficiency, and insulin requirement.

EIF2AK3. Autosomal recessive inheritance. It is a permanent form of neonatal diabetes. It is known as Wolcott-Rallison syndrome, which includes epiphyseal dysplasia, pancreatic exocrine insufficiency, and insulin requirement.

EIF2B1. Autosomal recessive inheritance. It causes a permanent form and can be associated with fluctuating liver function.

FOXP3. X-linked inheritance. It is a permanent form. The clinical features include immunodysregulation, polyendocrinopathy, enteropathy X-linked syndrome (autoimmune diabetes, autoimmune thyroid disease, and exfoliative dermatitis), and requires insulin for treatment.

Patients with the permanent forms could be treated with sulfonylureas rather than insulin. Sulfonylureas trigger beta cell membrane depolarization, electrical activity, calcium influx, and insulin release. Patients with neonatal diabetes require 0.5 mg/kg/day on average, although some patients may need higher doses of up to 2.3 mg/kg/day [4, 13].

Mitochondrial diabetes. Some mitochondrial DNA mutations are strongly associated with diabetes, with the most common mutation being the A3243G mutation in the mitochondrial DNA-encoded tRNA gene. A gradual development of pancreatic beta cell dysfunction upon aging, rather than insulin resistance, is the main mechanism of glucose intolerance development. This mutation affects insulin secretion and may involve an attenuation of cytosolic ADP/ATP levels, which leads to a resetting of the glucose sensor in the pancreatic beta cells. Unlike MODY-2, mitochondrial diabetes shows a pronounced age-dependent deterioration of pancreatic function. In clinical practice, mitochon-

drial diabetes is suspected when a strong familial clustering of diabetes is present. Mitochondrial diabetes can be discriminated from MODY based on the presence of maternal transmission in conjunction with a bilateral hearing impairment in most carriers, although the final proof is provided by genetic analysis [14].

MODY. This is the most common form of monogenic diabetes and is caused by the autosomal dominant transmission of a genetic defect in insulin secretion. It is characterized by impaired insulin secretion with minimal or no defects in insulin action. The clinical characteristics of patients are heterogeneous, and MODY is often misdiagnosed as type 1 or 2 diabetes mellitus. MODY has many subtypes (Table 64.1). MODY-2 is the most common type occurring during childhood, and MODY-3 is the most common type after puberty [15, 16].

MODY should be considered in the following situations [7, 8]:

Individuals with mild stable fasting hyperglycemia.

Multiple family members with diabetes without type 1 characteristics (no islet autoantibodies and low or no insulin requirements 5 years after diagnosis) or T2D (marked obesity and acanthosis nigricans).

In the above-mentioned situations, children and those diagnosed in early adulthood with diabetes not characteristic of type 1 or 2 that occurs in successive generations should have genetic testing for MODY [4]. These individuals should be referred for further evaluation and genetic testing confirmation. Some forms of MODY, such as *HNF1A* and *HNF4A*, are sensitive to sulfonylureas. Mild fasting hyperglycemia due to CGK is not progressive during childhood, does not develop complications, and does not respond to low-dose insulin or oral agents, so these patients should not receive treatment [4, 7].

Genetic defects in insulin action. There are rare genetic abnormalities in the insulin receptor or signal transduction. One of them is Donohue syndrome (leprechaunism), a genetic autosomal recessive disorder that results from the presence of homozygous or compound heterozygous mutations in the insulin receptor gene (*INSR*; 19p13.3-p13.2). The incidence of this pathology is 1 in 1,000,000 births. The characteristics of this syndrome include severe intrauterine and postnatal growth retardation, multiple endocrine dysfunction, hypertrichosis, virilization, emaciation, acanthosis nigricans, lipoatrophy, genitomegaly, postprandial hyperglycemia, fasting hypoglycemia, insulin resistance, hyperinsulinemia, and eventual ketoacidosis. Infants with Donohue syndrome also have distinc-

Table 64.1 Classification of MODY (adapted from references [4, 7, 15])

MODY type	Gene and locus	Age at diagnosis	Primary defect	Associated features	Severity of diabetes
1	*HNF-4a* 20q	Post-puberty	Gene transcription defects in beta cells	Macrosomia and/or neonatal hypoglycemia. It is characterized by a progressive insulin secretory defect with presentation in adolescence or early adulthood. It is sensitive to sulfonylureas	Severe
2	*GCK* 7p	Childhood	Impairment of beta cell sensitivity to glucose and defect in hepatic glycogenesis	Reduced birth weight. This is the most common cause in the absence of symptoms or marked hyperglycemia. This is a stable form with nonprogressive elevated fasting blood glucose levels. Typically, it does not require treatment; microvascular complications are rare	Mild
3	*HNF-1a* 12q	Post-puberty	Similar to MODY-1	Renal glycosuria. This form occurs with a progressive insulin secretory defect with presentation in adolescence or early adulthood; decreased renal threshold for glucosuria; and marked increase in postprandial glucose levels. It is sensitive to sulfonylureas	Severe
4	*PDF1 (IPF-1)* 13q	Early adulthood	Defects in transcription factors during embryogenesis lead to abnormal beta cell development and function	–	Mild
5	*HNF-1b* 17cen-q21.3	Post-puberty	Similar to MODY-1 and MODY-3	Glomerulocystic kidney disease, female genital malformations, hyperuricemia, gout, abnormal liver function tests, and atrophy of the pancreas	Mild
6	*NeuroD1/ BETA2* 2	Early adulthood	Abnormal development and function of beta cells	–	Unknown
7	*KLFA11* 2p25	Early adulthood	Reduced glucose sensitivity of beta cells	Phenotype similar to T2D	Unknown
8	*CEL* 9q24	<20 years	Impaired endocrine and exocrine pancreatic function	Exocrine pancreatic dysfunction	Unknown
9	*PAX4* 7q32	<20 years	Impaired transcription of apoptosis- and proliferation-related genes in pancreatic beta cells	–	Diabetic ketoacidosis is possible
10	*INS* 11p15.5	<20 years	Loss of beta cell mass through apoptosis	–	Unknown
11	*BLK* 8p23	<20 years	Decreased insulin synthesis and secretion in response to glucose	Higher incidence in obese individuals	Unknown

tive characteristics, with elfin facies, low birth weight, skin abnormalities, and large, low-set ears. The diagnosis is based on a combination of typical dysmorphic characteristics and clinical evaluation supported by glycemic and insulin results and genetic analysis. The treatment of these patients is supportive and requires a multidisciplinary team. For instance, blood glucose levels may be maintained with frequent or continuous feeds and complex carbohydrates. Currently, treatment with recombinant insulin-like growth factor 1 has demonstrated effectiveness. The prognosis for this disorder is complicated and fatal; most fetuses with the disorder are either aborted or die within the first year of life [17].

- **Endocrinopathies.** Several hormones such as cortisol, growth hormone, epinephrine, and glucagon antagonize the action of insulin. Over-secretion of these hormones can result in glucose intolerance or diabetes mellitus [18].

- **Drug- or chemical-induced diabetes.** Drugs may induce hyperglycemia through different mechanisms, including alterations in insulin secretion and sensitivity, direct cytotoxic effects on pancreatic cells, and increases in glucose production. The drugs included in this list are antihypertensive drugs, lipid-modifying agents, protease inhibitors, nucleoside reverse transcriptase inhibitors, phenytoin, valproic acid, second-generation antipsychotics, antidepressant agents, glucocorticoids, chemotherapeutic agents, some oral contraceptives, growth hormone, and somatostatin analogs [19].

- **Cystic fibrosis-related diabetes.** Diabetes is the most common comorbidity in patients with cystic fibrosis, occurring in approximately 20% of adolescents and 40–50% of adults with cystic fibrosis. Insulin insufficiency is the primary defect, although genetically determined beta cell function and insulin resistance associated with infection and inflammation may also contribute.

Annual screening for cystic fibrosis-related diabetes with an oral glucose tolerance test beginning at age 10 years is recommended. HbA1c test is not recommended. Screening for cystic fibrosis-related diabetes should be performed using the 2-h (1.75 g/kg maximum 75 g) oral glucose tolerance test [20].

- Patients with cystic fibrosis should be treated with insulin. For patients with impaired glucose tolerance, prandial insulin therapy should be considered to maintain weight. Oral diabetes agents are not as effective as insulin in improving nutritional and metabolic outcomes in cystic fibrosis-related diabetes and are not recommended [20].
- Annual monitoring for complications of diabetes beginning 5 years after the diagnosis of cystic fibrosis-related diabetes is recommended [4].
- **Post-transplantation diabetes mellitus.** In this type of diabetes, individuals develop new-onset diabetes after transplantation. Patients should be screened after organ transplantation for hyperglycemia once they are stabilized with an immunosuppressive regimen and in the absence of an acute infection. Oral glucose tolerance test is the preferred diagnostic test [4].

The main types of diabetes mellitus are types 1 and 2, which will be discussed in detail below.

Type 1 Diabetes Mellitus

Epidemiology

Type 1 diabetes is one of the most common chronic diseases of childhood and affects males and females equally, with a slight male predominance in younger children. Type 1 diabetes has increased in recent years in both sexes, all age and race/ethnic subgroups, except for those with the lowest prevalence (age 0–4 years and American Indians) [21]. Globally, type 1 diabetes represents approximately 2% of the estimated total cases of diabetes, ranging from <1 to >15% [22]. The incidence and prevalence of type 1 diabetes mellitus vary according to the following factors:

- Age. The highest incidence occurs between 10 and 14 years of age [23].
- Season. Type 1 diabetes appears mostly in autumn and winter [23].
- Geographic location. The lowest incidence was reported in Pakistan and Venezuela (0.1 per 100,000 per year); and the highest incidence, in Finland and Sardinia [24].
- Racial and ethnic groups. In the United States, the highest prevalence was in white youths, and the lowest prevalence was in American Indian youths [21].

The incidence of type 1 diabetes mellitus has been increasing at an annual rate of approximately 2.8% [24]. The increasing incidence of type 1 diabetes in children across the world over a short period cannot be explained by genetic factors; environmental risk factors have been suggested to contribute to the increasing trend in its incidence. Several risk factors have been associated with type 1 diabetes mellitus (e.g., infections, dietary factors, air pollution, and vaccines); however, most have been inconclusive [25].

Pathogenesis of Type 1 Diabetes Mellitus

Type 1 diabetes is an autoimmune disease. The pathogenesis of type 1 diabetes begins with the appearance of beta cell autoimmunity, which is primarily directed against insulin, glutamic acid decarboxylase (GAD), or both. Subsequently, other autoantibodies against islet antigen-2, tyrosine phosphatase-like insulinoma antigen 2, or the ZnT8 transporter may also appear. Dysglycemia and the symptoms of diabetes appear later [10, 26].

The rate of beta cell destruction is quite variable, but it is usually faster in infants and children than in adults. Pediatric patients may present with ketoacidosis as the first manifestation of the disease; other patients have modest hyperglycemia, which may increase with infection or other stressors. By contrast, adults may retain sufficient beta cell function to prevent ketoacidosis and eventually become insulin dependent [4].

Progression to diabetes occurred in 14–44% of children with persistent single insulin autoantibodies or GAD autoantibodies within 10 years. The incidence of progression in children with multiple islet autoantibodies was 50–70% within 10 years and 84% within 15 years. The progression to type 1 diabetes was faster in children younger than 3 years, children with the human leukocyte antigen genotype DR3/DR4-DQ8, and girls [27, 28]. Although accepted screening programs for type 1 diabetes are lacking, screening for type 1 diabetes risk with islet autoantibodies is recommended as an option for first-degree family members of a proband with type 1 diabetes. Individuals who test positive will be counseled about the risk of developing diabetes [4, 29].

Type 1 diabetes includes the following stages [4, 29]:

- Stage 1. A presymptomatic stage with autoimmunity (multiple autoantibodies) with normoglycemia
- Stage 2. A presymptomatic stage with autoimmunity but with dysglycemia (impaired fasting glucose or glucose tolerance), or HbA1c levels of 5.7–6.4% or ≥10% increase in HbA1c level
- Stage 3. A symptomatic stage and new-onset hyperglycemia according to the standard diabetes criteria
- Stage 4. Long-standing type 1 diabetes

Genetic Risk Factors of Type 1 Diabetes Mellitus

The primary risk factor of beta cell autoimmunity is genetic and mainly occurs in individuals with HLA-DR3-DQ2 and/ or HLA-DR4-DQ8 haplotypes. The region encoding HLA contributes approximately 50% of the genetic risk. Although non-HLA genetic factors have a slight individual effect, 58 genomic regions show substantial genome-wide evidence of a type 1 diabetes association. Some candidate genes with likely functional effects are *IL27*, *BAD*, *CD69*, *PRKCQ*, *CLEC16A*, *ERBB3*, and *CTSH* [26].

Environmental Risk Factors of Type 1 Diabetes Mellitus

The increase in the incidence of type 1 diabetes mellitus can be explained by changes in environment or lifestyle. A trigger from the environment in an autoimmunity-genetically susceptible individual is generally needed. These factors may be present in both the prenatal and postnatal life stages. Candidate triggers with the strongest evidence include maternal or postnatal enteroviral infection, older maternal age, infant weight gain, serious life events, overweight or increased height velocity, puberty, insulin resistance, and psychological stress. Other suggested triggers include the following: congenital rubella; cesarean section; higher birthweight; low maternal intake of vegetables; frequent respiratory or enteric infections; abnormal microbiome; early exposure to cereals, root vegetables, eggs, or cow milk; persistent or recurrent enteroviral infections; high glycemic load, fructose intake, dietary nitrates, or nitrosamines; and steroid treatment [30].

By contrast, evidence shows that higher omega-3 fatty acids are a postnatal protective factor, and higher maternal vitamin D intake or concentrations in late pregnancy, probiotics in the first month of life, and the introduction of solid food while breastfeeding after age 4 months have also been suggested to be protective factors [30].

Clinical Presentation

Children with type 1 diabetes typically present with symptoms of polyuria, polydipsia, and diabetic ketoacidosis. However, children often do not present with the classical signs and symptoms of diabetes. Physicians should be aware of other presentations such as the following: bedwetting in children who had no previous night bedwetting episodes, unintended weight loss, irritability and other mood changes, fatigue, weakness, blurred vision, candida diaper dermatitis, and vaginal yeast infection.

The prevalence of diabetic ketoacidosis in youths with type 1 diabetes is nearly 30%, and a higher prevalence has been associated with younger age at diagnosis, minority race/ethnicity, and low income [31]. The frequency of diabetic ketoacidosis at diagnosis ranges from 12.8 to 80% among countries. This variation may be explained, at least in part, by different levels of disease awareness and health-care provision [32].

Situations that cause diagnostic difficulties that may delay diagnosis include the following [33]:

- The hyperventilation of ketoacidosis may be misdiagnosed as pneumonia or asthma (cough and breathlessness distinguish these conditions from diabetic ketoacidosis).
- Abdominal pain associated with ketoacidosis may simulate an acute abdomen and lead to referral to a surgeon.
- Polyuria and enuresis may be misdiagnosed as a urinary tract infection.
- Polydipsia may be thought to be a psychogenic disorder.
- Vomiting may be misdiagnosed as gastroenteritis or sepsis (Codner limited care).

Management of Type 1 Diabetes Mellitus

Diabetes Self-Management Education and Support

All people with diabetes should participate in diabetes self-management education and receive support to obtain the knowledge and skills for diabetes self-care. The four critical time points to promote education skills are at diagnosis, annually, or when treatment targets are not met, in cases of medical, physical, or psychosocial complicating factors, and in transitions in life and care [34]. The treatment of patients with diabetes can only be effective if the family implements it. Health-care providers must be capable of evaluating individual and family psychosocial factors to overcome barriers to treatment plans. In addition, other people who participate in the patient's care must be involved. As a large portion of a child's day is spent in school, communication and cooperation with school personnel is essential for optimal diabetes management [2]. Optimal management of diabetes at school is a prerequisite for optimal school performance and the prevention of diabetes-related complications. Schools should facilitate prescribed medical interventions, including support of insulin administration, and manage appropriately the effects of low and high blood glucose levels according to parent and health-care team instructions [35].

Diabetes Education

Pediatric patients and caregivers should receive culturally sensitive and developmentally appropriate individualized diabetes education [2]. Education is key to the successful management of diabetes and maximizes the effectiveness of diabetes treatment. Structured educational programs should be aimed at the patient's achievement of diabetes care goals, improved psychosocial adaptation, and enhanced self-efficacy, in addition to implementing measures of glycemic control.

Educational interventions shown to be effective include the following [36]:

- Clear theoretical psycho-educational principles
- Integration into routine clinical care
- Ongoing provision of individualized self-management and psychosocial support
- Involvement of the continuing responsibility of parents and other caregivers
- Making use of cognitive behavioral techniques most often related to problem-solving, goal setting, communication skills, motivational interviewing, family conflict resolution, coping skills, and stress management
- Utilizing new technologies in diabetes care as one of the vehicles for educational motivation

Glycemic Control

Sufficient glycemic control must be achieved to prevent diabetes-related complications; however, strict glucose levels carry the risk of hypoglycemia. Although young children were previously thought to be at risk of cognitive impairment after episodes of hypoglycemia, current data have not confirmed this notion. Hence, current standards recommend lowering glucose levels to the safest possible level to prevent chronic complications. The blood glucose and HbA1c goals for type 1 diabetes across all pediatric age groups are as follows [2, 8, 37]:

- Blood glucose goal range before meals: 90–130 mg/dL
- Bedtime/overnight: 90–150 mg/dL
- HbA1c level: <7%, with an emphasis on target personalization

Goals should be individualized, and lower goals may be reasonable if they can be achieved without excessive hypoglycemia. Blood glucose goals should be modified in children with frequent hypoglycemia or hypoglycemia unawareness. A higher HbA1c level <7.5% may be more suitable for youth who cannot identify symptoms of hypoglycemia, with hypoglycemia unawareness, without access to analog insulins, or who cannot monitor blood glucose regularly. Even less stringent HbA1c targets (e.g., <8%) may be recommended for children with a history of severe hypoglycemia, severe morbidities, or short life expectancy. On the contrary, a lower goal (HbA1c level of 6.5%) may be appropriate if achievable without excessive hypoglycemia, impairment of quality of life, and undue burden of care. A

lower goal may also be appropriate during the honeymoon phase of type 1 diabetes [2, 8, 38].

Assessment of glycemic status (HbA1c or other glycemic measurement) should be performed at least two times a year in patients who meet treatment goals and at least quarterly in patients whose therapy recently changed or who do not meet glycemic goals [37].

Continuous glucose monitoring devices are rapidly improving diabetes management and could estimate the time in range as a useful metric of glycemic control. These devices report the number of days they are worn, the percentage of time they are active, and the mean glucose levels. The glycemic variability target recommended is ≤36%, with a target range of 70–180 mg/dL at >70%, <70 mg/dL at <4%, <54 mg/dL at <1%, >180 mg/dL at <25%, and >250 mg/dL at <5% [37, 39].

Blood Glucose Monitoring

Glucose monitoring enables patients, parents, and clinicians to evaluate the efficacy of current therapy, make treatment adjustments, and ensure that glucose levels are within the safe goal ranges [40, 41]. Glucose monitoring allows decisions about the insulin dose in patients with intensive management. Sleep is a time of particular risk for severe and asymptomatic hypoglycemia; hence, overnight routine testing is recommended [42].

Increased daily frequency of self-monitoring of blood glucose levels is associated with lower HbA1c levels (−0.2% per additional test per day) and fewer acute complications. When children are old enough, they should be encouraged to auto-self-monitor their glucose levels. All children and adolescents with type 1 diabetes should self-monitor glucose levels up to 6–10 times/day with a glucometer or by continuous glucose monitoring, including prior to meals and snacks, at bedtime, and as needed (during exercise, when driving, and when symptoms of hypoglycemia occur) [2].

Capillary blood and continuous glucose monitoring enable patients to detect the impacts of diet, exercise, illness, stress, and medications on glucose levels. Both types of devices allow patients to recognize hypoglycemia and hyperglycemia. Continuous glucose monitoring has become a standard of care in patients with type 1 diabetes. The advantages of using this technology are the high number of glucose readings per day (up to 288), the alert provided when the blood glucose threshold has been crossed, and the impact on glucose levels (lower HbA1c level, less hypoglycemia, and more time and time in range). However, this benefit is mediated by adherence to sensor therapy, with at least 60% use being associated with these findings [33, 43, 44]. Intermittently scanned continuous glucose monitoring devices may also be available at lower costs than traditional meter-based testing, do not require calibration, and are safe for the pediatric population [44, 45].

Insulin Therapy

Patients with type 1 diabetes mellitus lack sufficient insulin to maintain normoglycemia. Intensive insulin regimens delivered by combinations of multiple daily injections or pump therapy with differential substitution of basal and prandial insulin to obtain optimal metabolic control has become the gold standard for all age groups in pediatric diabetology [46]. The insulin requirement is 0.25–0.5 units/kg/day for children 9 months–2 years of age, 0.5–0.6 units/kg/day for children between 1 and 6 years of age, 0.75 units/kg/day for children ≥7 years until the onset of puberty, and 0.75–1.5 units/kg/day for children starting puberty. For patients with diabetic keto-acidosis, the starting dose may be 1 unit/kg/day. Insulin dose adjustments are based on blood glucose [41]. Daily insulin dosage varies greatly between individuals and changes over time. It therefore requires regular review and reassessment [46]. The pharmacokinetic parameters of insulin commonly used in pediatric patients are shown in Table 64.2.

Intensive management with multiple-dose insulin and/or continuous subcutaneous insulin infusion in children and adolescents with type 1 diabetes mellitus showed marked declines in HbA1c level and chronic complications [47].

The primary goal of treatment is to mimic natural insulin secretion. To achieve this, patients require administration of the following [41, 42]:

1. Basal insulin to maintain near-normal blood glucose levels to prevent starvation between meals and suppress hepatic glucose production. Patients can use continuous subcutaneous insulin infusion or intermediate- or long-acting insulin to mimic basal insulin secretion.

2. Short-acting insulin to cover the carbohydrates consumed during meals and normalize blood glucose levels by intermittent injections based on glycemic corrections and carbohydrate foods throughout the day. As a normal daily diet includes three meals per day, short-acting insulin should be administered at least three times daily. Patients using this regimen need to establish the following parameters:

- The units of rapid-acting insulin to be injected per gram of carbohydrates (insulin-to-carbohydrate ratio)
- The amount of glucose that decreases with 1 unit of rapid-acting insulin (sensitivity factor)

Although no insulin injection regimen satisfactorily mimics normal physiology, premixed insulins are not recommended for pediatric use. When the option is to use regular and NPH insulins, the recommendation should be to provide them as separate insulins, not premixed. Delivering prandial insulin before each meal is superior to postprandial injection and should be preferred if possible [46].

Insulin pumps have become increasingly available to patients with diabetes, and experts highlight their use as the chosen treatment option for many people across all age groups with type 1 diabetes. In adolescents, continuous use of subcutaneous insulin infusion was associated with lower rates of retinopathy (OR, 0.66; 95% CI, 0.045–0.95) and peripheral nerve abnormality (OR, 0.63; 95% CI, 0.42–0.95), suggesting an apparent benefit of continuous subcutaneous insulin infusion over multiple daily injections independent of glycemic control [48]. Insulin pump therapy can assist with reducing episodes of hypoglycemia and is appropriate for youth with diabetes regardless of age. Automated insulin delivery (closed loop) systems improve time in range, including minimizing hypoglycemia and hyperglycemia. Low-glucose suspend systems reduce the severity and duration of hypoglycemia while not leading to deterioration of glycemic control, as measured by HbA1c level. Predictive low-glucose suspend systems can prevent episodes of hypoglycemia and have been shown to be useful for reducing hypoglycemic exposure [44].

Nutritional Management

Nutritional management is one of the fundamental elements of care and education in type 1 diabetes and should be provided at diagnosis and reviewed at least annually by a specialist pediatric diabetes dietitian to increase dietary knowledge and adherence [49]. This management should focus on interventions to ensure normal growth and development, promote lifelong healthy eating habits, optimize glycemic control, prevent associated complications, and avoid overweight and underweight [39, 50]. To establish a nutritional program, health-care providers should consider an individual's energy needs and insulin regimen. In addition, nutritional management and education should be individualized, considering family habits, food preferences, religious or cultural needs, schedules, physical activity, and the patient's and family's abilities in numeracy, literacy, and self-management. The best approach to healthful eating is within the context of the family, focusing on healthy eating for all members [39, 50].

Table 64.2 Pharmacokinetic parameters of insulin commonly used in pediatric patients (adapted from Beck and Cogen [41])

Insulin	Action profile		
	Onset	Peak	Duration
Rapid-acting			
Lispro	15–30 min	30–90 min	3–6 h
Aspart	10–20 min	40–50 min	3–5 h
Glulisine	20–30 min	30–90 min	3–4 h
Short-acting			
Regular	30 min–1 h	2–5 h	5–8 h
Intermediate-acting			
NPH	2–4 h	4–12 h	12–18 h
Long-acting			
Glargine	1–1.5 h	No peak	20–24 h
Detemir	1–2 h	No peak	14–24 h

Healthy eating principles targeting an increased consumption of vegetables, fruits, legumes, whole grains, and dairy products are important, with an emphasis on foods with higher fiber contents and lower glycemic loads [50]. Decreased saturated fat intake underlies education; thus, the aim of improving diabetes outcomes and reducing cardiovascular risk is achieved [49, 51]. Recent studies have shown that meals with protein, fat, and more complex carbohydrates delay glucose level increases [52, 53]. Therefore, patients should be taught about all components of food intake and their respective contributions to the daily intake of calories [39, 50].

Matching insulin to the carbohydrate intake in patients receiving intensive insulin therapy requires comprehensive education in carbohydrate counting or experience-based estimation. Regular dietetic assessments by a specialist pediatric diabetes dietitian are necessary to adapt nutritional advice to growth, diabetes management, and lifestyle changes and to permit the identification and treatment of disordered eating patterns [49].

Patients with type 1 diabetes require specialized dietetic support, especially when eating disorders and celiac disease occur, which are more common in type 1 diabetes mellitus [49, 51].

Key dietary behaviors have been associated with improved glycemic outcomes such as the following [49]:

- adherence to an individualized meal plan, particularly carbohydrate intake recommendations;
- avoidance of frequent snacking episodes or large snacks without adequate insulin coverage;
- intake of regular meals and avoidance of skipping meals; and
- avoidance of overtreatment of hypoglycemia and insulin boluses before meals.

At diagnosis, appetite and energy intake are often high to compensate for catabolic weight loss; however, energy intake should be reduced when appropriate weight is restored to prevent overweight or obesity. Energy intake should be sufficient to achieve optimal growth and maintain an ideal body weight [49, 51].

In general, the nutritional recommendations for child and adolescent diabetics are the same as those for children and adolescents without diabetes. No single ideal dietary distribution of calories among carbohydrates, fats, and proteins has been established for people with diabetes, including children; therefore, macronutrient distribution should be individualized while keeping total calorie and metabolic goals in mind [50].

A guide to the distribution of macronutrients that reflects guidelines for healthy eating among children without diabetes could be used when individualizing the dietary management, distributed as follows [49, 51]:

- Carbohydrate, 45–65%
  - Moderate sucrose intake (up to 10% of the total energy intake)
- Fat, 30–35%
  - <10% saturated fat + trans-fatty acids; ≤7% when hyperlipidemia management is required
  - <10% polyunsaturated fat
  - >10% monounsaturated fat (up to 20% of total energy)
- Protein 15–20% (up to 25% in overweight or obese adolescents)

Carbohydrate intake should not be restricted, as it is essential for growth, and as internationally agreed, an excessive restriction of carbohydrates may result in deleterious effects on growth, a higher cardiovascular risk metabolic profile, and increased risk of disordered eating behaviors, as it also may increase the risk of hypoglycemia or potentially impair the effect of glucagon in hypoglycemia treatment. The mean requirement for carbohydrate if a child is consuming 45% energy from carbohydrates is up to 170 g at the age of 10 years and approximately 213 g in adolescents aged 14 years. However, high-quality carbohydrates are important. With a lower carbohydrate intake, children tend to consume more saturated fat. Carbohydrate intake should come predominantly from whole-grain breads and cereals, legumes, fruits, vegetables, and low-fat dairy foods (except for children aged <2 years), preferring those over other sources, especially those containing added sugars [50, 54].

Children and adolescents with type 1 diabetes require education regarding the amount, type, and distribution of carbohydrates over the day. Day-to-day consistency in carbohydrate intake using serving sizes or 15-g carbohydrate exchanges is encouraged for those receiving fixed mealtime insulin doses. A more flexible carbohydrate intake can be achieved using the insulin-to-carbohydrate ratio for children receiving intensive insulin therapy [49, 51].

Carbohydrate counting is a key nutritional intervention for patients with an intensive insulin regimen focused on carbohydrate as the primary nutrient affecting postprandial glycemic response. It aims to improve glycemic control, allows flexibility of food choices, and enables adjustment of the prandial insulin dose according to carbohydrate consumption. The commonly used methods of quantifying carbohydrate include the following: (1) gram increments of carbohydrate, (2) 10- to 12-g carbohydrate portions, and (3) 15-g carbohydrate exchanges. Research has not yet demonstrated a superior method of teaching carbohydrate counting [49].

Nutrition education begins with carbohydrate counting, where consistency rather than accuracy results in optimal glycemic outcomes. Over- or under-calculation by up to 10 g and 15% of the carbohydrate amount is unlikely to yield substantial hypoglycemia and hyperglycemia, respectively [50].

These programs should also consider the glycemic index of foods, which is a ranking of foods based on their acute glycemic impacts. The use of the glycemic index has been shown to provide additional benefit to glycemic control over that observed when only the amount of carbohydrates is considered. Low-glycemic-index foods decrease postprandial glucose excursion compared with carbohydrates with higher glycemic index values [50, 54].

As mentioned earlier, fat and protein are becoming increasingly recognized to also contribute to postprandial hyperglycemia. Both have been found to further delay the increase in postprandial glucose level. Consideration of the impact of fat and protein on glucose levels involves the application of advanced nutritional concepts that are best taught after basic carbohydrate counting skills have been established [54].

The primary goal regarding dietary fat intake in clinical practice is usually to decrease the intakes of saturated fat and trans-fatty acids. Saturated fat is the principal dietary determinant of plasma low-density lipoprotein (LDL) cholesterol. These types of fats are found in full-fat dairy products, fatty meats, and high-fat snacks, which should be avoided. Trans-fatty acids are formed when vegetable oils are processed and solidified. They are found in margarines, deep-frying fat, cooking fat, and manufactured products. Conversely, monounsaturated fatty acids and polyunsaturated fatty acids, which are found in vegetable oils, nuts, nut butters, and oily fish, can be used as substitutes to improve the lipid profile [54].

Recommendations for decreasing protein intake during childhood range from approximately 2 g/kg/day in early infancy to 1 g/kg/day for 10-year-olds and to 0.8–0.9 g/kg/day in later adolescence. Protein intake promotes growth only when sufficient total energy is available. High-protein diets (>25% total energy) are not generally advised for children with type 1 diabetes, as they may impact growth and vitamin and mineral intakes, except for obese adolescents. Inclusion of sources of vegetable proteins, such as legumes, in diets should be encouraged, as well as that of sources of animal protein, such as fish, lean cuts of meat, and low-fat dairy products [51, 55].

Children with type 1 diabetes have the same vitamin and mineral requirements as healthy children [51], so their intake should be as recommended in nutritional guidelines for the general pediatric population [56]. No clear evidence of the benefit from vitamin or mineral supplementation has been found in children diagnosed with type 1 diabetes who do not have underlying deficiencies [51].

High dietary sodium intake in children with type 1 diabetes is common and relates to vascular dysfunction. Sodium intake should be limited to at least that recommended for the general population. The guidelines for sodium intake in children 1–3 years are as follows: 1000 mg/day (2.5 g salt/day); 4–8 years, 1200 mg/day (3 g salt/day); and 9 years and older, 1500 mg/day (3.8 g salt/day) [54].

Antioxidants are strongly recommended for cardiovascular protection in young people with type 1 diabetes. Many fresh fruits and vegetables are naturally rich in antioxidants (tocopherols, carotenoids, vitamin C, and flavonoids), so their intake should be encouraged [51].

Estimates of dietary fiber intakes in children in many countries are lower than those recommended (3.3 g of fiber per megajoule or 14 g/1000 kcal in children aged >1 year). Intake of a variety of fiber-containing foods such as legumes, vegetables, fruits, and whole-grain cereals should be encouraged, as it promotes healthy bowel function, helps reduce lipid levels, and may be useful for enhancing protection against cardiovascular disease. Fiber-containing foods may also help improve satiety and replace more energy-dense foods. Processed foods tend to be lower in fiber; hence, unprocessed fresh foods should be encouraged. Fiber in the diet should be increased slowly to prevent abdominal discomfort, and any increase in fiber intake should be accompanied by an increase in fluid intake [49].

The dietary recommendations for specific insulin regimes include the following [54]:

Twice daily insulin regimens: Day-to-day consistency in carbohydrate intake to balance the insulin action profile and prevent hypoglycemia during periods of peak insulin action. The carbohydrate content consumed in the meals eaten at the time of insulin doses can be flexible if the patient or the family is taught to adjust the short/rapid-acting insulin to the carbohydrate eaten. Most of the time, this type of regimen requires carbohydrate intake before bed to help prevent nocturnal hypoglycemia.

- Intensive insulin regimens: individualized insulin-to-carbohydrate ratios should be used, as they enable the pre-prandial insulin dose to be matched to the carbohydrate intake. Snacks without meal boluses should be avoided, as it results in deterioration in glycemic control.

Exercise Management in Type 1 Diabetes

Regular exercise is important because it promotes and improves health and well-being, physical fitness, strength building, weight management, social interaction, self-esteem building, and creation of healthful habits for adulthood, and can help patients achieve their target lipid profile, body composition, fitness, and glycemic goals. However, barriers to exercise include fear of hypoglycemia and hyperglycemia, loss of glycemic control, and inadequate knowledge around exercise management [57].

Children and adolescents with diabetes have the same physical activity requirements as their peers without diabetes. The physical activity targets for toddlers (1–2 years) and preschoolers (3–4 years) are a minimum of 180 min of physical activity of any intensity throughout the day with an emphasis on movement-developing skills and varied activities throughout the day. Preschool physical activity should progress toward at least 60 min of energetic play near the age of 5 years. The recommendations for children (5–11 years) and youths (12–17 years) are a minimum of 60 min of moderate- to vigorous-intensity physical activity daily to achieve health benefits (at least 420 min/week of exercise); vigorous-intensity aerobic activities at least 3 days/week, with ≤2 consecutive days between aerobic activities; and muscle- and bone-strengthening activities (resistance training) at least 3 days/week in the absence of contraindications [58–60].

Overall, youths with type 1 diabetes are recommended to participate in ≥60 min of daily physical activity, including resistance and flexibility training. Although comorbid conditions or diabetes complications are uncommon in the pediatric population, patients should be medically evaluated for these conditions, which may restrict participation in an exercise program [50].

Sedentary time should also be minimized to achieve health benefits. Recreational screen time (television, computer, and video games) is not recommended for infants and toddlers, should be limited to <1 h/day for preschoolers, and should not exceed 2 h/day for older children. Patients should also minimize the time spent indoors, prolonged sitting, and sedentary transport [61].

To avoid hypoglycemia, patients should take the following precautions [57]:

- Decrease the prandial insulin level for the meal/snack before exercise and/or increasing food intake. Patients on insulin pumps can lower basal rates by approximately 10 to ≥50% or suspend the increase in basal rates for 1–2 h during exercise.
- Decreasing basal rates or long-acting insulin doses by approximately 20% after exercise may reduce delayed exercise-induced hypoglycemia.
- If patients are unable to lower their insulin levels through exercise, they should consider increasing their carbohydrate intake at a rate of approximately 0.5 g/kg/h of activity.
- If patients are able to lower their insulin levels, they should consider the timing of exercise relative to their last meal.
  - If activity occurs ≤3 h after a meal, they should consider bolus insulin reduction. In case of <60 min duration, the reduction will depend on the exercise intensity as follows: light, 25%; moderate, 50%; or heavy, 75%. In case of ≥60 min duration, they should consider a 50% reduction in light-intensity exercise and 75% reduction in moderate/heavy-intensity exercise.

  - If activity occurs >3 h after a meal, patients must consider basal insulin reduction. Patients with multiple-dose insulin should consider a 20% reduction in basal insulin on days with prolonged activity. Patients with continuous subcutaneous insulin infusion may reduce their basal insulin levels by 50–90% in the 60–90 min before the start of exercise until the exercise ends or even consider pump suspension at the start of exercise.
- Aerobic exercise may require an initial carbohydrate intake (15–20 g). The response to a downward trend in glucose during exercise should be the ingestion of 8–20 g of rapidly acting carbohydrate.
- Consider an overnight basal rate reduction of 10–40% on evenings after prolonged aerobic exercise or resistance training.

Blood glucose targets prior to exercise should be 90–250 mg/dL (5.0–13.9 mmol/L). Additional carbohydrate intake during and/or after exercise should be considered, depending on the duration and intensity of physical activity, to prevent hypoglycemia. Prior to exercise (1–3 h), a low-fat, 1- to 1.5-g/kg carbohydrate containing meal should be consumed to maximize glycogen stores and the availability of carbohydrate for exercise without prior insulin adjustment. If the patient has a blood glucose level of <5 mmol/L, engages in low- to moderate-intensity aerobic activities, and is fasting, 10–15 g of carbohydrate may prevent hypoglycemia. After exercise, carbohydrate intake must be sufficient to ensure replacement of both muscle and hepatic glycogen stores and prevent post-exercise hypoglycemia. Consuming as high as 1.5 g/kg of carbohydrate mixed with protein and low-fat snack after training ensures muscle recovery, requiring carefully adjusted insulin doses. Exercise lasting ≥60 min may require additional carbohydrate to maintain performance [50, 54].

Effect of Treatment on the Honeymoon Period of Type 1 Diabetes

A beneficial effect of intensive early insulin therapy on the protection of pancreatic beta cell function in newly diagnosed type 1 diabetes mellitus has been demonstrated [62, 63]. This protective effect results in better glycemic control and fewer complications [62, 64]. Early small doses of insulin have been observed to be effective to prevent beta cell failure in slowly progressive type 1 diabetes and have been recommended for patients with positive antibodies [65, 66]. During the honeymoon phase, the insulin requirement decreases, and basal insulin doses of 0.2–0.6 units/g/day during this phase may preserve beta cell function [41].

Immunomodulatory agents have been used to preserve beta cell function, with promising results reported for anti-CD3, Diapep277, oral insulin, and GAD65 treatments. The possibility of beta cell function (high residual C-peptide secretion) preservation in individuals within the first months of diagnosis has been shown in clinical trials with these immunomodulators [63, 64, 66, 67].

Glucagon

Intensive insulin treatment in type 1 diabetes reduces the incidence of complications but has an increased risk of hypoglycemia and weight gain. The main goal of type 1 diabetes treatment has been the simulation of physiological insulin secretion in healthy people. However, type 1 diabetes is a dual-hormone disease, for which the combination of insulin and glucagon might be more appropriate. Glucagon substitution in response to hypoglycemia as an alternative to carbohydrate consumption could potentially reduce the risk of weight gain. Closed-loop dual-hormone treatment could potentially benefit the treatment of type 1 diabetes. Until now, the use of glucagon has been limited by the need for reconstitution immediately before use. However, it can be expected that stable compounds available for dual-hormone treatment in the future will improve metabolic control for patients with type 1 diabetes [68, 69].

Islet Transplantations and Stem Cell Therapy

The only possible cure for patients with type 1 diabetes is the possibility of replacement pancreatic beta cells. Hence, transplantation strategies have gained much interest. Research into the replacement of beta cells has had significant advances in islet isolation, engraftment, and immunosuppressive strategies. However, the main remaining limitations are the insufficient supply of human tissue and the need for lifelong immunosuppression therapy [70, 71]. In an effort to find sources of insulin-producing beta cells, alternatives such as nonhuman donor cells (mainly porcine beta cells) or the possibility of deriving pluripotent stem cells from somatic cells have been encouraged. Cell reprogramming and differentiation to obtain patient-specific beta cells have allowed the possibility of cell therapy without immunosuppression [71].

Addition of Metformin for Children with Type 1 Diabetes Mellitus

Frequently, the metabolic control of patients with type 1 diabetes mellitus worsens during adolescence secondary to increases in weight and insulin resistance as a result of puberty hormones. Therefore, the use of metformin to improve insulin sensitivity in this group of patients has been considered. In a recent meta-analysis (6 clinical trials, $n = 325$), the addition of metformin in the treatment of pediatric patients with type 1 diabetes resulted in a modest decrease in total insulin daily dose (mean difference, −0.15 unit/kg/day; 95% CI, −0.24 to 0.06) and body mass index (mean difference, −1.46; 95% CI, −2.54 to 0.38). In addition, metformin was not superior to placebo in other metabolic control variables such as HbA1c level, lipid profile, and ketoacidosis events. The authors noted that the current evidence does not support the use of metformin in type 1 diabetes mellitus in pediatric patients to improve HbA1c. Future studies are needed to evaluate the long-term durability of the reductions in total insulin daily dose and body mass index achieved by adding metformin to insulin [72].

Management of Hypoglycemia in Children and Adolescents with Diabetes

Hypoglycemia is the most common acute complication of type 1 diabetes and is the major barrier to achieving optimal glycemic control [40, 73].

Hypoglycemia is defined as a decrease in the blood glucose level that exposes the patient to potential harm. Blood glucose levels <65 mg/dL have been often accepted as the cutoff level for defining hypoglycemia. However, a threshold of 70 mg/dL is used to start treatment because of the possibility of further decreases [40, 74].

Hypoglycemia is also classified as symptomatic or asymptomatic. The signs and symptoms in children are as follows [40, 75]:

- **Autonomic:** shakiness, sweatiness, trembling, palpitations, and pallor
- **Neuroglycopenic:** poor concentration, blurred or double vision, disturbed color vision, difficulty hearing, slurred speech, poor judgment and confusion, problems with short-term memory, dizziness and unsteady gait, loss of consciousness, seizure, and death
- **Behavioral:** irritability, erratic behavior, agitation, nightmares, and inconsolable crying
- **Nonspecific symptoms:** hunger, headache, nausea, and tiredness

Symptoms of hypoglycemia may occur at higher glucose levels in children compared with adults, and the thresholds may be altered by chronic hypoglycemia. Children have a higher risk of severe hypoglycemia than adults. In this age group, severe hypoglycemia is most often defined as an event associated with seizure or loss of consciousness [40].

Milder hypoglycemia should be treated with 10–15 g of oral glucose (approximately 0.3 g/kg) to increase blood glucose to approximately 54–70 mg/dL. This can be achieved by glucose tablets or sweetened fluids such as juice. After initial treatment, blood glucose should be retested in 10–15 min. In case of an inadequate response, treatment should be repeated, and the blood glucose level must be retested in another 10–15 min to confirm that a glucose level of 100 mg/dL has been reached. In some circumstances, this should be followed by additional complex carbohydrates (fruit, bread, cereal, or milk) to prevent the recurrence of hypoglycemia [40].

However, if the child is semiconscious/unconscious, sugar or any other powdery substance or thin liquids such as a glucose solution or honey should not be given forcibly to the child. The child should be put in a lateral position to prevent aspiration, and a thick paste of glucose (glucose powder with a few drops of water or table sugar crushed into powdered sugar with the consistency of thick cake icing) should be smeared inside the cheek; the efficacy of this practice is anecdotal [33].

Severe hypoglycemia requires urgent treatment. In a hospital setting, patients should be treated with intravenous glucose. The recommended dose is 10–30%, for a total of 200–500 mg/kg of glucose (10% glucose, 2–3 mL/kg). Rapid administration or excessive concentration (i.e., glucose 50%) may result in an excessive rate of osmotic change and risk of cerebral edema [40].

In settings outside the hospital, intramuscular or subcutaneous glucagon should be given (<12 years: 0.5 mg, >12 years: 1.0 mg or 10–30 μg/kg body weight). Caregivers should always have glucagon available and receive training in using it [40, 75].

Hypoglycemia should be prevented because it is associated with psychosocial dysfunction and, in rare cases, leads to permanent long-term sequelae and may be potentially life-threatening. Diabetes education is critical for preventing hypoglycemia. Patients, parents, and caregivers should be alert to situations in which increased glucose monitoring is required and when treatment regimens need to be changed. They should be alert to recognize the early signs of hypoglycemia, have a glucometer available for confirmation, and provide some source of glucose. Sleep is a time of particular risk for severe hypoglycemia, and asymptomatic hypoglycemia is common; for this reason, glucose levels are recommended to be monitored overnight, particularly in the presence of an additional risk factor that may predispose to nocturnal hypoglycemia. Currently available technologies such as continuous glucose monitoring and automated insulin suspensions have reduced the duration of hypoglycemia [75].

Children and adolescents with type 1 diabetes should wear some form of identification to alert others of their diabetes. If unexplained hypoglycemia occurs frequently, evaluation for unrecognized celiac and Addison's disease should be considered [40].

Sickness

Children and adolescents whose diabetes is under good metabolic control should not experience more illness or infections than children without diabetes. However, when any illness occurs, someone with diabetes potentially experiences hyperglycemia, hyperglycemia with ketosis, hyperglycemia with ketoacidosis, or hypoglycemia, and requires education and treatment to prevent exacerbation or even possible death [76, 77].

Many illnesses are associated with higher levels of stress hormones, which promote gluconeogenesis and insulin resistance. Severe illness increases ketone body production because of the inadequate provision of insulin under such circumstances and thus can contribute to acidosis, nausea, and vomiting, worsening dehydration and ultimately compromising the acid-base balance, resulting in metabolic decompensation, ketoacidosis, coma, and death. Illnesses associated with vomiting and diarrhea, such as gastroenteritis, often lower blood glucose levels rather than cause hyperglycemia while simultaneously producing a type of starvation ketosis, which exacerbates the situation [76].

Education about the effects of sick days is a critical component of diabetes management at home. The general sick-day diabetes management principles include the following [76, 77]:

- More frequent blood glucose and ketone (urine or blood) monitoring, at least every 3–4 h and sometimes every 1–2 h, including throughout the night.
- During sick days, do not stop insulin, even in the fasting state.
- During sick days, the insulin dose may need to be temporarily increased or decreased.
- When vomiting occurs, it should always be considered a sign of insulin deficiency until proven otherwise.
- Monitor and maintain salt and water balance.
- Treat the underlying precipitating illness.
- Sick-day guidelines, including insulin adjustment, should be taught soon after diagnosis and reviewed at least annually with patients and family members with a goal of minimizing and/or avoiding diabetic ketoacidosis and similarly minimizing and/or avoiding illness-associated hypoglycemia.

In case of loss of appetite, replacing meals with easily digestible food and sugar-containing fluids provides energy (carbohydrates) and may help prevent further ketosis. Necessary sick-day management supplies at home include glucose tablets, sweets, or candies, as well as dried fruit to prevent hypoglycemia; clean cool water to provide hydration and prepare salty soups; sugar- and electrolyte-containing fluids such as sports drinks or electrolyte mixtures to provide hydration, glucose, and salts; and easy-to-digest carbohydrates such as crackers or rice [76, 77].

Additional doses of short/rapid-acting insulin are required, with careful monitoring to reduce blood glucose levels, prevent ketoacidosis, and avoid hospital admission. The dose and frequency of injection will depend on the level and duration of hyperglycemia and the severity of ketosis (Table 64.3). Such supplemental doses are usually given subcutaneously but may also be given intramuscularly with health-care professional advice.

In the case of a patient who is a pump user, the previously mentioned key points of sick-day management are the same as those for a patient on insulin injections; however, specific management is recommended as follows [77]:

Hyperglycemia with negative ketones

- Give a correction bolus using a pump, and perform a blood glucose test hourly.
- Drink low-carbohydrate fluids or salty liquids.
- If the blood glucose level is decreased after 1 h, recheck again in 1–2 h to decide whether another bolus is needed.
- If the blood glucose level has not decreased, then give a bolus by syringe or pen.

Hyperglycemia with blood ketone levels >0.6 mmol/L or positive urine ketones

- Give a sick-day bolus by injection with pen or syringe using the guidelines in Table 64.3.
- Change the catheter, and check to be sure the pump is working.
- Reestablish insulin infusion with a new insulin infusion set and a cannula, with a temporary basal rate increase of 120–150%.
- Monitor blood glucose levels hourly, and recheck ketone levels at least every 4 h.
- Drink extra high-carbohydrate fluids if ketone levels are elevated and the blood glucose level is low or low-carbohydrate fluids if the blood glucose is elevated with or without elevated ketone levels.
- If the blood glucose level remains high; ketones persist; nausea, vomiting, or abdominal pain develops; or confusion or problems of staying awake and alert develop, proceed to the hospital for assessment.

If hypoglycemia (<65–70 mg/dL) and nausea or food refusal persists, a "mini glucagon treatment" (if available) may reverse the hypoglycemia and enable oral fluid intake. The recommended doses are as follows [77]:

Table 64.3 Fast-acting insulin dose calculation on sick days (adapted from Brink et al. [77])

Ketones		Blood glucose				
Blood (mmol/L)	Urine ketones	<100 mg/dL	100–180 mg/dL	180–250 mg/dL	250–400 mg/dL	400 mg/dL
<0.6	Negative or trace	Do not give extra insulin	No need to worry	Increase the insulin dose in the next meal if the blood glucose level is still elevated	Give extra 5% of the total daily dose or 0.05 U/kg	Give extra 10% of the total daily dose or 0.1 U/kg. Repeat if needed
0.6–0.9	Trace or small	Extra carbohydrates and fluids are needed	Extra carbohydrates and fluids are needed	Give extra 5% of the total daily dose or 0.05 U/kg	Give extra 5–10% of the total daily dose or 0.05–0.1 U/kg	Give extra 10% of the total daily dose or 0.1 U/kg. Repeat if needed
1.0–1.4	Small or moderate	Extra carbohydrates and fluids are needed	Extra carbohydrates and fluids are needed. Give an ordinary bolus dose	Extra carbohydrates and fluids are needed. Give 5–10% of the total daily dose or 0.05–0.1 U/kg	Give extra 5–10% of the total daily dose or 0.05–0.1 U/kg	Give extra 10% of the total daily dose or 0.1 U/kg. Repeat if needed
1.5–2.9	Moderate or high	Extra carbohydrates and fluids are needed	Extra carbohydrates and fluids are needed. Give 5% of the total daily dose or 0.05 U/kg. Repeat when the blood glucose level has increased	Extra carbohydrates and fluids are needed. Give 10% of the total daily dose or 0.1 U/kg	Give extra 10–20% of the total daily dose or 0.1 U/kg. Repeat the dose after 2 h if the ketone levels do not decrease	Consider evaluation at the emergency department
>3.0	High	Extra carbohydrates and fluids are needed. May need IV glucose if the child cannot eat or drink	Extra carbohydrates and fluids are needed. Give 5% of the total daily dose or 0.05 U/kg. Repeat when the blood glucose level has increased	Extra carbohydrates and fluids are needed. Give 10% of the total daily dose or 0.1 U/kg	Give extra 10–20% of the total daily dose or 0.1 U/kg. Repeat the dose after 2 h if the ketone levels do not decrease	Consider evaluation at the emergency department

- <2 years old = 0.02 mg = 2 units on insulin syringe
- 2–15 years old = 0.01 mg per year of age = 1 unit on insulin syringe per year of age
- >15 years old = 0.15 mg = 15 units on insulin syringe

Diabetes may also be an important risk factor for increased severity of illness and mortality in COVID-19 infections. An association between COVID-19 and new-onset type 1 diabetes and severe metabolic complications of preexisting diabetes, including DKA and hyperosmolarity, for which exceptionally high doses of insulin have been needed, has been reported. In the context of the COVID-19 pandemic, telephone consultations for sick-day management and routine diabetes care should be encouraged. This may help in the identification of children at risk of DKA, prevention of DKA, and avoiding urgent hospital visits. Families should be educated to not omit insulin, maintain hydration, treat the underlying symptoms of an intercurrent illness, and follow the general advice regarding healthy eating and continuing physical activity at home [78].

Surgery

When children with diabetes require surgery or other procedures requiring sedation or anesthesia, optimal management should maintain adequate hydration and near-normal glycemia while minimizing the risk of hypoglycemia [76]. The safe management of patients with type 1 diabetes in the perioperative period requires a consideration of each child's specific treatment, glycemic control, intended surgery, and anticipated postoperative course [79].

The presurgical assessment should be performed several days before surgery to allow an assessment of glycemic control, electrolyte status, and ketone levels. If glycemic control is known to be poor and surgery is not urgent, the procedure should be delayed until glycemic control has improved. If surgery cannot be delayed, admission to the hospital before surgery should be considered for stabilization of glycemic control [79].

Intravenous access, infusion of glucose, and frequent blood glucose monitoring are essential whenever general anesthesia is given. Glucose 5% is usually sufficient, but glucose 10% may be necessary when the risk of hypoglycemia is high. To minimize the risk of hypoglycemia, children should receive a glucose infusion when fasting for >2 h before general anesthesia [76, 79, 80].

The glucose target during surgical procedures is 90–180 mg/dL [79]. The appropriate glycemic targets during the perioperative period remain controversial and are less clear than that for surgery or postoperative control. However, studies in adults have not demonstrated any adverse effects of maintaining perioperative glycemic levels between 90 and 200 mg/dL [76, 80].

The stress from surgery leads to a complex neuroendocrine stress response characterized by hyperglycemia and a catabolic state [80]. In addition, hyperglycemia has been associated with an increased risk of postoperative infection, so it must be avoided. To achieve optimal glycemic control, the insulin dosage may need to be increased on the day of a major surgery and for approximately 2 days after surgery. This is best achieved by continuous IV insulin infusion even after the resumption of oral feeding [76, 80].

Before emergency surgery, the blood glucose, blood ß-hydroxybutyrate (if available), or urinary ketone concentration, serum electrolyte levels, and blood gases should always be checked if ketone or blood glucose levels are high. If ketoacidosis is present, the established treatment protocol for diabetic ketoacidosis should be followed and surgery should be delayed, if possible, until circulating volume and electrolyte deficits are corrected. If no ketoacidosis is observed, IV fluids and insulin management are started for elective surgery [79, 80].

Pediatric patients with type 1 diabetes need insulin, even while fasting, to avoid ketoacidosis and require careful blood glucose monitoring (hourly) before the procedure to detect hypoglycemia and hyperglycemia. At least 2 h before surgery, an IV insulin infusion (dilute 50 units regular [soluble] insulin in 50 mL of normal saline; 1 unit = 1 mL) and administration of glucose 5% (10% if increased risk of hypoglycemia is a concern) are started. If the blood glucose level is high (>250 mg/dL), 0.45 or 0.9% NaCl without glucose is used and the insulin supply is increased, but 5% dextrose should be added if the blood glucose level decreases to <250 mg/dL. Infusion is started at the following blood glucose levels: 0.025 mL/kg/h for <100–140 mg/dL, 0.05 mL/kg/h for 141–215 mg/dL, 0.075 mL/kg/h for 220–270 mg/dL, and 0.1 U/kg/h for >270 mg/dL [76, 79].

Blood glucose level should be monitored every 30–60 min during the operation and until the child recovers from anesthesia. The dextrose infusion and insulin must be adjusted to maintain the blood glucose levels within 90–180 mg/dL. Insulin infusion is continued if the blood glucose level is <90 mg/dL, as this will cause rebound hyperglycemia; instead, the rate of infusion is reduced. The IV insulin infusion may be stopped temporarily if the blood glucose level is <55 mg/dL, but only for 10–15 min [33, 76, 80].

Patients may initially receive an intravenous (IV) infusion without dextrose for minor surgeries or procedures lasting for <2 h if treated with basal/bolus insulin regimen or continuous subcutaneous insulin infusion. They should initially receive an IV infusion with dextrose for major surgeries or procedures (lasting for at least 2 h) or if treated with NPH insulin [80].

Once the child is able to resume oral nutrition, the child's usual diabetes treatment regimen should be continued. Short- or rapid-acting insulin (based on the child's usual insulin:

carbohydrate ratio and correction factor) should be administered, if needed, to reduce hyperglycemia or to match the food intake [79, 80].

Diabetic Ketoacidosis and Hyperglycemic Hyperosmolar State

Diabetic ketoacidosis results from a deficiency of circulating insulin and increased levels of counter-regulatory hormones. Several risk factors lead to diabetic ketoacidosis in newly diagnosed cases, such as younger patients (<2 years), delayed diagnosis, lower socioeconomic status, and countries with low prevalence rates of type 1 diabetes. In the case of patients with a known diagnosis, the risk factors include insulin omission, poor metabolic control, previous episodes of diabetic ketoacidosis, gastroenteritis with persistent vomiting, inability to maintain hydration, psychiatric and eating disorders, challenging social and family circumstances, peripubertal and adolescent girls, limited access to medical services, and failures of insulin pump therapy [81].

The combination of absolute or relative insulin deficiency and high counter-regulatory hormone concentrations results in an accelerated catabolic state with increased glucose production, resulting in hyperglycemia and hyperosmolality; it also increases lipolysis and ketogenesis and causes ketonemia and metabolic acidosis. If this cycle is not interrupted by exogenous insulin and fluid and electrolyte therapies, fatal dehydration and metabolic acidosis will ensue [81].

The clinical signs of diabetic ketoacidosis include the following: dehydration, tachycardia, tachypnea, deep respiration (Kussmaul respiration), ketone smell on the breath (odor of nail polish remover or rotten fruit), nausea, vomiting, abdominal pain (which may mimic an acute abdominal condition), confusion, drowsiness, progressive reduction in the level of consciousness, and eventually, loss of consciousness [81].

The biochemical criteria for the diagnosis of diabetic ketoacidosis are as follows [81]:

- Hyperglycemia (blood glucose level >200 mg/dL)
- Venous pH < 7.3 or bicarbonate level <15 mmol/L
- Ketonemia and ketonuria

The criteria for hyperglycemic hyperosmolar state (HHS) include the following [81]:

- Plasma glucose concentration >600 mg/dL
- Venous pH > 7.25; arterial pH > 7.30
- Serum bicarbonate level >15 mmol/L
- Low ketonuria and absent-to-mild ketonemia
- Effective serum osmolality >320 mOsm/kg
- Altered consciousness (e.g., obtundation and combativeness) or seizures

Emergency assessment should follow the general guidelines for Pediatric Advanced Life Support and include the following: immediate measurement of blood glucose level, blood or urine ketone levels, serum electrolyte levels, blood gases, and full blood count, and assessment of the severity of dehydration and level of consciousness [81].

The goals of therapy are to correct dehydration, correct acidosis, and reverse ketosis; slowly correct hyperosmolality and restore blood glucose to near-normal; monitor for complications of diabetic ketoacidosis and its treatment; and identify and treat any precipitating event. Management should be conducted in centers that are experienced in the treatment of diabetic ketoacidosis in children and adolescents and where vital signs, neurological status, and laboratory results can be monitored frequently [81].

Fluid replacement should begin before starting insulin therapy. Expand the volume, as required, to restore peripheral circulation. For patients who are severely volume depleted but not in shock, volume expansion should begin with 0.9% saline with 10- to 20-mL/kg doses over 1–2 h and may need to be repeated until tissue perfusion is adequate. In patients with diabetic ketoacidosis in shock, circulatory volume with isotonic saline in 20-mL/kg boluses should be infused as quickly as possible [82].

The subsequent rate of fluid administration, including the provision of maintenance fluid requirements, to replace the estimated fluid deficit evenly over 48 h should be calculated. Subsequent fluid management should include an isotonic solution for at least 4–6 h. Deficit replacement after 4–6 h should be with a solution with a tonicity of ≥0.45% saline with added potassium [82].

Insulin therapy should begin with 0.05–0.1 U/kg/h at least 1 h after starting fluid replacement therapy. In HHS, insulin administration should begin at a dose of 0.025–0.05 U/kg/h once plasma glucose is no longer declining at a rate of at least 3 mmol/L (50 mg/dL) per hour with fluid alone [81, 82].

During volume expansion and after commencing insulin therapy, the plasma glucose concentration typically decreases. To prevent a rapid decrease and hypoglycemia, 5% glucose should be added to the IV fluid when the plasma glucose level decreases to approximately 250–300 mg/dL or sooner if the rate of decrease is precipitous. Dextrose at 10% or even 12.5% may be needed to prevent hypoglycemia while continuing the insulin infusion to correct metabolic acidosis [81].

If the patient is hyperkalemic, potassium replacement therapy is deferred until the urine output is documented. Otherwise, 40-mmol potassium/L is started in the infusion or 20-mmol potassium/L in a patient receiving fluid at a rate of >10 mL/kg/h [81].

Bicarbonate administration is not recommended, except for the treatment of life-threatening hyperkalemia. The warning signs and symptoms of cerebral edema, including headache and slowing of heart rate, a change in neurological status (restlessness, irritability, increased drowsiness, or incontinence), specific neurological signs, increasing blood pressure, and decreased oxygen saturation, should be monitored. In patients with multiple risk factors of cerebral edema, mannitol or hypertonic saline should be available at bedside, and the dose to be given should be calculated beforehand. If the patient's neurological status deteriorates acutely, hyperosmolar therapy should be given immediately [81].

Management of an episode of DKA is not complete until an attempt has been made to identify and treat the cause so that it could be prevented. Recurrent DKA without a preceding febrile or vomiting illness is almost always the result of psychosocial problems and failure to take insulin [81].

In cases with uncomplicated mild to moderate ketoacidosis, subcutaneous rapid-acting insulin analogs are effective and can be used if IV insulin is not feasible. Subcutaneous regular insulin is also an alternative if rapid-acting insulin analogs and IV regular insulin infusion are not available. The suggested starting dose is 0.15 U/kg every 2–4 h. Subcutaneous insulin therapy may not be appropriate in youths with severe dehydration or young children (aged <2 years) [78].

Autoimmune Conditions

Patients with type 1 diabetes have an increased frequency of other autoimmune diseases. Autoimmune thyroid disease is the most common (17–30%). At the time of diagnosis, approximately 25% of patients have thyroid autoantibodies, and their presence is predictive of thyroid dysfunction (most commonly hypothyroidism). Thyroid dysfunction can alter glycemic control and linear growth rate. Therefore, thyroid function tests should be performed soon after a period of metabolic stability. Testing for anti-thyroid peroxidase and anti-thyroglobulin antibodies and measurement of thyroid-stimulating hormone concentrations soon after diagnosis are recommended. If the values are normal, rechecking should be performed every 1–2 years or sooner if the patient presents symptoms of thyroid dysfunction, goiter, abnormal growth rate, or unexplained glycemic variation [2, 83]. Hyperthyroidism is less common than hypothyroidism in association with type 1 diabetes but is still more common than in the general population. Hyperthyroidism may be due to Graves' disease or the hyperthyroid phase of Hashimoto's thyroiditis [83].

Celiac disease occurs in 1.6–16.4% of patients with type 1 diabetes. Screening by measuring serum levels of IgA and anti-tissue transglutaminase antibodies is recommended and should be performed at the time of diabetes diagnosis and at 2 and 5 years thereafter, as it is frequently asymptomatic [83]. In cases of IgA deficiency, IgG tissue transglutaminase antibodies or IgG deamidated gliadin peptide antibodies should be measured. Repeat screening within 2 years of diabetes diagnosis and then again after 5 years is recommended. More frequent screening is recommended for patients with first-degree relatives with celiac disease, growth failure, weight loss, failure to gain weight, gastrointestinal symptoms (diarrhea, flatulence, abdominal pain, or signs of malabsorption), unexplained hypoglycemia, or uncontrolled glycemia. The diagnosis could be confirmed with a small bowel biopsy, and patients should be placed on a gluten-free diet to reduce symptoms and frequency rates of hypoglycemia [2].

Addison's disease is suspected on the basis of the clinical picture of frequent hypoglycemia, unexplained decrease in insulin requirements, increased skin pigmentation, lassitude, weight loss, hyponatremia, and hyperkalemia. The diagnosis is confirmed by the demonstration of low morning cortisol levels in the presence of elevated basal ACTH levels, with an inadequate response to an ACTH stimulation test and positive anti-adrenal (21-hydroxylase) antibodies. Treatment with a glucocorticoid is urgent and lifelong. In some cases, the therapy must be supplemented with a mineralocorticoid such as fludrocortisone [83].

Another rare disorder is autoimmune gastritis, which includes chronic inflammation with destruction of parietal cells of the corpus and fundus of the stomach as a consequence of parietal cell antibodies as the principal immunological marker. Chronic damage to the proton pump may result in hypochlorhydria/achlorhydria, hypergastrinemia, and iron deficiency anemia due to decreased gastric secretion and decreased iron absorption. Parietal cell antibodies may also inhibit intrinsic factor secretion, which leads to vitamin B12 deficiency and pernicious anemia. The prevalence rates of parietal cell antibodies in children with type 1 diabetes range from 5.3 to 7.5%. Physicians should be aware of the possibility of parietal cell antibodies in cases of unclear anemia (microcytic and macrocytic) or gastrointestinal symptoms [83].

Psychosocial Issues

Type 1 diabetes places a substantial behavioral and psychological burden on young people and their families. Approximately one-third of adolescents with type 1 diabetes need mental health support, and their parents are also at increased risk of psychological distress [84]. Youth with diabetes should be assessed for psychosocial and diabetes-related distress, generally starting at 7–8 years. The offering to Adolescents should be offered the opportunity to interact with their care providers strting at the age of 12, or when developmentally appropriate [2]. Diabetes management in pediatric patients confers challenges that require family teamwork to maintain adherence and glycemic control. During follow-up, health-care providers should be alert to psychosocial issues and stresses that could affect adherence to treatment. Diabetes can impact mental health problems such as distress, fear of hypoglycemia and hyperglycemia, anxiety, disordered eating behaviors, or depression [2, 34]. In case of hospitalization, children with type 1 diabetes have higher odds (3.5) of being discharged from the hospital with a comorbid mood or anxiety disorder than other children [85]. These psychosocial factors are related to nonadherence, poor glycemic control and quality of life, and diabetes complications. Thus, screening for psychosocial distress and mental health problems is important, and referrals to trained mental health professionals as integral members of the pediatric diabetes multidisciplinary team should be provided to ensure optimal clinical care and long-term outcomes for these children [2, 34].

Young people with diabetes, especially those with a background of early diabetes onset, severe hypoglycemia, or chronic hyperglycemia, are at increased risk of mild decrements in general cognitive ability, information processing skills, executive functions, and academic achievement. Therefore, assessment of developmental progress in all domains of functioning (physical, intellectual, academic, emotional, and social development) should be conducted on a routine basis. Children with learning difficulties should be referred for a psycho-educational or neuropsychological evaluation to determine if learning disabilities are present [86].

Routine assessment should be performed with developmental adjustment to and understanding of diabetes management, including diabetes-related knowledge, insulin adjustment skills, goal setting, problem-solving abilities, regimen adherence, and self-management autonomy and competence. This is especially important during late childhood and prior to adolescence, when in many families, the child may take on diabetes management responsibilities without adequate maturity for effective self-management. The interdisciplinary team should provide interventions to emphasize appropriate family involvement and support in diabetes management, effective problem-solving and self-management skills, and realistic expectations about glycemic control [86].

Vaccination

Patients with diabetes mellitus are more susceptible to infections, for which immune system deficiency could be a reason. Routine vaccinations are recommended for children with diabetes, as for the general population, according to age [87]. However, the antibody responses to pertussis, diphtheria, tetanus, mumps, and hepatitis B vaccines are similar between patients with and without diabetes, although the response to measles and rubella vaccinations could be lower [88].

Pregnancy Prevention

Pre-pregnancy counseling is an important tool in chronic endocrine conditions to reduce the risk to mother and fetus. Starting at puberty, preconception counseling should be incorporated for all girls [2]. The management of pregnancies complicated by diabetes mellitus requires coordination among the team of obstetricians, endocrinologists, dietitians, and psychologists. The prevention of unintended pregnancies among teens with diabetes mellitus is critically important because these patients are as likely as healthy teens, in whom 83% pregnancies are unintended, to be sexually involved. Implants and intrauterine devices represent the most effective, safest, and most successful contraceptive options for adolescents [89].

Management of Cardiovascular Risk Factors

Pediatric patients with type 1 diabetes are at higher risk of early adult-onset cardiovascular disease. Adolescents with type 1 diabetes exhibit early changes in blood pressure, peripheral vascular function, and left ventricular myocardial deformation indexes, and detection could benefit from early therapeutic interventions [90].

Hypertension

Blood pressure should be measured at each consultation using an appropriate-size cuff, with the patient seated and relaxed. The result should be compared with normal levels for age, sex, and height. Children with high normal blood pressures ($\geq$90th percentile, or in adolescents aged $\geq$13 years, systolic blood pressure 120–129 mmHg with diastolic blood pressure <80 mmHg) or hypertension ($\geq$95th percentile or in adolescents $\geq$13 years systolic blood pressure >130 mmHg with diastolic blood pressure $\geq$80 mmHg) should have blood pressure confirmed on three separate days. Initial treatment includes dietary modification, increased exercise, and weight control. If high normal blood pressure persists for 3–6 months or in cases of hypertension, pharmacological treatment with angiotensin-converting enzyme inhibitors (ACE inhibitors) or angiotensin receptor blockers should be considered if ACE inhibitor is not tolerated. The goal of treatment is to maintain blood pressures consistently at <90th percentile or <120/80 mmHg in children $\geq$13 years of age [2, 33].

Dyslipidemia

The atherosclerotic process begins in childhood, and youths with type 1 diabetes may have subclinical cardiovascular disease abnormalities within the first decade of diagnosis. Screening for dyslipidemia should be performed soon after diagnosis and when initial glycemic control has been achieved in all children with type 1 diabetes from age 11 years. If normal results are obtained, this should be repeated every 5 years. If there is a family history of hypercholesterolemia or early cardiovascular disease, or if the family history is unknown, screening should commence as early as the age of 2 years. If LDL cholesterol is <100 mg/dL, a lipid profile testing is suggested every 3 years [2, 91].

The first step of therapy is optimizing glucose control and medical nutrition therapy. For patients aged >10 years, the addition of statin is suggested if despite medical nutrition therapy and lifestyle changes, the patient continues to have LDL cholesterol levels >160 mg/dL or LDL cholesterol levels >130 mg/dL and one or more cardiovascular disease risk factors. (The American Heart Association categorizes children with type 1 diabetes in the highest tier for cardiovascular risk.) The goal of therapy is to achieve a LDL cholesterol value of <100 mg/dL [2].

Nephropathy

Diabetic nephropathy (e.g., albuminuria) most commonly occurs after the onset of puberty and after 5–10 years of diabetes duration. Good glycemic and blood pressure control, mainly as the diabetes duration increases, is important to reduce the risk of nephropathy. Routine screening is important to ensure timely detection and treatment. Annual screening for albuminuria with a random (morning sample to avoid the effects of exercise) spot urine sample for albumin-to-creatinine ratio should be considered at puberty or at >10 years, once the child has had diabetes for 5 years [2]. Estimation of the glomerular filtration rate using equations for serum creatinine level, height, age, and sex at baseline is also recommended and should be repeated on the basis of clinical status. Treatment with an ACE inhibitor or an angiotensin receptor blocker titrated to normalization of albumin excretion should be considered when an elevated urinary albumin-to-creatinine ratio (>30 mg/g) is documented with at least two of three urine samples over a 6-month interval after efforts to improve glycemic control and normalize blood pressure [2].

Retinopathy

Diabetic retinopathy most commonly occurs after the onset of puberty and after 5–10 years of diabetes duration; however, it has been reported in pre-pubertal children and after a diabetes duration of only 1–2 years [2]. Early subclinical retinopathy may exist and can be detected through corneal confocal microscopy by the identification of corneal cellular pathology (lower epithelial and endothelial densities and higher keratocyte density) and small nerve fiber pathology in young patients with type 1 diabetes [92].

An initial dilated and comprehensive eye examination must be performed once youths with type 1 diabetes are aged ≥11 years or after puberty has started, whichever is earlier, in patients with a diabetes duration of 3–5 years. After the initial examination, patients must undergo repeat dilated and comprehensive eye examinations every 2 years or less frequently (every 4 years) on the advice of an eye care professional based on risk factor assessment, including a history of glycemic control with HbA1c levels <8%. Eye examinations could be more frequent if high-risk factors of vision loss are present [2, 33, 91].

Neuropathy

Diabetic neuropathy rarely occurs in pre-pubertal children or after 1–2 years of diabetes. Screening for peripheral neuropathy should start from the age of 11 years with 2–5 years of diabetes duration and annually thereafter [91]. A foot inspection at each medical visit is important to educate youths regarding the importance of foot care [33] (Codner limited care). A comprehensive foot examination should include an assessment of symptoms of neuropathic pain, inspection, palpation of pulses, assessment of reflexes, and determination of proprioception, vibration, and monofilament sensation [2].

Smoking

Smoking is a well-recognized cardiovascular disease risk. In youths with diabetes, additional cardiovascular disease risk factors must be avoided. Smoking increases microvascular and macrovascular complications. For these reasons, smoking avoidance (including cigarettes, other tobacco products, e-cigarettes, and secondhand smoke) is important to prevent microvascular and macrovascular complications and should be part of routine diabetes care [2, 34].

Quality of Life

Although the health-related quality of life of children/adolescents with type 1 diabetes may not be adversely affected compared with that of siblings without diabetes [93], burdens are imposed on children and their parents by a diagnosis of type 1 diabetes mellitus, which affects their health-related quality of life [94]. In general, type 1 diabetes is associated with lower health-related quality of life, higher unemployment rates, and additional sick leaves in adults [95]. Health-related quality of life is a critical diabetes outcome, but discrepancies exist between youth and parent-proxy reports in the Pediatric Quality of Life Inventory. Parents often underestimate their child's health-related quality of life, except in the youngest children. Although examining both reports is optimal, the youth report should be prioritized, particularly for young children and adolescents [96]. Although no correlation may exist between metabolic control and health-related quality of life in children, lower numbers of hypoglycemic and hyperglycemic episodes were associated with an increase in psychosocial and physical health scores [94].

Type 2 Diabetes

Over the last three decades, the incidence and prevalence of T2D have markedly increased in the pediatric population. Before the 1990s, T2D was rare in children and adolescents in the United States. However, by 1994, T2D had represented up to 16% of new cases of diabetes in children in urban areas; after 1999, the range of new cases of T2D was 8–45%, mainly among minority populations [97]. In the United States, the estimated T2D prevalence per 1000 youths aged 10–19 years increased significantly from 0.34 in 2001 to 0.46 in 2009 to 0.67 in 2017, an absolute increase of 0.32 per 1000 youths and a 95.3% relative increase over 16 years. The greatest absolute increases were observed among non-Hispanic Black and Hispanic youths. The projections of the Centers for Disease Control and Prevention assume a 2.3% annual increase in the prevalence of T2D in people aged <20 years, which will quadruple in 40 years [4].

The diagnosis of childhood T2D is based on the presence of diabetes mellitus in a child who typically shows the following characteristics:

- Overweight or obese (body mass index ≥85th to 94th percentile and >95th percentile for age and sex, respectively)
- A strong family history of T2D
- Residual insulin secretory capacity at diagnosis (reflected by normal or elevated insulin and C-peptide concentrations)
- Insidious onset of disease
- Demonstrated insulin resistance, including polycystic ovarian syndrome or acanthosis nigricans
- Lacking evidence of diabetic autoimmunity
- Higher likelihood of having hypertension and dyslipidemia

Although diabetic ketoacidosis is more frequent in type 1 diabetes, patients with T2D may occasionally have this presentation [31].

Testing to detect prediabetes or T2D should be considered in the following cases [2, 4]:

- Children and adolescents aged 10 years or at onset of puberty (if it occurs at a younger age)

- Children and adolescents who are overweight or obese (body mass index ≥85th percentile for age and sex, weight for height >85th percentile, or weight >120% of the ideal for height)
- Children and adolescents with one or more of the following additional risk factors for diabetes:

  - Family history of T2D in first- or second-degree relatives
  - Native American, African–American, Latino, Asian American, or Pacific Islander
  - Signs of insulin resistance or conditions associated with insulin resistance (acanthosis nigricans, hypertension, dyslipidemia, polycystic ovary syndrome, or small-for-gestational-age birth weight)
  - Maternal history of diabetes or gestational diabetes mellitus during gestation

If the test results are normal, repeat testing at a minimum of 3-year intervals or more frequently if BMI is increasing. Fasting plasma glucose level, 2-h plasma glucose level during oral glucose tolerance test, and HbA1c level can be used to test for prediabetes or diabetes in children and adolescents. Pediatric patients with overweight or obesity in whom T2D is considered should have a panel of pancreatic autoantibodies to exclude the possibility of type 1 diabetes [2, 98].

Pathophysiology of T2D Mellitus

Insulin resistance in muscle, fat, and liver, with progressive beta cell failure, and ongoing loss of insulin secretion in response to glucose characterize T2D mellitus. The following risk factors associated with this disorder can affect individuals beginning in childhood:

- **Obesity and insulin resistance.** Insulin resistance produces hyperinsulinism, and unsuccessful compensation from increased insulin secretion results in glucose intolerance and T2DM [99].
- **Intrauterine environment.** Poor intrauterine growth is associated with the subsequent development of metabolic syndrome and T2D. The effects of poor nutrition in early life produce changes in glucose-insulin metabolism, such as reduced capacity for insulin secretion and insulin resistance [100].
- **Exposition to gestational diabetes.** Maternal gestational diabetes is independently associated with a subsequent risk of T2D in offspring in the first 30 years of life; the risk is approximately threefold higher than among offspring of mothers without diabetes [101].
- **Ethnicity.** Ethnic differences in diabetes prevalence persist, even after adjustment for lifestyle and other risk fac-

tors. Diabetes mellitus is more likely (relative to Caucasians) among Asians, Native Americans, and Hispanics [102].

- **Sex and puberty.** Puberty represents a state of insulin resistance. This developmental stage is accompanied by a 30% decrease in insulin sensitivity and a compensatory increase in insulin secretion. The mean age at diagnosis of T2D in children is between 12 and 16 years, corresponding to the peak of adolescent growth. Girls are 1.5- to 3-fold more likely than boys to develop T2D as children or adolescents [103].
- **Family history.** Between 74 and 100% of children with T2D have a first- or second-degree relative with T2D. The lifetime risk is 40% if one parent is affected and 70% if both parents are affected [104].
- **Genetics.** The identification of the genetic factors involved in pediatric T2D has been a great challenge. In adults, several association studies have been conducted in which numerous SNPs have been shown to contribute to the risk of the disease; however, these SNPs currently account for only approximately 20% of heritability. By contrast, only few studies have involved pediatric patients, in whom the early onset of the disease may be due in part to greater genetic susceptibility, which makes them less tolerant of environmental aggressors. In this sense, a strong familial history of the disease suggests the involvement of genetic factors. We reported that the heritability of pediatric-onset T2D in Mexican youths was as high as 0.50 [105]. Likewise, the most important diabetes susceptibility variants reported to date are SNPs in the *TCF7L2* gene, which have strong associations with T2D in multiple ethnic populations [106]. Dabalea et al. identified *TCF7L2* variants associated with an increased risk of T2D among African–American youths [107]. In addition, we recently reported an association between SNPs in *SLC16A11* (rs13342232) and pediatric-onset T2D in the Mexican population. Our research group reported that SNPs previously associated with obesity, such as *ADORA/rs903361*, *CADM2/rs13078807*, *GNPDA2/rs10938397*, *VEGFA/rs6905288*, and *FTO/rs9939609*, were associated with an increased risk of pediatric-onset T2D in the Mexican population [108].

- The combination of multiple SNPs improves the prediction of the risk of T2D in youths with a modest significance. On the contrary, clinical factors such as body mass index and family history of T2D continue to have the highest predictive value in some populations [109].

Treatment

The treatment goals for T2D are the same as those for type 1 diabetes. In addition to blood glucose control, treatment must include attention to metabolic disorders such as obesity, hypertension, and dyslipidemia [2]. Lifestyle changes should be initiated at the time of diagnosis of T2D [110]. Education should focus on behavioral changes (diet and activity) and education on the administration of oral hypoglycemic agents and insulin as needed. The education and treatment team for a patient with T2D should ideally include a nutritionist, psychologist and/or social worker, and an exercise physiologist [3, 110].

The entire family will need education to understand the principles of the treatment of T2D and the critical importance of lifestyle changes for the entire family to successfully manage a youth with T2D [110].

Nutritional and Exercise Management

The aims of nutritional management must be focused on a multidisciplinary, family-centered, culturally appropriate approach that promotes the achievement of normal glycemia and HbA1c levels, preventing further weight gain in patients with a body mass index in the 85th–95th percentile or achieving weight loss for those with a body mass index >95th percentile while maintaining a normal linear growth. Physicians and dietitians should focus on nutritional counseling for children with T2D at the time of diagnosis and as a part of ongoing management [49, 51].

The entire family should be included in the education because caregivers influence the child's food intake and physical activity. The dietary recommendations should target dietary modifications and should be culturally appropriate, sensitive to family resources, and provided to all caregivers [49, 51, 110].

Healthy eating patterns should be encouraged, with an emphasis on consuming nutrient-dense, high-quality foods and reducing calorie-dense, nutrient-poor foods [111]. The dietary modifications should include the following:

- Eliminating sugar-containing soft drinks and juices and substitution of water, diet soft drinks, and other calorie-free beverages, which can result in substantial weight loss [110, 112]. FDA-approved non-nutritive sweeteners can be used, as they may help consumers limit their carbohydrate and energy intake as a tactic to manage blood glucose and/or weight [113].
- Increasing fruit and vegetable intake, which is known to confer several health benefits [110, 114].
- Reducing the use of processed, prepackaged, and convenience foods and the intake of foods made from refined, simple sugars, such as processed candy and high-fructose corn syrup [110].
- Control portions. Food and snacks should be served in a plate or bowl and not eaten directly from a box or can [110].

- Reducing the number of meals eaten away from home [110].
- Changing staple foods from enriched white rice and white flour to brown rice and whole-grain items with lower glycemic index values to promote gradual and sustainable energy elevations with meals [110].
- Changing family diet behaviors: limiting the availability of high-fat, high-caloric-density foods and drinks in the home; teaching families to interpret nutrition fact labels; emphasizing healthy parenting practices related to diet and activity; encouraging positive reinforcement of all goals achieved and avoiding blame for failure; and promoting that meals should be eaten on schedule, in one place, preferably as a family unit, and with no other activities (e.g., television, computer, or studying) [110].

In addition to following the above-mentioned recommendations, an individualized meal plan incorporating low-fat energy choices and carbohydrate management and the substitution of high- for low-glycemic-index foods may help control appetite, weight loss, blood glucose targets, and lipid levels [51].

Increasing daily physical activity to 60 min of moderate-to-vigorous exercise is an important component of treatment and a key strategy to increase energy expenditure; exercise can be completed in multiple shorter sessions. Promoting physical activity as a family event, including daily efforts to be more physically active, such as using stairs instead of elevators, walking or bicycling to school and shopping, and doing house and yard work, can help promote adherence to the plan. Limiting sedentary behaviors such as television viewing and computer use to <1 h a day has been shown to be an effective way of increasing daily physical activity and help maintain or achieve a healthy weight in children [51, 110].

Youth with overweight/obesity and T2D and their families should be provided with developmentally and culturally appropriate comprehensive lifestyle programs that are integrated with diabetes management to achieve a 7–10% decrease in excess weight [98].

Smoking and Tobacco Use

Cigarette smoking is damaging to all youths, but patients with diabetes are especially vulnerable to the negative health costs of smoking as a result of their compromised health status and disease and treatment-related complications [110, 114].

Additional research is needed to develop and study the efficacy of interventions specifically targeting smoking among youths with T2D within health-care settings. Patients should be asked at each visit if they smoke and counseled against beginning smoking. Youths who do smoke should be counseled on the importance of smoking cessation and provided resources for support [110].

Glycemic Monitoring

Limited evidence shows that self-monitored blood glucose has an impact on glycemic control in individuals with T2D. Blood glucose self-monitoring should be performed regularly, and the frequency should be individualized and include a combination of fasting and postprandial glucose measurements with a regularity based on the degree of glycemic control and available resources. Once glycemic goals have been achieved, limited at-home testing is needed; at most, several fasting and postprandial values per week are satisfactory. If values consistently exceed the target range, more frequent testing should be recommended because a change in therapy might be needed. During acute illness or when symptoms of hyperglycemia or hypoglycemia occur, patients should undergo more frequent testing and be in contact with their diabetes care team for advice [110].

Glycemic Targets

Glycemic status should be assessed every 3 months. A reasonable HbA1c target for most children and adolescents with T2D is <7% (53 mmol/mL). More stringent targets (e.g., <6.5% [48 mmol/mol]) may be appropriate for selected individual patients if they can be achieved without significant hypoglycemia or other adverse effects of treatment. Appropriate patients might include those with a short diabetes duration and less severe β-cell dysfunction and those treated with lifestyle or metformin alone and achieve significant weight improvement [2]. Self-monitoring of blood glucose needs to be individualized depending on the intervention for T2D [98, 115].

Pharmacological Treatment

The treatment of diabetes in children and adolescents cannot simply be derived from the pharmacological management that is routinely provided to adults with diabetes. The epidemiology, pathophysiology, developmental considerations, and response to therapy in pediatric-onset diabetes are different from those of adult diabetes [2]. A more aggressive phenotype of T2D exists in the pediatric population, which predisposes patients to an earlier dependence on insulin treatment and a presentation of chronic complications in an earlier term [98].

The aims of therapy for pediatric-onset T2D are to improve glycemia, prevent acute and chronic complications, prevent metabolic decompensation, improve insulin sensitivity and endogenous insulin secretion, and if possible, restore glucagon and incretin physiology [98].

Great uncertainty remains about the use of many novel drug treatments in the pediatric population, in whom the absence of information about safety limits their use [116]. The glycemic goals can usually be accomplished with metformin and basal insulin, alone, or in combination. The initial treatment is determined by symptoms, severity of hyperglycemia, and presence or absence of ketosis/ketoacidosis [76, 110].

Metformin

Metformin is a biguanide that increases insulin-mediated glucose uptake in the peripheral tissues and decreases hepatic glucose production, thereby promoting a decrease in plasma glucose levels [117, 118]. Currently, metformin is the only oral hypoglycemic agent approved for use in children with T2D [119].

Metformin monotherapy treatment should begin at 500 mg daily. The dose should be titrated by 500 mg once per week over 3–4 weeks to the maximal dose of 1000 mg twice daily. Blood glucose self-monitoring should be performed regularly and should be individualized on the basis of the degree of glycemic control and available resources [98, 110].

Metformin is associated with several gastrointestinal side effects, mainly nausea, abdominal pain, and headache; therefore, some patients may require slower dose escalation or may not be able to tolerate the maximum dose. Extended-release metformin preparations may have less frequent gastrointestinal side effects and are now currently available in tablet and suspension forms. Contraindications for metformin include renal and hepatic insufficiency, cirrhosis, hepatitis, and cardiopulmonary insufficiency, as metformin can lead to lactic acidosis in this setting. In addition, the absorption of vitamin B12 and folic acid can be impaired in patients taking metformin, and vitamin B12 deficiency may frequently occur in patients with anemia and peripheral neuropathy. Therefore, children and adolescents taking metformin should be advised to take multivitamins daily [115, 120].

For children on oral treatment, discontinuation of metformin 24 h before a major surgery (lasting at least 2 h) and on the day of surgery for a minor surgery is recommended. Hourly blood glucose monitoring is also recommended. If the blood glucose level is >180 mg/dL, IV insulin should be administered (as for elective surgery) to normalize levels; or subcutaneous insulin, if the patient is to undergo a minor procedure [76, 80].

In patients with ketosis, ketonuria, or ketoacidosis, treatment with subcutaneous or intravenous insulin should be initiated to rapidly correct the metabolic abnormality. Once a day of intermediate-acting or basal insulin (0.25–0.5 units/kg starting dose) is generally effective in attaining metabolic control. Metformin can be started along with insulin; once acidosis is resolved, the transition to metformin monotherapy can usually be achieved safely over 2–6 weeks [98].

If the patient fails to achieve a target HbA1c of <6.5% within 3–4 months on metformin monotherapy, the addition of basal insulin should be considered. If the target is not achieved on a combination of metformin and basal insulin (up to 1.2 units/kg), prandial insulin should be initiated and titrated to reach a target HbA1c level of <6.5% [110].

Glucagon-like peptide-1 analogs

Glucagon-like peptide-1 (GLP-1) is a hormone produced by the gut enteroendocrine cells, specifically the L cells of the small intestine, and is secreted after the ingestion of nutrients. Therefore, it controls meal-related glycemic excursions through augmentation of insulin levels and inhibition of glucagon secretion. GLP-1 also improves insulin biosynthesis and secretion and decreases β-cell apoptosis. In addition, it inhibits gastric emptying and food intake, actions maximizing nutrient absorption while limiting weight gain [120].

Liraglutide, a GLP-1 analog, has been recently approved by the Food and Drug Administration (FDA) and European Medicines Agency (EMA) for children and adolescents aged ≥10 years who have T2D according to the ELLIPSE Study data [121]. Liraglutide is efficacious for improving glycemic control and is started at a dose of 0.6 mg subcutaneously once daily, with incremental doses every 1–2 weeks or longer until fasting glucose targets are achieved to a maximum of 1.8 mg daily [115, 121]. Adverse effects with the use of liraglutide include nausea, vomiting, diarrhea, addominal pain and headache. In addition, a higher frequency of mild hypoglycemic episodes was also found [121].

If glycemic targets are no longer met with metformin (with or without basal insulin), liraglutide therapy should be considered in children 10 years of age or older if they have no past medical history or family history of medullary thyroid carcinoma or multiple endocrine neoplasia type 2 [39].

Insulin

When the individualized glycemic target can no longer be met with metformin alone or if metformin intolerance or renal or hepatic insufficiency develops, insulin therapy should be initiated alone or in combination with metformin unless metformin is contraindicated. The long-acting insulin analogs (glargine, detemir, or degludec) may be preferred [122].

Patients with ketosis, ketoacidosis, or a glucose concentration ≥200 mg/dL or HbA1c level ≥8.5% require a period of insulin therapy until glycemia has been restored to near-normal [2]. These patients require basal insulin (0.25–0.5 units/kg/day), and the dose can be adjusted according to the blood glucose values. Long-acting once daily insulin preparations could be administrated at bedtime [110]. Multiple daily injections with prandial short-acting insulin should be recommended in youths receiving high doses of basal insulin (up to 1.5 units/kg/day) [115, 122, 123].

Ongoing trials are evaluating the effects of sodium-glucose co-transporter 2 (SGLT2) inhibitors, dipeptidyl peptidase-4 (DPP-4) inhibitors, and sulfonylureas in children and adolescents with T2D. The results from these trials would soon expand the availability of pharmacological options to youths with T2DM [115, 122, 124].

Bariatric Surgery

Bariatric surgery, also called metabolic surgery, including Roux-in Y gastric bypass, vertical sleeve gastrectomy, laparoscopic adjustable gastric banding, laparoscopic gastric plication, and biliopancreatic, has been shown to significantly reduce weight, BMI, and cardiovascular comorbidities [2]. In addition, bariatric surgery has been shown to improve glucose metabolism in adolescents and adults with morbid obesity, which seems to be independent of weight loss, suggesting a direct hormonal effect [125].

The selection criteria for adolescent bariatric surgery include BMI $\geq$35 kg/m^2 and severe comorbidities such as T2D mellitus [98, 125, 126]. Recent results have demonstrated the remission of T2D and other comorbidities in nearly all youths after undergoing bariatric surgery [126–128], with attainment of HbA1c targets exceeding that observed with medical therapy [129]. A study conducted in México in adolescents with morbid obesity and T2D with gastric sleeve presented complete remission [130].

All bariatric procedures have an effect on glucose metabolism. The mechanisms responsible for improved glycemic control after bariatric surgery are thought to be associated with decreased nutritional intake, weight loss, and/or hormonal changes. The metabolic abnormalities associated with T2D mellitus can be reversed by bariatric surgery in most patients [125]. Roux-in-Y gastric bypass, the traditional surgical procedure for weight loss, can cause significant morbidity and mortality; however, newer techniques, which appear to be safer, include gastric banding and sleeve gastrectomy [110, 128].

Comorbidities

In children and adolescents with T2D and insulin resistance, the presence of multiple cardiovascular risk factors is likely to be associated with earlier severe complications [51]; thus, regular follow-up is essential to monitor weight and glycemic control and to prevent and address the development of diabetes-related complications such as hypertension and dyslipidemia [49, 51]. Hyperglycemia, dyslipidemia, and hypertension are contributors to the acceleration of atherosclerosis in T2D, along with oxidative stress, glycation of vascular proteins, and abnormalities in platelet function and coagulation. Endothelial dysfunction is an early sign of increased risk of cardiovascular disease, is predictive of cardiovascular events, and occurs in obese children relative to their level of obesity and degree of insulin resistance [110].

Blood pressure measurements, lipid panel, liver enzymes, albumin excretion, and dilated eye examinations should be performed at diagnosis because comorbidities may already be present at the time of diagnosis in youths with T2D. Then, the screening guidelines and treatment recommendations are similar to those for patients with type 1 diabetes. In addition, patients with T2D may need attention to other disorders, including polycystic ovary disease, obesity, sleep apnea, hepatitis steatosis, orthopedic disorders, and psychosocial concerns [2, 98].

Obesity

Weight loss and exercise both improve insulin resistance and glycemia, so the assessment of body mass index and pattern of weight gain should be considered a routine part of monitoring in youths with T2D, as obesity has deleterious associations with morbidity independent of insulin resistance and diabetes [110].

Hypertension

Hypertension is associated with endothelial dysfunction, arterial stiffness, and increased risk of both cardiovascular and kidney disease [131]. According to the TODAY study [132], hypertension was present in 13.6% of 699 US youths at a median diabetes duration of 7 months. Higher rates have been reported in Australia, with 36% of youths with T2D having hypertension within 1.3 years of diagnosis [133].

Several recommendations should be followed, such as measuring blood pressure with an appropriate-sized cuff at every clinic visit and normalizing the results for sex, height, and age. The initial treatment for blood pressure that is consistently $\geq$95th percentile at three visits should consist of efforts at weight loss, dietary salt restriction, and increased physical activity [110]. If blood pressure is still $\geq$95th percentile after 6 months, initiation of angiotensin-converting enzyme inhibitor therapy should be considered to achieve blood pressure values <90th percentile [134]. If the angiotensin-converting enzyme inhibitor is not tolerated due to adverse effects, an angiotensin receptor blocker is often used as a second-line therapy [98, 110].

Nephropathy

Early diabetic kidney disease (microalbuminuria and renal hyperfiltration) is common in adolescents with T2D and carries a higher risk of progression than the adult-onset type. Diabetic kidney disease is characterized by a long period with no signs of disease. One challenge in preventing the disease is the difficulty of identifying it at an early stage [135].

Albuminuria should be evaluated at diagnosis and annually thereafter. The definition of microalbuminuria used by the American Diabetes Association is either an albumin-to-creatinine ratio (ACR) of 30–299 mg/g in a spot urine or timed overnight sample or 24-h sample collections, with an albumin excretion rate of 20–199 μg/min. An elevated value may be secondary to exercise, smoking, menstruation, or orthostasis [110]. Abnormal screening tests should be repeated, as albuminuria may be transient. Therefore, the diagnosis of persistent abnormal microalbumin excretion requires the documentation of two of three consecutive abnormal values obtained on different days [91, 98, 110].

Non-diabetes-related causes of renal disease should be excluded, and consultation must be sought, especially if macroalbuminuria (ACR > 300 mg/g) is present [110]. Angiotensin-converting enzyme inhibitors are the agents of choice because of their beneficial effects for preventing diabetic nephropathy, even with normal blood pressures [103]. Albumin excretion should be monitored at 3- to 6-month intervals, and therapy doses should be titrated to achieve normal albumin-to-creatinine ratios as much as possible [110]. Non-diabetes-related causes of renal disease especially in the presence of ACR >300 mg/g can be referred to nephrologists [98].

Dyslipidemia

Hypertriglyceridemia and decreased HDL cholesterol levels are hallmarks of dyslipidemia, which is characteristic of insulin resistance and T2D in children and adolescents. Testing for dyslipidemia should be performed soon after diagnosis when blood glucose control has been achieved and annually thereafter. The target levels are as follows [110]:

- LDL cholesterol <100 mg/dL (2.6 mmol/L)
- HDL cholesterol >35 mg/dL (0.91 mmol/L)
- Triglycerides <150 mg/dL (1.7 mmol/L)

In the case of persistent dyslipidemia despite dietary and exercise counseling, pharmacotherapy may be initiated. Statin therapy has been shown to be as safe and effective in children as in adults and should be the first pharmacological intervention, beginning with the lowest available dose. Treatment with a fibric acid medication should also be considered when fasting triglycerides are >400–600 mg/dL [98, 110].

Polycystic Ovarian Syndrome

Polycystic ovarian syndrome (PCOS) is increasingly recognized in adolescents as part of insulin resistance syndrome. Adolescents with PCOS had an approximately 40% reduction in insulin-stimulated glucose disposal compared with body composition-matched non-hyperandrogenic control subjects [98, 136].

Reducing insulin resistance with weight loss, exercise, and metformin therapy improves ovarian function and increases fertility. Menstrual history taking should be performed for all girls with T2D at diagnosis and at each visit. An evaluation for PCOS should be considered if primary or secondary amenorrhea, hirsutism, and/or significant acne are found. PCOS is diagnosed on the basis of the presence of oligomenorrhea or amenorrhea with biochemical or clinical evidence of hyperandrogenism, with or without evidence of polycystic ovaries. Girls receiving diabetes treatment should also be counseled that fertility may improve as a result and that proper birth control should be used to prevent any unwanted pregnancy [98, 110].

Non-alcoholic Fatty Liver Disease

Hepatic steatosis is present in 25–50% of adolescents with T2D, and more advanced forms of non-alcoholic fatty liver disease (NAFLD), such as non-alcoholic steatohepatitis (NASH), have become increasingly common and are associated with progression to cirrhosis, portal hypertension, and liver failure. NAFLD is now the most frequent cause of chronic liver disorders among obese youths [110].

Interpretation of ALT levels should be based upon the sex-specific upper limits of normal in children (22 U/L for girls and 26 U/L for boys) and not on individual laboratory upper limits of normal. NAFLD/NASH or other causes of chronic hepatitis should be considered for persistently (>3 months) elevated ALT levels >3 times the upper limit of normal. The patients should be referred to the gastroenterology department if liver enzymes remain elevated >3 times [98].

Weight loss improves NAFLD, and metformin has been shown to improve liver enzymes and liver steatosis in insulin-resistant adolescents [137]. T2D therapies that improve insulin resistance appear to improve NAFLD and are therefore the standard approach to youths with both NAFLD and T2D. However, owing to the potential for progression to NASH, fibrosis, and cirrhosis, ongoing monitoring of liver enzymes is recommended in youths with T2D. Referral for biopsy is recommended if enzymes remain markedly elevated despite weight loss and/or diabetes therapies [110].

Obstructive Sleep Apnea

Obstructive sleep apnea is common in obese youths, but its prevalence in pediatric T2D has not yet been well documented. However, the prevalence is likely high, as the prevalence in adults is between 70 and 90% [138, 139]. Obstructive sleep apnea not only causes poor sleep quality and daytime sleepiness but also has clinical consequences, including hypertension, left ventricular hypertrophy, and increased risk of renal and cardiovascular disease [98, 110].

Youths with T2D can be screened for obstructive sleep apnea by questioning them about snoring, sleep quality, apnea, morning headaches, daytime sleepiness, and enuresis. If symptoms are suggestive, a diagnosis is made through a formal sleep study and referral to a sleep specialist [110].

Depression

Youths with T2D are at increased risk of major clinical depression, which is associated with poor adherence to diabetic treatment recommendations. Signs include depressed mood, markedly diminished interest or pleasure, increased or decreased appetite, insomnia or hypersomnia, psychomotor agitation or retardation, fatigue or loss of energy, feelings of worthlessness, and recurrent thoughts of death [98, 110].

Youths with T2D, particularly those with frequent emergency department visits or poor glycemic control, should be assessed for depression at diagnosis and periodically thereafter [110]. Patients identified as depressed should be referred to appropriate mental health-care providers experienced in addressing depression in youths [140].

Additional Health Problems Related to Obesity and T2D

All patients with T2D may have additional health problems related to the disease, such as orthopedic problems resulting in diminishing physical activity, pancreatitis, cholecystitis, pseudotumor cerebri, and deep tissue ulcers. These additional health problems should be screened at diagnosis and rescreened periodically [110].

Transition from Pediatric to Adult Care

The care and close supervision of diabetes management are increasingly shifted from parents and other adults to the youth with type 1 or 2 diabetes over the course of childhood and adolescence [141]. The shift from pediatric to adult health care is inevitable, and the transition is always difficult regardless of age. However, in some places, more than half of patients continued to receive pediatric care even after the age of 30 years [142].

The transition often occurs abruptly as older teens enter the next developmental stage, referred to as emerging adulthood, and a lack of consistent care may follow the transition in 30–40% of patients [76, 141]. The transition is a period associated with deterioration in glycemic control; increased occurrence of acute complications, psychosocial, emotional, and behavioral challenges; and the emergence of chronic complications [76, 141].

During this period, youths with T2D often struggle with becoming fully responsible for their diabetes care; therefore, discussion about the transition during the several visits before it occurs may help prepare the patient [76, 141]. Health-care providers and families should begin to prepare youths with diabetes in early- to mid-adolescence and at least 1 year before the transition to adult health care, and both pediatricians and adult health-care providers should assist in providing support for the teen and emerging adult [141].

Concluding Remarks

- The pathophysiology and diagnostic criteria for diabetes mellitus are the same in children and adults.
- However, issues specific to early childhood diabetes include changes in insulin sensitivity due to growth and development, dependence on care, and neurological susceptibility to changes in glucose.
- The younger age of presentation of diabetes in pediatric patients causes a longer disease exposure, with the development of chronic complications at an early age; therefore, close surveillance is required.
- Children are not small adults; thus, treatment should be adapted to age-related physiological changes.
- The only pharmacological treatments approved for children and adolescents are insulin for type 1 diabetes mellitus, metformin, liraglutide, and insulin for T2D mellitus and sulfonylureas for some types of neonatal diabetes. Pediatric patients with T2D could also be candidates for bariatric surgery.

Multiple-Choice Questions

1. What is the most common type of diabetes mellitus in children and adolescents?
   (a) **Type 1 diabetes mellitus**
   (b) Type 2 diabetes mellitus
   (c) Monogenic diabetes
   (d) MODY
   (e) Neonatal diabetes
   Although type 2 diabetes is occurring more frequently in pediatric patients and other forms such as neonatal diabetes are unique to this age range, type 1 diabetes is the predominant form in this age group.

2. Which of the following clinical features raises the suspicion of monogenic diabetes?
   (a) Diabetic ketoacidosis in a school-age child
   (b) A random plasma glucose level ≥200 mg/dL in a child with obesity, acanthosis nigricans, and a family history of type 2 diabetes
   (c) **Diabetes in the first 6 months of life, a strong family history of type 2 diabetes in a nonobese patient or low-risk ethnic group, and fasting glycemia of 100–150 mg/dL**
   (d) Neonatal hyperglycemia in infants with elfin facies, low birth weight, and skin abnormalities
   (e) Diabetes mellitus associated with autoantibodies
   Monogenic diabetes is characterized by impaired insulin secretion by pancreatic beta cells caused by a single gene mutation. These forms of diabetes represent less than 5% of patients with diabetes and are charac-

terized by onset generally before age 25 years, without clinical features of insulin resistance in type 2 diabetes and with negative associated autoantibodies.

3. What are the blood glucose and HbA1c goals for type 1 diabetes mellitus across all pediatric age groups?

   (a) Blood glucose level of 100–150 mg/dL before a meal and 100–125 mg/dL at bedtime/overnight, and HbA1c level of <8.5% in infants, <8.0% in school-children, and <7.5% in adolescents

   (b) **Blood glucose of 90–130 mg/dL before a meal and 90–150 mg/dL at bedtime/overnight, and HbA1c level of <7.5% across all pediatric age groups**

   (c) Blood glucose level of <100 mg/dL before a meal, <140 mg/dL after a meal, and 100–125 mg/dL at bedtime/overnight, and HbA1c level of <6.5% across all pediatric age groups

   (d) The lowest HbA1c level is possible regardless of the degree of hypoglycemia

   (e) Blood glucose level of <200 mg/dL after a meal and HbA1c level of <8.5% across all pediatric age groups

   Glycemic control needs to be of a sufficient degree to prevent diabetes-related complications; however, strict glucose levels carry the risk of hypoglycemia. Although young children were previously thought to be at risk of cognitive impairment after episodes of hypoglycemia, current data have not confirmed this notion. Hence, current standards recommend lowering glucose to the safest possible level to prevent chronic complications.

4. In an oral glucose tolerance test, what is the glucose load used to diagnose diabetes mellitus in children and adolescents?

   (a) 1.75 g of anhydrous glucose per kg body weight, with a maximum of 50 g

   (b) 1.50 g of anhydrous glucose per kg body weight, with a maximum of 75 g

   (c) 1.50 g of anhydrous glucose per kg body weight, with a maximum of 50 g

   (d) 1.75 g of anhydrous glucose per kg body weight, with a maximum of 65 g

   (e) **1.75 g of anhydrous glucose per kg body weight, with a maximum of 75 g**

   The loading of anhydrous glucose in the oral glucose tolerance test must be calculated per body weight, with a maximum adult load of 75 g. In the absence of unequivocal hyperglycemia, results should be confirmed by repeat testing.

5. Which of the following is the best treatment option for mild hypoglycemia in pediatric patients with type 1 diabetes?

   (a) Intravenous 10% glucose, 2–3 mL/kg

   (b) 10–15 g of oral glucose using complex carbohydrates

   (c) **10–15 g of oral glucose using simple carbohydrates**

   (d) Glucagon 10–30 µg/kg of body weight

   (e) Switching off the insulin pump

   Milder hypoglycemia should be treated with 10–15 g of oral glucose in the form of simple carbohydrates such as glucose tablets or sweetened fluids such as juice. Subsequently, blood glucose levels should be retested in 10–15 min. In case of an inadequate response, treatment should be repeated and blood glucose levels should be retested in another 10–15 min to confirm that a glucose level of 100 mg/dL has been reached. In some circumstances, this should be followed by administration of additional complex carbohydrates to prevent the recurrence of hypoglycemia. Intravenous glucose and glucagon are used in more severe hypoglycemia.

6. Which treatment has been observed to be effective at preventing beta cell failure in the honeymoon phase?

   (a) **Insulin**

   (b) Glucagon

   (c) Metformin

   (d) Sulfonylureas

   (e) None of the above

   Early small doses of insulin have been observed to be effective at preventing beta cell failure in slowly progressive type 1 diabetes, and they have been recommended for patients with positive antibodies. During the honeymoon phase, the insulin requirement decreases, and basal insulin of 0.2–0.6 units/g/day during this phase may preserve beta cell function.

7. If diabetes occurs at puberty and the patient has obesity, insulin resistance data, and a genetic background for T2DM, what type of diabetes are we required to rule out?

   (a) Neonatal diabetes

   (b) Type 1 diabetes mellitus

   (c) Monogenic diabetes

   (d) MODY

   (e) **Type 2 diabetes mellitus**

   The clinical data that usually support the presence of T2DM are overweight or obesity, first- or second-degree relatives with diabetes, presence of acanthosis nigricans, hypertension, dyslipidemia, non-alcoholic fatty liver, exposure to gestational diabetes, low height or macrosomia at birth, obstructive sleep apnea syndrome, and polycystic ovary syndrome. C-peptide levels ≥0.5 ng/dL may be an indirect marker that endogenous insulin secretion still exists and therefore lead to T2DM. However, this may be decreased at the beginning of diagnosis and late illness.

8. Which of the following is true regarding insulin therapy in patients with type 1 diabetes mellitus?

   (a) The insulin requirements are the same across all age groups (0.5 units/kg/day).

(b) Treatment regimens with two doses of insulin, multiple doses of insulin, or continuous infusion are equally effective.

(c) To avoid hypoglycemia, the short-acting dose of insulin should consider the amount of food to be consumed without taking into account glucose levels.

(d) The insulin pump is indicated only in patients for whom control with multiple injections is not achieved.

(e) **The insulin scheme should mimic natural production, with basal insulin to maintain glucose levels between meals and rapid insulin to cover carbohydrates and normalize glucose.**

Insulin requirements range from 0.25 to 1.5 units/kg/day according to age and pubertal development. Intensive management with the use of multiple-dose insulin and/or continuous subcutaneous insulin infusion in children and adolescents with type 1 diabetes mellitus showed a marked decline in HbA1c level and chronic complications. The primary goal of treatment is to mimic natural insulin secretion, with basal insulin to maintain near-normal blood glucose levels between meals and short-acting insulin to cover the carbohydrates consumed during meals and normalize blood glucose levels. Insulin pumps have become increasingly available to patients with diabetes, and experts highlight their use as the chosen treatment option for many people across all age groups living with type 1 diabetes.

9. How should the total energy intake be distributed in the management of type 1 diabetes mellitus?
   (a) Restricted energy intake with carbohydrate 50%, fat 30%, and protein 20%
   (b) Normal energy intake with a low-carbohydrate intake of 20% to prevent hyperglycemia
   (c) Normal energy intake with low fat to prevent ketosis
   (d) **Normal energy intake with carbohydrate 45–65%, fat 30–35%, and protein 15–25%**
   (e) Restricted energy intake with carbohydrate 60%, fat 25%, and protein 15%

Energy intake should be sufficient to achieve optimal growth and maintain an ideal body weight. The total daily energy intake should be distributed as follows: carbohydrate 45–65%, fat 30–35%, and protein 15–25%. Carbohydrates should not be restricted, as they are essential for growth.

10. Which pharmacological treatment(s) is/are approved to treat type 2 diabetes in children and adolescents?
    (a) **Liraglutide, metformin, and insulin**
    (b) Thiazolidinedione and metformin
    (c) Same as in adults
    (d) Insulin only

(e) SGLT2 inhibitor and metformin

Metformin is the only oral hypoglycemic agent approved for daily use in children with type 2 diabetes. Treatment with metformin monotherapy should begin at 500 mg daily. The dose should be titrated by 500 mg once per week over 3–4 weeks to the maximal dose of 1000 mg twice daily. If the patient fails to achieve a target HbA1c level of <6.5% within 3–4 months on metformin monotherapy, the addition of basal insulin should be considered. Liraglutide is a GLP-1 analog approved by the FDA and EMA in 2019 for children and adolescents aged ≥10 years with T2DM.

11. Which of the following is true about follow-up for pediatric patients with type 2 diabetes?
    (a) Nutritional management must be focused on achieving normal glycemia regardless of the body mass index.
    (b) Moderate-to-vigorous exercise for 15–30 min twice per week is recommended.
    (c) **The examination of comorbidities should be performed at diagnosis.**
    (d) Patients with type 2 diabetes do not need to self-monitor their blood glucose levels.
    (e) The target levels for dyslipidemia are LDL-C <200 mg/dL, HDL-C >35 mg/dL, and triglycerides <150 mg/dL.

Nutritional management must be focused on achieving normal glycemia and HbA1c levels, preventing further weight gain, or achieving weight loss while maintaining normal linear growth. Patients should increase their daily physical activity to 60 min of moderate-to-vigorous exercise. Blood pressure measurements, lipid panel, albumin excretion, and dilated eye examinations should be performed at diagnosis because comorbidities may already be present at that time. Blood glucose self-monitoring should be performed regularly. The target levels for dyslipidemia are LDL-C <100 mg/dL, HDL-C >35 mg/dL, and triglycerides <150 mg/dL.

References

1. Menke A, Casagrande S, Cowie CC. Prevalence of diabetes in adolescents aged 12 to 19 years in the United States, 2005-2014. JAMA. 2016;316(3):344–5.
2. 13. Children and adolescents: standards of medical care in diabetes-2021. Diabetes Care. 2021;44(Suppl 1):S180–99.
3. Springer SC, Silverstein J, Copeland K, Moore KR, Prazar GE, Raymer T, et al. Management of type 2 diabetes mellitus in children and adolescents. Pediatrics. 2013;131(2):e648–64.
4. American Diabetes Association. 2. Classification and diagnosis of diabetes: standards of medical care in diabetes-2021. Diabetes Care. 2021;44(Suppl 1):S15–s33.
5. Nowicka P, Santoro N, Liu H, Lartaud D, Shaw MM, Goldberg R, et al. Utility of hemoglobin A(1c) for diagnosing prediabetes

and diabetes in obese children and adolescents. Diabetes Care. 2011;34(6):1306–11.

6. Buse JB, Kaufman FR, Linder B, Hirst K, El Ghormli L, Willi S. Diabetes screening with hemoglobin A(1c) versus fasting plasma glucose in a multiethnic middle-school cohort. Diabetes Care. 2013;36(2):429–35.

7. Rubio-Cabezas O, Hattersley AT, Njolstad PR, Mlynarski W, Ellard S, White N, et al. ISPAD Clinical Practice Consensus guidelines 2014. The diagnosis and management of monogenic diabetes in children and adolescents. Pediatr Diabetes. 2014;15(Suppl 20):47–64.

8. Redondo MJ, Libman I, Maahs DM, Lyons SK, Saraco M, Reusch J, et al. The evolution of hemoglobin A(1c) targets for youth with type 1 diabetes: rationale and supporting evidence. Diabetes Care. 2021;44(2):301–12.

9. Hattersley AT, Greeley SAW, Polak M, Rubio-Cabezas O, Njølstad PR, Mlynarski W, et al. ISPAD Clinical Practice Consensus guidelines 2018: the diagnosis and management of monogenic diabetes in children and adolescents. Pediatr Diabetes. 2018;19(Suppl 27):47–63.

10. Mayer-Davis EJ, Kahkoska AR, Jefferies C, Dabelea D, Balde N, Gong CX, et al. ISPAD Clinical Practice Consensus guidelines 2018: definition, epidemiology, and classification of diabetes in children and adolescents. Pediatr Diabetes. 2018;19(Suppl 27):7–19.

11. Polak M, Cave H. Neonatal diabetes mellitus: a disease linked to multiple mechanisms. Orphanet J Rare Dis. 2007;2:12.

12. Greeley SA, Naylor RN, Philipson LH, Bell GI. Neonatal diabetes: an expanding list of genes allows for improved diagnosis and treatment. Curr Diab Rep. 2011;11(6):519–32.

13. Ashcroft FM, Puljung MC, Vedovato N. Neonatal diabetes and the KATP channel: from mutation to therapy. Trends Endocrinol Metab. 2017;28:377. https://doi.org/10.1016/j.tem.2017.02.003.

14. Maassen JA, T'Hart LM, Van Essen E, Heine RJ, Nijpels G, Jahangir Tafrechi RS, et al. Mitochondrial diabetes: molecular mechanisms and clinical presentation. Diabetes. 2004;53(1):S103–9.

15. Ergun-Longmire B, Maclaren NK. Management of type-1 and type-2 diabetes mellitus in children. In: De Groot LJ, Chrousos G, Dungan K, et al, editors. South Dartmouth: MDTextcom; 2000. Last Update 9 Dec 2013.

16. Shields BM, Hicks S, Shepherd MH, Colclough K, Hattersley AT, Ellard S. Maturity-onset diabetes of the young (MODY): how many cases are we missing? Diabetologia. 2010;53(12):2504–8.

17. Nijim Y, Awni Y, Adawi A, Bowirrat A. Classic case report of Donohue syndrome (Leprechaunism; OMIM *246200): the impact of consanguineous mating. Medicine (Baltimore). 2016;95(6):e710.

18. Resmini E, Minuto F, Colao A, Ferone D. Secondary diabetes associated with principal endocrinopathies: the impact of new treatment modalities. Acta Diabetol. 2009;46(2):85–95.

19. Fathallah N, Slim R, Larif S, Hmouda H, Ben SC. Drug-induced hyperglycaemia and diabetes. Drug Saf. 2015;38(12):1153–68.

20. Moran A, Pillay K, Becker D, Granados A, Hameed S, Acerini CL. ISPAD clinical practice consensus guidelines 2018: management of cystic fibrosis-related diabetes in children and adolescents. Pediatr Diabetes. 2018;19(Suppl 27):64–74.

21. Dabelea D, Mayer-Davis EJ, Saydah S, Imperatore G, Linder B, Divers J, et al. Prevalence of type 1 and type 2 diabetes among children and adolescents from 2001 to 2009. JAMA. 2014;311(17):1778–86.

22. Green A, Hede SM, Patterson CC, Wild SH, Imperatore G, Roglic G, et al. Type 1 diabetes in 2017: global estimates of incident and prevalent cases in children and adults. Diabetologia. 2021;64:2741.

23. Roche EF, McKenna AM, Ryder KJ, Brennan AA, O'Regan M, Hoey HM. Is the incidence of type 1 diabetes in children and adolescents stabilising? The first 6 years of a National Register. Eur J Pediatr. 2016;175(12):1913–9.

24. DIAMOND Project Group. Incidence and trends of childhood Type 1 diabetes worldwide 1990-1999. Diabet Med. 2006;23(8):857–66.

25. Butalia S, Kaplan GG, Khokhar B, Rabi DM. Environmental risk factors and type 1 diabetes: past, present, and future. Can J Diabetes. 2016;40(6):586–93.

26. Pociot F, Lernmark A. Genetic risk factors for type 1 diabetes. Lancet. 2016;387(10035):2331–9.

27. Giannopoulou EZ, Winkler C, Chmiel R, Matzke C, Scholz M, Beyerlein A, et al. Islet autoantibody phenotypes and incidence in children at increased risk for type 1 diabetes. Diabetologia. 2015;58(10):2317–23.

28. Ziegler AG, Rewers M, Simell O, Simell T, Lempainen J, Steck A, et al. Seroconversion to multiple islet autoantibodies and risk of progression to diabetes in children. JAMA. 2013;309(23):2473–9.

29. Couper JJ, Haller MJ, Greenbaum CJ, Ziegler AG, Wherrett DK, Knip M, et al. ISPAD clinical practice consensus guidelines 2018: stages of type 1 diabetes in children and adolescents. Pediatr Diabetes. 2018;19(Suppl 27):20–7.

30. Rewers M, Ludvigsson J. Environmental risk factors for type 1 diabetes. Lancet. 2016;387(10035):2340–8.

31. Dabelea D, Rewers A, Stafford JM, Standiford DA, Lawrence JM, Saydah S, et al. Trends in the prevalence of ketoacidosis at diabetes diagnosis: the SEARCH for diabetes in youth study. Pediatrics. 2014;133(4):e938–45.

32. Usher-Smith JA, Thompson M, Ercole A, Walter FM. Variation between countries in the frequency of diabetic ketoacidosis at first presentation of type 1 diabetes in children/adolescents: a systematic review. Diabetologia. 2012;55(11):2878–94.

33. Codner E, Acerini CL, Craig ME, Hofer SE, Maahs DM. ISPAD clinical practice consensus guidelines 2018: limited care guidance appendix. Pediatr Diabetes. 2018;19(Suppl 27):328–38.

34. 5. Facilitating behavior change and well-being to improve health outcomes: standards of medical care in diabetes-2021. Diabetes Care. 2021;44(Suppl 1):S53–72.

35. Bratina N, Forsander G, Annan F, Wysocki T, Pierce J, Calliari LE, et al. ISPAD clinical practice consensus guidelines 2018: management and support of children and adolescents with type 1 diabetes in school. Pediatr Diabetes. 2018;19(Suppl 27):287–301.

36. Phelan H, Lange K, Cengiz E, Gallego P, Majaliwa E, Pelicand J, et al. ISPAD clinical practice consensus guidelines 2018: diabetes education in children and adolescents. Pediatr Diabetes. 2018;19(Suppl 27):75–83.

37. 6. Glycemic targets: standards of medical care in diabetes-2021. Diabetes Care. 2021;44(Suppl 1):S73–84.

38. DiMeglio LA, Acerini CL, Codner E, Craig ME, Hofer SE, Pillay K, et al. ISPAD clinical practice consensus guidelines 2018: glycemic control targets and glucose monitoring for children, adolescents, and young adults with diabetes. Pediatr Diabetes. 2018;19(Suppl 27):105–14.

39. Standards of medical care in diabetes-2021 abridged for primary care providers. Clin Diabetes 2021;39(1):14–43.

40. Ly TT, Maahs DM, Rewers A, Dunger D, Oduwole A, Jones TW. ISPAD clinical practice consensus guidelines 2014. Assessment and management of hypoglycemia in children and adolescents with diabetes. Pediatr Diabetes. 2014;15(Suppl 20):180–92.

41. Beck JK, Cogen FR. Outpatient management of pediatric type 1 diabetes. J Pediatr Pharmacol Ther. 2015;20(5):344–57.

42. Phillips A. Advances in infusion sets and insulin pumps in diabetes care. Br J Community Nurs. 2016;21(3):124–7.

43. Haviland N, Walsh J, Roberts R, Bailey TS. Update on clinical utility of continuous glucose monitoring in type 1 diabetes. Curr Diab Rep. 2016;16(11):115.

44. Sherr JL, Tauschmann M, Battelino T, de Bock M, Forlenza G, Roman R, et al. ISPAD clinical practice consensus guidelines 2018: diabetes technologies. Pediatr Diabetes. 2018;19(Suppl 27):302–25.

45. Codner E, Acerini C, Craig ME, Hofer S, Maahs DM. ISPAD clinical practice consensus guidelines 2018: introduction to the limited care guidance appendix. Pediatr Diabetes. 2018;19(Suppl 27):326–7.

46. Danne T, Phillip M, Buckingham BA, Jarosz-Chobot P, Saboo B, Urakami T, et al. ISPAD clinical practice consensus guidelines 2018: insulin treatment in children and adolescents with diabetes. Pediatr Diabetes. 2018;19(Suppl 27):115–35.

47. Downie E, Craig ME, Hing S, Cusumano J, Chan AK, Donaghue KC. Continued reduction in the prevalence of retinopathy in adolescents with type 1 diabetes: role of insulin therapy and glycemic control. Diabetes Care. 2011;34(11):2368–73.

48. Zabeen B, Craig ME, Virk SA, Pryke A, Chan AK, Cho YH, et al. Insulin pump therapy is associated with lower rates of retinopathy and peripheral nerve abnormality. PLoS One. 2016;11(4):e0153033.

49. Smart C. Nutritional management of diabetes in childhood. In: Koletzko B, Bhatia J, Bhutta ZA, Cooper P, Makrides M, Uauy R, et al., editors. Pediatric nutrition in practice. 2nd ed. Basel: Karger; 2015.

50. Chiang JL, Maahs DM, Garvey KC, Hood KK, Laffel LM, Weinzimer SA, et al. Type 1 diabetes in children and adolescents: a position statement by the American Diabetes Association. Diabetes Care. 2018;41(9):2026–44.

51. Smart CE, Annan F, Bruno LPC, Higgins LA, Acerini CL. ISPAD clinical practice consensus guidelines 2014 compendium. Nutritional management in children and adolescents with diabetes. Pediatr Diabetes. 2014;15(S20):135–53.

52. Bell KJ, Smart CE, Steil GM, Brand-Miller JC, King B, Wolpert HA. Impact of fat, protein, and glycemic index on postprandial glucose control in type 1 diabetes: implications for intensive diabetes management in the continuous glucose monitoring era. Diabetes Care. 2015;38(6):1008–15.

53. Smart CE, Evans M, O'Connell SM, McElduff P, Lopez PE, Jones TW, et al. Both dietary protein and fat increase postprandial glucose excursions in children with type 1 diabetes, and the effect is additive. Diabetes Care. 2013;36(12):3897–902.

54. Smart CE, Annan F, Higgins LA, Jelleryd E, Lopez M, Acerini CL. ISPAD clinical practice consensus guidelines 2018: nutritional management in children and adolescents with diabetes. Pediatr Diabetes. 2018;19(Suppl 27):136–54.

55. FAO, World Health Organization, United Nations University. Energy and protein requirements. Estimates of energy and protein requirements of adults and children. Geneva: World Health Organization; 1985.

56. World Health Organization, United Nations FAO. Vitamin and mineral requirements in human nutrition. 2nd ed. Hong Kong: World Health Organization; 2004.

57. Riddell MC, Gallen IW, Smart CE, Taplin CE, Adolfsson P, Lumb AN, et al. Exercise management in type 1 diabetes: a consensus statement. Lancet Diabetes Endocrinol. 2017;5:377. https://doi.org/10.1016/S2213-8587(17)30014-1.

58. Pivovarov JA, Taplin CE, Riddell MC. Current perspectives on physical activity and exercise for youth with diabetes. Pediatr Diabetes. 2015;16(4):242–55. https://doi.org/10.1111/pedi.12272.

59. Tremblay MS, Warburton DE, Janssen I, Paterson DH, Latimer AE, Rhodes RE, et al. New Canadian physical activity guidelines. Appl Physiol Nutr Metab. 2011;36(1):36–46; 47–58.

60. Tremblay MS, Leblanc AG, Carson V, Choquette L, Connor Gorber S, Dillman C, et al. Canadian physical activity guidelines for the early years (aged 0-4 years). Appl Physiol Nutr Metab. 2012;37(2):345–69.

61. Tremblay MS, Carson V, Chaput JP, Connor Gorber S, Dinh T, Duggan M, et al. Canadian 24-hour movement guidelines for children and youth: an integration of physical activity, sedentary behaviour, and sleep. Appl Physiol Nutr Metab. 2016;41(6 Suppl 3):S311–27.

62. Brown RJ, Rother KI. Effects of beta-cell rest on beta-cell function: a review of clinical and preclinical data. Pediatr Diabetes. 2008;9(3pt2):14–22.

63. Herold KC, Gitelman SE, Masharani U, Hagopian W, Bisikirska B, Donaldson D, et al. A single course of anti-CD3 monoclonal antibody hOKT3gamma1(Ala-Ala) results in improvement in C-peptide responses and clinical parameters for at least 2 years after onset of type 1 diabetes. Diabetes. 2005;54(6):1763–9.

64. Raz I, Elias D, Avron A, Tamir M, Metzger M, Cohen IR. β-cell function in new-onset type 1 diabetes and immunomodulation with a heat-shock protein peptide (DiaPep277): a randomised, double-blind, phase II trial. Lancet. 2004;358(9295):1749–53.

65. Ryan EA, Imes S, Wallace C. Short-term intensive insulin therapy in newly diagnosed type 2 diabetes. Diabetes Care. 2004;27(5):1028–32.

66. Agardh C-D, Cilio CM, Lethagen ÅL, Lynch K, Leslie RDG, Palmér M, et al. Clinical evidence for the safety of GAD65 immunomodulation in adult-onset autoimmune diabetes. J Diabetes Complications. 2005;19(4):238–46.

67. Alleva DG, Gaur A, Jin L, Wegmann D, Gottlieb PA, Pahuja A, et al. Immunological characterization and therapeutic activity of an altered-peptide ligand, NBI-6024, based on the immunodominant type 1 diabetes autoantigen insulin B-chain (9-23) peptide. Diabetes. 2002;51(7):2126–34.

68. Reiband HK, Schmidt S, Ranjan A, Holst JJ, Madsbad S, Norgaard K. Dual-hormone treatment with insulin and glucagon in patients with type 1 diabetes. Diabetes Metab Res Rev. 2015;31(7):672–9.

69. Davidson JA, Holland WL, Roth MG, Wang MY, Lee Y, Yu X, et al. Glucagon therapeutics: dawn of a new era for diabetes care. Diabetes Metab Res Rev. 2016;32(7):660–5.

70. Xiang H, Yang C, Xiang T, Wang Z, Ge X, Li F, et al. Residual beta-cell function predicts clinical response after autologous hematopoietic stem cell transplantation. Stem Cells Transl Med. 2016;5(5):651–7.

71. Pellegrini S, Cantarelli E, Sordi V, Nano R, Piemonti L. The state of the art of islet transplantation and cell therapy in type 1 diabetes. Acta Diabetol. 2016;53(5):683–91.

72. Al Khalifah RA, Alnhdi A, Alghar H, Alanazi M, Florez ID. The effect of adding metformin to insulin therapy for type 1 diabetes mellitus children/adolescents: a systematic review and meta-analysis. Pediatr Diabetes. 2017;18(7):664. https://doi.org/10.1111/pedi.12493.

73. Juvenile Diabetes Research Foundation Continuous Glucose Monitoring Study Group. Prolonged nocturnal hypoglycemia is common during 12 months of continuous glucose monitoring in children and adults with type 1 diabetes. Diabetes Care. 2010;33(5):1004–8.

74. Seaquist ER, Anderson J, Childs B, Cryer P, Dagogo-Jack S, Fish L, et al. Hypoglycemia and diabetes: a report of a workgroup of the American Diabetes Association and the Endocrine Society. Diabetes Care. 2013;36(5):1384–95.

75. Abraham MB, Jones TW, Naranjo D, Karges B, Oduwole A, Tauschmann M, et al. ISPAD Clinical Practice Consensus Guidelines 2018: assessment and management of hypoglycemia in children and adolescents with diabetes. Pediatr Diabetes. 2018;19(Suppl 27):178–92.

76. International Diabetes Federation, International Society for Pediatric and Adolescent Diabetes. Global IDF/ISPAD guideline for diabetes in childhood and adolescence. Brussels: International Diabetes Federation; 2011. https://www.idf.org/sites/default/files/Diabetes-in-Childhood-and-Adolescense-Guidelines.pdf.

77. Brink S, Joel D, Laffel L, Lee WWR, Olsen B, Phelan H, et al. ISPAD Clinical Practice Consensus Guidelines 2014. Sick day management in children and adolescents with diabetes. Pediatr Diabetes. 2014;15(S20):193–202.

78. Priyambada L, Wolfsdorf JI, Brink SJ, Fritsch M, Codner E, Donaghue KC, et al. ISPAD Clinical Practice Consensus Guideline: diabetic ketoacidosis in the time of COVID-19 and resource-limited settings-role of subcutaneous insulin. Pediatr Diabetes. 2020;21(8):1394–402.

79. Jefferies C, Rhodes E, Rachmiel M, Agwu JC, Kapellen T, Abdulla MA, et al. ISPAD Clinical Practice Consensus Guidelines 2018: management of children and adolescents with diabetes requiring surgery. Pediatr Diabetes. 2018;19(Suppl 27):227–36.

80. Rhodes ET, Gong C, Edge JA, Wolfsdorf JI, Hanas R. ISPAD Clinical Practice Consensus Guidelines 2014. Management of children and adolescents with diabetes requiring surgery. Pediatr Diabetes. 2014;15(S20):224–31.

81. Wolfsdorf JI, Allgrove J, Craig M, Edge JA, Glaser N, Jain V, et al. ISPAD Clinical Practice Consensus Guidelines 2014 Compendium. Diabetic ketoacidosis and hyperglycemic hyperosmolar state. Pediatr Diabetes. 2014;15(Suppl. 20):154–79.

82. Wolfsdorf JI, Glaser N, Agus M, Fritsch M, Hanas R, Rewers A, et al. ISPAD Clinical Practice Consensus Guidelines 2018: diabetic ketoacidosis and the hyperglycemic hyperosmolar state. Pediatr Diabetes. 2018;19(Suppl 27):155–77.

83. Mahmud FH, Elbarbary NS, Fröhlich-Reiterer E, Holl RW, Kordonouri O, Knip M, et al. ISPAD Clinical Practice Consensus Guidelines 2018: other complications and associated conditions in children and adolescents with type 1 diabetes. Pediatr Diabetes. 2018;19(Suppl 27):275–86.

84. Hagger V, Trawley S, Hendrieckx C, Browne JL, Cameron F, Pouwer F, et al. Diabetes MILES Youth-Australia: methods and sample characteristics of a national survey of the psychological aspects of living with type 1 diabetes in Australian youth and their parents. BMC Psychol. 2016;4(1):42.

85. Sztein DM, Lane WG. Examination of the comorbidity of mental illness and somatic conditions in hospitalized children in the United States using the kids' inpatient database, 2009. Hosp Pediatr. 2016;6(3):126–34.

86. Delamater AM, de Wit M, McDarby V, Malik JA, Hilliard ME, Northam E, et al. ISPAD Clinical Practice Consensus Guidelines 2018: psychological care of children and adolescents with type 1 diabetes. Pediatr Diabetes. 2018;19(Suppl 27):237–49.

87. American Diabetes Association. 3. Foundations of care and comprehensive medical evaluation. Diabetes Care. 2016;39(Suppl 1):S23–35.

88. Dashti AS, Alaei MR, Musavi Z, Faramarzi R, Mansouri F, Nasimfar A. Serological response to vaccines in children with diabetes. Roum Arch Microbiol Immunol. 2015;74(3-4):112–7.

89. Hillard PJ. Prevention and management of pregnancy in adolescents with endocrine disorders. Adolesc Med State Art Rev. 2015;26(2):382–92.

90. Bradley TJ, Slorach C, Mahmud FH, Dunger DB, Deanfield J, Deda L, et al. Early changes in cardiovascular structure and function in adolescents with type 1 diabetes. Cardiovasc Diabetol. 2016;15(10):31.

91. Donaghue KC, Marcovecchio ML, Wadwa RP, Chew EY, Wong TY, Calliari LE, et al. ISPAD Clinical Practice Consensus Guidelines 2018: microvascular and macrovascular complications in children and adolescents. Pediatr Diabetes. 2018;19(Suppl 27):262–74.

92. Szalai E, Deak E, Modis L Jr, Nemeth G, Berta A, Nagy A, et al. Early corneal cellular and nerve fiber pathology in young patients with type 1 diabetes mellitus identified using corneal confocal microscopy. Invest Ophthalmol Vis Sci. 2016;57(3):853–8.

93. Mills SA, Hofman PL, Jiang Y, Anderson YC. Health-related quality of life of Taranaki children with type 1 diabetes. N Z Med J. 2015;128(1427):25–32.

94. Caferoglu Z, Inanc N, Hatipoglu N, Kurtoglu S. Health-related quality of life and metabolic control in children and adolescents with type 1 diabetes mellitus. J Clin Res Pediatr Endocrinol. 2016;8(1):67–73.

95. Nielsen HB, Ovesen LL, Mortensen LH, Lau CJ, Joensen LE. Type 1 diabetes, quality of life, occupational status and education level - a comparative population-based study. Diabetes Res Clin Pract. 2016;121:62–8.

96. Yi-Frazier JP, Hilliard ME, Fino NF, Naughton MJ, Liese AD, Hockett CW, et al. Whose quality of life is it anyway? Discrepancies between youth and parent health-related quality of life ratings in type 1 and type 2 diabetes. Qual Life Res. 2016;25(5):1113–21.

97. Pinhas-Hamiel O, Zeitler P. Clinical presentation and treatment of type 2 diabetes in children. Pediatr Diabetes. 2007;8(Suppl 9):16–27.

98. Zeitler P, Arslanian S, Fu J, Pinhas-Hamiel O, Reinehr T, Tandon N, et al. ISPAD Clinical Practice Consensus Guidelines 2018: type 2 diabetes mellitus in youth. Pediatr Diabetes. 2018;19(Suppl 27):28–46.

99. Druet C, Tubiana-Rufi N, Chevenne D, Rigal O, Polak M, Levy-Marchal C. Characterization of insulin secretion and resistance in type 2 diabetes of adolescents. J Clin Endocrinol Metab. 2006;91(2):401–4.

100. Hales CN, Barker DJ. The thrifty phenotype hypothesis. Br Med Bull. 2001;60:5–20.

101. Sellers EA, Dean HJ, Shafer LA, Martens PJ, Phillips-Beck W, Heaman M, et al. Exposure to gestational diabetes mellitus: impact on the development of early-onset type 2 diabetes in Canadian First Nation and Non-First Nation Offspring. Diabetes Care. 2016;39:2240.

102. Rosenbaum M, Fennoy I, Accacha S, Altshuler L, Carey DE, Holleran S, et al. Racial/ethnic differences in clinical and biochemical type 2 diabetes mellitus risk factors in children. Obesity (Silver Spring). 2013;21(10):2081–90.

103. American Diabetes Association. Type 2 diabetes in children and adolescents. Diabetes Care. 2000;23(3):381–9.

104. Valdez R, Greenlund KJ, Khoury MJ, Yoon PW. Is family history a useful tool for detecting children at risk for diabetes and cardiovascular diseases? A public health perspective. Pediatrics. 2007;120(2):S78–86.

105. Miranda-Lora AL, Vilchis-Gil J, Molina-Díaz M, Flores-Huerta S, Klünder-Klünder M. Heritability, parental transmission and environment correlation of pediatric-onset type 2 diabetes mellitus and metabolic syndrome-related traits. Diabetes Res Clin Pract. 2017;126(4):151–9.

106. Peng S, Zhu Y, Lü B, Xu F, Li X, Lai M. TCF7L2 gene polymorphisms and type 2 diabetes risk: a comprehensive and updated meta-analysis involving 121 174 subjects. Mutagenesis. 2013;28(1):25–37.

107. Dabelea D, Dolan LM, D'Agostino R Jr, Hernandez AM, McAteer JB, Hamman RF, et al. Association testing of TCF7L2 polymorphisms with type 2 diabetes in multi-ethnic youth. Diabetologia. 2011;54(3):535–9.

108. Miranda-Lora AL, Cruz M, Aguirre-Hernández J, Molina-Díaz M, Gutiérrez J, Flores-Huerta S, et al. Exploring single nucleotide polymorphisms previously related to obesity and metabolic traits in pediatric-onset type 2 diabetes. Acta Diabetol. 2017;54:653.

109. Miranda-Lora AL, Vilchis-Gil J, Juárez-Comboni DB, Cruz M, Klünder-Klünder M. A genetic risk score improves the prediction of type 2 diabetes mellitus in Mexican youths but has lower predictive utility compared with non-genetic factors. Front Endocrinol. 2021;12:647864.

110. Zeitler P, Fu J, Tandon N, Nadeau K, Urakami T, Bartlett T, et al. ISPAD Clinical Practice Consensus Guidelines 2014 Compendium. Type 2 diabetes in the child and adolescent. Pediatr Diabetes. 2014;15(Suppl. 20):26–46.

111. Xu H, Verre MC. Type 2 diabetes mellitus in children. Am Fam Physician. 2018;98(9):590–4.

112. Barlow SE. Expert committee recommendations regarding the prevention, assessment, and treatment of child and adolescent overweight and obesity: summary report. Pediatrics. 2007;120(Suppl 4):S164–S92.

113. Fitch C, Keim KS. Position of the Academy of Nutrition and Dietetics: use of nutritive and nonnutritive sweeteners. J Acad Nutr Diet. 2012;112(5):739–58.

114. Mays D, Streisand R, Walker LR, Prokhorov AV, Tercyak KP. Cigarette smoking among adolescents with type 1 diabetes: strategies for behavioral prevention and intervention. J Diabetes Complications. 2012;26(2):148–53.

115. Singhal S, Kumar S. Current perspectives on management of type 2 diabetes in youth. Children. 2021;8(1):37.

116. Lascar N, Brown J, Pattison H, Barnett AH, Bailey CJ, Bellary S. Type 2 diabetes in adolescents and young adults. Lancet Diabet Endocrinol. 2018;6(1):69–80.

117. Jones KL, Arslanian S, Peterokova VA, Park JS, Tomlinson MJ. Effect of metformin in pediatric patients with type 2 diabetes: a randomized controlled trial. Diabetes Care. 2002;25(1):89–94.

118. Lentferink YE, van der Aa MP, van Mill E, Knibbe CAJ, van der Vorst MMJ. Long-term metformin treatment in adolescents with obesity and insulin resistance, results of an open label extension study. Nutr Diabetes. 2018;8(1):47.

119. Kelsey MM, Geffner ME, Guandalini C, Pyle L, Tamborlane WV, Zeitler PS, et al. Presentation and effectiveness of early treatment of type 2 diabetes in youth: lessons from the TODAY study. Pediatr Diabetes. 2016;17(3):212–21.

120. Urakami T. Pediatric type 2 diabetes in Japan: similarities and differences from type 2 diabetes in other pediatric populations. Curr Diab Rep. 2018;18(6):29.

121. Tamborlane WV, Barrientos-Pérez M, Fainberg U, Frimer-Larsen H, Hafez M, Hale PM, et al. Liraglutide in children and adolescents with type 2 diabetes. N Engl J Med. 2019;381(7):637–46.

122. Arslanian S, Bacha F, Grey M, Marcus MD, White NH, Zeitler P. Evaluation and management of youth-onset type 2 diabetes: a position statement by the American Diabetes Association. Diabetes Care. 2018;41(12):2648–68.

123. Jensen ET, Dabelea D. Type 2 diabetes in youth: new lessons from the SEARCH study. Curr Diab Rep. 2018;18(6):36.

124. Barrett JS, Bucci-Rechtweg C, Amy Cheung SY, Gamalo-Siebers M, Haertter S, Karres J, et al. Pediatric extrapolation in type 2 diabetes: future implications of a workshop. Clin Pharmacol Ther. 2020;108(1):29–39.

125. Brandt ML, Harmon CM, Helmrath MA, Inge TH, McKay SV, Michalsky MP. Morbid obesity in pediatric diabetes mellitus: surgical options and outcomes. Nat Rev Endocrinol. 2010;6(11):637–45.

126. Inge TH, Zeller M, García VF, Daniels SR. Surgical approach to adolescent obesity. Adolesc Med Clin. 2004;15:429–53.

127. Kelly AS, Barlow SE, Rao G, Inge TH, Hayman LL, Steinberger J, et al. Severe obesity in children and adolescents: identification, associated health risks, and treatment approaches. A scientific statement from the American Heart Association. Circulation. 2013;128(15):1689–712.

128. Bondada S, Jen HC, DeUgarte DA. Outcomes of bariatric surgery in adolescents. Curr Opin Pediatr. 2011;23(5):552–6.

129. Michalsky MP, Inge TH, Teich S, Eneli I, Miller R, Brandt ML, et al. Adolescent bariatric surgery program characteristics: The Teen Longitudinal Assessment of Bariatric Surgery (Teen-LABS) study experience. Semin Pediatr Surg. 2014;23(1):5–10.

130. Nieto-Zermeño J, Flores RO, Río-Navarro BD, Salgado-Arroyo B, Molina-Díaz JM. [Efectos sobre el perfil metabólico, el índice de masa corporal, la composición corporal y la comorbilidad en adolescentes con obesidad mórbida, que han fallado al manejo conservador para bajar de peso, operados de manga gástrica laparoscópica. Reporte del primer grupo de cirugía bariátrica pediátrica en México]. Gac Med Mex. 2018;154(Suppl 2):S22–9.

131. Williams CL, Hayman LL, Daniels SR, Robinson TN, Steinberger J, Paridon S, et al. Cardiovascular health in childhood. a statement for health professionals from the Committee on Atherosclerosis, Hypertension, and Obesity in the Young (AHOY) of the Council on Cardiovascular Disease in the Young, American Heart Association. Circulation. 2002;106(1):143–60.

132. Copeland KC, Zeitler P, Geffner M, Guandalini C, Higgins J, Hirst K, et al. Characteristics of adolescents and youth with recent-onset type 2 diabetes: the TODAY cohort at baseline. J Clin Endocrinol Metab. 2011;96(1):159–67.

133. Eppens MC, Craig ME, Cusumano J, Hing S, Chan AKF, Howard NJ, et al. Prevalence of diabetes complications in adolescents with type 2 compared with type 1 diabetes. Diabetes Care. 2006;29(6):1300–6.

134. Batisky DL. What is the optimal first-line agent in children requiring antihypertensive medication? Curr Hypertens Rep. 2012;14(6):603–7.

135. Bjornstad P, Cherney DZ, Maahs DM, Nadeau KJ. Diabetic kidney disease in adolescents with type 2 diabetes: new insights and potential therapies. Curr Diab Rep. 2016;16(2):11.

136. Norman RJ, Dewailly D, Legro RS, Hickey TE. Polycystic ovary syndrome. Lancet. 2007;370(9588):685–97.

137. Nadeau KJ, Zeitler PS, Bauer TA, Brown MS, Dorosz JL, Draznin B, et al. Insulin resistance in adolescents with type 2 diabetes is associated with impaired exercise capacity. J Clin Endocrinol Metab. 2009;94(10):3687–95.

138. Rice TB, Foster GD, Sanders MH, Unruh M, Reboussin D, Kuna ST, et al. The relationship between obstructive sleep apnea and self-reported stroke or coronary heart disease in overweight and obese adults with type 2 diabetes mellitus. Sleep. 2012;35(9):1293–8.

139. Foster GD, Sanders MH, Millman R, Zammit G, Borradaile KE, Newman AB, et al. Obstructive sleep apnea among obese patients with type 2 diabetes. Diabetes Care. 2009;32(6):1017–9.

140. Walders-Abramson N. Depression and quality of life in youth-onset type 2 diabetes mellitus. Curr Diab Rep. 2014;14(1):449.

141. American Diabetes Association. 8. Pharmacologic approaches to glycemic treatment. Diabetes Care. 2017;40(Suppl 1):S64–74.

142. Onda Y, Nishimura R, Morimoto A, Sano H, Utsunomiya K, Tajima N. Age at transition from pediatric to adult care has no relationship with mortality for childhood-onset type 1 diabetes in Japan: Diabetes Epidemiology Research International (DERI) Mortality Study. PLoS One. 2016;11(3):e0150720.

Suggested Reading

ISPAD Clinical Practice Consensus Guidelines 2018. https://www.ispad.org/page/ISPADGuidelines2018. This compendium of consensus guidelines contains updates about significant advances in scientific knowledge and clinical care for pediatric and adolescent patients with diabetes mellitus.

13. Children and adolescents: standards of medical care in diabetes-2021. Diabetes Care. 2021;44(Suppl 1):S180–S199.

Pregnancy: Pregestational and Gestational Management

65

María Isabel García Argueta, Maricela González Espejel, and Joel Rodriguez-Saldana

Introduction

Gestational diabetes (GD) is defined as an alteration in carbohydrate metabolism diagnosed for the first time in the second or third trimester of gestation, it being clear that the diagnosis of same during the first trimester indicates pre-existing type 1 or 2 diabetes. The growing index of obesity is a global problem, where the main factors that unleash it are bad eating habits and sedentary lifestyle. Obesity in pregnancy is a risk factor for developing diabetes, which goes hand in hand with an increased maternal and fetal risk and hypertensive disorders. Women of a reproductive age are not the exception in regard to obesity; the U.S. National Health and Nutrition Survey (1999–2008) reveals that more than one third of the women of reproductive age are obese, and 7.6% of these women are extremely obese, with body mass indices (BMIs) equal or greater than 40; the percentage of pregnant women with obesity is estimated between 18 and 38% [1, 2]. In regard to Mexico, we have one of the highest prevalence of overweight, obesity, and diabetes in the world. Studies based on the Encuesta Nacional de Salud y Nutrición (ENSANUT, National Health and Nutrition Survey, in English) 2012 show that in the last decades, an increase has been observed in body mass and waist perimeter in the population, with a higher prevalence among young Mexican women of reproductive age, compared with other populations [3], and these changes evidently have attention-getting metabolic repercussions, above all because the female reproductive population is implicated. In consequence, pregnancy-associated diabetes is more and more frequent, and it is estimated that it significantly complicates around 1–16% of all births worldwide, depending on the population studied. The prevalence of GD has a variation directly proportional to the prevalence of type 1 diabetes (T1D) and type 2 diabetes (T2D), depending on the population under study. Other estimates indicate that 6–7% of pregnancies are complicated by this disease and that approximately 90% of the cases are represented by women with T1D and T2D. It has also been established that the highest prevalence is found among Hispanics, Afro-Americans and natives of America, Asia, and the Pacific islands [4]. Suffering GD significantly increases the risk of adverse results of the pregnancy compared with normal pregnancy: congenital malformations in 5% against 2% in the general population, perinatal mortality in 2.7% against 0.72%, premature birth in 25% against 6%, and fetal macrosomia in 54% against 10% [5]. This pregnancy complication is a growing problem for public health, with genetic, environmental, and social determinants; but obesity has a major importance as a risk factor. There exists the hypothesis that fetal overnutrition during maternal exposure GD is associated with increased overall abdominal adiposity, and a more central fat distribution pattern in 6- to 13-year-old children from a multi-ethnic population [6]. Therefore, the combination of diabetes and pregnancy is not a desirable situation due to the possible complications it incurs, so that it is necessary to detect and treat it in a timely fashion. Recent evidence suggests that there is an intrauterine programming related to hyperglycemia during pregnancy, which could explain the increased risk of metabolic alterations, obesity, and diabetes among the offspring of mothers who had a pregnancy associated with diabetes [7]. Epertise by health personnel who care pregnant women is essential primordial, and is fundamental for reducing maternal and fetal morbimortality in the pregnant diabetic. It is of vital importance to identify, from the first level of care, patients with risk factors and to implement strategies that include pre-conception and dietary counseling, promoting lifestyle changes that combat a sedentary lifestyle, and timely medical intervention with the various alternatives available [8]. Luckily the current panorama for the gestating individual has improved dramatically, since in the past a pregnant woman with diabetes was inconceivable. The dis-

M. I. G. Argueta · M. G. Espejel
72 Regional Hospital, Mexican Institute of Social Services, Mexico City, Mexico

J. Rodriguez-Saldana (✉)
Multidisciplinary Diabetes Center Mexico, Mexico City, Mexico

© The Author(s), under exclusive license to Springer Nature Switzerland AG 2023
J. Rodriguez-Saldana (ed.), *The Diabetes Textbook*, https://doi.org/10.1007/978-3-031-25519-9_65

covery of insulin in 1921 by the investigators Banting, MacLeod and Bets from the University of Toronto radically changed the prognosis for those ill with diabetes, as well as for gestating diabetes. Likewise, the use of glyburide and metformin during pregnancy, accepted in recent years, is one more tool in the treatment of pregestational and gestational diabetes. However, the pregnant woman with diabetes is exposed to high obstetric risk and elevated perinatal morbi-mortality, so it has not ceased to be a health problem.

Classification and Diagnosis

For many years, GD has been defined as an alteration in glucose metabolism, first recognized during pregnancy. In the 2016 publication of the American Diabetes Association (ADA), diabetes is classified in four general categories [9, 10]. This new classification, in contrast to the old classification by White, has greater clinical usefulness, since it is concrete, easy to remember, and applicable to diabetes during pregnancy.

1. Type 1 diabetes (T1D) which is secondary to the destruction of the beta cells of the pancreas, and in general leads to absolute insulin deficiency.
2. Type 2 diabetes (T2D) due to a progressive loss of insulin secretion.
3. GD, which is diabetes diagnosed in the second or third trimester of pregnancy and which is clearly not a previously manifested diabetes.
4. Specific diabetes, which is due to other causes, such as monogenic diabetes syndrome (such as the neonatal appearance and that in Young adults—MODY), diseases of the exocrine pancreas (like cystic fibrosis), and diabetes induced by chemical products (use of glucocorticoids after transplant or drugs for treating HIV/AIDS).

In this category, it is given as fact that both T1D and T2D may be pre-existing or pre-established in pregnancy, and that in both types there may or may not be vascular complications such as chronic hypertension, retinopathy, or nephropathy.

GD carries risks for the mother and neonate, and these risks increase with the levels of maternal glycemia after the period of pre-conception and throughout the pregnancy. GD is diagnosed based on the general criteria of the World Health Organization (WHO) of plasma glucose, or better the fasting plasma glucose and plasma glucose 2 h postprandial, or with the glucose tolerance test after ingesting 75 g of glucose orally or with the criteria of glycosylated hemoglobin (Table 65.1).

Fasting is understood as null consumption of foods for a period of 8 h; the glucose intolerance test is performed with 75 g of anhydrous glucose dissolved in water. In regard to the

Table 65.1 WHO criteria for diagnosing diabetes

Criteria	
Fasting plasma glucose	Equal or greater than 126 mg/dL (7.0 mmol/L)
Plasma glucose 2 h postprandial	Equal or greater than 200 mg/dL (11.1 mmol/L)
Glycosylated hemoglobin (A1c)	Equal or greater than 6.5% (48 mmol/L)
Random plasma glucose	Equal or greater than 200 mg/dL (11.1 mmol/L)

determination of A1c, it is worth noting that it requires standardized methods and certification for this determination.

The ADA recommends a selective screening in the first prenatal visit, where the patient risk of developing GD is stratified. The risk criteria are the following: over 25 years of age, weight above normal, first-degree family history of diabetes, background of glucose tolerance disorders, background of adverse obstetric events such as stillbirths, premature or macrosomic birth, and belonging to racial-ethnic groups at high risk for diabetes (Hispano-Americans). Patients with high risk should submit to an oral glucose tolerance test. In case of not agreeing with the diagnosis at that time, the test should be repeated between 24 and 28 weeks of gestation.

The Hyperglycemia and Adverse Pregnancy Outcomes (HAPO) study in 2008 showed evidence that the increase in just one standard deviation in fasting glucose and 2-h post-prandial levels is associated with a higher risk of birth weight above the 90 percentile, cesarean birth, neonatal hypoglycemia, blood levels of C-peptide above the 90 percentile (related to fetal hyperinsulinemia and neonatal hypoglycemia), birth before 37 weeks, shoulder dystocia or damage to the newborn, requiring intensive neonatal care, hyperbilirubinemia, and preeclampsia [11]. Consequently, after the International Association of Diabetes in Pregnancy Study Groups (IADPSG 2010) and the American Diabetes Association (ADA), proposed reducing the parameters in plasma glucose levels for the diagnosis of diabetes and a universal screening where in the first prenatal evaluation baseline glucose, glycosylated hemoglobin or casual glycemia should be determined for early detection of diabetes not recognized previously, and to start treatment and follow-up as done with previously recognized diabetes (Tables 65.2 and 65.3). It should be mentioned that ADA and the American College of Obstetricians and Gynecologists (ACOG) support the two-step strategy proposed by the National Institutes of Health (NIH) in 2013, which consists of performing a first glucose tolerance test with 50 g and in positive cases a second test with 100 g of oral glucose.

Despite differences regarding glucose levels, these diagnostic approaches have been accepted to establish the diagnosis of gestational diabetes. The results of meta-analysis comparing diagnostic criteria show similar associations in both systems, but it is evident that with the IADPSG

Table 65.2 IADPSG 2010 criteria for GD diagnosis during a glucose tolerance test with 75 g of glucose anhydrate dissolved in water

Baseline or fasting glucose	≥92 mg/dL (5.1 mmol/L)
First hour glucose	≥180 mg/dL (10.0 mmol/L)
Glucose at 2 h	≥153 mg/dL (8.5 mmol/L)

One or more of these values should be equal or greater to establish the diagnosis of diabetes

Table 65.3 Two-step strategy for the diagnosis of GD

Step 1. Perform the glucose tolerance test between weeks 24 and 28 of gestation with 50 g, without considering fasting, with determination of glucose at 1 h, in women not previously diagnosed with diabetes

    1 h ≥140 mg/dLᵃ (7.8 mmol/L), proceed to glucose tolerance curve with 100 g of glucose

Step 2. Glucose tolerance curve considering fasting, with 100 g of glucose and determinations of the first, second, and third hour

    Fasting 95–105 mg/dL (5.3–5.8 mmol/L)

    1 h 180–190 mg/dL (10.0–10.6 mmol/L)

    2 h 155–165 mg/dL (8.6–9.2 mmol/L)

    3 h 140–145 mg/dL (7.8–8.0 mmol/L)

The diagnosis is established when at least two of the four values are equal or greater

ᵃThe ACOG recommends levels below 135 mg/dL (7.5 mmol/L) in populations ethnically at high risk for GD; some experts recommend values of at least 130 mg/dL (7.2 mmol/L)

criteria, more patients are diagnosed with GD, which may lead to over-diagnosis and overtreatment. Putting the differences to one side, we do not adhere to the recommendations of ADA and IADPSG 2010, where it is established that every patient receiving prenatal care should be screened from the first prenatal visit for diabetes, preferably during the first trimester of gestation, since patients at low risk of developing GD represent barely a low percentage of the population and repeating the plasma glucose test between weeks 24 and 28 if the diagnosis is not established previously [12–14]. It is obvious that its practice will have a benefit in results that favor the pregnant woman.

Recommendations for the Diagnosis of Diabetes in the Pregnant Woman (American Diabetes Association, 2016)

1. Perform on every pregnant woman in her first visit for prenatal control a determination of fasting glucose using the standard diagnostic criteria, above all in pregnancies with risk factors in which there is not a previous diagnosis of T2D.
2. Test for a diagnosis of diabetes between weeks 24 and 28 of gestation in pregnant women not known to have previous diabetes.

3. Screening with a glucose tolerance test between weeks 6 and 12 post-partum for all women who had GD, with the object of detecting persistence of hyperglycemia and establishment of T2D.
4. Women with background of GD should have a permanent follow-up for developing diabetes or pre-diabetes at least every 3 years, since it is estimated that a considerable percentage (15–50%) of women that suffer GD develop T2D in a period of no more than 10 years.
5. All women with established history of GD or a pre-diabetic condition should receive interventions to change lifestyle or to use of metformin to prevent or delaying the development of diabetes.

Changes in Carbohydrate Metabolism in the Pregnant Woman

The metabolic changes natural in pregnancy have the object of creating an environment that allows embryogenesis, the growth of the fetus, its maturity and survival. In a normal pregnancy, directly or indirectly, the growth of the fetal placental unit increases levels of cortisol, growth hormone, human placental lactogens, estrogens, progesterone, and prolactin. In the first week of gestation, the increase in the production of estrogens and progesterone produces hyperplasia of the β cells of the pancreas, followed by an increase in the production of insulin and increased tissue sensitivity to same. This anabolism is translated into an increase in the response to insulin, which leads to fasting hypoglycemia, increased plasma lipids, hypoaminoacidemia, and a marked sensitivity to starvation. During the second half of pregnancy (particularly weeks 24–28), carbohydrate metabolism is affected by the increased production of human placental chorion gonadotropin, tumor necrosis factor α, prolactin, cortisol, and glucagon. These changes contribute to improved glucose tolerance, greater insulin resistance, reduced reserves of hepatic glycogen, and increased hepatic glycogenesis. As the gestation progresses, this response comes to be inadequate and insulin resistance is presented, which promotes a lipolysis and fasting ketonemia, as well as postprandial hyperglycemia, in which there is a greater supply of nutrients for the fetus. Placental transport of glucose is carried out through facilitated diffusion, so that maternal serum levels determine fetal levels; in a pregnancy with diabetes there is elevated fetal insulin, promoting the growth of same with increased fatty tissue and increased reserves of hepatic glycogen, which is associated with macrosomia, lipogenesis, organomegaly, polyhydramnios, etc. [15, 16]. Recently, there has been talk of leptin, which is a hormone produced mainly by fatty tissue cells, and its circulating levels are proportionate to adipose tissue mass; in the second and third trimesters of pregnancy its levels increase substantially; its role is related to mitogenic and angiogenic processes, in the regulation of immune response and in the transportation of nutrients, all important processes during placentation and embryonic development [17].

Treatment

The handling of diabetes should comprise a preventive focus in all senses; that is why it is determinant that all women of reproductive age have access to health services, information regarding reproductive health, a family planning method, methods to prevent sexually transmitted diseases, and that they are informed of the risk a pregnancy implies in association with overweight and obesity, nutritional advice during pregnancy, and the promotion of breastfeeding since abandoning this practice increases the risk of maternal overweight and obesity. Weight gain during pregnancy should be inversely proportional to the body mass index (BMI) previous to the pregnancy, so the intervention of nutritionists and dieticians is recommended in nutritional advice to achieve objectives regarding expected weight gain during pregnancy (Table 65.4).

In patients with pregestational diabetes, it is of vital importance that the pregnancy occurs in a euglycemic environment to avoid fetal complications that accompany peri-conception hyperglycemia, congenital malformations, and miscarriages being frequent. In the patient that debuts with diabetes in pregnancy, education regarding self-monitoring of glucose and the presence of ketonuria is primordial, as well as educating families in the identification of hypoglycemia data. Opportune treatment of GD will significantly reduce perinatal complications such as fetal death, congenital malformations, fetal macrosomia, shoulder dystocia, bone fractures secondary to obstetric trauma, nerve lesions, and newborns with delayed intrauterine growth; it will even be a factor that will influence the future reduction in risk of juvenile obesity in the children of mothers with diabetes. The main objective in treatment is the strict control of blood glucose levels; Table 65.5 lists the main care to which every patient with pre-existing diabetes should have access. It is worth mentioning that if the healthcare model is applied by levels, the first contact doctors are in charge of detecting those patients of reproductive age with risk factors, especially patients with pre-existing diabetes (T1D or T2D) sus-

ceptible to getting pregnant, so the pregnancy is in conditions of metabolic control, and they are referred timely to second or third level care for its management.

In countries like Mexico, it has been established that women represent an intermediate-risk group from an ethnic point of view, for developing diabetes, and therapeutic goals have been established for the treatment of GD, recommended in national Clinical Practice Guides—Guías de Práctica Clínica 2009 (GPC 2009), where the objective is to achieve blood glucose levels described in Table 65.6. The implementation of the GPC in recent years in Mexico has the goal of unifying medical criteria in the diagnosis and treatment of various pathologies.

ADA, in its publication in 2016 [18], proposes the following general recommendations for the management of patients with diabetes:

1. Offer pre-conception advice that covers the importance of glycemia control as normally and safely as possible; ideally A1c should be <6.5% with the object of reducing the risk of congenital anomalies. For the area of pregnancy in the peri-conception period and an adequate prenatal control, the gynecologist and obstetrician should recommend to the woman with pregestational type 1 and type 2 diabetes, fasting glucose levels ≤90 mg/dL (5.0 mmol/L), in the first postprandial hour ≤130–140 mg/dL (7.2–7.8 mmol/L), and at 2 h postprandial ≤120 mg/dL (6.7 mmol/L).
2. Family planning is an obligatory subject, prescribing a safe, efficient anti-conceptive method until the woman is prepared and ready to be pregnant.

Table 65.4 Expected weight gain during pregnancy in relation to BMI

Total gain at the end of pregnancy	BMI
12–18 kg (28–40 lb)	<18.5
11.5–16 kg (25–35 lb)	18.5–25
6.8–11 kg (15–25 lb)	25–30
5–9 kg (11–20 lb)	>30

Table 65.5 Pregestational and antenatal care in women with pre-existing diabetes

Pregestational
Prophylactic folic acid 3–5 mg a day
Optimization of glucose levels
Retina examination
Urine examination in search of albuminuria
Blood pressure control in the case of hypertension
Advice regarding the increase in the incidence of fetal morphological malformations and increase in the risk of severe hypoglycemia events during the first trimester of gestation
Antenatal
Adequate glucose control during pregnancy
Advice for optimum weight gain during the pregnancy, based on the mother's body mass index
Ultrasound examination in search of fetal malformations between weeks 12 and 14 and around 20 weeks
Evaluation of fetal growth (cephalic and abdominal circumference) every 4 weeks after 20 weeks and every 2 weeks after 28 weeks. Determinations of amniotic fluid
Advice on the incidence of fetal movement (perceived by the mother)
Determination of the time and birth type based on gestational age, glucose control, and estimated fetal weight

Table 65.6 Therapeutic goals in the management of GD in Mexico

Fasting glucose	60–90 mg/dL (3.3–5 mmol/L)
1 h postprandial	≤140 mg/dL (7.7 mmol/L)
2 h postprandial	≤120 mg/dL (6.6 mmol/L)
If fetal growth is equal to or greater than the 90 percentile, glycemia goals will be more strict:	
Fasting	≤80 mg/dL (4.4 mmol/L)
2 h postprandial	≤110 mg/dL (6.1 mmol/L)

Table 65.7 Dietary portions in relation to the body mass index (BMI)

Caloric portion	BMI
36–40 kcal/kg of current weight	<19.8
30 kcal/kg of current weight	19.8–26
24 kcal/kg of current weight	26–29
And should be personalized	>29

Of the total kilocalories, 40 m to 45% should correspond to carbohydrates, 20–25% proteins, and 40% or less fats, of which less than 10% should be saturated fats

3. Women with pre-existing type 1 or type 2 diabetes who plan to get pregnant or are pregnant should be advised of the risk of developing and/or the progression of diabetic retinopathy. Vision examinations before the pregnancy or in the first trimester of gestation, then every trimester, every year after the birth, and as suggested by the specialist according to the degree of retinopathy.

4. Change in lifestyle is an essential component in the management of GD and can be the first pattern for treatment.

5. Medications should be added if necessary with the goal of reaching glycemic objectives. The pharmaceuticals broadly accepted in GD are insulin and metformin; glyburide can be used, but it has a higher rate of neonatal hypoglycemia and macrosomia compared with insulin or metformin. Other agents have not been adequately studied. The majority of the oral agents cross the placenta, and all lack long-term safety data.

6. The change in lifestyle means reducing to a minimum the sedentary lifestyle and promoting adequate diet. It is of vital importance to have nutritional counseling for the patient with pre-existing diabetes or diabetes which is manifested during pregnancy, since in the majority of cases it can be sufficient to reach adequate control of glucose levels. Nutritional counseling is not exclusive to a nutritionist, since from the first office visit the doctor or prenatal nurse can orient the pregnant patient, whether or not she has diabetes. And when conditions allow it, every pregnant patient with diabetes or risk factors should be referred to a nutritionist. The recommended dietary portions are the following (Table 65.7).

Insulin

Insulin does not cross the placental barrier and has been, for many decades, the basis of treatment for glycemic control in pregnant women, and it has the consensus of various international organizations such as the American College of Obstetricians and Gynecologists (ACGO), the American Diabetes Association (ADA), and the Food and Drug Administration (FDA). It is the pharmacological intervention of first choice in GD, accepted by various organizations and countries. The insulins approved for use during pregnancy are immediate and rapid (INPH and IR), along with short-action analogues such as lispro and aspart. Not approved for use during pregnancy are long-term insulin analogues such as glargine and determir. Insulin schema may be somewhat complex to indicate to the patient, and the success of their administration depends on various factors, among them the ability of the patient and skill given before application. The total dose may vary from patient to patient, which is calculated by kilo of weight per day; if the patient is thin 0.1–0.3 IU per kilo of weight per day is considered, and if obese 0.4–0.7 IU per kilo of weight per day. At the start of pharmacotherapy, it is important to start with lower dosage, in order to avoid unexpected hypoglycemia. One common strategy for dosing consists in dividing the total dose into two applications in which 2/3 will be applied in the morning before breakfast and 1/3 before dinner. IR is added when the therapeutic goal of postprandial glycemia is not reached, in which case the morning 2/3 dose would be INPH and 1/3 rapid action, and at dinner it would be ½ INPH and ½ rapid action. This schema can be adjusted with dosage up to 1.5 IU/Kg of weight/day, according to the evolution of the patient and the time of gestation, since in the second and third trimester a greater need for insulin is expected due to the resistance found in this stage of pregnancy [19].

The Use of Oral Hypoglycemic Drugs in Pregnancy

In the United States, oral hypoglycemic drugs have not been specifically approved by the FDA for treatment in GD. However, in the last decade there has been growing scientific evidence in favor of oral hypoglycemic drugs, which, compared with insulin, have the advantage of not requiring multiple injections and therefore fewer events of hypoglycemia, as well as a lower cost. Their use during pregnancy is increasing, above all in women with GD and pre-existing T2D, and especially in women with excess weight. Glyburide and metformin are within group B of the FDA as medications for use during pregnancy. This means that reproduction studies in animals have not demonstrated risks to the fetus. There are no studies in pregnancies, but their use has been approved in pregnancy. Before prescribing any oral hypoglycemic drugs, one should remember that they cross the fetal placental barrier and, although no adverse effects to the fetus have been reported, long-term studies are scarce. Therefore, we will concentrate on the details of only two oral antidiabetics: glyburide and metformin.

Glyburide

Glyburide is a potent anti-diabetic agent belonging to the second generation of sulfonylureas and also known as glybenclamide. Its hypoglycemic drugs action is due to stimulation of beta cells in the pancreatic islets that cause an increase in the secretion of insulin. Also considered a secretagogue, it is absorbed orally and does not depend on food; it is metabolized in the liver and reaches maximum concentrations in approximately 3 h, with a half-life of 8 h. Sulfonylureas join the receptors in the ATP-dependent potassium channels, reducing the passage of potassium and producing depolarization of the membrane. This depolarization stimulates the entry of calcium through the calcium channels, increasing intracellular calcium concentrations, which in turn induces the secretion and/or exocytosis of insulin. For this drug to be effective, it requires a minimum number of viable beta cells. Prolonged administration of glyburide also causes extra-pancreatic effects that contribute to its hypoglycemic drugs activity, such as reduction of hepatic glucose production and improved insulin sensitivity in peripheral tissues, the latter due to an increase in the number of insulin receptors and more efficient union of insulin with its receptor. Glyburide reduces the circulating levels of glucose by 20% and is most efficient in patients with normal weight or slight overweight. It was the first oral hypoglycemic drugs tested and used prospectively to manage GD, and its effectiveness is similar to insulin. In comparison with insulin, it is less likely to experience maternal hypoglycemia, and only 1–15% experience symptomatic hypoglycemia. The most common side effects are at the gastrointestinal level, and include slight nausea, epigastric burning, or the sensation of fullness; dermatological ones such as a slight itch or rash and increasement in hepatic function tests that are rarely associated with icterus. The current recommended dosage is 2.5–5 mg a day or twice a day, with a maximum dose of 20 mg. Its use is not recommended if the patient is lactating, although this is not an indication for suspending lactation since lactation at the maternal breast has many benefits for both fetus and mother [20].

Metformin

This is a biguanide that has the effect of reducing insulin sensitivity. Like glyburide, metformin and other biguanides require residual function of the pancreatic β cells in order to be effective. It reduces fasting and postprandial glucose. It acts through three mechanisms: (1) it reduces hepatic production of glucose by inhibiting gluconeogenesis and glycogenolysis, (2) in muscle it increases insulin sensitivity and improves the capture of peripheral glucose, as well as its use, and (3) it delays intestinal absorption of glucose. It does not stimulate insulin secretion, so it does not provoke hypoglycemia. It is used alone or in combination with glybenclamide or with insulin. The dose is 1000–2000 mg a day, divided into two doses with food or after it. The commonly reported side effects are nausea, vomiting, and increase in intestinal movement. Its widespread use in women with pregestational diabetes, with polycystic ovary syndrome and low fertility, marked the pattern for its use in pregnant patient with diabetes. When metformin use continued into the end of the third trimester, no side effects were observed to mother or fetus associated with its consumption. Recent studies have evaluated glycemic control in women with GD treated with metformin vs. insulin and have demonstrated that metformin is an effective agent for adequate glycemic control; it was also observed that women treated with metformin have less weight gain during pregnancy [21]. Meta-analysis studies have established that metformin has efficacy and safety similar to insulin in terms of neonatal hypoglycemia; the frequency of products with higher weight for gestational age, newborn entry into phototherapy, respiratory stress syndrome, and perinatal death. Metformin is safe in regard to incidence of peaks in hypoglycemia. However, it is necessary to state that there is a need for additional studies, with greater sample sizes that evaluate the long-term effect on children born to women with GD treated with metformin [22, 23]. Metformin is excreted in human mother's milk. No adverse effects have been observed in newborns or breastfed babies. However, as there is only limited data available, breastfeeding is not recommended during treatment with metformin. Each individual case should be decided as to interruption of breastfeeding, taking into account that the benefits of maternal breastfeeding are greater compared with the potential risk of adverse effects in the breastfed.

Management of Pregnancy

To date there is no consensus regarding how to solve pregnancy of the patient with diabetes, and most is based on recommendations and points of good practice. Every patient with GD should be referred for its control and treatment from the moment this diagnosis is known, to a second or third level hospital that has a multidisciplinary team that includes the services of obstetrics, perinatology, endocrinology, nutrition and diet, social work, psychology, etc. Structural ultrasound should be performed between weeks 18 and 22, to discard fetal malformations, and series of ultrasounds every 4 weeks with measurement of fetal abdominal perimeter at the start of the third trimester to identify fetuses with greater risk of macrosomia. At week 32 of gestation cardiotocographic tests should start without stress once a week and increase to twice a week from week 36. There should be evaluations by ultrasound of amniotic fluid levels, estimated weight, and fetal abdominal perimeter. There is no evidence-based medication regarding the decision to induce labor or keep waiting, but this is a decision that worries the obstetrician since in these patients there is a higher rate of intrauterine fetal death and higher risk of shoulder dystocia associated with fetal macrosomia. In addition, the fetus may have greater weight for gestational age, situation that can cause confusion at the time of deciding the time for interruption and conditions a premature birth that has hyaline membrane and respiratory stress. These patients have four times more mortality compared with nondiabetic pregnancy. Scheduling the birth by cesarean to avoid obstetric trauma is normally offered to patients with GD in order to prevent cases of obstetric trauma in newborns with macrosomia. Induced labor at term may have a success rate of 80%, but with a significantly higher rate of cesareans compared with uncomplicated pregnancies. Studies recommend the induction of labor at 39 weeks of gestation for women with glucose levels controlled with insulin or oral hypoglycemic drugs [24, 25]. During labor in patients with pre-existing or gestational diabetes, glucose levels should be monitored and maintained at a range between 70 and 110 mg/dL (3.6–6.1 mm/L), ranges that are recommended by ACOG and the American College of Endocrinology (ACE) [26], since high levels of glucose during labor have been associated with a greater risk of neonatal hypoglycemia. Achieving this goal requires glucose intravenous solutions and continuous insulin infusions or else rapid action insulin previous to capillary glucose medication. The demands for glucose as a source of energy increase during labor, contrary to the many institutions that restrict caloric consumption due to the risk of maternal aspiration. Women with T1D require glucose supplements to maintain adequate blood values in order to reduce cetoacidosis. Women with T2D and GD may have sufficient reserves of glycogen to maintain glucose levels around 70 mg/dL, during the latent phase of labor, without the need for glucose supplementation. However, glucose requirements increase during the prolonged induction of labor, active labor, and during the expulsion phase. Neonate should be monitored regarding hypoglycemia, hypocalcemia, and hyperbilirubinemia. In the post-labor phase, women should be able to restart normal diet. After birth, the hyperglycemic effects of placental hormones quickly disappear and plasma glucose levels return to normal, but it is recommended to test glucose concentrations for the first 24–72 h with capillary glucose to exclude persistent hyperglycemia in the post-birth period. Women with a background of GD should have follow-up for the next 6–12 weeks' post-birth with a glucose tolerance test to discard diabetes or carbohydrate intolerance, since it is estimated that 70% of these women have a risk of developing T2D up to 10 years later [27]. Maternal breastfeeding alone the first 6 months and complementary until 2 years offers benefits that prolong the effects of intrauterine hyperglycemic environment in newborns and infants of mothers with obesity or diabetes; likewise, it has benefits in maternal glucose metabolism that prevents or delays the establishment of metabolic syndrome or T2D [28, 29].

Conclusions

Women in whom GD is diagnosed should be treated with nutrition therapy and, when necessary, medication for both fetal and maternal benefit. Insulin and oral antidiabetics have equivalent in efficacy, and either can be an appropriate first-line therapy in GD. During the first trimester of gestation all pregnant women should be screened for GD, whether by the patients medical history, clinical risk factors, or laboratory screening test results to determine blood glucose levels. Women with GD should be counseled regarding the option of scheduled cesarean delivery when the estimated fetal weight is 4500 g or more. Women with GD with good glycemic control and no other complications can be managed expectantly. In most cases, women with good glycemic control who are receiving medical therapy do not require delivery before 39 weeks of gestation. Postpartum screening at 6–12 weeks is recommended for all women who had GD to identify women with T2D, impaired fasting glucose, or glucose tolerance test repeat testing at least every 3 years.

Multiple-Choice Questions

1. Gestational diabetes is defined as:
   (a) The lipid metabolism disorder during all of pregnancy.
   (b) **Carbohydrate metabolism alteration first diagnosed in the second or third trimester of gestation.**
   (c) Amino acid metabolism alteration after the second half of pregnancy.
   (d) Carbohydrate metabolism alteration first diagnosed in the first or second trimester of gestation.
   (e) Carbohydrate metabolism alteration first diagnosed in the third trimester of gestation.
2. The growing index of obesity is a global problem; bad dietary habits and sedentary lifestyle are the main factors unleashing the development of GD.
   (a) False.
   (b) **True.**
   (c) Only obesity is a factor.

(d) Only bad dietary habits.

(e) Only a sedentary lifestyle.

3. What percentage of pregnancies are complicated by diabetes?

    (a) **6–7%**

    (b) 50%

    (c) 1%

    (d) 90%

    (e) 20%

4. In GD, it is known that there is a risk factor related to ethnicity. Which populations are most susceptible to suffering GD?

    (a) **Hispanics, Afro-Americans, Native Americans, Asians and Pacific Islanders.**

    (b) Nordics and Africans.

    (c) Asians, French and Russians.

    (d) Muslims.

5. The following is true in regard to the classification of diabetes, as published by ADA 2016.

    (a) Type 1 diabetes (T1D) is secondary to the destruction of the beta cells of the pancreas and leads to absolute insulin deficiency.

    (b) Type 2 diabetes (T2D) is due to a progressive loss of insulin secretion.

    (c) GD is diabetes diagnosed in the second or third trimester of pregnancy which is not a clearly manifested diabetes.

    (d) Specific diabetes is due to other causes, such as monogenic diabetes syndrome (such as neonatal appearance diabetes and in youths—MODY), diseases of exocrine pancreas (such as cystic fibrosis), and diabetes induced by chemical products (use of glucocorticoids after transplant or drugs for HIV/AIDS).

    (e) **All of the above.**

6. Are risk factors for developing GD?

    (a) Age under 25 years, weight below normal, family history of breast cancer.

    (b) Age over 35 years, history of stillbirth and sterility.

    (c) **Age over 25 years, weight above normal, first-degree family history of diabetes, background of glucose intolerance, history of adverse obstetric events such as stillbirth, prematurity or macrosomies and belonging to ethno-racial groups at high risk for diabetes (Hispano-Americans).**

    (d) Background of previous pregnancies with fetal microsomia.

    (e) Background of previous births with intrauterine death.

7. What percentage of women that suffer GD develop type 2 diabetes in a lapse of no more than 10 years?

    (a) **15–50%**

    (b) 1%

    (c) 0%

    (d) 100%

    (e) 3%

8. Diagnosis criteria for GD during a glucose tolerance test with 75 g of glucose dissolved in water of the IADPSG 2010:

    (a) Fasting glucose equal or greater than 200 mg/dL (5.1 mmol/L), glucose at the first hour equal or greater than 180 mg/dL (10.0 mmol/L), glucose at 2 h equal or greater than 153 mg/dL (8.5 mmol/L), one or more of these values to establish diagnosis.

    (b) **Fasting glucose equal or greater than 92 mg/dL (5.1 mmol/L), glucose at 1 h equal or greater than 180 mg/dL (10.0 mmol/L), glucose at 2 h equal or greater than 153 mg/dL (8.5 mmol/L), one or more of these values to establish the diagnosis.**

    (c) Fasting glucose equal or greater than 300 mg/dL (5.1 mmol/L), glucose at 1 h equal or greater than 180 mg/dL (10.0 mmol/L), glucose at 2 h equal or greater than 153 mg/dL (8.5 mmol/L), one or more of these values to establish diagnosis.

    (d) Fasting glucose equal or greater than 400 mg/dL (5.1 mmol/L), glucose at 1 h equal or greater than 180 mg/dL (10.0 mmol/L), glucose at 2 h equal or greater than 153 mg/dL (8.5 mmol/L), one or more of these values to establish diagnosis.

    (e) Fasting glucose equal or greater than 500 mg/dL (5.1 mmol/L), glucose at 1 h equal or greater than 180 mg/dL (10.0 mmol/L), glucose at 2 h equal or greater than 153 mg/dL (8.5 mmol/L), one or more of these values to establish diagnosis.

9. The insulin dose for GD is:

    (a) **The total dose may vary from patient to patient, which is calculated for kilo of weight per day; if the patient is thin use 0.1–0.3 IU per kilo of weight per day and if obese, 0.4–0.7 IU per kilo of weight per day.**

    (b) The total dose may vary from patient to patient, which is calculated for kilo of weight per day; if the patient is thin use 1–2 IU per kilo of weight per day and if obese, 0.4–0.7 IU per kilo of weight per day.

    (c) The total dose may vary from patient to patient, which is calculated for kilo of weight per day; if the patient is thin use 0.1–0.3 IU per kilo of weight per day and if obese, 1–2 IU per kilo of weight per day.

    (d) The total dose may vary from patient to patient, which is calculated for kilo of weight per day; if the patient is thin use 3 IU per kilo of weight per day and if obese, 4 IU per kilo of weight per day.

    (e) The total dose may vary from patient to patient, which is calculated for kilo of weight per day; if the patient is thin use 5 IU per kilo of weight per day and if obese, 3 IU per kilo of weight per day.

10. Of oral hypoglycemic drugs, the following is false:

    (a) In the last decade, there is growing scientific evidence in favor of oral hypoglycemic drugs to manage GD, which in comparison with insulin have the advantage of not requiring multiple injections; there are fewer events of hypoglycemia and the cost is lower.

    (b) Glyburide is a potent anti-diabetic agent belonging to a second generation of sulfonylureas and also known as glybenclamide. It is a biguanide that reduces insulin sensitivity.

    (c) Like glyburide, metformin and other biguanides require residual function of the beta cells of the pancreas to be effective in managing GD and T2D.

    (d) The current recommended dose of glyburide is 2.5–5 mg a day or twice a day, with a maximum dose of 20 mg. The recommended dose of metformin is 1000–2000 mg a day, divided into two doses with food or after same.

    (e) **No oral hypoglycemic drugs should be used in treating GD.**

Glossary

ACOG The American College of Obstetricians and Gynecologists.

ADA The American Diabetes Association.

BMI is the result of dividing the weight of a person in kilograms by the square of his height in meters.

Congenital malformations are anatomic alterations that occur in the intrauterine stage and may be alterations in organs, extremities, or systems, due to environmental, genetic factors, deficiencies in nutrient capture, or consumption of noxious substances.

ENSANUT 2012 National health and nutrition survey 2012 (Mexico).

FDA The Food and Drug Administration.

Fetal macrosomia Traditionally, fetal macrosomia has been defined as arbitrary weight at birth, such as 4000, 4100, 4500, or 4536 g. It is currently defined as a fetus that is large for gestational age (>90 percentile).

GD Gestational diabetes, which is defined as alteration in carbohydrate metabolism diagnosed for the first time in the second or third trimester of gestation.

HAPO Study Hyperglycemia and Adverse Pregnancy Outcomes study.

IADPSG The International Association of Diabetes in Pregnancy Study Groups.

Insulin From the Latin "isla." It is a polypeptide hormone formed by 51 amino acids, produced and secreted by the beta cells of the Isles of Langerhans of the pancreas. Discovered by Frederick Grant Banting, Charles Best, James Collip, and J.J.R. Macleod of the University of Toronto, Canada, in 1921.

NIH National Institutes of Health.

Obesity Obesity and overweight are defined as abnormal or excessive accumulation of fat that may prejudice health. A simple way to measure obesity is the body mass index (BMI), which is the weight of a person divided by height in meters squared. A person with BMI equal or above 30 is considered obese and with a BMI equal or greater than 25 is considered overweight.

Oral hypoglycemic drugs Anti-diabetes drugs which are classified as sulfonylureas, biguanides, alpha-glucosidase inhibitors, meglytinids (Repaglinide, Nateglinide), and thiazolidinediones.

Perinatal mortality is the fetus and newborn risk of dying as a consequence of the reproductive process.

Premature birth According to WHO, birth that occurs after week 20 and before 37 complete weeks.

T1D Type 1 diabetes, which is secondary to the destruction of the beta cells of the pancreas, and in general leads to absolute insulin deficiency.

T2D Type 2 diabetes, which is due to a progressive loss of insulin secretion.

WHO World Health Organization.

Women of reproductive age Women between 15 and 44 years.

References

1. Liat S, Cabrero L, Hod M, Yogev Y. Obesity in obstetrics. Best Pract Res Clin Obstet Gynaecol. 2015;29:79–90.
2. Aviram A, Hod M, Yogev Y. Maternal obesity: implications for pregnancy outcome and long-term risks—a link to maternal nutrition. Int J Gynecol Obstet. 2011;115(Suppl. 1):S6–S10.
3. Albrecht SS, Barquera S, Popkin BM. Exploring secular changes in the association between BMI and waist circumference in Mexican-origin and white women: a comparison of Mexico and the United States. Am J Hum Biol. 2014;26:627–34.
4. Practice Bulletin. Gestational diabetes mellitus. Obstet Gynecol. 2013;122(2 Part 1):406–16.
5. McCance DR. Diabetes in pregnancy. Best Pract Res Clin Obstet Gynaecol. 2015;29:685–99.
6. Lawrence JM. Women with diabetes in pregnancy: different perceptions and expectations. Best Pract Res Clin Obstet Gynaecol. 2011;25:15–24.
7. Crume TL, Ogden L, West NA, et al. Association of exposure to diabetes in utero with adiposity and fat distribution in a multiethnic population of youth: The Exploring Perinatal Outcomes among Children (EPOCH) Study. Diabetologia. 2011;54:87–92.
8. Hadar E, Ashwal E, Hod M. The preconceptional period as an opportunity for prediction and prevention of non-communicable disease. Best Pract Res Clin Obstet Gynaecol. 2015;29:54–62.
9. American Diabetes Association. Classification and diagnosis of diabetes. Sec. 2. In standards of medical care in diabetes 2016. Diabetes Care. 2016;39(Suppl 1):S13–22.
10. Sacks DA, Metzger BE. Classification of diabetes in pregnancy. Time to reassess the alphabet. Obstet Gynecol. 2013;121(2):345–8.
11. The HAPO Study Cooperative Research Group. Hyperglycemia and adverse pregnancy outcomes. N Engl J Med. 2008;358(19):1991–2002.

12. Ogunyemi DA, Fong A, Rad S, Fong S, Kjos SL. Attitudes and practices of health care providers regarding gestational diabetes: results of a survey conducted at the 2010 meeting of the International Association of Diabetes in Pregnancy Study Group (IADPSG). Diabet Med. 2011;28(8):976–86.

13. Wendland EM, Torloni MR, Falavigna M, et al. Gestational diabetes and pregnancy outcomes – a systematic review of the World Health Organization (WHO) and the International Association of Diabetes in Pregnancy Study Groups (IADPSG) diagnostic criteria. BMC Pregnancy Childbirth. 2012;12:23. https://doi.org/10.1186/1471-2393-12-23.

14. McIntyre HD, Metzger BE, Coustan DR, et al. Counterpoint: establishing consensus in the diagnosis of GDM following the HAPO study. Curr Diab Rep. 2014;14:497.

15. Buchanan TA. Intermediary metabolism during pregnancy: implication for diabetes mellitus. In: Le Roith D, Olefsky JM, Tyalor SI, editors. Diabetes mellitus: a fundamental and clinical text. 3rd ed. Philadelphia: Wolters Kluwer Health; 2003. p. 1237–50. Pro Quest Library.

16. Thomas A. Buchanan. Effects of maternal diabetes mellitus on intrauterine development. In: Le Roith, Derek, Olefsky, Jerrold M., and Tyalor, Simeon I. Diabetes mellitus: a fundamental and clinical text (3). Philadelphia: Wolters Kluwer Health, 2003: p. 1251–1264. Pro Quest Library.

17. Tessier DR, Ferraro ZM, Gruslin A. Role of leptin in pregnancy: consequences of maternal obesity. Placenta. 2013;34:205–11.

18. American Diabetes Association. Management of diabetes in pregnancy. Sec.12. In standards of medical care in diabetes. Diabetes Care. 2016;39(Suppl 1):S94–8.

19. Guía de Práctica Clínica. Diagnóstico y Tratamiento de la Diabetes en el Embarazo. México: Secretaria de Salud; 2009.

20. Berggren EK, Boggess KA. Oral agents for the management of gestational diabetes. Clinical Obstet Gynecol. 2013;56(4):827–36.

21. Spaulonci CP, Bernardes LS, Trindade TC, et al. Randomized trial of metformin vs insulin in the management of gestational diabetes. Am J Obstet Gynecol. 2013;209:34.e1–7.

22. Zhao LP, Sheng XY, Zhou S, Yang T, Ma LY, Zhou Y, Cui YM. Metformin versus insulin for gestational diabetes mellitus: a metaanalysis. Br J Clin Pharmacol. 2015;80(5):1224–34.

23. Singh AK, Singh R. Metformin in gestational diabetes: an emerging contender. Indian J Endocrinol Metab. 2015;19(2):236–44.

24. Korkmazer E, Solak N, Tokgöz VY. Gestational diabetes: screening, management, timing of delivery. Curr Obstet Gynecol Rep. 2015;4:132–8.

25. Benhalima K, Devlieger R, Van Assche A. Screening and management of gestational diabetes. Best Pract Res Clin Obstet Gynaecol. 2015;29:339–49.

26. Garrison EA, Jagasia S. Inpatient management of women with gestational and pregestational diabetes in pregnancy. Curr Diab Rep. 2014;14:457.

27. Theodoraki A, Baldeweg SE. Symposium on diabetes. Gestational diabetes mellitus. Br J Hosp Med. 2008;69(10):562–7.

28. Gunderson EP. Breastfeeding after gestational diabetes pregnancy. Diabetes Care. 2007;30(S2):S161–8.

29. Trout KK, Averbuch T, Barowski M. Promoting breastfeeding among obese women and women with gestational diabetes mellitus. Curr Diab Rep. 2011;11(7):7–12.

Further Reading

American Diabetes Association. 14. Management of diabetes in pregnancy: standards of medical Care in diabetes – 2021. Diabetes Care. 2021;44(Supp 1):S200–10.

NICE. National Institute of Clinical Excellence. Diabetes in pregnancy: management from preconception to the postnatal period. nice.org.uk. Last updated 16 Dec 2021.

Priya G, Bajaj S, Kalra B, Coetzee A, Kalra S, Dutta D, et al. Clinical practice recommendations for the detection and management of hyperglycemia in pregnancy from South Asia, Africa and Mexico during COVID-19 pandemic. J Family Med Prim Care. 2021;10:4350–63.

Willy Marcos Valencia

Diabetes in Older Adults

Diabetes is chronic and progressive, with increasing prevalence in older age groups [1]. Moreover, with longer disease duration, there is greater risk to develop its complications. In parallel, aging itself increases the risk for age-related or age-dependent chronic diseases, such as cardiovascular [2], cancer [3], depression [4], dementia [5], and frailty (increased vulnerability and poor health outcomes) [6]. Ultimately, the scenario of diabetes in the older adult is more complex and complicated than in younger age groups, with heterogeneous presentations at the real clinic setting, even for subjects of the same age and similar comorbidities [7].

There will be two billion people older than 60 by the year 2050, from which 434 million will be older than 80, and about 1 out of 4 will have diabetes [8]. Therefore, we need to increase our understanding and dissemination toward better, safer, effective, and efficient approaches to this group.

To accomplish this goal, it is necessary to enhance the understanding of diabetes and aging in the older population. Figure 66.1 offers a magnified visual perspective, aiming to summarize the multiple factors that ought to be considered when evaluating an older patient with diabetes.

Geriatric Considerations in the Management of Diabetes in the Older Adult

The guidelines from the American Diabetes Association (ADA, Chap. 11) [14] provide multiple recommendations and considerations to expand the approach to diabetes especially for this age group. Notably, this approach was built upon a consensus by experts from both the ADA and the American Geriatrics Society (AGS) [15]. What might be the most valuable contribution is the framework to stratify patients according to their health status and disease burden (summarized in the form of a table), which was then adopted by the ADA guidelines.

The framework (presented as a table) provides clinicians with a practical framework how to stratify their patients, and from there, individualize targets and therapies. This approach offers a tool to disseminate the need for individualization of targets and therapies based on factors that go beyond the presence of macrovascular complications.

Nevertheless, while there can be other suggested approaches, including those for specific settings such as long-term care [16], we recommend clinicians to take advantage from this framework, especially intended to those teams without formal training in geriatrics.

The approach stratifies patients in three settings. A reasonable approach to present this information would be as follows:

The healthy older adult: As long as there are no major multiple and/or life-threatening diseases, and in the absence of functional or cognitive deficit, these older adults could potentially benefit from approaches similar to those of younger age. We recommend considering factors such as life expectancy, in addition to patient-centered discussions for preferences and feasibility of implementing escalating strategies to achieve the desired targets. As with everything in geriatrics, the principle of "start low, and go slow" will also apply in this setting. On the other hand, having such patient with uncontrolled diabetes and not providing further interventions would be consistent with clinical inertia, which can also be observed in this population.

The older adult with severely complex health scenario: This is the third situation, in which older patients are enduring multiple severe chronic diseases, with impairment in physical function (activities of daily living) and memory disorders. Many are already in long-term care, or palliative care, or are eligible for those services.

W. M. Valencia (✉)
Medical University of South Carolina, Charleston, SC, USA
e-mail: valenciw@musc.edu

© The Author(s), under exclusive license to Springer Nature Switzerland AG 2023
J. Rodriguez-Saldana (ed.), *The Diabetes Textbook*, https://doi.org/10.1007/978-3-031-25519-9_66

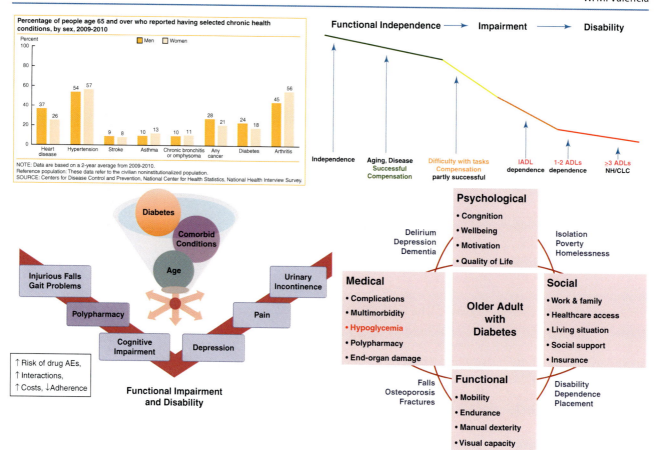

Fig. 66.1 A geriatrics approach to understanding diabetes in the older adult. On the left upper corner, the prevalence of chronic diseases increases in the older population [9]. Beyond the traditional diabetes-related complications, older adults with diabetes will also have a variety of multiple other chronic diseases, increasing their pharmacologic needs and regimens, the risk for drug-to-drug and drug-to-disease interactions. Thus, their diabetes care will start at a higher level of burden, complexity, and impact to their lives. On the right upper corner, a simplified yet powerful depiction on how function changes, and declines, throughout the lifespan of a person (slide courtesy of Hermes Florez, based on literature from Verbrugge et al. [10]). Younger patients will usually be considered as independent and able to compensate for the disease burden (granted there will be a spectrum of reactions). In this setting, providers would usually give for granted the young patients' ability to take care of themselves. On the other hand, with accumulating/worsening chronic diseases, all human beings go through an aging process that culminates with certain death. Excluding those who may suffer an acute fatal event (e.g., sudden cardiac death or accidents), the rest will go through a progressive course of functional decline (some earlier, other later). Clinicians must recognize that these processes are very heterogeneous, and for those unable to compensate, there will be a loss of the ability to carry the instrumental activities of daily living (or IADLs), which include managing medications. On the left lower corner, the additive effects of diabetes, aging, and multimorbidity can be associated with a variety of geriatric syndromes, further increasing the risk for progressive functional decline and disability (slide courtesy of Hermes Florez, based on literature from Laiteerapong et al. [11]). Hence, considering the physical/mental decline, in the setting of multiple diseases and complex regimens, the negative consequences also include greater risks for adverse complications (e.g., hypoglycemia), poor quality of life, and increased social and economic burden [12]. Finally, on the right lower corner, a previously presented visual summary of our geriatrics approach to the older adult with diabetes [7]. The four geriatric domains are intertwined, especially in the setting of this chronic disease, causing complications of its own (within the medical domain), and also interacting with the functional, mental/psychological, and social domains. The arrows go in both directions. From one side, diabetes fosters new medical issues (e.g., diabetes leading to depression leading to poor motivation and poor quality of life), and on the other direction, situations that hinder diabetes management (e.g., poor family support leading to social isolation leading to poor diabetes control). In summary, the clinical scenario of an older adult with diabetes, and multimorbidity, impaired physical and cognitive function (both a consequence from diabetes itself, or associated with age-related diseases), will have implications and consequences for diabetes self-management and self-efficacy, quality of life, and increasing vulnerability [13]. Hence, the need to implement strategies that can counter the challenges, while adjusting therapeutic targets and interventions. To do so, provider caring for older adults with diabetes will benefit from gaining insights to the "geriatrics field"

Then, the scenario in between, defined for older patients with chronic diseases but still independent, without severe physical or cognitive dysfunction, and preserved activities of daily living, but might have issues with instrumental activities of daily living (which include management of medications).

One of the most striking points from this framework is that geriatric syndromes (falls and urinary incontinence) are determinant factors and need to be incorporated in the assessment and plan. Note that clinicians need not become Geriatricians, but rather incorporate some geriatric approaches to the care of older patients with diabetes.

Geriatric Syndromes and Assessments for Older Patients with Diabetes

In order to effectively apply the framework from ADA/AGS as discussed in the prior section, we need to expand the description of geriatric syndromes and the comprehensive geriatrics assessment. Noteworthy, addressing, assessing, and incorporating these factors into the care of an older patient with diabetes will be feasible to conduct, even at a busy clinic setting.

As previously established, older age and the aging process lead to greater risk for developing chronic medical diseases, functional and cognitive decline, and then, the geriatric syndromes. These geriatric syndromes, while being syndromes, can have multifactorial etiologies, but usually share common risk factors and pathophysiologic mechanisms. Screening and detection is a key factor for management, even if the final diagnosis is not ultimately defined [17].

Considering the setting of diabetes, we can map them all to the heightened burden produced by long-standing disease, especially if complications presented. The geriatric syndromes include polypharmacy, urinary incontinence, impaired mobility, falls, frailty, persistent pain, cognitive impairment, and depression, and they add further complexity to older patient with diabetes [17–19]. Progression in these syndromes lead to poor quality of life and loss of independence, a situation where patients will require assistance to care for themselves, and even transition to institutionalization of different types (assisted living facilities, community living centers, or nursing homes).

The connection between diabetes and geriatric syndromes has been described. For example, a French study of 987 older patients (age ≥ 70) with diabetes found that both macrovascular [20] and microvascular [21] complications were associated with cognitive function, nutritional risk, and evidence for self-care deficit. The authors highlighted the multiple and potential bidirectional pathways between cardiovascular disease and geriatric syndromes.

Table 66.1 presents a distribution of geriatric syndromes within each of the four geriatric domains. This operationalization is solely for practical purposes, since in reality, there will be significant overlap (one syndrome connected to more than one domain), related to pathophysiology and outcomes.

Medical Domain

Polypharmacy: There are several ways to define polypharmacy (based on the total number of medications, the number of medications for one condition and the use of medications that are not justified by benefits over risks) [22]. However, it is easy to understand how an older person with diabetes and diabetes-associated complications will likely meet the first two definitions, just by following the standard-of-care treatment [23]. The issue is that as these medications accumulate, polypharmacy leads to increased costs and non-adherence [24], and non-adherence leads to uncontrolled glycemic control. Moreover, increased economic costs lead to mental preoccupation/anxiety as well as socioeconomic burden.

Each visit is an opportunity to review the medication profile, and ensure (1) patient knowledge and justification for each medication, (2) advise against non-required over the counter, and (3) promptly adjust therapeutic interventions, striving to reduce medications when there is no certainty that the benefits outweigh the risks. Moreover, the patient can be further engaged in self-management as improvements in lifestyle could be clinically significant enough and warrant fewer medications, ultimately improving diabetes and patient-centered goals.

Unfortunately, polypharmacy will be quite prevalent in the older population with diabetes, and will often be related to other geriatric syndromes such as falls [25, 26], which will be further reviewed in a subsequent section. Additionally, a vast majority of older patients with diabetes will have an indication for an antihypertensive medication, with indications ranging from primary/secondary prevention of diabetic nephropathy in normotensive patients, all the way to established hypertension, heart disease, and others. The key factor will be to ensure the patients do not have orthostatic hypotension, and to adjust pharmacologic therapies accordingly. Most notably, these changes can greatly benefit the patient. Decreasing psychotropic agents and polypharmacy reduces the risk for falls [27, 28].

Multimorbidity: The accumulation of multiple chronic diseases is a common scenario in the older patient [29], but not always associated with non-disease-based physical limitations [30]. Hence, their presentation and impact is highly variable, leading to different health status, between individuals, and over time. Most notably, different older persons with similar conditions may present with different clinical status.

Table 66.1 Geriatric syndromes within the four geriatric domains

Medical	Functional	Psychological	Social
Polypharmacy	Impaired mobility	Dementia	Social isolation
Multimorbidity	Falls	Depression	Homelessness
Malnutrition	Urinary incontinence	Poor quality of life	Food insecurity
	Frailty		
	Self-care deficit		

Researchers have modeled the disease clusters from 750 aging patients, and found that older patients with established cardiovascular disease and highest burden of comorbidities (≥6 per their study) will benefit less from intensive regimens [31]. From our standpoint, we agree with this concept, consistent with the different strata presented in the ADA/AGS framework, but emphasize that the "paper can be deceiving." Before meeting a new patient, most clinicians review the clinical information available in medical records, and we have found a very heterogeneous presentation of health status, beyond the records, based on physical and cognitive function. Notwithstanding, chronic medical conditions might impact daily functioning and health-related quality of life (HRQOL). Older adults with longer disease duration, or uncontrolled disease, with complications, will be at greater risk for impaired daily functioning and poor HRQOL.

Nutritional Status: While this is not a geriatric syndrome per se, we need to unveil, even if only briefly, the associated syndromes of frailty with sarcopenic obesity. Diabetes is associated with obesity as we age [32]. Many older patients with diabetes, as they age, and as they develop functional impairment due to the diabetes and its complications and other age-related problems, then remain with increased weight, but endure changes in body composition, with loss of lean mass. Obesity itself affects all four geriatric domains, and if left untreated, leads to a vicious cycle of progressive deterioration of physical activity, function, worsening of diseases, further weight gain, and further worsening of this "setting" [33]. Consequently, the success on diabetes management will be challenged by the persistence of such negative scenarios in the geriatric population.

Malnutrition

On the other hand, despite the obesity epidemic and the clear relationship between obesity, insulin resistance, and diabetes, the proportion of malnutrition risk is similar in subjects with diabetes than in others in the community [34] and in hospital [35]. In other words, older patients with obesity may suffer from macro- and micronutrient deficiency. Moreover, in connection to the aging process and concomitant chronic diseases, the risks for malnutrition are greater in this age group. It has even been shown that diabetes in stroke patients is a risk factor for malnutrition, probably due to dietary restriction and higher rate of dysphagia [36]. Thus, oral health and swallowing capacities must be checked. Particularly, oral candidiasis must be searched and treated and patient referred to dentist surgeon. Nutritional interventions and lifestyle changes need to be adapted to individualized nutritional risks.

Functional Domain

Diabetes is associated with early declines in physical function [37]. Hence, older patients with long-standing disease have been exposed to diabetes-related decline, apart from the "expected" age-related decline.

Moreover, dexterity and physical capacity are needed to perform diabetes self-management (for instance, visual loss can impair the ability to read glucose results and inject insulin units). Tools such as the insulin delivery systems, with training for those with visual impairment, can be implemented to allow the person to maintain independence in the management of diabetes.

Within this domain, we assess the geriatric syndromes of falls, impaired mobility, functional decline, vision loss, and hearing loss, which are among the most common geriatric syndromes. More recently, the frailty syndrome continues gaining increasing attention, and the future might have evidence to support that frailty ought to be included in the framework as well as falls and urinary incontinence.

Impaired Mobility

The most common risk factors are older age, low physical activity, strength or balance impairment, and chronic diseases such as obesity, diabetes, and osteoarthritis [38]. Hence, unsurprisingly, mobility impairment is common in older adults. Unfortunately, with diabetes and other diseases sharing mutual risk factors, and in itself, counters the potential for disease prevention. Clinicians need to assess and understand the impact from impaired mobility, dexterity, and function to define the most appropriate plan of care.

Self-Care Deficit and Functional Decline

The assessment of Instrumental Activities of Daily Living (IADLs) [39] explores capacities to live in an autonomous way at home. These activities include shopping, cooking, household cleaning/laundry, telephone use, managing medications, finances, and driving/using public transportation. The inability to carry at least two or more IADLs would place a patient in the second category from the ADA guidelines. Nevertheless, limitations on these IADLs can be supplemented through informal (family/friends) or formal support (e.g., home health nurse to assist with medication management). The assessment of Activities of Daily Living (ADLs) [40] explores the actions to take care of basic needs without help. These include dressing, toileting, bathing, eating, and getting around the home. Limitations in two or more ADLs are consistent with the highest complexity in the ADA model, and glycemic targets are further increased. These limitations are also consistent with nursing home level of care. However, again, these limitations can be supplemented by formal or informal support, with the main objective to keep the patient at home. Often, structural modifications are helpful.

The dependency in IADLs is mainly associated with cognitive troubles. Particular attention should be given to the capacities to self-manage medications. Care plan can be adjusted based on the outcomes from this assessment. Sensory loss, particularly but not only visual loss, can impact diabetes self-management and self-efficacy. When detected, referral to specialist and subsequent intervention may facilitate the management of diabetes in the older person.

Falls

Due to the strong connection between diabetes and falls, we decided to expand this section. Falls are generally driven by a combination of intrinsic (the person's characteristics) and extrinsic (exogenous, the environment) factors. Falls risk is already increased by age (without diabetes), due to age-related decline in gait, balance, proprioception, and sarcopenia [41, 42]. In addition, there are multiple mechanisms by which diabetes and its complications increase the risk for falls. Diabetes can contribute in several ways to the intrinsic factors, impairing gait (diabetic peripheral polyneuropathy, diabetic peripheral vascular disease and amputations, neuropathic pain), vision (diabetic retinopathy), judgment (dementia in diabetes), balance (autonomic dysfunction), and the combination of impaired judgment and balance (pharmacotherapy and hypoglycemia) [43–47]. Ultimately, the combination of older age and diabetes increases falls risk by 17-fold [42, 48], while the involved diabetes-related factors will have an additive effect and worsen this risk [49].

Falls are terribly under-detected, and it is imperative to understand its definition. A true fall is defined as a person coming to rest inadvertently on a level below their prior location [50]. Falling from a standing position to the ground is not the only scenario. An older patient might try to go from supine to sitting and from sitting to standing, and they might go back to supine or sitting, respectively, and these will qualify as falls too. Even without considering those scenarios (which are severely under-detected) "traditional" falls are more prevalent in older people, and this is the age group at the greatest risk for serious injury or even death [51], constituting a public health problem that is largely preventable [52]. Unfortunately, less than half of providers know that their patients are falling [53]. Furthermore, the quality of bone in diabetes is affected, making them more vulnerable for fragility fractures [54]. Patients receiving insulin therapy are at greater risk for falls (requiring hospi-

talization) compared to those without diabetes [55]. Additionally, a fall can be the presentation of hypoglycemia, requiring the clinician to purposely inquire about the occurrence of previous falls. It cannot be overstated how important this matter is, especially since it may lead to a life-changing injury [56]. Those at high risk for hypoglycemia should be screened for falls as a routine CGA to be added to the CDE. Then, a comprehensive fall risk assessment may follow if falls occur more than once per year, or if there are issues with gait and balance [57].

Urinary Incontinence

Urinary incontinence is frequent in older people with diabetes. It can worsen quality of life, depression, disability, morbidity, and mortality [58, 59]. Similar to other geriatric syndromes, it is rarely due to a single disease. Older patients with diabetes are exposed to diabetes-related factors, such as uncontrolled diabetes with hyperglycemia, leading to glycosuria, polyuria, and from there, urinary incontinence, which can then become a hazard if the patient has other detrimental ongoing issues, such as impaired mobility, or falls risk. In addition, the pharmacology of Sodium Glucose Co-Transporter 2 inhibitors would increase the risk for urinary incontinence, and also increase the risk for urinary infections, which are also associated with urinary incontinence.

A study of community-dwelling older adults with diabetes identified geriatric factors (e.g., inability to ambulate or transfer independently) as important predictors for urinary incontinence in the setting of diabetes and frailty [60].

The intervention is to inquire about symptoms, incorporate those into the clinical decision making, and refer the patient to the corresponding specialists. Nevertheless, we recommend ensuring that reversible factors are considered, such as glycemic control.

Psychological Domain

Depression, delirium, and dementia are the classic most common geriatric syndromes. Notably, personality disorders and addictions are increasing in prevalence in this age group. In addition, we incorporate the sphere of poor quality of life within this domain.

Dementia

Both obesity and diabetes are recognized as risk factors for cognitive decline [61]. While there is no clear pathophysiologic pathway (most likely, it is multifactorial), the epidemiological links between diabetes and dementia are quite strong. The current understanding of cognitive decline and dementia put them closer with diabetes and cardiometabolic dysfunction. Alzheimer's disease is the sixth leading cause of death in the United States and is the fifth leading cause among people aged 65 years and over [62]. Compared to those without diabetes, older adults with diabetes are 50–100% more likely to develop dementia, and the risk is greater with longer diabetes duration, poorer glycemic control, and coexistent chronic vascular complications [63]. Furthermore, as another example of the interconnection between geriatric domains, patients with dementia are at greater risk for falls [64].

Thus, the evaluation of cognitive function in older adults with diabetes is warranted, especially for the oldest and those with longer duration of disease [65]. We would suggest additional interest for those patients who volunteer symptoms of memory dysfunction, or who volunteer having issues managing their pharmacologic interventions for diabetes. Quite often, clinicians are used to developing very accurate and complex insulin regimens, but must realize that as plan of care that is not feasible to be effectively implement, will not be efficacious, and only look good on paper. Hence, understanding the cognitive function of the older patient with diabetes will facilitate strategizing targets and interventions. Notably, an earlier detection and diagnosis of dementia will provide additional benefits and opportunities, such as to address proper resources and support, and increase the understanding by providers and family to start dealing with the dementia disease.

Depression

The incidence of depression in diabetes is double than in the general population [66], and it becomes a greater problem in the older population. This is not only due to diabetes-related issues, such as the impact from diabetic complications [67], but also because of age-related issues, such as advancing age, personal loss of function, loss of friends and family support. Furthermore, depression as a separate disease in and of itself will often require pharmacologic therapy, which will further increase the complexity of the case, and negatively impacts diabetes outcomes, such as glycemic control [68], self-care [69], and greater risk for diabetes complications, creating a vicious cycle. Moreover, a study evaluating a survival analysis between younger and older adults with diabetes (and controlling for covariables) found that depression increased mortality risk in the group aged 65 and older (78% greater than in those without depression), while there was no major difference in the younger group [70].

Poor Quality of Life

Older adults have an increased prevalence of multimorbidity and lower QOL [71]. They also present greater coexistence of diabetes and depression [72], which as discussed, negatively impacts HRQOL, diabetes itself, and its outcomes [73].

The Action to Control Cardiovascular Risk in Diabetes (ACCORD) trial compared intensive versus standard glycemic control. They used SF-36 to evaluate HRQOL and found intensive glycemic control did not lead to QOL benefits (no change) [74].

Social Domain

Elder abuse, social isolation, poverty, lack of family or social support are common scenarios affecting the older person. The social network of people decreases, as family and friends may age and die, or become ill and dependent themselves, so that they are no longer part of the support system. In the general population with diabetes, the economic costs from diabetes are composed of direct (management-related costs) and indirect (work absenteeism, reduced productivity at work and at home, reduced labor force participation from chronic disability, and premature mortality) [75]. In the geriatric older person with diabetes, it is possible that the latter may be less frequent (since many have already retired). However, the costs of management may actually be higher than in younger patients, if we consider the natural history of the disease, which may require a greater number of medications to achieve control, as well as the development of complications and the increase in life expectancy [76–78]. The economic situation can be a major constraint for those who are depending on insurance status and family support, an important resource that could be lacking more in this age group.

Food Insecurity

While it appears that this scenario is gaining more prevalence, it is possible that what has increased is the detection and awareness for this social issue. Food insecurity increases the older patients' vulnerability and risk to develop hypoglycemia. A study reported that patients with limited income have 40% greater risk of having food insecurity and inadequate glucose control [79]. Another study evaluated food insecurity in patients with homelessness, and of those who screened positive and had diabetes, 43.5% reported hypoglycemia symptoms [80].

Table 66.2 Addressing geriatric syndromes in the assessment of older patients with diabetes

Domain	Syndrome	Assessment and intervention
Medical	Polypharmacy	Medication reconciliation at each visit. For each prescription, ask yourself the question: does the patient benefit from this medication (dose, frequency) at this moment?
	Multimorbidity	Older patients are at greater risk for new diseases or complications. A patient could have been in the healthy category by the last visit, but now present after a stroke. Then, his targets and approaches need to be adjusted accordingly
	Malnutrition	Involve the nutritionist team
Functional	Impaired mobility	Consider if the patient has the functional ability to carry the proposed plan of care
	Falls	Ask if the patient has fallen in the past year
		Observe gait and balance while the patient walks into the office
		If these issues are present, the patient has falls risk, refer to the local geriatrician, or falls clinic
		In addition, adjust the glycemic regimen. Avoid hypoglycemia. Avoid regimens with increased risk for hypoglycemia
	Urinary incontinence	Ask if the patient has any issues with urinary incontinence
		Offer referrals to the geriatrician, urologist, gynecologist
		Avoid hyperglycemia
		Consider caution with medications that increase glycosuria
	Frailty	If the patient reports involuntary weight loss, fatigue, weakness, muscle loss, decrease the intensity of the glycemic regimen, avoid hypoglycemia, and refer the patient to a geriatrician
	Self-care deficit	If the patient has ≥2 limitations for IADLs, suggested HbA1c target is between 7.5 and 8%
		If the patient has ≥2 limitations for ADLs, suggested HbA1c target is between 8 and 8.5%
		Ensure the primary care or geriatrician is involved, to facilitate support at home or living situation
		Adjust pharmacologic regimens accordingly. Especially, if the patient has issues with medication management, consider regimens compatible with home health nurse services
	Dementia	Counsel the patient on the potential role for diabetes, but once the dementia disease is established, the priorities shift toward patient safety, avoidance of hypoglycemia
		Refer the patient to the neurologist or geriatrician for further assessment
	Depression	Refer the patient to the geriatric psychiatrist team, aiming to improve depression, as its relationship with glycemic control is bidirectional
	Food insecurity	Adjust glycemic targets, avoiding agents with the highest risk for hypoglycemia. Counsel on strategies to decrease antihyperglycemic medications if eating less and/or losing weight. Refer the patient to the primary care team and social worker team, to address potential community resources

Special Consideration for Diabetes Management in Older Adults

This book offers separate chapters addressing lifestyle, nutrition and exercise, obesity, and pharmacologic interventions. We would emphasize the consideration for modest intentional weight loss as a desirable outcome, as long as it is compatible with the broad comprehensive plan of care for the management of an older patient with diabetes [33]. Exercise interventions in this age group are effective and feasible to implement, providing multiple health benefits beyond diabetes control [81].

Most notably, there are no large randomized clinical trials aiming to prove or disprove the expert-based recommendations (as summarized in this chapter) for the individualized care (targets and strategies) for older adults with diabetes, at different levels of disease burden and health status [82].

Prevention of hypoglycemia is a major priority that should be addressed as soon as detected, through an adjustment of the therapy required to accomplish the established target.

Nevertheless, treatment intensification should not be neglected, as macrovascular and microvascular complications should still be prevented in this age group.

Regarding geriatric syndromes, we do not suggest that all practices taking care of diabetes perform a complete geriatrics assessment. First of all, we recommend awareness to this geriatric issues, and then provide a few practical suggestions to address these issues (Table 66.2).

Hypoglycemia in Older Adults: Primary and Secondary Prevention

Hypoglycemia is associated with cognitive impairment, both acute (erratic and irrational behavior, confusion, impaired vision and balance, which can result in falls or accidents) and chronic (leading to dementia) [83]. A prospective cohort study that followed 16,667 patients with diabetes without dementia at study entry found that severe hypoglycemia was associated with greater risk of dementia [84]. However, in frail, elderly patients with diabetes, avoidance of hypoglycemia, hypotension, and drug interactions due to polypharmacy is of even greater concern [85].

Hypoglycemia events require a clear understanding of their etiology to avoid a recurrence. Details on the history may reveal that the patient accidentally injected the correct dose twice because of forgetting an earlier dose, or that the patient was interrupted during a meal that remained unfinished. In both scenarios, the regimen may remain effective and safe if the events are isolated and conditions do not change. However, recurrent events can be a sign of cognitive decline or early self-care deficits. Regardless of this, glycemic targets need to be adjusted, and further coordination of services (formal or informal) will be required in order to deliver the injectable therapeutic plan and to avoid hypoglycemia.

Secondary Prevention

While one isolated event of hypoglycemia due to a very specific and likely isolated scenario (e.g., patient describes that skipped a meal due to an urgent phone call, which ultimately led to a hypoglycemic event), it is feasible to continue the same regimen, and emphasize education to prevent any future events.

However, if there is evidence for recurrent events, the team needs to address:

- Patient-related factors.
- Modifications to the pharmacologic regimen.
- Reassess glycemic targets.

Primary Prevention

We recommend especial care for those patients at the highest risk (older, on insulin or sulfonylurea, low HbA1c). Considering the potential devastating consequence from even one adverse event (e.g., hypoglycemia leading to a fall, hip fracture, institutionalization, death), we recommend providers to consider strategies to identify patients in whom hypoglycemia has not been present, but who remain at high risk. Our Miami VA team collaborates with the leaders in diabetes care for the Veterans Administration in the USA, fostering the use of electronic tools to detect patients at high risk and avoid overtreatment [86]. While this specific approach might only apply to our healthcare system, the concept could be translated to other healthcare systems.

Pharmacotherapy

Finally, Table 66.3 presents a summary of considerations regarding specific pharmacologic agents and strategies for the management of diabetes in the older patient.

Table 66.3 Special considerations for pharmacologic therapy of diabetes in older adults [7, 14–16, 87]

Order of priority	Pharmacologic agents	Advantages	Disadvantages
Standard first line	Metformin	– No hypoglycemia	– GI side effects are easily countered by always taking with meals
		– Safe and effective	– Risk of vitamin B12 deficiency: monitor and supplement
		– Lowers CV and cancer risk	– The risk for lactic acidosis is actually very low
1	Dipeptidyl-4 inhibitors (Sitagliptin, Vildagliptin, Saxagliptin, Linagliptin, Alogliptin)	– Low hypoglycemia risk	– CV and heart failure risk (saxagliptin)
		– Weight neutral	– Increased upper respiratory infections
		– Safe and effective (especially when aiming for less than strong reductions in HbA1c)	– Expensive – Limited long-term data in older adults
1	Sulfonylureas (Glimeperide, Glipizide)	– Effective	– Moderate risk hypoglycemia (glyburide is contraindicated)
		– Long-term experience in this age group	– Weight gain
		– Lower CV risk	– Patients losing weight or doing exercise require close monitoring (increased risk for hypoglycemia)

Table 66.3 (continued)

Order of priority	Pharmacologic agents	Advantages	Disadvantages
1	Sodium Glucose co-transporter 2 inhibitors (Canagliflozin, Empagliflozin, Dapagliflozin, Ertugliflozin)	– Low hypoglycemia risk	– High cost
		– Lower weight	– GU infections and urinary incontinence, especial care is required in this age group
		– Lower systolic blood pressure	– Risk for volume depletion, orthostatic hypotension, possibly falls
		– Improve CV risk/mortality (empagliflozin, canagliflozin), renal (empagliflozin)	– Limited long-term data in older adults
1	Glucagon-like peptide 1 receptor agonists (Exenatide, Liraglutide, Albiglutide, Dulaglutide, Lixisenatide, Semaglutide)	– Low hypoglycemia risk	– High cost
		– Lower weight	– GI side effects
		– Reduce CV risk (liraglutide)	– Risk for acute pancreatitis (exenatide and liraglutide)
		– Convenient formulation (daily or weekly)	– Risk for acute kidney injury (exenatide)
2	Long-acting insulin (Glargine, Detemir, Degludec)	– Effective	– Hypoglycemia risk
		– Long-term experience in this age group	– Weight gain
2	GLP-1RA and insulin fixed combinations (insulin glargine + lixisenatide, insulin degludec + liraglutide)	– Effective	– Moderate hypoglycemia risk
		– Convenient formulation (daily or qod)	– High cost
			– Not applicable to all subjects (e.g., not for those who require high dosages)
3	Alpha-glucosidase inhibitors (Acarbose, Miglitol)	– Mild to moderate hypoglycemia risk	– Frequent dosing schedule
		– Effective (especially when aiming for less than strong reductions in HbA1c)	– GI side effects might not be countered easily
			– Contraindication with chronic renal failure (miglitol)
3	Thiazolidinediones (Pioglitazone)	– Low hypoglycemia risk	– Suspected CV risk, heart failure exacerbation
		– Convenient formulation (daily)	– Suspected risk for bladder cancer
4	Intermediate-acting insulin (NPH)	– Long-term experience in this age group	– High risk for hypoglycemia
			– Weight gain
			– Schedule requires at least two injections per day to cover basal needs
4	Pre-mixed insulin 70/30 (NPH + regular, NPH + aspart) 75/25 (lispro protamine + lispro)	– Long-term experience in this age group	– High risk for hypoglycemia
			– Risk for BID regimens would leave lunch time uncovered

Multiple-Choice Questions

1. Geriatric syndromes in diabetes management:
   (a) Are of exclusive competency of geriatricians
   (b) **Are determinant and essential in the assessment and plan**
   (c) Are only secondary to glycemic control
   (d) Are uncommon and irrelevant for the clinical outcomes

2. Geriatric syndromes include all of the following except:
   (a) Polypharmacy
   (b) **Type 2 diabetes**
   (c) Persistent pain
   (d) Urinary incontinence
   (e) Falls

3. Macrovascular and microvascular diabetes complications are associated with:
   (a) Cognitive function
   (b) Nutritional risk
   (c) Self-care deficit
   (d) **All of the above**
   (e) None of the above

4. Polypharmacy:
   (a) Is an expected consequence of aging
   (b) **Represents a geriatric syndrome by itself**
   (c) Supports the use of multiple anti-diabetic medications in this age group

    (d) Is essential to address patients' needs

    (e) Increases costs and non-adherence

5. Each medical visit is an opportunity to address the following aspect of drug treatment:

    (a) Patients' compliance with medical orders

    (b) **Striving to reduce medications when there is no certainty that benefits outweigh the risks**

    (c) The opportunity to add new medications

    (d) The adequate use of **over the** counter medications

    (e) Encourage the use of high-cost medications that these patients can afford

6. Patients who will benefit less from intensive regimens:

    (a) Are extremely rare

    (b) Are less years of education

    (c) Are the ones with less comorbidities

    (d) **Are the ones with six or more comorbidities**

    (e) Are the ones with cardiovascular disease

7. Diabetes in older patients is a risk factor of:

    (a) **Malnutrition**

    (b) Falls

    (c) Dehydration

    (d) Peripheral artery disease

    (e) All of the above

8. The functional domain in the elderly includes all of the following except:

    (a) **Intelligence**

    (b) Eating

    (c) Vision loss

    (d) Hearing loss

    (e) Cooking

9. The following factors account for the increased risk of falls in elderly with diabetes:

    (a) Impaired gait

    (b) Loss of vision

    (c) Cognitive impairment

    (d) Polypharmacy

    (e) **All of the above**

10. Intensive glycemic control in the elderly clearly and remarkably improves quality of life in the elderly with diabetes:

    (a) True

    (b) **False**

References

1. Ford ES, Giles WH, Dietz WH. Prevalence of the metabolic syndrome among US adults: findings from the third National Health and Nutrition Examination Survey. JAMA. 2002;287(3):356–9.

2. Bonora E, Kiechl S, Willeit J, et al. Insulin resistance as estimated by homeostasis model assessment predicts incident symptomatic cardiovascular disease in Caucasian subjects from the general population: the Bruneck study. Diabetes Care. 2007;30(2):318–24.

3. Djioque S, Nwabo Kamdje AH, Vecchio L, et al. Insulin resistance and cancer: the role of insulin and IGFs. Endocr Relat Cancer. 2013;20(1):R1–R17.

4. Stuart MJ, Baune BT. Depression and type 2 diabetes: inflammatory mechanisms of a psychoneuroendocrine comorbidity. Neurosci Biobehav Rev. 2012;36(1):658–76.

5. De Felice FG, Ferreira ST. Inflammation, defective insulin signaling, and mitochondrial dysfunction as common molecular denominators connecting type 2 diabetes to Alzheimer disease. Diabetes. 2014;63(7):2262–72.

6. Espinoza SE, Jung I, Hazuda H. Frailty transitions in the San Antonio Longitudinal Study of Aging. J Am Geriatr Soc. 2012;60(4):652–60.

7. Valencia WM, Florez H. Pharmacological treatment of diabetes in older people. Diabetes Obes Metab. 2014;16:1192–203.

8. World Health Organization (2015) Ageing and Health. Fact sheet N404. http://www.who.int/mediacentre/factsheets/fs404/en/. Accessed 1 March 2022.

9. Federal Interagency Forum on Aging-Related Statistics. Older Americans 2012. https://agingstats.gov/docs/PastReports/2012/OA2012.pdf. Accessed 1 March 2022.

10. Verbrugge LM, Yang L-S. Aging with disability and disability with aging. J Disabil Policy Stud. 2002;12(4):253–37.

11. Laiteerapong N, Karter AJ, Liu JH, et al. Correlates of quality of life in older adults with diabetes. The Diabetes & Aging Study. Diabetes Care. 2011;34(8):1749–53.

12. Redekop WK, Koopmanschap MA, Stolk RP, Rutten GE, Wolffenbuttel BH, Niessen LW. Health-related quality of life and treatment satisfaction in Dutch patients with type 2 diabetes. Diabetes Care. 2002;25:458–63. PMID: 11874930.

13. Valencia WM, Palacio A, Tamariz L, Florez H. Metformin and ageing. Diabetologia. 2017;60:1662. https://doi.org/10.1007/s00125-017-4349-5.

14. American Diabetes Association. Standards of medical care in diabetes–2018. Diabetes Care. 2018;41(Suppl 1):S1–159.

15. Kirkman SM, Briscoe VJ, Clark N, et al. Diabetes in older adults. Diabetes Care. 2012;35:2650–64.

16. Munshi MN, Florez H, Huang ES, et al. Management of diabetes in long-term care and skilled nursing facilities: a position statement of the American Diabetes Association. Diabetes Care. 2016;39(2):308–18.

17. Inouye SK, Studenski S, Tinetti ME, Kuchel GA. Geriatric syndromes : clinical, research and policy implications of a core geriatric concept. J Am Geriatr Soc. 2007;55(5):780–91.

18. Munshi M. Managing the "geriatric syndrome" in patients with type 2 diabetes. Consult Pharm. 2008;23(Suppl B):12–6.

19. Sinclair A, Dunning T, Rodriguez-Manas L. Diabetes in older people: new insights and remaining challenges. Lancet Diabetes Endocrinol. 2015;3(4):275–85.

20. Bauduceau B, Doucet J, Le Floch JP, et al. Cardiovascular events and geriatric scale scores in elderly (70 years old and above) type 2 diabetic patients at inclusion in the GERODIAB cohort. Diabetes Care. 2014;37(1):304–11.

21. Le Floch JP, Doucet J, Bauduceau B, et al. Retinopathy, nephropathy, peripheral neuropathy and geriatric scale scores in elderly people with type 2 diabetes. Diabet Med. 2014;31(1):107–11.

22. Valencia WM, Danet M, Florez H, Bourdel-Marchasson I. Assessment procedures including comprehensive geriatric assessment. In: Sinclair A, Dunning T, Rodríguez Mañas L, Munshi M, editors. Diabetes in old age. 4th ed. New York: Wiley-Blackwell; 2017. https://doi.org/10.1002/9781118954621.ch5.

23. Karter AJ, Laiteeranpong N, Chin MH, et al. Ethnic differences in geriatric conditions and diabetes complications among older, insured adults with diabetes: the diabetes and aging study. J Aging Health. 2015;27(5):894–918.

24. Barat I, Andrease F, Damsgaard EM. Drug therapy in the elderly: what doctors believe and patients actually do. Br J Clin Pharmacol. 2001;25:861–70.

25. Woolcott JC, Richardson KJ, Wiens MO, Patel B, Marin J, Khan KM, Marra CA. Meta-analysis of the impact of 9 medication classes on falls in elderly persons. Arch Intern Med. 2009;169:1952–60.

26. Peron EP, Ogbonna KC. Antidiabetic medications and polypharmacy. Clin Geriatr Med. 2015;31:17–27.

27. Lloyd BD, Williamson DA, Singh NA, Hansen RD, Diamond TH, Finnegan TP, Allen BJ, Grady JN, Stavrinos TM, Smith EU, Diwan AD, Fiatarone Singh MA. Recurrent and injurious falls in the year following hip fracture: a prospective study of incidence and risk factors from the Sarcopenia and Hip Fracture study. J Gerontol A Biol Sci Med Sci. 2009;64:599–609.

28. Hanlon JT, Boudreau RM, Roumani YF, Newman AB, Ruby CM, Wright RM, Hilmer SN, Shorr RI, Bauer DC, Simonsick EM, Studenski SA. Number and dosage of central nervous system medications on recurrent falls in community elders: the Health, Aging and Body Composition study. J Gerontol A Biol Sci Med Sci. 2009;64:492–8.

29. Boyd CM, Darer J, Boult C, Fried LP, Boult L, Wu AW. Clinical practice guidelines and quality of care for older patients with multiple comorbid diseases: implications for pay for performance. JAMA. 2005;294:716–24.

30. Rothrock NE, Hays RD, Spritzer K, Yount SE, Riely W, Cella D. Relative to the general US population, chronic diseases are associated with poorer health-related quality of life as measured by the Patient-Reported Outcomes Measurement Information System (PROMIS). J Clin Epidemiol. 2010;63(11):1195–204.

31. Laiteerapong N, Iveniuk J, John PM, Laumann EO, Huang ES. Classification of older adults who have diabetes by comorbid conditions, United States, 2005-2006. Prev Chronic Dis. 2012;9:E100.

32. Tyrovolas S, Koyanagi A, Garin N, et al. Diabetes mellitus and its association with central obesity and disability among older adults: a global perspective. Exp Gerontol. 2015;64:70–7.

33. Valencia WM, Stoutenberg M, Florez H. Weight loss and physical activity for disease prevention in obese older adults: an important role for lifestyle management. Curr Diab Rep. 2014;14:539–49.

34. Farre TB, Formiga F, Ferrer A, et al. Risk of being undernourished in a cohort of community-dwelling 85-year-olds: the Octabaix study. Geriatr Gerontol Int. 2014;14:702–9.

35. Vischer UM, Perrenoud L, Genet C, et al. The high prevalence of malnutrition in elderly diabetic patients: implications for anti-diabetic drug treatments. Diabet Med. 2010;27:918–24.

36. Finestone HM, Greene-Finestone LS, Wilson ES, et al. Malnutrition in stroke patients on the rehabilitation service and at follow-up: prevalence and predictors. Arch Phys Med Rehabil. 1995;76:310–6.

37. Fritschi C, Bronas UG, Park CG, Collins EG, Quinn L. Early declines in physical function among aging adults with type 2 diabetes. J Diabetes Complications. 2017;31(2):347–52.

38. Brown CJ, Flood KL. Mobility limitation in the older patient. A clinical review. JAMA. 2013;310:1168–77.

39. Lawton MP, Brody EM. Assessment of older people: self-maintaining and instrumental activities of daily living. Gerontologist. 1969;9:179–86.

40. Katz S, Downs TD, Cash HR, et al. Progress in development of the index of ADL. Gerontologist. 1970;10:20–30.

41. Richardson JK, Hurvitz EA. Peripheral neuropathy: a true risk factor for falls. J Gerontol A Biol Sci Med Sci. 1995;50:M211–5.

42. Lord S, Sherrington C, Menz H, Close J. Falls in older people: risk factors and strategies for prevention. Cambridge: Cambridge University Press; 2007.

43. Cavanagh PR, Derr JA, Ulbrecht JS, Maser RE, Orchard TJ. Problems with gait and posture in neuropathic patients with insulin-dependent diabetes mellitus. Diabet Med. 1992;9:469–74.

44. Schwartz AV, Hillier TA, Sellmeyer DE, et al. Older women with diabetes have a higher risk of falls: a prospective study. Diabetes Care. 2002;25:1749–54.

45. Schwartz AV, Vittinghoff E, Sellmeyer DE, et al. Diabetes-related complications, glycemic control, and falls in older adults. Diabetes Care. 2008;31:391–6.

46. Berlie HD, Garwood CL. Diabetes medications related to an increased risk of falls and fall-related morbidity in the elderly. Ann Pharmacother. 2010;44:712–7.

47. Pijpers E, Ferreira I, de Jongh RT, et al. Older individuals with diabetes have an increased risk of recurrent falls: analysis of potential mediating factors: the Longitudinal Ageing Study Amsterdam. Age Ageing. 2012;41:358–65.

48. Vinik AL, Vinik EJ, Colberg SR, Morrison S. Falls risk in older adults with type 2 diabetes. Clin Geriatr Med. 2015;31:89–99.

49. Vinik AI, Camacho P, Reddy S, et al. Aging, diabetes and falls. Endocr Pract. 2017;23(9):1117–39.

50. Gibson MJ, Andres K, Isaacs B, et al. Prevention of falls in later life. Dan Med Bull. 1987;34(Suppl b):1–24.

51. World Health Organization. Falls. Fact sheet N344. 2012. http://www.who.int/mediacentre/factsheets/fs344/en/. Accessed 1 March 2022.

52. Centers for Disease Control and Prevention (CDC). Falls among older adults: an overview. 2014. http://www.cdc.gov/HomeandRecreationalSafety/Falls/adultfalls.html. Accessed 1 March 2022.

53. Stevens JA, Ballesteros MF, Mack KA, Rudd RA, DeCaro E, Adler G. Gender differences in seeking care for falls in the aged Medicare Population. Am J Prev Med. 2012;43:59–62.

54. Gonnelli S, Caffarelli C, Giordano N, Nuti R. The prevention of fragility fractures in diabetic patients. Aging Clin Exp Res. 2015;27(2):115–24.

55. Yau RK, Strotmeyer ES, Resnick HE, et al. Diabetes and risk of hospitalized fall injury among older adults. Diabetes Care. 2013;36:3985–91.

56. Seaquist ER, Anderson J, Childs B, et al. Hypoglycemia and diabetes: a report of a workgroup of the American Diabetes Association and the Endocrine Society. Diabetes Care. 2013;36:1384–95.

57. American Geriatrics Society and British Geriatrics Society. Summary of the Updated American Geriatrics Society/British Geriatrics Society Clinical Practice Guideline for prevention of falls in older persons. J Am Geriatr Soc. 2011;59(1):148–57.

58. Aguilar-Navarro S, Navarrete-Reyes AP, Grados-Chavarria BH, Garcia-Lara JM, Amieva H, Avila-Funes JA. The severity of urinary incontinence decreases health-related quality of life among community-dwelling elderly. J Gerontol A Biol Sci Med Sci. 2012;67(11):1266–71.

59. Khatutsky G, Walsh EG, Brown DW. Urinary incontinence, functional status, and health-related quality of life among Medicare beneficiaries enrolled in the program for all-inclusive care for the elderly and dual eligible demonstration special needs plans. J Ambul Care Manage. 2013;36(1):35–49.

60. Hsu A, Conell-Price J, Stijacic Cenzer I, et al. Predictors of urinary incontinence in community-dwelling frail older adults with diabetes mellitus in a cross-sectional study. BMC Geriatr. 2014;14:137.

61. Alosco ML, Gunstad J. The negative effects of obesity and poor glycemic control on cognitive function: a proposed model for possible mechanisms. Curr Diab Rep. 2014;14:495.

62. Tejada-Vera B. Mortality from Alzheimer's disease in the United States: data for 2000 and 2010. NCHS data brief, no 116. Hyattsville: National Center for Health Statistics; 2013. http://www.cdc.gov/nchs/data/databriefs/db116.htm. Accessed 1 March 2022.

63. Mayeda ER, Whitmer RA, Yaffe K. Diabetes and cognition. Clin Geriatr Med. 2015;31:101–15.

64. van Dijk PT, Meulenberg OG, van de Sande HJ, Habbema JD. Falls in dementia patients. Gerontologist. 1993;33:200–4.

65. Barbagallo M, Dominguez LJ. Type 2 diabetes mellitus and Alzheimer's disease. World J Diabetes. 2014;5(6):889–93.

66. Anderson RJ, Freedland KE, Clouse RE, Lustman PJ. The prevalence of comorbid depression in adults with diabetes: a meta-analysis. Diabetes Care. 2001;24:1069–78.

67. De Groot M, Anderson R, Freedland KE, Closue RE, Lustam PJ. Association of depression and diabetes complications: a meta-analysis. Psychosom Med. 2001;63:619–30.

68. Lustman PJ, Anderson RJ, Freland KE, de Groot M, Carney RM, Clouse RE. Depression and poor glycemic control: a meta-analytic review of the literature. Diabetes Care. 2000;23:9347–2.

69. Gonzalez JS, Peyrot M, McCarl LA, et al. Depression and diabetes treatment nonadherence: a meta-analysis. Diabetes Care. 2008;31:2398–403.

70. Kimbro LB, Mangione CM, Steers WN, et al. Depression and all-cause mortality in persons with diabetes: are older adults at higher risk? Results from the Translating Research Into Action for Diabetes Study. J Am Geriatr Soc. 2014;62:1017–22.

71. Martin M, Battegay E, Rocke C. Editorial: quality of life in multimorbidity. Gerontology. 2014;60(3):247–8. https://doi.org/10.1159/000358797.

72. Amato L, Paolisso G, Cacciatore F, et al. Non-insulin-dependent diabetes mellitus is associated with a greater prevalence of depression in the elderly. Diabete Metab. 1996;22:314–8. PMID: 8896992.

73. Goldney RD, Phillips PJ, Fisher LJ, Wilson DH. Diabetes, depression, and quality of life: a population study. Diabetes Care. 2004;27:1066–70.

74. Anderson RT, Narayan KM, Feeney P, et al. Effect of intensive glycemic lowering on health-related quality of life in type 2 diabetes. ACCORD trial. Diabetes Care. 2011;34(4):807–12. https://doi.org/10.2337/dc10-1926.

75. American Diabetes Association (ADA). Economic costs of diabetes in U.S. in 2007. Diabetes Care. 2008;31(3):596–695.

76. Redekop WK, Koopmanschap MA, Rutten GE, Wolffenbuttel BH, Stolk RP, Niessen LW. Resource consumption and costs in Dutch patients with type 2 diabetes mellitus. Results from 29 general practices. Diabet Med. 2002;19(3):246–53.

77. Bourdel-Marchasson I. Diabetes mellitus care models for older people, The European perspective. In: Sinclair AJ, editor. Diabetes in old age. New York: Wiley-Blackwell; 2009. p. 453–8.

78. Romon I, Rey G, Mandereau-Bruno L, et al. The excess mortality related to cardiovascular diseases and cancer among adults pharmacologically treated for diabetes - the 2001-2006 ENTRED cohort. Diabet Med. 2014;31:946–53.

79. Waitman J, Caeiro G, Romero Gonzalez SA, et al. Social vulnerability and hypoglycemia among patients with diabetes. Endocrinol Diabetes Nutr. 2017;64(20):92–9.

80. O'Toole TP, Roberts CB, Johnson EE. Screening for food insecurity in six veteran administration clinics for the homeless, June-December 2015. Prev Chronic Dis. 2017;14:160375.

81. Mora JC, Valencia WM. Exercise and older adults. Clin Geriatr Med. 2018;34:145–62.

82. Huang ES. Management of diabetes mellitus in older people with comorbidities. BMJ. 2016;353:i2200.

83. Frier BM. Hypoglycaemia in diabetes mellitus: epidemiology and clinical implications. Nat Rev Endocrinol. 2014;10:711–22.

84. Whitmer RA, Karter AJ, Yaffe K, Quesenberry CP Jr, Selby JV. Hypoglycemic episodes and risk of dementia in older patients with type 2 diabetes mellitus. JAMA. 2009;301(15):1565–72.

85. Ligthelm RJ, Kaiser M, Vora J, Yale JF. Insulin use in elderly adults: risk of hypoglycemia and strategies for care. J Am Geriatr Soc. 2012;60:1564–70.

86. Wright SM, Hedin SC, McConnell M, et al. Using shared decision-making to address possible overtreatment in patients at high risk for hypoglycemia: the Veterans Health Administration's Choosing Wisely Hypoglycemia Safety Initiative. Clin Diabetes. 2018;36(2):120–7.

87. Aroda VR, Rosenstock J, Wysham C, et al. Efficacy and safety of LixiLan, a titratable fixed-ratio combination of insulin glargine plus lixisenatide in type 2 diabetes inadequately controlled on basal insulin and metformin: the LixiLan-L randomized trial. Diabetes Care. 2016;39:1972–80.

Further Reading

Abdelhafiz AH, Pennells D, Sinclair AJ. A modern approach to glucose-lowering therapy in frail older people with type 2 diabetes mellitus. Expert Rev Endocrinol Metab. 2022;17:95–8. https://doi.org/10.1080/17446651.2022.2044304.

Sinclair AJ, Addelhafiz AH. Challenges and strategies for diabetes management in community-living older adults. Clin Diabetes. 2020;33:217–27.

The Artificial Pancreas

Barry H. Ginsberg, Richard Mauseth,
and Joel Rodriguez-Saldana

Abbreviations

AP	Artificial pancreas
CGMS	Continuous glucose monitoring system
FDA	US Food and Drug Administration
HbA1c	Hemoglobin A11c
iOS	Apple operating system
MPC	Model predictive control. A controller algorithm
PID	Proportional integral derivative. A controller algorithm

Objectives

- Describe the need for an artificial pancreas.
- Describe the history of artificial pancreas.
- Describe the components of an artificial pancreas.
- Describe the algorithms used in an artificial pancreas.
- Describe the clinical testing of an artificial pancreas.
- Describe the current and future devices.

Introduction

The artificial pancreas is an imprecise term that can mean a bioengineered product, such as an islet cell transplant, gene therapy to replace the pancreas, or the combination of a continuous glucose sensor, an insulin pump (with or without a glucagon pump), and a computer with an algorithm to con-

B. H. Ginsberg
Diabetes Technology Consultants, Wyckoff, NJ, USA

R. Mauseth
Dose Safety, Redmond, WC, USA

J. Rodriguez-Saldana (✉)
Multidisciplinary Diabetes Center Mexico, Mexico City, Mexico

trol the delivery of insulin. In this chapter, we will consider only the last. This is an exciting topic with products being developed by an unusual consortium of academics, the JDRF, the NIH, the FDA, the Helmsley Foundation, and medical device companies. The first artificial pancreas was approved by the FDA in October of 2016 and was first marketed in June 2017 [1].

History

The first attempt at an artificial pancreas was a hybrid external device that measured venous glucose and delivered IV insulin. It was created by Kadish and colleagues in 1964 [2] and was followed over the next 10 years by a series of 5 hybrid devices, one of which, the Biostator, was commercially available [3, 4]. The Biostator worked with a complex, expensive dual lumen catheter, measuring venous glucose and delivering IV insulin. It drew some blood into its tubing, mixed with reagents and measured the glucose. It used the glucose value with an algorithm to deliver insulin and control the blood glucose. It did this very well. The Biostator was a tremendous research tool and had some medical therapy applications, but was too big, too complicated, too invasive, too expensive, and used too much blood to be used long term by individual patients (Fig. 67.1).

The pathway of development soon split, with some working on an implantable device, whereas others worked on a totally external device (Fig. 67.2). Implantable devices got an early start with the development of implantable insulin pumps by Infusaid, Siemens, and Minimed (1980–1981). In 1986 a fully automated artificial pancreas with an IV glucose monitor was tested by Minimed. Because of multiple problems including frequent catheter blockage, sensor fouling, and the invasiveness of the system, further work on the project was suspended.

© The Author(s), under exclusive license to Springer Nature Switzerland AG 2023
J. Rodriguez-Saldana (ed.), *The Diabetes Textbook*, https://doi.org/10.1007/978-3-031-25519-9_67

Fig. 67.1 The Biostator, the first commercially available artificial pancreas. (Courtesy of William Clarke, University of Virginia)

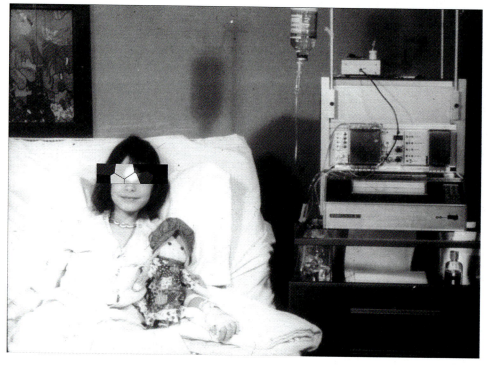

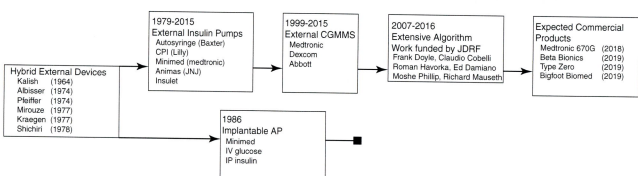

Fig. 67.2 Timeline of development of the Artificial Pancreas

Work on an external artificial pancreas progressed slowly, as the individual components, the insulin pump, and the subcutaneous continuous glucose monitor progressed. A major stimulus to the development was the decision by the Juvenile Diabetes Research Foundation in 2007 to extensively fund research on artificial pancreas algorithms. The project led by Aaron Kowalski set up 8 major artificial pancreas centers and funded research on three different types of algorithms: Proportional Integral Derivative (PID), Model Predictive Controller (MPC), and Fuzzy Logic systems. With their funding for the basic science and clinical studies and their coordination with the major stakeholders, the field progressed rapidly and the first artificial pancreas was approved in September 2016. Special thanks for helping this development should also go to the NIH which had multiple special award cycles for the artificial pancreas and to the FDA which set up a special committee to coordinate regulation of the artificial pancreas.

The Medtronic 670G, first marketed in June, 2017, is the first artificial pancreas, but many new systems are on their way with additions of a modular approach (Type Zero), addition of glucagon (Beta Bionics), and a leasing approach (Bigfoot). Second generation systems using better insulins, smaller devices, and extending the wear time are also in development.

Technology

Components of an Artificial Pancreas

Insulin Pump

An artificial pancreas consists of at least three components, an insulin pump, a continuous glucose monitoring system, and a computer, running an AP algorithm (Fig. 67.3). To understand the artificial pancreas, you need to fully under-

Fig. 67.3 Components of an Artificial Pancreas System

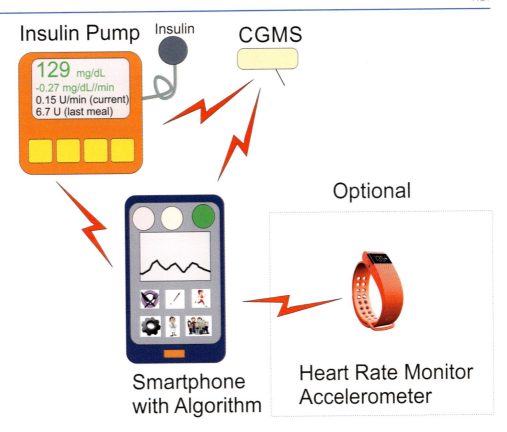

stand an insulin pump, continuous glucose monitoring (CGMS), and intensive insulin therapy. You should review those chapters before proceeding here.

Modern insulin pumps are fully digital. The digital motors are capable of infusion rates as low as 0.05 U/min and as high as 10 U/min with about 5% inaccuracy. They need to communicate with the controller and for an artificial pancreas they also need to communicate with the Computer/Smartphone and generally do so with Bluetooth 4.0 or later. In practice, they also often communicate with the CGMS system. The pumps can work without the artificial pancreas algorithm and should the AP fail, the patient can use the pump as an open loop system.

Continuous Glucose Monitoring

Continuous glucose monitoring (CGM) has been available in some form for almost 20 years but have only become very accurate in 2015. These systems monitor glucose frequently (every 1 to 5 min) rather than continuously and they do not measure blood glucose but rather the glucose in the interstitial space which lags blood glucose by 5–15 min. The best current systems work well in an artificial pancreas. They report glucose every 5 min, have median errors of about 10 percent, and can connect to a controller with Bluetooth 4 or later. Appropriate systems are available as a needle catheter lasting 1–2 weeks and an implantable system that lasts 6–12 months.

Most interesting is the development of a CGMS system built around the needle of an insulin pump catheter, expected to be released sometime in 2017.

Computer

Early experimental systems used laptop computers. As computers got smaller, some systems used netbook computers. Most algorithms for an artificial pancreas do not require extensive computing power and can easily be run by the best of current smartphones. There are experimental systems that run on the Apple iOS and others that run on the Google Android operating system. Additional advantages of running on a smartphone include availability of broadband internet connections and the ability to transmit directly over cellular networks (like texting). There are now smartphones with dual SIMs, so that the personal telephone system and the operating system of the AP are separate. The Medtronic 670G has a computer built into the insulin pump.

Algorithms

For an artificial pancreas, there are 3 common types of algorithms [5]. They differ in their basic approach to calculating the amount of insulin needed at any point.

PID

The first controllers for modern artificial pancreas systems are the PID or proportional, integral, derivative controllers.

These controllers, well established in industrial processes, assess the error in the system, *i.e.,* the difference between the current glucose and the desired glucose using three terms, as seen in Fig. 67.4.

The first term is *Proportional*, a function of the difference between the current glucose (in red) and the desired glucose (in green), shown in the figure as a black two headed arrow. The greater the discrepancy from the desired glucose, the more insulin the controller will suggest.

The second term is *Integral*, a function of the length of time the glucose has been different than the desired glu-

cose. This term is a function of the area under (or above the curve if hypoglycemic) the curve, *i.e.,* the integral of the difference over the past time (shown in yellow). The higher this term, the more insulin the controller will suggest.

The last term is *Derivative*, a function of the slope of the glucose curve (shown in orange). The more rapidly the current glucose is approaching the desired glucose, the less insulin the controller will suggest (if approaching from above).

Thus, the PID controller evaluates the current glucose (proportional), the past glucose (integral), and the future glucose (derivative).

PID controllers are very stable and have been incorporated into the first implanted artificial pancreas and the currently only FDA approved artificial pancreas, the Medtronic 670G.

Model Predictive Controller

Model Predictive Controllers are also very stable "industrial" controllers. Figure 67.5 shows a block diagram of a simple MPC, adapted from Lunze et al. [6]. In this controller, the glucose is separately evaluated to optimize the model parameter and to compare to the current glucose target. These feed the controller, which is based upon the model of diabetes with various food, glucose, and insulin compartments (glucagon too in some) and parameters for the movement among them. The MPC controller generates an insulin infusion rate, which is tested for safety then applied to the patient, altering the glucose value and the process repeats. Variations on this basic approach use glucagon, are modular, or learn from previous days.

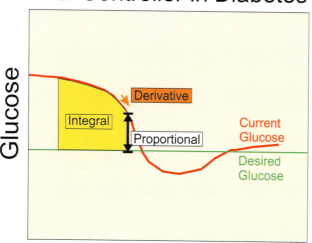

Fig. 67.4 PID control of glucose

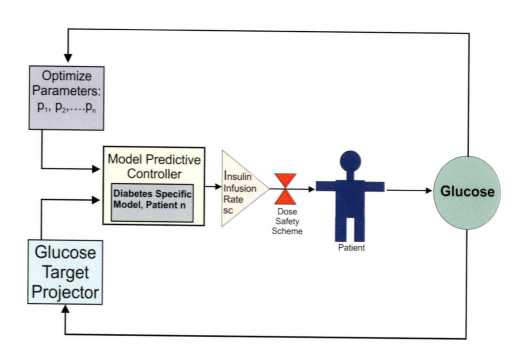

Fig. 67.5 Block diagram of a simple MPC

Fuzzy Logic

Fuzzy logic controllers use analog processes and fuzzy logic principles to mimic the approach a skilled diabetes caregiver would use to manage glucose levels. The MD Logic Artificial Pancreas was the first approved algorithm for an artificial pancreas, being cleared by the European Union in 2015, but there was no hardware approved with it, so there was no product. Another major fuzzy logic system is currently under development by Dose Safety.

Clinical Testing

Evaluating an Artificial Pancreas

Clinical Trial Structure

Clinical trials of the artificial pancreas go through 2 stages after individual components are validated. The first part is feasibility, usually done in 3 parts. The first trials are always done in a clinical research facility with medical personnel always readily available. The second set of trials are often done at a hotel or a diabetes summer camp with medical personnel nearby. The subjects can participate in activities of daily living although a nurse will generally accompany them the first time. The last part is usually a short home trial of 2–4 weeks. The subjects are often remotely monitored and medical personnel are available by phone at all times. Most of these trials will have 15–30 subjects. The second part is the pivotal trial, usually done at home. Twenty-five to 100 subjects are followed at home for 3–6 months.

Safety

Mild hypoglycemia is common in type 1 diabetes with about 20,000 to 40,000 episodes occurring daily in the USA [7]. Serious hypoglycemia occurs about once every two years. Thus, the most important safety feature of an artificial pancreas is no increase in hypoglycemia (a reduction in hypoglycemia would be considered an effectiveness outcome). Similarly, ketoacidosis occurs in about 2–4% of patients with type 1 diabetes each year and we would expect this and episodes of hyperglycemia to be no higher with an artificial pancreas [8, 9].

Effectiveness

Tests of effectiveness are tricky. The gold standard for effectiveness is hemoglobin A1c (HbA1c). This marker, however, is improved by hypoglycemia. Thus, a new therapy could eliminate hypoglycemia and result in an increased HbA1c. Thus, the time in the normal range as determined by CGMS is also important. Most clinical trials have reported normal values as Time in Range (TIR) of 70–140 mg/dL or 70–180, low values as time <70, and high values at time >180 as well as the number and severity of hypoglycemia and the number of hyperglycemic events.

Clinical Trials of Artificial Pancreas Devices

The clinical trials of the devices being currently tested are remarkably similar. All eliminate most of the hypoglycemic episodes in the tested patients. Hemoglobin A1c has generally fallen slightly but glucose time in range 70–180 mg/dL has increased, generally to the 70–80% range. This achievement is dramatic, since the trials are generally done in patients who are already in very good glucose control.

Available Devices

As of August 1, 2017, only a single device has been cleared by the FDA and marketed to patients with Type 1 diabetes, the Medtronic 670G. The AP uses a Medtronic insulin pump and CGMS and a PID algorithm that is built into the pump.

The major clinical trial had 124 participants who used the device for 3 months. The trial demonstrated a difference in the average glucose values and a decrease in HbA1c from 7.4 to 6.9. There was a dramatic decrease in hypoglycemia and time in hypoglycemia and an increase in time in range 70–140 and a corresponding decrease in time > 140. Overall it was an impressive demonstration of the power of the artificial pancreas, even compared to patients already using an insulin pump and a CGMS.

Future Devices

Other groups are close to reaching the market. Type Zero diabetes has taken a modular approach. They have built each part of the controller into a separate module. Thus, they test each module for safety and effectiveness and add new modules to the system as they are approved. The system is designed to be run on an Android phone but is otherwise hardware independent. Much like devices that work with your computer, every device that works with the Type Zero device will have a "driver" to allow the device to communicate with the algorithm. Some devices may also need a module to ensure proper use of the device.

Beta Bionics, a company commercializing the algorithms of Boston University, is developing a system using two pumps, delivering insulin and glucagon. Because there is currently no stable liquid glucagon formulation, their first device will be an insulin-only device.

The third company is Bigfoot Biomedical. They are using a proprietary algorithm developed by the company. Their commercial model, unique in many ways, is to lease the device and all disposables for a single monthly fee. This simplifies the usage of the device and the reimbursement.

Cyber-Security

A few years ago, it became clear the insulin pumps could be "hacked" and forced to deliver a lethal dose of insulin. The risk is much higher with an artificial pancreas. The Diabetes Technology Society set standards for diabetes medical devices to prevent such attacks. Using the Common Criteria, they suggested at least a level 4 security was needed. This level of security needs to be designed with the device and built into it. It cannot be added on later. Thus far, none of the companies creating an artificial pancreas had used these standards.

Concluding Remarks

- The artificial pancreas is now available after 20 years of promises.
- Current devices are hybrid devices. The patient still needs to enter information about diet and exercise.
- More systems are on their way with better algorithms and a larger choice of devices.

Questions

1. What are the components of an Artificial Pancreas?
2. What types of algorithms are available? How do they work?
3. Describe currently available devices.
4. How are AP systems clinically tested?
5. What are the advantages of an AP?

References

1. Weinzimer SA. Closed-loop systems: diversity and natural selection. Diabetes Care. 2012;35(11):2111–2.
2. Kadish AH. Automation control of blood sugar. I. A servomechanism for glucose monitoring and control. Am J Med Electron. 1964;3:82–6.
3. Cobelli C, Renard E, Kovatchev B. Artificial pancreas: past, present. Future Diabetes. 2011;60(11):2672–82.
4. Albisser AM, Leibel BS, Ewart TG, Davidovac Z, Botz CK, Zingg W. An artificial endocrine pancreas. Diabetes. 1974;23:389–96.
5. Doyle FJ III, Huyett LM, Lee JB, Zisser HC, Dassau E. Closed-loop artificial pancreas systems: engineering the algorithms. Diabetes Care. 2014;37(5):1191–7.
6. Lunze K, Singh T, Walter M, Brendel M, Leonhardt S. Blood glucose control algorithms for type 1 diabetic patients: A methodological review. Biomed Signal Process Control. 2013;8:107–19. https://doi.org/10.2016/j.bspc.2012.9.003.
7. Donnelly LA, Morris AD, Frier BM, Ellis JD, Donnan PT, Durrant R, Band MM, Reekie G, Leese P. Frequency and predictors of hypoglycaemia in type 1 and insulin-treated type 2 diabetes: a population-based study. Diabet Med. 2005;22:749–55.
8. FDA. The Content of Investigational Device Exemption (IDE) and Premarket Approval (PMA) Applications for Artificial Pancreas Device Systems 2012.
9. Moon SJ, Jung I, Park C-Y. Current advances of artificial pancreas systems: a comprehensive review of clinical evidence. Diabetes Metab J. 2021;45:813–39.

Unproven Therapies for Diabetes

68

Jothydev Kesavadev, Anjana Basanth, and Sanjay Kalra

Introduction

Prevalence and History of Diabetes

There has been a pronounced upsurge in worldwide diabetes prevalence during the past few decades, more notably in developing countries, owing to the rapid globalisation and changing lifestyles. Diabetes-associated complications such as coronary artery and peripheral vascular disease, stroke, diabetic neuropathy, amputations, renal failure, and blindness also add to this burden. According to the recent IDF estimates, one in 10 are living with diabetes. Diabetes-related deaths (6.7 million) were also higher than the total number of deaths caused by HIV (0.068.0 million), tuberculosis (1.5 million), and malaria (0.0627 million) combined. Nearly 537 million people worldwide are estimated to have diabetes, and IDF has raised the concern that by 2030 almost 643 million people and by 2045 almost 783 million adults will have diabetes [1, 2].

The history of diabetes dates back to 3500 years ago, where the first-ever mentioning of clinical features similar to diabetes mellitus is found to have been made in the greatest Egyptian medical document 'Ebers Papyrus' in 1500 BC (Ebbell 1937). Descriptions of this devastating disease have also been found in ancient Indian and Chinese medical literature, as well as in the work of ancient Greek and Arab physicians [3]. Indian physicians named the condition 'madhumeha' or 'honey urine' observing that the urine from diabetes affected individuals attracted ants and flies [4]. Apollonius of Memphis is believed to have coined the term 'diabetes' in 230 BC, meaning 'to pass through' and it was Aretaeus of Cappadocia (second century AD) who provided the first accurate description of diabetes [5]. Later on the Indian physician Sushruta and the surgeon Charaka (400–500 AD) differentiated between the two types of diabetes primarily based on their occurrence in lean or overweight individuals [5, 6].

Remarkable advancements in understanding and management of diabetes took place in the nineteenth century, mostly attributable to the significant progress achieved in various scientific disciplines. Until the discovery of insulin in the 1920s by Banting and colleagues, diabetes treatments mostly adapted highly crude methods for which the success rates were extremely poor [5] and physicians of those times used to make interesting recommendations such as 'oil of roses, dates, raw quinces and gruel, jelly of viper's flesh, broken red coral, sweet almonds and fresh flowers of blind nettles' which represented a variety of beliefs and practices of the times [7]. There are also mentions of opium being prescribed liberally [7, 8] (probably for easing the symptoms of complications like gangrene). Of note, in 1897, the average life expectancy for a 10-year-old child diagnosed with diabetes was 1.3 years, compared with 4.1 years for a 30-year-old person [9].

The first-ever scientific remedy, discovered in 1922, and awarded the Nobel Prize in 1923, insulin turned out to be a major advancement in treating diabetes and enabled patients to live near-normal life [3, 10]. The first-ever oral scientific remedy Sulphonylurea was added to the treatment armamentarium, only in the 1950s. Consequently, other oral scientific remedies with diverse mechanisms of action such as metformin, glucosidase inhibitors, and insulin sensitizers were discovered, enabling better management of the disease. Currently, our treatment armamentarium consists of a vast array of technologies and therapeutic options to make individualised treatment more of a reality. Depending on the type of diabetes and its aetiology, patients may be treated with oral drugs or injectables or sometimes a combination of both. For absolutely insulin-deficient type 1 diabetes mellitus (T1DM) patients, insulin pump therapy or multiple daily insulin injections are the only scientifically recognised modalities of therapy; in the absence of them, subjects are likely to die. With such advances in modern medicine, a dra-

J. Kesavadev (✉) · A. Basanth
Jothydev's Diabetes Research Centers, Trivandrum, Kerala, India

S. Kalra
Department of Endocrinology, Barthi Hospital, Karnal, India

© The Author(s), under exclusive license to Springer Nature Switzerland AG 2023
J. Rodriguez-Saldana (ed.), *The Diabetes Textbook*, https://doi.org/10.1007/978-3-031-25519-9_68

matic improvement in life expectancy has been noted after 1940. As per WHO, the average lifespan of a child born in 2015 is predicted to be 71.4 years whereas earlier estimates of global life expectancy were 30.9 years in 1900, 46.7 in 1940, 61.13 in 1980 [11, 12].

Complementary and Alternative Medicine

Definition and Epidemiology

According to National Center for Complementary and Integrative Health (NCCIH), a subsidary of the National Institutes of Health (NIH), USA, Complementary and Alternative Medicine (CAM) are those healthcare approaches that have developed outside the realm of conventional medicine. Types of complementary and alternative health approaches fall into one of the 2 subgroups, viz. natural products or mind and body practices. Natural products (available widely and often sold as dietary supplements) consist of herbs (or botanicals), vitamins and minerals, and probiotics. Mind and body practices include a variety of procedures or techniques administered or taught by a trained practitioner or teacher (e.g. yoga, chiropractic and osteopathic manipulation, meditation, massage therapy, acupuncture, relaxation techniques, tai chi, etc.). However, some approaches may not neatly fit into either of these groups—e.g. the practices of traditional healers, Ayurvedic medicine, traditional Chinese medicine, homoeopathy, and naturopathy [13].

Of the various demographic descriptors and characteristics of users documented for an inclination towards CAM, more consistent ones include being female, more highly educated, wealthier, employed, and having private health insurance [14–17]. Research has also demonstrated that individuals who possess positive health behaviours and exhibit fewer health risk factors are more frequent CAM users [18].

According to the statistics from 2012 National Health Interview Survey (NHIS), 33.2% of US adults and 11.6% of US children aged 4 to 17 used complementary health approaches. The most commonly used approach was natural products (dietary supplements other than vitamins and minerals). The mind and body approaches most commonly used by adults included yoga, chiropractic or osteopathic manipulation, meditation, and massage therapy. The popularity of such practices might definitely increase in coming years as evident from the data on the percentage of adults who practice yoga. The percentage of followers of this system of practice was found to be increased substantially, from 5.1% in 2002 to 6.1% in 2007 and 9.5% in 2012. As per the survey, nearly 59 million Americans spend money out-of-pocket on complementary health approaches, and their annual spending totalled around 30 billion dollars [19, 20].

Possible Reasons Towards CAM Popularity

A vast majority of patients opt for CAM therapies as a complement to conventional care rather than as an alternative choice [21]. In a US-based study, total visits to complementary medical practitioners (629 million) exceeded total visits to US primary care physicians (386 million) [22]. Traditional CAM practices are extremely popular in South-Asian countries, where modern conventional medicines are often inaccessible and unaffordable to the majority of individuals. Therefore despite the perception about the efficacy of modern medicines, traditional medicine continues to relish acceptance among these populations [23].

Several factors have been noted as reasons for the extensive use of these rather scientifically unproven methods of CAM therapies (Table 68.1). Dissatisfaction arising from conventional therapies, at times, clubbed with higher treatment expenses, concern over side effects of drugs, an urge to have a grip on the course of the disease, and a notion of CAM therapies being compatible with patient's values and beliefs [17, 24–27] are some of them. Patients' expectations of their efficacy [27, 28], advanced stage of the disease [29, 30], experiences with conventional healthcare professionals and complementary medicine practitioners, and 'healthcare pluralism' are also identified as the reasons for this widespread acceptability of CAM therapies. The later term describes the fact that when people become ill they can opt for seeking assistance and treatment advice from diverse sources ranging from friends/family, conventional/CAM practitioners etc. which essentially will have an impact on their treatment choices [31, 32]. Analysis of the 2002 National Health Interview Survey pointed out that around six million American adults had opted CAM therapies predominantly because they found conventional medical treatments unaffordable. Among 63% of the individuals who faced such cost constraints, herbal remedies were found to be the most popular approach [33].

Table 68.1 Reasons for CAM popularity

- Belief that CAM practices are devoid of any side effects and are totally safe
- Non-invasive nature
- Easy accessibility
- Advanced stage of the disease and unpleasant experiences with conventional healthcare professionals
- As recommended by someone close (family members, friends, etc.)
- Pleasant therapeutic experience
- Modern conventional medicines being inaccessible and unaffordable
- Dissatisfaction arising from conventional therapies
- Poor doctor–patient relationship
- Insufficient time with doctor
- Concern over side effects of drugs
- An urge to have a grip on the course of disease
- Notion of CAM therapies being compatible with patient's values and beliefs

CAM Therapies for Diabetes Management

Many Anti-diabetic Medications Have a Natural Origin

Many of the standard conventional drugs have a history of natural origin. However, administering them in their natural form may not be of much benefit. Phytochemicals or compounds present in the natural sources often serve as 'lead' molecules for the synthesis of bioactive compounds and also newer analogues could be derived from some of them. This search for novel bioactive from nature plants, animals, or microflora still continues to widen our treatment armamentarium. Estimates suggest that around one-half of all licensed drugs that were registered worldwide in the 25 year period prior to 2007 were either natural products or their synthetic derivatives [34, 35].

Over 400 traditional plant treatments for diabetes have been reported and only a few of them have undergone valid scientific scrutiny to prove their safety and efficacy [36]. Metformin, a popular anti-diabetic drug and widely accepted first-line agent, was derived from a traditional anti-diabetic plant *Galega officinalis* (Goat's Rue or French Lilac) [37] whose active ingredient was found to be glargine or isoamylene guanidine. While guanidine and certain derivatives were found to have toxic effects, the biguanides (two linked guanidine rings) turned out beneficial and were available for therapeutic use since the 1950s [38]. Further research confirmed antihyperglycaemic efficacy of metformin without causing overt hypoglycaemia or weight gain. Metformin in addition to its antihyperglycaemic properties also stands out for its effects beyond glycaemic control such as improvements in endothelial dysfunction, haemostasis and oxidative stress, insulin resistance, lipid profiles, and fat redistribution [39, 40]. The United Kingdom Prospective Diabetes Study demonstrated that early use of metformin reduced cardiovascular mortality and increased survival in overweight and obese T2DM patients beyond that expected for the prevailing level of glycaemic control [41]. This proven efficacy, safety, beneficial cardiovascular and metabolic effects, and its capacity to be associated with other anti-diabetic agents make metformin the first line of choice for T2DM patients [42] and is included in the World Health Organization (WHO) list of essential medicines [43]. Phlorizin, isolated from the bark of apple trees, was found to cause glycosuria [44] but later led to the discovery of better analogues with SGLT2 inhibiting activity such as dapagliflozin, empagliflozin, and canagliflozin [45, 46].

The discovery of insulin by Frederick Banting and Charles Best in 1921 was indeed a major breakthrough in the treatment of diabetes and it all began with a murky concoction of canine pancreas extract [34, 47]. Likewise, Exenatide and highly accepted insulin with anti-diabetic activities have their origin from animals. Exenatide, a glucagon-like peptide-1 (GLP-1) agonist, is a synthetic version of exendin-4, a hormone found in the venom of Gila monster *Heloderma suspectum* which was isolated by Dr. John Eng in 1992 [48, 49]. This drug has been approved for use in T2DM management [50].

Apart from anti-diabetic compounds of plant and animal origin, some have been derived from microbes. Examples include Acarbose (from Actinoplanes sp.), Miglitol (from Bacillus and Streptomyces sp.), Voglibose (from Streptomyces hydroscopicus subsp. Limoneus) [46], etc. The alpha-glucosidase inhibitor Acarbose used in T2DM is a pseudo-oligosaccharide isolated from the culture broths of various actinomycetes [51]. It is probably the most widely used digestive enzyme inhibitor for the treatment of T2DM, acting on α-glucosidase, α-amylase, sucrase, and maltase, but without insulinotropic properties [52]. With regulated research and controlled clinical trials, there is a higher probability that many more natural agents could be incorporated into the modern stream of medicine.

Prevalence and Patterns of CAM Use Among Diabetes Patients

According to Villa-Caballero and colleagues, the presence of diabetes is a predictor of CAM use and ethnicity determines the types of CAM followed. Of the different CAM modalities, biologically based practices (e.g. dietary supplements, herbal products, and botanical products) are the most commonly used and studied for treating diabetes [53, 54] which is probably due to their wider and cheaper availability, and also being inherent in the cultures and ancestral beliefs of the individuals. Egede et al. using the data from the 1996 Medical Expenditure Panel Survey compared the prevalence and pattern of use of complementary and alternative medicine (CAM) in individuals with and without diabetes and identified factors associated with CAM use. Analysis revealed that diabetes affected individuals were 1.6 times more likely to use CAM than those without diabetes and the most commonly used CAM therapies among diabetes patients were found to be, in the order of importance, nutritional advice and lifestyle diets, spiritual healing, herbal remedies, massage therapy, and meditation training [55]. Another study from Israel reported that almost every fourth patient with diabetes uses CAM [56]. India, a country with a rich history of traditions, rituals, and healing practices, has a very high CAM use of 67% among its diabetic population, of which majority (97%) used Naturopathy, which often included herbalism [57]. An ethnographic study conducted in Kerala revealed that the patient's perceptions of disease as well as its management are influenced by their cultural background and environmental resources. Many of them frequently used Ayurvedic and traditional herbal medicines as supplements to conventional therapy [58].

The National Center for Complementary and Alternative Medicine (NCCAM now re-named as NCCIH) conducted an analysis of the data from National Center for Health Statistics, Centers for Disease Control and Prevention (CDC), and demonstrated that, among adults with T2DM, 30.9% used complementary medicine for any reason, but only 3.4% used complementary medicine to treat or manage their T2DM versus 7.1% of those with T1DM. Almost 77% of the T2DM patients, who used complementary medicine to treat/manage their disease, used it in conjunction with their conventional prescription medicine. Furthermore, individuals with more severe diabetes were predicted to be more likely to use complementary medicine. The most prevalent types of complementary medicine therapies followed included diet-based interventions and non-vitamin/non-mineral dietary supplements [30]. In a study that determined the nature and prevalence of dietary supplement use among chronically ill children, 60% of the patients with T1DM reported using supplements to manage their disease and 31% admitted non-prescribed use [59].

Concerns with CAM Therapies

The widespread use of CAM practices poses several risk factors (see Table 68.2) such as the patients getting overloaded with consecutive unsuccessful therapeutic measures owing to false diagnosis, running into life-threatening situations, adverse effects, and hidden costs of treatment. Opting for these unconventional practices might delay the initiation of effective modern conventional treatments and thereby increase the chances of treatment failures and unbearable treatment expenses [60–64]. Drug–herb interactions, compromised quality of the products due to adulteration or presence of inappropriate amounts of active ingredients, lack of proper regulations on various CAM practices and CAM practitioners, underdeveloped research, poor quality of clinical trials, false claims and fake publicity, absence of proper communication with health practitioners, etc., are all known to be the contributing risk factors towards the failure of CAM therapies [65–68].

Compromised Quality of CAM Products

Lack of proper adherence to manufacturing, marketing, and storage protocols might lead to deterioration in product quality, viz. contamination with undesirable substances; intra-product and inter-product variations; mislabelling of the contents, misidentification, etc., which leaves us highly unsure regarding their safety and efficacy [61, 69–71].

Table 68.2 General concerns associated with CAM therapies

- Adverse drug interactions
- Patient's belief of receiving optimum therapy and finally running into life-threatening conditions and increased treatment costs
- CAM products not meeting quality standards due to reasons such as:
  - Products being adulterated with modern medicines to achieve/enhance the efficacy
  - Inadvertent incorporation of unintended constituents due to errors with herb selection, good manufacturing procedures, etc.
    - Intra- and inter-product variations
    - Mislabelling of the contents
- Poor quality of the clinical trials making it difficult to arrive at a definite conclusion regarding efficacy and safety of CAM practices
- Patient's prejudice that CAM therapies are natural and safe, which increases their tendency towards self-treatment practices and use of over-the-counter products
- Lack of proper communication between the patients and health practitioners regarding CAM use
- Polypharmacy with CAM and conventional treatments resulting in decreased medication adherence and more negative quality of life
- Lack of stringent regulations to guard against quackery in CAM practices

Considering the example of herbs, they do not have a consistent, standardised composition and different plant parts have a different profile of constituents. Furthermore, several factors such as climate, growing conditions, time of harvesting, and post-harvesting factors such as storage conditions and processing are all known to influence the content and concentration of constituents. Although standardisation of many of these products has been implemented, it may not be always feasible since active constituents of many botanicals are still unknown [31]. In a meta-analysis conducted, high variability in ginsenosides levels in ginseng across different source parameters, viz. ginseng-type, assay technique, and ginsenoside type, was shown to result in high variability in their efficacy. This is a warning signal that the reported safety and efficacy data of a particular product may highly differ when compared to other over-the-counter batches, preparations, varieties, and species of the herb [72].

Many US-manufactured and Indian-manufactured Ayurvedic medicines that were sold over the Internet were adulterated with unacceptable levels of lead, mercury, or arsenic [73], and serious consequences were also reported with the use of 'herbal' products that contained 'hidden' active drug compounds or heavy metal contaminants [74–78]. The Centers for Disease Control and Prevention (CDC), USA, had reported lead intoxication from Ayurvedic medications among pregnant women [79]. Since 2007, the FDA has imposed an import alert on certain Ayurvedic products to prevent such products from entering the United States [80]. Accidental or intentional contamination of CAM products with conventional drugs (e.g. corticosteroids) or poisonous substances (e.g. heavy metals, pesticide residues) and microorganisms is also reported [81, 82]. Chinese 'herbal' creams were found to contain corticosteroids [83], and some Indian

Ayurvedic remedies contained heavy metals [74]. Likewise, deterioration in the quality of 'homoeopathic' remedies [84, 85] as well as that of therapeutic essential oils [86], is also a major concern. Another classic example is 'Chinese herb nephropathy' where weight reduction pills supposed to contain the herb *Sephania tetrandra* were inadvertently contaminated with nephrotoxic herb *Aristolochia fangchi,* causing nephropathy and/or cancer in women attending a slimming clinic in Belgium [87–89].

Complications from Drug Interactions

When CAM products such as herbal medicines or dietary supplements are used concomitantly with conventional drugs, a very common practice, there may be a potential for drug–product interactions. Product–product interactions may also occur when many of these products are used concurrently [90]. These interactions often alter the pharmacokinetics or pharmacodynamics of conventional drugs, thereby altering their absorption, distribution, metabolism, and/or excretion [66, 67]. Herbs possessing hypoglycaemic activity like ginseng, garlic, and bitter melon are all reported to have additive effects in patients taking oral hypoglycaemics or insulin [72, 91–93]. In contrast, dietary gums (e.g. gum guar) usually prescribed to overcome postprandial hyperglycaemia were found to reduce the absorption of hypoglycaemic agents like metformin and glibenclamide by prolonging gastric retention [92, 94, 95]. Since diabetes patients are often burdened with many other comorbidities, the majority of them would require lifelong polypharmacotherapy (multiple medications) and hence stand at increased risk of such harmful drug interactions [96].

Underdeveloped Research and Poor Quality of Clinical Trials

Unlike conventional medicine, CAM in general lacks an established research infrastructure and therefore many of the already available scientific evidence are methodologically weak or outright flawed [97–101]. Measures such as the implementation of CONSORT guidelines [102, 103] for reporting and the establishment of a 'field' for CAM in the Cochrane database [104] have allowed us to make a more reliable assessment of the safety and efficacy of these systems of medicinal practices [101].

False Claims and Fake Publicity

Alternative medicine is widely promoted among the public and some of them even claim these therapies to be highly effective with no side effects [105]. The inherent notion among the public that these therapies are 'natural' and hence 'completely safe' enables easier exploitation by advertisers and commerce. The absence of stringent regulations in many countries can allow exaggerated claims to be made and this is more pronounced in areas of commerce that are difficult to control, for example products sold over the internet [106]. It is often seen that the lay literature and even certain 'professional' texts based on some CAM practices make unsubstantiated medical claims as well as encourage self-treatment for even some serious conditions [31, 107].

In India, 'The Drugs and Magic Remedies (Objectionable Advertisements) Act', 1954, controls the advertising of drugs and restricts advertisements of such 'wonder-drugs or remedies' [108].

Lack of Proper Regulations and Policies

Among WHO's 194 countries 97 countries have a national policy on TM/CAM and only 124 countries regulate herbal medicines [109]. The WHO has published a series of technical guidelines and reviewed regulations on herbal medicines in the document 'Regulatory Situation of Herbal Medicines: a Worldwide Review' [110]. In the United States, national non-governmental organisations, such as the Accreditation Commission for Acupuncture and Oriental Medicine, the American Board of Medical Acupuncture, the Council of Chiropractic Education, etc., accredit education in some of them, while most other nations are devoid of these [68]. In the United States prior to 1994, CAM supplements were classified as either foods or drugs depending on the intended use and later Dietary Supplement Health and Education Act (DSHEA 1994) framed a better definition for 'dietary supplement'. It effectively took out any product containing a vitamin, mineral, herb, or amino acid marketed as a supplement to the normal diet from obtaining USFDA approval. This legislation allows such products to forego the stringent approval processes and does not require any proof of their safety and efficacy before being marketed. However, this has led to the situation where many of them are available over the counter even in grocery stores [61, 111].

Similar is the situation of CAM practitioners in many countries where they are not regulated in any manner. There are no systems in place to evaluate the training or expertise of these practitioners [68, 112–114]. In rural areas where timely access to treatment is challenging, this poses a major problem. Many of the times, local practitioners become the primary point of approach and thus the lack of authentic therapists can aggravate the situation [68, 114]. Therefore, imposing restrictions on CAM practitioners without any acceptable educational qualifications and adopting standards of practice should be given due priority to minimise such practice risks [115].

Absence of Proper Communication with Health Practitioners

When the extent of patients' utilisation of complementary medicine, and their knowledge and attitude regarding the same, was studied by Giveon et al., more than half of the respondents believed that natural drugs are safe with no side effects. Users may not relate their symptoms to CAM and not disclose its use to their physician, leading to complications such as delayed diagnosis and treatment, delaying or replacing a more effective form of treatment or even compromise the efficacy of certain conventional drugs. The situation becomes even worse when CAM users are advised by the healers to discontinue the use of prescription drugs, particularly in those with chronic disease conditions [116]. CAM practitioners usually do not encourage inquiries regarding the constituents of their preparations, and most patients are least interested to know about the same as they consider such preparations to be 'natural', otherwise 'safe'. Healthcare professionals are mostly unaware of CAM use by their patients and are not consulted prior to their use [117]. Unfortunately, there are also instances where even when the physicians are aware of their patients using such unproven remedies, they may not be trained to recognise potentially serious side effects [33]. Therefore, it becomes practically impossible to apprehend whether CAM therapy played any significant contributory role towards the efficacy or failure of conventional treatment [118].

In its Position Statement on 'Unproven Therapies', ADA raises the concern that most patients do not disclose the use of alternative medicine and hence conventional practitioners need to specifically ask their patients about the same. ADA continuously evaluates the usefulness of different CAM therapies, their potential risks to the patients and so on to characterise the effectiveness of such treatment modalities. They, however, do not recommend the use of any such unless their safety and efficacy has been established by current standards [119]. In the United Kingdom, the House of Lords' Select Committee on Science and Technology's report on CAM recommended statutory regulation of CAM practitioners and recommended regulatory bodies of healthcare professionals to develop guidelines on CAM competence and training. By this regulation, conventional healthcare professionals are expected to have a basic knowledge of such therapies, and conventional health providers may have interactions with state registered CAM practitioners [120].

Concerns with Other CAM Therapies

Homoeopathy, for example, even though accepted widely, the methodological quality of the trials based on this system of therapy is found to be very poor. Arguments are still on in the view whether homoeopathy is superior to the placebo as a treatment concept [121–123]. Adverse effects can occur if the remedies are not highly diluted since most but not all homoeopathic remedies are devoid of active molecules. Many of the homoeopathic prescriptions include remedies containing arsenic or other highly poisonous substances and in case such a remedy is used in its undiluted form by any chance, it could result in life-threatening consequences [124]. Therapies involving mechanical techniques might cause detrimental effects. Chiropractors, for example, apply a controlled force to a spinal joint and can cause vertebral arterial dissection after upper spinal manipulation [125]. Acupuncture (stimulates specific points on the body by inserting thin needles through the skin) can cause complications like pneumothorax [126, 127], cardiac tamponade [128–130], and central nervous system injuries [131]. Serious infectious complications (like hepatitis, HIV, sub-acute bacterial endocarditis, etc.) can also arise when the practitioners are not concordant with aseptic techniques [132, 133].

Impact of CAM on Diabetes Treatment Outcomes

In a survey conducted among participants of SEARCH for Diabetes in Youth, patients who followed a 'CAM diet' reported a better quality of life (QOL), whereas supplement use and stress reduction activities resulted in decreased QOL. Moreover, children who did not follow any CAM practices experienced lesser treatment barriers [134]. In another study among patients with T2DM and/or cardiovascular disease, higher CAM use was highly correlated with a decreased quality of life in. This was attributed to the negative effects of using multiple therapies where some of them could, in fact, interfere with conventional care [135]. CAM use was also found to decrease the adherence towards prescribed medications in different patient populations [136] including those with diabetes. Patients with T2DM who used CAM were almost 6.16 times less adherent to their prescribed diabetes medication than the non-CAM using counterpart [137, 138]. One of the major reasons postulated towards this diminished adherence is that CAM users are both logistically and psychologically burdened and may need to sacrifice part or all of their prescribed diabetes medication so as to continue using CAM. Another reason pointed out was that the patients believed in CAM healers more than the conventional practitioners [136].

In spite of branding 'natural' and a long history of use, most of these traditional medicines are not necessarily safe. As noted earlier, use of CAMs may delay the use of effective modern conventional treatments and cause adverse effects. Health risks can arise from issues such as drug–herb interactions, adulteration of the products, or the presence of inappropriate amounts of active ingredients in the products [65–67]. Diabetic patients frequently undergo treatment for associated diseases such as hypertension, neuropathy, cardiovascular disease, and so on. While evaluating the effect of CAMs, it is important to understand drugs and drug interactions in depth, and the failure to record the present history of CAM use may lead to problems with other medicines that the patient uses [65, 139]. Instances such as renal failure with use of the dietary supplement chromium picolinate, hepatotoxicity with ingestion of sheep bile, and poor outcomes in a group of patients after abrupt stopping of insulin injections to initiate various CAM therapies have been documented [140]. Another very common drawback noted with CAM products used in diabetes is that when combined with insulin or secretagogues, the patient may experience additive hypoglycaemia due to drug interactions [53]. Herbal medications that claimed to treat diabetes were found to illegitimately incorporate modern medicines with chlorpropamide [141], glibenclamide [142] etc. with a view to enhancing their efficacy and finally resulting in undesirable outcomes. Lead poisoning from herbal remedies is another grave concern [143, 144]. Furthermore, CAM practitioners, as well as manufacturers of such ethnic herbal remedies, even provide patients with fatal advice such as urging them to stop all medicines of diabetes and injections while following CAM therapies which makes the situation even worse [142, 145]. Nutritional advice and lifestyle modifications form essential components of diabetes management, and such recommendations are also often prescribed by many of the CAM providers. The risk lies with the fact that such advice often differs from those endorsed by conventional diabetes care providers and even does not adhere to the guidelines of ADA for diabetes management. Whether these additional nutritional advice and lifestyle diets complement and reinforce ADA guidelines or conflict with the conventional system is another matter of debate [55]. American Diabetes Association's Standards of Medical Care do not support the use of vitamin, mineral, or herbal supplements for diabetes management, due to the lack of sufficient evidence [146].

Fatty liver, non-alcoholic steatohepatitis (NASH), and subsequent cirrhosis are becoming very common in diabetes and associated disorders. Despite the lack of studies or evidence, more and more people are accepting natural remedies with the belief that they are effective with no side effects. But here, the dictum, 'medications with efficacy will also have side effects' stands true. However, those who are advising as well as using it are totally unaware of adverse events. Several observational studies have reiterated the potential hepatotoxic effects of herbal preparations, including asymptomatic minor transaminase elevations, acute and chronic hepatitis, granulomatous hepatitis, asymptomatic to severe cholestasis, sinusoidal obstruction syndrome, acute liver failure requiring transplantation as well as progression to cirrhosis and portal hypertension [194].

Several systematic reviews have been published that weighed the impact and efficacy of various CAM therapies on preventing and treating diabetes. Recently, the effect of Ayurveda on treating diabetes mellitus was studied by Sridharan et al., and the effect of Chinese herbal medicines on impaired glucose tolerance or impaired fasting blood glucose was assessed by Grant et al. Both these reviews pointed out the benefits of following these traditional systems of medicine in treating diabetes or pre-diabetic conditions. The authors, however, stop short of recommending such practices citing the biased nature of certain studies and lack of sufficient evidence [99, 147]. An overview of beneficial and adverse effects identified with some of the widely used herbs, herbal products, and supplements for diabetes management is provided in Table 68.3.

Table 68.3 Commonly used herbs and supplements for diabetes management [53, 64, 69, 95, 148–151, 194, 195]

Name of herb, herbal product, or supplement	Beneficial effects/ hypothesised mechanism of action	Side effects/drug interactions and contradictions
Cinnamomum zeylanicum	Increases insulin sensitivity by increasing PPAR (alpha and gamma) expression, increases cellular glucose entry by enhanced insulin receptor phosphorylation and translocation of GLUT4 glucose transporter to the plasma membrane, promotes glycogen synthesis	Skin irritations if used topically, interacts with secretagogues and causes hypoglycaemia, coumarins possess anticoagulant, carcinogenic, and hepatotoxic properties
Gymnema sylvestre	Insulin secretagogue, increases glucose uptake promoting enzymes, stimulates and increases beta cell number	May cause hypoglycaemia when combined with secretagogues
Bitter melon (*Momordica charantia*)	Hypoglycaemic action, insulin mimetic, enhances glucose uptake by tissues, inhibition of glucose producing enzymes, enhances glucose oxidation (G6PDH pathway)	Gastrointestinal discomfort, hypoglycaemic coma, favism, haemolytic anaemia in persons with G-6PDH deficiency, abortifacient activity of α and β momorcharin, hypoglycaemia when used with sulfonylureas
Fenugreek (*Trigonella foenum-graecum*)	Insulin secretagogue, hypoglycaemic activity, lipid-lowering effects, increases HDL cholesterol, slows carbohydrate absorption and delays gastric emptying, inhibits glucose transport, increases insulin receptors, improves utilisation of peripheral glucose	Diarrhoea, gas, uterine contractions, allergic reactions, drug interaction with hypoglycaemic agents, anticoagulant drugs, MAO inhibitors, contraindicated in pregnancy

(continued)

Table 68.3 (continued)

Name of herb, herbal product, or supplement	Beneficial effects/ hypothesised mechanism of action	Side effects/drug interactions and contradictions
Guar gum	Alters gastrointestinal transit and delays glucose absorption, lipid-lowering effects by decreasing its absorption and increasing bile excretion	Gastrointestinal upset, may delay the absorption of drugs, possibility of hypoglycaemia when combined with secretagogues, additive lipid lowering when used along with antihyperlipidemic agents
Noni (Morinda citrifolia)	Reduces fasting glucose, HbA1c, serum triglycerides, and LDL cholesterol and improves insulin sensitivity (data limited to in vivo and in vitro studies)	Severe acute liver failure; acute hepatitis with portal inflammation and periportal necrosis
Gurmar (Gymnema sylvestre)	Gymnemic acid type A, phytochemical compound present in shoot tips and seeds, is one of the most potent hypoglycaemic components. Some of the alkaloids and saponins in the plant also act as appetite suppressants	Hepatotoxicity, may cause acute hepatitis
Chromium	Lipid-lowering effects, insulin sensitising effect by decreasing tyrosine phosphatase activity or direct effect on insulin receptor by increasing tyrosine kinase activity at the insulin receptor, may promote glucose transport	Renal toxicity and dermatological reactions, potential hypoglycaemia with secretagogues, steroids may decrease chromium levels, vitamin C may increase chromium absorption
Alpha-lipoic acid	Improves insulin resistance and increases glucose effectiveness	Can affect thyroid function in patients with thyroid disease, might produce allergic skin reactions, abdominal pain, nausea, vomiting, diarrhoea, and vertigo
Omega-3 fatty acid/fish oil	Lowers triglycerides, anti-inflammatory, anti-platelet, hypotensive, slight increase in blood glucose	High intake might cause bleeding, fish meat to be eaten with caution due to contamination with high levels of methyl mercury; may increase LDL, drug interactions with anticoagulant and anti-hypertension drugs

Evidence regarding the use of other systems of CAM for diabetes is also in its infancy and in fact, the available little evidence cautions the patients and the practitioners regarding their safe and effective use. Studies which assess acupuncture are methodologically problematic mainly due to reasons such as the procedure has no adequate control condition, treatments in daily practice are mostly individualised, short duration of the studies, etc. [152–154]. None of the trials conducted in diabetes patients could provide convincing evidence on acupuncture for treating conditions like insulin resistance [154], diabetic gastroparesis [155], and diabetic peripheral neuropathy [156]. Practitioners and patients who support acupuncture for diabetic neuropathy may also bear in mind the increased risk of acupuncture needle site infection with high blood glucose levels [157]. Opting for acupuncture after discontinuing conventional therapy recently led to the death of a 30-year-old T1DM individual in India [158]. 'Sweet therapy' is another peculiar diabetes treatment practised in Kerala, which claims to stimulate the sleeping pancreas to secrete insulin by intake of glucose-rich foods such as sweet desserts. However, the long-term serious implications of such modalities on the health of the patients are not documented.

Trials that investigated the effects of tai chi [159–163] and qi gong [152, 164] on diabetes also could not reach any definitive conclusions. Such mind–body therapies which involve movements can at best be considered as alternative modes of exercise [165, 166]. The perceived advantage of these therapies is that they can be performed at almost any level of exercise tolerance when compared to traditional exercise, and thus might be helpful for increasing movement and activity especially for some persons with diabetes such as older and obese individuals [152]. They might also be helpful in imparting behavioural and psychological changes and thereby help patients to cope with the disease and increase their quality of life [167]. However, neither yoga [168, 169] nor tai chi [170–172] has been shown to have any significant impact on improving the glycaemic status. In diabetes patients who follow practices such as massage, Therapeutic Touch, Healing Touch, and Reiki, appropriate blood glucose monitoring and titration of anti-diabetes medications should be recommended when blood glucose levels become lower as pain and discomfort decrease. During energy therapy, catecholamines like epinephrine and norepinephrine get released which can increase lipolysis and thermogenesis, leading to increased energy expenditure and weight changes [157].

Recommendations for a Prospective CAM Use

Proper Patient–Physician Fit and Judicious Choice of Therapies

The current hypothesis is that treatment settings influence a patient's mindset and even influence the effects of interventions. This speaks volumes regarding the importance of maintaining a positive relationship between the patient and the caregiver in achieving commendable treatment efficacy [121]. Unfortunately, most of the times patients following conventional medicine were dissatisfied with the manner of communication by the practitioners, were worried about the side effects of pharmacotherapy, and also felt the lack of a holistic treatment approach. On the other hand, CAM seemed to reinforce a patient's own self-healing capacity. Alternative therapists tend to spend more time with their patients which help to develop a good patient–physician fit, and many of the patients appreciated this approach [173].

CAM use often remains underreported and thus a lack of proper communication between patients and healthcare providers can often end up in treatment failures or adverse events. Care providers should put in their efforts to understand the motivations behind a patient's CAM use and be prepared to counsel such patients, when needed, about the options available and should be able to assess, as well as present information to the patients regarding the expected risks, side effects, benefits, and choices regarding self-management and its cost to the patient, helping them to make an informed choice [53, 136, 174]. In patients who persist on following CAM, it is advisable to identify the effects of each of the components of these medications so that patients can be counselled regarding any contra-indications to any of the constituents. Patients should be adequately monitored and warned of the potential side effects, and healthcare practitioners should be aware of the potential interactions between the active components of the alternative medications and other prescribed medications [175]. For individuals exploring supplements, FDA's documents such as 'Tips for the savvy supplement user', 'Tips for Older Dietary Supplement Users', and 'Questions and Answers on Dietary Supplements' might turn helpful (accessible at http://www.fda.gov). A database of natural medicine available at 'www.prescribersletter.therapeuticresearch.com' provides necessary information regarding the usage of herbs and supplements and their safety issues [176]. The American Diabetes Association in two of its articles 'A Step-by-Step Approach to Complementary Therapies' and 'Guidelines for Using Vitamin, Mineral, and Herbal Supplements' has offhandedly acknowledged the popularity of CAM for diabetes and provides a set of approaches that could be undertaken in order to safely integrate complementary therapies into an individual's healthcare plan [177, 178]. In its position statement, ADA proposes to evaluate each questionable diagnostic or therapeutic modalities and recommends proving new and innovative, but unproven, diagnostic and therapeutic measures for patients based on certain preset criteria and also

encourages healthcare providers to ask patients about their alternative therapy practices [179].

Proper Regulations and Well-Conducted Research

Although anti-diabetic drugs used in modern medicine have a natural origin [34], administering them in their natural form may not be of much benefit. Randomised clinical trials of herbal medicine interventions too often underreport the crucial characteristics of the intervention, thereby deviating from the standards set by Consolidated Standards of Reporting Trials (CONSORT) [180, 181]. However, with regulated research, there is a higher probability that many more natural agents could be used in modern medicine. Experts recommend that CAM and dietary supplements should be subject to scrutiny similar to conventional medicines by organisations such as the NIH and FDA. Any measure to bypass these may render the healthcare system inefficient, incapable, and dangerous [182, 183]. Adequate or accepted research methodology for evaluating these healthcare practices needs to be developed. Consideration should also be given to increase the overall quality of research, avoid publication bias, protect intellectual property, and also to certify authentic CAM products and practices from illegitimate ones [184].

Integrating CAM into Conventional Care

Although CAM practices lack sufficient evidence, the popularity of such practices is ever increasing and its integration into mainstream health care is much looked at. In certain regions, CAM practices are included under health insurance coverage and certain 'integrated' delivery systems have also been established [15, 185]. While considering the integration of medical systems, apart from emphasising patients' expectations and needs, it should be prioritised that accepted standards of medical and scientific principles of practice remain unaltered [186]. With such integration, patients are believed to get benefited at multiple levels such as better decision-making, enhanced physical and emotional well-being, and gaining knowledge on health-promoting practices (Furnham 1996). Healthcare providers can also get benefitted in terms of greater satisfaction through learning new treatment strategies and developing skills to implement them [187]. Thus a more integrated system is expected to facilitate discussion and collaboration between the two systems of medicine to improve healthcare delivery [188]. A snapshot of the recommendations suggested towards a prospective CAM use is provided in Table 68.4.

Table 68.4 Recommendations for a prospective CAM use

Developing a proper patient–physician fit that can encourage patients to openly communicate regarding CAM use
- Healthcare providers should try to understand patient's motivations behind CAM use so as to choose an optimal treatment plan
- Healthcare providers can take efforts to assess, as well as present necessary information to the patients regarding different aspects of CAM use and thus help them make a more informed choice

Validating the safety and efficacy of CAM therapies through well-planned clinical trials that meet quality research standards

Impose proper regulations and scrutiny on CAM practices, products, and practitioners to ensure their safety, quality, and efficacy

Integration of CAM and conventional medical systems by giving emphasis to patient's expectations and needs, without altering the accepted standards of medical and scientific principles

CAM Therapy and COVID-19

The Coronavirus disease 2019 (COVID-19) caused by severe acute respiratory syndrome coronavirus 2 (SARS-CoV-2) has met international health systems with a low level of preparedness and emergency response [189]. A wide range of CAM therapies are being practised worldwide including acupuncture, acupressure, cupping, massage, gestalt therapy, reflexology, muscle therapy, etc. for the prevention and cure of COVID-19 [190]. With a rich history of traditional medicines, countries like China and India explored the effectiveness of their traditional medicines to prevent and cure COVID-19.

In India, the ministry of AYUSH (Ayurveda, Yoga and Naturopathy, Unani, Siddha, and Homoeopathy) to encourage research in various traditional drugs on COVID-19 established guidelines focusing on multi-pronged approach of Ayurvedic medications, which are already in use for a long time for ailments like fever, cough, and respiratory distress [191].

Evidence from several studies has shown that some plant preparations and spices such as pepper, ginger, cumin, and coriander seeds have anti-viral, anti-bacterial, and anti-microbial properties [192, 193]. Given that some of these preparations lack data related to efficacy, adverse events, manufacturing method, and quality control. However, many preparations are also being propagated without having any scientific evidence.

Currently, there is only limited research from human clinical trials in regard to the effectiveness of CAM in prevention, treatment, or symptom relief in COVID-19.

Conclusion

Even with the advancements achieved in modern conventional medicine, a lot many patients still continue to follow traditional CAM practices due to a variety of reasons such as their perceived safety and efficacy, easy availability or matching with their cultural beliefs and practices, and so on. However, the risk–benefit ratio of these CAM practices on the disease outcomes especially the chronic one like diabetes still remains unproven. Conventional healthcare providers in most cases are not aware of their patients following such modes of therapies and also are not in a position to comment on regarding the same. They should put in efforts to maintain a good rapport with the patients so as to enable open communication regarding CAM use so as to help them make a judicious choice of such therapies. Imposing stringent rules and regulations as well as conducting clinical trials that meet quality research standards can no doubt reveal the true potential of at least some of these age-old practices. With that achieved, the successful integration of reliable and safe CAM practices into mainstream health care can be thought of in order to improve the overall treatment experience and outcomes.

Multiple-Choice Questions

1. Complementary and alternative medicines:
   (a) Are essential additional elements of diabetes management
   (b) **Are healthcare approaches developed outside the realm of conventional medicine**
   (c) Are exclusively medicines
   (d) Include surgical interventions
   (e) Are evidence-based
2. Complementary health approaches:
   (a) Are rarely used
   (b) Are largely used by people with low economic resources
   (c) **Are used by 33.2% of adults in the United States**
   (d) Are used mostly by men
   (e) Represent a minimal amount of healthcare costs
3. Reasons for the popularity of complementary alternative medications include all of the following, except:
   (a) Easy accessibility
   (b) Dissatisfaction with conventional medical care
   (c) Belief of safety
   (d) **High costs**
   (e) Poor doctor–patient relationship
4. Many currently approved anti-diabetic medications have a natural origin:
   (a) **True**
   (b) False
5. Examples of anti-diabetic drugs with natural origin:
   (a) Insulin
   (b) Sulfonylureas
   (c) **Metformin**
   (d) **SGLT2 inhibitors**
   (e) **GLP-1 agonists**

6. The percentage of patients with type 2 diabetes using complementary medicine in addition to conventional prescriptions:
   (a) 15%
   (b) 27%
   (c) 48%
   (d) 60%
   (e) **77%**

7. The use of complementary alternative medications has several risks, including:
   (a) Adverse effects
   (b) Hidden costs
   (c) Overload with unsuccessful therapies
   (d) Lack of proper regulations
   (e) **All of the above**

8. The hypothesised mechanism of action of chromium:
   (a) Insulin secretagogue
   (b) **Insulin sensitizing agent**
   (c) Insulin mimetic
   (d) Inhibits glucose transport
   (e) Alters gastrointestinal transit

9. The hypothesised mechanism of action of guar gum:
   (a) Insulin secretagogue
   (b) Insulin sensitizing agent
   (c) Insulin mimetic
   (d) Inhibits glucose transport
   (e) **Alters gastrointestinal transit**

10. Recommendations for the prospective use of complementary alternative medications involve:
    (a) Recognition as essential elements of management
    (b) Learning about their effectiveness
    (c) **Judicious choice of therapies**
    (d) Combination with standard therapies
    (e) Discourage their use by patients

References

1. IDF diabetes atlas 2021. International diabetes federation. 10th ed; 2021.
2. https://www.who.int/. Accessed on 15 01 2022.
3. Karamanou M, Protogerou A, Tsoucalas G, Androutsos G, Poulakou-Rebelakou E. Milestones in the history of diabetes mellitus: the main contributors. World J Diabetes. 2016;7(1):1.
4. Papaspyros NS. The history of diabetes mellitus: G. Thieme; 1964.
5. Poretsky L. Principles of diabetes mellitus. New York: Springer US; 2010.
6. Frank LL. Diabetes mellitus in the texts of old Hindu medicine (Charaka, Susruta, Vagbhata). Am J Gastroenterol. 1957;27(1):76–95.
7. Lakhtakia R. The history of diabetes mellitus. Sultan Qaboos Univ Med J. 2013;13(3):368.
8. Allan FN. The writings of Thomas Willis, MD: diabetes three hundred years ago. Diabetes. 1953;2(1):74–8.
9. MacCracken J, Hoel D, Jovanovic L. From ants to analogues: puzzles and promises in diabetes management. Postgrad Med. 1997;101(4):138–50.
10. Ahmed AM. History of diabetes mellitus. Saudi Med J. 2002;23(4):373–8.
11. Life expectancy increased by 5 years since 2000, but health inequalities persist. Geneva: World Health Organization, Observatory GH; 2016 19 May 2016 Report No.
12. Mishra S. Does modern medicine increase life-expectancy: quest for the moon rabbit? Indian Heart J. 2016;68(1):19–27.
13. Complementary, Alternative, or integrative health: What's in a name? USA: National Center for Complementary and Integrative Health; 2016 [updated June 2016 cited 2016 27.09.16]. Available from: https://nccih.nih.gov/health/integrative-health
14. MacLennan AH, Wilson DH, Taylor AW. The escalating cost and prevalence of alternative medicine. Prev Med. 2002;35(2):166–73.
15. O'Brien K. Complementary and alternative medicine: the move into mainstream health care. Clin Exp Optom. 2004;87(2):110–20.
16. Lloyd P, Lupton D, Wiesner D, Hasleton S. Choosing alternative therapy: an exploratory study of sociodemographic characteristics and motives of patients resident in Sydney. Aust N Z J Public Health. 1993;17(2):135–44.
17. Astin JA. Why patients use alternative medicine: results of a national study. JAMA. 1998;279(19):1548–53.
18. Nahin RL, Dahlhamer JM, Taylor BL, Barnes PM, Stussman BJ, Simile CM, et al. Health behaviors and risk factors in those who use complementary and alternative medicine. BMC Public Health. 2007;7(1):217.
19. Nahin R, Barnes P, Stussman B. Expenditures on complementary health approaches: United States, 2012. Natl Health Stat Rep. 2016;95:1.
20. Clarke TC, Black LI, Stussman BJ, Barnes PM, Nahin RL. Trends in the use of complementary health approaches among adults: United States, 2002–2012. Natl Health Stat Rep. 2015;79:1.
21. Barnes PM, Bloom B, Nahin RL. Complementary and alternative medicine use among adults and children: United States, 2007. Centers for Disease Control and Prevention, National Center for Health Statistics Hyattsville, MD: US Department of Health and Human Services; 2008.
22. Eisenberg DM, Davis RB, Ettner SL, Appel S, Wilkey S, Van Rompay M, et al. Trends in alternative medicine use in the United States, 1990–1997: results of a follow-up national survey. JAMA. 1998;280(18):1569–75.
23. Amin F, Islam N, Gilani A. Traditional and complementary/alternative medicine use in a South-Asian population. Asian Pacific Journal of Health Sciences 2015;2:36–42.
24. Barnes PM, Powell-Griner E, McFann K, Nahin RL. Complementary and alternative medicine use among adults: United States, 2002. Sem Integr Med. 2004;2(2):54–71.
25. Naja F, Mousa D, Alameddine M, Shoaib H, Itani L, Mourad Y. Prevalence and correlates of complementary and alternative medicine use among diabetic patients in Beirut, Lebanon: a cross-sectional study. BMC Complement Altern Med. 2014;14(1):1.
26. Verhoef MJ, Balneaves LG, Boon HS, Vroegindewey A. Reasons for and characteristics associated with complementary and alternative medicine use among adult cancer patients: a systematic review. Integr Cancer Ther. 2005;4(4):274–86.
27. Ernst E. The role of complementary and alternative medicine. Br Med J. 2000;321(7269):1133.
28. Bauml JM, Chokshi S, Schapira MM, Im EO, Li SQ, Langer CJ, et al. Do attitudes and beliefs regarding complementary and alternative medicine impact its use among patients with cancer? A cross-sectional survey Cancer. 2015;121(14):2431–8.
29. Kim SH, Shin DW, Nam Y-S, Kim SY, Yang H-k, Cho BL, et al. Expected and perceived efficacy of complementary and alternative medicine: A comparison views of patients with cancer and oncologists. Complement Thr Med. 2016;28:29–36.
30. Nahin RL, Byrd-Clark D, Stussman BJ, Kalyanaraman N. Disease severity is associated with the use of complementary medicine to

treat or manage type-2 diabetes: data from the 2002 and 2007 National Health Interview Survey. BMC Complement Altern Med. 2012;12:193.

31. Barnes J. Quality, efficacy and safety of complementary medicines: fashions, facts and the future. Part I. regulation and quality. Br J Clin Pharmacol. 2003;55(3):226–33.

32. Furnharm A. Why do people choose and use complementary therapies? In complementary medicine an objective appraisal. Edited by: Ernst E. Oxford: Butterworth-Heinemann; 1996.

33. Tu H, Hargraves J. High cost of medical care prompts consumers to seek alternatives. Data Bullet. 2004;28:1.

34. Osadebe PO, Odoh EU. Natural products as potential sources of antidiabetic drugs. Br J Pharm Res. 2014;4(17):2075.

35. Newman DJ, Cragg GM. Natural products as sources of new drugs over the last 25 years⊥. J Nat Prod. 2007;70(3):461–77.

36. Bailey CJ, Day C. Traditional plant medicines as treatments for diabetes. Diabetes Care. 1989;12(8):553–64.

37. Oubre A, Carlson T, King S, Reaven G. From plant to patient: an ethnomedical approach to the identification of new drugs for the treatment of NIDDM. Diabetologia. 1997;40(5):614–7.

38. Biguanides SG. A review of history, pharmacodynamics and therapy. Diabete Metab. 1982;9(2):148–63.

39. Bailey CJ, Day C. Metformin: its botanical background. Practical Diabetes International. 2004;21(3):115–7.

40. Goodarzi MO, Bryer-Ash M. Metformin revisited: re-evaluation of its properties and role in the pharmacopoeia of modern antidiabetic agents. Diabetes Obes Metab. 2005;7(6):654–65.

41. Group UPDS. Effect of intensive blood-glucose control with metformin on complications in overweight patients with type 2 diabetes (UKPDS 34). Lancet. 1998;352(9131):854–65.

42. Rojas LBA, Gomes MB. Metformin: an old but still the best treatment for type 2 diabetes. Diabetol Metab Syndr. 2013;5(1):6.

43. WHO model lists of essential medicines [updated April 2015]. 19:[Available from: http://www.who.int/medicines/publications/essentialmedicines/en/

44. Ehrenkranz JR, Lewis NG, Kahn CR, Roth J. Phlorizin: a review. Diabetes Metab Res Rev. 2005;21(1):31–8.

45. White JR. Apple trees to sodium glucose co-transporter inhibitors: A review of SGLT2 inhibition. Clinical Diabetes. 2010;28(1):5–10.

46. Ríos JL, Francini F, Schinella GR. Natural products for the treatment of type 2 diabetes mellitus. Planta Med. 2015;81(12/13):975–94.

47. Karamitsos DT. The story of insulin discovery. Diabetes Res Clin Pract. 2011;93:S2–8.

48. Eng J, Kleinman W, Singh L, Singh G, Raufman J-P. Isolation and characterization of exendin-4, an exendin-3 analogue, from Heloderma suspectum venom. Further evidence for an exendin receptor on dispersed acini from Guinea pig pancreas. J Biol Chem. 1992;267(11):7402–5.

49. Furman BL. The development of Byetta (exenatide) from the venom of the Gila monster as an anti-diabetic agent. Toxicon. 2012;59(4):464–71.

50. Nathan DM, Buse JB, Davidson MB, Ferrannini E, Holman RR, Sherwin R, et al. Medical Management of Hyperglycemia in type 2 diabetes: A consensus algorithm for the initiation and adjustment of therapy. A consensus statement of the American Diabetes Association and the European Association for the Study of Diabetes. Diabetes Care. 2009;27(1):4–16.

51. Leroux-Stewart J, Rabasa-Lhoret R, Chiasson J-L. α-Glucosidase inhibitors. In: International textbook of diabetes mellitus. New York: John Wiley & Sons, Ltd; 2015. p. 673–85.

52. Wehmeier U, Piepersberg W. Biotechnology and molecular biology of the α-glucosidase inhibitor acarbose. Appl Microbiol Biotechnol. 2004;63(6):613–25.

53. Birdee GS, Yeh G. Complementary and alternative medicine Therapies for diabetes: A clinical review. Clin Diabetes. 2010;28(4):147–55.

54. Villa-Caballero L, Morello CM, Chynoweth ME, Prieto-Rosinol A, Polonsky WH, Palinkas LA, et al. Ethnic differences in complementary and alternative medicine use among patients with diabetes. Complement Thr Med. 2010;18(6):241–8.

55. Egede LE, Ye X, Zheng D, Silverstein MD. The prevalence and pattern of complementary and alternative medicine use in individuals with diabetes. Diabetes Care. 2002;25(2):324–9.

56. Koren R, Lerner A, Tirosh A, Zaidenstein R, Ziv-Baran T, Golik A, et al. The use of complementary and alternative medicine in hospitalized patients with type 2 diabetes mellitus in Israel. J Altern Complement Med. 2015;21(7):395–400.

57. Kumar D, Bajaj S, Mehrotra R. Knowledge, attitude and practice of complementary and alternative medicines for diabetes. Public Health. 2006;120(8):705–11.

58. Chacko E. Culture and therapy: complementary strategies for the treatment of type-2 diabetes in an urban setting in Kerala. India Soc Sci Med. 2003;56(5):1087–98.

59. Ball SD, Kertesz D, Moyer-Mileur LJ. Dietary supplement use is prevalent among children with a chronic illness. J Am Diet Assoc. 2005;105(1):78–84.

60. Niggemann B, Grüber C. Unconventional and conventional medicine: who should learn from whom? Pediatr Allergy Immunol. 2003;14(3):149–55.

61. Ventola CL. Current issues regarding complementary and alternative medicine (CAM) in the United States: part 2: regulatory and safety concerns and proposed governmental policy changes with respect to dietary supplements. P T. 2010;35(9):514.

62. Boström H, Rössner S. Quality of alternative medicine—complications and avoidable deaths. Int J Qual Health Care. 1990;2(2):111–7.

63. Sadikot SM, Das AK, Wilding J, Siyan A, Zargar AH, Saboo B, et al. Consensus recommendations on exploring effective solutions for the rising cost of diabetes. Diabetes Metab Syndr Clin Res Rev. 2017;11(2):141–7.

64. Kesavadev J, Saboo B, Sadikot S, Das AK, Joshi S, Chawla R, et al. Unproven Therapies for diabetes and their implications. Adv Ther. 2016:1–18.

65. Guthrie D, Guthrie R. Management of diabetes mellitus: A guide to the pattern approach. 6th ed. New York: Springer Publishing Company, LLC; 2008. 544 p.

66. Marchetti S, Mazzanti R, Beijnen JH, Schellens JH. Concise review: clinical relevance of drug–drug and herb–drug interactions mediated by the ABC transporter ABCB1 (MDR1, P-glycoprotein). Oncologist. 2007;12(8):927–41.

67. Rehman US, Choi MS, Choe K, Yoo HH. Interactions between herbs and antidiabetics: an overview of the mechanisms, evidence, importance, and management. Arch Pharm Res. 2015;38(7):1281–98.

68. Debas HT, Laxminarayan R. E. SS. Complementary and alternative medicine. In: Jamison DT, Breman JG, Measham AR, Alleyne G, Claeson M, Evans DB, Jha P, Mills A, Musgrove P, editors. Disease control priorities in developing countries. 2nd ed. Washington (DC): Co-published by Oxford University Press, New York; 2006.

69. Shane-McWhorter L. Complementary and alternative medicine (CAM) supplement use in people with diabetes: A clinician's guide. Arlington County, Virginia: American Diabetes Association; 2007.

70. Ko RJ. Adulterants in Asian patent medicines. N Engl J Med. 1998;339(12):847.

71. Grant KL. Patient education and herbal dietary supplements. Am J Health Syst Pharm. 2000;57(21):1997–2003.

72. Vuksan V, Sievenpiper JL. Herbal remedies in the management of diabetes: lessons learned from the study of ginseng. Nutr Metab Cardiovasc Dis. 2005;15(3):149–60.

73. Saper RB, Phillips RS, Sehgal A, Khouri N, Davis RB, Paquin J, et al. Lead, mercury, and arsenic in US-and Indian-manufactured ayurvedic medicines sold via the internet. JAMA. 2008;300(8):915–23.

74. Ernst E. Toxic heavy metals and undeclared drugs in Asian herbal medicines. Trends Pharmacol Sci. 2002;23(3):136–9.

75. Goudie AM, Kaye JM. Contaminated medication precipitating hypoglycaemia. Med J Aust. 2001;175(5):256.

76. Huang WF, Wen KC, Hsiao ML. Adulteration by synthetic therapeutic substances of traditional Chinese medicines in Taiwan. J Clin Pharmacol. 1997;37(4):344–50.

77. Ries CA, Sahud MA. Agranulocytosis caused by Chinese herbal medicines: dangers of medications containing aminopyrine and phenylbutazone. JAMA. 1975;231(4):352–5.

78. Shaw D, Leon C, Kolev S, Murray V. Traditional remedies and food supplements. Drug Saf. 1997;17(5):342–56.

79. Lead poisoning in pregnant women who used ayurvedic medications from India — new York City, 2011–2012. USA: Centers for Disease Control and Prevention, 2012 August 24. Report No.

80. FDA. Use caution with ayurvedic products USA U.S. Food and Drug Administration; 2008 [updated 07/15/2015]. Available from: http://www.fda.gov/ForConsumers/ConsumerUpdates/ucm050798.htm

81. Barnes J, Anderson LA, Phillipson JD. Herbal medicines: a guide for healthcare professionals. London: Pharmaceutical Press; 2003.

82. Bisset NG. Herbal drugs and phytopharmaceuticals: a handbook for practice on a scientific basis: Stuttgart: Medpharm Scientific Publishers xvi, 566p. ISBN 3887630254 En Originally published in German (1984).(EBBD, 190000550); 1994.

83. MKeane F, Munn S, Du Vivier A, Taylor N, Higgins E. Analysis of Chinese herbal creams prescribed for dermatological conditions. BMJ. 1999;318(7183):563–4.

84. Kerr HD, Saryan LA. Arsenic content of homeopathic medicines. J Toxicol Clin Toxicol. 1986;24(5):451–9.

85. Morice A. Adulterated. Lancet. 1986;327(8485):862–3.

86. Tisserand R, Young R. Essential oil safety: a guide for health care professionals. Elsevier Health Sciences; 2013.

87. Cosyns J-P, Jadoul M, Squifflet J-P, Wese F-X, de Strihou CvY. Urothelial lesions in Chinese-herb nephropathy. Am J Kidney Dis. 1999;33(6):1011–7.

88. Nortier JL, Martinez M-CM, Schmeiser HH, Arlt VM, Bieler CA, Petein M, et al. Urothelial carcinoma associated with the use of a Chinese herb (Aristolochia fangchi). N Engl J Med. 2000;342(23):1686–92.

89. Cosyns J-P. Aristolochic acid and 'Chinese herbs nephropathy'. Drug Saf. 2003;26(1):33–48.

90. Barnes J. Quality, efficacy and safety of complementary medicines: fashions, facts and the future. Part II: efficacy and safety. Br J Clin Pharmacol. 2003;55(4):331–40.

91. Gardiner P, Phillips R, Shaughnessy AF. Herbal and dietary supplement-drug interactions in patients with chronic illnesses. Am Fam Physician. 2008;77(1):73–8.

92. Izzo AA. Herb–drug interactions: an overview of the clinical evidence. Fundam Clin Pharmacol. 2005;19(1):1–16.

93. Aslam M, Stockley I. Interaction between curry ingredient (karela) and drug (chlorpropamide). Lancet. 1979;313(8116):607.

94. Gin H, Orgerie M, Aubertin J. The influence of guar gum on absorption of metformin from the gut in healthy volunteers. Horm Metab Res. 1989;21(02):81–3.

95. Neugebauer G, Akpan W, Abshagen U. Interaction of guar with glibenclamide and bezafibrate. Beitr Infusionther Klin Ernahr. 1983;12:40.

96. Caughey GE, Roughead EE, Vitry AI, McDermott RA, Shakib S, Gilbert AL. Comorbidity in the elderly with diabetes: identification of areas of potential treatment conflicts. Diabetes Res Clin Pract. 2010;87(3):385–93.

97. Hardy ML, Coulter I, Venuturupalli S, Roth EA, Favreau J, Morton SC, et al. Ayurvedic interventions for diabetes mellitus: A systematic review: summary. Evid REp Technol Assess (Summ) 2001;(41):2p.

98. Elder C. Ayurveda for diabetes mellitus: a review of the biomedical literature. Altern Ther Health Med. 2004;10(1):44.

99. Sridharan K, Mohan R, Ramaratnam S, Panneerselvam D. Ayurvedic treatments for diabetes mellitus. Cochrane Database Syst Rev. 2011;12:CD008288.

100. Linde K, Jonas WB, Melchart D, Willich S. The methodological quality of randomized controlled trials of homeopathy, herbal medicines and acupuncture. Int J Epidemiol. 2001;30(3):526–31.

101. Ernst E, Cohen M, Stone J. Ethical problems arising in evidence based complementary and alternative medicine. J Med Ethics. 2004;30(2):156–9.

102. Begg C, Cho M, Eastwood S, Horton R, Moher D, Olkin I, et al. Improving the quality of reporting of randomized controlled trials: the CONSORT statement. JAMA. 1996;276(8):637–9.

103. Moher D, Jones A, Lepage L, Group C. Use of the CONSORT statement and quality of reports of randomized trials: a comparative before-and-after evaluation. JAMA. 2001;285(15):1992–5.

104. Ezzo J, Berman BM, Vickers AJ, Linde K. Complementary medicine and the Cochrane collaboration. JAMA. 1998;280(18):1628–30.

105. Misra A, Gulati S, Luthra A. Alternative medicines for diabetes in India: maximum hype, minimum science. Lancet Diabetes Endocrinol. 2016;4(4):302–3.

106. Mukherjee PK, Houghton PJ. Evaluation of herbal medicinal products: perspectives on quality, Safety and Efficacy. London: Pharmaceutical Press; 2009.

107. Vickers A, Stevensen C, Van Toller S. Massage and aromatherapy: a guide for health professionals. New York: Springer; 2013.

108. Drugs and magic remedies (objectionable advertisements) act, Stat 21 (30th April 1954, 1954).

109. World Health Organization. WHO global report on traditional and complementary medicine 2019. World Health Organization. 2019. https://apps.who.int/iris/handle/10665/312342

110. Zhang X. Regulatory situation of herbal medicines A worldwide review. Geneva: World Health Organization; 1998. p. 26.

111. Berman JD, Straus SE. Implementing a research agenda for complementary and alternative medicine. Annu Rev Med. 2004;55:239–54.

112. Mills SY. Regulation in complementary and alternative medicine. Br Med J. 2001;322(7279):158.

113. Santé Omdl. WHO global atlas of traditional, complementary and alternative medicine: WHO Centre for Health Development; 2005.

114. Ries NM, Fisher KJ. Increasing involvement of physicians in complementary and alternative medicine: considerations of professional regulation and patient safety. Queen's Law J. 2013;39(1):273–300.

115. Myers SP, Cheras PA. The other side of the coin: safety of complementary and alternative medicine. Med J Aust. 2004;181(4):222–5.

116. Giveon SM, Liberman N, Klang S, Kahan E. Are people who use "natural drugs" aware of their potentially harmful side effects and reporting to family physician? Patient Educ Couns. 2004;53(1):5–11.

117. Tan AC, Mak JC. Complementary and alternative medicine in diabetes (CALMIND)--a prospective study. J Complement Integr Med. 2015;12(1):95–9.

118. Ezuruike UF, Prieto JM. The use of plants in the traditional management of diabetes in Nigeria: pharmacological and toxicological considerations. J Ethnopharmacol. 2014;155(2):857–924.

119. American Diabetes A. Unproven therapies. Diabetes Care. 2004;27(Suppl 1):S135.

120. House of lords- science and technology - sixth report. UK Parliament, 2000.

121. Shang A, Huwiler-Müntener K, Nartey L, Jüni P, Dörig S, Sterne JAC, et al. Are the clinical effects of homoeopathy placebo effects? Comparative study of placebo-controlled trials of homoeopathy and allopathy. Lancet. 366(9487):726–32.

122. Linde K, Clausius N, Ramirez G, Melchart D, Eitel F, Hedges LV, et al. Are the clinical effects of homoeopathy placebo effects? A meta-analysis of placebo-controlled trials. Lancet. 1997;350(9081):834–43.

123. Jonas WB, Anderson RL, Crawford CC, Lyons JS. A systematic review of the quality of homeopathic clinical trials. BMC Complement Altern Med. 2001;1(1):12.

124. Ernst E. The risks of homeopathy? 2012 [cited 2017 03 February]. Available from: http://edzardernst.com/2012/12/the-risks-of-homeopathy/.

125. Ernst E. Life-threatening complications of spinal manipulation. Stroke. 2001;32(3):809–10.

126. Brettel H. Akupunktur als Todesursache. Munch Med Wochenschr. 1981;123(3):97–8.

127. Mazal DA, King T, Harvey J, Cohen J. Bilateral pneumothorax after acupuncture. N Engl J Med. 1980;302(24):1365.

128. Cheng TO. Cardiac tamponade following acupuncture. Chest J. 2000;118(6):1836–7.

129. Kataoka H. Cardiac tamponade caused by penetration of an acupuncture needle into the right ventricle. J Thorac Cardiovasc Surg. 1997;114(4):674–6.

130. Kirchgatterer A, Schwarz CD, Holler E, Punzengruber C, Hartl P, Eber B. Cardiac tamponade following acupuncture. Chest J. 2000;117(5):1510–1.

131. Peuker ET, White A, Ernst E, Pera F, Filler TJ. Traumatic complications of acupuncture: therapists need to know human anatomy. Arch Fam Med. 1999;8(6):553.

132. Ernst E, White A. Life-threatening adverse reactions after acupuncture? A systematic review Pain. 1997;71(2):123–6.

133. Rampes H, James R. Complications of acupuncture. Acupunct Med. 1995;13(1):26–33.

134. McCarty RL, Weber WJ, Loots B, Breuner CC, Vander Stoep A, Manhart L, et al. Complementary and alternative medicine use and quality of life in pediatric diabetes. J Altern Complement Med. 2010;16(2):165–73.

135. Spinks J, Johnston D, Hollingsworth B. Complementary and alternative medicine (CAM) use and quality of life in people with type 2 diabetes and/or cardiovascular disease. Complement Thr Med. 2014;22(1):107–15.

136. Owen-Smith A, Diclemente R, Wingood G. Complementary and alternative medicine use decreases adherence to HAART in HIV-positive women. AIDS Care. 2007;19(5):589–93.

137. Alfian S, Sukandar H, Arisanti N, Abdulah R. Complementary and alternative medicine use decreases adherence to prescribed medication in diabetes patients. Annal Trop Med Public Health. 2016;9(3):174–9.

138. Haque M, Emerson SH, Dennison CR, Levitt NS, Navsa M. Barriers to initiating insulin therapy in patients with type 2 diabetes mellitus in public-sector primary health care centres in Cape Town. S Afr Med J. 2005;95(10):798–802.

139. White JR Jr, Hartman J, Campbell RK. Drug interactions in diabetic patients. The risk of losing glycemic control. Postgrad Med. 1993;93(3):131–2, 5–9

140. Yeh GY, Eisenberg DM, Davis RB, Phillips RS. Use of complementary and alternative medicine among persons with diabetes mellitus: results of a national survey. Am J Public Health. 2002;92(10):1648–52.

141. Wood D, Athwal S, Panahloo A. The advantages and disadvantages of a 'herbal' medicine in a patient with diabetes mellitus: a case report. Diabet Med. 2004;21(6):625–7.

142. Kulambil Padinjakara RN, Ashawesh K, Butt S, Nair R, Patel V. Herbal remedy for diabetes: two case reports. Exp Clin Endocrinol Diabetes. 2009;117(1):3–5.

143. Roche A, Florkowski C, Walmsley T. Lead poisoning due to ingestion of Indian herbal remedies. New Zealand Med J. 2005;118:1219.

144. Keen RW, Deacon AC, Delves HT, Moreton JA, Frost PG. Indian herbal remedies for diabetes as a cause of lead poisoning. Postgrad Med J. 1994;70(820):113–4.

145. Gill G, Redmond S, Garratt F, Paisey R. Diabetes and alternative medicine: cause for concern. Diabet Med. 1994;11(2):210–3.

146. American Diabetes Association. Standards of medical care in diabetes 2014. Diabetes Care. 2014;37(Suppl 1):S14–80.

147. Grant SJ, Bensoussan A, Chang D, Kiat H, Klupp NL, Liu JP, et al. Chinese herbal medicines for people with impaired glucose tolerance or impaired fasting blood glucose. Cochrane Database Syst Rev. 2009;4:CD006690.

148. Geil P, Shane-McWhorter L. Dietary supplements in the management of diabetes: Potential risks and benefits. J Acad Nutr Diet. 2008;108(4):S59–65.

149. Medagama AB, Bandara R. The use of complementary and alternative medicines (CAMs) in the treatment of diabetes mellitus: is continued use safe and effective? Nutr J. 2014;13:102.

150. Chang H-y, Wallis M, Tiralongo E. Use of complementary and alternative medicine among people living with diabetes: literature review. J Adv Nurs. 2007;58(4):307–19.

151. D'Huyvetter K. Complementary and alternative medicine in diabetes. In: Handbook of Diabetes Management. New York: Springer; 2006. p. 257–71.

152. DiNardo MM, Gibson JM, Siminerio L, Morell AR, Lee ES. Complementary and alternative medicine in diabetes care. Curr Diab Rep. 2012;12(6):749–61.

153. Ahn AC, Bennani T, Freeman R, Hamdy O, Kaptchuk TJ. Two styles of acupuncture for treating painful diabetic neuropathy–a pilot randomised control trial. Acupunct Med. 2007;25(1–2):11–7.

154. Liang F, Koya D. Acupuncture: is it effective for treatment of insulin resistance? Diabetes Obes Metab. 2010;12(7):555–69.

155. Camilleri M, Parkman HP, Shafi MA, Abell TL, Gerson L. Clinical guideline: management of gastroparesis. Am J Gastroenterol. 2013;108(1):18–37.

156. Bo C, Xue Z, Yi G, Zelin C, Yang B, Zixu W, et al. Assessing the quality of reports about randomized controlled trials of acupuncture treatment on diabetic peripheral neuropathy. PLoS One. 2012;7(7):e38461.

157. Guthrie DW, Gamble M. Energy Therapies and diabetes mellitus. Diabetes Spectrum. 2001;14(3):149–53.

158. Assary G Youth with congenital diabetes died after stopping insulin on a dubious prescription. Deccan Chronicle 2014 August 19.

159. Lee MS, Choi T-Y, Lim H-J, Ernst E. Tai chi for management of type 2 diabetes mellitus: a systematic review. Chin J Integr Med. 2011;17(10):789–93.

160. Kan Y, Zhao Y, Shao H. Affect the insulin sensitivity of tai chi exercise on obesity with type 2 diabetic patients. J Tradit Chin Med Chin Mater Med Jilin (Chin). 2004;24:11.

161. Wang J, Cao Y. Effects of tai chi exercise on plasma neuropeptide y of type 2 diabetes mellitus with geriatric obesity. J Sports Sci. 2003;24:67–8.

162. Wang P, Han Q, Li G, Liang R. Evaluation of varying aerobics interferential effects on type 2 diabetes patients in community. China Med Herald. 2009;6:34–5.

163. Song R-Y, Lee E-O, Bae S-C, Ahn Y-H, Lam P, Lee I-O. Effects of tai chi self-help program on glucose control, cardiovascular risks, and quality of life in type II diabetic patients. J Muscle Joint Health. 2007;14(1):13–25.

164. Xin L, Miller YD, Brown WJ. A qualitative review of the role of qigong in the management of diabetes. J Altern Complement Med. 2007;13(4):427–34.

165. Chao Y-FC, Chen S-Y, Lan C, Lai J-S. The cardiorespiratory response and energy expenditure of tai-chi-qui-gong. Am J Chin Med. 2002;30(04):451–61.

166. Hagins M, Moore W, Rundle A. Does practicing hatha yoga satisfy recommendations for intensity of physical activity which improves and maintains health and cardiovascular fitness? BMC Complement Altern Med. 2007;7(1):1.

167. Ospina M, Bond K, Karkhaneh M, Tjosvold L, Vandermeer B, Liang Y, et al. Meditation practices for health: state of the research. Rockville, Maryland: AHRQ; 2007.

168. Aljasir B, Bryson M, Al-shehri B. Yoga practice for the management of type II diabetes mellitus in adults: a systematic review. Evid Based Complement Alternat Med. 2010;7(4):399–408.

169. Innes KE, Vincent HK. The influence of yoga-based programs on risk profiles in adults with type 2 diabetes mellitus: a systematic review. Evid Based Complement Alternat Med. 2007;4(4):469–86.

170. Lam P, Dennis SM, Diamond TH, Zwar N. Improving glycaemic and BP control in type 2 diabetes: the effectiveness of tai chi. Aust Fam Physician. 2008;37(10):884.

171. Lee M, Pittler M, Kim MS, Ernst E. Tai chi for type 2 diabetes: a systematic review. Diabet Med. 2008;25(2):240–1.

172. Tsang T, Orr R, Lam P, Comino EJ, Singh MF. Health benefits of Tai Chi for older patients with type 2 diabetes: The "Move It for Diabetes Study"-A randomized controlled trial. Clin Interv Aging. 2007;2(3):429.

173. White P. What can general practice learn from complementary medicine? Br J Gen Pract. 2000;50(459):821–3.

174. MCNZ. Statement on complementary and alternative medicine 2011 13-09-2016; (March). Available from: https://www.mcnz.org.nz/assets/News-and-Publications/Statements/Complementary-and-alternative-medicine.pdf

175. Miller LG. Herbal medicinals: selected clinical considerations focusing on known or potential drug-herb interactions. Arch Intern Med. 1998;158(20):2200–11.

176. Association AD, Childs B, Cypress M, Spollett G. Complete Nurse's guide to diabetes Care. New York: McGraw-Hill Companies, Incorporated; 2009.

177. Guidelines for using vitamin, mineral, and herbal supplements. Diabetes Spectrum. 2001;14(3):160.

178. A step-by-step approach to complementary Therapies. Diabetes Spectr. 2001;14(4):225.

179. Unproven Therapies. Diabetes Care 2003;26(suppl 1):s142-s.

180. Gagnier JJ, Moher D, Boon H, Beyene J, Bombardier C. Randomized controlled trials of herbal interventions underreport important details of the intervention. J Clin Epidemiol. 2011;64(7):760–9.

181. Gagnier JJ, Boon H, Rochon P, Moher D, Barnes J, Bombardier C, et al. Recommendations for reporting randomized controlled trials of herbal interventions: explanation and elaboration. J Clin Epidemiol. 2006;59(11):1134–49.

182. Cohen K, Cerone P, Ruggiero R. Complementary/alternative medicine use: responsibilities and implications for pharmacy services. P T. 2002;27(9):440–7.

183. Kwan D, Hirschkorn K, Boon H. US and Canadian pharmacists' attitudes, knowledge, and professional practice behaviors toward dietary supplements: a systematic review. BMC Complement Altern Med. 2006;6(1):1.

184. Sarris J. Current challenges in appraising complementary medicine evidence. Med J Aust. 2012;196(5):310–1.

185. Barrett B. Alternative, complementary, and conventional medicine: is integration upon us? J Altern Complement Med. 2003;9(3):417–27.

186. Frenkel MA, Borkan JM. An approach for integrating complementary–alternative medicine into primary care. Fam Pract. 2003;20(3):324–32.

187. Mann D, Gaylord SA, Norton SK. Integrating complementary & alternative therapies with conventional care: program on integrative medicine, Department of Physical Medicine & Rehabilitation, UNC School of Medicine; 2004.

188. O'Connell BS. Complementary and integrative medicine: emerging Therapies for diabetes, part 2: preface. Diabetes Spectrum. 2001;14(4):196–7.

189. World Health Organization WHO coronavirus (COVID-19) dashboard | WHO coronavirus (COVID-19) dashboard with vaccination data. WHO. Published 2020. https://covid19.who.int/

190. Stub T, Jong MC, Kristoffersen AE. The impact of COVID-19 on complementary and alternative medicine providers: A cross-sectional survey in Norway. Adv Integr Med. 2021;8(4):247–55. https://doi.org/10.1016/j.aimed.2021.08.001. Epub 2021 Aug 11

191. Interdisciplinary AYUSH Research & Development Task Force. Ministry of AYUSH, Government of India. https://www.ayush.gov.in/docs/clinical-protocol-guideline.pdf. Accessed 16 Sep 2020.

192. Ogbole OO, Akinleye TE, Segun PA, Faleye TC, Adeniji AJ. In vitro antiviral activity of twenty-seven medicinal plant extracts from Southwest Nigeria against three serotypes of echoviruses. Virol J. 2018;15:110. https://doi.org/10.1186/s12985-018-1022-7.7.

193. Charan J, Bhardwaj P, Dutta S, Kaur R, Bist SK, Detha MD, Kanchan T, Yadav D, Mitra P, Sharma P. Use of complementary and alternative medicine (CAM) and home remedies by COVID-19 patients: A telephonic survey. Indian. J Clin Biochem. 2020;36(1):1–4. https://doi.org/10.1007/s12291-020-00931-4. Epub ahead of print

194. Philips CA, Ahamed R, Rajesh S, George T, Mohanan M, Augustine P. Comprehensive review of hepatotoxicity associated with traditional Indian ayurvedic herbs. World J Hepatol. 2020;12(9):574–95.

195. Nerurkar PV, Hwang PW, Saksa E. Anti-diabetic potential of noni: the yin and the Yang. Molecules. 2015;20(10):17684–719.

Insulin Delivery: An Evolution in the Technology

69

Jothydev Kesavadev, Gopika Krishnan, and Nelena Benny

Introduction

All patients with type 1 diabetes (T1DM) require insulin due to absolute deficiency, and most type 2 diabetes (T2DM) patients require insulin at one time or the other due to progressive β-cell failure, to sustain life [1, 2]. In people with diabetes, the most efficient therapeutic option available to reduce hyperglycemia continues to be insulin even though they experience numerous challenges with the use of insulin including interference with daily living, financial constraints, the complexity of regimens, injection discomfort, and public embarrassment for injecting insulin [3, 4]. Therefore, to avoid the complications related to diabetes such barriers have to be handled with advanced and proven technologies for insulin delivery [5].

Beginning with the syringe for injecting insulin, progressing to insulin pumps, insulin pens, and sensor-augmented pumps, the growth of diabetes technologies accelerated with the introduction of hybrid closed-loop systems, integration with consumer electronics, and cloud-based data systems [6, 7]. These devices have favorably improved patients' perceptions about insulin therapy along with improving their quality of life [8]. However, the right choice and application of diabetes technologies are essential for positive outcomes.

The first manufactured insulin pump was introduced as early as in the 1970s, whereas the first manufactured insulin pen was introduced only in 1985 [9].

Insulin Delivery Devices

Insulin Vial and Syringe

In 1924, 2 years after the discovery of insulin, Becton, Dickinson and Company (BD) made a syringe specifically designed for insulin injection [10] (Fig. 69.1). Initially, syringes were made of metals and/or glass, which were reusable and after each use, required boiling for sterilization. In 1925, Novo Nordisk launched the first insulin syringe, the "Novo Syringe" (Fig. 69.2). To reduce the extent of needle-associated infections, disposable syringes were developed. In 1954, BD mass-produced the first glass disposable syringes called the BD Hypak. In 1955, an all-plastic Monoject syringe (Roehr Products Inc) was introduced onto the market. In the 1960s, BD introduced the 1-mL LuerLok insulin syringe available with either a detachable needle or a permanently attached needle. Disposable plastic syringes from numerous vendors were available on the market by the mid-1960s [11]. These syringes reduced pain and the rate of needle-associated infections [12]. In spite of all these advances, many patients did not feel to inject insulin 3–4 times a day due to needle phobia.

By 1970, BD manufactured the first one-piece insulin syringe with an integral needle [13]. Following, U-100 plastic insulin syringes with units marking down the side of the syringe came into use [11]. In 1988, the BD Safety-Lok insulin syringe with advanced safety features was introduced. In 2012, BD introduced the BD Veo insulin syringe with an Ultra-Fine 6-mm needle, offering less pain and reduced plunger force to ease the flow of large insulin doses [14]. Due to the reduced risk of intramuscular injections, this syringe has been widely preferred [15]. The FDA approved a U-500 specific insulin syringe designed by BD to address the dosing errors while administering doses from a U-500 vial with a U-100 insulin syringe in 2016 [16]. Instead of the long, large bore-sized and reusable needles used in earlier years, nowadays, small bore-sized and short-length needles (8 mm, 6 mm, and 5 mm) are used for insulin injection.

J. Kesavadev (✉) · N. Benny
Jothydev's Diabetes Research Centre, Trivandrum, Kerala, India

G. Krishnan
Academics and Research, Jothydev's Diabetes Research Centre, Trivandrum, Kerala, India

© The Author(s), under exclusive license to Springer Nature Switzerland AG 2023
J. Rodriguez-Saldana (ed.), *The Diabetes Textbook*, https://doi.org/10.1007/978-3-031-25519-9_69

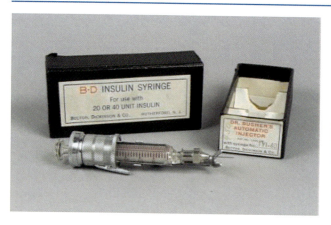

Fig. 69.1 First insulin syringe

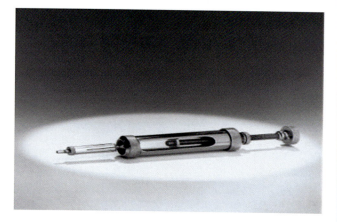

Fig. 69.2 Novo syringe

For more than 50 years, vials and syringes have remained as the only option for insulin delivery although "conventional" syringe technology has become less popular in the current era.

Insulin Pen

Due to inconvenience and inaccuracy in preparing the insulin dose, insulin shots using vial and syringe have a lot of challenges [9]. These issues contributed to the development of insulin pens. The introduction of insulin pens was a phenomenal achievement in insulin delivery. In 1985, the first insulin pen, the NovoPen, was launched by Novo Nordisk followed by NovoPen 2 in 1988. NovoPen 2 has a distinct dial-up setting to measure the required dose [17]. In common, pens provide more simple, accurate, and convenient insulin delivery over syringes (Table 69.1). An insulin pen has mainly three components: an insulin cartridge, a disposable short needle, and an incremental "one-click per unit" dosing. These devices can be either reusable or disposable. Reusable insulin pens have a replaceable cartridge whereas disposable pens have a prefilled cartridge and are discarded after use.

Table 69.1 Advantages and disadvantages of insulin delivery methods

Methods	Advantages	Disadvantages
Vial and syringe	• Less expensive compared to insulin pen and pump	• Increased pain at the site of injection versus pen • Inconvenience in carrying • Decreased accuracy when compared to pens • Less patient-friendly
Insulin pen	• Efficient and convenient delivery of insulin • Accurate dosing and flexible because of disposable and reusable options • Ease of injection and time saving • Easy to carry • Better treatment compliance and long-term cost-effectiveness	• More expensive than syringes • Does not allow the mixing of different insulin types • Low dosing
Insulin pumps	• Continuous delivery of insulin • Better glycemic control • Increased patient compliance and acceptance • Decreased hypoglycemia	• More expensive • Increased risk of DKA if pump fails • Injection site infection • Technical and safety issues with the cannula and infusion set (detach, crimp, or leakage) • Can cause skin irritability or hypersensitivity in patients
Intraperitoneal	• Direct insulin delivery to the portal vein • More physiological	• Invasive • More cost • Increased risk of infection and portal vein thrombosis
Inhaled insulin	• Noninvasive • Increased patient compliance • Rapid onset of action (10–15 min) • Better PPBG control	• Reduced bioavailability • Inhalational devices issues • Decreased lung function • Transient cough
Oral insulin	• Increased portal insulin concentration • Noninvasive • Patient-friendly	• Reduced bioavailability
Buccal insulin	• Relatively large surface for absorption • Presystemic metabolism in the GI and liver avoided • The level of vascularization is very high in some areas	• Great variations of permeability among the different areas of the oral mucosa • Reduced bioavailability
Nasal insulin	• No interference with pulmonary functions	• Reduced bioavailability (15–25%) • Local irritation • Nasal irritation
Transdermal insulin	• Needle-free	• Skin irritation, blister, pain and redness • Safety not established

PPBG Postprandial blood glucose

Novo presented the world's first disposable, prefilled insulin pen known as "Novolet" in 1989 [18]. Insulin adsorbs onto the plastic surface of these prefilled pens over time and a precise concentration can be accomplished by legitimate blending. Therefore, the dose accuracy and blood glucose (BG) stability between cartridge changes are increased by pens [19].

The newer insulin pens are more accurate and furnish with safety features such as audible clicks with each dose to improve accuracy and reduce the chances of human errors [9, 20]. Another achievement in the pen device (HumaPen® Memoir™) is integrated with recording the time and date of the last 16 injections [21].

Compared with syringes, pens offer more flexibility, accuracy, discreetness, and long-term cost-effectiveness, providing improved treatment continuity and adherence. Therefore, the use of insulin pens exhibits better glycemic control and has wider acceptance [22, 23]. Despite insulin pens being convenient, less painful, and patient-friendly, they are related with higher cost in comparison with vial and syringe [24, 25].

Technologic refinements over the fundamental features of the earlier versions have produced more advanced insulin pens. Finer and safer needles which are shorter and thinner (31–32 G × 4–5 mm) that offer reduced pain perception and require less thumb force and time to inject insulin have also been developed resulting in improved patient satisfaction [26, 27].

First Generation Insulin Pens

From the 1990s, first-generation insulin pens are available on the market. The prominent insulin pens in this category are multiple generations of durable pens of the NovoPen family, AllStar (Sanofi), and prefilled pens, such as FlexPen, FlexTouch (Novo Nordisk), Humalog Pen, Kwikpen (Eli Lilly), and SoloSTAR (Sanofi) (Fig. 69.3). NovoPen 3, a durable pen allowing a maximum dosage of 70 U, was launched in 1992 (Fig. 69.4). The essential feature of this device was less wastage of insulin while resetting the dose at the dial and push-up buttons. This pen was more economical and was further refined for patient subsegments, such as NovoPen 1.5 and NovoPen Junior. In 1996, NovoPen 1.5 was launched, a shorter version of NovoPen 3, which can hold smaller insulin cartridges. NovoPen3 Demi, the first Novo family member to allow half-unit dose increments, was advertised in 1999. In 2001, FlexPen, a prefilled insulin pen, was introduced. In 2003, NovoPen Junior, with vibrant colors, specifically designed for children with diabetes, was initiated [28]. The NovoPen 4 (dose increments of 1.0 U, maximum dose of 60 U) was launched in 2005. In 2007 and 2008, refiled insulin pens, Kwikpen (Eli Lilly) and SoloSTAR (Sanofi), were launched respectively [29].

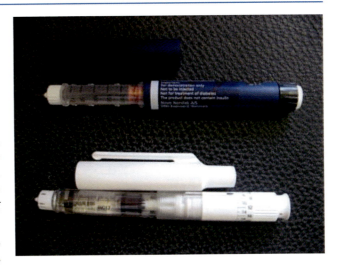

Fig. 69.3 First generation insulin pens

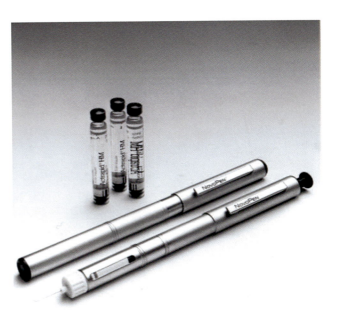

Fig. 69.4 NovoPen®

In 2011, Novo Nordisk introduced FlexTouch, a re-engineered version of the original FlexPen. It is the single prefilled insulin pen with an easy touch button, which improves the ease of use and device handling for the patients [30]. In 2012, Sanofi India launched its first indigenously developed reusable insulin pen, AllStar, specifically designed for diabetes patients in India. The key features of this pen are the slim and discreet design, clear dose magnification window, dose arrow on both sides, bayonet cartridge lock, short dial-out distance, penalty-free reverse dialing, audible click sound with every unit dialed and dispensed, and non-rotating dial button during dispensing [31]. In 2017, Junior KwikPen, a prefilled half-unit insulin pen, was considered to be lighter and smaller than other half-unit insulin pens and was approved on the market.

In 2021, Toustar Reusable Insulin Pen Sanofi was intended to be used in conjunction with the insulin glargine 300 U/mL in a dedicated cartridge (Toujeo® 1.5 mL cartridges) to deliver insulin through subcutaneous injection using commercially available needles. The key features are user can reverse dial without losing insulin and simple "push-to-reset" plunger (no screwing required) [32].

Insulin pen needles of 4 mm, 5 mm, 6 mm, 8 mm, and 12.7 mm lengths are used. The Nano 4-mm pen needle (BD), the shortest pen needle, is more comfortable and easiest to use. These needles require low thumb force and allow higher flow rate and insulin absorption [33].

Next-Generation Insulin Pens

Since 2007, second-generation pen devices or "smart pens" with a memory function were available on the market. These devices have a multidose memory feature that allows storing the date, time, and amount of the previous doses [34, 35]. These devices are unified with USB or Bluetooth features for efficient monitoring and data management. In 2007, Eli Lilly launched HumaPen MEMOIR, the world's first digital insulin pen with memory, and HumaPen LUXURA HD, a reusable pen for people who require insulin dosing in half-unit increments from 0.5 to 30 units. In 2010, Novo Nordisk launched NovoPen Echo, the first insulin pen with memory and half-unit dosing features [36]. In 2012, NovoPen 5, a successor to NovoPen 4 was launched with a simple memory function for use with the 3-mL Penfill cartridge [37].

The newer smart pens are designed to guide the individual with diabetes about the insulin dosage (by means of inbuilt calculators), memory functions to remember the amount and time of insulin dosage, and automatic transmission of insulin dose to the mobile logbook through Bluetooth technologies [12].

Connected Pens

Connected pens are next-generation insulin pens with characteristics that go beyond the memory function. In 2017, Pen System was launched by Companion Medical which consists of a Bluetooth-enabled wireless insulin pen with a smartphone interface and bolus advisor [38]. These pens will automatically record the dose of insulin injected, and the data can be shared with collaborating CGM devices and Glooko's Diasend digital diabetes management platforms and are expected to be synced with Roche's mySugr app [39]. Novo

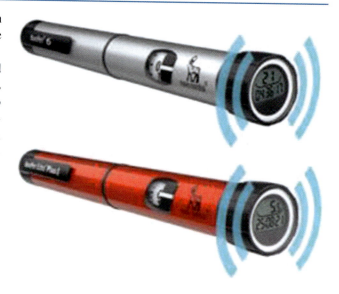

Fig. 69.5 NovoPen 6 and NovoPen Echo Connected pens

Nordisk's NovoPen 6 and NovoPen Echo Plus also fall into this category of pens (Fig. 69.5). These pens will automatically record the dose of insulin injected and the data will be shared with Dexcom G6 CGM, FreeStyle Libre system (Abbott), and Glooko's Diasend digital diabetes management platforms. Connected pens are furnished with NFC (near-field communication) technology that permits scanning of these devices to transfer the data off to another device [40]. Another advanced innovation in pen technology was Bluetooth/internet-connected insulin pen cap that aids the generation of smart dosing systems through a mobile app for the convenience of T1DM patients who do not use an insulin pump [41].

Even though insulin pens offer the convenience of use, less pain, and better treatment adherence and health outcomes, they have limitations such as difficulty in applying a mixture of insulins, higher cost, and lack of universal insurance coverage [42]. Regardless of the ease of use, pens are mechanically more complex than insulin syringes [43].

InPen Smart Insulin Pen

In 2020, Medtronic launched connected smart insulin pen, the InPen, acquired from Companion Medical. The InPen is the only FDA cleared, smart insulin pen system that combines the freedom of a reusable Bluetooth pen with the intelligence of an intuitive mobile app that helps users administer the right insulin dose, at the right time (Fig. 69.6). The InPen sends dose information to a mobile app and the app uses the glucose levels and a carbohydrate estimate to recommend the dose. It even considers the amount of insulin that is still working in the body, to help avoid low glucose.

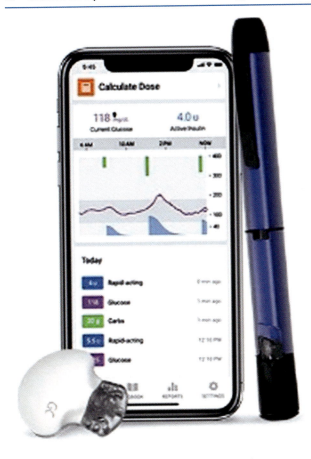

Fig. 69.6 InPen with Guardian connect and connected app

Injection Aids: I-Port Advance Injection Port

To reduce the frequency of multiple injections and needle phobia in patients with diabetes, injection aids are also used in practice. In 2016, an injection port was designed known as i-port Advance launched by Medtronic. It is a small and discrete patch, which can be attached to the skin and the device remains adhered to the skin for up to 72 h and allows multiple injections. It is the first device to combine an injection port and an inserter in one complete set which helps to eliminate the need for multiple injections without puncturing the skin for each dose. This device is useful for insulin requiring patients having needle phobia and helps them to accomplish glycemic control effectively [44, 45]. Although there was an initial excitement, this device remains unpopular probably because insulin shots with newer needles are virtually painless.

Insulin Pumps

Insulin pumps are small, computerized devices that imitate the way the human pancreas works by delivering small doses of short acting insulin continuously (basal rate). The device is also used to deliver variable amounts of insulin when a meal is eaten (bolus). Pumps are modernized gadgets for the delivery of insulin and can be used for dispensing insulin in any patient who exhibits the desire to initiate pump therapy and fulfills the criteria for a pump candidate [1].

Continuous Subcutaneous Insulin Infusion (CSII)

In normal physiology, a continuous small amount of insulin secretion from the beta cells of the pancreas reduces hepatic glucose output, and when food is ingested a larger amount of insulin is secreted to maintain euglycemia [46]. The CSII therapy was used by DCCT trial in nearly 40% of the participants in the intensive arm [47]. The current generation of insulin pumps are more patient-friendly due to its smaller size and smart features such as built-in-dose calculators and alarms [46]. The main components of an insulin pump are an insulin reservoir, infusion set, and tubing. The insulin reservoir is connected to the infusion set and a catheter helps to continuously deliver insulin to meet the daily requirement. The pump has user-specific inbuilt programs to dispense insulin at basal rates (slow, continuous) and in incremental (bolus) doses before meals [48]. This characteristic helps in the removal of the inherent variations associated with the injection depth and multiple injection sites that are typical of conventional subcutaneous injections. The infusion site needs to be changed only once every 2–3 days. Therefore, insulin pumps terminating the need for multiple injections on a daily basis can lead to less insulin variation [49, 50].

In 1963, the first portable insulin pump was invented by Dr.Arnold Kadish but it was limited by its size and technical issues [51](Fig. 69.7). In 1979, the first commercial insulin pump was introduced in the USA [20]. In 1976, Dean Kamen introduced the first wearable insulin pump, known as the "blue brick" and later the "autosyringe," and led to the introduction of insulin pump therapy in the same year [52]. The first SOOIL insulin pump was clinically evaluated at Seoul National University Hospital in 1979 [53]. In 1983, MiniMed introduced their first insulin pump, MiniMed 502. In 1986, MiniMed introduced the implantable insulin pump to deliver insulin intraperitoneally. Insulin delivered through this device was absorbed quickly and directly to the portal system [54]. In 2000, new versions of the pump with improved memory and battery life were launched on the market. Later in 2007, implantable insulin pump devices were discontinued by Medtronic.

In the 1990s, new-generation external pumps were released which are comparatively small, compact, handy, and effective. These "smart pumps" have characteristics as built-in bolus calculators, personal computer interfaces, and alarms [55]. The insulin pump models which are approved on the global market are Medtronic MiniMed,

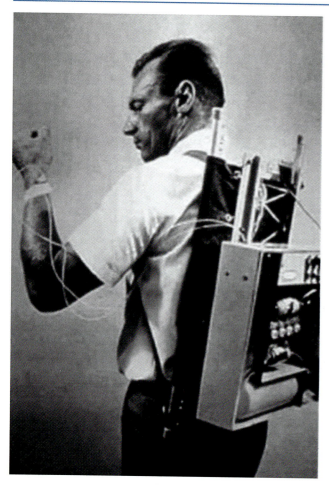

Fig. 69.7 Dr. Arnold Kadish with the first insulin pump

OmniPod (Insulet), T:Slim (Tandem), DANA R (SOOIL), Cellnovo, Accu-Chek Solo Micropump (Roche), and Ypsomed [56].

Medtronic introduced the first-ever "intelligent" insulin pump in 2003. The system comprises a MiniMed Paradigm 512 insulin pump and a Paradigm Link blood glucose monitor. Nowadays, BG readings from the glucometer are wirelessly and automatically transmitted to the insulin pump, and the required insulin doses are recommended by a Bolus Wizard calculator [57].

Insulin pumps are commonly used for insulin replacement in T1DM patients, but it has now been widely used by T2DM patients as well [58]. In patients with hyperglycemia, diabetes management with CSII provides better glycemic and metabolic control (reduces HbA1c, glycemic variation, and hypoglycemia) [59, 60]. The use of insulin pumps contributes to the patients' quality of life. However, the major limitations associated with the infusion sets are that they can exhibit handling issues and can detach, leak, or cause skin irritability, thus undermining the convenient use of insulin pumps [61]. Patient education before starting CSII therapy is of utmost importance to avoid the chances of a "pump failure" [62].

Patch Pumps

The barriers associated with infusion set have led to the development of "patch pumps." These pumps are free of infusion sets, small, lightweight, and attached to the skin through an adhesive. Patch pumps also offer additional comfort and flexibility to users, especially while traveling. Insulet introduced OmniPod, the first tubeless insulin pump in 2011. It consists of an integrated infusion set and automated inserter that converses wirelessly with an integrated BG meter. The Omnipod patch pump provides complete freedom to the users to engage in routine activities [63]. The specific simplified patch pump models available on the market are V-Go (Valeritas) and PAQ (CeQur) [64]. The second-generation Omnipod, which is smaller and more compact was launched in 2013. This version of the patch pump has modern features such as "human factor screens" and improvements in both correction and meal boluses for insulin dose calculation [65].

Continuous Intraperitoneal Insulin Infusion (CIPII)

Continuous intraperitoneal insulin infusion (CIPII) is considered to permit the infusion of insulin into the peritoneal cavity. The advantage of this method is that it more closely coincides the physiology than the other conventional therapies [66]. Two different technologies have been developed in CIPII: implanted intraperitoneal pumps such as MiniMed MIP2007C (Medtronic) and a percutaneous port attached to an external pump such as the Accu-Chek Diaport system (Roche Diabetes Care). The MIP 2007C is implanted under the subcutaneous tissue in the lower abdomen, and from this subcutaneous pocket, the peritoneum is opened, and the tip of the catheter is carefully inserted and directed towards the liver. After implantation, at least every 3 months the pump reservoir is refilled in the outpatient clinic with concentrated insulin transcutaneously. The Accu-Chek Diaport system permits insulin infusion into the peritoneal cavity through an Accu-Chek insulin pump and an infusion set. CIPII has been proven as a viable option for T1D patients with skin problems and unable to securely or efficiently control their diabetes with subcutaneous insulin [67].

The drawbacks of this route of insulin administration include the invasive nature, cannula blockage, higher cost, portal vein thrombosis, and peritoneal infection. Medtronic announced the worldwide termination of the implantable insulin pump in 2007.

Sensor-Augmented Pump Therapy (SAP)

The new generations of CGMs are more accurate, smaller in size, and shown to improve glycemic control in patients with T1DM [68]. When CGM readings are used to adjust insulin delivery through an insulin pump, it is known as sensor-augmented pump (SAP) therapy [69]. In patients with T1DM, SAP reduces A1c by 0.7–0.8% compared to baseline or MDI therapy. The introduction of real-time, sensor-augmented insulin pumps is considered a major turning point in the development of "closed-loop" insulin delivery or an artificial pancreas (AP) [1]. SAP therapy produces higher-level results in reducing hypoglycemia and achieving glycemic control to conventional therapies [70, 71].

Medtronic launched the MiniMed Veo System in 2009, with a Low-Glucose Suspend feature that automatically halts insulin delivery when sensor glucose levels reach a preset low threshold. This device has been considered the first stepping stone to an AP system [72].

The pump provides more accurate dosing, avoids the need for multiple daily injections, and thus provides convenience and a flexible lifestyle. They can also store a plethora of data that can be transmitted to computer programs or bolus insulin calculators and further analyzed to make insulin dose adjustments. The limitations of pump therapy are technical problems associated with the infusion set and higher acquisition costs. Patients also complained of skin irritations and infections at the insertion sites. Technical issues such as kinking, bending, or crimping of inserted cannulas and leakage of infusion sets have also been observed [61]. SAP requires patient involvement for using CGM glucose readings to adjust insulin pump delivery. This makes SAP susceptible to human errors.

Automation of Insulin Pump

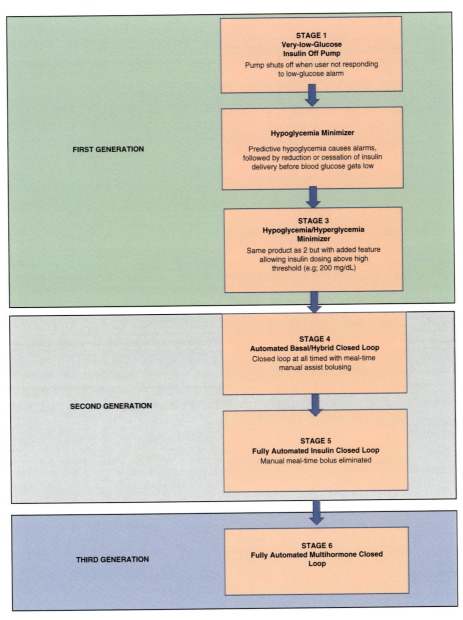

Artificial Pancreas (Closed Loop)

MiniMed 530G with an Enlite sensor has been acknowledged as a first-generation artificial pancreas (AP) device system with Threshold Suspend automation. In 2013, this device was approved by the FDA for diabetes patients >16 years of age [55]. In 2015, Medtronic introduced the MiniMed 640G system, which has been taking one step closer to the artificial pancreas system. This system has integrated smart characteristics such as active insulin tracking, a bolus progress bar, and predictive battery life [73] (Fig. 69.8).

Since the conception of CSII, the main aim was to design an artificial pancreas that mimics exquisite sugar control with minimal human interference. An artificial pancreas or a

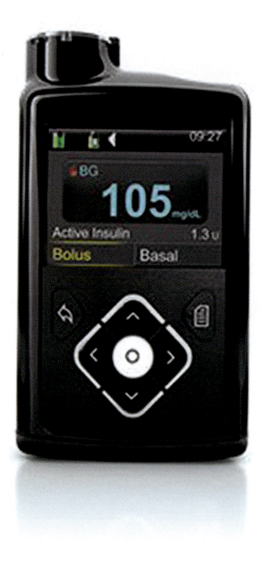

Fig. 69.8 A new-generation insulin pump: MiniMed 640G insulin pump system by Medtronic

"closed-loop" is a compilation of progressive technologies to engage automation to achieve glycemic targets. Generally, AP links three devices [74]:

1. A sensor like CGM that measures BG and sends data to a computer algorithm
2. A control algorithm to analyze the data and calculate the required insulin dose
3. An insulin infusion pump to deliver insulin as per the computer instructions

Since 2016, safety and efficacy studies have been conducted on the combinational use of the predictive low-glucose suspension algorithm (PLGM) (commercially, "SmartGuard technology") with the MiniMed 640G insulin pump that automatically suspends insulin delivery based on the prediction of low glucose levels [75]. In 2017, the first hybrid closed-loop system, the MiniMed 670G insulin pump with a Guardian 3 sensor, was approved by the FDA (Fig. 69.9). When in auto mode, it functions as a hybrid closed-loop system that automatically controls basal insulin delivery every 5 min based on the CGM values to hold BG levels tightly to the specific target [8]. These systems have been reported to enhance glycemic targets [BG, HbA1c, time-in-range (TIR)] and reduce the incidence of nocturnal hypoglycemia to improve better safety, treatment satisfaction, sleep quality, and cognition in T1D patients [76–78].

In 2018, the FDA approved Insulet's Omnipod Dash System, a CSII system comprising a tubeless, waterproof, Bluetooth wireless technology pump with a capacity of 200 units of U-100 insulin and an advanced personal diabetes manager (PDM) that regulates the pump [79] (Fig. 69.10).

In 2021, Medtronic launched new MiniMed 780G insulin pump designed to work with Medtronic's Guardian sensors to continuously monitor glucose levels throughout the day (Fig. 69.11). Basal insulin adjusts insulin dosage every five minutes as needed based on glucose levels. Bolus is delivered automatically up to every 5 min if maximum auto basal delivery is reached or if glucose level is above 120 mg/dL. This pump helps to achieve the Time in Range goal of >70% and HbA1c goal of 7.0%.

Future steps in the evolution of the artificial pancreas will be [80]:

1. Use of predictive algorithms to minimize hypoglycemia even before hypoglycemia occurs.
2. Use of algorithms to keep blood sugar in target range (hypoglycemia/hyperglycemia minimizer).
3. Automated basal and/or hybrid closed-loop.
4. Fully automated (insulin).
5. Dual (insulin + glucagon) hormonal closed-loop.

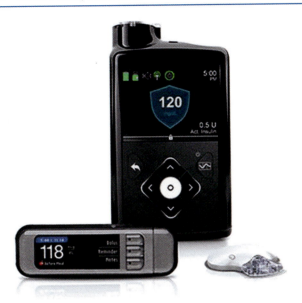

Fig. 69.9 First Artificial Pancreas: MiniMed 670G insulin pump system with Guardian 3 sensor

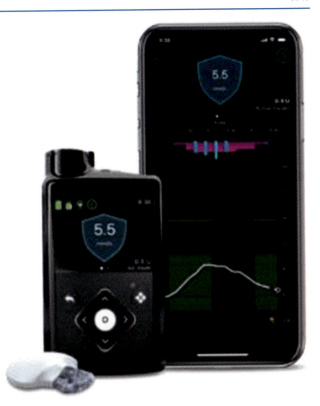

Fig. 69.11 MiniMed 780G System

Alternate Controller-Enabled Infusion (ACE) Pumps

Another modern technology in this area has been the arrival of alternate controller-enabled (ACE) infusion pumps. Despite the conventional stand-alone pumps, ACE pumps can be interoperable: used jointly with different components of diabetes technologies, permitting custom-made diabetes management for patients according to individual device preferences. The ACE insulin pump can be combined with automated insulin dosing (AID) systems, CGMs, BG meters, and other electronics. In 2019, the FDA approved the first interoperable t:Slim X2 insulin pump for subcutaneous insulin delivery for children and adults with diabetes [81]. The FDA approved a new-generation, interoperable, control-IQ artificial pancreas system (tandem diabetes) in 2020. A clinical trial that revealed that the use of the control-IQ AP system was linked with a greater percentage of TIR, over the use of SAP, paved the way for this approval [78].

Do-It-Yourself Artificial Pancreas (DIY-APS)

People affected by T1DM have been expecting an affordable and efficient solution for the management of this chronic disease for decades. Lack of accessible and actionable data, unaffordability of the current systems, and long timeline of

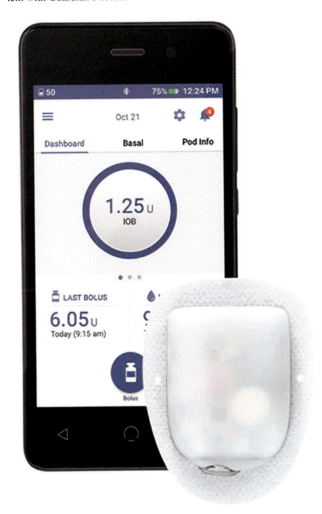

Fig. 69.10 Omnipod DASH pump

medical device development cycles have led to general annoyance in the T1DM community. The first Diabetes Mine D-Data Exchange gathering at Stanford University spotlighted the sentiments and frustrations of patients with T1D and their families/caregivers gathered online under the hashtag "#WeAreNotWaiting" in waiting for their needs to be addressed in 2013. This event marked the beginning of the DIY-APS movement. A major dimension of the #WeAreNotWaiting initiative was that the tech-savvy diabetes followers started self-building their closed-loop systems, also known as "looping." These automated insulin delivery systems are generally known as a "Do-it-yourself" artificial pancreas (DIY-APS) [82, 83]. The basic components of DIY-APS are:

(a) A real-time CGM.
(b) An insulin pump.
(c) A minicomputer or smartphone app.

The diabetes community shared DIY diabetes device-related projects on digital and social media platforms such as Facebook, Twitter, NightScout, and GitHub, which led to the merging of these projects [84]. Through a gradual and systematic method of assembling, merging, and processing data from patients' devices to deliver significant actionable information, there has been a rush in the propagation and convergence of DIY diabetes device-related projects. Dana Lewis, Scott Leibrand, and Ben West launched the OpenAPS project, providing the instructions and outline of a DIY patient-built artificial pancreas system (APS) in 2014. In 2015, the open-source version, also known as OpenAPS, was launched [85]. On January 31, 2020, more than 1776 PWD around the globe have implemented various layouts of DIY-APS [86]. DIY-APS uses individually made unauthorized algorithms to convert CGM data and calculate insulin doses, FDA approved communication devices and insulin pumps. Since it involves the use of unauthorized algorithms, these systems are not FDA approved, commercialized, or regularized. In 2017, another innovation in the DIY-APS evolution was "RileyLink," designed by Pete Schwamb for his daughter Riley, who had T1D. It is a translator device that allows easy communication between the insulin pump and iPhone. This device is considered more user-friendly, and it is easy to set up and maintain procedures [87]. Real-life experiences from patients and caregivers, unscientific data, and published reports from selected cohorts have highlighted the clinical benefits and reductions in self-management burden with DIY-APS [88].

In India, Jazz Sethi, a 26-year-old professional dancer from Ahmedabad, who has been living with T1D since the age of 13, is the first user of Do-It-Yourself (DIY) artificial pancreas. *Diabetes and Metabolic Syndrome: Clinical Research and Review* has narrated her experience with this breakthrough technology, why she decided to use the system,

and how the device has produced significant improvement in her quality of life and management of T1D [89].

There are mainly three types of DIY-APS:

1. OpenAPS
2. AndroidAPS
3. Loop

OpenAPS

OpenAPS is a safe, powerful, and easily understandable system that proposes to adjust insulin dosage to manage the BG levels in the recommended range, overnight and between meals. The first Open APS was developed by Dana Lewis, Scott Leibrand, and Ben West, and the code written with the help of Chris Hannemann was on a Raspberry Pi computer and a communication stick to connect to an old Medtronic pump.

Generally, an OpenAPS consists of an insulin pump, a CGM system, and an algorithm running on a microcomputer. The algorithms used in OpenAPS are oref0 (OpenAPS Reference Design Zero), Adjusting for unexpected BG deviation, and Bolus snooze. Recently, an "Advanced Meal Assist (AMA)" feature has been integrated into the OpenAPS algorithm. AMA gives an extremely adaptable algorithm for securely dosing insulin after meals, regardless of broadly differing meal types, and the high variations in rates of digestion between individuals, making it the most widely used postprandial insulin dosing algorithm. The ultimate aim of the OpenAPS system is to completely automate insulin dosing in all situations. In that regulation, an oref1 algorithm has been developed that utilizes small "supermicroboluses (SMB)" of insulin at mealtimes and ensures more rapid and secure insulin delivery in response to BG rises [90].

OpenAPS reads the CGM data every 5 min and queries the insulin pump every few minutes for recent settings and activities such as current and maximum basal rates, recent boluses, insulin on board (IOB), insulin sensitivity factor (ISF), carb ratio (CR), duration of insulin acting (DIA), and BG target/ range. Based on the communication from the insulin pump, OpenAPS updates the bolus wizard calculation and decides upon whether to cancel or supply a temporary basal. OpenAPS accomplishes this function through a physical piece of hardware called a "rig" that implement a sequence of commands to collect the CGM data, runs it through Oref0, and performs the dose calculations based on the pump setting values. The system can guide on changes in insulin to carbohydrate ratios and ISF settings through either Autosens (checking back 8–24 h) or Autotune (check back either 24 h or a user-specified period). However, this was the first developed system; recent users have been preferring AndroidAPS which offers more combinations of compatible devices and in-warranty pumps.

AndroidAPS

AndroidAPS is an open-source app with all properties of OpenAPS but runs on Google Android smartphones. The smartphone receives data from a CGM and transmits it with the insulin pump via Bluetooth. In 2017, the first AndroidAPS was developed in Europe by Milos Kozak and Adrian Tappe and it works with modern in-warranty pumps with Bluetooth capability. The algorithms used here are Oref0 and Oref1. The app is available in different versions particular to geographic locations and languages. The basic elements of the profile include basal rates (BR), ISF, CR, and DIA. AndroidAPS supplies multiple possibilities for remote monitoring of adults and pediatric patients with T1D. NSClient app can be used to check the relevant data by parents and caregivers of kids with T1D on their Android phones. Features like alarms using the xDrip+ app in follower mode, remote monitoring and control with SMS commands, and remote profile switch and temperature targets through the NSClient app provide the kid-friendly convenience of this system.

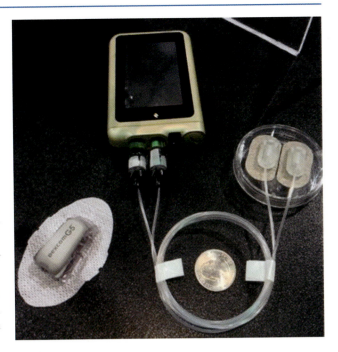

Fig. 69.12 iLet Bionic Pancreas

Loop

The Loop algorithm is different from OpenAPS and runs on an iOS operating system. The Apple iPhone receives CGM data and communicates with the insulin pump via Bluetooth. In 2016, the first loop was developed by Nate Racklyeft and a D-Dad, Pete Schwamb. Loop makes use of a free application, Xcode, to convert the raw code into an iOS application and install it on an iPhone. Loop documentation is available on GitHub and the builders need to register as Apple developers to install the necessary software. The loop makes a forecast using BG values every 5 min from 30 min ago and integrates between that value and the current glucose value to make adjustments in insulin dose and to provide bolus recommendations and temporary basal rates. The app communicates with a small translator device called RileyLink that ensures interaction between the pump, iPhone, and CGM [90]. It is almost the size of a tic-tac box and needs to be carried with you at all times. In a loop system, the pump speaks via radio language and the iPhone speaks via Bluetooth, and RileyLink acts as a translator to loop these parts together.

Bionic Pancreas (BP)

The "bionic pancreas" is a type of closed-loop system consisting of two infusion pumps (separately for insulin and glucagon) and connected to a CGM via a smartphone app. In 2015, the first bionic pancreas, "iLet" (Beta Bionics), exclusively for T1D treatment, was innovated by Dr. Edward Damiano. In this system, based on the appraised CGM data

automated dosing assessments of insulin and glucagon levels are made every 5 min (Fig. 69.12). These data are transmitted to pumps to control insulin or glucagon delivery [91]. In 2019, the FDA approved iLet BP as the "breakthrough device designation" [92].

D-Dads

D-Dads are fathers whose fatherhood has been challenged by T1D. Unsatisfied with the disruption and unpredictability of diabetes care, some D-dads thought "outside the box" to ease the burden of diabetes management.

Dr. Edward R. Damiano, a professor of biomedical engineering at Boston University, was determined to develop a bionic pancreas when his 11-month-old son, David, was diagnosed with T1D. Frustrated with the absence of reliable technologies, he created a bionic pancreas with the help of physicians and researchers [93]. The US Food and Drug Administration (FDA) conferred "breakthrough device designation" to the iLet bionic pancreas in 2019 [94]. Pete Schwamb, a software engineer, made innovatory contributions in the field of diabetes technologies. Pete's effort to gain access to the insulin pump data of his 6-year-old daughter, Riley, led to the development of RileyLink, a translator device used to communicate between the insulin pump and iPhone. Later, he developed the first iOS-based automated insulin delivery system, "loop," in association with Nathan Racklyeft [95]. Bryan Mazlish, a Wall Street quantitative analyst and one of the cofounders of Bigfoot Biomedical, made a fully functional homebrew artificial pancreas to manage his son's T1D. Being a hacker by profession, he has been recognized as a standard-bearer for the DIY-APS hacking mission [93]. Jeffrey Brewer, a past president of the Juvenile Diabetes Research Foundation (JDRF), also known as "the father of the artificial pancreas," has commenced research projects on automated insulin delivery systems. Later, he co-founded Bigfoot Biomedical accompanying Bryan Mazlish to develop its own closed-loop system, the Bigfoot smartloop system [96]. John Costik, the father of a 4-year-old boy, Evan, who had T1D, designed a code to hack his son's CGM, to upload the values into the cloud and remotely acquire those data using a web-based or android interface. He later made the code available as open-source and initiated "Nightscout CGM in the Cloud Project" for wider dissemination of the technology [85, 97]. Lane Desborough, D-Dad of Hayden is the name of an engineer from Medtronic, one of the so-called D-dads in diabetes technology by Nightscout CGM in the Cloud. He was a chief engineer at Medtronic and was one of the advocates of the #WeAreNotWaiting movement. Lane was the first person to get involved in the DIY-APS movement from the industry and later co-founded Bigfoot Biomedical [98]. Tidepool, a non-profitable organization was started by the D-Dads Howard Look and Steve McCanne and has been creating a regulated loop version of DIY-APS. Tidepool is currently on a venture to release a regulated version of the DIY-APS in collaboration with Omnipod and Dexco [99, 100].

D-Dads have been making significant contributions to turn the artificial pancreas dream into reality while focusing on its equitable access and affordability.

Bolus Calculator Apps

Bolus calculator/bolus advisor mobile apps are used for insulin dose calculation available in smartphones. These can function independently or can be integrated into pumps to calculate the accurate insulin dose by incorporating expected carbohydrate intake, measured blood glucose values, and previous insulin doses [101]. The most commonly used bolus calculator apps are Diabetes: M, mySugr (Roche), and PredictBGL. Bolus wizards are built-in automated bolus calculators specific to insulin pumps for insulin dose recommendations. The use of bolus wizards has been correlated with better glycemic control and treatment satisfaction [102]. In 2016, Endocrine Society Clinical Practice Guidelines have strongly promoted patients to use suitably adjusted built-in bolus calculators in CSII to improve glycemic control [103].

Implanted Pancreas

Another novel AP technology was the implanted artificial pancreas, a fully implantable insulin delivery device, which is under development at De Montfort University. It is a gel-based system that responds to BG variation by changing the insulin delivery rate. The performance of this system in glycemic control is well tested in a diabetic domestic pig [104]. It reduces hourly management and human interference to improve user acceptance and quality of life in diabetes patients [105].

Insulin Inhalers

Insulin delivery to the lungs was the first reported substitute for subcutaneous injection. It has long been estimated that insulin delivery by aerosol reduces blood glucose [106]. Insulin inhalers permit patients to breathe fine-inhalable insulin (pulmonary insulin) (either dry powder-based formulations or solution) into their lungs [12].

Advantages of the pulmonary route include a broad and well-perfused absorptive surface, the absence of certain peptidases that are present in the gastrointestinal (GI) tract that breaks down insulin, and the ability to bypass the "first-pass metabolism" [107]. Although the exact mechanism of insulin absorption across the pulmonary epithelium remains unclear, it is believed to involve transcytotic and paracellular mechanisms [106].

When introduced to the market, inhalable insulin was considered a remarkable innovation to address needle phobia and incorrect insulin injection techniques pertained to systemic insulin delivery methods [108]. In 2006, the first inhaled product Exubera® was approved by the US FDA. Exubera® was a dry power formulation available as 1 mg and 3 mg doses to be taken with the help of an Inhance™ inhaler device [109]. Exubera® was found to have pharmacokinetic and pharmacodynamic (PK/PD) properties similar to insulin aspart with a faster onset of action (10–15 min) [110]. In clinical trials in patients with uncontrolled T1DM and T2DM, Exubera® was found to reduce postprandial blood glucose and A1c markedly [111] although Exubera® was contraindicated in smokers as it increased the risk of hypoglycemia due to greater absorption compared to nonsmokers [112]. Along with this, patients were required to undergo pulmonary function tests before treatment initiation, after 6 months, and annually thereafter [109, 112]. This product did not flourish well commercially despite the noninvasive route possibly due to higher cost, the bulky delivery device, concerns related to decline in pulmonary function, and less preference by the patients and physicians. In 2007, this product was withdrawn from the market due to poor sales volume.

Another promising inhaled insulin is Afrezza (Sanofi and MannKind) based on Technosphere® dry powdered formulation. The onset of action of Afrezza inhaled insulin is 15 min and duration is 2–3 h, which is ideal for postprandial blood glucose control [113]. Initially, the common side effects are transient non-productive cough and a modest reduction in lung function [114]. In 2014, Afrezza got FDA approval for prandial insulin therapy [115]. The delivery system of Afrezza is small, handy, and displays the dose in units [116]. The use of Afrezza has provided remarkable glycemic control and reduction of hypoglycemia in T1DM patients [117, 118]. The recognition of inhalable insulins is further limited by insurance barriers, safety concerns, and competing products [116].

Jet Injectors

Another possible innovation to the market could be jet injectors, a type of syringe that dispenses insulin subcutaneously with the use of a high-pressure air mechanism. In the 1860s, Pioneer jet injector technology was introduced. Later, it was reintroduced in the 1940s as the "Hypospray," focusing on patients' self-management of insulin. In the 1950s, the US military designed a high-speed system, "Ped-O-Jet" (Keystone Industries), in the category of a multiuse nozzle jet injector (MUNJI) for mass vaccination programs. In 1997, the Ped-O-Jet was discontinued as a result of contamination issues built with the use of MUNJI [119]. During the 1990s, the new-generation, disposable-syringe jet injectors (DSJIs) with disposable dose chambers (insulin cartridge) and nozzles were launched. Even though the idea is not firsthand to the market, the wider acceptance of these devices has been interrupted by the cost, low absorption with the repeated use, and high contamination rates of the previous systems [120]. The jet injectors are a solution for patients with needle phobia [121]. Recent safety and feasibility studies have assessed the treatment efficiency and pharmacokinetic and pharmacodynamic (PK-PD) profiles of the insulin administered by the new-generation jet injectors [122].

Oral Insulin

The oral route of insulin administration may be the most patient-friendly way of taking insulin and it could more closely imitate physiological insulin delivery (more portal insulin concentration than peripheral) [123]. Despite this, the limitations in making oral insulin include inactivation by proteolytic enzymes in the GI tract and low permeability through the intestinal membrane due to the larger size and hydrophobicity of insulin resulting in poor bioavailability. Several pharmaceutical companies are engaged in developing carriers to protect insulin from GI degradation and facilitate intestinal transport of insulin to deliver insulin to the circulation with sufficient bioavailability.

Natural and synthetic nanoparticles have been used as a carrier or vehicle for insulin such as chitosan, liposomes, polymeric nanovesicles, polylactides, poly-ε, poly-alkyl cyanoacrylate, and various polymeric hydrogels [124–129].

Certain oral insulin preparations such as Capsulin, ORMD-0801, IN-105, oral hepatic directed vesicles, and Eligen have undergone phase 1 and phase 2 trials with promising results [130].

Colonic Insulin Delivery

Oral colon delivery is currently considered of importance not only for the treatment of local pathologies, such as primarily inflammatory bowel disease but also as a means of achieving systemic therapeutic goals. The large intestine is preferably not suited for absorption processes for drugs but it has certain advantages over the small intestine like long transit time, lower levels of peptidases (prevent the destruction of peptides), and higher responsiveness to permeation enhancers. Accordingly, it has been under extensive inquisition as a possible strategy to enhance the oral bioavailability of peptide and protein drugs. Oral delivery systems intended for colonic release of insulin were devised according to microflora-, pH-, and time-dependent strategies [131].

Bioavailability and pharmacological availability data are generally still far from being reliable in terms of magnitude, onset, duration, and above all, consistency for this route of administration and it is under investigation and despite its progress, there is still a long way to go before these products will be available on the market.

Nasal Insulin

In theory, intranasal delivery has several advantages over oral (bypass GI peptidases), subcutaneous (noninvasive and painless), and inhalation route (no issue with lung function) which makes this route appealing for the delivery of insulin. However, intranasal delivery has disadvantages such as limited permeability of a large molecule through the nasal mucosa and rapid mucociliary clearance resulting in variable absorption [132].

Significantly, intranasal delivery with early porcine and bovine insulins was studied in patients with T1DM [133, 134]. Currently, two technologies are under investigation: Nasulin™ (CPEX Pharmaceuticals) and nasal insulin by Nastech Pharmaceutical Company Inc. Both insulin preparations have a bioavailability of about 15–25% with the onset of action approximately 10–20 min [135, 136]. The substances such as bile salt, surfactant, and fatty acid derivatives are being investigated to improve mucosal permeability of insulin but they increase the risks for local irritation, nasal secretion, sneezing, or burning sensation [137].

Nasal insulin crosses the blood-brain barrier since it has a hypothesized effect on memory function [138]. Treatment with intranasal insulin improved memory, preserved caregiver-rated functional ability, and preserved general cognition without any remarkable hypoglycemic event. These improvements in cognitive functions were combined with changes in the Aβ42 level and in the tau protein-to-Aβ42 ratio in cerebrospinal fluid [139]. Based on these, investigations are ongoing to evaluate the usefulness of this agent for the treatment of Alzheimer's disease.

Buccal Insulin

Buccal delivery of insulin has similar efficacy as oral insulin with the advantage of bypassing GI degradation. In addition, the relatively large surface area results in better bioavailability [140]. Initially, Generex Biotechnology developed Orallyn™ which is a liquid formulation of short acting insulin that is administered using Generex's metered dosage aerosol applicator (RapidMist™). Eli Lilly and Generex conducted phase 1 and phase 2 trials in patients with T1DM and T2DM with favorable results [141]. Another fragment being developed by Shreya Life Sciences Pvt. Ltd., India, is oral Recosulin® [142].

Another technique for the delivery of insulin is fast dissolving films as a substitute to oral tablets for rapid drug delivery [143]. The Monosol Rx (Pharm Film Drug delivery technology) in collaboration with Midatech Company developed Midaform™ insulin, which is delivered by buccal route.

Transdermal

Transdermal insulin delivery terminates the problems associated with needles and injections and the large surface area of the skin makes it an appropriate route for insulin delivery. Although the perforation of insulin is halted by the stratum corneum, the outermost layer of the skin, numerous methods have been explored to overcome the barrier of the stratum corneum [144].

There are several strategies insulin can be delivered transdermally such as:

(a) Iontophoresis, the technique that uses small electric currents [145].
(b) Sonophereis or phonopheresis uses ultrasound waves [146].
(c) Microdermal ablation by removing the stratum corneum [147].
(d) Electroporation utilizes high voltage pulses that are applied for a very short time [148].
(e) Transfersulin is the insulin encapsulated in transferosome, an elastic, flexible vesicle, which squeezes by itself to deliver drugs through skin pores [149].

(f) Insupatch™, a device developed as an add-on to an insulin pump that applies local heat to the skin in order to increase the absorption of insulin [150].
(g) Recombinant human hyaluronidase (rHuPH20) to increase insulin absorption from subcutaneous tissue [151].

Moreover, microneedles with a 1 μm diameter and of various lengths can deliver insulin in an effective, accurate, and precise manner [152]. Microneedle technology also can be combined as a transdermal patch.

The transdermal insulin delivery techniques are limited by skin injury, burn or blister formation, and rarely significant pain and discomfort.

Other Non-conventional Routes

Ocular Route

No human trial has been reported with this route and an animal study failed to achieve significant plasma insulin concentration [153].

Rectal Route

Rectal gels [154] and suppositories [155] showed fair results. However, this route is not commercially viable.

Intra-Tracheal

In 1924, the administration of insulin was reported [156] but is not practical so not taken up for further development.

Conclusion

There is a long history of research focusing on recognizing a route of administration for insulin that is minimally or non-invasive, effective, safe, convenient, and cost-effective for patients. Each route and delivery method has its own potential advantages and disadvantages. There has been a high-speed evolution in diabetes technologies to improve the quality of life and to extend the endurance of subjects with diabetes. Though there were commendable developments in the currently available devices, many of those were prohibitively expensive. Additionally, there were serious issues associated with cannula blockages, infusion set handling, Bluetooth connectivity, and user-friendliness. As the search for more accurate and user-friendly methods continues, advances in pumps, CGMs, and predictive algorithms can make the closed-loop system as physiologic as possible with >90–95% TIR and the least time spent in hypoglycemia. Some of the promising experiences are shared by subjects using DIY-APS. The DIY revolution has prompted all device manufacturers to introduce ACE pumps and compatible sensors. The ultimate dream is to develop an artificial pancreas capable of 100% TIR and 0% time below range and affordable to everyone. Even though the mission demands enormous commitment and time, it has the potential to transform diabetes therapy.

References

1. Kesavadev J, Das AK, Unnikrishnan R, Joshi SR, Ramachandran A, Shamsudeen J, Krishnan G, Jothydev S, Mohan V. Use of insulin pumps in India: suggested guidelines based on experience and cultural differences. Diabetes Technol Ther. 2010;12(10):823–31.
2. Garg SK, Rewers AH, Akturk HK. Ever-increasing insulin-requiring patients globally. Diabetes Technol Ther. 2018;20:S21–S2424.
3. Knutsen PG, Voelker CQ, Nikkel CC. Clinical insights into a new, disposable insulin delivery device. Diabetes Spectrum. 2015;28(3):209–13.
4. Home P, Riddle M, Cefalu WT, Bailey CJ, Bretzel RG, Del Prato S, Leroith D, Schernthaner G, van Gaal L, Raz I. Insulin therapy in people with type 2 diabetes: opportunities and challenges? Diabetes Care. 2014;37(6):1499–508.
5. Kesavadev J, Saboo B, Krishna MB, Krishnan G. Evolution of insulin delivery devices: from syringes, pens, and pumps to DIY artificial pancreas. Diabetes Therapy. 2020;11:1251–69.
6. Rex J, Jensen KH, Lawton SA. A review of 20 years' experience with the NovoPen family of insulin injection devices. Clin Drug Investig. 2006;26:367–401.
7. Weaver KW, Hirsch IB. The hybrid closed-loop system: evolution and practical applications. Diabetes Technol Ther. 2018;20:S216–S223223.
8. Technology D. Standards of medical care in diabetes-2020. Diabetes Care. 2020;43:S77–88.
9. Selam JL. Evolution of diabetes insulin delivery devices. J Diabetes Sci Technol. 2010;4(3):505–13. https://doi.org/10.1177/193229681000400302.
10. Milestones BD. Available from: http://www.bd.com/aboutbd/history/.
11. Fry A. Insulin delivery device technology 2012: where are we after 90 years? J Diabetes Sci Technol. 2012;6:947–53.
12. Shah RB, Patel M, Maahs DM, Shah VN. Insulin delivery methods: past, present and future. Int J Pharm Investig. 2016;6:1–9.
13. Exchange Supplies. The history of injecting, and the development of the syringe. https://www.exchangesupplies.org/article_history_of_injecting_and_development_of_the_syringe.php
14. Aronson R, Gibney MA, Oza K, Berube J, KasslerTaub K, Hirsch L. Insulin pen needles: effects of extra-thin wall needle technology on preference, confidence, and other patient ratings. Clin Ther. 2013;35:933.e4.
15. BD. BD VeoTM insulin syringes with BD UltraFineTM 6mm 9 31G needle. https://www.bd.com/en-us/offerings/capabilities/diabetes-care/insulinsyringes/bd-veo-insulin-syringe-with-ultra-fine6mm-needle (2020).
16. Shaw KF, Valdez CA. Development and implementation of a U-500 regular insulin program in a federally qualified health center. Clin Diabetes. 2017;35:162–7.
17. Novo Nordisk Blue sheet. Quarterly perspective on diabetes and chronic diseases. 2010. Available from: http://www.press.novonordisk-us.com/bluesheet-issue2/downloads/NovoNordisk_Bluesheet_Newsletter.pdf.
18. Novo Nordisk History. Novo Nord. https://www.novonordisk.co.in/content/dam/Denmark/HQ/aboutus/documents/HistoryBook_UK.pdf (2020).
19. Dunne T, Whitaker D. Prefilled insulin syringes. Anaesthesia. 2016;71:349–50.
20. Penfornis A, Personeni E, Borot S. Evolution of devices in diabetes management. Diabetes Technol Ther. 2011;13(Suppl 1):S93–102.
21. Ignaut DA, Venekamp WJ. HumaPen Memoir: a novel insulin-injecting pen with a dose-memory feature. Expert Rev Med Devices. 2007;4:793–802.
22. Singh R, Samuel C, Jacob JJ. A comparison of insulin pen devices and disposable plastic syringes - simplicity, safety, convenience and cost differences. Eur Endocrinol. 2018;14:47–51.
23. Guerci B, Chanan N, Kaur S, Jasso-Mosqueda JG, Lew E. Lack of treatment persistence and treatment nonadherence as barriers to glycaemic control in patients with type 2 diabetes. Diabetes Ther. 2019;10:437–49.
24. Pfützner A, Bailey T, Campos C, Kahn D, Ambers E, Niemeyer M, et al. Accuracy and preference assessment of prefilled insulin pen versus vial and syringe with diabetes patients, caregivers, and healthcare professionals. Curr Med Res Opin. 2013;29:475–81.
25. Xue L, Mikkelsen KH. Dose accuracy of a durable insulin pen with memory function, before and after simulated lifetime use and under stress conditions. Expert Opin Drug Deliv. 2013;10:301–6.
26. Hirsch IB. Does size matter? Thoughts about insulin pen needles. Diabetes Technol Ther. 2012;14:1081.
27. Aronson R, Gibney MA, Oza K, Bérubé J, Kassler-Taub K, Hirsch L. Insulin pen needles: effects of extra-thin wall needle technology on preference, confidence, and other patient ratings. Clin Ther. 2013;35:923–33.e4.
28. Hyllested-Winge J, Sparre T, Pedersen LK. NovoPen Echo() insulin delivery device. Med Devices. 2016;9:11–8.
29. Ignaut DA, Opincar M, Lenox S. FlexPen and KwikPen prefilled insulin devices: a laboratory evaluation of ergonomic and injection force characteristics. J Diabetes Sci Technol. 2008;2:533–7.
30. Wielandt JO, Niemeyer M, Hansen MR, Bucher D, Thomsen NB. FlexTouch: a prefilled insulin pen with a novel injection mechanism with consistent high accuracy at low-(1 U), medium-(40 U), and high-(80 U) dose settings. J Diabetes Sci Technol. 2011;5:1195–9.
31. Sanofi. launches specially designed 'made in India' re-usable insulin pen-AllStarTM Press Release. Diabetes in Control, Mar 9, 2019, https://www.diabetesincontrol.com/new-smart-pens-hoped-to-change-the-waywe-treat-diabetes/Sanofi, accessed April 13, 2023,
32. Veasey R, Ruf CA, Bogatirsky D, Westerbacka J, Friedrichs A, Abdel-Tawab M, Adler S, Mohanasundaram S. A review of reusable insulin pens and features of TouStar—a new reusable pen with a dedicated cartridge. Diabetol Metab Syndr. 2021;13(1):1–7.
33. Whooley S, Briskin T, Gibney MA, Blank LR, Berube J, Pflug BK. Evaluating the user performance and experience with a re-engineered 4 mm 9 32G pen needle: a randomized trial with similar length/− gauge needles. Diabetes Ther. 2019;10:697–712.
34. Healthworld.com. Eli Lilly launches 200 U/mL prefilled insulin pen. Econ Times.
35. Gudiksen N, Hofstätter T, Rønn BB, Sparre T. FlexTouch: an insulin pen-injector with a low activation force across different insulin formulations, needle technologies, and temperature conditions. Diabetes Technol Ther. 2017;19:603–7.
36. Olsen BS, Lilleøre SK, Korsholm CN, Kracht T. Novopen Echo for the delivery of insulin: a comparison of usability, functionality

and preference among pediatric subjects, their parents, and health care professionals. J Diabetes Sci Technol. 2010;4:1468–75.

37. Review EP. Novo Nordisk's award-winning NovoPen 5 with easy-to-use memory function approved in China.

38. Bailey TS, Stone JY. A novel pen-based Bluetooth-enabled insulin delivery system with insulin dose tracking and advice. Expert Opin Drug Deliv. 2017;14:697–703.

39. Freed S. New smart pens hoped to change the way we treat diabetes. Diabetes Control. https://www.diabetesincontrol.com/new-smart-pens-hoped-to-change-the-waywe-treat-diabetes/. Accessed 13 Apr 2023.

40. DiaTribeLearn. NovoPen 6 and NovoPen Echo Plus: connected insulin pens to launch in early 2019.

41. Sangave NA, Aungst TD, Patel DK. Smart connected insulin pens, caps, and attachments: a review of the future of diabetes technology. Diabetes Spectr. 2019;32:378–84.

42. MedicalNewsToday. What are insulin pens and how do we use them?

43. Pearson TL. Practical aspects of insulin pen devices. J Diabetes Sci Technol. 2010;4:522–31.

44. Khan AM, Alswat KA. Benefits of using the i-port system on insulin-treated patients. Diabetes Spectr. 2019;32:30–5.

45. Burdick P, Cooper S, Horner B, Cobry E, McFann K, Chase HP. Use of a subcutaneous injection port to improve glycemic control in children with type 1 diabetes. Pediatr Diabetes. 2009;10:116–9.

46. Polonsky KS, Given BD, Hirsch L, Shapiro ET, Tillil H, Beebe C. Quantitative study of insulin secretion and clearance in normal and obese subjects. J Clin Invest. 1988;81:435–41.

47. Maniatis AK, Klingensmith GJ, Slover RH, Mowry CJ, Chase HP. Continuous subcutaneous insulin infusion therapy for children and adolescents: an option for routine diabetes care. Pediatrics. 2001;107:351–6.

48. Medtronic. What is insulin pump therapy. Medtronic.

49. Al-Tabakha MM, Arida AI. Recent challenges in insulin delivery systems: a review. Indian J Pharm Sci. 2008;70:278–86.

50. Al Hayek AA, Robert AA, Babli S, Almonea K, Al Dawish MA. Fear of self-injecting and self-testing and the related risk factors in adolescents with type 1 diabetes: a cross-sectional study. Diabetes Ther. 2017;8:75–83.

51. Kadish AH. A servomechanism for blood sugar control. Biomed Sci Instrum. 1963;1:171–6.

52. Allen N, Gupta A. Current diabetes technology: striving for the artificial pancreas. Diagnostics. 2019;9:31.

53. SOOIL. SOOIL history. https://sooil.com/eng/about/history.php. Accessed 13 Apr 2023.

54. Duckworth WC, Saudek CD, Henry RR. Why intraperitoneal delivery of insulin with implantable pumps in NIDDM? Diabetes. 1992;41:657–61.

55. Skyler JS, Ponder S, Kruger DF, Matheson D, Parkin CG. Is there a place for insulin pump therapy in your practice? Clin Diabetes. 2007;25:50–6.

56. Magennis C The different types of insulin pumps available in 2019.

57. Medtronic. Innovation milestones Hieronymus Laura GS. Insulin delivery devices.

58. Hieronymus Laura GS. Insulin delivery devices.

59. Kesavadev J, Shankar A, Sadasrian Pillai PB, et al. CSII as an alternative therapeutic strategy for managing type 2 diabetes: adding the Indian experience to a global perspective. Curr Diabetes Rev. 2016;12:312–4.

60. Maiorino MI, Bellastella G, Casciano O, et al. The effects of subcutaneous insulin infusion versus multiple insulin injections on glucose variability in young adults with type 1 diabetes: the 2-year follow-up of the observational METRO study. Diabetes Technol Ther. 2018;20:117–26.

61. Heinemann L, Krinelke L. Insulin infusion set: the Achilles heel of continuous subcutaneous insulin infusion. J Diabetes Sci Technol. 2012;6:954–64.

62. Moser EG, Morris AA, Garg SK. Emerging diabetes therapies and technologies. Diabetes Res Clin Pract. 2012;97:16–26.

63. Heinemann L, Waldenmaier D, Kulzer B, Ziegler R, Ginsberg B, Freckmann G. Patch pumps: are they all the same? J Diabetes Sci Technol. 2019;13:34–40.

64. Ginsberg BH. Patch pumps for insulin. J Diabetes Sci Technol. 2019;13:27–33.

65. DiaTribeLearn. Insulet's second generation omnipod patch pump approved by FDA.

66. Garcia-Verdugo R, Erbach M, Schnell O. A new optimized percutaneous access system for CIPII. J Diabetes Sci Technol. 2017;11:814–21.

67. Gimenez M, Purkayajtha S, Moscardo V, Conget I, Oliver N. Intraperitoneal insulin therapy in patients with type 1 diabetes. Does it fit into the current therapeutic arsenal? Endocrinol Diabet Nutr. 2018;65(3):182–4.

68. Garg SK, Voelmle MK, Beatson CR, Miller HA, Crew LB, Freson BJ, et al. Use of continuous glucose monitoring in subjects with type 1 diabetes on multiple daily injections versus continuous subcutaneous insulin infusion therapy: a prospective 6-month study. Diabetes Care. 2011;34:574–9.

69. Steineck I, Ranjan A, Nørgaard K, Schmidt S. Sensor-augmented insulin pumps and hypoglycemia prevention in type 1 diabetes. J Diabetes Sci Technol. 2017;11:50–8.

70. Matsuoka A, Hirota Y, Urai S, et al. Effect of switching from conventional continuous subcutaneous insulin infusion to sensor augmented pump therapy on glycemic profile in Japanese patients with type 1 diabetes. Diabetol Int. 2018;9:201–7.

71. Oviedo S, Contreras I, Bertachi A, et al. Minimizing postprandial hypoglycemia in type 1 diabetes patients using multiple insulin injections and capillary blood glucose self-monitoring with machine learning techniques. Comput Methods Prog Biomed. 2019;178:175–80.

72. Medtronic. Innovation milestones.

73. Medtronic. Minimed TM 640G insulin pump system. Medtronic.

74. NIDDK.NIH: Story of discovery: artificial pancreas for managing type 1 diabetes: cutting-edge technology 50 years in the making. https://www.niddk.nih.gov/news/archive/2017/story-discovery-artificial-pancreas-managing-type1-diabetes. Accessed 13 Apr 2023.

75. Biester T, Kordonouri O, Holder M. "Let the algorithm do the work": reduction of hypoglycemia using sensor-augmented pump therapy with predictive insulin suspension (SmartGuard) in pediatric type 1 diabetes patients. Diabetes Technol Ther. 2017;19:173–82.

76. Garg SK, Weinzimer SA, Tamborlane WV, et al. Glucose outcomes with the in-home use of a hybrid closed-loop insulin delivery system in adolescents and adults with type 1 diabetes. Diabetes Technol Ther. 2017;19:155–63.

77. Sharifi A, De Bock MI, Jayawardene D, et al. Glycemia, treatment satisfaction, cognition, and sleep quality in adults and adolescents with type 1 diabetes when using a closed-loop system overnight versus sensor-augmented pump with low-glucose suspend function: a randomized crossover study. Diabetes Technol Ther. 2016;18:772–83.

78. Brown SA, Kovatchev BP, Raghinaru D, et al. Six-month randomized, multicenter trial of closed-loop control in type 1 diabetes. N Engl J Med. 2019;381:1707–17.

79. Home Insulet. https://www.insulet.com/. Accessed 13 Apr 2023.

80. Shah VN, Shoskes A, Tawfik B, Garg SK. Closed-loop system in the management of diabetes: past, present, and future. Diabetes Technol Ther. 2014;16:477–90.

81. FDA. FDA authorizes first interoperable insulin pump intended to allow patients to customize treatment through their individual diabetes management devices. FDA.

82. Omer T. Empowered citizen 'health hackers' who are not waiting. BMC Med. 2016;14:118.

83. Marshall DC, Holloway M, Korer M, Woodman J, Brackenridge A, Hussain S. Do-it-yourself artificial pancreas systems in type 1 diabetes: perspectives of two adult users, a caregiver and three physicians. Diabetes Ther. 2019;10:1553–644.

84. White K, Gebremariam A, Lewis D, et al. Motivations for participation in an online social media community for diabetes. J Diabetes Sci Technol. 2018;12:712–8.

85. Lewis DM. Do-it-yourself artificial pancreas system and the OpenAPS movement. Endocrinol Metab Clin N Am. 2020;49:203–13.

86. OPENAPS.ORG. OpenAPS Outcomes. OPENAPS. ORG. 2020.

87. Mine D. Homegrown closed loop technology: mom connects to RileyLink.

88. Lewis D, Leibrand S. Real-world use of open source artificial pancreas systems. J Diabetes Sci Technol. 2016;10:1411.

89. Kesavadev J, Saboo B, Kar P, Sethi J. DIY artificial pancreas: a narrative of the first patient and the physicians' experiences from India. Diabetes Metab Syndr Clin Res Rev. 2021;15(2):615–20.

90. Kesavadev J, Srinivasan S, Saboo B, Krishna B, M. and Krishnan, G. The do-it-yourself artificial pancreas: a comprehensive review. Diabetes Therapy. 2020;11(6):1217–35.

91. Bux Rodeman K, Hatipoglu B. Beta-cell therapies for type 1 diabetes: transplants and bionics. Cleve Clin J Med. 2018;85:931–7.

92. JDRF. FDA grants breakthrough device status: iLet bionic pancreas.

93. Idlebrook C. The diabetes dads behind 3 type 1 breakthroughs. Insulin Nation; 2015.

94. JDRF. FDA Grants breakthrough device status: iLet bionic pancreas. 2019.

95. Racklyeft N. The history of loop and LoopKit reflecting on the past in celebration of version 1.0. Medium.

96. Bevan A "Not Good Enough": how one dad led the change in diabetes devices through grassroots research and collaboration.

97. Gavrila V, Garrity A, Hirschfeld E, Edwards B, Lee JM. Peer support through a diabetes social media community. J Diabetes Sci Technol. 2019;13:493–7.

98. AAMI. Linkedin. Advancing safety in health technology. https://www.linkedin.com/company/aami_2. Accessed 13 Apr 2023.

99. Glu. An interview with Tidepool CEO Howard Look. glu.

100. Snider C. Tidepool loop, one year in: a development update. Tidepool.

101. Huckvale K, Adomaviciute S, Prieto JT, Leow MK-S, Car J. Smartphone apps for calculating insulin dose: a systematic assessment. BMC Med. 2015;13:106.

102. Shashaj B, Busetto E, Sulli N. Benefits of a bolus calculator in pre- and postprandial glycaemic control and meal flexibility of paediatric patients using continuous subcutaneous insulin infusion (CSII). Diabet Med. 2008;25:1036–42.

103. Peters AL, Ahmann AJ, Battelino T, et al. Diabetes technology-continuous subcutaneous insulin infusion therapy and continuous glucose monitoring in adults: an endocrine society clinical practice guideline. J Clin Endocrinol Metab. 2016;101:3922–37.

104. Taylor MJ, Gregory R, Tomlins P, Jacob D, Hubble J, Sahota TS. Closed-loop glycaemic control using an implantable artificial pancreas in diabetic domestic pig (sus scrofa domesticus). Int J Pharm. 2016;500:371–8.

105. Peyser T, Dassau E, Breton M, Skyler JS. The artificial pancreas: current status and future prospects in the management of diabetes. Ann N Y Acad Sci. 2014;1311:102–23.

106. Gänsslen M. Über inhalation von insulin. Klin Wochenschr. 1925;4:71.

107. Heinemann L. Alternative delivery routes: inhaled insulin. Diabetes Nutr Metab. 2002;15:417–22.

108. Santos Cavaiola T, Edelman S. Inhaled insulin: a breath of fresh air? A review of inhaled insulin. Clin Ther. 2014;36:1275–89.

109. FDA Approved Drug Products.

110. Patton JS, Bukar JG, Eldon MA. Clinical pharmacokinetics and pharmacodynamics of inhaled insulin. Clin Pharmacokinet. 2004;43:781–801.

111. Alabraba V, Farnsworth A, Leigh R, Dodson P, Gough SC, Smyth T. Exubera inhaled insulin in patients with type 1 and type 2 diabetes: the first 12 months. Diabetes Technol Ther. 2009;11:427–30.

112. Flood T. Advances in insulin delivery systems and devices: beyond the vial and syringe. Insulin. 2006;1:99–108.

113. Richardson PC, Boss AH. Technosphere insulin technology. Diabetes Technol Ther. 2007;9(Suppl 1):S65–72.

114. Neumiller JJ, Campbell RK, Wood LD. A review of inhaled technosphere insulin. Ann Pharmacother. 2010;44:1231–9.

115. Heinemann L, Baughman R, Boss A, Hompesch M. Pharmacokinetic and pharmacodynamic properties of a novel inhaled insulin. J Diabetes Sci Technol. 2017;11:148–56.

116. Oleck J, Kassam S, Goldman JD. Commentary: why was inhaled insulin a failure in the market? Diabetes Spectr. 2016;29:180–4.

117. Seaquist ER, Blonde L, McGill JB, et al. Hypoglycaemia is reduced with use of inhaled Technosphere((R)) insulin relative to insulin aspart in type 1 diabetes mellitus. Diabet Med. 2019;37(5):752–9.

118. Akturk HK, Snell-Bergeon JK, Rewers A, et al. Improved postprandial glucose with inhaled technosphere insulin compared with insulin aspart in patients with type 1 diabetes on multiple daily injections: the STAT study. Diabetes Technol Ther. 2018;20:639–47.

119. Papania MJ, Zehrung D, Jarrahian C. In: Plotkin SA, Orenstein WA, Offit PA, KMBT-PV E, Seventh E, editors. Technologies to improve immunization. Amsterdam: Elsevier; 2018. p. 1320. e17–53.e17.

120. Al-Tabakha M. Recent advances and future prospects of non-invasive insulin delivery systems. Int J Appl Pharm. 2019;11:16–24.

121. Guo L, Xiao X, Sun X, Qi C. Comparison of jet injector and insulin pen in controlling plasma glucose and insulin concentrations in type 2 diabetic patients. Medicine. 2017;96:e5482.

122. Hu J, Shi H, Zhao C, et al. Lispro administered by the QS-M needle-free jet injector generates an earlier insulin exposure. Expert Opin Drug Deliv. 2016;13:1203–7.

123. Arbit E, Kidron M. Oral insulin: the rationale for this approach and current developments. J Diabetes Sci Technol. 2009;3:562–7.

124. Abdel-Moneim A, Ramadan H. Novel strategies to oral delivery of insulin. Current progress of noncarriers for diabetes management. Drug Des Dev. 2022;83:301–16.

125. Sonia TA, Sharma CP. An overview of natural polymers for oral insulin delivery. Drug Discov Today. 2012;17:784–92.

126. Ramesan RM, Sharma CP. Challenges and advances in nanoparticle-based oral insulin delivery. Expert Rev Med Dev. 2009;6:665–76.

127. Damgé C, Reis CP, Maincent P. Nanoparticle strategies for the oral delivery of insulin. Expert Opin Drug Deliv. 2008;5:45–68.

128. Chaturvedi K, Ganguly K, Nadagouda MN, Aminabhavi TM. Polymeric hydrogels for oral insulin delivery. J Control Release. 2013;165:129–38.

129. Geho WB, Geho HC, Lau JR, Gana TJ. Hepatic-directed vesicle insulin: a review of formulation development and preclinical evaluation. J Diabetes Sci Technol. 2009;3:1451–9.

130. Heinemann L. New ways of insulin delivery. Int J Clin Pract Suppl. 2010;166:29–40.

131. Maroni A, Zema L, Del Curto MD, Foppoli A, Gazzaniga A. Oral colon delivery of insulin with the aid of functional adjuvants. Adv Drug Deliv Rev. 2012;64:540–56.

132. Yaturu S. Insulin therapies: current and future trends at dawn. World J Diabetes. 2013;4:1–7.

133. Salzman R, Manson JE, Griffing GT, Kimmerle R, Ruderman N, McCall A. Intranasal aerosolized insulin. Mixed-meal studies and long-term use in type I diabetes. N Engl J Med. 1985;312:1078–84.

134. Frauman AG, Cooper ME, Parsons BJ, Jerums G, Louis WJ. Long-term use of intranasal insulin in insulin-dependent diabetic patients. Diabetes Care. 1987;10:573–8.

135. Leary AC, Stote RM, Cussen K, O'Brien J, Leary WP, Buckley B. Pharmacokinetics and pharmacodynamics of intranasal insulin administered to patients with type 1 diabetes: a preliminary study. Diabetes Technol Ther. 2006;8:81–8.

136. Illum L. Nasal drug delivery — recent developments and future prospects. J Control Release. 2012;161:254–63.

137. Stote R, Marbury T, Shi L, Miller M, Strange P. Comparison pharmacokinetics of two concentrations (0.7% and 1.0%) of Nasulin, an ultra-rapid-acting intranasal insulin formulation. J Diabetes Sci Technol. 2010;4:603–9.

138. Benedict C, Frey WH 2nd, Schiöth HB, Schultes B, Born J, Hallschmid M. Intranasal insulin as a therapeutic option in the treatment of cognitive impairments. Exp Gerontol. 2011;46:112–5.

139. Craft S, Baker LD, Montine TJ, Minoshima S, Watson GS, Claxton A, et al. Intranasal insulin therapy for Alzheimer disease and amnestic mild cognitive impairment: a pilot clinical trial. Arch Neurol. 2012;69:29–38.

140. Heinemann L, Jacques Y. Oral insulin and buccal insulin: a critical reappraisal. J Diabetes Sci Technol. 2009;3:568–84.

141. Kumria R, Goomber G. Emerging trends in insulin delivery: buccal route. J Diabetol. 2011;2:1–9.

142. World's First Oral Insulin Spray Launched in India. Asia Pacific Biotech News. 2008;12:60.

143. Bala R, Pawar P, Khanna S, Arora S. Orally dissolving strips: a new approach to oral drug delivery system. Int J Pharm Investig. 2013;3:67–76.

144. Prausnitz MR, Langer R. Transdermal drug delivery. Nat Biotechnol. 2008;26:1261–8.

145. Kanikkannan N. Iontophoresis-based transdermal delivery systems. BioDrugs. 2002;16:339–47.

146. Rao R, Nanda S. Sonophoresis: recent advancements and future trends. J Pharm Pharmacol. 2009;61:689–705.

147. Andrews S, Lee JW, Choi SO, Prausnitz MR. Transdermal insulin delivery using microdermabrasion. Pharm Res. 2011;28:2110–8.

148. Charoo NA, Rahman Z, Repka MA, Murthy SN. Electroporation: an avenue for transdermal drug delivery. Curr Drug Deliv. 2010;7:125–36.

149. Malakar J, Sen SO, Nayak AK, Sen KK. Formulation, optimization and evaluation of transferosomal gel for transdermal insulin delivery. Saudi Pharm J. 2012;20:355–63.

150. Freckmann G, Pleus S, Haug C, Bitton G, Nagar R. Increasing local blood flow by warming the application site: beneficial effects on postprandial glycemic excursions. J Diabetes Sci Technol. 2012;6:780–5.

151. Vaughn DE, Muchmore DB. Use of recombinant human hyaluronidase to accelerate rapid insulin analogue absorption: experience with subcutaneous injection and continuous infusion. Endocr Pract. 2011;17:914–21.

152. Bariya SH, Gohel MC, Mehta TA, Sharma OP. Microneedles: An emerging transdermal drug delivery system. J Pharm Pharmacol. 2012;64:11–29.

153. Morgan RV. Delivery of systemic regular insulin via the ocular route in cats. J Ocul Pharmacol Ther. 1995;11:565–73.

154. Ritschel WA, Ritschel GB, Ritschel BE, Lücker PW. Rectal delivery system for insulin. Methods Find Exp Clin Pharmacol. 1988;10:645–56.

155. Yamasaki Y, Shichiri M, Kawamori R, Kikuchi M, Yagi T, Ara S, et al. The effectiveness of rectal administration of insulin suppository on normal and diabetic subjects. Diabetes Care. 1981;4:454–8.

156. Laqueur E, Grevenstuk A. Uber die wirkung intratrachealer zuführung von insulin. Klin Wochenschr. 1924;3:1273–4.

Index

© The Editor(s) (if applicable) and The Author(s), under exclusive license to Springer Nature Switzerland AG 2023
J. Rodriguez-Saldana (ed.), *The Diabetes Textbook*, https://doi.org/10.1007/978-3-031-25519-9